Medical Radiology

Diagnostic Imaging

Series Editors

Hans-Ulrich Kauczor
Paul M. Parizel
Wilfred C. G. Peh

The book series *Medical Radiology – Diagnostic Imaging* provides accurate and up-to-date overviews about the latest advances in the rapidly evolving field of diagnostic imaging and interventional radiology. Each volume is conceived as a practical and clinically useful reference book and is developed under the direction of an experienced editor, who is a world-renowned specialist in the field. Book chapters are written by expert authors in the field and are richly illustrated with high quality figures, tables and graphs. Editors and authors are committed to provide detailed and coherent information in a readily accessible and easy-to-understand format, directly applicable to daily practice.

Medical Radiology – Diagnostic Imaging covers all organ systems and addresses all modern imaging techniques and image-guided treatment modalities, as well as hot topics in management, workflow, and quality and safety issues in radiology and imaging. The judicious choice of relevant topics, the careful selection of expert editors and authors, and the emphasis on providing practically useful information, contribute to the wide appeal and ongoing success of the series. The series is indexed in Scopus.

Benoît Ghaye
Catherine Beigelman-Aubry
Rodrigo Salgado
Editors

Measurements in Cardiopulmonary Imaging: When, How, Why

Springer

Editors
Benoît Ghaye
Department of Radiology
Université Catholique de Louvain
Brussels, Belgium

Catherine Beigelman-Aubry
Radiodiagnostic & Intervent. Radiology
University Hospital of Lausanne
Lausanne, Vaud, Switzerland

Diagnostic Imaging
Foch Hospital
Suresnes, France

Rodrigo Salgado
Department of Radiology
Antwerp University Hospital
Edegem, Belgium

ISSN 0942-5373 ISSN 2197-4187 (electronic)
Medical Radiology
ISSN 2731-4677 ISSN 2731-4685 (electronic)
Diagnostic Imaging
ISBN 978-3-030-81073-3 ISBN 978-3-030-81074-0 (eBook)
https://doi.org/10.1007/978-3-030-81074-0

This Springer imprint is published by the registered company Springer Nature Switzerland AG
The registered company address is: Gewerbestrasse 11, 6330 Cham, Switzerland

Preface

A comprehensive book dedicated to measurements in cardiothoracic imaging has been lacking for decades. Many of us fondly remember *Repères et mesures en imagerie médicale* by Alain Coussement and *An Atlas of Roentgenographic Measurement* by Theodore Keats—both with their final editions published in 1990—as indispensable companions during and well beyond our residency training. These classic references, however, were predominantly based on conventional radiographic measurements.

The thorax represents a body region where measurements are particularly numerous and clinically impactful. Unlike many other anatomical areas, the diagnostic workup of certain lesions, a pulmonary nodule for instance, relies fundamentally on quantitative assessment, primarily density and size, to guide clinical decision-making.

The goal of this work has been to emphasize current measurements that may be used as a guide in routine practice within each chest and cardiovascular compartment according to the imaging modality used.

The journey toward completing *Measurements in Cardiopulmonary Imaging: When, How, Why* has been a long one, marked by the COVID-19 pandemic that profoundly affected the professional and personal lives of so many. As a consequence, some authors departed from the project while others joined along the way. We are deeply grateful to all contributors for their unwavering commitment and perseverance despite these challenging circumstances.

We also wish to express our sincere thanks to Prakash Balasubramanian and Nathalie Lhorset-Poulain from Springer for their invaluable support throughout the production of this book.

Brussels, Belgium — Benoît Ghaye
Lausanne, Switzerland — Catherine Beigelman-Aubry
Edegem, Belgium — Rodrigo Salgado

Contents

Introduction: When, How and Why?

Cornelia Schaefer-Prokop and Esther Pompe

Contents

Quantitative or qualitative research? Which position would you support? Why?
Nick's answer on Quora.com

> *On the one hand, quantitative research is often seen as more objective and scientific, while qualitative research is seen as more subjective and interpretive. On the other hand, quantitative research can sometimes be too reductionist, while qualitative research can sometimes be too unfocused*

Medical imaging has revolutionized the diagnosis and management of cardiopulmonary diseases, providing invaluable insights into both structure and function. As imaging technology advances, so does the ability to quantify physiological and pathological changes using radiological biomarkers. Knowing when, how, and why to apply these measurements is essential for radiologists, cardiologists, pulmonologists, surgeons, oncologists, and researchers to ensure accurate diagnosis, disease monitoring, and treatment evaluation.

This book, *Measurements in Cardiopulmonary Imaging: When, How, and Why*, aims as a guide to radiological quantitative biomarkers in cardiothoracic imaging. It serves to provide a structured and practical reference for clinicians and imaging specialists, ensuring that quantitative imaging biomarkers are applied effectively to enhance diagnostic accuracy and patient management. By integrating the latest research with clinical scenarios, it offers a roadmap for the use of cardiopulmonary imaging measurements. Therefore, it is designed to bridge the gap between technical

C. Schaefer-Prokop (✉)
Department of Radiology, Meander Medical Centre (MMC) Amersfoort and Diagnostic Image Analysis Group (DIAG), Radboud University Nijmegen, Nijmegen, The Netherlands

E. Pompe
Department of Radiology, University Medical Centre (UMC) Utrecht, Utrecht, The Netherlands

Med Radiol Diagn Imaging (2026)
https://doi.org/10.1007/174_2025_681,
Published Online: 23 January 2026

advancements and clinical application, offering a comprehensive approach to measurement-based imaging in cardiac, pulmonary, and vascular diseases.

The book is divided into four main sections:

- *Part I: Technical Aspects* explores imaging modalities such as cardiac CT and MRI, nuclear medicine, and radiation dose considerations.
- *Part II: Clinical Part—Lung, Pleura, and Mediastinum* describes measurement-based imaging techniques covering conditions such as pulmonary nodules, infiltrative lung disease, and post-therapeutic follow-ups.
- *Part III: Clinical Part—Vessels* focuses on vascular imaging, addressing pulmonary hypertension, embolism, thoracic aorta assessment, and interventional radiology.
- *Part IV: Clinical Part—Heart* provides an in-depth look at cardiac imaging, including coronary artery evaluation, hemodynamic, heart chamber assessments, and myocardial tissue characterization. The final chapter critically examines the opportunities and limitations of measurement-based cardiovascular imaging.

1 Why Is Quantification of Image Information Desirable?

Interpretation of medical images relies on visual assessment. Over time accumulated knowledge about anatomical—meaning morphological—variations enables the radiologist or clinician to differentiate abnormal structures or patterns from normal.

It is still daily practice that instead of exact quantification, semiquantitative descriptions are used such as "beginning, some, moderate or extensive" to describe the extent of disease. While these descriptions have a clinical value in indicating the clinical seriousness or the tendency of longitudinal behavior, they are hampered by ambiguity and subjectivity. Workload and inherent limitations of morphology restrict the number of manual measurements. While structured reporting helps to harmonize disease evaluation, it still suffers from differences in radiological interpretation and restrictions of human visual assessment.

There is an increasing desire for reliable, reproducible, and more accurate assessment of disease in our community, and this holds true for the individual patient as well as healthcare politicians and insurances. With the emergence of new, yet highly expensive drugs (e.g., immunomodulatory medication), there is an increasing need to assess a patient's likely response to therapy, ideally before treatment begins. While this predictive information often lies beyond the limits of human visual assessment, it may be embedded within the image data and accessible through advanced computer-based analysis. Techniques involving machine learning and deep learning have shown to be able to extract such image-based biomarkers, potentially bridging this gap.

While the majority of imaging biomarker development is situated in oncological applications, it especially concerns cardiothoracic imaging, where the literature lists a broad range of non-oncologic applications of imaging-based quantification including COPD, interstitial lung disease or the assessment of extent, and functional impairment in myocardial ischemia. In that context, it has been shown that features that established in qualitative image assessment and already known to correlate with outcome, e.g., bronchial wall thickness in COPD exacerbations, represent important assets also in computer-based quantification.

2 Definition and Criteria for Imaging Biomarkers

An *imaging biomarker* is a quantifiable characteristic extracted from medical images that serves as an objective indicator of a biological or pathological process, patient risk stratification, evaluation of treatment response, and patient outcome.

Quantitative imaging biomarkers are typically expressed as continuous variables. In contrast, ordinal classifications, such as CAD-RADS or

LU-RADS, consist of a limited set of predefined categories. There are various levels of quantitative measures ranging from manual diameter or distance measurements done in 2D images to volumetry obtained in 3D imaging or functional assessment using advanced image processing and taking 4D information into account. Each level of quantification has its own merits and limitations as being outlined in each of the following chapters. While manual measurements may suffer from limited reproducibility and quantitative accuracy, they are relatively simple, cheap, and quick tools that represent an important parameter in patient assessment in many clinical situations also today. In that respect, the book aims to inform the reader about the whole spectrum of measurement options ranging from the "classic" manual diameter assessment to the development of advanced computer-based biomarkers that provide information beyond visually accessible evaluation.

Biomarkers play an increasingly important role in healthcare to guide individualized treatment strategies, often referred to as precision or personalized medicine. This personalized approach is most advanced in oncology but is expanding across other healthcare domains. Quantitative imaging enables the evaluation of disease presence and progression over time and facilitates risk assessment, prognosis, and prediction of therapeutic outcomes. Compared to invasive biopsies, imaging offers a faster, less invasive, and more repeatable method of evaluation.

Moreover, imaging biomarkers can help detect subclinical disease, enhancing our understanding of the continuum between normal and pathological states. Reliable imaging biomarkers can support the development of medical products in regulatory settings. This is especially evident in chronic pulmonary conditions such as emphysema, asthma, or interstitial lung disease, where the development of targeted therapies has been closely linked to advancements in quantitative imaging.

3 Requirements for and Limitations of Imaging Biomarkers

The reliability of imaging biomarkers is influenced by a range of factors, including variability in imaging hardware, software algorithms, acquisition protocols, measurement techniques, and the degree of human involvement. Each of these elements can introduce inconsistencies, potentially affecting the precision and compatibility of quantitative imaging results across, time, settings, and institutions.

For an imaging biomarker to be considered clinically useful, several requirements must be met. First and foremost is reproducibility—the ability to produce consistent results under similar conditions. A robust biomarker must demonstrate low variability across repeated measurements within the same subject (intra-subject reproducibility) but must also align with established reference standards or known true values.

In addition to technical consistency, an imaging biomarker must be clinically relevant. This means that an imaging biomarker should be sensitive to biological changes and reflect disease progression, treatment response, or risk. In addition, validation of the biomarker against established clinical endpoints or gold-standard indicators of disease activity is essential.

Despite their potential, several limitations of imaging biomarkers should be considered. These mainly include challenges in standardizing protocols across different imaging centers, making cross-study or cross-center comparison difficult. Limited external validation can lead to decreased performance when applied to different patient populations, imaging systems, or clinical scenarios. Moreover, certain biomarkers are highly sensitive to imaging parameters, such as slice thickness, reconstruction kernel, and contrast timing—factors that may vary widely between institutions.

In recent years, there have been substantial international efforts toward standardization of image acquisition to achieve robust and repeatable imaging biomarkers, and recommendations for quality assurance have been published. In 2007, the Radiological Society of North America launched the Quantitative Imaging Biomarkers Alliance (QIBA), which represents a collaboration of researchers, health care professionals, and industry with the goal to foster quantitative imaging research and its translation into clinical practice.

With machine learning-driven biomarkers, there are additional concerns regarding overfitting, particularly in small or homogeneous datasets. Without robust validation strategies, such models may demonstrate high performance during developments but fail in real-world clinical application. Lastly, lack of interpretability, especially in deep learning models, can make it difficult for radiologists and clinicians to understand how decisions are made, reducing trust and limiting practical use.

In spite of these challenges, imaging biomarkers continue to hold great promise. With increased efforts toward multi-site validation and technological accessibility, they are thought to enhance precision diagnostics and support personalized patient care.

4 Conclusion

Imaging biomarkers offer quantifiable insights beyond traditional visual assessment and enhance the diagnostic, prognostic, and therapy response capabilities of diagnostic imaging. Chest imaging occupies a strategic position in this endeavor anatomically encompassing the leading causes of mortality worldwide with heart disease, lung cancer, and COPD.

As cardiopulmonary diseases grow in complexity and treatments become increasingly personalized—and costly—the role of quantitative imaging continues to expand. Moving beyond visual estimation toward measurable, reproducible, and biologically meaningful image-derived data empowers radiologists and clinicians to make well-informed decisions. While limitations and challenges remain, ongoing advancements in imaging technology and AI are rapidly pushing the field forward.

The book is intended to support radiologists and imaging specialists in understanding and applying imaging biomarkers in clinical practice. By integrating quantitative imaging into routine practice, we can improve diagnostic precision, enhance prognostic assessment, and contribute to more personalized patient management in cardiothoracic care.

All these quantitative measurements successively validated by researchers and clinicians represent a huge amount of data. Nowadays, numerous tasks—some of them time-consuming—are becoming progressively relieved by AI. Nevertheless, before our final acceptance of these tools in clinical settings, radiologists and clinicians need to be familiar not only with their potential but also with their susceptibility to influencing aspects and subsequent potential limitations to be able to appropriately interpret the results. The knowledge of quantitative criteria detailed in this book ensures a solid base in this important task.

Disclaimer All measurements in this book have been obtained from peer-reviewed papers and guidelines from professional organizations, unless explicitly stated otherwise. While the authors, editors, and publisher have gone through a rigorous process to establish their correct reproduction from the original source, each measurement must be interpreted in the correct clinical context, this along with an accurate way of measurement, and taking into account all technical variables, this including follow-up exams with various equipment or software. Neither the authors, the editors, nor the publisher can accept any legal responsibility for any improper application or interpretation of these measurements as well as their potential consequences.

Part I
Technical Part - Technical Requirements

Radiation Dose

Denis Tack

Contents

D. Tack (✉)
Department of Radiology, Epicura Hospital, Baudour, Belgium

Abbreviations

ALARA	As low as reasonably achievable
BRR	Benefit/risk ratio
CTDI	Computed tomography dose index
DAP	Dose area product
DLP	Dose length product
DRL	Diagnostic reference level
DSB	DNA double-strand break
FANC	Federal Agency for Nuclear Control
Gy	Gray
ICRP	International Commission on Radiological Protection
LNT	Linear-no-threshold model
mGy	Milligrays
mSv	Millisievert
PACS	Picture archiving and communication system
Sv	Sievert

1 Origins and Foundation of Radiation Risks

1. X-rays used in medical imaging are ionizing radiations and may induce cancers, an effect known as stochastic and cumulative. Based on studies on nuclear bomb survivors in Japan, the carcinogenic effect of ionizing radiation is definite with exposures above 100 mSv (RERF 2022; National Research Council 2006). Below this threshold, although no

Med Radiol Diagn Imaging (2026)

https://doi.org/10.1007/174_2024_504,
Published Online: 24 July 2024

direct effect of radiations as used by medical imaging for the chest can be observed and measured, it is considered that repeated individual exposures induce cumulative risks that are proportional to the dose. Thus, risks can be extrapolated from high doses at which increased cancer incidence has been observed to lower doses as used in medical imaging. This extrapolation from high to low doses used as a rule by all authorities around the world is known as the linear-no-threshold (LNT) model of carcinogenesis and remains a matter of debate in the scientific community (Hendee and O'Connor 2012). Indeed, the LNT model of carcinogenesis can be opposed to a hormetic model in which low exposures could indeed bring a protection against cancer (Cohen 2002; Tubiana et al. 2009).

2. The physiologic foundation of X-ray toxicity is based on the fact that any radiation—even if very low—induces DNA double-strand breaks (DSBs). These breaks have been proven to be able to initiate mutations within cells and subsequently a cancer (Chadwick and Leenhouts 2014). DSBs can be quantified in blood cells and are influenced by numerous factors such as radiation, but also iodine injection without radiation, stress, tissue oxidative reactions such as during infection, etc.
3. Legislation aim to protect populations against risks. The LNT has been considered as a conservative approach to radiation risks in the low-level radiation field as used in diagnostic radiology (Euratom 1997, 2014). Thus, the general rule when using radiations in medicine is that any radiation should be justified and minimized according to the as low as reasonably achievable (ALARA) principle.
4. Some rules also mention that the benefit from performing a diagnostic test should exceed the risk of radiation (AFCN 2020a). They may even state that any radiation without a benefit higher than the risk is not allowed. Data on benefit/risk ratios (BRRs) are available in screening programs of asymptomatic people for breast cancer (Pashayan et al. 2018) or for lung cancer screening (Mascalchi et al. 2006, 2012). The BRR is estimated by establishing the ratio between the number of lives extrapolated and 100,000 individuals saved by screening as compared to the number of induced cancer by X-rays calculated using the LNT model and the BEIR VII tables of risks (Hendee and O'Connor 2012).
5. Because no randomization can be made for testing the use of medical imaging in symptomatic patients, e.g., for suspected pneumonia, no estimation of BRR can be made in clinical settings. In symptomatic patients, the use of imaging is supposed to be "by far" superior to the risk of radiation.
6. Things become even more complex to handle/evaluate when the benefit from using ionizing radiation is not directly related to each patient's health but is related to the whole population (e.g., screening of tuberculosis with chest X-ray). Benefit could also be of legal, medicolegal, or financial nature as when one has to prove an injury that is to be compensated by an insurance (Euratom Directive 2013/57).
7. Interventional radiology may result in exposures that are no more in the low-level radiation field. Deterministic effects of radiations such as skin burn or necrosis may occur after interventional therapeutic procedures using X-rays. In the chest, these doses could be seen after cardiac procedures such as in electrophysiology, in particularly obese patients. The threshold used in these procedures to prevent injuries is explained below.
8. Because any exposure induces a cumulative risk during lifetime, it is considered important to measure the radiation doses emitted—even if very small—and to quantify the risks they induce.

2 How Is the Radiation Dose Measured?

- Methods for quantifying radiation exposure to patients depend on the modality and device used for imaging (e.g., radiographs versus CT).
- For radiographic and fluoroscopic examinations, the radiation dose can be measured

either at tube output with a dose area product (DAP) meter or at the patient's skin with thermoluminescent dosimeters.

- For CT examinations, the radiation dose delivered to the patient is estimated/calculated from CT parameters and from measurements performed on standardized cylindrical plastic phantoms. From these measurements, organ doses can be estimated based on conversion factors established by the ICRP (Deak et al. 2010).
- With both radiographic and CT devices, anthropomorphic phantoms can be used to better estimate organ doses, but this is still pure research.
- The standard device used nowadays in radiographic examinations is the DAP meter that is placed directly at the tube output. The X-ray beam goes through an ionizing chamber, and the measured exposure is expressed as the product of energy and surface. The unit is the mGy cm^2. The emitted radiation dose is thus directly measured for each exposure.
- The standard method used in CT is indirect. Measurements are performed by the vendor on a computed tomography dose index (CTDI) phantom—either 16 cm in diameter for the head or 32 cm in diameter for the body—prior to delivering the scanner device on the market (McNitt-Gray 2002). Based on these measurements, the device can calculate and display any dose before a planned acquisition or that delivered immediately after the acquisition. The $CTDI_{vol}$ represents the dose per slice, takes the helical pitch into account, and is expressed in mGy (Fig. 1). The total dose delivered by an acquisition that takes the scan length into account is named dose length product (DLP) and corresponds to the product of the dose per slice by the scan length, expressed in mGy cm. The total dose of an examination eventually corresponds to the sum of DLP of all exposures.
- According to international rules, all exposures are stored in the patients' medical chart, usually together with images or on separate IT servers. A dose report in image format can be sent into the PACS together with the clinical images. It is usually named "dose report." An example of dose report is shown in Fig. 2 for a

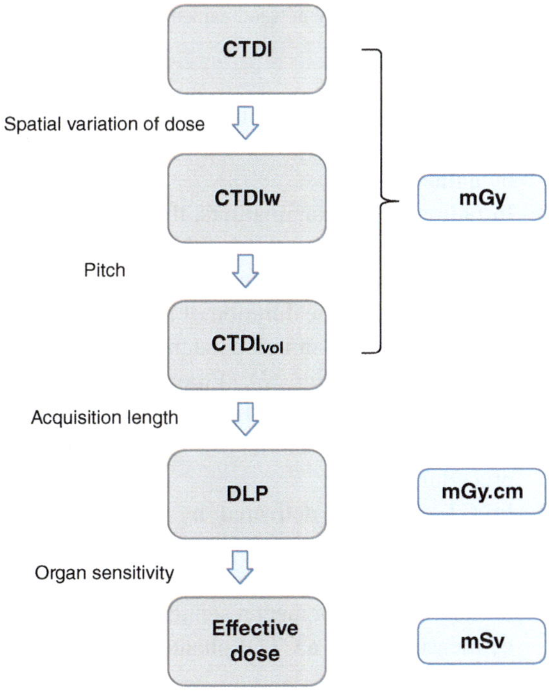

Fig. 1 Transition of CT doses from CTDI to effective dose. (Modified from https://www.radiologycafe.com/frcr-physics-notes/ct-imaging/ct-dose/)

a

• Sexe	M	• Méd. Praticien		•+ Temps scopie (min)	0:03
• Service		• Etablissement	Centre Hospitalier Epicura ATH S2	•+ Produit dose x surface (µGy*m²)	55.35
				•+ Dose à l'entrée(mGy)	0.60

kV	mAs	ms	Niveau ...	Longueur ...	Chp d...	Filtre Cu	Format	Corr. de noirc.	Caractéris...	Date et heure	Programme anatomique	DAP	EXI	Dose ...	Foyer	Grille	N° image
124.9	1.2	3.5	2.500	1	lr	Cu 0.1 mm	RAD	0		26-10-2022 11:37:02	RAD Thorax Face PA (THORAX ...	6.40	59	61	Petit	125	1
124.9	6.9	13.2	2.500	1	c	Cu 0.1 mm	RAD	0		26-10-2022 11:37:38	*RAD Thorax Prof (THORAX /RTH)	40.08	174	391	Grand	125	2

b

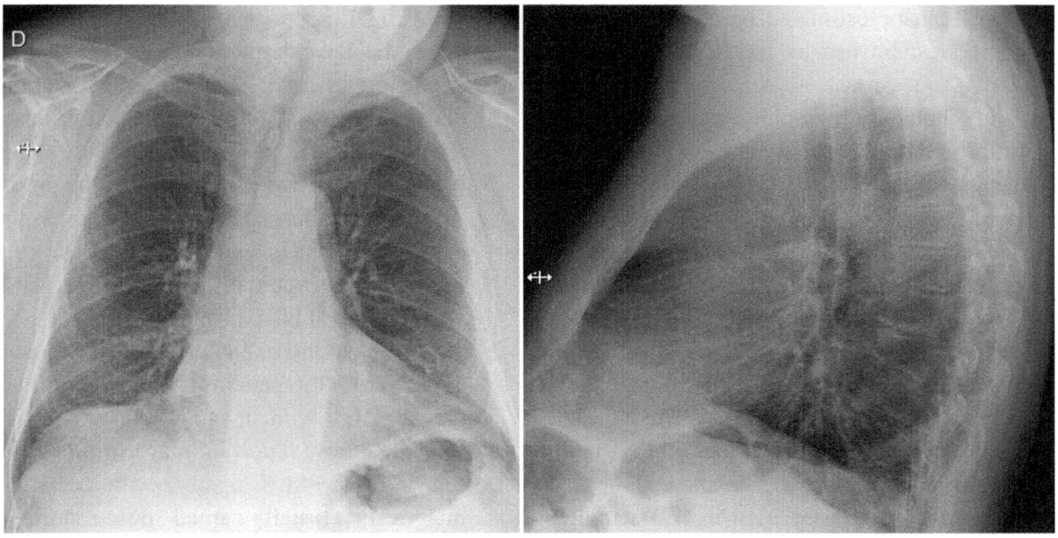

Fig. 2 PA and lateral chest X-rays and their corresponding dose report. (**a**) Dose report: two exposures were obtained, one PA (first line) and one lateral (second line). DAP is expressed in µGy m² (and named "Produit Dose-Surface"). Fluoroscopy was used during 3 s (named "temps de scopie"). Total DAP is 55.55 µGy m². (**b**) PA and lateral X-ray corresponding to the dose report displayed in (**a**)

chest X-ray and in Fig. 3 for a CT of the chest. In such reports, any exposure is represented by a line.

- In radiographic examinations, the dose delivered during fluoroscopy is added to that of each radiography and included in the total dose displayed. The duration of fluoroscopy is also displayed as an independent information in this report (Fig. 2). Fluoroscopy dose should be null in standard chest X-ray. It could be however substantial in interventional procedures.
- In CT, the dose delivered by the localizer radiograph—also named scout views or topograms—is not displayed by some CT vendors, because it does not meet a standard method to be measured with a CTDI phantom. With one vendor however, the dose of the localizer is converted into $CDTI_{vol}$ and DLP as well and is thus considered for the calculation of the total delivered dose. It is calculated as a simulation of a helical acquisition using the parameters of the scout. As the localizer dose represents only a small percentage of the dose delivered during helical acquisitions, it does not significantly impact the total dose delivered with the one and important restriction that is reduced-dose chest CT achieving DLP as low as 10 mGy cm. Some users therefore scan patients at reduced dose without obtaining first a localizer and thus with fixed tube current and no tube current modulation. Importantly, such acquisition protocols are not suited for large (obese) patients.

a

No.	Protocol	#of scan(s)	kVp	CTDIvol (mGy)	DLP (mGy.cm)	Body Size AP/LA	Total mAs	Range (mm)
1	DualScano	1	80	0.02 (Body)	0.64 (Body)	***	80	***
2	DualScano	1	80	0.02 (Body)	0.96 (Body)	***	120	***
3	Helical	1	100	1.70 (Body)	65.30 (Body)	27.53/ 28.41	555	315.0

SURE **Exposure**

No.	Name	SD	SUREIQ	Image Thickness	Recon FC	Recon Process	XY
3	20.00	20.00	Aice:Thorax	5.0	-	OFF	3DOEM

b

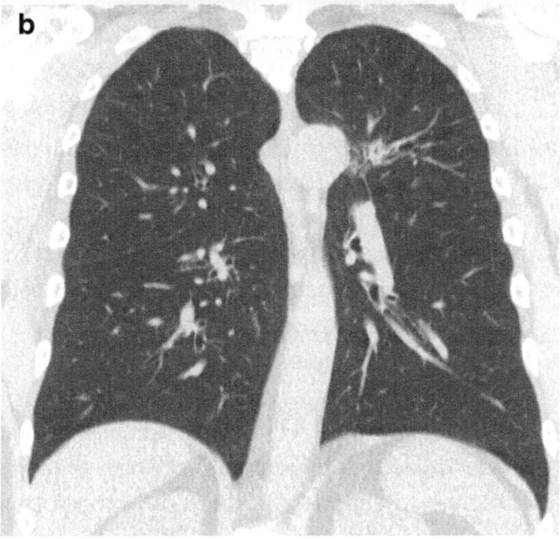

Fig. 3 CT dose report of a standard-dose chest CT examination. (**a**) Three exposures were obtained. The two first ones are the scout views in PA and lateral orientations. The corresponding calculated DLPs are 0.64 and 0.96 mGy cm, respectively. The helical acquisition is the third exposure. The DLP is 65.30 mGy cm in this patient with an average diameter of 28 cm (body size is calculated by the scanner device and displayed in this table). (**b**) This figure easily shows ground glass opacities next to a nodular density lateral to the aortic arch and mild emphysema in the two apices

- The dose measured by radiographic and/or CT devices represents absorbed doses, that is, the energy absorbed (in Joule) per kilogram. The unit is the Gray (Gy), and it is usually expressed in milligrays (mGy). These doses do not represent a patient risk, nor an organ dose. To estimate the risk, the absorbed dose must be converted into effective dose, expressed in sievert (Sv) usually in millisievert (mSv) (Fig. 1).
- The conversion factors of DAP into mSv in chest X-ray depend on the tube voltage used and the incidence, frontal or lateral (Wall et al. 2011).
- The conversion of DLP into mSv for CT of the chest has been studied by several sources and may also depend on several parameters, i.e., if the entire chest is scanned or only the heart (that is located at the level of the breast). These factors, as are risks, also depend on gender

and age, being higher in young patients and in females (Deak et al. 2010; Paul et al. 2014). In the radiological literature, 0.014 mSv/mGy cm has been proposed in 1999 (Paul et al. 2014) and is the most frequently used conversion factor, probably because it is the lowest one, and because authors always tried to prove that the dose delivered by reduced-dose CT of the chest is close to that of a chest X-ray with two exposures. A value of 0.017 mSv/mGy cm has been proposed by the European Commission in 2000 (Euratom 2000), but is less used, probably because it is less favorable for comparing reduced-dose CT and chest X-ray. As there is no reference method for establishing these conversion factors, any of them is acceptable.

- Conversion factors consider the radiosensitivity of organs located in the chest such as lungs, breast, bone marrow, and thyroid. The relative radiosensitivity of each organ as compared to all others being exposed during a full-body radiation has been defined by the ICRP and has varied from one report to the other (ICRP 1990, 2007; Paul et al. 2014). The last version is dated from 2007.
- Once absorbed doses have been measured and converted into effective doses, the risks from CT and radiographs can be compared.

3 Management of Radiation Values in Chest Dosimetry

1. As a general rule, there is no limit of radiation doses delivered in medicine. Legal limits only address the exposure to workers using radiation or exposed to radiations (radiology departments, operating rooms, cath lab, nuclear medicine, or workers of nuclear plants).
2. According to point 1, it does not make sense to set alarms in the CT devices if the dose to be delivered is higher than a diagnostic reference level (DRL). The reasons for higher dose values to individuals are obesity, arms along the torso, ventilation devices set next to the patient (intensive care patients), etc.
3. To provide images of adequate quality, devices are tuned to adapt the dose to the patient's absorptions. Thus, the dose delivered to a small patient for a chest X-ray can be up to 100 times lower than that delivered to an extremely obese patient. Similarly, a tenfold ratio can be observed in CT between such patients.
4. Therefore, there is no normal dose range available for individual patients.
5. In order to address possible dose excesses delivered to patients, a method used in microbiology was applied to radiation protection, that is, benchmarking through surveys. Dose surveys were introduced in the 1990s in the United Kingdom on chest X-ray, with the following method described in point 6.
6. Doses delivered to ten consecutive standard-weight patients (70 ± 3 kg) were collected for each device in participating centers. The average dose per device was calculated. The dose repartition between devices showed tenfold differences between extremes. The 75th percentile of dose repartition was then defined as the DRL. DRL was used as a benchmark of normal/abnormal practice, indicating that those devices delivering higher doses than the DRL were supposed to require optimization to achieve a lower dose than 75th percentile.
7. Optimization per definition consists of suppressing the dose excess, that is, the one that is not going to provide a better diagnosis capability than a lower dose.
8. According to the Euratom 97/43 directive, this method was later applied to CT dose descriptors ($CTDI_{vol}$ and DLP). Please see below confounding factors regarding the survey methods and results. Adaptations of the EU directives may depend on each EU member state. Thus, normal values depend on the area where devices are installed. Typical values for these procedures including comparisons with neighboring countries are provided by the Belgian Federal Agency for Nuclear Control (FANC) (2021).

4 Confounding Factors

1. At the individual level, the radiation dose should deeply vary between patients because devices are designed to provide a standard constant image quality and not a standard dose. Provided that the device settings are correctly set to do so, the energy absorbed by the patient is adapted to its absorption in correlation to its weight. As stated above, a tenfold ratio could be observed between doses delivered in small individuals as compared to larger ones.
2. Importantly, patients' individual doses should not be compared to DRL, which represents a benchmark of median doses between devices. A high individual dose does not represent good or bad practice since it is determined mainly through the patient's habitus.
3. For survey purposes, a local dose value should be obtained by sampling a very large amount of data in order to reduce uncertainties related to interindividual variability, which is extremely high for chest X-ray and very high for CT (Taylor et al. 2017, 2019).
4. For chest X-ray, to determine the median value representative of the local practice with less than 25% variability, the number of data to be collected approximates 1000 per device (a number being collected over a long period (months or years)) (Taylor et al. 2019). Interestingly, as local dose values show high variabilities, these also impact the variability of the DRL at a national level, with variability values larger than 25% of actual dose values, regardless of the number of centers participating in the survey, provided that more than 60 devices/centers participate in the survey (Vanaudenhove et al. 2020).
5. For chest CT, the minimum sample size to provide a local value of DLP with variability lower or equal to 10% is 300 examinations (Taylor et al. 2017). The uncertainty on the DRL level is of at least 20% (Vanaudenhove et al. 2019).
6. Nevertheless, there could be dose differences between devices as high as tenfold for chest X-ray obtained with flat panels, just because of the device and detector types (Taylor et al. 2019).
7. Reference values may change and be reduced each time a survey is conducted. This is predictable since 25% of centers/devices with dose values exceeding the DRL should be optimized. To note, the frequency of surveys for CT as recommended by the EU is once every 5 years. The main reasons for dose reductions are technology improvements through new devices, equipped with new detectors, generators, filters, and reconstruction algorithms. This was observed in the 15 first years of multidetector CT technique, between 1999 and 2015. The usual life of a CT device in that period was 7 years. Since then, technology improvements have dramatically improved clinical diagnoses, and one observed that CT lives increased up to 10–15 years. This impacted the results of dose surveys (see below next paragraph).
8. In Belgium, since 2008, CT dose surveys have been conducted every year. It was hypothesized that increasing the survey frequency would accelerate the CT optimization process. Indeed, DRLs were reduced between surveys, in particular in the first surveys (AFCN 2021). This reduction decreased however over time, and the dose values now reach an asymptote. This is the reason why the frequency of CT surveys was recently increased to the reference one (5 years) by the AFCN.
9. Current levels of DAP values in adults' chest X-rays are 100 mGy cm^2 for the PA view and 250 mGy cm^2 for the lateral view. DRLs are, respectively, at 150 and 400 mGy cm^2 (AFCN 2020b).
10. Corresponding typical effective doses are 0.03 mSv for PA chest view and 0.10 mSv for both PA and lateral views (Radiologyinfo.org 2022).
11. For chest CT, three acquisition protocols are typically used:
    - A full dose protocol (unenhanced) is used with median DLP values ranging from 60 to 300 mGy as reported in surveys, with

the corresponding effective dose ranging from 1.0 to 5.1 mSv using the 0.017 mSv/mGy cm conversion factor (Paul et al. 2014). Owing a scan length of 30 cm for the entire chest, the corresponding $CTDI_{vol}$ values ranged from 2 to 10 mGy.

- In selected cases, a reduced-dose protocol (unenhanced) with DLP was usually reported between 10 and 30 mGy cm, with the corresponding effective dose ranging from 0.17 to 0.51 mSv using a 0.017 mSv/mGy cm conversion factor. The corresponding $CTDI_{vol}$ values ranged from 0.33 to 1 mGy.
- To note, reduced-dose chest CT protocols are also named "low-dose" or even "ultralow-dose" protocols. These terms relate to relativistic comparisons with a standard-dose protocol that itself results from local choices in acquisition protocol optimization options. Terms such as "ultralow-dose" should not be used (Bankier and Kressel 2012).

5 Clinical Implementation of the Measurement

1. Radiation dose quantifications and values have strictly no impact on clinical practice if protocols are used for appropriate indications:
   - It is to note that reduced-dose protocols with DLP ranging from 10 to 30 mGy cm could disable assessing emphysema adequately (Bankier and Tack 2010).
   - Reduced-dose protocols have been proven efficient to demonstrate ground glass opacities in SARS-CoV-2 pulmonary infections (Desmet et al. 2021).
   - Reduced-dose protocols are typically used for nodule detection in lung cancer screening (Bankier and Tack 2010).
2. Dose optimization of CTPA examinations, in particular in pregnant women, should also include reductions of acquisition extent, with the lung volume to be scanned being located between the aortic arch and the top of the diaphragms. Such dose reduction has no impact on the diagnosis of pulmonary embolism but yields a 50% dose reduction (Litmanovich et al. 2014; Michalakis et al. 2014).
3. Appropriate optimization of CT parameters is a complex and multidisciplinary process that has been described earlier (Tack 2014).

6 Summary of What Should Be Done with Dose Measurements

1. Chest X-rays:
   - Make sure that dose reports are collected electronically and sent in the medical charts and to a dose monitoring software.
   - Compute this software to display median doses of PA and of PA + lateral views.
   - Compare your local median doses with the reference of your national agency.
   - Bear in mind that the exactness of your local data depends on the number of examinations. Sample high numbers of data on long time periods.
   - Bear in mind that even DRLs have their own uncertainties.
2. Unenhanced chest CT:
   - Make sure that dose reports are collected electronically and sent in the medical charts and to a dose monitoring software.
   - Collect $CTDI_{vol}$ to compare your median value to that of the national agency.
   - Compare your local DLP with DRLs and, if provided, with target values (usually 50th percentile of dose distributions).
3. For both chest X-rays and CT, do not set alerts at levels of DRLs, since it does not make sense. Doses should go as high as needed in obese patients.

Disclaimer All measurements in this book have been obtained from peer-reviewed papers and guidelines from professional organizations, unless explicitly stated otherwise. While the authors, editors, and publisher have gone through a rigorous process to establish their correct reproduction from the original source, each measurement must be interpreted in the correct clinical context, this along with an accurate way of measurement, and taking into account all technical variables, this including follow-up exams with various equipment or software. Neither the authors, the editors, nor the publisher can accept any legal responsibility for any improper application or interpretation of these measurements as well as their potential consequences.

References

AFCN (2020a) Arrêté royal du 13 février 2020 relatif aux expositions médicales et aux expositions à des fins d'imagerie non médicale avec des équipements radiologiques médicaux Chapitre I Définitions et champ d'application. Available at: https://etaamb.openjustice.be/fr/arrete-royal-du-13-fevrier-2020_n2020200179.html. Accessed 1 Nov 2022

AFCN (2020b) Niveaux de référence diagnostiques en radiologie conventionnelle adultes. https://afcn.fgov.be/fr/professionnels/professions-medicales/applications-radiologiques/nrd/radiologie-conventionnelle

AFCN (2021) Niveaux de référence diagnostiques en scanner adultes. https://www.icrp.org/publication.asp?id=ICRP%20Publication%20103

Bankier AA, Kressel HY (2012) Through the Looking Glass revisited: the need for more meaning and less drama in the reporting of dose and dose reduction in CT. Radiology 265(1):4–8. https://doi.org/10.1148/radiol.12121145

Bankier AA, Tack D (2010) Dose reduction strategies for thoracic multidetector computed tomography: background, current issues, and recommendations. J Thorac Imaging 25(4):278–288. https://doi.org/10.1097/RTI.0b013e3181eebc49

Chadwick KH, Leenhouts HP (2014) In: Tack D, Kalra MK, Gevenois PA (eds) Risks from ionising radiation in radiation dose from multidetector CT. Springer. e-ISBN: 978-3-642-24535-0

Cohen BL (2002) Cancer risk from low-level radiation. AJR Am J Roentgenol 179(5):1137–1143. https://doi.org/10.2214/ajr.179.5.1791137

Deak PD, Smal Y, Kalender WA (2010) Multisection CT protocols: sex- and age-specific conversion factors used to determine effective dose from dose-length product. Radiology 257(1):158–166. https://doi.org/10.1148/radiol.10100047

Desmet J, Biebaû C, De Wever W et al (2021) Performance of low-dose chest CT as a triage tool for suspected COVID-19 patients. J Belg Soc Radiol 105(1):9. https://doi.org/10.5334/jbsr.2319

Euratom (1997) Council Directive 97/43/Euratom on health protection of individuals against the dangers of ionizing radiation in relation to medical exposure. Available at: http://eur-lex.europa.eu/legal-content/EN/TXT/?uri=celex:31997L0043

Euratom (2000) European Commission—radiation protection 140 report. Available at: https://energy.ec.europa.eu/system/files/2014-11/140_0.pdf

Euratom (2014) Council Directive 2013/59/Euratom of 5 December 2013 laying down basic safety standards for protection against the dangers arising from exposure to ionising radiation, and repealing Directives 89/618/Euratom, 90/641/Euratom, 96/29/Euratom, 97/43/Euratom and 2003/122/Euratom. Available at: http://eur-lex.europa.eu/legal-content/EN/ALL/?uri=OJ:L:2014:013:TOC. Published 17 Jan 2014

Hendee WR, O'Connor MK (2012) Radiation risks of medical imaging: separating fact from fantasy. Radiology 264(2):312–321. https://doi.org/10.1148/radiol.12112678

ICRP Publication 103 (2007) The 2007 recommendations of the International Commission on Radiological Protection. https://www.icrp.org/publication.asp?id=ICRP%20Publication%20103

ICRP Publication 60 (1990) Recommendations of the International Commission on Radiological Protection. https://www.icrp.org/publication.asp?id=ICRP%20Publication%2060

Litmanovich DE, Tack D, Lee KS et al (2014) J Thorac Imaging 29(1):38–49. https://doi.org/10.1097/RTI.0000000000000064

Mascalchi M, Belli G, Zappa M et al (2006) Risk-benefit analysis of X-ray exposure associated with lung cancer screening in the Italung-CT trial. AJR Am J Roentgenol 187(2):421–429. https://doi.org/10.2214/AJR.05.0088

Mascalchi M, Mazzoni LN, Falchini M et al (2012) Dose exposure in the ITALUNG trial of lung cancer screening with low-dose CT. Br J Radiol 85(1016):1134–1139. https://doi.org/10.1259/bjr/20711289. Epub 2011 Oct 5

McNitt-Gray MF (2002) AAPM/RSNA physics tutorial for residents: topics in CT. Radiographics 22(6):2002. https://doi.org/10.1148/rg.226025128

Michalakis N, Keyzer C, De Maertelaer V et al (2014) Reduced z-axis coverage in multidetector-row CT pulmonary angiography decreases radiation dose and diagnostic accuracy of alternative diseases. Br J Radiol 87(1033):20130546. https://doi.org/10.1259/bjr.20130546. Epub 2013 Nov 20

National Research Council (2006) Health risks from exposure to low levels of ionizing radiation: BEIR VII—phase 2. Committee to assess health risks from exposure to low levels of ionizing radiation. National Academies Press, Washington, DC

Pashayan N, Morris S, Gilbert FJ, Pharoah PDP (2018) Cost-effectiveness and benefit-to-harm ratio of risk-stratified screening for breast cancer: a life-table model. JAMA Oncol 4(11):1504–1510. https://doi.org/10.1001/jamaoncol.2018.1901. Erratum in: JAMA Oncol. 2022 Mar 1;8(3):484

Paul JF, Keyzer C, Williams M (2014) Radiation dose optimisation of cardiac and vascular MDCT in adults and pediatric patients. In: Tack D, Kalra MK, Gevenois PA (eds) Radiation dose from multidetector CT. Springer. e-ISBN: 978-3-642-24535-0

Radiologyinfo.org (2022) Effective doses in adults. https://www.radiologyinfo.org/en/info/safety-xray

RERF (2022) Radiation Effects Research Foundation, Hiroshima, Japan. https://www.rerf.or.jp/en/programs/. Accessed 1 Nov 2022

Tack D (2014) ALARA concept for MDCT optimization: what is reasonable, what is achievable? In: Tack D, Kalra MK, Gevenois PA (eds) Radiation dose from multidetector CT. Springer. e-ISBN: 978-3-642-24535-0

Taylor S, van Muylem A, Howarth N et al (2017) CT dose survey in adults: what sample size for what precision? Eur Radiol 27(1):365–373. https://doi.org/10.1007/s00330-016-4333-3

Taylor S, Van Muylem A, Howarth N et al (2019) X-ray examination dose surveys: how accurate are my results? Eur Radiol 10:5307–5313. https://doi.org/10.1007/s00330-019-06055-5

Tubiana M, Feinendegen LE, Yang C, Kaminski JM (2009) The linear no-threshold relationship is inconsistent with radiation biologic and experimental data. Radiology 251(1):13–22. https://doi.org/10.1148/radiol.2511080671

Vanaudenhove T, Van Muylem A, Howarth N et al (2019) CT diagnostic reference levels: are they appropriately computed? Eur Radiol 295(10):5264–5271. https://doi.org/10.1007/s00330-019-06141-8

Vanaudenhove T, Van Muylem A, Howarth N et al (2020) Variabilities in X-ray diagnostic reference levels. Eur Radiol 30(8):4641–4647. https://doi.org/10.1007/s00330-020-06819-4

Wall BF, Haylock R, Jansen JTM (2011) Radiation risks from medical X-ray examinations as a function of the age and sex of the patient. Health Protection Agency Centre for Radiation. Available at: https://assets.publishing.service.gov.uk/government/uploads/system/uploads/attachment_data/file/340147/HPA-CRCE-028_for_website.pdf. Accessed 2 Feb 2023

Technical Aspects of Cardiac CT

Ana Ezponda and Gorka Bastarrika

Contents

Abstract

Rapid technological advances in hardware and post-processing techniques have increased the use of computed tomography (CT) of the heart in multiple clinical scenarios. Coronary computed tomography angiography (CCTA) is commonly accepted as a clinically useful noninvasive imaging modality for the diagnosis and exclusion of obstructive coronary artery disease (CAD), particularly in patients with intermediate pretest probability of coronary artery disease. However, CCTA is technically complex. In this chapter, we review technical and patient-related factors that may adversely affect the image quality and discuss potential measures that can be taken to avoid or mitigate these artifacts. In addition, future improvements in cardiac CT are described.

Abbreviations

CAD	Coronary artery disease
CCTA	Coronary computed tomography angiography
CMR	Cardiac magnetic resonance
CT	Computed tomography
DECT	Dual-energy CT
DSCT	Dual-source CT
ECG	Electrocardiogram
FFR_{CT}	Fractional flow reserve computed tomography

A. Ezponda · G. Bastarrika (✉)
Department of Radiology, Clínica Universidad de Navarra, Pamplona, Spain
e-mail: aezponda@external.unav.es; bastarrika@unav.es

Med Radiol Diagn Imaging (2026)
https://doi.org/10.1007/174_2023_450,
Published Online: 02 November 2023

ICA	Invasive coronary angiography
IHD	Ischemic heart disease
kV	Kilovoltage
MDE	Myocardial delayed enhancement
MPI	Myocardial perfusion imaging
mSv	Millisievert
PET	Positron emission tomography
SDCT	Single-detector CT
SPECT	Single-photon emission CT

1 Introduction

Coronary artery disease (CAD) is the leading cause of death worldwide (World Health Organization, WHO 2021). CAD is defined by the stenosis or blockage of the coronary arteries, generally secondary to atherosclerosis. Early detection of CAD is essential to reduce the morbidity and mortality rate associated with the disease. Although invasive coronary angiography (ICA) is the primary diagnostic tool and the standard of reference to evaluate CAD, the use of coronary computed tomography angiography (CCTA) has significantly increased in the last two decades, particularly since the advent of multidetector-row CT systems (Reeves 2021; Schoepf et al. 2004). In fact, a recent study has demonstrated that the rate of CCTA exams performed in hospital outpatient departments has increased markedly over the last decade (Reeves 2021). One of the factors which have contributed substantially to the rapid rise of CCTA is the advancements of CT technology in hardware and software solutions, which have allowed better temporal and spatial resolutions and reduced radiation doses. As a matter of fact, since the introduction of dual-source CT (DSCT) scanners, current effective radiation doses can even approach to 1 mSv (Akers et al. 2017; Ananthasubramaniam et al. 2017; Visseren et al. 2021).

With the ongoing evolution of ever faster and more sophisticated multidetector-row CT technologies, CT of the heart has evolved into an examination that is applied to a broad variety of clinical situations. CCTA has traditionally constituted an excellent imaging technique to *rule out hemodynamically significant coronary artery disease* (CAD) owing to its *high negative predictive value* (Ghekiere et al. 2017).

> **Increasing Relevance of Cardiac CT**
> *With the ongoing evolution of sophisticated multidetector-row CT technologies, CT of the heart has evolved into an examination that is applied to a broad variety of clinical situations. The high negative predictive value of CCTA in patients with low to intermediate risk of CAD makes it superior to stress testing.*

CCTA also provides high accuracy for the detection of significant coronary stenoses and has emerged as a useful noninvasive tool to predict cardiac events (Visseren et al. 2021). The Coronary CT Angiography EvaluatioN For Clinical Outcomes: An InteRnational Multicenter (CONFIRM) registry found that both the burden and severity of CAD in CCTA were important in predicting subsequent events (Hadamitzky et al. 2013). In this cohort, higher degrees of coronary stenosis (i.e., higher CAD-RADS scores) were associated with decreased event-free survival.

Guidelines recommend the use of *noninvasive imaging tests as the first-line method in patients in whom CAD cannot be excluded by clinical assessment* alone (Neumann et al. 2020) (Table 1). Selection of the initial noninvasive diagnostic test (CCTA, stress echocardiography, stress CMR, SPECT or PET) should be based on the clinical likelihood of CAD, patient's characteristics, local expertise, and availability of tests. Similar to these guidelines, recently revised American College of Radiology (ACR) criteria also consider appropriate the first-line use of noninvasive functional and anatomical imaging tests in patients with chronic chest pain and high probability of CAD (with or without previously known IHD) (Akers et al. 2017).

Table 1 Recommendations of the use of noninvasive imaging tests in the initial diagnostic management in symptomatic patients with suspected CAD (adapted from 2019 ESC Guidelines)

Class of recommendation I (B level of evidence)
• Noninvasive functional imaging for myocardial ischemia or CCTA is recommended as the initial test for diagnosing CAD in symptomatic patients in whom obstructive CAD cannot be excluded by clinical assessment alone. • Functional imaging for myocardial ischemia is recommended if CCTA has shown CAD of uncertain functional significance or is not diagnostic.
Class of recommendation IIa (C level of evidence)
• CCTA should be considered as an alternative to ICA if another noninvasive test is equivocal or nondiagnostic.
Class of recommendation III (C level of evidence)
• CCTA is not recommended when extensive coronary calcification, irregular heart rate, significant obesity, inability to cooperate with breath-hold commands, or any other conditions make good image quality unlikely.

CAD coronary artery disease, *CCTA* coronary computed tomography angiography, *ICA* invasive coronary angiography

Expert consensus recommendations consider it appropriate to perform CCTA as a *first-line* test for evaluating patients *with known or not known CAD history who present with stable typical or atypical chest pain* or other symptoms indicating possible anginal equivalent. According to the results of the ISCHEMIA Trial, CCTA may also be performed when considering evaluation for *revascularization strategies* (Narula et al. 2021). Other CCTA indications are summarized in Fig. 1. In *asymptomatic* individuals, CCTA may be appropriate when there is high risk for presenting a large amount of noncalcified plaque. In contrast, CCTA is rarely appropriate in low- to intermediate-risk asymptomatic patients (Narula et al. 2021).

In order to overcome the less specificity and positive predictive value of CCTA, other CT strategies like fractional flow reserve derived from CT (FFR_{CT}) and CT perfusion have been developed (Narula et al. 2021).

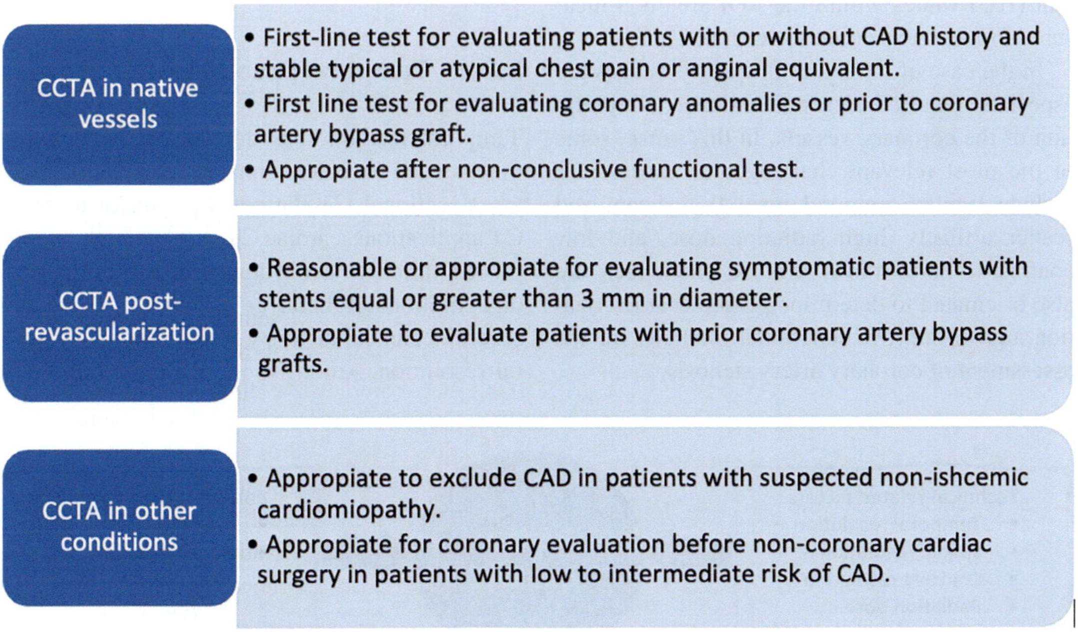

Fig. 1 Role of CCTA in chronic coronary artery disease. (Adapted from “SCCT 2021 Expert Consensus Document on Coronary Computed Tomographic Angiography: A Report of the Society of Cardiovascular Computed Tomography” (J Cardiovasc Comput Tomogr., 2021))

2 Challenges in Cardiac CT and Source of Artifacts

Cardiac CT is technically more complex and challenging than other types of CT exams, as it demands high performance requirements (Goldman 2008; Schoepf et al. 2004). In radiological examinations, *image quality* is a subjective entity determined both by *technical aspects* and by *patient-related factors* (image noise, spatial resolution, image contrast, and artifacts) (Fig. 2).

In CCTA examinations, the goal is to achieve a motion-free volumetric dataset through the heart during the peak coronary artery enhancement (Ghekiere et al. 2017). Thus, the two principal determinants of *image quality* in CCTA are *image noise* and *vascular enhancement*. These two parameters are usually evaluated in practice with the "image-to-noise" and "contrast-to-noise" ratios (Ghekiere et al. 2017), which are determined by placing a region of interest (ROI) in contrast-enhanced structures (i.e., left ventricular cavity). Standard deviation of the Hounsfield unit (HU) values within the ROI area is a measure of image noise (Ghekiere et al. 2017).

In the case of CCTA, high-quality images are especially required for accurate image interpretation of the coronary vessels. In this sense, some of the most relevant challenges of cardiac CT include limited temporal resolution, beam and scatter artifacts, high radiation dose, and low contrast-to-noise ratios. Future challenges are also orientated to determine plaque characterization and to improve functional methods for the assessment of coronary artery stenosis.

Remember
Knowledge of challenges of CCTA and potential artifacts is essential to develop methods for avoiding or mitigating them.

2.1 Cardiac Motion Artifact and ECG Gating

Continuous movement of the heart is one of the main technical challenges in cardiac CT. To "freeze" cardiac motion and to visualize the coronary arteries, image acquisition and reconstruction are synchronized with the electrocardiogram (ECG) (Mahesh and Cody 2007). It is known that, in most cases, the diastolic phase is the time of the cardiac cycle with least movement. Therefore, scanning or reconstructing projection data during this relatively motionless time window (mid-diastole occurring at approximately 65–75% of the R-R interval) will minimize cardiac motion artifacts (Fig. 3) (Goldman 2008).

2.2 Temporal Resolution

Temporal resolution is defined as the minimal time needed for calculating or reconstructing one cross-sectional CT dataset. In contrast to other CT applications, cardiac CT requires high temporal resolution to avoid image distortion by cardiac motion (Roberts et al. 2008). There are several technical factors which determine temporal resolution. Among them, the most important

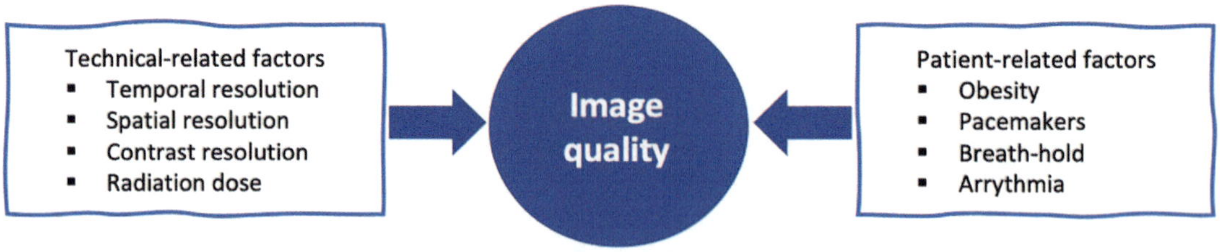

Fig. 2 Factors affecting image quality in cardiac CT studies

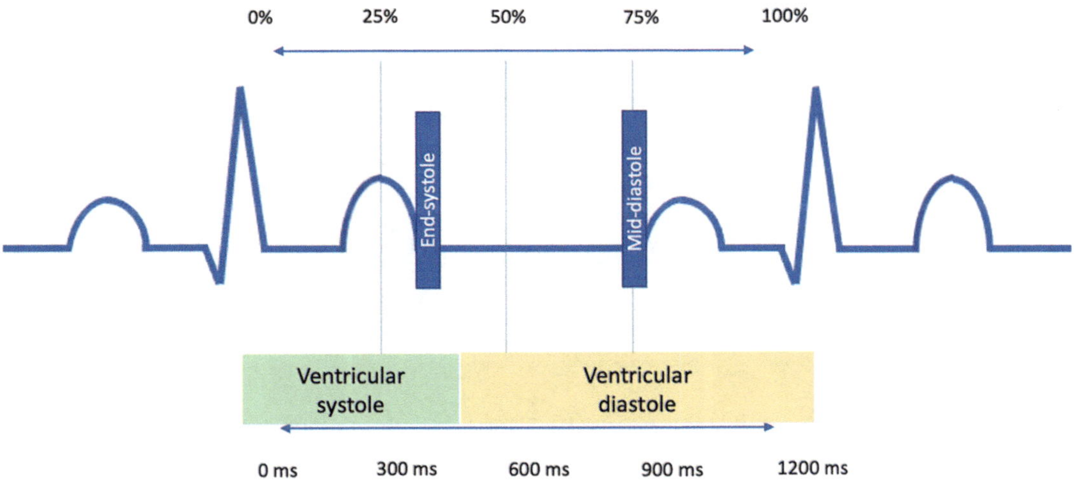

Fig. 3 Relationship between cardiac cycle and ECG. Cardiac CT studies are generally reconstructed in mid-diastole in individuals with a low resting heart rate, whereas the end systole is preferred in patients with a high heart rate

one is *gantry rotation time or speed*. Progressive advances in CCTA over the first decade of the twenty-first century have played an essential role in reducing gantry rotation time. Because of faster gantry rotation, temporal resolution has been improved from 250 ms with the first generation of 4-slice CT systems to 66 ms with the latest generation of DSCT systems (Flohr et al. 2009). Nowadays, the entire heart volume can be imaged in a single beat, eliminating motion artifact associated with the beating heart (Fig. 4).

Temporal Resolution

The larger the number of detectors in the z-direction, the fewer the gantry rotations required to completely image the heart.

Other factors influencing the temporal resolution achieved with MDCT scanners include the *acquisition mode*, the *type of image reconstruction*, and the *pitch* (Mahesh and Cody 2007). These methods have been developed to overcome the limited temporal resolution of certain CT scanners.

As said, data acquisition in CCTA is synchronized with the patient's ECG. The principal acquisition modes include the following:

Retrospective ECG gating (Fig. 5): In a retrospectively gated exam, continuous CT projections are acquired throughout the cardiac cycle in a helical mode, with continuous table movement (Menke et al. 2013). Each position of the heart is covered by a detector row at every point of the cardiac cycle. The images are afterwards reconstructed at the required cardiac phases. With current MDCT scanners, the study length can be covered in 3–4 heartbeats. Low pitch values (<1) are required in this acquisition technique to cover the heart during all phases. The pitch is adapted to the HR: the higher the HR, the faster the table moves. Due to the repeated radiation of the same anatomical area, *higher radiation doses* are obtained with this acquisition mode compared to other ECG gating techniques. The radiation dose is modulated along the cardiac cycle. Full tube current is used in those phases in which coronary artery reconstructions are expected (that is, the diastole in low HR and the systole in high HR), while radiation will be kept to a minimum in the rest of the phases of the cardiac cycle (Jakobs et al. 2002; Menke et al. 2013). The main advantage of retrospective gating is the ability to create *cine reconstructions* to evaluate cardiac and valvular function.

Prospective ECG triggering (Fig. 6): Currently, there are two major acquisition modes when

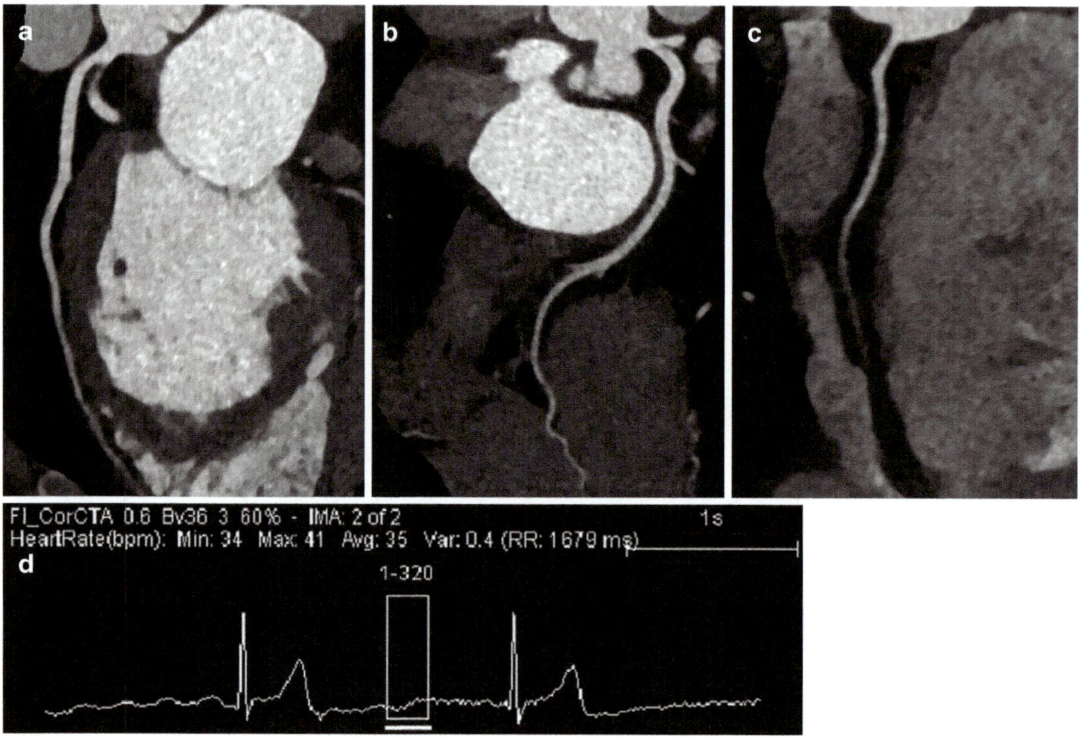

Fig. 4 CCTA acquisition with high pitch in a single heartbeat in a 42-year-old male with atypical chest pain. (**a–c**) Curved multiplanar images of the left anterior descending artery (**a**), circumflex (**b**), and right coronary (**c**) arteries. (**d**) ECG scheme of the acquisition mode. Dose-length product (DLP) of the examination was 26.8 mGy cm

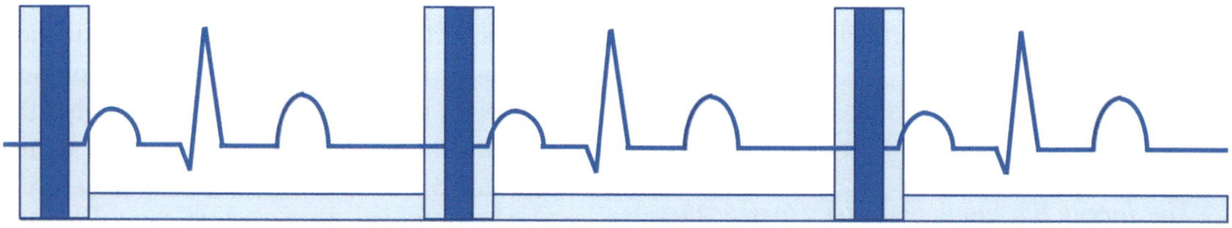

Fig. 5 Retrospective ECG gating with tube modulation

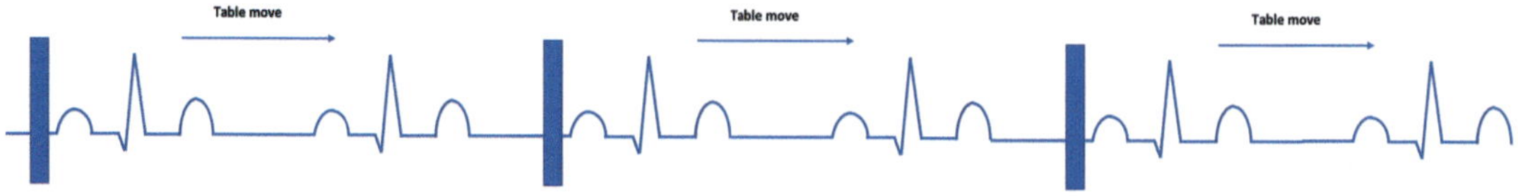

Fig. 6 Prospective ECG gating (step-and-shoot acquisition)

prospective ECG triggering is considered: the *sequential mode* (also known as *"step-and-shoot" mode*) and the single heartbeat *high-pitch mode* (Murphy et al. 2017). The ECG is used to trigger image acquisition at a specific time in the cardiac cycle, so the patient is exposed to radiation only during this interval. In the sequential mode, the table is stationary during data acquisition and moves in between data acquisition. Since the patient does not receive continuous irradiation throughout the cardiac cycle, the main advantage of this method is its lower radiation dose compared to the retrospective acquisition mode (Naoum et al. 2015; Leschka et al. 2010). However, as only one interval of the cardiac cycle is acquired, it is not possible to perform cine reconstructions or assess left ventricular function. The time point for scanning is defined prior to data acquisition. The number of heartbeats required to complete the study will depend on the detector width. With the *padding technique* that slightly increases the full radiation dose window, the images can be reconstructed in additional phases of the cardiac cycle (Schmermund et al. 1998).

The *prospective ECG gating with high pitch* is a recently developed spiral acquisition mode, which is inherent to DSCT systems (Choi et al. 2004; Lewis et al. 2016). With this acquisition mode, the second X-ray tube acquires scan data at the same angular position at a quarter rotation time and the pitch can be as high as 3.4. This technique enables entire heart acquisition within one heartbeat, thus significantly reducing the radiation dose.

The *pitch* plays a significant role in increasing both the temporal and the spatial resolution. Increasing the pitch will reduce the radiation dose, as the patient is exposed to radiation for a shorter time. The classical definition of pitch (or *detector pitch*) refers to the ratio of the table distance traveled in one gantry rotation and the total X-ray beam collimation. In the first helical CT scanners (single-source CT, SSCT), the slice thickness and X-ray beam width were equivalent. As a result, a pitch of 1.0 meant that the X-ray beams from adjacent rotations were contiguous. Pitch values less than 1 implied overlapping of the X-ray beam (and higher radiation dose) and greater than 1, a gapped X-ray beam (Goldman 2008; Mahesh and Cody 2007). With the development of MDCT scanners, a new definition of pitch was adopted (Goldman 2008). *Pitch or beam pitch* is now defined as the ratio between the table distance traveled in one gantry rotation and the total thickness of all simultaneously acquired slices. In this new definition, the denominator (total width) is the product of the number and thickness of simultaneously acquired slices (Goldman 2008). Pitch values range from 0.2 to 0.4 with SSCT and up to 3 with DSCT (Ghekiere et al. 2017).

2.3 Short Acquisition Time

The time required to cover an area depends on the area covered by the detector array, the gantry rotation time, and the pitch. To increase the speed at which the heart can be scanned, CT scanners have an array of X-ray detectors that cover a large area, allowing data collection from multiple "slices" in each rotation of the gantry. In MDCT scanners, the size of the array depends on the size and number of individual detectors. Detector arrays range from about 40 to 160 mm. As increasing the size of the detectors would result in a worse spatial resolution, larger arrays require more detectors to maintain the spatial resolution.

As previously mentioned, the *most quiescent part of the heart cycle is the diastolic phase* (Mahesh and Cody 2007). At rest, the normal heart rate (HR) in adults can range from 60 to 100 beats per minute (bpm). With an HR of 60–70 bpm, diastole occurs for two-thirds of the R-R′ interval (lasting for about 175 ms), whereas one-third of the time is spent in systole. As the HR increases, both systolic and diastolic phases shorten. However, the duration of the diastole is disproportionately reduced compared with the systole. For this reason, the required temporal resolution of CT scanners increases with higher heart rates. For heart rates of less than 70 bpm, a temporal resolution of less than 250 ms may be sufficient for motion-free imaging in diastole. In contrast, the desired temporal resolution in the systolic phase or for high heart rates is approximately of 50–100 ms.

In addition to the use of CT scanners with high temporal resolution and ECG-synchronized acquisition, *optimal patient preparation* is essential to avoid motion artifacts. Although there are fewer requirements for HR reduction in CT scanners with improved temporal resolution, there is still a tangible benefit with HR control, including better image quality and reduced effective dose. A target heart rate of 60 bpm or less is desired for CCTA (Abbara et al. 2016). This is generally achieved with pharmacologic intervention using *beta-adrenergic blocking agents* (beta-blockers) prior to the CCTA (Sheth et al. 2015). Most protocols involve the administration of oral beta-blockers (most frequently metoprolol) 1 h prior to the scan. The premedication dose (50–100 mg of metoprolol) depends on the patient's baseline HR at rest and the patient's weight (Abbara et al. 2016). In patients with resting HR of <60 bpm, some experts advocate that the administration of 50 mg of metoprolol might also be adequate to reduce HR variability and improve image quality.

> **Remember**
> *The diastole is the phase of the cardiac cycle with the least heart motion. The duration of the diastolic phase shortens with increasing HR. Optimal patient preparation with beta-blockers is essential for HR control prior to CCTA.*

2.4 Small Structures and Spatial Resolution

The coronary arteries are difficult to image because of their small caliber and displacement both during the cardiac cycle and with respiration (Ghekiere et al. 2017; Roberts et al. 2008). Indeed, degrees of motion of each coronary artery vary during the cardiac cycle (Table 2) (Ghekiere et al. 2017). To achieve an optimal visualization of the coronary arteries, high spatial resolution (at best submillimeter) is demanded (Flohr et al. 2009).

Table 2 Intervals of the cardiac cycle with the less likelihood of motion for each coronary artery

Coronary artery	Cardiac phase
Right coronary artery	40% of R-R interval
Left anterior descending	60–70% of R-R interval
Circumflex artery	50–60% of R-R interval

The spatial resolution defines the ability of a CT scanner to distinguish high-contrast anatomical details. It is usually defined in terms of line pairs per centimeter obtained from phantom scans. Both the scan *x–y* plane (*in-plane resolution*) and the *z*-direction (*through-plane resolution*) must be considered. The detector *z*-axis dimension is a major determinant of through-plane (*z*-axis) resolution. This type of resolution has improved since thinner collimated slices became available for routine use.

Regarding the *number of active detector channels*, the development of MDCT scanners has allowed to increase the spatial resolution by widening the volume coverage in the *z*-axis direction (Murphy et al. 2017). Larger volume coverage with multidetector CT has also led to reduced overall scan time (higher temporal resolution).

The spatial resolution not only depends on the *detector properties*, but also on the *reconstruction filter* used, the *contrast of the object* that is imaged, and the *image noise*. Since this information is not available on images, the voxel size is often used as an alternative surrogate marker. The *voxel size* is defined by the matrix and field of view (FOV). The image obtained on the monitor is made of a series of voxels (or three-dimensional pixels), the size of which depends on the spatial resolution of the CT scanner (Abbara et al. 2016). The average attenuation of the tissue within the voxel determines the displayed shade of gray (from black to white). If a voxel within a coronary artery contains tissues with widely different absorption rates (calcium and a fatty plaque), the whole of the voxel will be displayed as white, and useful information about plaque characteristics will be lost. The occurrence of this phenomenon ("*partial volume*" artifact) has been reduced with the employment of latest generation CT scanners. The smaller the voxel size, the less partial volume effects will be seen, and the spatial resolution will be better.

In addition to beta-blockers, nitroglycerin administration is desired for optimal coronary artery visualization. The most commonly used regimen consists of sublingual spray (1–2 puffs)

administered 1–2 min prior to the contrast-enhanced data acquisition. Nitroglycerin should be withheld in the presence of absolute contraindications, including recent intake of phosphodiesterase inhibitor or severe arterial hypotension (Abbara et al. 2016).

Thinner slice reconstructions, filtering kernels, and *iterative reconstruction* (IR) are factors that also affect the spatial resolution. Convolution filters are applied to reduce the blurring that occurs with back projection alone. Kernel filters can be roughly classified into standard, smooth, and sharp. The type of filters determines the spatial resolution and the noise: noise increases with sharp kernels, while spatial resolution improves with sharp kernels and worsens with the smooth ones.

2.5 Contrast Resolution

Contrast resolution is the ability to distinguish two different adjacent objects based on their attenuation values. A sufficient contrast-to-noise ratio is also required to resolve small and low-contrast structures such as plaques (Mahesh and Cody 2007). Several factors determine both image noise and contrast resolution: patient features, detector type, tube current and voltage, slice thickness, convolution filters, IR, and contrast media administration protocols. In the field of CCTA, high intra-arterial opacification (>250 HU) is required to evaluate the coronary vasculature. This is achieved with iodinated contrast media. The overall contrast volume is a function of the injection rate and the injection duration. Usually, high injection rates are employed (5 cc/s). Dual-head power injectors enable the mixture of contrast to reduce streak artifacts caused by dense contrast material in right cavities. The use of a saline bolus is useful to compact the contrast bolus and to optimize the amount of contrast. Bolus tracking or test bolus protocols are acceptable to trigger acquisition during peak arterial enhancement. Suboptimal contrast enhancement is associated with low image quality and inaccurate coronary stenosis assessment (Kalisz et al. 2016).

In selected patients, reducing the tube voltage to 100 kVp or even to 80 kVp allows significantly reducing the amount of contrast volume to obtain high-quality examinations at low radiation doses. When image noise and vascular enhancement are adequate, the remaining interpretability factors are motion related.

2.6 Radiation Dose

As in any radiological examination, a further important aspect in CCTA studies is keeping the radiation dose "as low as reasonably achievable" (ALARA principle) while maintaining image quality.

As explained above, there are three approaches to ECG-synchronized image acquisition: *retrospective ECG gating* with *spiral* data acquisition, *prospective ECG gating* with *sequential* ("step-and-shoot") data acquisition, and *prospective ECG gating* with *spiral data acquisition and high pitch* (Goldman 2008; Jakobs et al. 2002). The choice of the ECG gating technique has a great impact on the radiation dose to the patient. From the technical perspective, high pitch values reduce the radiation dose, as the patient is exposed to radiation for a shorter period. In third-generation DSCT scans, the effective radiation dose can even be below 1 mSv (Feng et al. 2018). The effective radiation dose (in millisieverts, mSv) is estimated by multiplying the dose-length product (DLP) by the correspondent conversion factor. Recent studies recommend using cardiac-specific conversion factors that range between 0.0229 and 0.0277 mSv/mGy cm, instead of the traditionally employed (0.017 mSv/mGy cm) applicable to chest CT exams (Trattner et al. 2018).

In order to reduce the effective radiation dose, *tube current modulation* and *tube voltage adaptation* can be added to the acquisition modes described above (Abada et al. 2006; Jakobs et al. 2002; Park et al. 2012). This is particularly important in retrospectively ECG-gated CCTA, in which tube current must be modulated in order to keep radiation dose at reasonable levels. In this acquisition mode, the tube output is raised to the nominal level during a limited interval in each cardiac cycle where the data are most likely to be reconstructed (i.e., in the systolic or diastolic phase, depending on the HR). During the remaining part of the cardiac cycle, the tube output can decrease even more than 95% of the nominal dose (Jakobs et al. 2002).

> **Dose Reduction**
> *For dose reduction in CCTA, ECG-controlled tube current modulation is recommended, especially in retrospectively ECG-gated acquisitions.*

Reducing the tube voltage is another effective method of lowering the radiation dose. In fact, the radiation dose is proportional to the square of the tube voltage. More interestingly, contrast and signal-to-noise ratios remain unaffected as the photoelectric effect is predominant with low kV (Park et al. 2012). This strategy results in higher attenuation of the iodine contrast material within the vessels and enables to optimize the use of contrast. However, low tube voltage acquisition is only recommended in certain individuals, for example in nonobese patients and in patients without significant coronary artery calcification or prior stent placement (von Ballmoos et al. 2011).

Iterative reconstruction (IR) algorithms selectively remove image noise by frequent comparison of the acquired dataset with an expected one (Naoum et al. 2015). Although this technology has been available since the early 1980s, technical advances in CT allowed its reintroduction into routine CT exams in 2008 (Naoum et al. 2015). When using IR instead of the traditional filtered back projection (FBP) reconstructions, diagnostic images can be achieved at low tube currents and voltages. In retrospectively ECG-gated studies, tube voltage and tube current modulation combined with IR have allowed to reduce radiation doses from 21 mSv to 4–6 mSv.

Another important aspect to reduce the effective radiation dose is to limit the *scan length* to exactly encompass the heart and the coronary arteries (Flohr et al. 2009; Leschka et al. 2010). The scan length can be planned in the scout view, in a range extending from the pulmonary artery bifurcation (at the level of the carina) to the cardiac apex. The scan length can also be determined in the prior calcium scoring acquisition. Adding 1 cm to the estimated scan length ensures inclusion of the heart and avoids incomplete acquisitions due to possible changes in inspiration depth between calcium score and CCTA. In patients with a history of prior bypass grafting, the examination should start at the thoracic inlet in order to include the origin of the left internal mammary graft.

> **Message**
> *Automated tube current modulation, tube voltage optimization, and iterative reconstruction along with the optimal ECG gating acquisition mode reduce effective radiation doses in CCTA.*

3 Image Quality Failures and Artifacts in CCTA

Despite improvements in cardiac CT technology, examinations are still vulnerable to a number of artifacts. Most common artifacts in CCTA are listed in Table 3. Patient-related factors such as tachycardia or arrhythmia, and technical factors such as inappropriate scanning delay with retrospective ECG gating, can result in artifacts that may obscure or simulate pathologic conditions. Cardiac cycle phase misregistration artifacts for example are caused by ECG signal failure, heart rate variation, or patient breathing during the acquisition (Fig. 7).

Table 3 CCTA artifacts, causes, and solutions. Adapted from *"Image quality in coronary CT angiography: Challenges and technical solutions" (Br J Radiol. 2017)*

Artifact	Problem	Cause	Solution
Blurring	Motion	• HR > acquisition speed • Breathing during acquisition • Inappropriate cardiac cycle phase reconstruction	• HR control (beta-blockers) • Breath-hold instructions • Optimal cardiac cycle phase reconstruction • Multisegment acquisition/ reconstruction
Stairstep or banding	Motion Cardiac cycle phase misregistration	• HR variation (tachycardia/ arrhythmia) • ECG signal failure • Breathing during acquisition	• HR control (beta-blockers) • Optimal cardiac cycle phase reconstruction • ECG editing • Pre-scan ECG quality check • Breath-hold instructions
Streak	Beam-hardening effect (attenuating low-energy photons by dense structures)	• Metallic implants, surgical clips, and coronary stents • Vessel filled with high iodine concentration	• Contrast injection followed by a mixture of contrast and saline • Use a high-kV monoenergetic X-ray beam (DSCT)
Blooming	High-attenuation objects appear larger than they are	• Coronary calcifications • Stents	• High spatial resolution reconstruction algorithms + iterative reconstruction • Use the smallest available focal spot • Use a high-kV monoenergetic X-ray beam (DSCT)
Windmill	Highly attenuating structures are surrounded by low-attenuating rims, and low-attenuating structures appear larger and have a "fanlike" appearance	• Moving structures during acquisition • HR > temporal resolution > spiral acquisition pitch	• Sequential acquisition is preferred • HR control (beta-blockers) • Optimize spiral scanning pitch
Low attenuating	Air bubbles	• Air within the contrast material bolus • Surgery	Check i.v. line before contrast injection

Motion artifacts are common in CCTA and result either from respiratory motion or from voluntary motion. Respiratory motion artifacts frequently affect the depiction of the inferior aspect of the heart and occur in studies with long scanning times (especially in patients with coronary grafts) (Fig. 8). It is important to note that these artifacts cannot be corrected with image data reconstruction methods or during the post-processing. Therefore, practicing the breath-hold with the patient prior to the actual acquisition is encouraged to prevent these artifacts.

Coronary calcifications and *in-stent evaluation* remain a challenge in CCTA. Improving spatial resolution is considered the best technique to reduce artifacts related to coronary calcification and stents. "*Blooming artifacts*" resulting from heterogeneous attenuation coefficients within the voxels (partial volume effect) may lead to an artificial increase in the size of high-density structures (calcified plaques) (Fig. 9). The use of thin slices and small field of views (FOVs) is crucial to improve spatial resolution. DSCT, IR, and sharp kernels are also able to facilitate in-stent evaluation.

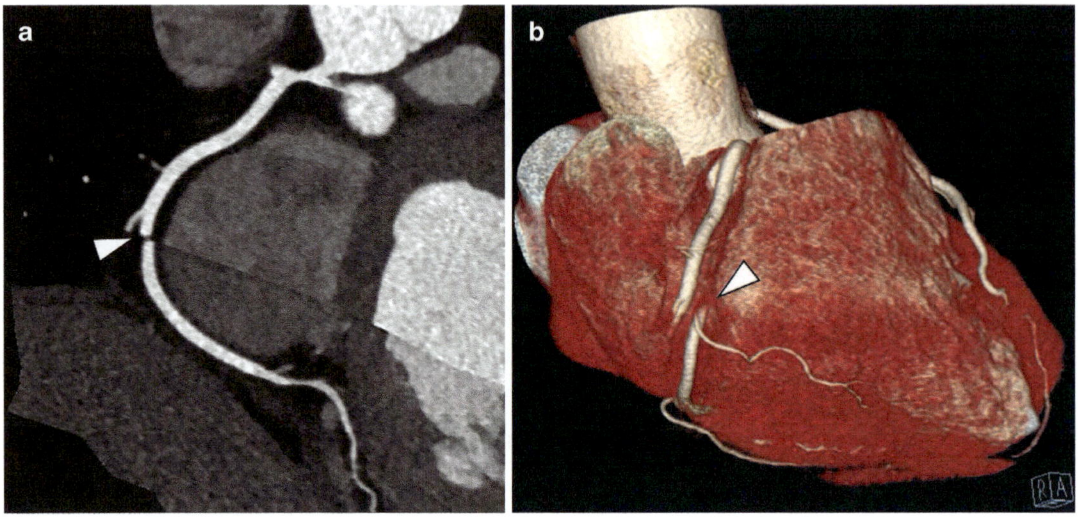

Fig. 7 Stair-step artifact. Curved planar (**a**) image of the right coronary artery and volume rendering (**b**) reconstruction. A linear band of misregistration affecting the mid-right coronary artery is clearly seen (arrowheads)

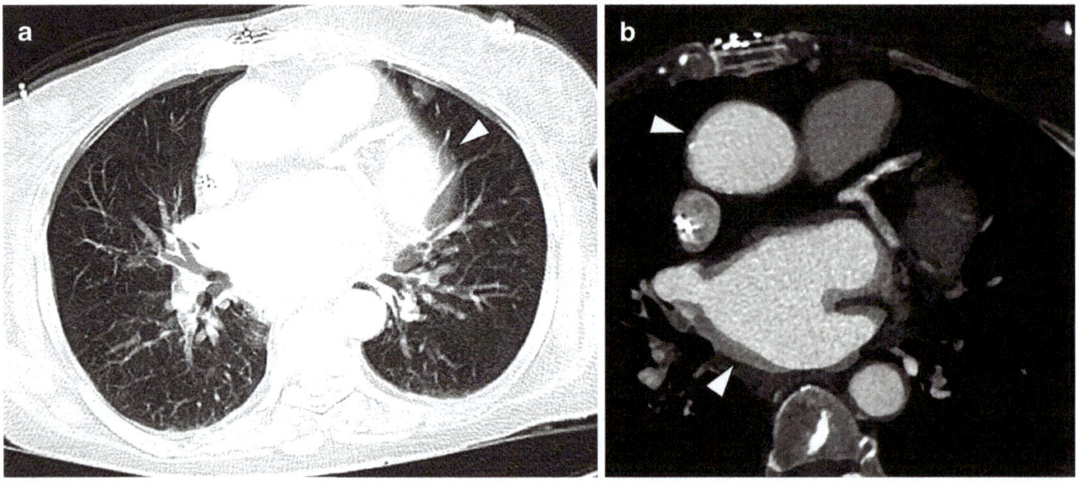

Fig. 8 Respiratory motion-related artifact. On axial CCTA images obtained with lung (**a**) and mediastinal (**b**) windows, this artifact is shown as blurring and double contouring of the heart (arrowhead in **a**), ascending aorta, and left atrium (arrowheads in **b**)

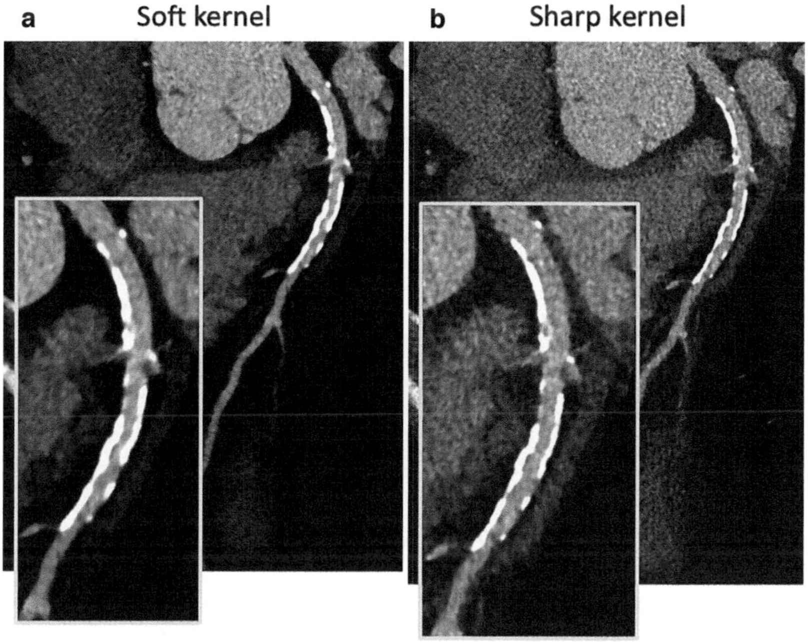

Fig. 9 Curved planar images of a markedly calcified left anterior descending coronary artery. Blooming artifact reduction is observed with the sharp filter reconstruction kernel

4 Solutions

4.1 CT Generations: Configuration of Detector Arrays

Since the performance of the first CCTA in the 1990s using electron-beam CT, CT technology has rapidly evolved (Schmermund et al. 1998). Major leaps in spiral acquisition, *gantry rotation speed*, and *increased number of detectors* have allowed to shorten scan duration (Ghekiere et al. 2017).

One of the essential components of CT scanners is the detector array. This element is responsible for sensing the X-ray radiation partially attenuated by body tissues and for converting them into a digital signal. The first helical scans consisted of a single-row (slice) detector CT (SDCT or SSCT), that is, a large number of detector elements in a single row across the irradiated slice (Goldman 2008). In SDCT, slice thickness was determined by the X-ray beam collimation.

Multidetector or multislice CT scanners (MDCT or MSCT) have an array of X-ray detectors that cover a larger area enabling collecting data from multiple "slices" for each rotation of the scanner. The size of the array depends on the size and number of individual detectors (Goldman 2008). Increasing the size of the detectors would result in a worse spatial resolution. Thus, larger arrays require more detectors to maintain the spatial resolution. In MDCT, the slice thickness depends on detector configuration and not on X-ray beam collimation. A greater number of thinner detector arrays has improved the spatial resolution from the initial 5–10 mm with the SDCT systems to less than 0.5 mm with the DSCT systems.

As analyzed when talking about temporal resolution, the time it takes to cover an area depends not only on the area covered by the detector array but also on the gantry rotation speed and the pitch. The maximal gantry rotation speed of current scanners is within the range of 250–350 ms.

Another advantage of MDCT over previous CT generations is the sophisticated algorithms they use for reconstructing partial scan data or recombining data from various phases. *Partial scan reconstruction* is widely used in CCTA for both prospective and retrospective gating acquisitions, as it achieves short effective exposure

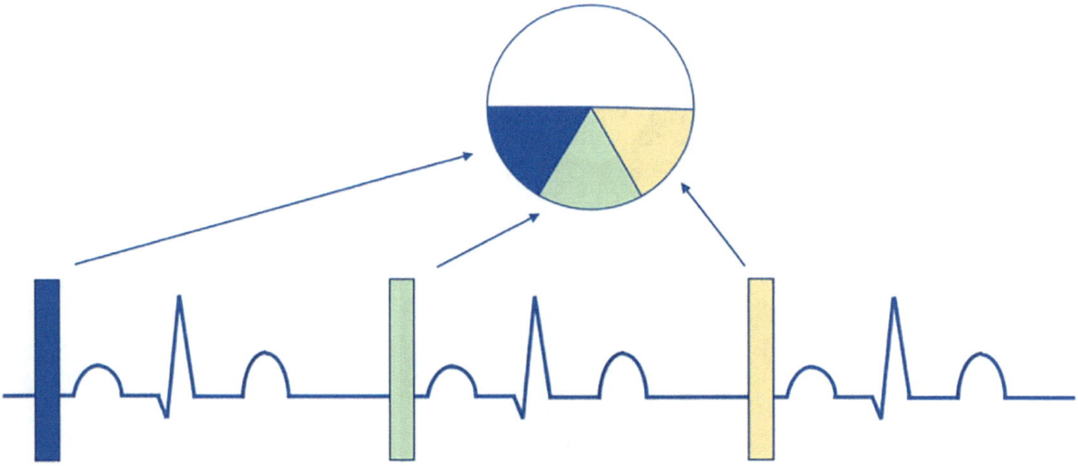

Fig. 10 Multisegment reconstruction. Image acquisitions (colored boxes) in mid-diastole during successive cardiac cycles. The circle represents the angular range

times (Choi et al. 2004; Mahesh and Cody 2007). To generate an image, only 180° of the projection data (plus the fan angle, which ranges from 30° to 60°) are needed. The remaining 180° is a mirror image of the first. Hence, the temporal resolution is approximately one-half of the gantry rotation speed for a single-source CT scanner and one-fourth for a dual-source CT scanner (Kalisz et al. 2016). This type of reconstruction even allows to acquire data during a single heartbeat with more advanced systems (Goldman 2008).

Monosegment and multisegment reconstructions also determine the temporal resolution. In multisegment reconstructions, the image is reconstructed from projection data from the same phase of the cardiac cycle at successive heartbeats, as the scan utilizes only a short data window in each cycle (Fig. 10). This is possible only with retrospective ECG gating, and the best results are achieved in patients with a regular heart rhythm. Whereas partial scan employs mid-rotation (180°) for data acquisition, multisegment reconstruction employs less than 180° of rotation. Monosegment reconstruction is usually applied with HR of less than 75 bpm. In contrast, the multisegment acquisition is usually employed when HR increases and better temporal resolution is required (Ghekiere et al. 2017).

Another requirement for CCTA is the isotropic sub-millimetric spatial resolution. To differentiate a 10–20% coronary stenosis, an isotropic spatial resolution of at least 0.3 mm is required (Lewis et al. 2016). *Isotropic spatial resolution* means that the spatial resolution in the transaxial plane (*x*–*y* plane) and in the longitudinal direction (*z* direction) is equivalent. Isotropic data implies cube-shaped voxels of equal length on each side.

Even prior to the multislice era, CT scanners presented an in-plane spatial resolution of 0.3 mm. However, through-plane resolution was limited due to the wider slices that were required to complete the acquisition within a breath-hold. Advances in MDCT scanners have made isotropic data acquisition feasible for nearly every application. This uniform image quality in all planes results in improved multiplanar and 3D imaging. Improvements in in-plane resolution have also reduced partial volume artifacts. Furthermore, since the development of 64-row CT scanners, isotropic acquisitions can now be achieved routinely with virtually no penalty in increased radiation dose and scan time.

4.2 Dual-Source CT Systems

Dual-source CT scanners have two X-ray sources (tubes) oriented 90° to each other. With these systems, each tube needs to rotate 90° to obtain a complete dataset (with half-scan reconstruction), allowing temporal resolution to be increased up to 66 ms (Goldman 2008). As an example, third-generation dual-source 192-slice CT scan (SOMATOM Force, Siemens, Healthineers, Forchheim, Germany) has a rotation time of 250 ms and a temporal resolution of 66 ms. This fast acquisition speed allows to "freeze" the heart more effectively at the end systole in patients with high HR (Feng et al. 2018).

5 New Developments

Important technological advances in CT include *wider detectors* for greater coverage with less gantry rotation times, *dual-energy CT* with simultaneous imaging at different energy levels to increase the contrast difference between tissues, and emergence of *spectral CT* to enhance atherosclerotic plaque imaging through nanoparticle technology (Ananthasubramaniam et al. 2017).

5.1 Dual Energy

Dual-energy CT principles are largely based on the photoelectric effect and can be achieved by analyzing intrinsic variations in attenuation when materials are exposed to beams with different energy levels (kV). DECT examinations are performed with low and high energy levels of photons (80 and 140 kVp). The most relevant applications of DECT in cardiac imaging include the following:

Myocardial perfusion imaging. DECT allows to differentiate photon energy levels and to map the iodine distribution in the myocardium as a quantitative marker for perfusion. Different studies have demonstrated that the combination of CCTA and DECT-MPI improves the accuracy of the test, with less false-positive CCTAs.

Myocardial delayed enhancement. DECT acquisition may provide a feasible alternative for myocardial viability assessment in patients with contraindications to CMR. Prospectively ECG-gated axial acquisition 5–7 min after the actual CCTA can help to assess *myocardial delayed enhancement* (MDE). The pooling of iodine in the interstitial space of the myocardial scar follows the same principles as the pooling of gadolinium on late gadolinium-enhanced MRI images. Due to better contrast-to-noise ratio, the combination of monoenergetic images at low energy levels with iodine density images has improved the diagnostic performance of DECT compared to MDE with SSCT (Mukai-Yatagai et al. 2020). On the other hand, different studies have demonstrated that MDE on CT can also be used to reflect myocardial fibrosis in cardiomyopathy. Compared to MRI, MDE with DSCT has the disadvantage of increments of radiation exposure and less spatial resolution. Ideally, 80–100 cc of contrast material should be administered to improve the image quality in MDE.

Coronary atherosclerotic plaque characterization. Differentiating components of noncalcified plaques (lipid vs. fibrous) is a challenge owing to the limited spatial resolution of CT technology. In a near future, DECT may overcome this problem by means of tissue decomposition.

Minimizing artifacts and contrast dose requirements. Virtual monoenergetic images at low photon energy levels can be generated to boost the iodine signal and reduce the amount of iodinated contrast. High keV monoenergetic images *reduce blooming* and *beam-hardening artifacts* and may allow the generation of calcium-free angiograms to improve the assessment of the vessel lumen.

Message

DECT-delayed myocardial enhancement is useful to identify postischemic fibrotic changes, especially when myocardial perfusion images are also acquired. This acquisition mode may also be used to reveal other myocardial diseases, such as the fibrotic changes occurring in the hypertrophic myocardium.

5.2 Spectral Imaging and Photon Counting CT Systems

Novel spectral CT systems are equipped with photon-counting detectors that enable differentiation of photons from multiple energy levels. These detectors convert the incoming X-ray photon into electrical charges. In contrast to DECT, which is performed with only two photon energy levels, spectral CT employs multiple energy levels to provide more detailed tissue information.

Photon-counting detectors allow reduction of electronic noise, beam-hardening, and metal artifacts with increased contrast-to-noise ratio and an extremely high spatial resolution. Implementation of these features will improve visualization of cardiovascular structures.

5.3 Myocardial Perfusion Imaging

CCTA allows noninvasive evaluation of the coronary vasculature and assesses the degree of coronary stenosis. However, a coronary stenosis (especially those visually estimated to be 50–69%) does not always induce myocardial ischemia (Neumann et al. 2020). Therefore, CCTA alone is limited to predict the hemodynamic significance of coronary stenosis.

Myocardial perfusion imaging (MPI) with CT offers the advantage of combining anatomical and functional information. Technical developments have improved the spatial coverage and allowed the implementation of CT myocardial perfusion techniques in the clinical practice. The international CORE320 study was the first to demonstrate that the combination of static CT-MPI and CCTA can correctly identify coronary stenosis associated with myocardial ischemia on SPECT (Rochitte et al. 2014). Single-center studies have demonstrated high accuracy of CT-MPI compared to SPECT, CMR, ICA, PET, and invasive FFR (van Assen et al. 2020). Growing evidence also establishes the incremental diagnostic value of the combination of CT-MPI and CCTA over CCTA alone (Dewey et al. 2020). In fact, MPI is particularly accurate when interpreted in the context of CCTA findings. However, like any other technique, CT-MPI presents advantages, disadvantages, and technical challenges (Table 4).

Table 4 Challenges, advantages, and disadvantages of radiological tools (CMR and CT) for the assessment of myocardial ischemia

	CMR	CT
Technical challenges	Spatial resolution for stenosis quantification and coronary hemodynamic assessment Nonlinear association between contrast agent signal and ischemia quantification Free-breathing perfusion MRI Quantification of myocardial blood flow	Beam hardening in stenosis quantification Contrast agent dynamics, noise, and dose for ischemia quantification
Advantages	Assessment of function, perfusion, and viability without ionizing radiation	Quantitative scale and high spatial resolution for coronary stenosis and plaque analysis
Disadvantages	Limited coronary stenosis analysis	Radiation dose Low contrast-to-noise ratio

According to most recent recommendations, CT-MPI together with CCTA should be performed in patients at high atherosclerotic risk for obstructive CAD, including those with prior coronary intervention or significant calcification, or when there is a stenosis of indeterminate functional significance and if knowledge of the presence and severity of ischemia would impact patient management.

For CT-MPI, there are three main approaches: static MPI, dynamic MPI, and dual-energy CT perfusion (Table 5). *Static CT-MPI* evaluates myocardial perfusion by analyzing the distribution of contrast (in SDCT) or the iodine concentration (in DECT) throughout the myocardium

Table 5 Description of CT perfusion imaging modalities. Adapted from "Society of cardiovascular computed tomography expert consensus document on myocardial computed tomography perfusion imaging." *J Cardiovasc Comput Tomogr, 2020*

Modality	Description	Advantages	Disadvantages
Static MPI	Simple image taken at peak myocardial perfusion to visualize hypoattenuation	Technically simple CCTA images can be used for rest MPI Low radiation exposure	Dependent on good image quality: susceptible to artifacts Timing of acquisition is critical Visual analysis of perfusion defects: need normal segment to identify abnormal perfusion Semiquantitative analysis: unclear if added value over qualitative
Dynamic MPI	Repeated images over time (transit of contrast) to create time-attenuation curves	Fully quantifiable flow (MBF): higher quantification accuracy Potential to detect balanced and microvascular ischemia	Increased CT hardware requirements Susceptible to artifacts Longer scan. Higher radiation doses compared to static MPI Additional software requirements
DECT perfusion	Separate energy X-ray beams to distinguish myocardium, contrast attenuation	Higher contrast differentiation than the other modalities Possible beam-hardening correction Different quantitative approaches possible	Specific CT hardware and software requirements

during a single period as the contrast transits the myocardium (Fig. 11). To acquire high spatial resolution images of the entire heart in a short time interval, at least 64 MDCT systems are required. *Static CT-MPI* can be performed with or without the administration of a vasodilator stressor. This technique provides qualitative or semiquantitative assessment of myocardial perfusion. In contrast, *dynamic CT-MPI* acquires multiple images over a specific time period, visualizing the entire in- and outflow of contrast medium (Celeng et al. 2019). With this acquisition, myocardial perfusion can be determined quantitatively (absolute myocardial blood flow, MBF) (Fig. 12). Challenges associated with dynamic technique include *increased radiation dose*, *motion artifacts*, and *image quality limitations*.

DECT perfusion allows for two types of analysis: monoenergetic (or monochromatic) examination and material decomposition. In the first type, an optimal energy level must be chosen to study the myocardial perfusion. Iodine contrast, with a high atomic number, has higher density at lower energy levels (higher contrast enhancement in the myocardium). However, these lower energy levels are associated with increased beam-hardening artifacts and noise. On the other hand, material decomposition yields information about the tissue atomic number and provides iodine density maps. Visual analysis as well as measurements of iodine concentration in a voxel can be performed.

In stress myocardial perfusion CT, *beam hardening* arising from high-density iodine contrast material in the cardiac chambers hampers accurate assessment of myocardial perfusion. This artifact can be eliminated with specific beam-hardening correction algorithms (Kitagawa et al. 2010). Different software solutions have been developed to mitigate this artifact. Some of them, for example, identify high-enhancing fluid-filled chambers when the cavity presents an attenuation >250 HU. Other challenges include limited temporal resolution with the consequent *cardiac motion artifacts* and *low contrast-to-noise ratios* (Dewey et al. 2020). Scanning with low voltage (70–80 kV) during perfusion enables

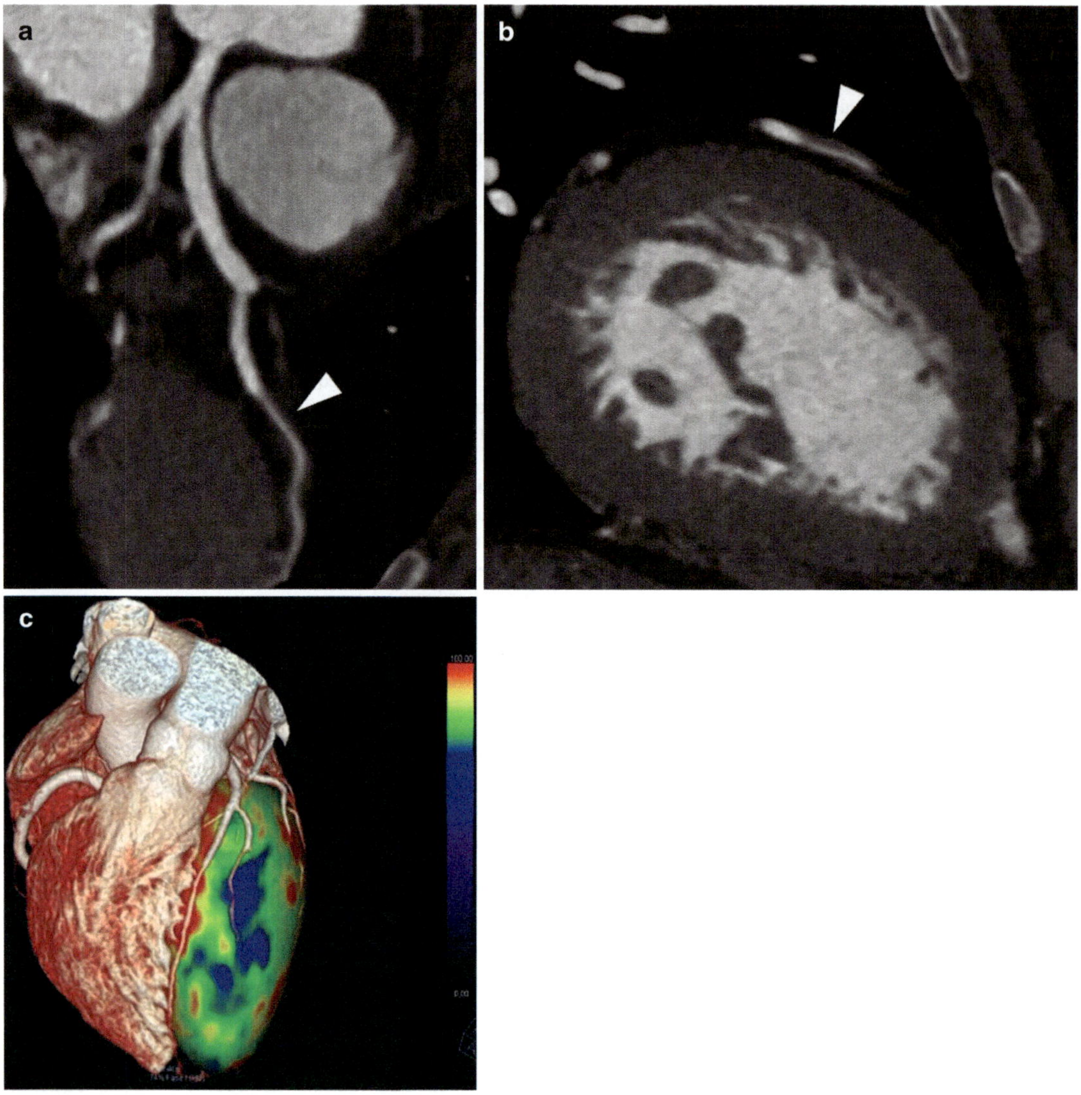

Fig. 11 CCTA performed in a 45-year-old woman with chest pain. Curved and multiplanar images (**a**, **b**) showed spontaneous dissection of the second diagonal branch (arrowheads). Static perfusion data represented into a 3D volume-rendered reconstruction (**c**) demonstrated reduced myocardial perfusion in the vascular territory of the diagonal branch (in blue)

a substantial reduction in radiation dose while increasing contrast-to-noise ratio.

> **Perfusion**
> *Myocardial CT perfusion challenges include limited temporal resolution, beam artifacts, low contrast-to-noise ratios, and increased radiation doses.*

As in CMR studies, image acquisition during systole has improved CT perfusion analysis. It is thought, however, that beta-blockers might reduce the vasodilator effect of stressor agents and underestimate the ischemic burden. Expert committees suggest the initial assessment of factors impairing the exclusion of obstructive CAD on CCTA (previously known CAD or significant coronary calcium). Patients with known significant CAD or severe CAC should undergo CT-MPI

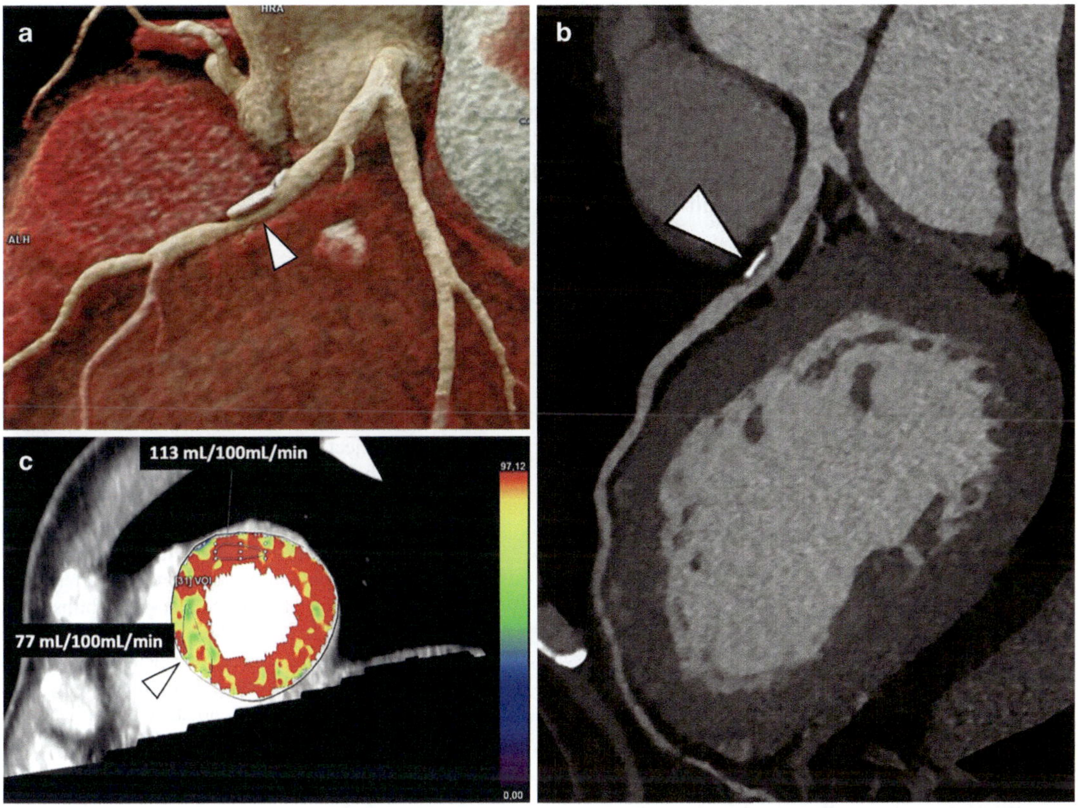

Fig. 12 CCTA performed in a 53-year-old man with atypical chest pain. Cinematic volume-rendered (**a**) and curved planar reconstructions (**b**) showed an intermediate stenosis in the midsegment of the left anterior descending coronary artery (arrowheads). (**c**) Dynamic CT-myocardial perfusion imaging demonstrated a significant reduction of the myocardial blood flow in the mid-anteroseptal segment of the left ventricle (77 mL/100 mL/min) compared to the remote myocardium (113 mL/100 mL/min)

prior to CCTA. In the rest of the patients, CCTA should be performed first (Patel et al. 2020).

5.4 FFR_{CT} and ECV Derived from CT

Invasive fractional flow reserve (FFR) is considered the gold standard for estimating ischemia and for guiding coronary revascularization. Advances in computational fluid dynamics and image-based modeling allowed the measurement of *FFR derived from CT* (*FFR_{CT}*). The indications are summarized in Fig. 13.

To what extent the implementation of FFR_{CT} will translate into improved patient outcomes still needs to be elucidated. Of note, a meta-analysis showed that CT myocardial perfusion has a higher specificity than FFR_{CT} (86% versus 78%) (Dewey et al. 2020).

Myocardial extracellular volume fraction (*ECV*) derived from CT delayed enhancement (CTDE) allows assessment of diffuse myocardial fibrosis. The principle is based on the extracellular distribution and pharmacokinetics of iodinated contrast media, which is similar to gadolinium-based contrast media. Good correlations between CT-derived ECV and both histology and LGE-MRI have been demonstrated (Takafuji et al. 2020). Calculation of ECV_{CT} is classically performed with the acquisition of unenhanced cardiac CT images prior to CCTA. Development of DECT provides a new strategy to estimate ECV, which does not require

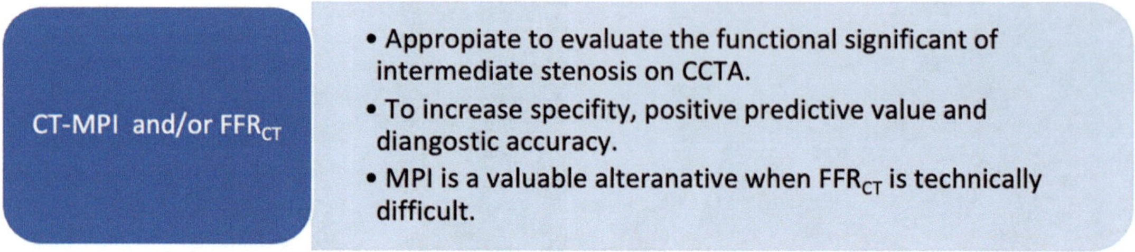

Fig. 13 Indications of CCTA with FFR$_{CT}$ and/or CT-MPI in chronic coronary artery disease

the previous performance of non-contrast CT (Qi et al. 2021). Therefore, radiation dose can be reduced. One of the main challenges related to estimating ECV$_{CT}$ is the amount of iodinated contrast medium required. Although it appears that ECV$_{CT}$ can be achieved accurately with the contrast doses used for conventional CCTA, further investigation is needed.

Acknowledgments and Funding None.

Disclaimer All measurements in this book have been obtained from peer-reviewed papers and guidelines from professional organizations, unless explicitly stated otherwise. While the authors, editors, and publisher have gone through a rigorous process to establish their correct reproduction from the original source, each measurement must be interpreted in the correct clinical context, this along with an accurate way of measurement, and taking into account all technical variables, this including follow-up exams with various equipment or software. Neither the authors, the editors, nor the publisher can accept any legal responsibility for any improper application or interpretation of these measurements as well as their potential consequences.

References

Abada HT, Larchez C, Daoud B, Sigal-Cinqualbre A, Paul JF (2006) MDCT of the coronary arteries: feasibility of low-dose CT with ECG-pulsed tube current modulation to reduce radiation dose. Am J Roentgenol 186(6 SUPPL. A):387–390. https://doi.org/10.2214/AJR.05.0216

Abbara S, Blanke P, Maroules CD, Cheezum M, Choi AD, Han BK, Marwan M, Naoum C, Norgaard BL, Rubinshtein R, Schoenhagen P, Villines T, Leipsic J (2016) SCCT guidelines for the performance and acquisition of coronary computed tomographic angiography: a report of the society of Cardiovascular Computed Tomography Guidelines Committee: endorsed by the North American Society for Cardiovascular Imaging (NASCI). J Cardiovasc Comput Tomogr 10(6):435–449. https://doi.org/10.1016/j.jcct.2016.10.002

Akers SR, Panchal V, Ho VB, Beache GM, Brown RKJ, Ghoshhajra BB, Greenberg SB, Hsu JY, Kicska GA, Min JK, Stillman AE, Stojanovska J, Abbara S, Jacobs JE (2017) ACR Appropriateness Criteria ® chronic chest pain-high probability of coronary artery disease. J Am Coll Radiol 14(5):S71–S80. https://doi.org/10.1016/j.jacr.2017.01.034

Ananthasubramaniam K, Sareen N, Rudin G (2017) Advances in cardiac computed tomography. In: Computed tomography - advanced applications. IntechOpen, pp 3–26. https://doi.org/10.5772/intechopen.68554

Celeng C, Leiner T, Maurovich-Horvat P, Merkely B, de Jong P, Dankbaar JW, van Es HW, Ghoshhajra BB, Hoffmann U, Takx RAP (2019) Anatomical and functional computed tomography for diagnosing hemodynamically significant coronary artery disease: a meta-analysis. JACC Cardiovasc Imaging 12(7):1316–1325. https://doi.org/10.1016/j.jcmg.2018.07.022

Choi HS, Choi BW, Choe KO, Choi D, Yoo K, Kim M, Kim J (2004) Pitfalls, artifacts, and remedies in multidetector row CT coronary angiography. Radiographics 24(3):787–800. https://doi.org/10.1148/rg.243035502

Dewey M, Siebes M, Kachelrie BM, Kofoed KF, Maurovich-Horvat P, Nikolaou K, Bai W, Kofler A, Manka R, Kozerke S, Chiribiri A, Schaeffter T, Michallek F, Bengel F, Nekolla S, Knaapen P, Lubberink M, Senior R, Tang MX, Piek JJ, van de Hoef T, Martens J, Schreiber L, Quantitative Cardiac Imaging Study Group (2020) Clinical quantitative cardiac imaging for the assessment of myocardial ischaemia. Nat Rev Cardiol 17(7):427–450. https://doi.org/10.1038/s41569-020-0341-8

Feng R, Mao J, Liu X, Zhao Y, Tong J, Zhang L (2018) High-pitch coronary computed tomographic angiography using the third-generation dual-source computed tomography: initial experience in patients with high heart rate. J Comput Assist Tomogr 42(2):248–255. https://doi.org/10.1097/RCT.0000000000000678

Flohr TG, Raupach R, Bruder H (2009) Cardiac CT: how much can temporal resolution, spatial resolution, and volume coverage be improved? J Cardiovasc Comput

Tomogr 3(3):143–152. https://doi.org/10.1016/j.jcct.2009.04.004
Ghekiere O, Salgado R, Buls N, Leiner T, Mancini I, Vanhoenacker P, Dendale P, Nchimi A (2017) Image quality in coronary CT angiography: challenges and technical solutions. Br J Radiol 90(1072):20160567. https://doi.org/10.1259/bjr.20160567
Goldman LW (2008) Principles of CT: multislice CT. J Nucl Med Technol 36(2):57–68. https://doi.org/10.2967/jnmt.107.044826
Hadamitzky M, Achenbach S, Al-Mallah M, Berman D, Budoff M, Cademartiri F, Callister T, Chang HJ, Cheng V, Chinnaiyan K, Chow BJW, Cury R, Delago A, Dunning A, Feuchtner G, Gomez M, Kaufmann P, Kim YJ, Leipsic J, Fay YL, Hausleiter J (2013) Optimized prognostic score for coronary computed tomographic angiography: results from the CONFIRM registry (COronary CT angiography evaluation for clinical outcomes: an international multicenter registry). J Am Coll Cardiol 62(5):468–476. https://doi.org/10.1016/j.jacc.2013.04.064
Jakobs TF, Becker CR, Ohnesorge B, Flohr T, Suess C, Schoepf UJ, Reiser MF (2002) Multislice helical CT of the heart with retrospective ECG gating: reduction of radiation exposure by ECG-controlled tube current modulation. Eur Radiol 12(5):1081–1086. https://doi.org/10.1007/s00330-001-1278-x
Kalisz K, Buethe J, Saboo SS, Abbara S, Halliburton S, Rajiah P (2016) Artifacts at cardiac CT: physics and solutions. Radiographics 36(7):2064–2083. https://doi.org/10.1148/rg.2016160079
Kitagawa K, George RT, Arbab-Zadeh A, Lima JAC, Lardo AC (2010) Characterization and correction of beam-hardening artifacts during dynamic volume CT assessment of myocardial perfusion. Radiology 256(1):111–118. https://doi.org/10.1148/radiol.10091399
Leschka S, Kim CH, Baumueller S, Stolzmann P, Scheffel H, Marincek B, Alkadhi H (2010) Scan length adjustment of CT coronary angiography using the calcium scoring scan: effect on radiation dose. Am J Roentgenol 194(3):272–277. https://doi.org/10.2214/AJR.09.2970
Lewis MA, Pascoal A, Keevil SF, Lewis CA (2016) Selecting a CT scanner for cardiac imaging: the heart of the matter. Br J Radiol 89(1065):1–11. https://doi.org/10.1259/bjr.20160376
Mahesh M, Cody DD (2007) AAPM/RSNA physics tutorial for residents multiple-row detector CT. Radiographics 27(5):1495–1510. https://doi.org/10.1148/rg.275075045
Menke J, Unterberg-Buchwald C, Staab W, Sohns JM, Seif Amir Hosseini A, Schwarz A (2013) Head-to-head comparison of prospectively triggered vs retrospectively gated coronary computed tomography angiography: meta-analysis of diagnostic accuracy, image quality, and radiation dose. Am Heart J 165(2):154. https://doi.org/10.1016/j.ahj.2012.10.026
Mukai-Yatagai N, Ohta Y, Amisaki R, Sasaki N, Akasaka T, Watanabe T, Kishimoto J, Kato M, Ogawa T, Yamamoto K (2020) Myocardial delayed enhancement on dual-energy computed tomography: the prevalence and related factors in patients with suspicion of coronary artery disease. J Cardiol 75(3):302–308. https://doi.org/10.1016/j.jjcc.2019.08.004
Murphy DJ, Keraliya A, Himes N, Aghayev A, Blankstein R, Steigner ML (2017) Quantification of radiation dose reduction by reducing z-axis coverage in 320-detector coronary CT angiography. Br J Radiol 90(1076):20170252. https://doi.org/10.1259/bjr.20170252
Naoum C, Blanke P, Leipsic J (2015) Iterative reconstruction in cardiac CT. J Cardiovasc Comput Tomogr 9(4):255–263. https://doi.org/10.1016/j.jcct.2015.04.004
Narula J, Chandrashekhar Y, Ahmadi A, Abbara S, Berman DS, Blankstein R, Leipsic J, Newby D, Nicol ED, Nieman K, Shaw L, Villines TC, Williams M, Hecht HS (2021) SCCT 2021 expert consensus document on coronary computed tomographic angiography: a report of the Society of Cardiovascular Computed Tomography. J Cardiovasc Comput Tomogr 15(3):192–217. https://doi.org/10.1016/j.jcct.2020.11.001
Neumann FJ, Sechtem U, Banning AP, Bonaros N, Bueno H, Bugiardini R, Chieffo A, Crea F, Czerny M, Delgado V, Dendale P, Knuuti J, Wijns W, Flachskampf FA, Gohlke H, Grove EL, James S, Katritsis D, Landmesser U, Clapp B (2020) 2019 ESC guidelines for the diagnosis and management of chronic coronary syndromes. Eur Heart J 41(3):407–477. https://doi.org/10.1093/eurheartj/ehz425
Park YJ, Kim YJ, Lee JW, Kim HY, Hong YJ, Lee HJ, Hur J, Nam JE, Choi BW (2012) Automatic Tube Potential Selection with Tube Current Modulation (APSCM) in coronary CT angiography: comparison of image quality and radiation dose with conventional body mass index-based protocol. J Cardiovasc Comput Tomogr 6(3):184–190. https://doi.org/10.1016/j.jcct.2012.04.002
Patel AR, Bamberg F, Branch K, Carrascosa P, Chen M, Cury RC, Ghoshhajra B, Ko B, Nieman K, Pugliese F, Schoepf J, Blankstein R (2020) Society of cardiovascular computed tomography expert consensus document on myocardial computed tomography perfusion imaging. J Cardiovasc Comput Tomogr 14(1):87–100. https://doi.org/10.1016/j.jcct.2019.10.003
Qi RX, Shao J, Jiang JS, Ruan XW, Huang S, Zhang Q, Hu CH (2021) Myocardial extracellular volume fraction quantitation using cardiac dual-energy CT with late iodine enhancement in patients with heart failure without coronary artery disease: a single-center prospective study. Eur J Radiol 140:109743. https://doi.org/10.1016/j.ejrad.2021.109743
Reeves RA (2021) Cardiac imaging trends from 2010 to 2019 in the in the Medicare population. Radiol Cardiothorac Imaging 3(5):e210156. https://doi.org/10.1148/ryct.2021210156

Roberts WT, Bax JJ, Davies LC (2008) Cardiac CT and CT coronary angiography: technology and application. Heart 94(6):781–792. https://doi.org/10.1136/hrt.2007.116392

Rochitte CE, George RT, Chen MY, Arbab-Zadeh A, Dewey M, Miller JM, Niinuma H, Yoshioka K, Kitagawa K, Nakamori S, Laham R, Vavere AL, Cerci RJ, Mehra VC, Nomura C, Kofoed KF, Jinzaki M, Kuribayashi S, de Roos A, Laule M, Tan SY, Hoe J, Paul N, Rybicki FJ, Brinker JA, Arai AE, Cox C, Clouse ME, Di Carli MF, Lima JA (2014) Computed tomography angiography and perfusion to assess coronary artery stenosis causing perfusion defects by single photon emission computed tomography: the CORE320 study. Eur Heart J 35(17):1120–1130. https://doi.org/10.1093/eurheartj/eht488

Schmermund A, Rensing BJ, Sheedy PF, Bell MR, Rumberger JA (1998) Intravenous electron-beam computed tomographic coronary angiography for segmental analysis of coronary artery stenoses. J Am Coll Cardiol 31(7):1547–1554. https://doi.org/10.1016/S0735-1097(98)00132-6

Schoepf UJ, Becker CR, Ohnesorge BM, Yucel EK (2004) CT of coronary artery disease. Radiology 232(1):18–37. https://doi.org/10.1148/radiol.2321030636

Sheth PJ, Danton GH, Siegel Y, Kardon RE, Infante JC, Ghersin E, Fishman JE (2015) Cardiac physiology for radiologists: review of relevant physiology for interpretation of cardiac MR imaging and CT. Radiographics 35(5):1335–1351. https://doi.org/10.1148/rg.2015140234

Takafuji M, Kitagawa K, Nakamura S, Hamdy A, Goto Y, Ishida M, Sakuma H (2020) Feasibility of extracellular volume fraction calculation using myocardial CT delayed enhancement with low contrast media administration. J Cardiovasc Comput Tomogr 14(6):524–528. https://doi.org/10.1016/j.jcct.2020.01.013

Trattner S, Halliburton S, Thompson CM, Xu Y, Chelliah A, Jambawalikar SR, Peng B, Peters MR, Jacobs JE, Ghesani M, Jang JJ, Al-Khalidi H, Einstein AJ (2018) Cardiac-specific conversion factors to estimate radiation effective dose from dose-length product in computed tomography. JACC Cardiovasc Imaging 11(1):64–74. https://doi.org/10.1016/j.jcmg.2017.06.006

van Assen M, Vonder M, Pelgrim GJ, Von Knebel Doeberitz PL, Vliegenthart R (2020) Computed tomography for myocardial characterization in ischemic heart disease: a state-of-the-art review. Eur Radiol Exp 4(1):1–13. https://doi.org/10.1186/s41747-020-00158-1

Visseren FLJ, Mach F, Smulders YM, Carballo D, Koskinas KC, Bäck M, Benetos A, Biffi A, Boavida JM, Capodanno D, Cosyns B, Crawford C, Davos CH, Desormais I, Di Angelantonio E, Franco OH, Halvorsen S, Hobbs FDR, Hollander M, Williams B (2021) 2021 ESC Guidelines on cardiovascular disease prevention in clinical practice. Eur Heart J 42(34):3227–3337. https://doi.org/10.1093/eurheartj/ehab484

von Ballmoos MW, Haring B, Juillerat P, Alkadhi H (2011) Meta-analysis: diagnostic performance of low-radiation-dose coronary computed tomography angiography. Ann Intern Med 154(6):413–420. https://doi.org/10.7326/0003-4819-154-6-201103150-00007

World Health Organization, WHO (2021) WHO

Cardiac MR Technique

Juerg Schwitter

Contents

Abstract

The unique ability of MRI to assess function, flow, and tissue characteristics makes it very attractive for cardiac assessment. However, to this aim, two major problems have to be addressed. First, cardiac motion correction must be performed which is straight forward by using the ECG. Second, respiratory motion must be dealt with in order to allow for sufficient spatial and temporal resolution. The most popular approach is the application of breath holds which allows to address all current standard cardiac evaluations. Investigations during stress are of particular importance in the work-up of cardiac patients. To further improve tissue characterization, temporal and spatial resolution are pushed to their limits by free-breathing approaches which are under intense investigation. Some are close to routine application.

Finally, novel techniques are ready for use in humans. Hyperpolarized ^{13}C-carbon molecules allow for near real-time metabolic studies of the heart. ^{19}F-fluroine molecules feature ideal properties to detect and track macrophages and to target noninvasively specific cell surface epitopes or other molecular structures such as fibrin.

J. Schwitter (✉)
Centre de la RM Cardiaque du CHUV,
Centre IRM interventionnelle du CHUV,
Centre Hospitalier Universitaire Vaudois—CHUV,
Lausanne, Switzerland

Faculté de Biologie et Médicine, Université de Lausanne, UniL, Lausanne, Switzerland
e-mail: jurg.schwitter@chuv.ch;
https://www.cardiologie.chuv.ch

Med Radiol Diagn Imaging (2026)

https://doi.org/10.1007/174_2023_404,
Published Online: 27 May 2023

1 Challenges of Cardiac vs. Noncardiac MRI

MRI is an excellent technique for visualization of anatomical structures, but it yields its most important contribution to establish a patient's diagnosis, when used for tissue characterization, functional analyses, and flow measurements. These unique aspects of MRI make it also a very attractive method for cardiac assessment (Schwitter 2020). However, in comparison to noncardiac MRI, the application of MRI to the heart comes with several additional obstacles. First, cardiac and respiratory motion must be dealt with. In addition, the position of the heart close to the lungs but also to solid organs of the upper abdomen impacts negatively on magnetic field homogeneity. And finally, many cardiac diseases such as coronary artery disease or some valvular diseases are not detectable at rest and the heart must be stressed to evaluate its reserve. Cardiac investigations during stress impose particularly high demands on scanner hardware and software and may be challenging also for the technicians and doctors that perform such stress cardiac MRI studies.

2 Heart Motion

With state-of-the-art MR machines, the heart can be imaged in real time. However, this approach suffers from relatively low spatial and temporal resolution as an entire image is acquired in a "single shot." For details, see Fig. 1 and Table 1. To improve temporal and/or spatial resolution, however, the acquisitions should be spread over several heartbeats which requires correction of heart motion. Fortunately, this motion information is relatively easy to get via the ECG, particularly at 1.5 T, and its correction is straight forward. From the ECG, the R wave is detected and used to trigger the various pulse sequences. The most popular type of triggered acquisition is the so-called segmented k-space acquisition, which acquires a predefined portion of the lines in k-space during each cardiac cycle, see Fig. 2 (Chien et al. 1991). The portions of k-space lines that are acquired at the same trigger delay after the R wave are then combined to yield a completely filled k-space which then allows to reconstruct a full image. With this technique, the time to acquire such a portion of k-space lines determines the temporal resolution

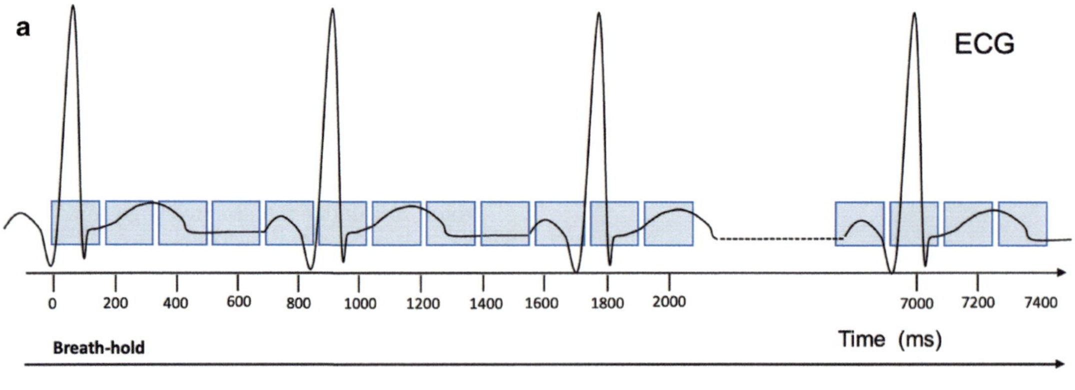

Fig. 1 (**a**) Real-time acquisition—no triggering and no respiratory motion control. This acquisition is "free-running," and no ECG triggering is applied. Each blue box represents the acquisition of a full image (i.e., full k-space data, or reduced k-space in case of acceleration methods, which are generally used for this kind of acquisition). An example of real-time function imaging is given in Fig. 6. This type of acquisition can also be combined with bipolar gradients preceding each read-out to allow for phase-contrast flow measurements. (**b**) Real-time acquisition for perfusion—with triggering. To achieve strong T_1-weighting, a 90° saturation pulse (black line) is played out after the ECG trigger (red line). Saturation preparation is followed by a saturation recovery time TS to allow for relaxation evolution and for timing the acquisition window to fall into phases of minor cardiac motion during the cardiac cycle (in this example in late systole and in mid-diastole). The blue box indicates acquisition of a full image (full k-space data). This sequence runs during contrast medium administration to monitor signal increase in the myocardium during hyperemic stress. S1–S4 indicates short-axis slices 1–4. The dashed QRS complexes and red trigger lines indicate as many heartbeats as needed to fully cover the first pass of the contrast medium

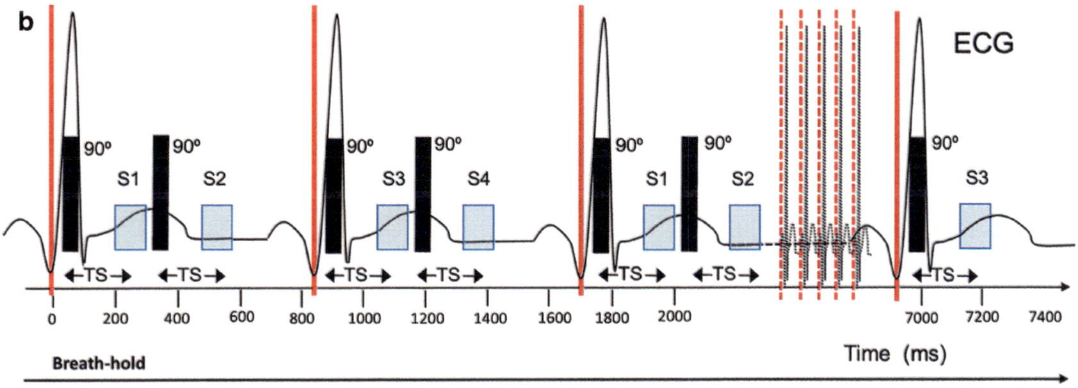

Fig. 1 (continued)

Table 1 Cardiac MRI pulse sequences and reconstructions in clinical routine cardiology/radiology and under development

Acquisition strategy	Real time	Segmented acquisition	Free breathing
Applications in clinical cardiology routine			
	Function (constriction)	**Volumes/function**	
	Perfusion stress	**Dobutamine stress**	
		Flow	
		LGE	
		Mapping (T_1, T_2, T_2^*)	
		Tagging	
Applications under evaluation in specialized centers			
	Interventional (catheter guidance)	**Interventional** (lesion characterization)	**Interventional** (roadmap generation)
	Metabolism: hyperpolarized ^{13}C	**Mapping** ($T_1\rho$)	**Coronary MR angiography**
			Flow (4D and 5D)
			High-resolution 3D LGE
			Metabolism: spectroscopy (^{1}H, ^{31}P)
			^{19}F-fluorine MRI
Technical aspects			
Typical acquisition duration per image	50–100 ms	Several heartbeats	Several minutes
Cardiac motion compensation	No	ECG	ECG
Respiratory motion compensation	No	Breath-hold	Navigation • Diaphragmatic • Self-navigation • Pilot tone • Image-based
Typical data representation	2-Dimensional	2-Dimensional	3-Dimensional
Typical reconstruction strategies	Parallel imaging	Parallel imaging	Parallel imaging
	Compressed sensing	Compressed sensing	Compressed sensing
	Spatially selective excitation		Artificial intelligence

ECG electrocardiogram, *LGE* late-gadolinium enhancement

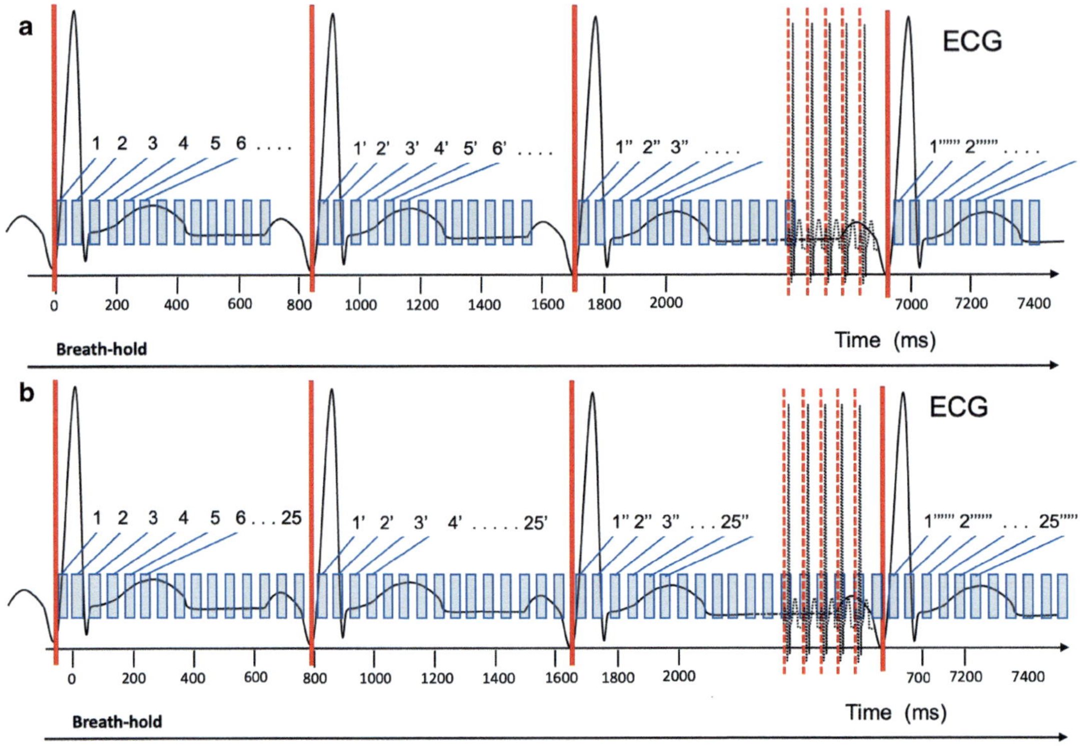

Fig. 2 (**a**) Segmented acquisition—with prospective triggering. In this acquisition scheme, several portions of k-space lines are acquired (1, 2, 3, etc.) every cardiac cycle. The ECG trigger is used as the timing reference. Portions **1**, **1″**, **1‴**, etc. are combined to yield a full image (i.e., full k-space data) for phase 1 of the cardiac cycle and so on. The combination of these multiple phases yields the cine loop information for functional assessment. This prospectively triggered acquisition is typically used in patients with irregular heartbeats. An example of this prospective acquisition scheme is given in Fig. 7. This acquisition does not cover the late diastolic period of the cardiac cycle. The dashed QRS complexes and red trigger lines indicate as many heartbeats as needed to acquire a full k-space (i.e., to allow for full image reconstruction per phase). (**b**) Segmented acquisition—with retrospective triggering. Widely used sequence: In this retrospective scheme, again portions of k-space lines are acquired, this time, however, in "free running" mode. This acquisition is therefore not interrupted to wait for the next trigger. Instead, the trigger time points are recorded and used to retrospectively divide up the acquired k-space lines into, e.g., 25 portions per cardiac cycle. The combination of these multiple phases yields the cine loop information for functional assessment. With this pulse sequence, the entire cardiac cycle is covered. Portions **1**, **1″**, **1‴**, etc. are then combined to yield a full image (i.e., full k-space data) for phase 1 of the cardiac cycle and so on (see example in Fig. 7). The dashed QRS complexes and red trigger lines indicate as many heartbeats as needed to acquire a full k-space (i.e., to allow for full image reconstruction per phase). This type of acquisition can also be combined with bipolar gradients preceding each read-out to allow for phase-contrast flow measurements. An example for a phase-contrast flow measurement is shown in Fig. 10. (**c/d**) Segmented LGE acquisition in late systole and mid-diastole—with triggering. Widely used breath-hold LGE sequence: In this segmented scheme, again portions of k-space lines (blue box) are acquired. This time, however, a non-slice selective 180° inversion pulse (black box) is played out to achieve strong T_1-weigthting. After the inversion time TI, the portions **1**, **1″**, **1‴**, etc. are then combined to yield a full LGE image (i.e., full k-space data). The trigger delay after the ECG trigger can be chosen such that the data acquisition occurs in late systole (top) or in mid-diastole (bottom). Late systolic LGE is particularly useful in patients with irregular heartbeats. The dashed QRS complexes and red trigger lines indicate as many heartbeats as needed to acquire a full k-space (i.e., to allow for full LGE image reconstruction). Examples of this acquisition scheme are given in Figs. 5 and 8. The inversion time TI can also cover a certain range to generate images with different TIs allowing to calculate the longitudinal relaxation constant T_1, i.e., to create T_1 maps acquired in a breath hold (see Fig. 9 as an example). In analogy, a T_2-weighting prepulse can replace the 180° inversion pulse to get T_2-weighting. By covering a range of echo times TE, the transverse relaxation constant T_2 can be calculated to obtain T_2 maps in a breath hold

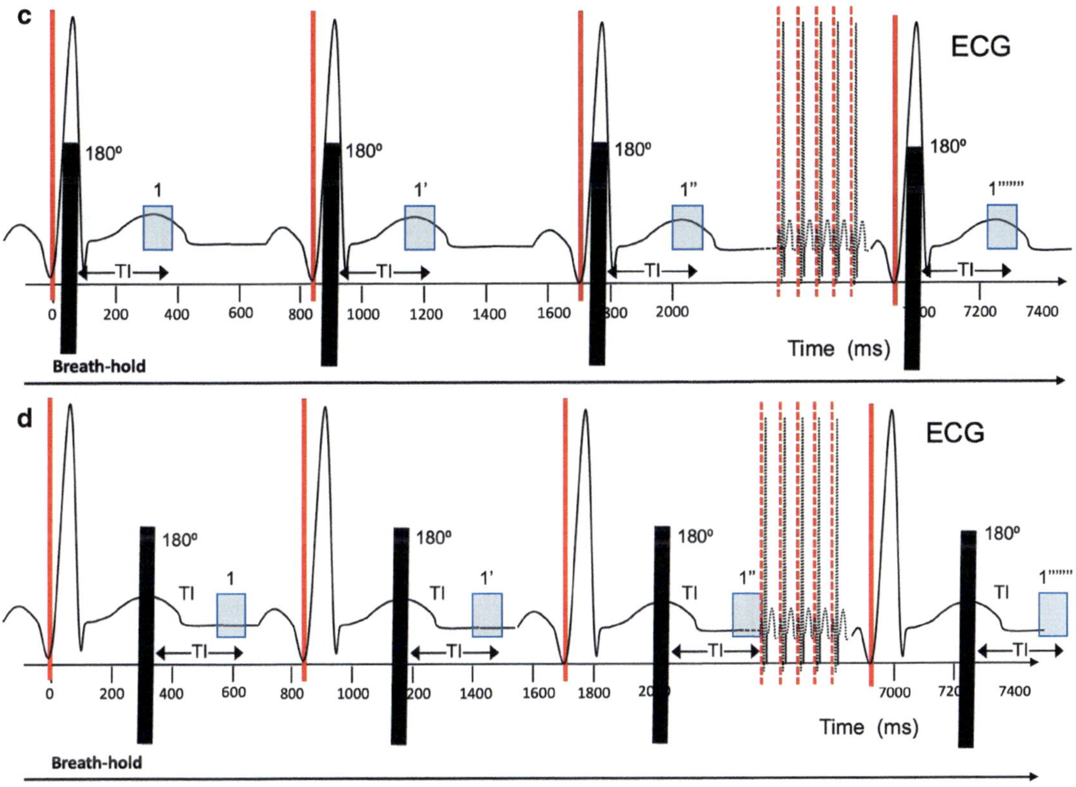

Fig. 2 (continued)

of the image series constructed, i.e., the temporal resolution of the cine loop, e.g., if the goal is to assess changes of chamber volumes over time. If, e.g., a portion of k-space lines consists of 8 lines and the matrix to fill is 256, 32 heartbeats are needed to fill the k-space for that image (=256 lines/8 lines per heartbeat = 32 heartbeats). If, e.g., the acquisition for that portion of k-space lines lasts 32 × 1.5 ms = 48 ms, the temporal resolution for this time series is 48 ms. A cardiac cycle length of 1000 ms would then yield 21 images or phases to cover the entire cardiac cycle. This is a very attractive strategy, as such an acquisition can be completed within a breath hold. Such segmented k-space techniques are therefore often called "breath-hold"-techniques. This strategy of triggered acquisition is nowadays typically combined with parallel imaging (Pruessmann et al. 1999) and compressed sensing (Lustig et al. 2007) techniques to further speed up the acquisition to fit it into a comfortable breath-hold duration. With a parallel-imaging acceleration by a factor of 2, 16 heartbeats are needed to fill the complete k-space. If compressed sensing techniques are added, a cine loop can be acquired within 1–2 heartbeats. When pushed to the limits, the entire heart can be covered with several short- and long-axis acquisitions during a single breath hold (Vincenti et al. 2014). Importantly, to achieve short repetition times per k-space line, high-performance gradient systems are required (see below). Of paramount importance for reliable measurements is its triggering with a good and artifact-free ECG signal. A reliable and artifact-free ECG is not only a prerequisite for good image quality, but also a condition "sine qua non" for the safe performance of stress tests in the magnet (see also paragraph below). If the ECG signal is not reliable, it is strongly advised to reposition the electrodes until the R wave is constantly detected. With the robust vector-ECG techniques installed on all MR scanner brands today, it is in general a straightforward procedure, certainly on 1.5 T machines.

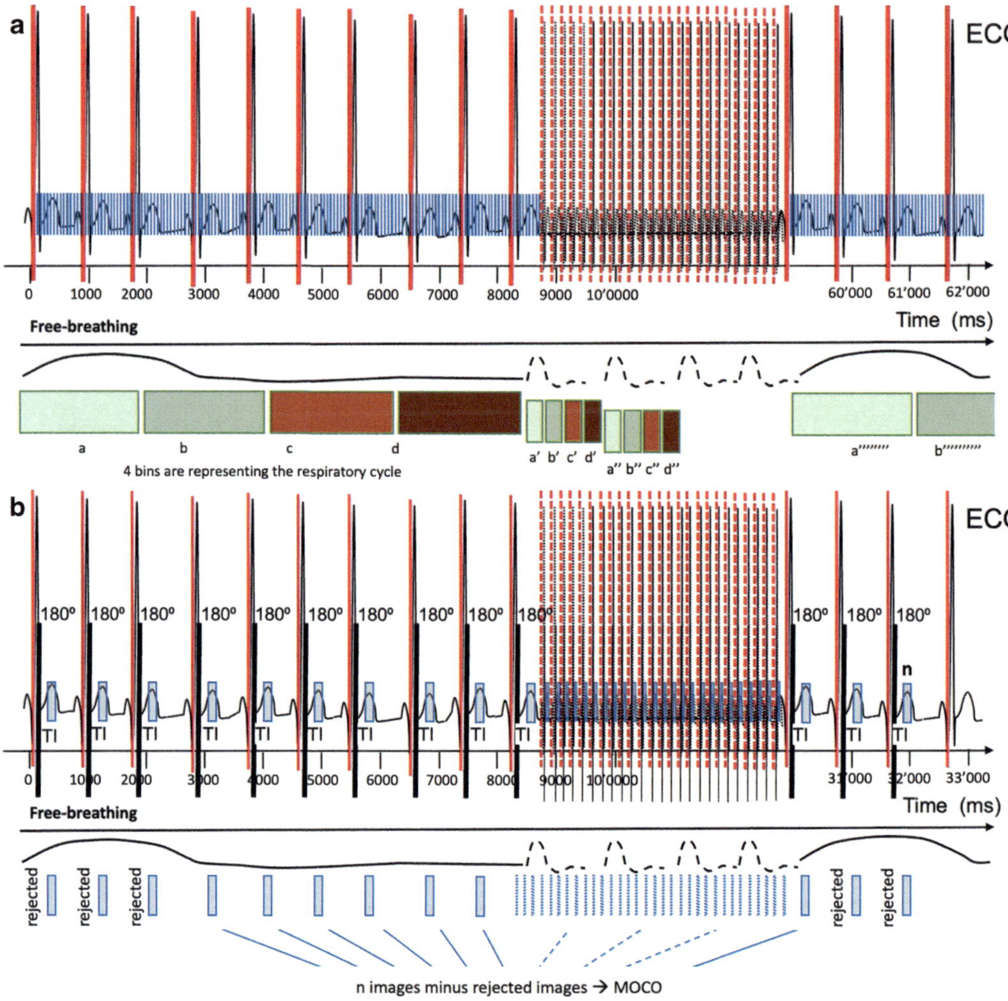

Fig. 3 (**a**) Free-breathing acquisition—with retrospective triggering. This free-breathing scheme acquires small portions of k-space lines as in the segmented approach; however, many more small portions are acquired over several minutes to acquire images with higher spatial and temporal resolutions (than in a single breath hold). Portions are combined to create a full image for a particular phase in the cardiac cycle. The combination of these multiple phases yields the cine loop information for functional assessment. The ECG trigger (red lines) is used as the timing reference. In addition, respiratory motion is represented by portions or bins **a–d** in this example. In analogy to combine portions of k-space lines to create a full image for that portion, i.e., phase of the cardiac cycle, corresponding bins, e.g., **a** to **a**″″′ are combined to create a full image for that particular phase of the respiratory cycle. Information to create bins can be obtained by several different techniques (e.g., self-navigation, image-based navigation, pilot tone technology, or by the "old-fashioned" diaphragmatic navigator technique). The diaphragmatic navigator often uses only one bin for reconstruction (=bin acquired in the acceptance window) and rejects the other bins. Free-breathing acquisitions can be modified by bipolar gradients to yield phase-contrast flow images. This acquisition type can also be limited to a single portion to cover a single phase of the cardiac phase only to yield a still-frame anatomical image (see example in Fig. 4). This single frame version can be combined with magnetization preparation to yield T_1, T_2, or LGE images. The dashed QRS complexes and red trigger lines indicate as many heartbeats as needed to acquire a full k-space (i.e., to allow for full image reconstruction per phase). (**b**) Free-breathing LGE acquisition—with triggering. This free-breathing LGE scheme acquires a full image per heartbeat (blue box = full k-space; single-shot acquisition) with high spatial resolution but low signal-to-noise. A given number of images n is acquired during free breathing. A fixed portion of these *n* images, e.g., 25% with the most distant position with relation to the mean position of all *n* images is rejected, the remaining images undergo a motion-correction procedure to yield one high-resolution LGE image with adequate signal-to-noise. Black box: non-slice selective180° inversion pulse followed by inversion time TI (to set normal myocardium to zero signal). The trigger delay is chosen in this example to place the read-out into late systole to allow for good image quality in patients with irregular heartbeats. Several examples are given in Fig. 5

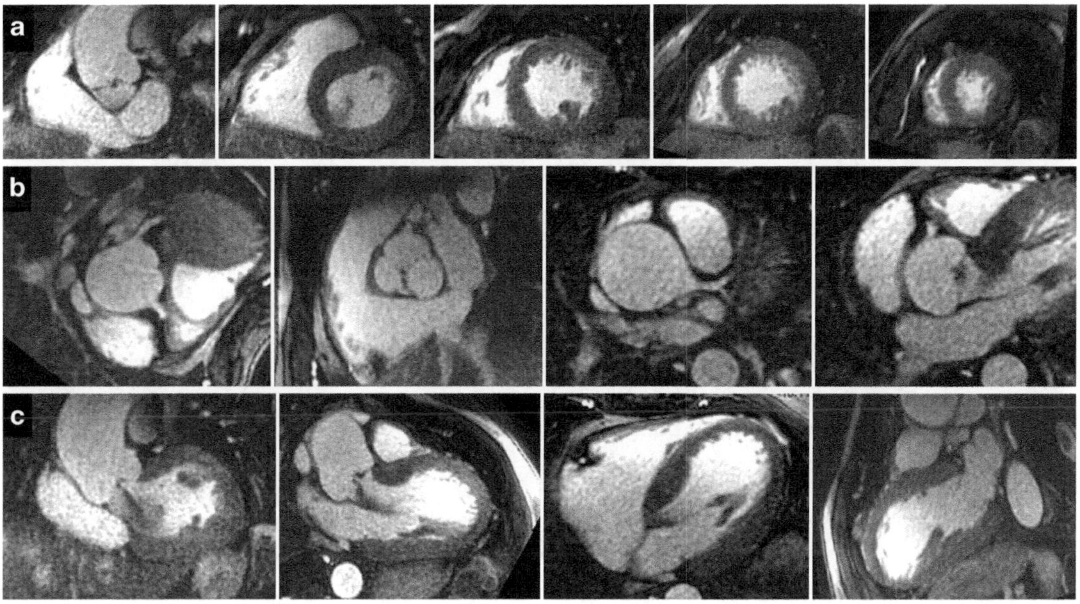

Fig. 4 Example of free-breathing acquisition with self-gating and ECG triggering for anatomical information. Example of a free-breathing technique that acquires a single cardiac phase as explained in Fig. 3a. Cardiac anatomy can be investigated at any desirable plane in this 3D acquisition. (**a**) Short-axis views of the RV and LV; (**b**) investigation of the aortic root showing a bicuspid aortic valve with fusion of the left and noncoronary cusp and calcifications in this location. (**c**) Long-axis views visualize an aortic regurgitation jet toward the anterior mitral valve leaflet

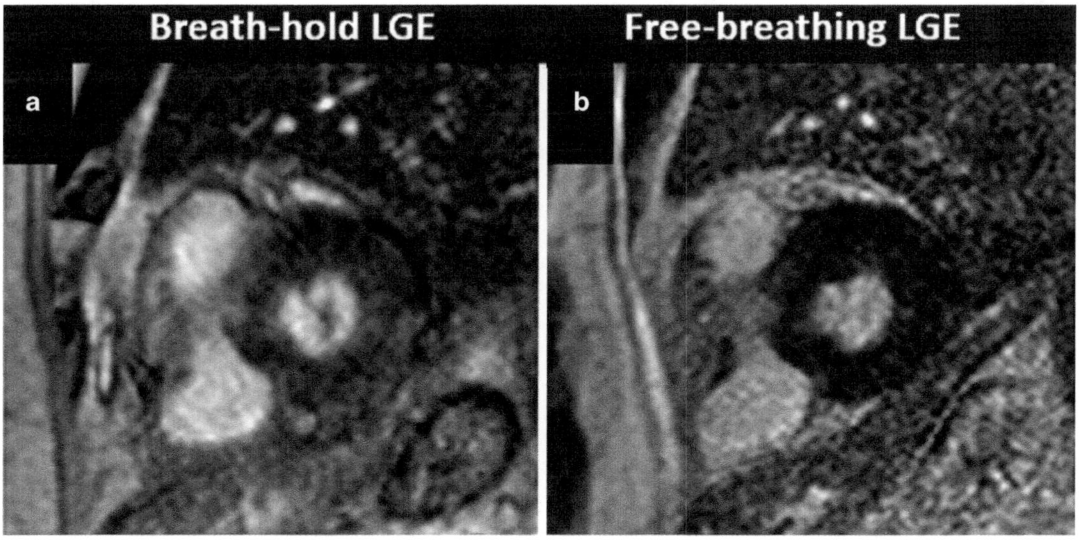

Fig. 5 Examples of breath-hold segmented and free-breathing LGE acquisitions with ECG triggering. Example of a segmented LGE acquisition with ECG triggering on the left column (as explained in Fig. 2d) and free-breathing LGE acquisition on the right column (as explained in Fig. 3b). Suboptimal and severely reduced LGE image quality in **a**, **e**, and **c**, respectively, due to difficulties in breath-holding. The free-breathing technique yields better image quality at the same high in-plane spatial resolution (1.3 mm × 1.3 mm) in **b**, **d**, and **f**

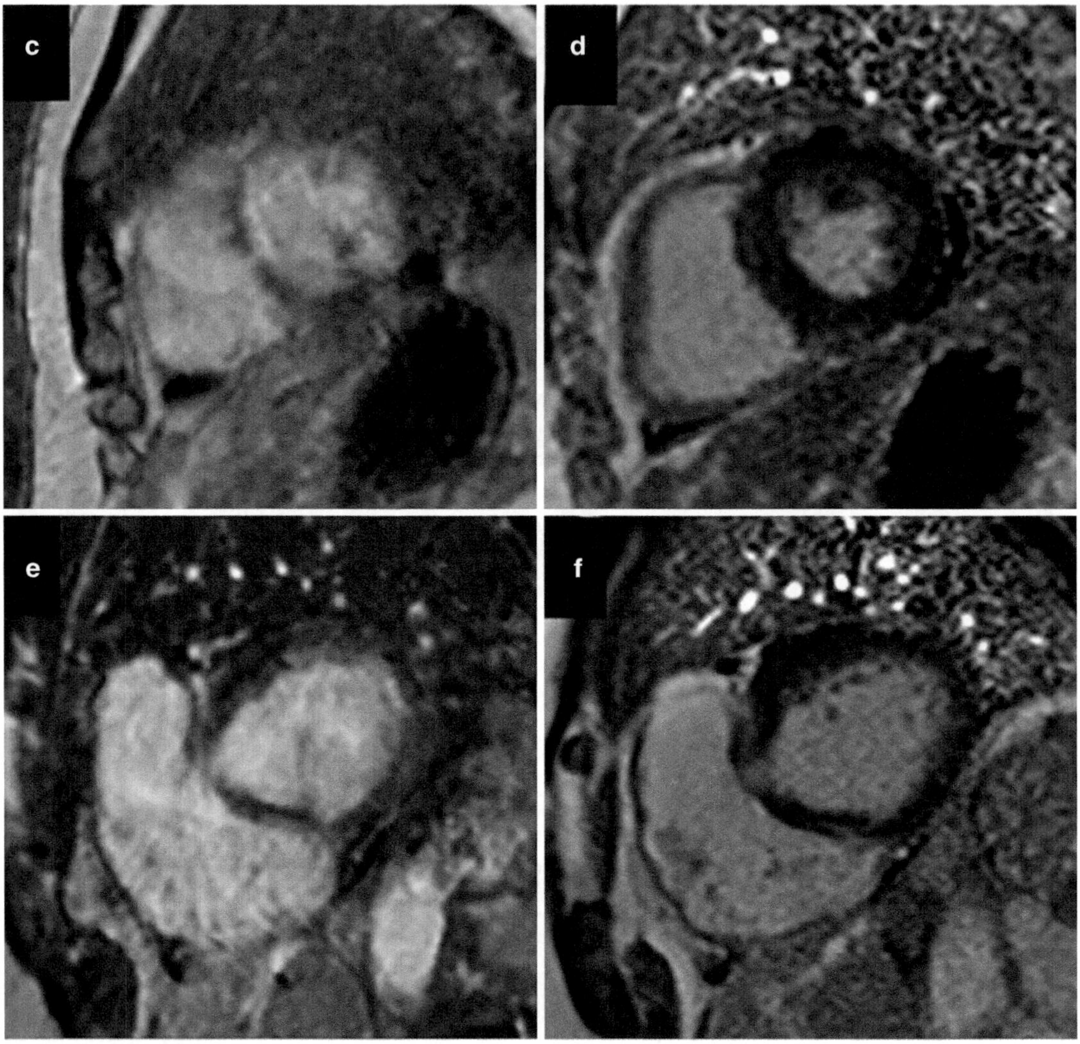

Fig. 5 (continued)

In some cardiac conditions, e.g., for some pericardial diseases, systolic and diastolic function can depend on the respiratory phase. To assess this function-respiration dependence, real-time acquisitions can be used. These acquisitions allow to assess cardiac function during deep inspiration and expiration as shown in Fig. 6. With these pulse sequences, the complete k-space is acquired in a single shot (Fig. 1). These images are acquired one after the other without ECG triggering, and the temporal resolution of the time series corresponds to the length of acquisition to fill the complete k-space. Such single-shot real-time acquisitions can yield anatomical, i.e., functional information (Francone et al. 2006) but also flow information in real time (Eichenberger et al. 1995). These sequences are typically combined with high acceleration factors of parallel imaging and compressed sensing. As the change in heart position during free breathing is not corrected for by these real-time pulse sequences, quantitative measurements are difficult to obtain, while a qualitative visual evaluation of cardiac function during breathing can be very helpful for the diagnoses of pericardial diseases, e.g., to discriminate restrictive vs. constrictive conditions (example in Fig. 6).

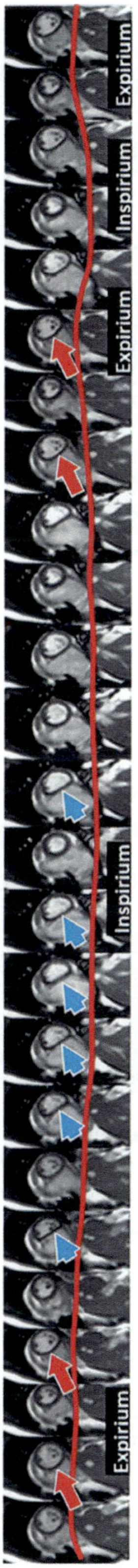

Fig. 6 Example of real-time acquisition without ECG triggering. Example for a real-time acquisition without ECG triggering (free running, Fig. 1a) to assess the loading conditions of the RV and LV during respiration in a patient with acute pericarditis. During inspiration, venous return to the heart is increased and the volume overload to the impaired RV causes a shift of the interventricular septum toward the LV (blue arrows). During expiration, the RV can handle the reduced load and the septum demonstrates a normal shape (red arrows). The series of images shows every fifth image (out of 800 images acquired over 1 min, temporal resolution per image 75 ms)

A very different approach for real-time imaging is not focusing on sophisticated reconstruction thereby accepting compromises in temporal/spatial resolution and signal-to-noise, but speeds up spatial encoding by limiting the acquisition volume to a volume of interest. This so-called spatially selective excitation can reduce the volume down to a few centimeters. For example, reducing a volume of $40 \times 40\ \text{cm}^2$ to $10 \times 10\ \text{cm}^2$ equals an acceleration factor of 16 while preserving spatial and temporal resolution. This technique yielded arterial flow information in real time with a spatial and temporal resolution of $0.7 \times 0.7\text{mm}^2$ and 22 ms, respectively (Schwitter et al. 2006).

3 Respiratory Motion

In clinical routine cardiac MRI, the preferred method to suppress respiratory motion during data acquisition is the so-called breath-hold technique (for details, see also Table 1). This procedure is applicable in most cardiac patients. In severely dyspneic patients, the number of k-space lines "per portion" can be increased to shorten the breath-hold duration (Fig. 2). If, e.g., the number of lines "per portion" is doubled, the breath-hold duration is half and the temporal resolution of this acquisition will be half. As the iso-volumetric end-systolic phase of the LV lasts for approximately 50 ms, it is advisable to keep the temporal resolution below 50 ms (Figs. 7 and 8). Breathhold techniques are also used for T1 and T2 mapping (see example in Fig. 9; pulse sequence in Fig. 2b). In this context, it should be noted that high acceleration factors of compressed sensing techniques (when utilizing the time domain for sparsity) can result in artificially low temporal resolution and underestimation of cardiac function. With these limitations, breath-hold techniques cannot yield very high temporal and spatial resolution simultaneously and alternative strategies might be required. Accordingly, considerable efforts are undertaken to develop free-breathing techniques.

The principle to correct for respiratory motion during free breathing is to obtain a signal that correlates with respiratory motion and then to

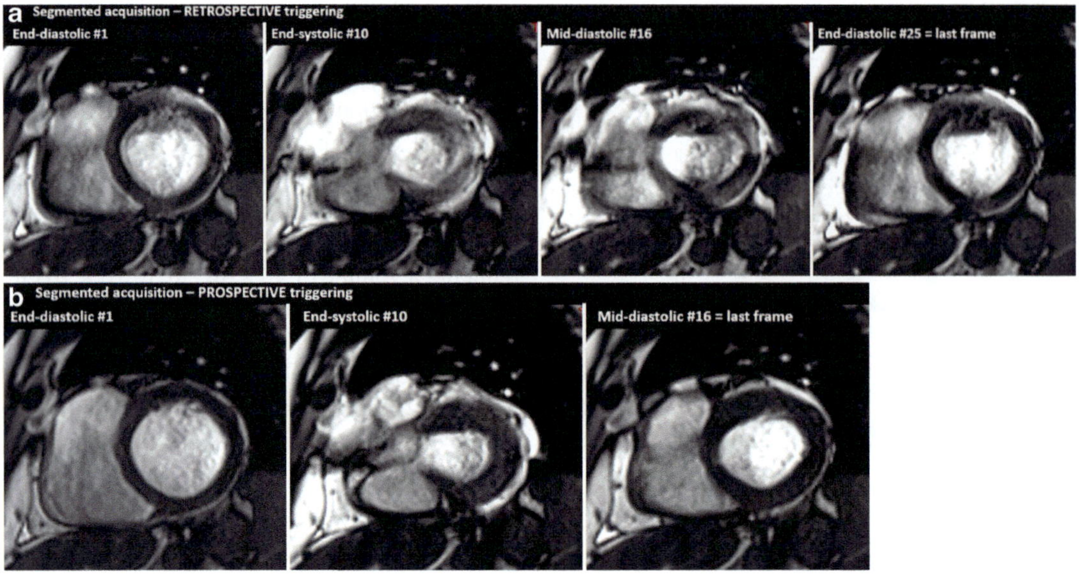

Fig. 7 Example of breath-hold segmented cine acquisition with ECG triggering. Example for a segmented acquisition with retrospective and prospective ECG triggering (Fig. 2a, b, respectively) in a patient with frequent extrasystoles. (**a**) End-systolic frames show blurred endocardial borders with retrospective ECG triggering (top row **a**), while prospective triggering preserves sharp endocardial borders even during irregular heartbeats (bottom row, **b**). Note, prospective triggering does not cover late diastolic phases of the cardiac cycle

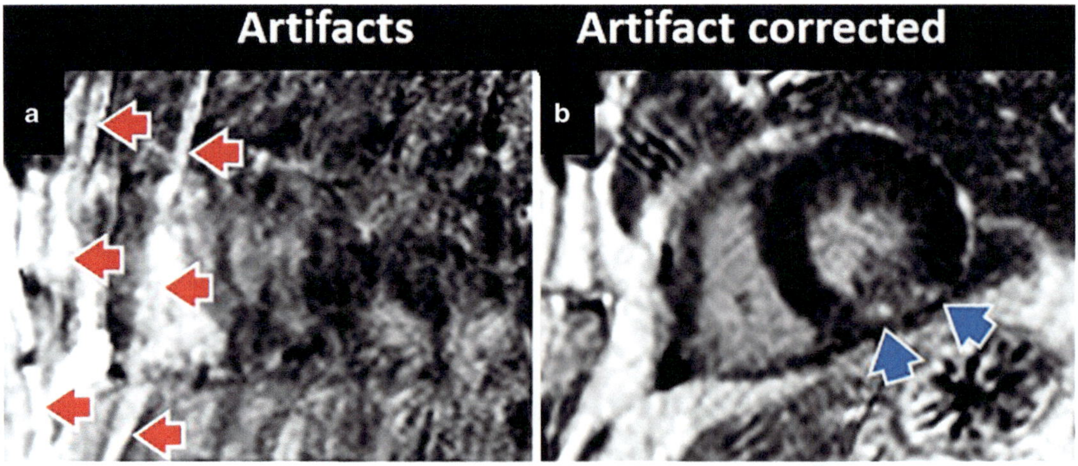

Fig. 8 Example of breath-hold segmented LGE acquisition with ECG triggering. Example for a segmented late-gadolinium enhancement (LGE) acquisition with ECG triggering and acquisition in late systole (Fig. 2d). Even when acquired in late systole to guarantee good image quality in patients with irregular heartbeats, other artifacts can occur. (**a**) This patient was unable to hold his breath >12 s resulting in ghosts along the phase-encoding direction (red arrows). (**b**) Phase encoding is changed to minimize respiratory artifacts, and the portion of k-space lines is increased to reduce the number of heartbeats to yield a full k-space. With these measures, LGE image quality is good and an inferior infarct is shown (blue arrows). (**c**) Mis-triggering results in blurred endocardial borders in this LGE image (red arrows). (**d**) ECG is repositioned to yield a reliable trigger and LGE image quality is good. (**e**) At 3 T, suboptimal shimming results in inhomogeneous energy deposition by the non-slice selective 180° inversion pulse and incomplete inversion in the lateral LV wall (red arrow). (**f**) Shimming of a smaller volume over the heart yields adequate quality

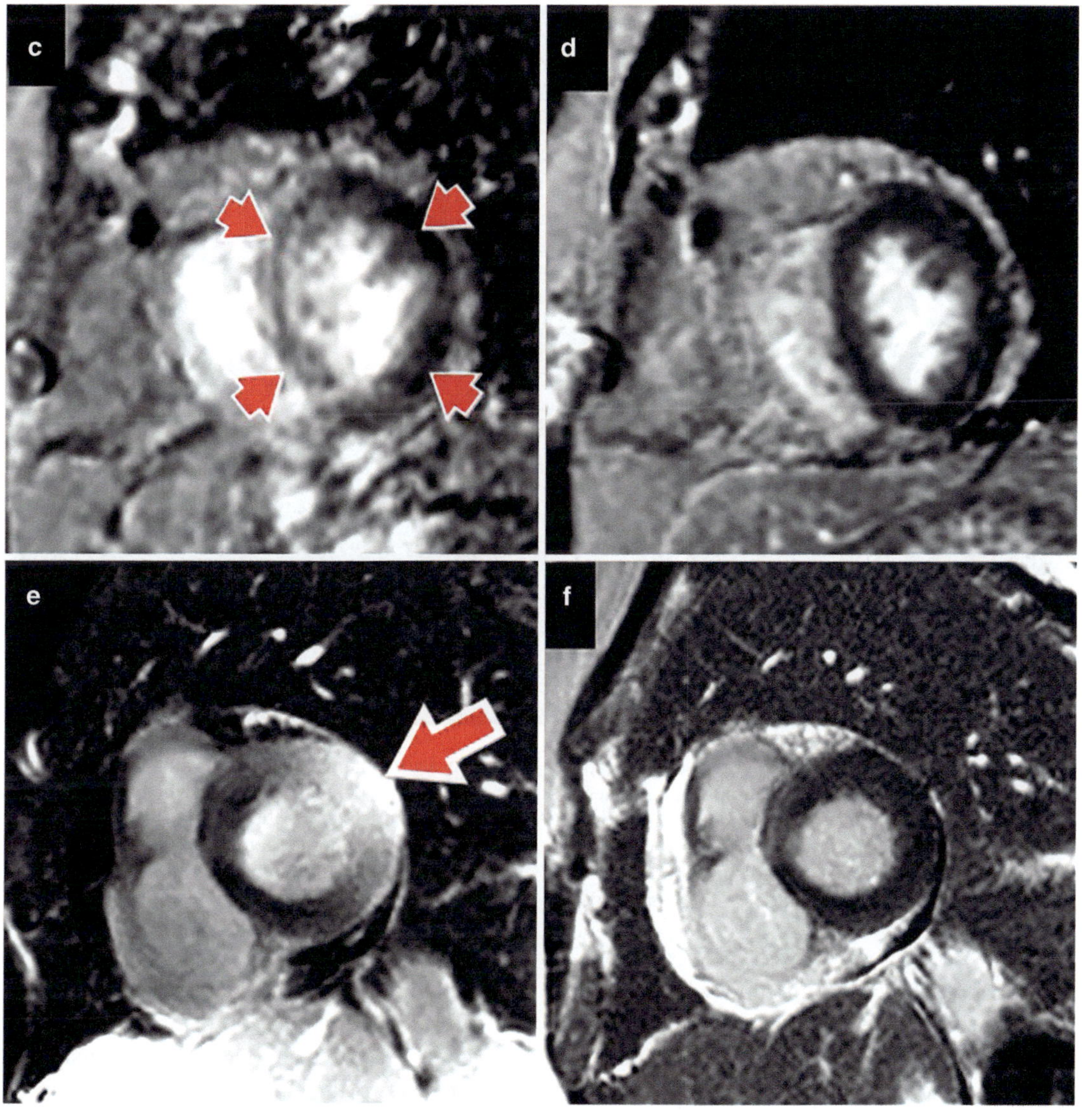

Fig. 8 (continued)

gate the data acquisition (which is typically ECG triggered). For more details, see Fig. 3a and Table 1. Gating is the acceptance of acquired data, if the respiratory position is in a predefined range (e.g., within 5 mm of the position of the diaphragm). If respiration is outside this predefined range, data are not acquired (or acquired data outside this range are rejected and not used for image reconstruction). A popular and simple method in the past was the use of an abdominal belt. The stretching of the belt during respiration provided a signal for acquisition gating. Later, pencil beam-like excitations were used and are still in use that can measure the foot-head displacement of the right hemidiaphragm (Wang et al. 1996; Nagel et al. 1999; Stuber et al. 1999). For images acquired within the gating window (of, e.g., 5 mm), displacement can be corrected for. Often a conversion is used so that 5 mm displacement of the diaphragm is converted to 0.6×5 mm = 3 mm displacement of the acquired image position. This approach, however, requires

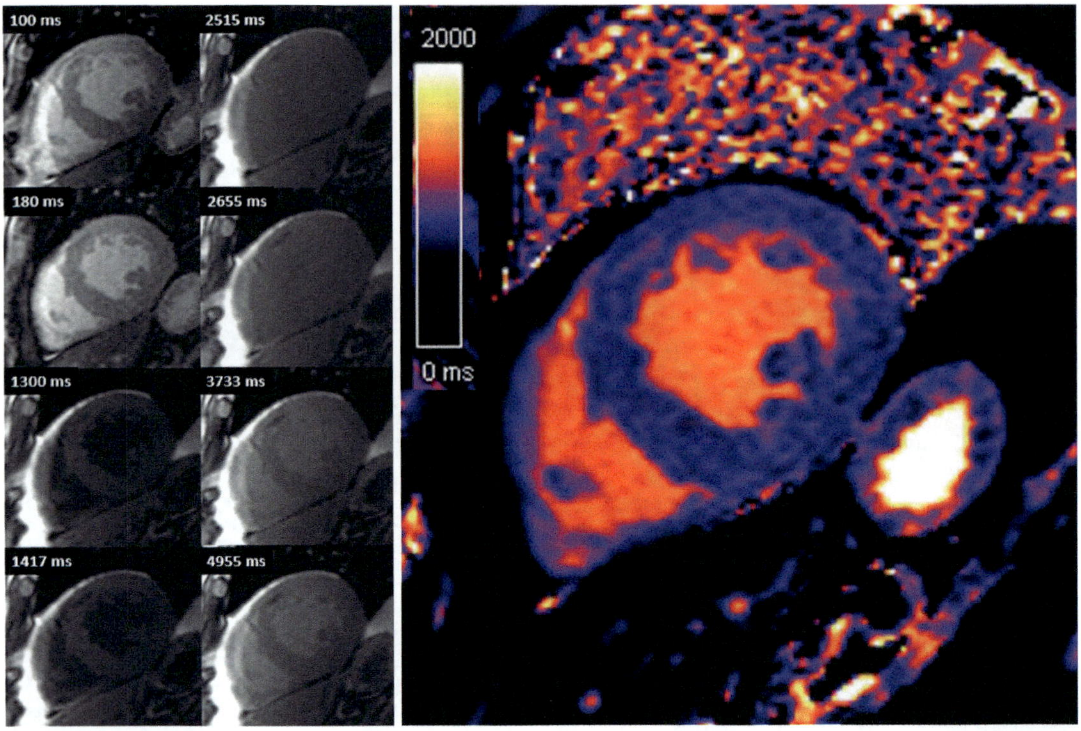

Fig. 9 Example of breath-hold segmented T_1-mapping acquisition with ECG triggering. Example of a segmented acquisition with ECG triggering and magnetization preparation (Fig. 2d). In this example, the inversion time between the non-slice selective 180° inversion pulse and the read-out is varied (as indicated on the images to the left) in order to obtain a series of LGE images from which the T_1 can be calculated, i.e., from which the T_1 map is calculated. In this Fabry patient native T_1 was reduced to 838 ms and 856 ms in the septum and the lateral LV wall, respectively, a typical finding in this disease

an unpredictable acquisition time, which depends on the pattern of respiration of a given patient, and it assumes a constant correlation between diaphragm and heart motion, which is not necessarily constant over the full range for respiratory positions. Therefore, novel strategies aim to directly track the motion of the heart during respiration. A promising technique is called "self-navigation." This technique exploits the fact that the central signal in k-space is correlated with the respiratory motion. Once this information is collected, the data in k-space can be corrected for the displacement in foot-head direction and are then used for image reconstruction (Stehning et al. 2005). Also, with radial k-line acquisitions, the k-lines acquired in the foot-head direction can be used to track the respiratory displacement of the heart and can be used to correct the k-space data for this displacement (Monney et al. 2015). Most of these approaches correct for the foot-head direction only, which is known to account for approximately 80% of the respiratory displacement of the heart but more sophisticated approaches are under development (Roy et al. 2021). Another self-gated approach acquires low-resolution images of the heart which allow for displacement calculation and high-resolution images are then acquired based on this displacement information (Munoz et al. 2019). Many of these novel approaches are promising but are not yet mature enough for clinical application. A different approach is not correcting for free-respiration cardiac displacement during data acquisition, but acquires data continuously to correct then the acquired images for respiratory displacement (Fig. 3).

Finally, a very different approach is not correcting for cardiac displacement during free respiration, but tries to control, or better tries to directly suppress respiratory motion. High-frequency or pulsatile flow ventilation applies very small tidal volumes at high frequencies. This allows for efficient CO_2 elimination and almost completely suppresses respiratory motion. As a result, the patient remains in end-inspiratory position for up to 20 min without the need to breath. This technique is applicable to conscious patients. For a pilot study, a pulsatile flow ventilator was modified to become MRI compatible, and full cardiac MRI protocols could be applied without any pause yielding motion-free images (Beigelman-Aubry et al. 2017).

4 Magnetic Field Strength and Field Inhomogeneities

Magnetic field homogeneity is important for precise spatial encoding, i.e., for image quality. The position of the heart is close to air at the lateral wall of the left ventricle but also close to solid organs at the inferior wall of the heart. This particular location is demanding regarding shimming, and the shim volume should be restricted to the heart. The left ventricular inferolateral wall, where the liver reaches the lung structures, is particularly difficult to shim, and artifacts of pulse sequences with long echo times are typically encountered at this location. For these reasons, a magnetic field strength of 1.5 T is less problematic for cardiac imaging than higher field strengths such as 3 T. Also, there is less distortion of the ECG by magnetohydrodynamic effects at 1.5 T compared to 3 T. A higher field strength generates an improved signal-to-noise ratio, but state-of-the-art steady-state free-precession sequences are excellent for preserving magnetization and thus signal. The utilization of 3 T machines also results in a quadruple increase in RF power absorption which impedes the application of some of pulse sequences that need magnetization preparation. In order to monitor CMR image quality in research, but also in clinical routine, produced on 1.5 T and 3 T systems, standardized and easy to apply quality criteria tested in the large EuroCMR registry are available (Klinke et al. 2013).

A small number of studies report good image quality of cardiac acquisitions at 0.55 T (Bandettini et al. 2020). At 0.55 T using the same high-performance gradient system as on a 1.5 T scanner of 45 mT/m and slew rate of 200 T/m/s, robust quantification of LV and RV function was shown (Bandettini et al. 2020). However, all large multicenter, multivendor cardiac MRI trials are conducted on 1.5 T systems, and such trials should provide the basis for recommendations.

Magnetic field homogeneity is also crucial for accurate flow measurements (Gatehouse et al. 2010). Accordingly, phase-contrast flow data should be acquired near the isocenter of the magnet (e.g., within a radius of 5 cm) to guarantee optimal accuracy (Gatehouse et al. 2010). Even in high-quality homogeneous magnetic fields, a background phase-offset correction should be performed. To this end, it is recommended to retain a large enough field-of-view with only small wrap-around artifacts to allow for nonmoving tissue to serve as reference regions (see Fig. 10).

New generation implanted devices like pacemakers and implantable cardiac defibrillators (ICDs) are nowadays MR conditional, i.e., implanted patients can safely undergo CMR examinations (Gimbel et al. 2013; Gold et al. 2015). However, these devices, particularly, ICDs, can cause relevant magnetic field inhomogeneities with reduced image quality. Pacemaker-implanted patients can be investigated in general with steady-state free-precession pulse sequences which yield diagnostic quality in 95% and 98% of LV and RV function assessment, respectively (Schwitter et al. 2013). ICDs are substantially more demanding with respect to cardiac studies, and diagnostic quality with steady-state free-precession pulse sequences is achieved in only 50% and 70%, respectively (Schwitter et al. 2016). Therefore, fast gradient echo read-out pulse sequences are recommended in ICD patients that yield diagnostic quality in up to 74% and 84% for the LV and RV function assessment, respectively. LGE imaging is sometimes difficult in ICD patients even with the use of fast gradient read-outs, as the energy deposition of the 180° inversion pulse is not homogeneous across the field-of-view (the metallic composition of the device can cause strong frequency off-resonances in its vicinity). In fact, the B1+ variation can be as high as 25% at 1.5 T and even higher at 3 T. A cardiac pulse generator at

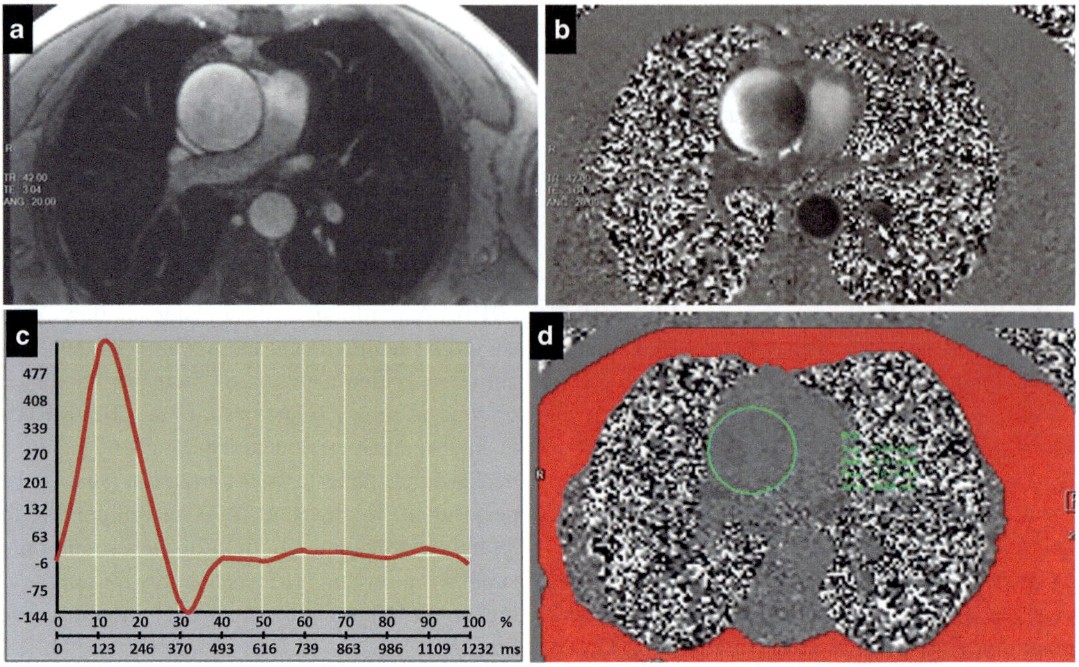

Fig. 10 Example of breath-hold segmented phase-contrast acquisition with ECG triggering for flow quantification. Example of a segmented acquisition with retrospective ECG triggering and bipolar gradient magnetization preparation to yield a phase-contrast pulse sequence for flow measurement (Fig. 2b). The magnitude and the corresponding phase-contrast image of one phase of the cardiac cycle is given in **a** and **b**, respectively. To minimize the effect of field inhomogeneities, target vessel should be located close to the magnet isocenter. Nevertheless, phase-offset errors can still occur and a phase-offset correction is recommended as applied in **d**. Of note, this phase correction should consider stationary tissue located "on all sides" of the target vessel for precise correction. Thus, wrap-around artifacts should be avoided with this acquisition. (**c**) The measurement yielded a mild aortic regurgitation with regurgitation fraction of 16% (15 mL per beat) at a heart rate of 46 bpm

5–10 cm from the heart results in a 2–6 kHz resonance frequency offset in the myocardium (Rashid et al. 2014). Therefore, it is recommended to use wideband inversion-recovery techniques that adjusts for inversion pulse bandwidth and frequency offset. With this technique frequency bandwidth and frequency offset adjustments are typically in the ranges of 2000–4000 Hz and −1500 to 1500 Hz, respectively (Ibrahim et al. 2018).

5 Stress Test to Assess Cardiac Function and Perfusion Reserve

Cardiovascular disease causes more deaths in the United states than all forms of cancer and chronic respiratory disease combined with ischemic heart disease being the leading cause accounting for 43% of all cardiovascular deaths. Therefore, ischemia testing is of paramount importance, and pulse sequences nowadays are easy to use for this purpose. The basic component of the pulse sequence is a real-time acquisition yielding one complete image or slice (without any segmentation) in one "shot" (see also Fig. 1b, Table 1). With this technique, several slices are acquired per heartbeat to cover the LV repetitively during the wash-in of contrast medium into the myocardium. This concept is called first-pass perfusion acquisition (see Fig. 1b). Typically, myocardial perfusion is sufficient to meet myocardial oxygen demand during resting conditions. If this condition is not met, the myocardium undergoes resting ischemia which generally ends in myocardial infarction. Accordingly, to test the significance of coronary artery stenoses, i.e., whether they can cause myocardial ischemia, perfusion by first-pass MR techniques is tested during pharmacologically induced hyperemia of the myocardium. During pharmacological hyperemia, perfusion of the myocardium increases about 2–4 times above resting values in the presence of healthy non-stenosed coronary arteries (Schwitter et al. 2000). However, in the case of critical coronary artery stenosis, resting flow cannot be increased and contrast medium wash-in is not increased in such territories compared to territories supplied by non-stenosed coronary arteries. This testing during hyperemia and associated tachycardia is challenging for scanner hardware and software. Nowadays, all state-of-the-art 1.5 T MR machines are equipped with hardware and software that allow for accelerated acquisitions during stress perfusion tests. As an alternative to perfusion stress testing, myocardial ischemia can be induced by dobutamine administration. To monitor the contractile response to dobutamine, a fast segmented breath-hold acquisition is used (Nagel and Bruder 2020). As stress testing is the backbone of every ischemic heart disease CMR evaluation, physicians performing these examinations must be trained to manage acute complications, mainly arrhythmias and side effects of vasodilators. Adenosine is a frequently used stressor for first-pass perfusion CMR. Its short half-life leads to a benign risk profile. Frequent side effects are dyspnea and flushing, while severe side effects of higher degree AV block or bronchospasm are rare. In a large registry reporting on >37,000 patients, stress CMR was associated with mild and severe side effects in 0.04% and 0.01% of examinations, respectively (Bruder et al. 2015). The infrastructure of a CMR center must allow for monitoring of blood pressure, heart rate, cardiac rhythm, and breathing as well as patients' symptoms during a CMR stress test. MRI conditional equipment is available for this purpose. In addition, a defibrillator and drugs for emergency treatment and resuscitation must be available. Importantly, the CMR physicians must provide competency in basic and advanced life support.

The diagnostic performance of perfusion CMR is best documented for 1.5 T systems. The high robustness and reliability at 1.5 T also translate into excellent economic characteristics with substantial cost savings in the management of ischemic heart disease by CMR vs. coronary angiography (Moschetti et al. 2022).

6 Nonproton MR Imaging

6.1 Hyperpolarized ^{13}C-Carbon Cardiac MRI

Hyperpolarization techniques for ^{13}C-carbon compounds show great potential to assess myocardial metabolism in near-real-time acquisitions. Compared to polarizations of 3–4 ppm for conventional ^{1}H-imaging at 1.5 T, with current hyperpolarization techniques, polarizations in the range of 30–50% can be produced and thus offer an unprecedented increase in signal (Ardenkjær-Larsen et al. 2003). This technique requires a MR scanner system that can receive the ^{13}C-carbon signal, and a polarizer is also required on site to produce the hyperpolarized ^{13}C-carbon contrast medium. This technique is readily available in animals (Schwitter 2006; Seymour et al. 2015; Yoshihara et al. 2015; Fuetterer et al. 2017) and is now also applicable in humans on clinical MR scanners. In diabetic patients, it measured noninvasively a reduced Krebs cycle activity in the myocardium by assessing the conversion of injected hyperpolarized ^{13}C-pyruvate to lactate and ^{13}C-bicarbonate (Cunningham et al. 2016; Rider et al. 2020).

6.2 ^{19}F-Fluorine Cardiac MRI

Another nucleus, ^{19}F-fluorine, is also a candidate for clinical MRI (Schwitter 2015). Contrast media containing ^{19}F-fluorine atoms, known as perfluorocarbons, can be administered intravenously and after phagocytosis through macrophages, the ^{19}F-fluorine signal allows to visualize the macrophage load of organs, e.g., of the heart affected by myocarditis (van Heeswijk et al. 2013). The micelles containing the perfluorocarbons can also be covered by antibodies to target, e.g., fibrin. These antibody-covered perfluorocarbon-containing micelles are then used as noninvasive probe to visualize thrombi in vivo with extraordinary specificity as no natural fluorine compounds are present in the body (Temme et al. 2015). This technique is available on clinical 3 T machines (Bönner et al. 2015), and a first application in patients was recently reported for ^{19}F-based ventilation measurements (Obert et al. 2020; Pippard et al. 2021).

Disclaimer All measurements in this book have been obtained from peer-reviewed papers and guidelines from professional organizations, unless explicitly stated otherwise. While the authors, editors, and publisher have gone through a rigorous process to establish their correct reproduction from the original source, each measurement must be interpreted in the correct clinical context, this along with an accurate way of measurement, and taking into account all technical variables, this including follow-up exams with various equipment or software. Neither the authors, the editors, nor the publisher can accept any legal responsibility for any improper application or interpretation of these measurements as well as their potential consequences.

References

Ardenkjær-Larsen JH, Fridlund B, Gram A, Hansson G, Hansson L, Lerche MH et al (2003) Increase in signal-to-noise ratio of >10,000 times in liquid-state NMR. Proc Natl Acad Sci 100(18):10158–10163

Bandettini WP, Shanbhag SM, Mancini C, McGuirt DR, Kellman P, Xue H et al (2020) A comparison of cine CMR imaging at 0.55 T and 1.5 T. J Cardiovasc Magn Reson 22(1):37

Beigelman-Aubry C, Peguret N, Stuber M, Delacoste J, Belmondo B, Lovis A et al (2017) Chest-MRI under pulsatile flow ventilation: a new promising technique. PLoS One 12:e0178807

Bönner F, Merx MW, Klingel K, Begovatz P, Flögel U, Sager M et al (2015) Monocyte imaging after myocardial infarction with 19F MRI at 3 T: a pilot study in explanted porcine hearts. Eur Heart J Cardiovasc Imaging 16(6):612–620

Bruder O, Schneider S, Pilz G, van Rossum AC, Schwitter J, Nothnagel D et al (2015) Update on acute adverse reactions to gadolinium based contrast agents in cardiovascular MR. Large multi-national and multi-ethnical population experience with 37788 patients from the EuroCMR Registry. J Cardiovasc Magn Reson 17(1):58

Chien D, Atkinson DJ, Edelman RR (1991) Strategies to improve contrast in turboFLASH imaging: reordered phase encoding and K-space segmentation. J Magn Reson Imaging 1(1):63–70

Cunningham C, Lau J, Chen A, Geraghty B, Perks W, Roifman I et al (2016) Hyperpolarized 13C metabolic MRI of the human heart: initial experience. Circ Res 119(11):1177–1182

Eichenberger AC, Schwitter J, McKinnon GC, Debatin JF, von Schulthess GK (1995) Phase-contrast echo-planar MR imaging: real-time quantification of flow and velocity patterns in the thoracic vessels induced by Valsalva's maneuver. J Magn Reson Imaging 5(6):648–655

Francone M, Dymarkowski S, Kalantzi M, Rademakers FE, Bogaert J (2006) Assessment of ventricular coupling with real-time cine MRI and its value to differentiate constrictive pericarditis from restrictive cardiomyopathy. Eur Radiol 16(4):944–951

Fuetterer M, Busch J, Peereboom SM, von Deuster C, Wissmann L, Lipiski M et al (2017) Hyperpolarized 13C urea myocardial first-pass perfusion imaging using velocity-selective excitation. J Cardiovasc Magn Reson 19(1):46

Gatehouse P, Rolf M, Graves M, Hofman M, Totman J, Werner B et al (2010) Flow measurement by cardiovascular magnetic resonance: a multi-centre multi vendor study of background phase offset errors that can compromise the accuracy of derived regurgitant or shunt flow measurements. J Cardiovasc Magn Reson 12:5–13

Gimbel RJ, Bello D, Schmitt M, Merkely B, Schwitter J, Hayes DL et al (2013) Randomized trial of pacemaker and lead system for safe scanning at 1.5 Tesla. Heart Rhythm 10:685–691

Gold MR, Sommer T, Schwitter J, Al Fagih A, Albert T, Merkely B et al (2015) Full-body MRI in patients with an implantable cardioverter-defibrillator: primary results of a randomized study. J Am Coll Cardiol 65(24):2581–2588

Ibrahim E, Runge M, Stojanovska J, Agarwal P, Ghadimi-Mahani M, Attili A et al (2018) Optimized cardiac magnetic resonance imaging inversion recovery sequence for metal artifact reduction and accurate myocardial scar assessment in patients with cardiac implantable electronic devices. World J Radiol 10(9):100–107

Klinke V, Muzzarelli S, Lauriers N, Locca D, Vincenti G, Monney P et al (2013) Quality assessment of cardiovascular magnetic resonance in the setting of the European CMR registry: description and validation of standardized criteria. J Cardiovasc Magn Reson 15(1):55

Lustig M, Donoho D, Pauly JM (2007) Sparse MRI: the application of compressed sensing for rapid MR imaging. Magn Reson Med 58(6):1182–1195

Monney P, Piccini D, Rutz T, Vincenti G, Coppo S, Koestner S et al (2015) Single centre experience of the application of self navigated 3D whole heart CMR for the assessment of cardiac anatomy in congenital heart disease. J Cardiovasc Magn Reson 17:55

Moschetti K, Kwong R, Petersen S, Lombardi, Garot J, Atar D et al (2022) Cost-minimization analysis for cardiac revascularization in 12 healthcare systems based on the EuroCMR/SPINS Registries. JACC Cardiovasc Imaging 15(4):607–625

Munoz C, Cruz G, Neji R, Botnar RM, Prieto C (2019) Motion corrected water/fat whole-heart coronary MR angiography with 100% respiratory efficiency. Magn Reson Med 82(2):732–742

Nagel E, Bruder O (2020) CAD: ischemia - stress dobutamine-CMR. In: Schwitter J (ed) CMR update, 3rd edn. Herz-MRI. www.herz-mri.ch, Lausanne, Switzerland, pp 84–91

Nagel E, Bornstedt A, Schnackenburg B, Hug J, Oswald H, Fleck E (1999) Optimization of realtime adaptive navigator correction for 3D magnetic resonance coronary angiography. Magn Reson Med 42(2):408–411

Obert AJ, Gutberlet M, Kern AL, Kaireit TF, Grimm R, Wacker F et al (2020) 1H-guided reconstruction of 19F gas MRI in COPD patients. Magn Reson Med 84(3):1336–1346

Pippard BJ, Neal MA, Maunder AM, Hollingsworth KG, Biancardi A, Lawson RA et al (2021) Reproducibility of 19F-MR ventilation imaging in healthy volunteers. Magn Reson Med 85(6):3343–3352

Pruessmann KP, Weiger M, Scheidegger MB, Boesiger P (1999) SENSE: sensitivity encoding for fast MRI. Magn Reson Med 42(5):952–962

Rashid S, Rapacchi S, Vaseghi M, Tung R, Shivkumar K, Finn JP et al (2014) Improved late gadolinium enhancement MR imaging for patients with implanted cardiac devices. Radiology 270(1):269–274

Rider OJ, Apps A, Miller J, Lau JYC, Lewis AJM, Peterzan MA et al (2020) Noninvasive in vivo assessment of cardiac metabolism in the healthy and diabetic human heart using hyperpolarized (13)C MRI. Circ Res 126(6):725–736

Roy CW, Heerfordt J, Piccini D, Rossi G, Pavon AG, Schwitter J et al (2021) Motion compensated whole-heart coronary cardiovascular magnetic resonance angiography using focused navigation (fNAV). J Cardiovasc Magn Reson 23(1):33

Schwitter J (2006) Myocardial perfusion imaging by cardiac magnetic resonance. J Nucl Cardiol 13(6):841–854

Schwitter J (2015) Cellular imaging – a bright future for 19F-CMR. Eur Heart J Cardiovasc Imaging 16(6):606–608

Schwitter J (2020) CMR-Update, 3rd edn. Herz-MRI, Lausanne, Switzerland. www.herz-mri.ch

Schwitter J, DeMarco T, Kneifel S, von Schulthess GK, Jorg MC, Arheden H et al (2000) Magnetic resonance-based assessment of global coronary flow and flow reserve and its relation to left ventricular functional parameters: a comparison with positron emission tomography. Circulation 101(23):2696–2702

Schwitter J, Oelhafen M, Wyss BM, Kozerke S, Amann-Vesti B, Luscher TF et al (2006) 2D-Spatially-selective real-time magnetic resonance imaging for the assessment of microvascular function and its relation to the cardiovascular risk profile. J Cardiovasc Magn Reson 8(5):759–769

Schwitter J, Kanal E, Schmitt M, Anselme F, Albert T, Hayes DL et al (2013) Impact of the Advisa MRI™ Pacing System on the diagnostic quality of cardiac MR images and contraction patterns of cardiac muscle during scans: Advisa MRI randomized clinical multicenter study results. Heart Rhythm 10:864–872

Schwitter J, Gold MR, Al Fagih A, Lee S, Peterson M, Ciuffo A et al (2016) Image quality of cardiac magnetic resonance imaging in patients with an implantable cardioverter defibrillator system designed for the magnetic resonance imaging environment. Circ Cardiovasc Imaging 9(5):e0040252

Seymour AM, Giles L, Ball V, Miller JJ, Clarke K, Carr CA et al (2015) In vivo assessment of cardiac metabolism and function in the abdominal aortic banding model of compensated cardiac hypertrophy. Cardiovasc Res 106(2):249–260

Stehning C, Börnert P, Nehrke K, Eggers H, Stuber M (2005) Free-breathing whole-heart coronary MRA with 3D radial SSFP and self-navigated image reconstruction. Magn Reson Med 54(2):476–480

Stuber M, Botnar RM, Danias PG, McConnell MV, Kissinger KV, Yucel EK et al (1999) Contrast agent-enhanced, free-breathing, three-dimensional coronary magnetic resonance angiography. J Magn Reson Imaging 10(5):790–799

Temme S, Grapentin C, Quast C, Jacoby C, Grandoch M, Ding Z et al (2015) Noninvasive imaging of early venous thrombosis by 19F magnetic resonance imaging with targeted perfluorocarbon nanoemulsions. Circulation 131(16):1405–1414

van Heeswijk RB, De Blois J, Kania G, Gonzales C, Blyszczuk P, Stuber M et al (2013) Selective in-vivo visualization of immune-cell infiltration in a mouse model of autoimmune myocarditis by fluorine-19 cardiac magnetic resonance. Circ Cardiovasc Imaging 6:277–284

Vincenti G, Monney P, Chaptinel J, Rutz T, Coppo S, Zenge MO et al (2014) Compressed sensing single-breathhold multi-slice magnetic resonance for fast quantification of left ventricular function, volumes, and mass. JACC Cardiovasc Imaging 7(9):882–892

Wang Y, Rossman PJ, Grimm RC, Wilman AH, Riederer SJ, Ehman RL (1996) 3D MR angiography of pulmonary arteries using realtime navigator gating and magnetization preparation. Magn Reson Med 36(4):579–587

Yoshihara HA, Bastiaansen JA, Berthonneche C, Comment A, Schwitter J (2015) An intact small animal model of myocardial ischemia-reperfusion: characterization of metabolic changes by hyperpolarized 13C MR spectroscopy. Am J Physiol Heart Circ Physiol 309(12):H2058–H2066

Quantitative Nuclear Medicine in Cardiopulmonary Imaging

Mario Jreige and John O. Prior

Contents

M. Jreige · J. O. Prior (✉)
Department of Nuclear Medicine and Molecular Imaging, Lausanne University Hospital and University of Lausanne, Lausanne, Switzerland
e-mail: john.prior@chuv.ch

Abstract

Advances in nuclear medicine imaging, particularly positron emission tomography (PET/CT) and single-photon emission computed tomography (SPECT/CT), have played a crucial role in routine clinical practice, allowing the quantification of disease processes with high accuracy using intrinsic quantitative evaluation techniques (Bateman et al. 2016; Kusmirek et al. 2020). The contribution of nuclear medicine to noninvasive cardiothoracic imaging covers a wide range of indications. This chapter focuses on the quantitative aspects of nuclear medicine applied to routine diagnosis and clinical research, particularly in thoracic neoplasms, myocardial perfusion, and cardiac inflammation imaging.

1 Origins and Physiological Foundation

1.1 Tracers Used in Clinical Routine in Cardiopulmonary Imaging

Advances in nuclear medicine imaging, particularly positron emission tomography (PET/CT) and single-photon emission computed tomography (SPECT/CT), have played a crucial role in routine clinical practice, allowing the quantification of disease processes with high accuracy

Med Radiol Diagn Imaging (2026)

https://doi.org/10.1007/174_2024_521,

Published Online: 15 December 2024

using intrinsic quantitative evaluation techniques (Bateman et al. 2016; Kusmirek et al. 2020). The contribution of nuclear medicine to noninvasive cardiothoracic imaging covers a wide range of indications. This chapter focuses on the quantitative aspects of nuclear medicine applied to routine diagnosis and clinical research, particularly in thoracic neoplasms, myocardial perfusion, and cardiac inflammation imaging.

2-[^{18}F] fluorodeoxyglucose (^{18}F-FDG) is the most widely used radiotracer for detecting lung and other thoracic neoplasms. However, its applications extend beyond cancer imaging to include the evaluation of inflammatory processes such as sarcoidosis (Treglia et al. 2014) or infectious disorders (Casali et al. 2021). Cancer cells have a higher uptake of glucose and FDG than normal cells due to their increased levels of glucose transporters (GLUTs) and hexokinase. Once inside the cell, glucose is converted into glucose-6-phosphate by hexokinase, whereas FDG is converted into FDG-6-phosphate (Fig. 1). Glucose-6-phosphate has more metabolic pathways available than FDG-6-phosphate, which cannot be metabolized. Cancer cells also show reduced expression of glucose-6-phosphatase, leading to the accumulation of both glucose-6-phosphate and FDG-6-phosphate within the cell. This accumulation of FDG-6-phosphate allows its use in visualizing tumors on PET/CT scans. The metabolic intensity of a malignant tumor's PET scan is related to its histology and number of cancer cells present. Some cancers, such as Hodgkin's lymphoma and melanoma, show high intensity on ^{18}F-FDG PET/CT, while others, such as low-grade adenocarcinoma, mucinous adenocarcinomas, or MALT lymphomas, have low FDG activity. Additionally, FDG can also be taken up by benign processes, such as infection and inflammation, due to the strong affinity of white blood cells and fibroblasts for FDG (Wong et al. 2016).

Recently, several radiopharmaceutical tracers have been developed to assess cardiovascular diseases (CVD) by targeting myocardial perfusion, metabolism, and inflammation. The inorganic compounds ^{13}N-ammonia ($^{13}N\text{-}NH_3$) and ^{15}O-water ($^{15}O\text{-}H_2O$) are tracers labeled with short-lived positron emitters (^{13}N: 10 min; ^{15}O: 2 min) that are produced using an on-site cyclotron and have been used for cardiac perfusion imaging (Manabe et al. 2018). $^{15}O\text{-}H_2O$ diffuses freely into cardiomyocytes. With respect to ^{13}N-

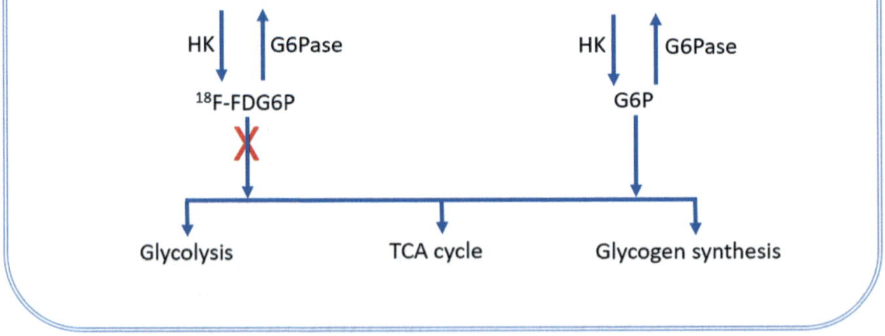

Fig. 1 Both glucose and fluorine-18-fluorodeoxyglucose (^{18}F-FDG) are accumulated in tumor cells via the glucose transporter (GLUT) and are phosphorylated by hexokinase (HK) to G6P and ^{18}F-FDG6P, respectively. G6P is consumed for energy production, whereas ^{18}F-FDG6P is not metabolized. *G6P* glucose-6-phosphate, *G6Pase* glucose-6-phosphatase, *GLUT* glucose transporter, *HK* hexokinase, *TCA* tricarboxylic acid, *^{18}F-FDG* fluor-18-fluorodeoxyglucose, *^{18}F-FDG6P* fluor-18-fluorodeoxyglucose-6-phosphate

NH_3, although the exact mechanism of its transport across the cardiac membrane has not been clearly elucidated, it has been suggested that ^{13}N-ammonia may cross cellular membranes by diffusion (Kitsiou et al. 1999). On the other hand, several radiometal ions have also been used as cardiac imaging tracers, especially in myocardial perfusion imaging. The most widely used in clinical practice is the monovalent cation thallium-201 ($^{201}Tl^+$), a gamma ray emitter suitable for scintigraphy and SPECT/CT, and the monovalent cationic rubidium ($^{82}Rb^+$), a positron emitter suitable for PET/CT. Both tracers have an ionic radius comparable to that of K^+ and are therefore substrates of the Na^+/K^+ pump, which actively transports K^+ across the cell membrane into myocytes (Yoshinaga et al. 2010). Radiometal complex tracers have also been used for myocardial perfusion imaging, in which technetium-99m (^{99m}Tc) forms a complex with six methoxyisobutylisonitrile (^{99m}Tc-sestamibi) and two 1,2-bis(di(2-ethoxyethyl)phosphino) ethane (^{99m}Tc-tetrofosmin) molecules, which are positively charged, lipophilic, monovalent, and capable of diffusing into myocytes (Manabe et al. 2018). [^{18}F]-FDG is also widely used for imaging of cardiac inflammation. Somatostatin receptor imaging with [^{68}Ga]Ga-DOTATATE has also been used to detect cardiac inflammation (Tarkin et al. 2017).

1.2 Quantitative Methods in PET/CT and SPECT/CT

PET/CT allows noninvasive in vivo assessments of regional tissue function and measurement of molecular pathways and interactions in vivo. Quantifying the data acquired by PET/CT is a multistep procedure that needs to be addressed at the data acquisition, processing, and analysis levels. For data acquisition, scanner normalization, injected dose control, correction of activity remaining in the syringe, and cross-calibration with the well counter (blood) and/or dose calibrator (injected dose) are the main points to be checked. Finally, data analysis focuses on the quantification methods used. The standardized uptake value (SUV) is the most widely used method. However, other methods are also available for special applications, including the arterial input function, tissue time-activity curves, compartment models, and linearizations, such as the Patlak plot (Lammertsma 2019; Patlak et al. 1983). Assessment of myocardial blood flow (MBF) in cardiology is an example of a compartment model analysis (Yoshinaga et al. 2018).

Advances in image reconstruction algorithms, such as the 3D ordered-subset expectation maximization iterative protocol, have enabled the absolute quantification of SPECT/CT by incorporating compensations for attenuation, scatter, and collimator-detector response, thus allowing the calculation of SUV values (Halim et al. 2021).

2 Measurement Process Overview

2.1 Units Used in Clinical Practice and Research in NM

The standardized uptake value (SUV) is a semiquantitative measure of tissue uptake, which is the ratio of the concentration of radioactivity in the tissue to the dose administered at the time of injection divided by body weight. Many factors affect the SUV, including the accuracy of dose calibration, time elapsed between injection and imaging (dose-to-scan time), motion artifacts, patient weight, and blood glucose levels (Adams et al. 2010):

$$\mathrm{SUV}\left(\mathrm{g/mL}\right)=\frac{\text{Activity concentration in tissue}\left(\mathrm{kBq/mL}\right)}{\text{Injected activity}\left(\mathrm{MBq}\right)/\text{body weight}\left(\mathrm{kg}\right)}$$

The administered dose may also be corrected by the lean body mass (LBM) or body surface area (BSA), thus allowing to calculate SUV_{LBM} or SUL (standard uptake lean body mass) and SUV_{BSA}, respectively (Tahari et al. 2014; Kim et al. 1994).

When SUV is calculated, the result can be reported as the mean measured value or SUV_{mean}, which represents the average SUV of voxels within the volume of interest (VOI); the maximum measured value or SUV_{max}, which is obtained by PET by calculating the SUV at the highest image pixel in the ROI; or the SUV_{peak}, which is measured in a spherical VOI with a volume of 1 mL at a position that provides the maximum VOI average (Zaidi and Karakatsanis 2018). The advantage of SUV_{peak} over SUV_{max} is that it avoids the noise bias, but on the other hand, SUV_{peak} is more susceptible to partial volume effects (Lodge et al. 2012).

SUV_{max} can be affected by various image acquisition and reconstruction parameters; in addition, it can also vary among different PET scanners, which has become particularly marked in recent years with the introduction of digital PET/CT systems. Enhanced photon-counting technology in digital PET/CT and the impact of delayed higher uptake and retention resulted in notably elevated SUV_{max} (Fuentes-Ocampo et al. 2019). The European Association of Nuclear Medicine (EANM) has developed reconstruction guidelines to standardize SUV measurements across different imaging systems, known as the EARL harmonization program. The aim of this process is to decrease the discrepancy in SUV values and enhance the comparability of PET images obtained from diverse scanners and protocols by utilizing a reference phantom and a standard SUV normalization method (Boellaard et al. 2015).

Metabolic volume, or metabolic tumor volume (MTV), as applied in oncology studies, is the lesion volume within a delineated boundary that can be calculated using various thresholding or region-growing techniques, the most common being relative thresholding based on a specific voxel SUV per SUV_{max} or SUV_{peak}. The MTV is expressed in cm^3. Total glycolytic volume (TGV) is the product of the mean SUV within the region and the metabolic tumor volume and is expressed in cm^3 g/mL. These volumetric parameters have valuable clinical applications; for example, MTV and total lesion glycolysis (TLG) applied to ^{18}F-FDG PET/CT have been shown to predict prognosis in patients with non-small cell lung cancer (NSCLC) (Im et al. 2015). A 50% decrease in TLG in patients with NSCLC can predict treatment response after chemotherapy with high sensitivity (100%) and negative predictive value (100%), better than decreases in MTV (83% and 90%) and response evaluation criteria in solid tumors (RECIST) (75% and 89%, respectively) (Moon et al. 2013).

2.2 Standard Uptake Value (SUV) in Oncologic Thoracic Neoplasia

2.2.1 SUV in Lung Cancer

Standardized uptake value (SUV) is a crucial quantitative measure in oncology PET/CT imaging that is widely used to assess the metabolic activity of lung lesions and help differentiate benign from malignant nodules. In oncological lung assessments, the SUV provides a measure of FDG uptake, reflecting the metabolic activity of the tissue. The use of SUV in ^{18}FDG PET/CT scans has been widely studied and proven to be a valuable tool in the assessment and monitoring of lung cancer. A study conducted by Sun et al. showed that SUV_{max} was significantly associated with the T stage, grade of malignancy, and pathological subtype of lung adenocarcinoma. In the same T-stage group, the SUV_{max} of lung adenocarcinoma was highest in patients with high-grade malignancy and solid-predominant invasive adenocarcinoma (Sun et al. 2022).

Increased FDG uptake by lung cancer cells, as measured by SUV_{max}, is thus considered predictive of the biological aggressiveness of NSCLC (Sun et al. 2022; Paesmans et al. 2010). The SUV_{max} of the primary lung lesion has also been shown to be significantly correlated with patient survival, with a higher SUV_{max} being associated with lower overall survival and relapse-free survival, even in the early stages of NSCLC (Qiu et al. 2021; Downey et al. 2016; Davies et al. 2007; Yoo et al. 2014). In most cases, malignant lesions show higher SUVs than benign lesions and normal lung tissue due to increased glucose metabolism. The reference range for SUV in oncological assessments may vary depending on factors such as patient demographics, scanner calibration, and imaging protocols. However, an SUV of 2.5 is often cited as a threshold value, beyond which a lung nodule is more likely to be malignant, although this value is not absolute and is limited to lung lesions measuring more than 1 cm (Khalaf et al. 2008).

Furthermore, a prospective multicenter trial by Weir-McCall et al., comparing qualitative and semiquantitative PET/CT criteria for solitary pulmonary nodules, found that SUV_{max} was the most accurate technique for diagnosing these nodules. The accuracy of the diagnosis should be adjusted based on the size of the nodule; for nodules smaller than 12 mm, an SUV_{max} of 1.75 or visual uptake equal to the mediastinum had the highest accuracy to differentiate malignant from benign nodules. For nodules larger than 16 mm, an SUV_{max} of 3.6 or visual PET uptake greater than the mediastinum was the most accurate for this purpose (Weir-McCall et al. 2021). The use of ^{18}F-FDG PET in differentiating metastatic disease from second primary tumors in patients with synchronous pulmonary lesions has been found to be helpful, although no study has provided a clear absolute cutoff for making this distinction. Instead, the relative difference in SUV values between the lesions was measured (Dijkman et al. 2010). Regarding the characterization of lymph node involvement, SUV_{max} proved to have high specificity but limited sensitivity, thus preserving an essential valuable contribution to endoscopic endobronchial ultrasound-guided fine needle aspiration in lymph node staging, particularly for lymph nodes with low tracer uptake. In a retrospective study, the sensitivity, specificity, and accuracy of PET/CT for detecting metastatic lymph nodes were 48.1%, 88.1%, and 82.6% in the squamous cell carcinoma group and 57.5%, 95.9%, and 86.3% in the adenocarcinoma group, respectively. Lymph nodes were considered malignant when their SUV_{max} was higher than that of the normal background (Wang et al. 2015). In the same study, using a cutoff of 2.5 g/mL for SUV_{max} was reported to degrade the sensitivity of PET/CT to 37% and 40%, respectively (Wang et al. 2015). False-positive PET findings of lymph node involvement can be attributed to granulomatous infections, such as tuberculosis, or inflammatory lesions, such as sarcoidosis.

With regard to the detection of metastasis, FDG PET/CT is considered the modality of choice for the evaluation of extra-encephalic metastases in patients with NSCLC with a sensitivity of 93% and a specificity of 96% (Kandathil et al. 2018). In the specific case of adrenal metastases, the combination of mean CT attenuation greater than 10 Hounsfield units (HU) and SUV_{max} greater than 3.1 g/mL had a sensitivity and specificity of 97% and 86%, respectively, for the identification of metastatic disease. The ratio of the SUV_{max} of the adrenal nodule to the SUV_{mean} of the liver, set at 2.5, has a negative predictive value of 100% for malignancy (Brady et al. 2009). Adrenal adenomas have been shown to exhibit lower uptake compared to adrenal metastases, with a mean SUV_{max} of 2.9 ± 1.0 and an adrenal-to-liver SUV ratio of 0.9 ± 0.3, respectively. In contrast, adrenal metastases demonstrate significantly higher values, with a mean SUV_{max} of 8.4 ± 3.8 and an adrenal-to-liver SUV ratio of 3.0 ± 1.3 (Watanabe et al. 2013).

Nevertheless, it remains essential to consider the whole clinical context when evaluating oncological diseases, as inflammatory conditions and infections can also lead to high SUVs. Moreover, advances in imaging technology and standardized protocols continue to refine SUV measurements, improving their reliability as a diagnostic tool in the evaluation of lung cancer. For instance, dynamic whole-body (WB) ^{18}F-FDG PET is a promising technique for quantifying dynamic values in lung lesions using a two-compartment linear Patlak model (FDG influx rate constant = Ki, metabolic rate = MR-FDG, distribution volume = DV-FDG) that may help differentiate between malignant and inflammatory lesions (Skawran et al. 2022; Weissinger et al. 2023).

In addition, false-negative FDG images are due to the technical limitations of PET/CT and inherent characteristics of neoplasms. Lesions less than 2–3 times the spatial resolution of the scanner appear less active and have a lower SUV owing to the partial volume effect. Lesions with small cells, neoplasms with low metabolism, and highly differentiated tumors can lead to false-negative results, such as low-grade malignancies, such as carcinoma in situ and minimally invasive or some other adenocarcinoma (Chao and Zhang 2012; Kim et al. 1998; Greenspan 2017). False-negative PET/CT results may also occur in cases of metastases with hemorrhage or necrosis. For pulmonary carcinoid tumors, ^{68}Ga-DOTA-peptides (^{68}Ga-DOTA-TOC, ^{68}Ga-DOTA-TATE, etc.) have been shown to outperform ^{18}F-FDG in terms of detection rate. In particular, ^{68}Ga-DOTA-peptides demonstrate superior diagnostic efficiency in cases involving adjacent atelectasis. The combination of ^{68}Ga-DOTA-peptides and ^{18}F-FDG PET/CT findings is regarded as a highly reliable tool for preoperative assessment (Jiang et al. 2019).

2.2.2 MTV and TLG in Lung Cancer

In addition to the SUV, metabolic tumor volume (MTV) and total lesion glycolysis (TLG) have emerged as important volumetric and metabolic parameters in oncologic imaging. MTV quantifies the volume of tumor tissue with increased FDG uptake, providing a measure of tumor burden, whereas TLG combines both the volume (MTV) and metabolic activity of the tumor using SUV_{mean}, offering a more comprehensive assessment of tumor aggressiveness. Studies have shown that the MTV and TLG are valuable prognostic indicators of lung cancer. Liao et al. found that higher MTV and TLG values were significantly associated with poorer overall survival in non-small cell lung cancer patients (Liao et al. 2012). Similarly, Huang et al. demonstrated that the MTV of the primary lung tumor has the potential to become a valuable prognostic biomarker for survival outcomes in NSCLC patients (Huang et al. 2014). Wen et al. demonstrated that stage I/II NSCLC with increased TLG was associated with an increased mortality risk (Wen et al. 2021). These findings underscore the role of MTV and TLG in PET/CT quantification as they provide additional prognostic information that can guide treatment planning and improve patient management. Their integration into the clinical routine must be thoroughly considered and evaluated to maximize the benefits for patient care.

2.2.3 PERCIST Applications

PET response criteria in solid tumors (PERCIST) is a set of PET-based evaluation criteria for assessing tumor response to treatment, as detailed in Table 1 (Wahl et al. 2009). A volume of interest (VOI) is placed in the center of the hottest

Table 1 PET response criteria in solid tumor (PERCIST) evaluation

Complete metabolic response (CMR)	• Complete resolution of ^{18}F-FDG uptake within the measurable target lesion so that it is less than mean liver activity and at the level of surrounding background blood pool activity • Disappearance of all other lesions to background blood pool levels • No new suspicious ^{18}F-FDG avid lesions • If progression according to RECIST criteria, must verify with follow-up
Partial metabolic response (PMR)	• Reduction of a minimum of 30% in target measurable tumor ^{18}F-FDG SUL peak, with absolute drop in SUL of at least 0.8 SUL units • No increase >30% of SUL or size in all other lesions • No new lesions
Stable metabolic disease (SMD)	• Not CMR, PMR, or progressive metabolic disease (PMD) • No new lesions
Progressive metabolic disease (PMD)	• >30% increase in ^{18}F-FDG SUL peak, with >0.8 SUL unit increase in tumor SUV_{peak} from the baseline scan in pattern typical of tumor and not of infection/treatment effect • Or visible increase in the extent of ^{18}F-FDG tumor uptake • Or new ^{18}F-FDG-avid lesions which are typical of cancer and not related to treatment effect or infection

tumor, and semiquantitative standardized uptake value corrected for lean body mass (SUL) in the tumor and background reference normal structures is used. Measurement is recommended after visual inspection of PET images to help identify FDG-avid foci that best match the tracer uptake in malignant lesions. The SUL_{peak} is measured by averaging the SUL values of all pixels contained in a 1 mL sphere volume centered on the single hottest pixel of the lesion. Important points to consider are the following: For a lesion to be considered measurable, its SUL_{peak} must be greater than or equal to one and a half times the mean SUL of the reference liver plus two times the standard deviation. If the blood pool reference activity is used instead of the liver, the lesion should be at least twice the mean SUL plus two times its standard deviation, because the blood pool activity is typically less than that of the liver. The target lesion does not have to be the same lesion between the two time points; rather, the hottest lesion is selected at each evaluation time point (Marcus et al. 2022).

The following imaging conditions are essential to allow comparison of multiple PET/CT scans: (a) The difference between the injection-to-imaging time of the baseline scan and the follow-up scan should be less than or equal to 15 min. (b) The injection-to-imaging start time for both baseline and follow-up scans should be greater than or equal to 50 min and less than or equal to 70 min. (c) The same imager should be used at the same location. (d) The same acquisition and reconstruction protocols, as well as the same software version, are used. (e) The difference between the injected dose of ^{18}F-FDG (in MBq) for the baseline study and that for the follow-up study should be less than or equal to 20%. (f) Patients should fast for at least 4 h before the administration of ^{18}F-FDG with serum glucose levels less than 200 mg/dL (Hyun O et al. 2016).

RECIST 1.1 is currently the standard imaging method used in clinical trials. However, RECIST and PERCIST measure two different tumor characteristics, and because ^{18}F-FDG PET/CT can detect more metastatic lesions, including bone metastases (particularly isodense bone metastasis), than enhanced CT, it is not uncommon for the two criteria to yield different responses. In a prospective study of patients with NSCLC, PERCIST showed a difference in PFS between the groups of patients with a partial metabolic response and those with stable metabolic disease after chemotherapy, whereas RECIST 1.1 was not able to show this difference (Shang et al. 2016).

2.3 Cardiac Myocardial Perfusion Imaging

Cardiac myocardial perfusion imaging (MPI) using SPECT/CT and PET/CT is a valuable diagnostic tool for assessing and monitoring various cardiac conditions, particularly when quantitative techniques and specific tracers are used. This imaging technique provides critical information regarding myocardial perfusion, viability, and function, which aids in accurate diagnosis, treatment planning, and prognostic assessment, ultimately leading to improved patient care.

In guidelines developed collaboratively by SNMMI with the American Society of Nuclear Cardiology (ASNC) and the Society of Cardiovascular CT (SCCT), MPI was proposed as a diagnostic tool with high accuracy in the evaluation of coronary artery disease, showing that it provides important information about myocardial perfusion and can aid in the detection of significant coronary artery stenosis (Dorbala et al. 2013). Quantitative analysis of PET/CT images with the use of radiotracers such as rubidium-82 or N-13 ammonia allows for precise measurement of myocardial blood flow and ejection fraction, providing valuable insights into the extent and severity of coronary artery disease. A study conducted by Naya et al. demonstrated that the combination of PET/CT myocardial perfusion imaging and quantitative analysis using tracers, such as ^{18}F-flurpiridaz, can accurately determine myocardial viability and predict the likelihood of functional recovery after revascularization in patients with ischemic cardiomyopathy. This finding underscores the potential value of this quantitative imaging approach in treatment planning and prognostic assessment (Naya et al. 2014). The use of quantitative techniques with specific tracers has enabled the precise evaluation of myocardial viability and function, guiding clinical decision-making and improving patient outcomes. A meta-analysis showed that both cardiac magnetic resonance (CMR) and PET/CT MPI are highly accurate in detecting hemodynamic cardiovascular disease, with an AUC of 0.94 (95% CI 0.92–0.96) and 0.92 (95% CI 0.89–0.94), a pooled sensitivity of 0.88 (95% confidence interval [CI]: 0.80–0.93) and 0.83 (95% CI: 0.70–0.91), and a pooled specificity of 0.89 (95% CI: 0.85–0.93) and 0.89 (95% CI, 0.86–0.91) for CMR and PET/CT, respectively (Yang et al. 2019).

Cardiac PET MPI uses quantitative techniques that employ mathematical models to determine both absolute and relative measures of myocardial blood flow (MBF) and myocardial flow reserve (MFR). The method most commonly used to evaluate MBF and MFR is tracer kinetic modeling, which involves the administration of tracers such as ^{82}rubidium chloride (^{82}Rb) or ^{13}N-ammonia ($^{13}NH_3$). It measures its uptake and clearance in the myocardium over time, as well as MFR, which is the ratio of stress MBF to rest MBF (Bateman et al. 2021).

Quantitative techniques can provide more accurate and reproducible measures of MBF and MFR than visual interpretation, which can be subjective and influenced by observer variability. These quantitative techniques allow for standardization and application across different positron emission tomography (PET) scanners and imaging protocols, leading to more reliable results between institutions. Quantitative techniques have been shown to improve diagnostic accuracy for the detection of coronary artery disease (CAD) and other myocardial perfusion abnormalities. As a result, these techniques are increasingly employed in clinical practice to guide treatment decisions, evaluate prognosis, and monitor treatment response in patients with CAD and other cardiovascular conditions. Cardiac myocardial perfusion PET/CT is highly effective for diagnosing coronary microvascular dysfunction (CMD) by quantifying myocardial blood flow and flow reserve, enabling the detection of impaired perfusion even in the presence of normal coronary arteries. In contrast, cardiac magnetic resonance (CMR) imaging is valuable for assessing myocardial tissue changes and can complement PET/CT findings by offering additional insights into myocardial health. Future research focusing on further exploring the complementary roles of both modalities will be essential for improving early detection and stratification of CMD.

2.4 Cardiac Sarcoidosis

Cardiac sarcoidosis (CS) is a serious form of sarcoidosis that accounts for 13–25% of sarcoidosis-related fatalities (Doughan and Williams 2006). Despite the increased risk of death and disability associated with cardiac involvement, diagnosing CS remains a challenge owing to its broad and nonspecific symptoms, ranging from asymptomatic electrocardiogram abnormalities to sudden death, progressive heart failure, and arrhythmias. While clinical manifestations of cardiac involvement are obvious in approximately 25% of sarcoidosis patients, myocardial granulomas can be detected in nearly 25–79% of autopsy examinations (Matsui et al. 1976). An endomyocardial biopsy can provide a definitive histologic diagnosis of CS, but this invasive procedure carries risks and lacks sensitivity owing to the heterogeneous distribution of myocardial involvement. Recent advances in PET using ^{18}F-FDG have emerged as promising tools for managing patients with CS and are most commonly used for imaging myocardial inflammation in clinical practice (Skali et al. 2013).

Cellular uptake of ^{18}F-FDG in sarcoidosis is associated with inflammatory cell infiltrates, which are characterized by high levels of glycolytic activity to meet their significant energy demands. This results in active inflammatory cells with ATP levels approximately eight times higher than normal (Mehta et al. 2008). Visualization of active sarcoid lesions in various organs is achieved through increased ^{18}F-FDG uptake on PET imaging in areas where the tracer accumulates in the active inflammatory lesions.

To prevent false-positive results, it is important for patients to follow an additional dietary regimen along with fasting before the examination, as normal muscle cells rely on glucose as a key energy source. Therefore, it is essential to suppress physiological uptake of ^{18}F-FDG in the heart. During fasting, free fatty acids account for up to 90% of oxygen consumption by normal muscle cells. A high-fat, high-protein, low-carbohydrate diet has been shown to reduce glucose uptake by normal heart tissue, thereby shifting metabolism in favor of fatty acids and suppressing glucose utilization and ^{18}F-FDG uptake by normal heart tissue. To achieve this, it is recommended to follow these dietary modifications for at least 36 h prior to the examination and up to 72 h if possible; otherwise, a 24-h fasting protocol can be used as an alternative to dietary preparation. Additionally, some protocols involve pre-administration of unfractionated intravenous (IV) heparin to suppress myocardial ^{18}F-FDG uptake. IV unfractionated heparin activates lipoprotein and hepatic lipases, increasing plasma free fatty acid levels and ultimately reducing glucose consumption in normal muscle cells. Doses as high as 50 IU/kg can be used, provided that there are no contraindications for intravenous heparin injections. Quality control steps include confirmation of adequate suppression of myocardial physiological ^{18}F-FDG uptake, defined as no visible ^{18}F-FDG uptake or uptake that is lower than that of the blood pool (Osborne et al. 2017).

Kim and colleagues analyzed 17 studies involving 891 patients, reporting a pooled sensitivity of 84% and a specificity of 83% in the detection of CS (Kim et al. 2020). In a study of 38 patients who underwent ^{18}F-FDG PET/CT for CS, Ahmadian et al. found that cardiac metabolic activity, measured by SUV, was a predictor of adverse events, providing further evidence for the prognostic value of ^{18}F-FDG PET/CT in the evaluation of CS (Ahmadian et al. 2014). Meta-analyses have shown that cardiac MRI boasts a higher sensitivity than ^{18}F-FDG PET/CT for diagnosing cardiac sarcoidosis (95% vs. 84%, $p = 0.002$), while both modalities have similar specificity (85% vs. 82%, $p = 0.85$) (Aitken et al. 2022). Additionally, PET/CT offers the advantage of a comprehensive assessment of sarcoidosis throughout the entire body in a single examination.

Subramanian et al. demonstrated that a novel SUV-based metric, the ^{18}F-FDG uptake index (UI), defined as the product of the maximum left ventricular SUV and the number of left ventricular segments with abnormal uptake, was an independent predictor of treatment response (Subramanian et al. 2021). In a study of 23 patients undergoing treatment with CS, Osborne et al. found that a reduction in myocardial inflammation, as measured by SUV, on serial ^{18}F-FDG PET/CT scans was associated with an improvement in the left ventricular ejection fraction with an expected increase in EF of 7.9% per SUV reduction of 10 g/mL (Osborne et al. 2014).

3 Common Artifacts: Confounding Factors and Technical Improvements

3.1 Oncologic Measurements with PET/CT: Respiratory Motion Artifacts

Respiratory motion artifacts significantly impact the accuracy and reliability of PET/CT FDG imaging, posing a substantial challenge for the quantification of metabolic activity. These artifacts are caused by the natural motion of the lungs, diaphragm, and chest wall during breathing, which leads to misregistration between the PET and CT images and blurring of the PET signal, particularly in the lung bases. This results in erroneous standardized uptake values (SUVs), potentially masking small lesions or falsely elevating SUV measurements, thereby compromising the diagnostic accuracy and treatment planning. Various methods have been developed to mitigate these artifacts, including respiratory gating, which synchronizes image acquisition with the patient's breathing cycle, and advanced image reconstruction algorithms that correct for motion. Studies have shown that these techniques significantly improve the image quality and quantification accuracy. Breath-hold (BH) PET/CT, a recently introduced acquisition consisting of lung PET/CT acquisition performed during a single breath-hold averaging 20 s for PET and 10 s for CT, has been shown to identify a significantly greater number of lung nodules than free-breath PET/CT (n = 422 versus n = 191, $p < 0.001$) (Jreige et al. 2023) (Fig. 2). BH PET/CT has also been shown to reduce background lung uptake and provide better registration and SUV quantification of lesions, particularly in the lower thorax (Cui et al. 2024). In addition, advances in post-processing algorithms, such as data-driven gating (DDG), which enables the automatic extraction of respiratory signals from PET data without the need for external monitoring devices, using signals derived from the raw PET data, make it possible to generate motion-corrected images (Pan et al. 2022; Schleyer et al. 2018). This advanced technique improves the clarity and sharpness of PET/CT images, resulting in increased sensitivity and specificity for the detection of lung nodules. Studies such as those by Büther et al. and Sigfridsson et al. have demonstrated that DDG can significantly improve the detection rate of small lung nodules and provide more accurate SUV measurements than uncorrected images (Büther et al. 2016; Sigfridsson et al. 2021). Consequently, DDG has the potential to significantly enhance diagnostic confidence and aid in the early detection and management of pulmonary malignancies.

3.2 Cardiac MPI Quality Control

The sources of errors in SPECT and PET radionuclide imaging include patient motion, poor signal-to-noise ratio, attenuation artifacts, and reconstruction artifacts. In hybrid imaging, the primary sources of error are related to artifacts resulting from the misregistration of the transmission and emission scans and motion during the attenuation-correction CT scan or coronary artery calcium scoring (Holly et al. 2010; Nakazato et al. 2013).

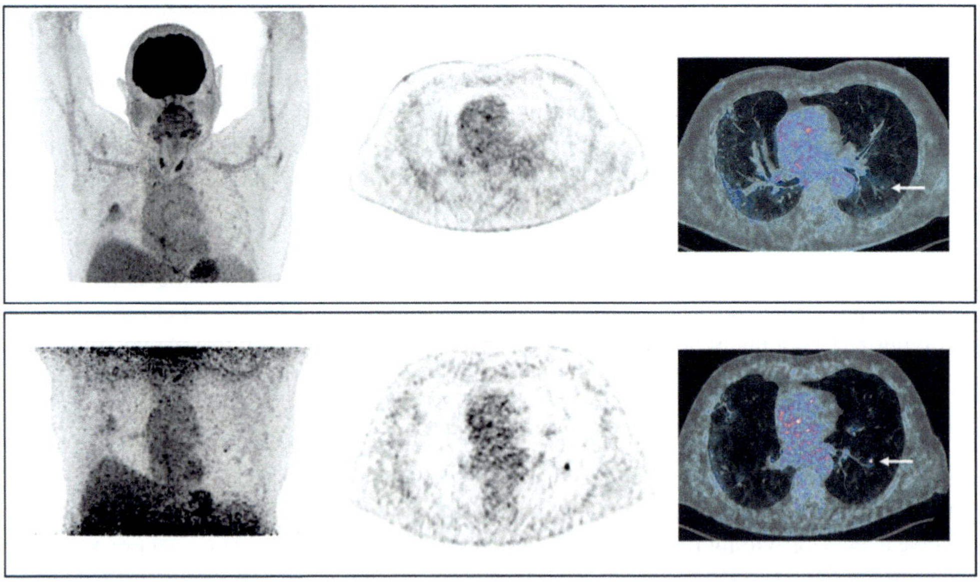

Fig. 2 A 77-year-old patient with lung adenocarcinoma straddling the middle and upper right lobes was classified as pT2 pN0 cM0 in 2006 stage IB and treated by upper right and middle lobectomy in 2006 followed by adjuvant chemotherapy. New appearance of a single 6 mm solid pulmonary nodule of an undetermined nature in the apical segment of the left lower lobe. ^{18}F-FDG PET/CT with both free-breathing (FB) and breath-hold (BH) acquisitions showed nodule tracer uptake with better visualization and higher SUVmax (8.4 g/mL) in BH than in FB (1.9 g/mL)

Misregistration is the primary cause of artifacts in PET or SPECT/CT imaging, which can occur because the heart's position on MPI is different from that on CT, resulting from vasodilator stress or imaging for attenuation-correction CT during a specific phase of the respiratory cycle when the myocardium is not at its average heart position, as represented by the PET image. To ensure accurate measurement of myocardial blood flow, patients should be advised to remain stationary during PET MPI, and any involuntary movements such as coughing or sneezing should be documented. Patient motion can be difficult to detect during image acquisition and should be controlled during post-processing to avoid artifacts that may alter the MBF measurement. With PET, the dynamic image file can be processed to exclude frames with motion and to sum the remaining frames. However, this approach may not be optimal for short-lived radiotracers, particularly during the initial 1–3 min of ^{82}Rb image acquisition. A patient's motion during a CT scan can also result in streak artifacts that can affect the accuracy of coronary artery calcium scoring.

4 Conclusion and Future Perspectives

This chapter provides a comprehensive overview of nuclear medicine imaging techniques, particularly PET/CT and SPECT/CT, in cardiopulmonary imaging and emphasizes the clinical applications of these imaging techniques in diagnosing and monitoring various cardiopulmonary conditions, including lung cancer, coronary artery disease, and cardiac sarcoidosis. Various radiotracers, including ^{18}F-FDG and ^{82}Rb, for imaging thoracic neoplasms, myocardial perfusion, and cardiac inflammation are covered. Key quantitative methods, including SUV, MTV, TLG, and the PERCIST criteria, are recognized as essential metrics for evaluating metabolic activity and tumor burden in oncological imaging. Challenges and artifacts in nuclear imaging, including respiratory motion and misregistration, are addressed, along with potential solutions like respiratory gating and breath-hold techniques. Future perspectives suggest ongoing improvements in image acquisition, reconstruction, and analysis techniques to enhance diagnostic accuracy and patient care. Overall, this chapter underscores the significant contributions of nuclear medicine imaging to cardiopulmonary diagnostics and highlights the importance of continued research and development in this field to improve patient outcomes.

Disclaimer All measurements in this book have been obtained from peer-reviewed papers and guidelines from professional organizations, unless explicitly stated otherwise. While the authors, editors, and publisher have gone through a rigorous process to establish their correct reproduction from the original source, each measurement must be interpreted in the correct clinical context, this along with an accurate way of measurement, and taking into account all technical variables, this including follow-up exams with various equipment or software. Neither the authors, the editors, nor the publisher can accept any legal responsibility for any improper application or interpretation of these measurements as well as their potential consequences.

References

Adams MC, Turkington TG, Wilson JM, Wong TZ (2010) A systematic review of the factors affecting accuracy of SUV measurements. Am J Roentgenol 195(2):310–320

Ahmadian A, Brogan A, Berman J, Sverdlov AL, Mercier G, Mazzini M et al (2014) Quantitative interpretation of FDG PET/CT with myocardial perfusion imaging increases diagnostic information in the evaluation of cardiac sarcoidosis. J Nucl Cardiol 21(5):925–939

Aitken M, Chan MV, Urzua Fresno C, Farrell A, Islam N, McInnes MDF et al (2022) Diagnostic accuracy of cardiac MRI versus FDG PET for cardiac sarcoidosis: a systematic review and meta-analysis. Radiology 304(3):566–579

Bateman TM, Dilsizian V, Beanlands RS et al (2016) American Society of Nuclear Cardiology and Society of Nuclear Medicine and Molecular Imaging joint position statement on the clinical indications for myocardial perfusion PET. J Nucl Cardiol 23(5):1227–1231

Bateman TM, Heller GV, Beanlands R, Calnon DA, Case J, deKemp R et al (2021) Practical guide for interpreting and reporting cardiac PET measurements of myocardial blood flow: an information statement from the American Society of Nuclear Cardiology, and the Society of Nuclear Medicine and Molecular Imaging. J Nucl Med 62(11):1599–1615

Boellaard R, Delgado-Bolton R, Oyen WJG, Giammarile F, Tatsch K, Eschner W et al (2015) FDG PET/CT: EANM procedure guidelines for tumour imaging: version 2.0. Eur J Nucl Med Mol Imaging 42(2):328–354
Brady MJ, Thomas J, Wong TZ, Franklin KM, Ho LM, Paulson EK (2009) Adrenal nodules at FDG PET/CT in patients known to have or suspected of having lung cancer: a proposal for an efficient diagnostic algorithm. Radiology 250(2):523–530
Büther F, Vehren T, Schäfers KP, Schäfers M (2016) Impact of data-driven respiratory gating in clinical PET. Radiology 281(1):229–238
Casali M, Lauri C, Altini C, Bertagna F, Cassarino G, Cistaro A et al (2021) State of the art of 18F-FDG PET/CT application in inflammation and infection: a guide for image acquisition and interpretation. Clin Translat Imaging 9(4):299–339
Chao F, Zhang H (2012) PET/CT in the staging of the non-small-cell lung cancer. J Biomed Biotechnol 2012:783739 [cited 2023 Aug 28]. https://www.ncbi.nlm.nih.gov/pmc/articles/PMC3346692/.
Cui Y, Jia J, Yan Q, He X, Yuan K, Li Z et al (2024) The impact of deep-inspiration breath-hold total-body PET/CT imaging on thoracic 18F-FDG avid lesions compared with free-breathing. Eur J Radiol 177:111549
Davies A, Tan C, Paschalides C, Barrington SF, O'Doherty M, Utley M et al (2007) FDG-PET maximum standardised uptake value is associated with variation in survival: analysis of 498 lung cancer patients. Lung Cancer (Amsterdam, The Netherlands) 55(1):75–78
Dijkman BG, Schuurbiers OCJ, Vriens D, Looijen-Salamon M, Bussink J, Timmer-Bonte JNH et al (2010) The role of 18F-FDG PET in the differentiation between lung metastases and synchronous second primary lung tumours. Eur J Nucl Med Mol Imaging 37(11):2037–2047
Dorbala S, Di Carli MF, Delbeke D, Abbara S, DePuey EG, Dilsizian V et al (2013) SNMMI/ASNC/SCCT guideline for cardiac SPECT/CT and PET/CT 1.0. J Nucl Med 54(8):1485–1507
Doughan AR, Williams BR (2006) Cardiac sarcoidosis. Heart 92(2):282–288
Downey RJ, Akhurst T, Gonen M, Vincent A, Bains MS, Larson S et al (2016) Preoperative F-18 fluorodeoxyglucose-positron emission tomography maximal standardized uptake value predicts survival after lung cancer resection. J Clin Oncol [cited 2023 Aug 28]. https://ascopubs.org/doi/pdf/10.1200/JCO.2004.11.109?role=tab.
Fuentes-Ocampo F, López-Mora DA, Flotats A, Paillahueque G, Camacho V, Duch J et al (2019) Digital vs. analog PET/CT: intra-subject comparison of the SUVmax in target lesions and reference regions. Eur J Nucl Med Mol Imaging 46(8):1745–1750
Greenspan BS (2017) Role of PET/CT for precision medicine in lung cancer: perspective of the Society of Nuclear Medicine and Molecular Imaging. Transl Lung Cancer Res 6(6):617–620
Halim F, Yahya H, Jaafar KN, Mansor S (2021) Accuracy assessment of SUV measurements in SPECT/CT: a phantom study. J Nucl Med Technol 49(3):250–255
Holly TA, Abbott BG, Al-Mallah M, Calnon DA, Cohen MC, DiFilippo FP et al (2010) Single photon-emission computed tomography. J Nucl Cardiol 17(5):941–973
Huang W, Fan M, Liu B, Fu Z, Zhou T, Zhang Z et al (2014) Value of metabolic tumor volume on repeated 18F-FDG PET/CT for early prediction of survival in locally advanced non-small cell lung cancer treated with concurrent chemoradiotherapy. J Nucl Med 55(10):1584–1590
Hyun O J, Lodge MA, Wahl RL (2016) Practical PERCIST: a simplified guide to PET response criteria in solid tumors 1.0. Radiology 280(2):576–584
Im HJ, Pak K, Cheon GJ, Kang KW, Kim SJ, Kim IJ et al (2015) Prognostic value of volumetric parameters of 18F-FDG PET in non-small-cell lung cancer: a meta-analysis. Eur J Nucl Med Mol Imaging 42(2):241–251
Jiang Y, Hou G, Cheng W (2019) The utility of 18F-FDG and 68Ga-DOTA-peptide PET/CT in the evaluation of primary pulmonary carcinoid. Medicine (Baltimore) 98(10):e14769
Jreige M, Darçot E, Lovis A, Simons J, Nicod-Lalonde M, Schaefer N et al (2023) Lung CT stabilization with high-frequency non-invasive ventilation (HF-NIV) and breath-hold (BH) in lung nodule assessment by PET/CT. Eur J Hybrid Imaging 7:16
Kandathil A, Kay FU, Butt YM, Wachsmann JW, Subramaniam RM (2018) Role of FDG PET/CT in the eighth edition of TNM staging of non-small cell lung cancer. Radiographics [cited 2023 Aug 28]. https://pubs.rsna.org/doi/10.1148/rg.2018180060.
Khalaf M, Abdel-Nabi H, Baker J, Shao Y, Lamonica D, Gona J (2008) Relation between nodule size and 18F-FDG-PET SUV for malignant and benign pulmonary nodules. J Hematol Oncol 1:13
Kim CK, Gupta NC, Chandramouli B, Alavi A (1994) Standardized uptake values of FDG: body surface area correction is preferable to body weight correction. J Nucl Med 35(1):164–167
Kim BT, Kim Y, Lee KS, Yoon SB, Cheon EM, Kwon OJ et al (1998) Localized form of bronchioloalveolar carcinoma: FDG PET findings. AJR Am J Roentgenol 170(4):935–939
Kim SJ, Pak K, Kim K (2020) Diagnostic performance of F-18 FDG PET for detection of cardiac sarcoidosis; a systematic review and meta-analysis. J Nucl Cardiol 27(6):2103–2115
Kitsiou AN, Bacharach SL, Bartlett ML, Srinivasan G, Summers RM, Quyyumi AA et al (1999) 13N-ammonia myocardial blood flow and uptake: relation to functional outcome of asynergic regions after revascularization. J Am Coll Cardiol 33(3):678–686
Kusmirek JE, Magnusson JD, Perlman SB (2020) Current applications for nuclear medicine imaging in pulmonary disease. Curr Pulmonol Rep 9(3):82–95
Lammertsma AA (2019) Quantification of PET studies. J Nucl Cardiol 26(6):2045–2047

Liao S, Penney BC, Wroblewski K, Zhang H, Simon CA, Kampalath R et al (2012) Prognostic value of metabolic tumor burden on 18F-FDG PET in nonsurgical patients with non-small cell lung cancer. Eur J Nucl Med Mol Imaging 39(1):27–38

Lodge MA, Chaudhry MA, Wahl RL (2012) Noise considerations for PET quantification using maximum and peak standardized uptake value. J Nucl Med 53(7):1041–1047

Manabe O, Kikuchi T, Scholte AJHA, El Mahdiui M, Nishii R, Zhang MR et al (2018) Radiopharmaceutical tracers for cardiac imaging. J Nucl Cardiol 25(4):1204–1236

Marcus C, Tajmir SH, Rowe SP, Sheikhbahaei S, Solnes LB (2022) 18F-FDG PET/CT for response assessment in lung cancer. Semin Nucl Med 52(6):662–672

Matsui Y, Iwai K, Tachibana T, Fruie T, Shigematsu N, Izumi T et al (1976) Clinicopathological study of fatal myocardial sarcoidosis. Ann N Y Acad Sci 278:455–469

Mehta D, Lubitz SA, Frankel Z, Wisnivesky JP, Einstein AJ, Goldman M et al (2008) Cardiac involvement in patients with sarcoidosis: diagnostic and prognostic value of outpatient testing. Chest 133(6): 1426–1435

Moon SH, Cho SH, Park LC, Ji JH, Sun JM, Ahn JS et al (2013) Metabolic response evaluated by 18F-FDG PET/CT as a potential screening tool in identifying a subgroup of patients with advanced non-small cell lung cancer for immediate maintenance therapy after first-line chemotherapy. Eur J Nucl Med Mol Imaging 40(7):1005–1013

Nakazato R, Berman DS, Alexanderson E, Slomka P (2013) Myocardial perfusion imaging with PET. Imaging Med 5(1):35–46

Naya M, Murthy VL, Taqueti VR, Foster CR, Klein J, Garber M et al (2014) Preserved coronary flow reserve effectively excludes high-risk coronary artery disease on angiography. J Nucl Med 55(2):248–255

Osborne MT, Hulten EA, Singh A, Waller AH, Bittencourt MS, Stewart GC et al (2014) Reduction in ^{18}F-fluorodeoxyglucose uptake on serial cardiac positron emission tomography is associated with improved left ventricular ejection fraction in patients with cardiac sarcoidosis. J Nucl Cardiol 21(1):166–174

Osborne MT, Hulten EA, Murthy VL, Skali H, Taqueti VR, Dorbala S et al (2017) Patient preparation for cardiac fluorine-18 fluorodeoxyglucose positron emission tomography imaging of inflammation. J Nucl Cardiol 24(1):86–99

Paesmans M, Berghmans T, Dusart M, Garcia C, Hossein-Foucher C, Lafitte JJ et al (2010) Primary tumor standardized uptake value measured on fluorodeoxyglucose positron emission tomography is of prognostic value for survival in non-small cell lung cancer: update of a systematic review and meta-analysis by the European Lung Cancer Working Party for the International Association for the Study of Lung Cancer Staging Project. J Thorac Oncol 5(5):612–619

Pan T, Thomas MA, Luo D (2022) Data-driven gated CT: an automated respiratory gating method to enable data-driven gated PET/CT. Med Phys 49(6):3597–3611

Patlak CS, Blasberg RG, Fenstermacher JD (1983) Graphical evaluation of blood-to-brain transfer constants from multiple-time uptake data. J Cereb Blood Flow Metab 3(1):1–7

Qiu X, Liang H, Zhong W, Zhao J, Chen M, Zhu Z et al (2021) Prognostic impact of maximum standardized uptake value on 18F-FDG PET/CT imaging of the primary lung lesion on survival in advanced non-small cell lung cancer: a retrospective study. Thorac Cancer 12(6):845–853

Schleyer P, Hong I, Jones J, Hamill J, Panin V, Fuerst S (2018) Data-driven respiratory gating whole body PET using continuous bed motion. In: 2018 IEEE nuclear science symposium and medical imaging conference proceedings (NSS/MIC), pp 1–5 [cited 2024 Sep 10]. https://ieeexplore.ieee.org/document/8824401.

Shang J, Ling X, Zhang L, Tang Y, Xiao Z, Cheng Y et al (2016) Comparison of RECIST, EORTC criteria and PERCIST for evaluation of early response to chemotherapy in patients with non-small-cell lung cancer. Eur J Nucl Med Mol Imaging 43(11):1945–1953

Sigfridsson J, Lindström E, Iyer V, Holstensson M, Velikyan I, Sundin A et al (2021) Prospective data-driven respiratory gating of [68Ga]Ga-DOTATOC PET/CT. EJNMMI Res 11:33

Skali H, Schulman AR, Dorbala S (2013) 18F-FDG PET/CT for the assessment of myocardial sarcoidosis. Curr Cardiol Rep 15(4):352

Skawran S, Messerli M, Kotasidis F, Trinckauf J, Weyermann C, Kudura K et al (2022) Can dynamic whole-body FDG PET imaging differentiate between malignant and inflammatory lesions? Life 12(9):1350

Subramanian M, Swapna N, Ali AZ, Saggu DK, Yalagudri S, Kishore J et al (2021) Pre-treatment myocardial 18FDG uptake predicts response to immunosuppression in patients with cardiac sarcoidosis. JACC Cardiovasc Imaging 14(10):2008–2016

Sun X, Chen T, Xie C, Liu L, Lei B, Wang L et al (2022) Relationships between SUVmax of lung adenocarcinoma and different T stages, histological grades and pathological subtypes: a retrospective cohort study in China. BMJ Open 12(5):e056804

Tahari AK, Chien D, Azadi JR, Wahl RL (2014) Optimum lean body formulation for correction of standardized uptake value in PET imaging. J Nucl Med 55(9):1481–1484

Tarkin JM, Joshi FR, Evans NR, Chowdhury MM, Figg NL, Shah AV et al (2017) Detection of atherosclerotic inflammation by 68Ga-DOTATATE PET compared to [18F]FDG PET imaging. J Am Coll Cardiol 69(14):1774–1791

Treglia G, Annunziata S, Sobic-Saranovic D, Bertagna F, Caldarella C, Giovanella L (2014) The role of 18F-FDG-PET and PET/CT in patients with sarcoidosis: an updated evidence-based review. Acad Radiol 21(5):675–684

Wahl RL, Jacene H, Kasamon Y, Lodge MA (2009) From RECIST to PERCIST: evolving considerations for PET response criteria in solid tumors. J Nucl Med 50 Suppl 1:122S–150S

Wang Y, Ma S, Dong M, Yao Y, Liu K, Zhou J (2015) Evaluation of the factors affecting the maximum standardized uptake value of metastatic lymph nodes in different histological types of non-small cell lung cancer on PET-CT. BMC Pulm Med 15(1):20

Watanabe H, Kanematsu M, Goshima S, Kondo H, Kawada H, Noda Y et al (2013) Adrenal-to-liver SUV ratio is the best parameter for differentiation of adrenal metastases from adenomas using 18F-FDG PET/CT. Ann Nucl Med 27(7):648–653

Weir-McCall JR, Harris S, Miles KA, Qureshi NR, Rintoul RC, Dizdarevic S et al (2021) Impact of solitary pulmonary nodule size on qualitative and quantitative assessment using 18F-fluorodeoxyglucose PET/CT: the SPUTNIK trial. Eur J Nucl Med Mol Imaging 48(5):1560–1569

Weissinger M, Atmanspacher M, Spengler W, Seith F, Von Beschwitz S, Dittmann H et al (2023) Diagnostic performance of dynamic whole-body Patlak [18F]FDG-PET/CT in patients with indeterminate lung lesions and lymph nodes. J Clin Med 12(12):3942

Wen W, Piao Y, Xu D, Li X (2021) Prognostic value of MTV and TLG of 18F-FDG PET in patients with stage I and II non-small-cell lung cancer: a meta-analysis. Contrast Media Mol Imaging 2021:7528971

Wong TZ, Khandani AH, Sheikh A (2016) Chapter 11: Nuclear medicine. In: Gunderson LL, Tepper JE (eds) Clinical radiation oncology, 4th edn. Elsevier, Philadelphia, pp 206–216 [cited 2023 Nov 12]. https://www.sciencedirect.com/science/article/pii/B9780323240987000113.

Yang K, Yu S-Q, Lu M-J, Zhao S-H (2019) Comparison of diagnostic accuracy of stress myocardial perfusion imaging for detecting hemodynamically significant coronary artery disease between cardiac magnetic resonance and nuclear medical imaging: a meta-analysis. Int J Cardiol 293:278–285

Yoo IR, Chung SK, Park HL, Choi WH, Kim YK, Lee KY et al (2014) Prognostic value of SUVmax and metabolic tumor volume on 18F-FDG PET/CT in early stage non-small cell lung cancer patients without LN metastasis. Biomed Mater Eng 24(6):3091–3103

Yoshinaga K, Klein R, Tamaki N (2010) Generator-produced rubidium-82 positron emission tomography myocardial perfusion imaging-from basic aspects to clinical applications. J Cardiol 55(2):163–173

Yoshinaga K, Manabe O, Tamaki N (2018) Absolute quantification of myocardial blood flow. J Nucl Cardiol 25(2):635–651

Zaidi H, Karakatsanis N (2018) Towards enhanced PET quantification in clinical oncology. Br J Radiol 91(1081):20170508

Part II
Clinical Part - Lung, Mediastinum, Pleura, and Chest Wall

Chest X-Ray

Mathieu Lederlin

Contents

M. Lederlin (✉)
Department of Radiology, University Hospital of Rennes, Rennes, France
e-mail: Mathieu.LEDERLIN@chu-rennes.fr

Abstract

Chest X-ray is still nowadays the most commonly used imaging modality worldwide. Paradoxically, it is less and less taught today. As cross-sectional imaging has become increasingly efficient, rapid, and accessible, education in chest radiography has declined proportionately, both in quantity and quality. Furthermore, in institutions where chest X-ray is still taught, students are hardly trained to make measurements on plain radiographs. The only measure that is still universally performed is the cardiothoracic ratio, though it is often roughly estimated in clinical routine practice. This chapter proposes to revisit a certain number of measurements and indexes of frontal and lateral chest X-rays, some still used, and others somewhat fallen into disuse. It is an opportunity to discuss the diagnostic value of each of these metrics, and tentatively raise renewed interest in some of them.

1 Introduction

Chest X-ray is still nowadays the most commonly used imaging modality worldwide (United Nations Scientific Committee on the Effects of Atomic Radiation 2008). Paradoxically, it is less and less taught today (Fabre et al. 2018). As cross-sectional imaging

Med Radiol Diagn Imaging (2026)

https://doi.org/10.1007/174_2024_513,
Published Online: 01 December 2024

has become increasingly efficient, rapid, and accessible, education in chest radiography has declined proportionately, both in quantity and quality. Furthermore, in institutions where chest X-ray is still taught, students are hardly trained to make measurements on plain radiographs. The only measure that is still universally performed is the cardiothoracic ratio, though it is often roughly estimated in clinical routine practice. In addition, the spread of computed tomography (CT), performed for any equivocal frontal chest X-ray, has somewhat pushed aside the lateral view of chest X-ray. Currently, radiologists who still know how to read lateral chest X-ray are becoming rare (and old!), and even rarer are those who know its measurements.

Reading chest X-ray is one of the most difficult tasks for a radiologist. It may be very tricky, even for experienced readers. Normal aspects may vary greatly between patients depending on gender, age, height, weight, and morphology of individuals. This variability explains, for example, why some mediastinal lines may not be always visible. In addition, there may be within-subject variability depending on technical conditions. For example, there are significant differences between posteroanterior (PA) and anteroposterior (AP) views. In any case, it is essential to ensure that the films comply with strict quality criteria, especially if measurements have to be obtained.

This chapter proposes to revisit a certain number of measurements and indexes of frontal and lateral chest X-rays, some still used, and others somewhat fallen into disuse. It is an opportunity to discuss the diagnostic value of each of these metrics and tentatively raise renewed interest in some of them.

2 Cardiac Measurements

Cardiac measurements on chest X-ray are dominated by the measurement of the cardiothoracic ratio, which is performed universally.

2.1 Cardiac Diameter

The measurement of cardiac diameter is quite simple but is mainly influenced by patient's age, gender, height, and weight (Pfaffenberger et al. 2013; Brakohiapa et al. 2017).

Measurement: It is performed on a frontal PA view by drawing a horizontal line at the level of the maximal transverse diameter of the cardiac silhouette. Alternatively, the two largest right and left heart half-diameters from the midline can be added together (Fig. 1).

Threshold values: The upper limit values, beyond which cardiomegaly is suggested, are **14.5 cm** in adult women and **15.5 cm** in adult men (Morales et al. 2012). These values offer the best compromise between sensitivity and specificity. However, cardiac diameter remains a rather crude marker. Higher thresholds, e.g., 17 cm in women and 19 cm in men, allow specificity >90% but at the cost of decreased sensitivity (Torres et al. 2021). Some authors also have proposed threshold values for anteroposterior (AP) view: 15 cm in women and 16.5 cm in men (Kabala and Wilde 1987).

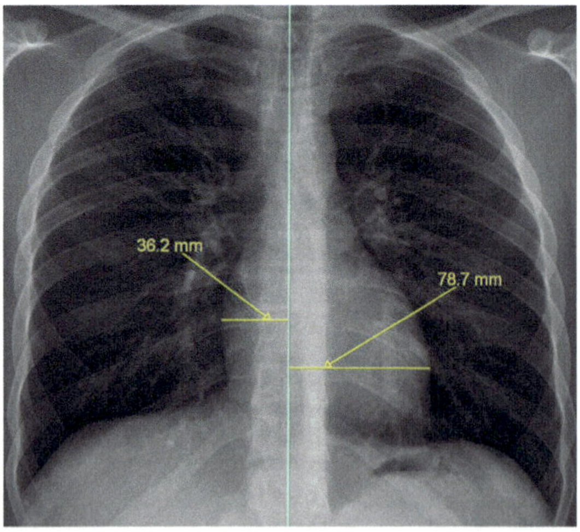

Fig. 1 Normal cardiac diameter. Normal frontal chest X-ray in a 27-year-old man. The cardiac diameter is measured at 11.5 cm

Comments and differential diagnosis: An increase in cardiac diameter is most often related to cardiomegaly, mainly secondary to left ventricle (LV) dilation, but it may also correspond to a pericardial effusion, a prominent epipericardial fat pad, or an anterior mediastinal mass resulting in a silhouette sign with the heart. Note that a chest X-ray obtained in poor inspiration may also result in an increase of the cardiac diameter. As a recall, epipericardial fat presents as a slightly lower opacity than that of the heart. The difference related to acquisitions in diastole or in systole is negligible and in the order of 2% (Yamazaki et al. 2002).

2.2 Cardiothoracic Ratio

First described in 1919 (Danzer 1919), the cardiothoracic ratio is the most widely used metric on chest X-ray. Compared to the absolute value of the cardiac diameter, it is a relative measure and therefore less dependent on the patient's body size and gender, even though the threshold differs for young children.

Measurement: It is calculated on a PA frontal X-ray as the ratio of the cardiac diameter (i.e., the widest heart width as described above) to the largest thoracic diameter, taking the inner margins of the ribs as limits (Fig. 2). The ratio is usually presented with two decimals (so 0.52 is used rather than 0.5).

Threshold values: In upright PA view, the upper limit of the ratio is usually set at **0.50** in female and male adults and children older than 5 years (Kearney et al. 2002). However, as with cardiac diameter, the cardiothoracic ratio is a broad index that shows many limitations (Truszkiewicz et al. 2021). It actually correlates weakly with the true size of cardiac cavities, and some authors have suggested an upper threshold of 0.55 for heart chamber enlargement (Simkus et al. 2021). A small cardiothoracic ratio **<0.40**, also termed microcardia or "small heart syndrome," may be related to pulmonary emphysema (Wigh 1978; Xu et al. 2017) or some rare conditions such as adrenal insufficiency, malnutrition, or chronic fatigue syndrome (Miwa and Fujita 2008).

Supine AP views performed with a smaller focus-film distance result in a cardiothoracic ratio 12.5% larger compared to upright PA view (Milne et al. 1988). Therefore, higher threshold values ranging from 0.55 to 0.58 have been proposed for AP view (Kabala and Wilde 1987).

Finally, in children under 5 years, for whom a supine AP radiograph is usually performed, the upper limit is usually 0.55 and may be as high as 0.60 in newborns (Maresh and Washburn 1938; Edwards et al. 1981).

Comments and differential diagnosis: A high cardiothoracic ratio corresponds to the same conditions as those related to a high cardiac diameter, mainly represented by cardiomegaly with LV dilatation, but also pericardial effusion, cardiac tumor, or anterior mediastinal mass resulting in a silhouette sign with the heart (Fig. 3).

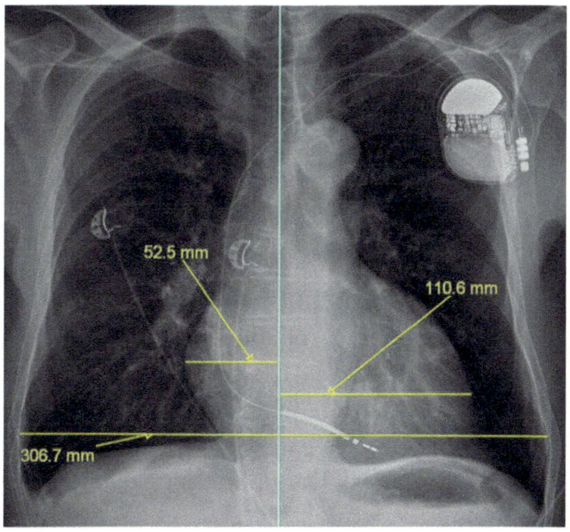

Fig. 2 Increased cardiothoracic ratio. Frontal chest X-ray in a 62-year-old man with left ventricular failure. The cardiothoracic ratio is 0.53. Other measurements in the same patient are shown in Fig. 6

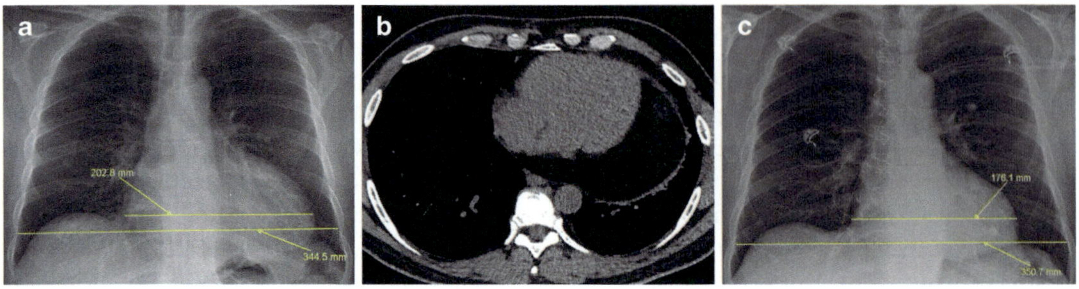

Fig. 3 Increased cardiothoracic ratio. (**a**) Chest X-ray performed for chest pain in a 60-year-old man revealing a cardiac enlargement with a cardiothoracic ratio measured at 0.59. (**b**) Corresponding CT scan showing a pericardial fatty mass. (**c**) After resection of a pericardial lipoma, the postoperative radiograph shows a cardiothoracic ratio measured at 0.50

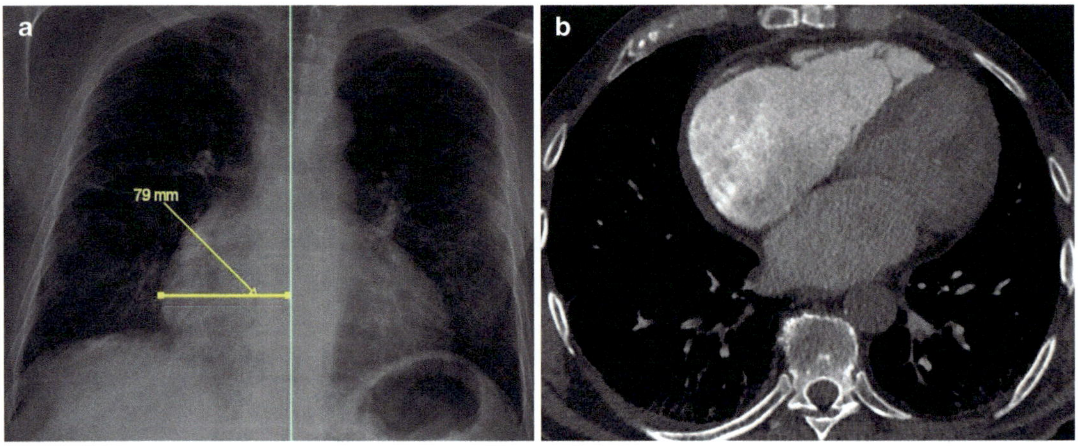

Fig. 4 Right atrial enlargement. (**a, b**) Dilation of right atrium in a 63-year-old man with a history of tricuspid regurgitation

2.3 Right Atrial Enlargement

Dilation of the right atrium is often visually recognized as a more prominent and convex right lower heart border.

Measurement: It is obtained on a frontal PA view by drawing a horizontal line from the midline to the right lateral edge of the cardiac silhouette (Fig. 4).

Threshold values: The upper limit of the measure is **5.5 cm**.

Comments and differential diagnosis: Quantitative assessment of this lateral protrusion may not be reliable due to substantial anatomical variability in this area. In addition, other conditions such as prominent epicardial fat pad, right middle lobe disease, or cardiac/paracardiac tumors may result in a bulging right cardiac border.

2.4 Left Atrial Enlargement

Left atrium (LA) enlargement is usually detected visually, as the classic "double-density sign," i.e., the right border of LA bulging and then leading to a double right heart border. From this sign, an oblique diameter of LA can be measured. Furthermore, when LA enlargement is severe, an indirect sign may be a widening of the subcarinal angle.

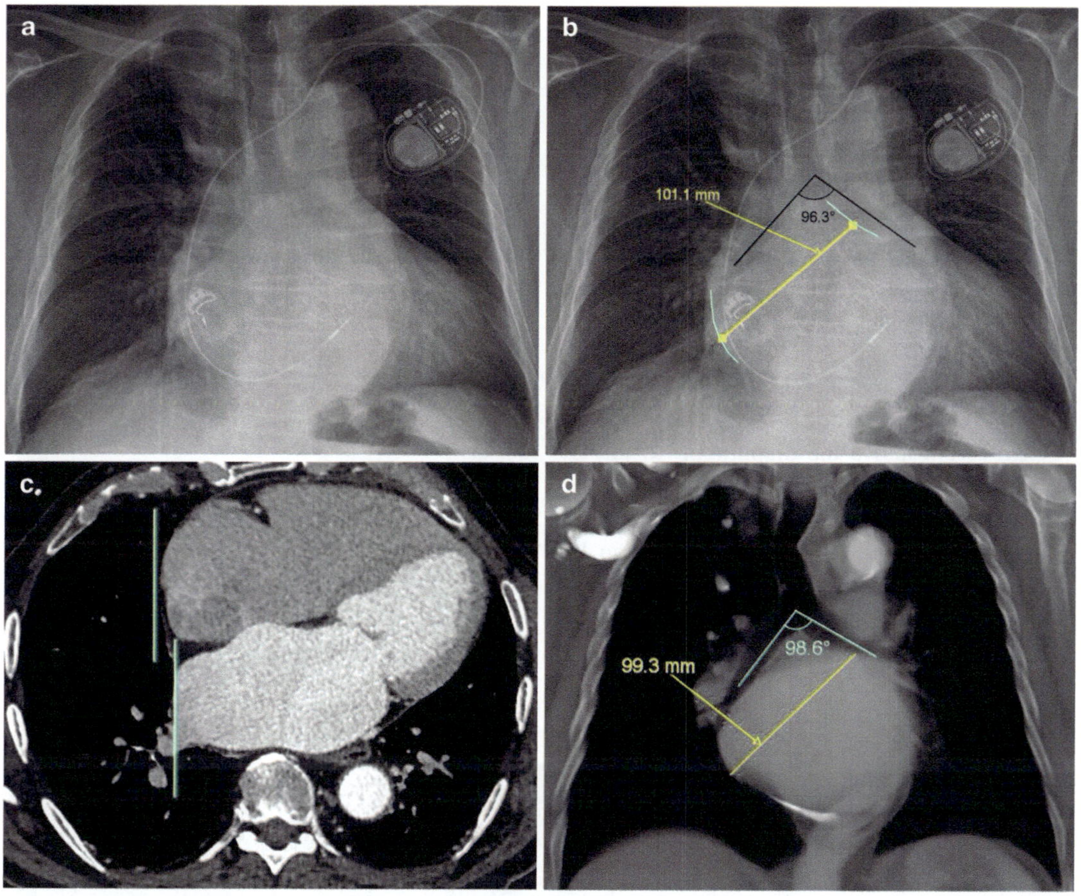

Fig. 5 Left atrial enlargement. (**a**, **b**) Chest X-ray showing direct (yellow line) and indirect (black angle) signs of LA dilation. LA oblique diameter is drawn between the right lateral edge of LA (curved blue line in **b**) and the midpoint of the left main bronchus (straight blue line in **b**). (**c**) Corresponding axial CT slice showing the right borders of the right and left atria, explaining the double-density sign on frontal chest X-ray. (**d**) Coronal CT view (average MPR, 70 mm thick slab) showing LA oblique diameter and increased subcarinal angle

Measurement: It is performed on a frontal view and requires the double-density sign to be first detected. The diameter of LA is measured as an upward and leftward line joining the right lateral edge of LA to the midpoint of the inferior wall of the left main bronchus (Fig. 5). The measurement of the subcarinal angle is detailed below in this chapter.

Threshold values: An oblique measurement greater than **7 cm** indicates LA enlargement (Webb and Higgins 2010; Brant and Helms 2012). A subcarinal angle greater than **80°** may reflect a severe LA dilation.

Causes: A variety of heart diseases can lead to LA enlargement (e.g., mitral stenosis and regurgitation, left ventricular failure, atrial fibrillation).

Comments and differential diagnosis: The LA diameter measurement would be more accurate than the simple double-density sign. Splaying of the carina may indicate severely enlarged LA, but also mediastinal lymph node or other subcarinal masses (see below).

2.5 Left Ventricular Enlargement

Diagnosis of left ventricle (LV) enlargement on chest X-ray is primarily visual, based on the cardiothoracic ratio and possibly on more subtle signs to identify LV or RV dilation. On a frontal chest view, there is no other measurement than the cardiothoracic ratio. On a lateral chest view, the Hoffman-Rigler sign was described in 1965 (Hoffman and Rigler 1965; Freeman et al. 2003).

Measurement: On a lateral view, a line is drawn from the posterior border of the inferior vena cava (2 cm above the diaphragm) to the LV posterior border (Fig. 6).

Threshold values: A distance above **1.8 cm** indicates a posterior shift of the LV, i.e., an LV dilation.

Comments: Although most heart diseases can cause LV enlargement, this measurement is rarely used nowadays.

3 Measurements of the Mediastinum

3.1 Mediastinothoracic Ratio

The mediastinothoracic ratio was used until the 1990s to detect and quantify enlargement of the upper mediastinum, particularly in Hodgkin's lymphoma. With the spread of CT, this index has progressively fallen into disuse. Currently, visual analysis of mediastinal borders as well as mediastinal opacity on chest X-ray remains essential to detect early-stage diseases.

Measurement: It is calculated on a PA frontal view as the ratio of the maximum width of the mediastinum (generally the middle or upper one) divided by the internal thoracic diameter at T5–T6 level, which corresponds roughly to the carina level.

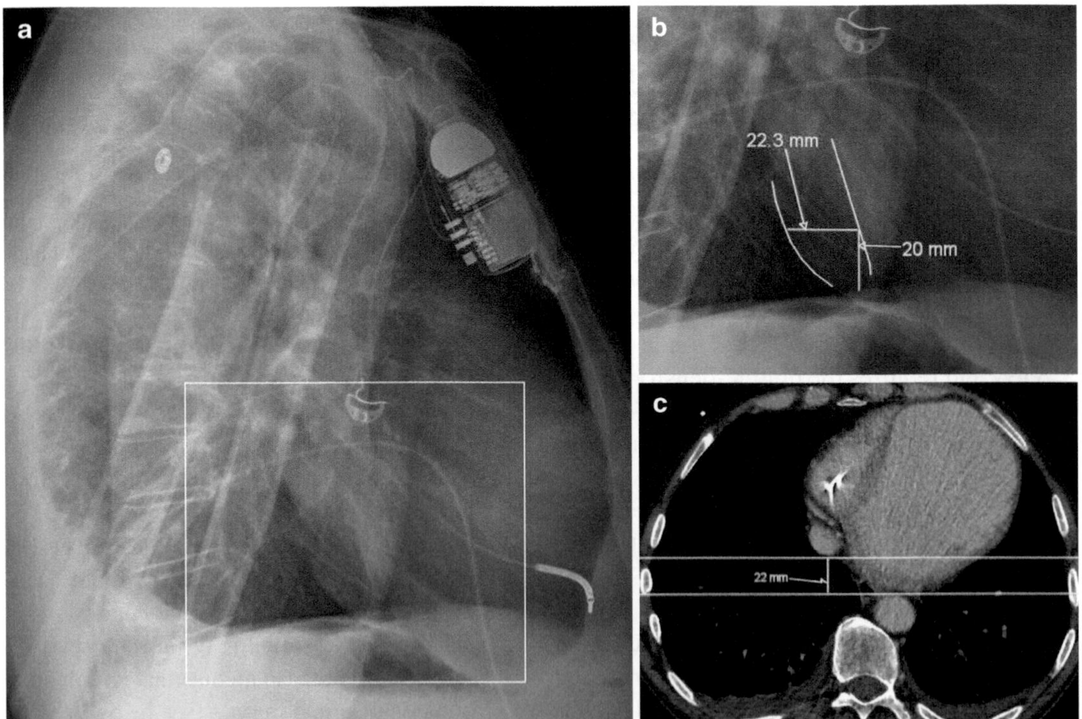

Fig. 6 The Hoffman-Rigler sign (same patient as in Fig. 2). Lateral chest X-ray with arms backward (**a**) showing a posterior pleural effusion that was not visible on the frontal view. Close-up view (**b**) showing a 22 mm distance between the posterior border of the inferior vena cava (straight blue line) and the posterior border of the left ventricle (curved blue line). Corresponding CT scan (**c**) that helps to understand the measurement

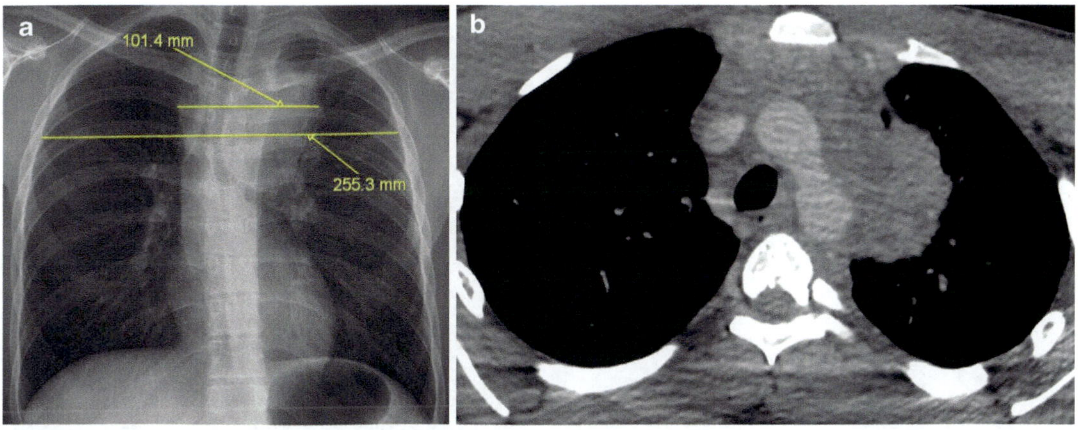

Fig. 7 Increased mediastinothoracic ratio due to Hodgkin's lymphoma. Chest X-ray (**a**) and corresponding CT scan (**b**) in a 22-year-old man showing a tumoral enlargement of the upper mediastinum. The mediastinothoracic ratio is measured at 0.40. Note the abnormal left paravertebral line related to pleural/extrapleural fat involvement in the left paravertebral area

Threshold values: The upper limit value of this ratio is **0.33** (Lister et al. 1989; Bradley et al. 1999). Alternatively, a mediastinal width greater than 10 cm also indicates a bulky mediastinal disease by default.

Comments and differential diagnosis: An increase of the mediastinothoracic ratio usually reflects a large soft tissue mass occupying the middle mediastinum (Fig. 7). Before the era of CT and PET/CT, a ratio >0.33 in Hodgkin's lymphoma defined a mediastinal bulk, which suggested an aggressive disease with a poor prognosis. Less frequently, an increased mediastinothoracic ratio may correspond to an aneurysm of thoracic aorta, but generally, a visual analysis of mediastinal borders and lines makes it possible to establish its vascular origin (Fig. 8). Mediastinal lipomatosis will be suspected when the mediastinal enlargement shows a lower opacity than a hydric one.

3.2 Vascular Pedicle Width

The vascular pedicle corresponds to the leash of large mediastinal vessels extending from the thoracic inlet to the heart. Milne and Pistolesi introduced it in 1970 in order to assess physiologic vascular changes, such as the circulating blood volume (Milne et al. 1984, 1985).

Normal: Acute cardiac failure

Normal or narrowed: Increased capillary permeability

Enlarged: Fluid overload, e.g., renal failure, chronic heart failure

Measurement: On a frontal chest view.

The vascular pedicle width (VPW) is measured by adding the distance from the lateral wall of the right brachiocephalic vein to the midline and the distance from the midline to the origin of the left subclavian artery from the aortic arch.

Threshold values: The normal VPW is 4.8 cm ± 5 mm and correlates with BMI and BSA. However, sequential changes in the same patient are more accurate than comparison between different patients.

It is estimated that a change of 1 cm of the VPW corresponds to change of the systemic blood volume of 2 L.

Comments: Any sequential modification of the VPW should reflect variations in volume or pressure of the systemic venous system (Fig. 9). Widening of the VPW is mainly linked to an increase of the circulating blood volume and less strongly to an increase of the right atrial pressure.

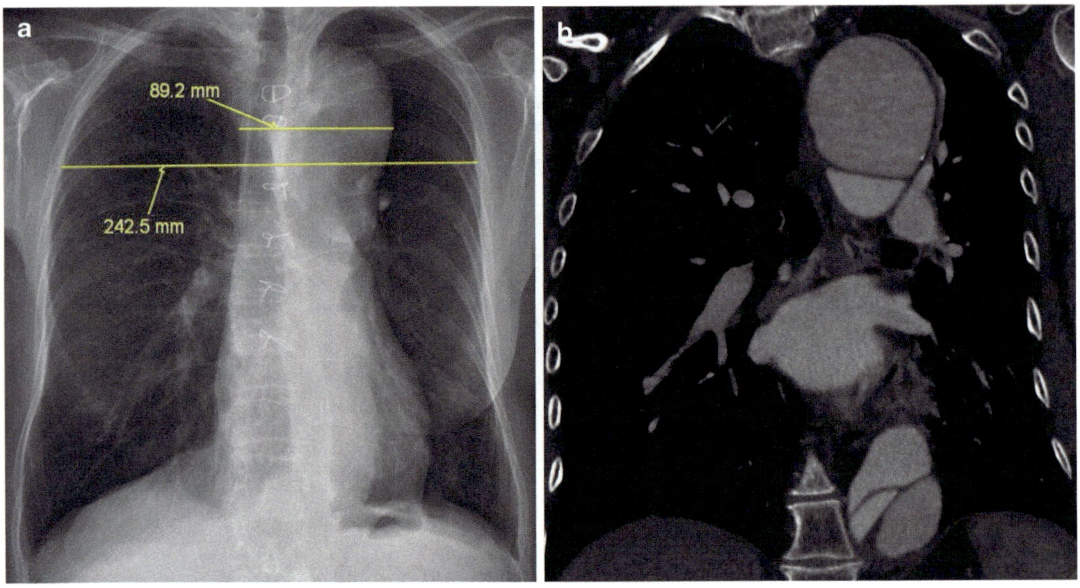

Fig. 8 Increased mediastinothoracic ratio of vascular origin. Chest X-ray (**a**) and coronal CT angiography of aorta (**b**) in a 63-year-old woman with a history of type A aortic dissection previously operated (sternotomy wires). Chest X-ray shows an enlargement of the upper mediastinum (mediastinothoracic ratio measured at 0.37), involving the aortic knob. Postcontrast coronal CT reconstruction confirms the dilatation of the transverse and descending aorta with a persistent patent false lumen

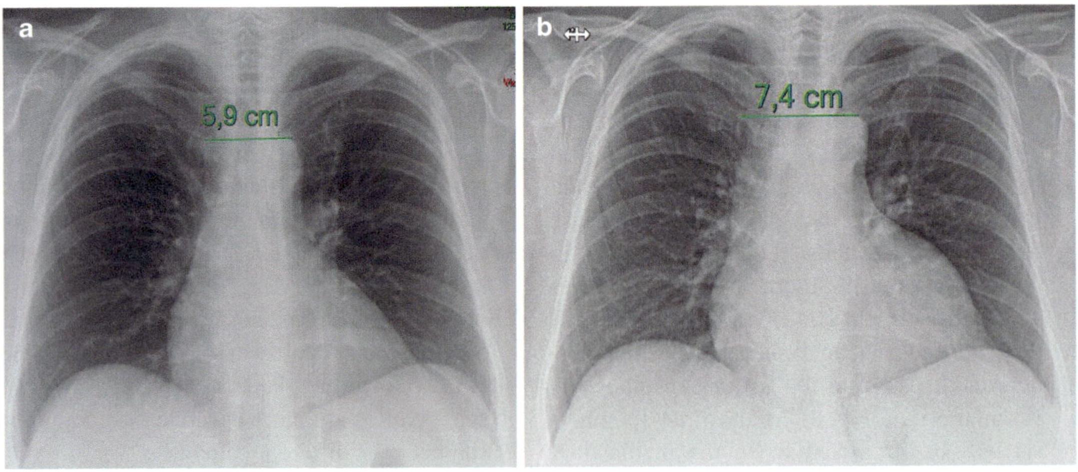

Fig. 9 Increase of vascular pedicle width. Frontal chest X-ray in erect position. Enlargement of the vascular pedicle width from 59 (**a**) to 74 (**b**) mm over a few days. The patient showed a 5 kg over 1 week secondary to acute renal insufficiency responsible for increase of the systemic blood volume

The VPW is minimally affected by inspiration/expiration acquisitions although it may be altered by mechanical ventilation with positive end-expiratory pressure. Also, erect AP or PA acquisition and tube-to-detector distance will minimally affect the VPW. On the other hand, gravity will be a major factor, and therefore, only chest X-rays obtained in erect or in supine position can be compared.

The VPW can also help to differentiate different causes of pulmonary edema:

3.3 Lines and Stripes

Mediastinal lines and stripes are sometimes inconsistent or difficult to recognize, and most do not require measurement: left paraspinal lines, left paratracheal stripe, aortic-pulmonary stripe, aortopulmonary window, and azygo-esophageal recess (Gibbs et al. 2007; Marano et al. 2011). The main point is to be able to detect a change in their appearance. Some of them can however be measured: anterior and posterior junction lines, right paratracheal stripe and posterior tracheal stripe, and right paraspinal line, the latter being better defined than the left one, with a thickness until 5 mm (Marano et al. 2011). Although a *line* corresponds theoretically to a thin double interface <1 mm, while a *stripe* or a *band* is thicker, the classical denomination of the various lines and stripes as presented in literature will be used in the following paragraphs.

3.3.1 Anterior Junction Line

The anterior junction line corresponds to the anterior and superior interface between the right and left lungs. It is visible in approximately 40% of patients and appears as a thin oblique line projecting through the sternum, the spine (T4–T6 level), and the lower part of the trachea (Fig. 10).

Measurement: On a frontal chest view.

Threshold values: The upper limit value is **1 cm** thickness.

Comments: Thickening of the anterior junction line may be caused by the normal thymus in young patients, by anterior mediastinal masses, or by fat (Fig. 11).

3.3.2 Posterior Junction Line

The posterior junction line is located slightly above the previous one, above the clavicle and projecting through the trachea and the spine (T3–T4 level). It is formed by the posterior apposition of the pleural layers of the upper lobes, posterior to the trachea and esophagus. It is visible in approximately 30% of patients.

Measurement: On a frontal chest view.

Threshold values: The upper limit value is 1 cm thickness.

Comments and differential diagnosis: Thickening of the posterior junction line is

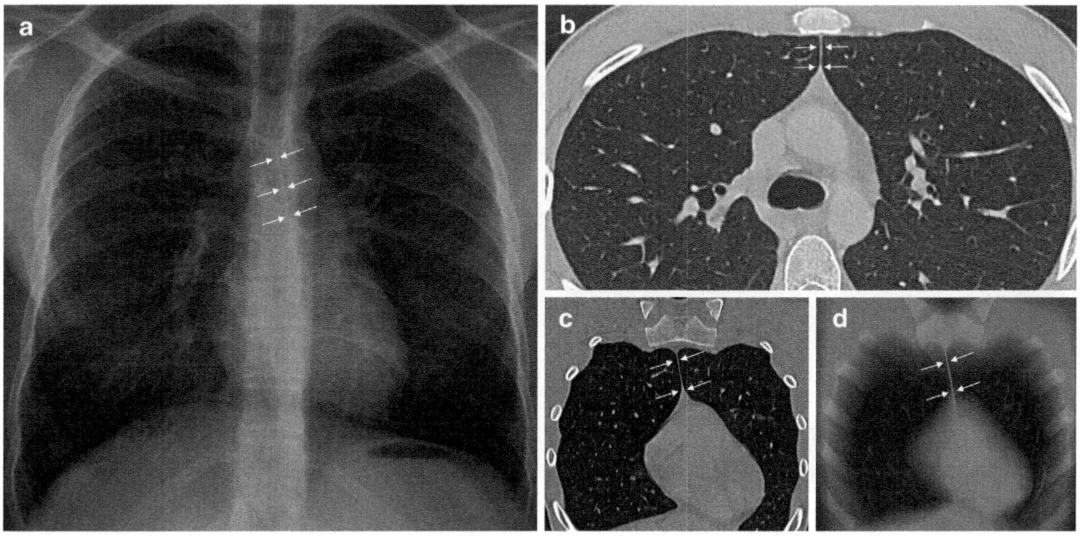

Fig. 10 Anterior junction line. Chest X-ray (**a**) and corresponding CT scan (**b–d**) in an 18-year-old man showing a thin anterior junction line

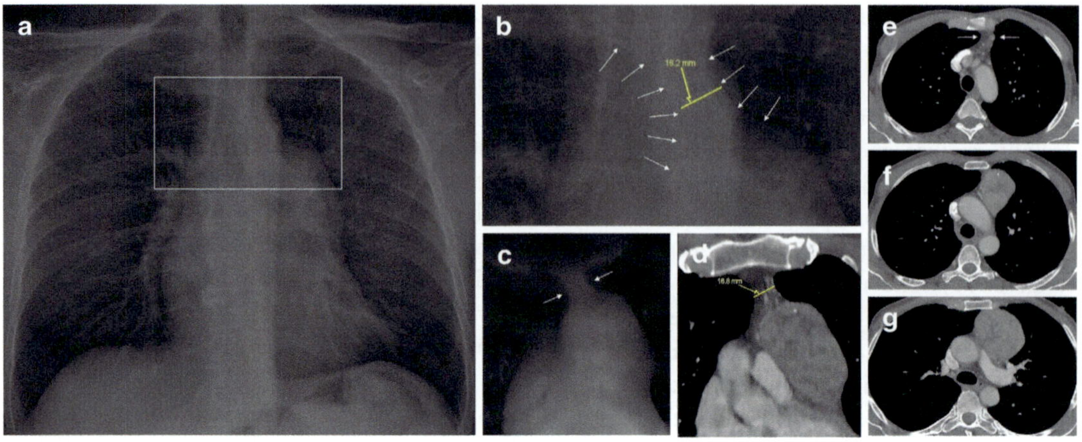

Fig. 11 Thickening of the anterior junction line. (**a**, **b**) Chest X-ray in a 55-year-old man showing deformity and thickening of the anterior junction line, as measured at 16.2 mm. (**c**–**g**) Chest CT scan confirming the thickened anterior junction line extending downwards with a mediastinal mass that turned out to be a type B thymoma

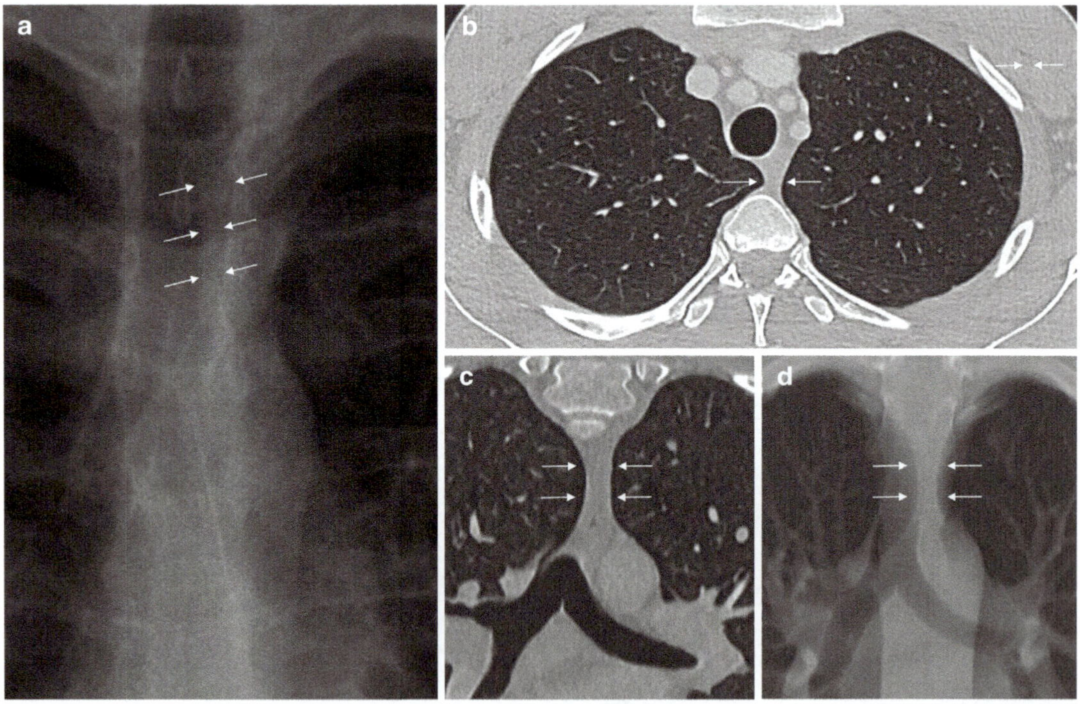

Fig. 12 Posterior junction line. Chest X-ray (**a**) and CT (**b**–**d**) showing a normal posterior junction line in the same patient as in Fig. 10

typically due to posterior mediastinal masses. Nevertheless, varying amount of intervening mediastinal fat may result in a stripe (Fig. 12).

3.3.3 Right Paratracheal Stripe

The right paratracheal stripe is visible in approximately 90% of patients on a frontal chest view and corresponds to the layer between the trachea medially and the right lung laterally. In practice, its lateral border is not always sharply defined because of variable vascular and bone superimpositions.

Measurement: On a frontal chest view.

Threshold values: The upper limit value is **4 mm** thickness.

Comments: Thickening of the right paratracheal stripe may be due to a variety of diseases such as tracheal tumors, thyroid tumors, paratracheal lymphadenopathy, paramediastinal pleural effusion, right upper lobe atelectasis, etc. (Figs. 13 and 14).

3.3.4 Para-Azygo-Esophageal Line

In a prevertebral location, this line presents with an upper third straight or concave relative to the right lung, a variable middle third straight or convex toward the right, and a straight lower third (Whitten et al. 2007).

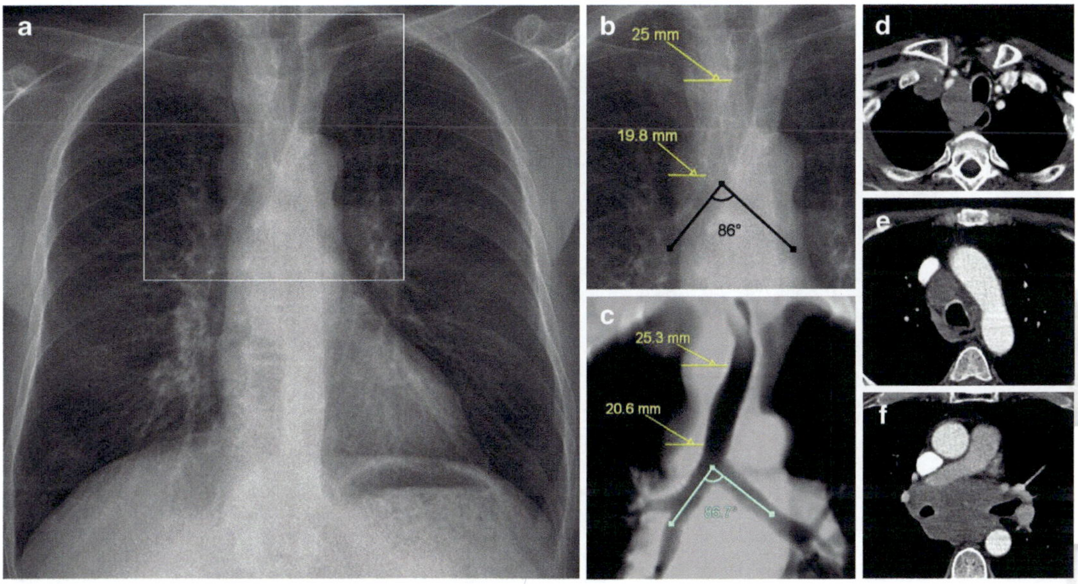

Fig. 13 Thickening of the right paratracheal stripe. Frontal chest X-ray (**a**, **b**) and corresponding CT scan (**c**–**f**) in a 58-year-old man with small cell lung cancer. Lymph node involvement of the stations 2R and 4R is responsible for the lobulated thickening of the right paratracheal stripe with leftward displacement of the trachea. Note also the large tissue mass within the lymph node station 7 (**f**), which accounts for the widening of the subcarinal angle (see also Fig. 20)

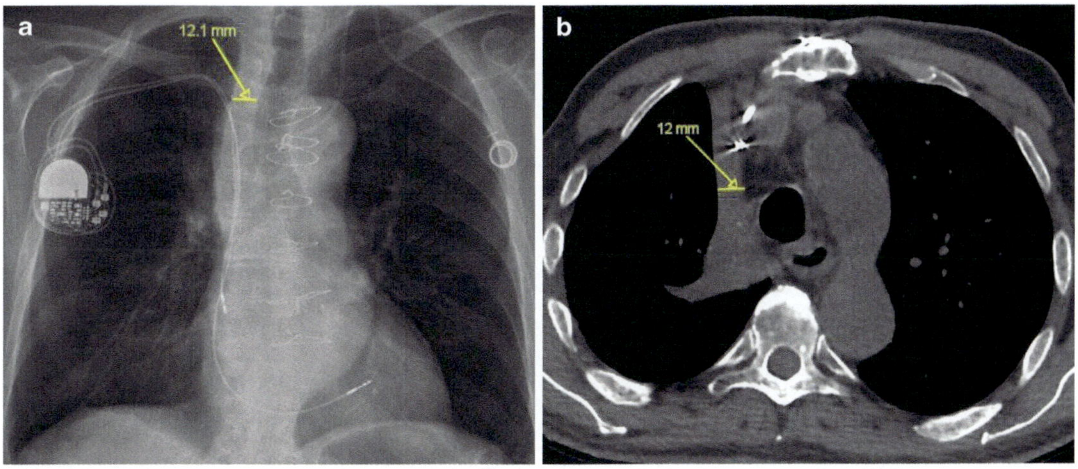

Fig. 14 Thickening of the right paratracheal stripe. Frontal chest X-ray (**a**) and CT scan (**b**) showing a regularly thickened right paratracheal stripe related to a right upper lobe atelectasis

Comments: Displacement of this line may be related to left atrial enlargement, lymph node enlargement, hiatal hernias, esophageal disorders, gastroesophageal varices, bronchopulmonary foregut malformations, or pleural disease (Gibbs et al. 2007; Marano et al. 2011).

3.3.5 Posterior Tracheal Stripe

The posterior tracheal stripe (or tracheoesophageal stripe) is always visible on a lateral view. It is formed by air in the trachea and air in the right lung outlining the posterior wall of the trachea.

Measurement: On a lateral chest view (Fig. 15).

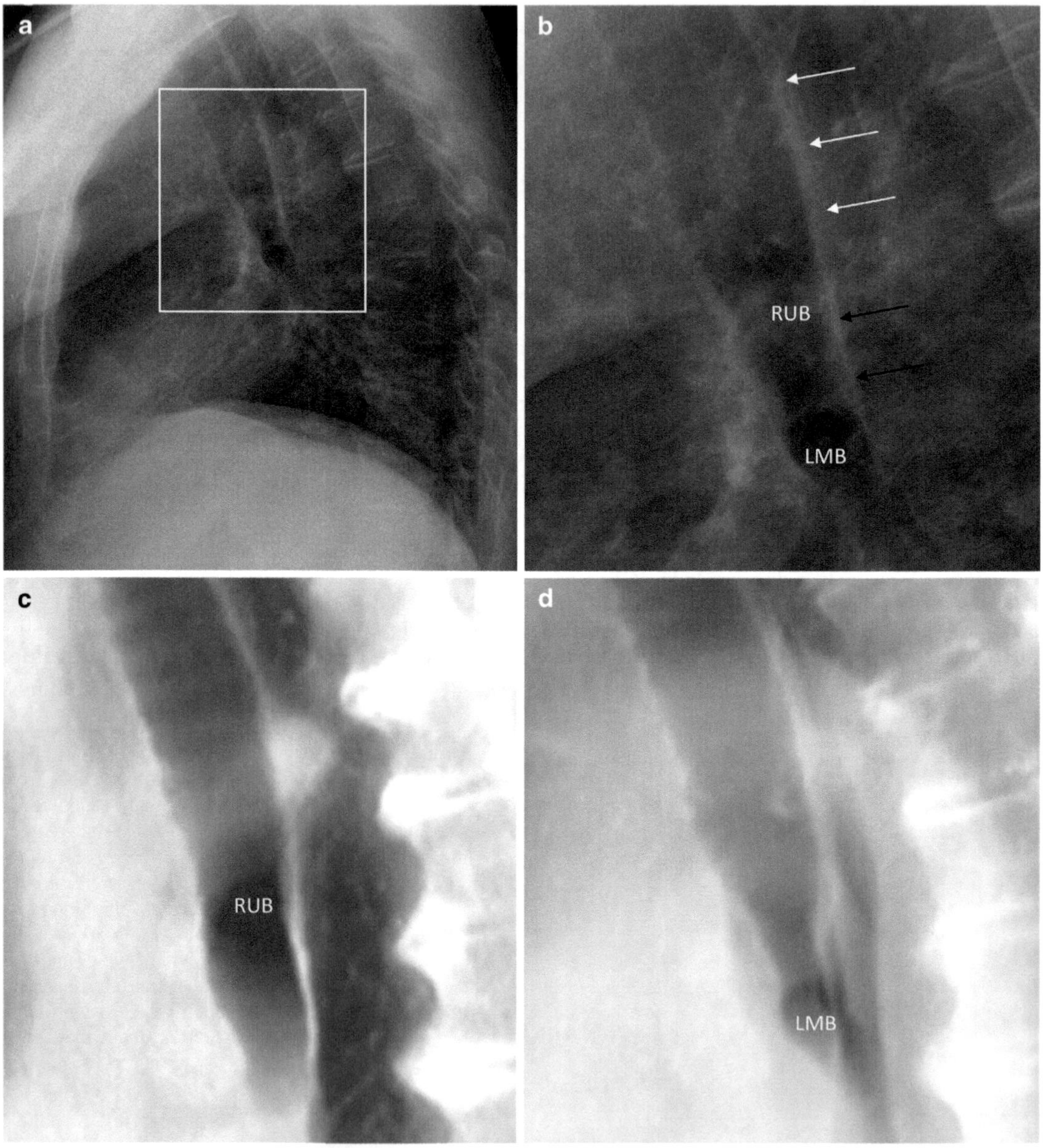

Fig. 15 Normal posterior tracheal stripe and intermediate stem line. (**a**) Lateral chest X-ray in a healthy 62-year-old man. (**b**) Close-up view showing the posterior tracheal stripe (white arrows) appearing as a vertical band posterior to the trachea, in continuity with the intermediate stem line (black arrows) below the level of the right upper lobe bronchus (RUB). (**c**, **d**) Average density MPR 30 mm (**c**) and 70 mm thick slab (**d**) sagittal CT views in the same patient. *LMB* left main bronchus

Threshold values: The posterior tracheal stripe is normally less than 2.5 mm thick (Franquet et al. 2002). It should not be confused with the tracheoesophageal stripe that may be formed when the esophagus is filled by air, with the interface lying between the trachea and the anterior wall of the esophagus instead of the right lung. The tracheoesophageal stripe is superior to **5.5 mm** in thickness.

Comments: Thickening of the posterior tracheal stripe may be caused by numerous diseases including aortic arch abnormalities, esophageal tumors or other causes of thickening, mediastinal abscess, or hematoma.

4 Measurements of Proximal Airways

The examination of the proximal airways should not be omitted on chest X-ray. Admittedly, this analysis can be tricky and has largely been supplanted by CT. However, an optimal reading of chest X-ray requires systematic analysis of trachea, proximal bronchi, and sometimes obtaining some measurements (Collins and Stern 2008).

4.1 Trachea

Measurement: On frontal (2 cm above the aortic arch) and lateral views (Fig. 16).

Threshold values: In men, the lower and upper limits of normal diameter are **13–25 mm** on frontal and **13–27** mm on lateral views, respectively. In women, these values are **10–21 mm** on frontal and **10–23 mm** on lateral views, respectively (Webb and Higgins 2010; Breatnach et al. 1984).

Comments:

- A diameter larger than **3 cm** generally corresponds to a tracheobronchomegaly or Mounier-Kuhn disease (Fig. 17) and should be completed by the measurement of proximal bronchi to confirm the diagnosis.
- A reduction in tracheal diameter may be related to various neoplastic (Fig. 18)

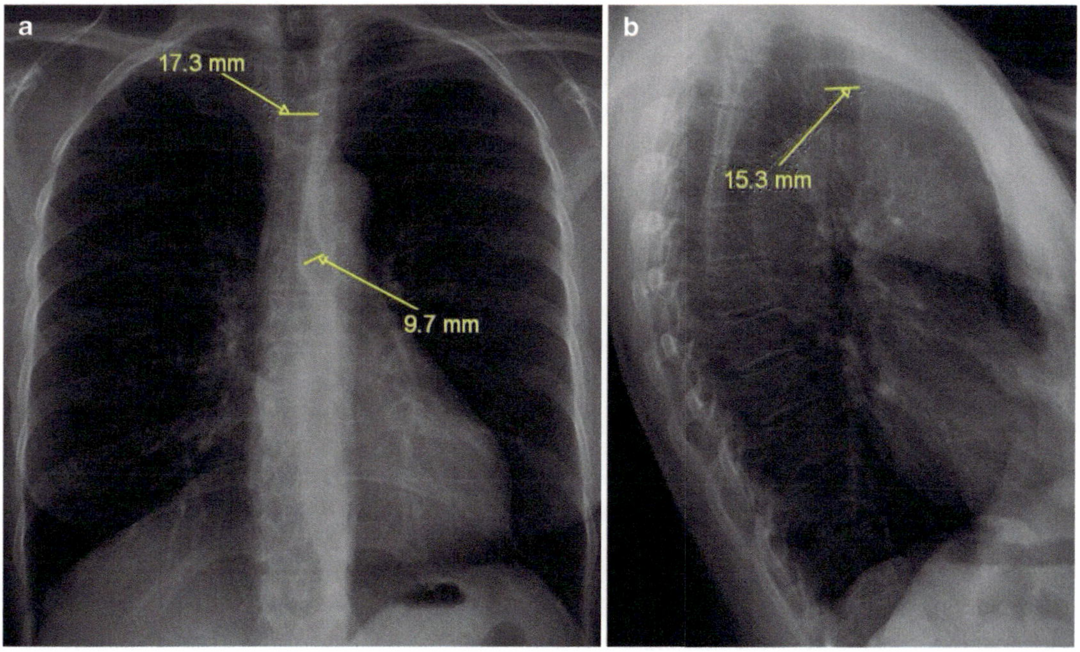

Fig. 16 Normal diameters of the trachea. Frontal and lateral chest X-rays in a healthy 60-year-old woman. Note that the borders of the left main bronchus are visible allowing its measurement, whereas the right main bronchus is not well identified and cannot be measured accurately

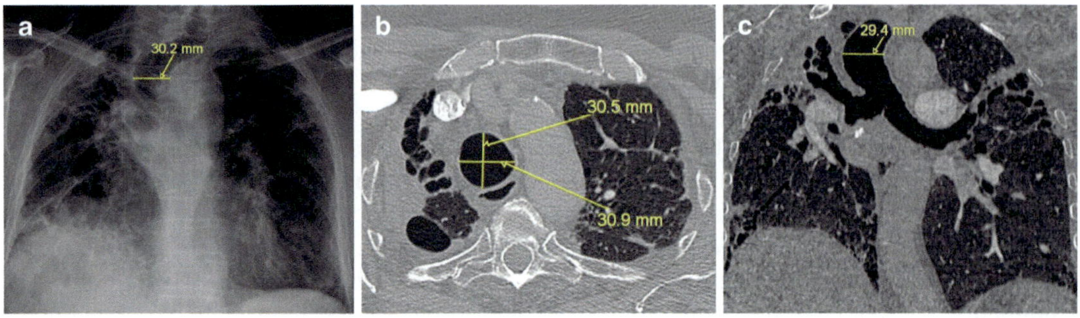

Fig. 17 Tracheal dilation. Chest X-ray (**a**) and corresponding CT scan (**b**, **c**) in a 76-year-old man with a history of idiopathic bronchiectasis and pulmonary fibrosis. The coronal and sagittal diameters of the trachea exceed the 30 mm threshold, suggesting tracheobronchomegaly. However, the normal diameters of the right and left stem bronchi (measuring 19 mm and 16 mm, respectively) do not support this diagnosis

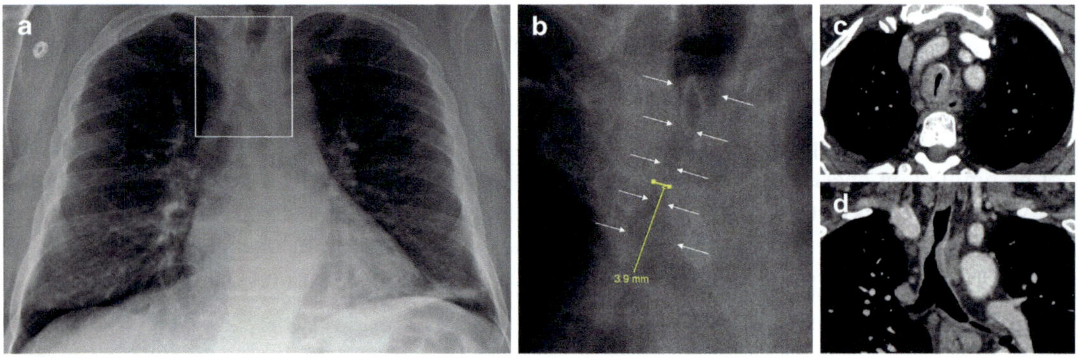

Fig. 18 Tracheal stenosis. Chest X-ray (**a**, **b**) in a 57-year-old man with a history of COPD and dyspnea, revealing a reduction in the coronal diameter of the trachea (arrows). Corresponding CT scan showing irregular and circumferential thickening of tracheal wall related to squamous cell carcinoma

and nonneoplastic conditions (e.g., granulomatosis with polyangiitis, amyloidosis, relapsing polychondritis, tuberculosis).

– A reduction in coronal diameter combined with an increase in sagittal diameter defines the so-called saber-sheath trachea, which strongly suggests a chronic obstructive pulmonary disease (see below).

4.2 Right and Left Main Bronchi

The main bronchi may not be easily visible as they are often obscured by vascular and skeletal superimpositions (Fig. 16).

Measurement: On a frontal chest view.

Threshold values: The upper limits of normal for right and left main bronchi are **24 mm** and **23 mm**, respectively (Webb and Higgins 2010).

Comments: An increase in main bronchi diameters, together with trachea enlargement, is suggestive of tracheobronchomegaly.

4.3 Intermediate Stem Line

Also called *intermediate stripe*, the intermediate stem line corresponds to the posterior wall of the bronchus intermedius, which is outlined posteriorly by the azygo-esophageal recess. It is visible in approximately 60% of patients.

Measurement: On lateral chest view, the intermediate stem line is continuous with the posterior wall of the trachea and appears as a vertical or oblique stripe bounded posteriorly by the azygo-esophageal recess (Fig. 15).

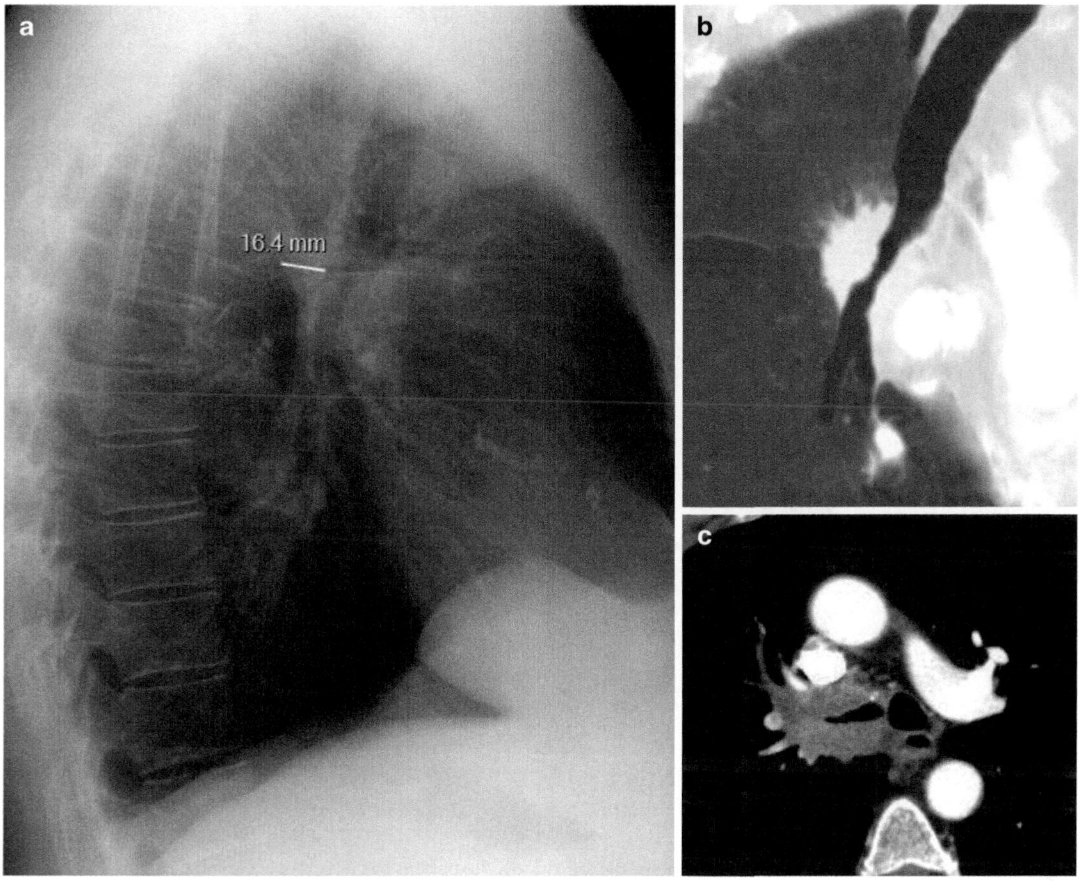

Fig. 19 Thickening of intermediate stem line. Lateral chest X-ray (**a**) in a 62-year-old man showing a thickened intermediate stem line. The corresponding CT views (**b**, **c**) reveal a bronchial wall thickening and stenosis of the right main bronchus extending to the bronchus intermedius secondary to a squamous cell carcinoma and responsible for the thickened intermediate stem line. (*Courtesy Catherine Beigelman*)

Threshold values: The upper limit value is **3 mm** thickness. Thickening may be tricky to detect.

Causes: A thickened intermediate stem line may be caused by primary lung malignancy, lymphadenopathy, or pulmonary edema (Fig. 19).

4.4 Subcarinal Angle

The subcarinal angle corresponds to the angle of the tracheal bifurcation. Normal values may vary substantially between individuals.

Measurement: On a frontal chest view.

Threshold values: The normal value is between **40° and 80°** (Haskin and Goodman 1982; Chen et al. 1982; Alavi et al. 1970; Taskin et al. 1991; Murray et al. 1995).

Comments: In addition to left atrial enlargement (Fig. 5), the subcarinal angle may be mechanically widened when there is a large pathological process within the subcarinal space including, among others, lymphoma, lung cancer (Fig. 20), bronchogenic cyst, pericardial effusion, etc.

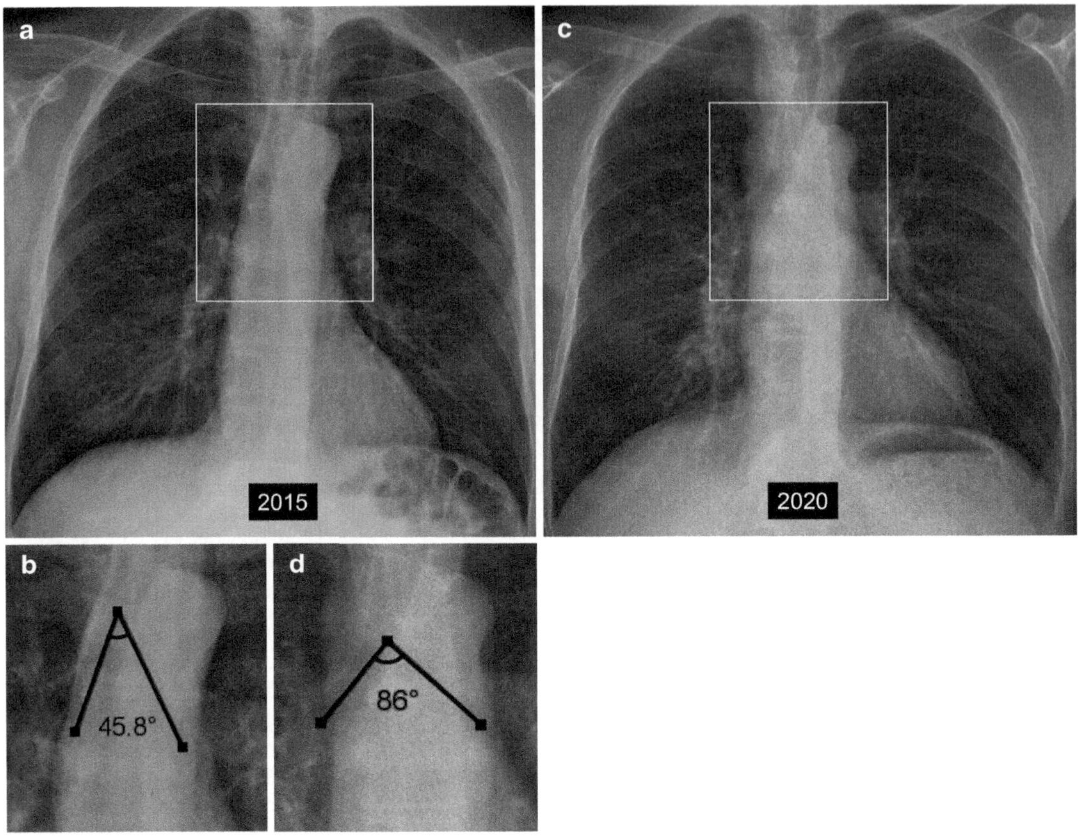

Fig. 20 Subcarinal angle. Evolution over time of the subcarinal angle (same patient as in Fig. 13). In 2015 (**a**, **b**), the patient is healthy with a normal radiograph and a subcarinal angle within the normal range. Five years later (**c**, **d**), the patient has developed a small cell lung cancer with a large subcarinal opacity, which widens the subcarinal angle

5 Measurements of the Diaphragm

Normal difference of highness between both hemidiaphragms should be around 2 cm, higher on the right side (Simon 1971; Simon et al. 1973). If the right hemidiaphragm is more than 3 cm higher than the left, or if the left hemidiaphragm is higher than the right, a specific cause must be sought (e.g., phrenic nerve palsy, diaphragmatic eventration, diaphragmatic rupture, cervical myelopathy).

The top of the normal diaphragm should be located at the junction between its medial third and middle third. Any lateral displacement of this point should suggest a subpulmonic pleural effusion, usually associated with an increased opacity at the level of the diaphragmatic dome (Petersen 1960) (Fig. 21). An abdominal disorder such as subphrenic abscess or a hepatic disease should also be looked for, the latter on the right side, when in the appropriate clinical setting.

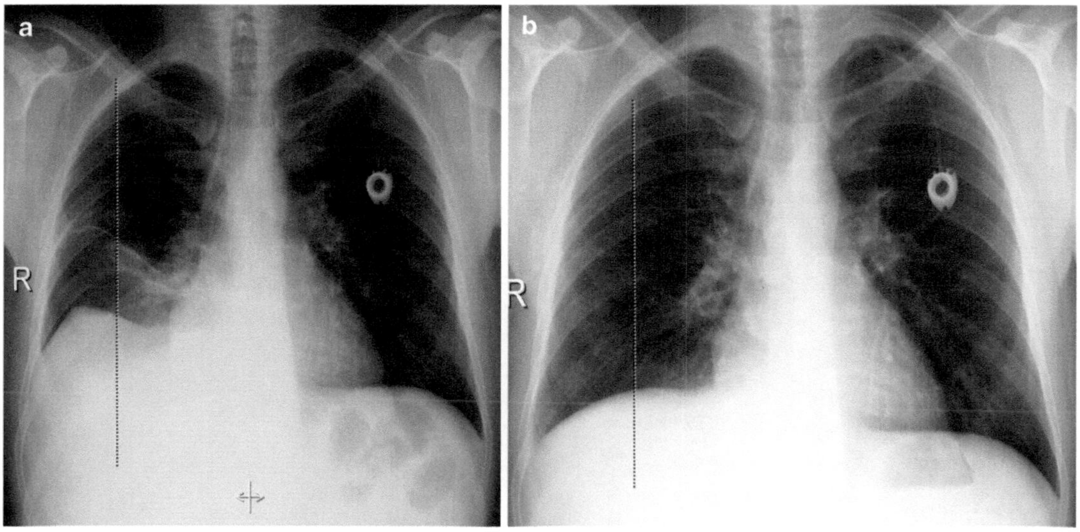

Fig. 21 Subpulmonic pleural effusion. (**a**) Frontal chest X-ray showing that the top of the « opacity of the diaphragm » is located in its lateral half, in other words, external to the vertical red line separating the diaphragmatic opacity into two equal parts. This finding is consistent with the diagnosis of a subpulmonic pleural effusion. (**b**) Chest X-ray obtained after thoracocentesis of 350 ml of pleural fluid shows that the appearance of the diaphragmatic opacity returned to normal with its top located in the internal half of the diaphragmatic opacity

6 Measurements Related to Lung Hyperinflation

Hyperinflation is a detrimental consequence of emphysema and COPD. Although CT is much more sensitive for identifying emphysema, chest X-ray can be valuable to detect signs of hyperinflation on plain radiographs (Thurlbeck and Simon 1978).

6.1 Flattening of the Diaphragm

Flattening of the diaphragm is the most sensitive sign on chest X-ray to detect lung hyperinflation.

Measurement: The best incidence for measuring diaphragmatic flattening is the lateral view. A straight line must be drawn from the sternophrenic angle anteriorly to the costophrenic angle posteriorly, allowing the height of hemidiaphragm convexity to be measured. Flattening of the right hemidiaphragm may also be measured on a PA view by taking as reference a straight line joining the costophrenic angle laterally and the cardiophrenic angle medially (Fig. 22).

Threshold values: On a lateral view, the diaphragm is considered flat if the maximum curvature of the dome is less than **2.7 cm** (Webb and Higgins 2010). On a frontal view, this value is **1.5 cm**.

Comments and differential diagnosis: The loss of height of the convexity of the hemidiaphragm is a sensitive indicator of lung hyperinflation and correlates well with airflow obstruction in COPD (Fig. 23). It is commonly associated with a scalloped aspect. Caution should be taken as pleural effusion in the posterior costophrenic recess may hamper the measurement and create a false impression of diaphragmatic flattening.

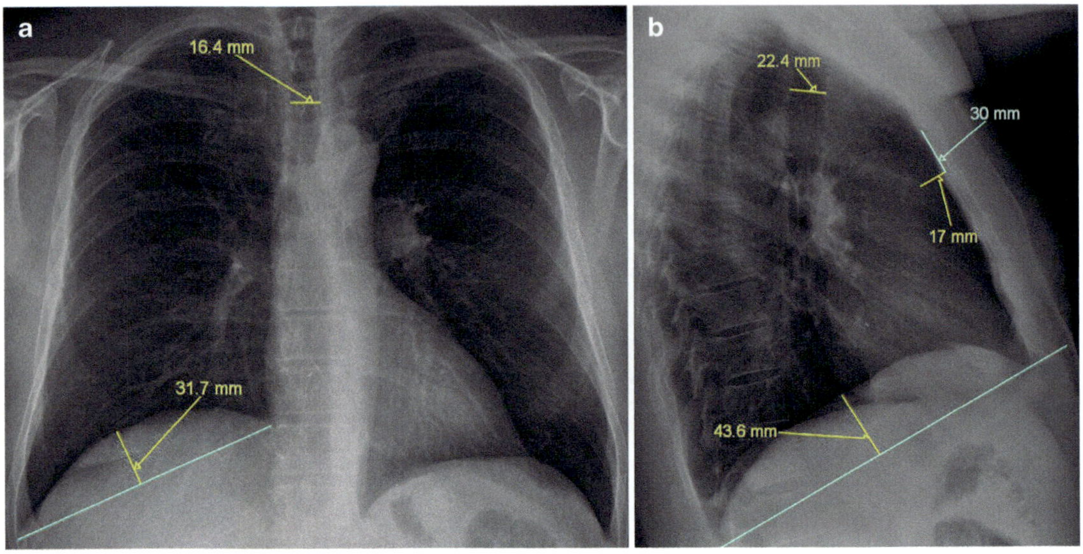

Fig. 22 Normal diaphragmatic dome. Frontal and lateral chest X-rays in a 58-year-old man with no history of COPD. On the frontal view, the dome of the right hemidiaphragm rises to more than 1.5 cm. On the lateral view, both hemidiaphragms rise to more than 2.7 cm, and the retrosternal space is less than 4.4 cm. There is no saber-sheath trachea as the coronal/sagittal diameter ratio is 0.73, which is greater than 0.66

6.2 Retrosternal Clear Space

The retrosternal clear space is a physiologic lucency located behind the sternum on a lateral chest view.

Measurement: On lateral view, a horizontal line must be drawn 3 cm below the manubriosternal angle of Louis, from the posterior cortex of the sternum to the anterior border of the ascending aorta (Fig. 22).

Threshold values: The retrosternal space normally measures less than **4.4 cm** in width (Webb and Higgins 2010).

Differential diagnosis: Increased retrosternal airspace is a sign of hyperinflation and pulmonary emphysema (Fig. 23). Conversely, obliteration of the retrosternal space indicates an anterior mediastinal mass, e.g., thymoma or lymphoma.

6.3 Saber-Sheath Trachea

Saber-sheath trachea refers to a decrease in the coronal diameter of the trachea associated with an increase in its sagittal diameter. This measurement is usually done on CT but was originally described in chest X-ray (Greene and Lechner 1975).

Measurement: It requires both frontal and lateral views (Fig. 22). The measurements should normally be made 1 cm above the aortic arch (Ciccarese et al. 2014).

Threshold values: The saber-sheath trachea is defined by a coronal/sagittal diameter ratio **<2:3**.

Comments: This sign is quite common and almost pathognomonic for COPD (Fig. 23), provided that the extrathoracic part of the trachea is not narrowed.

6.4 Other Signs of Hyperinflation

Other features of lung hyperinflation include:

- Increase of the anteroposterior diameter of the chest ("barrel chest")
- More than six anterior or ten posterior ribs visible above the diaphragm on frontal view
- Horizontalization of the ribs
- Increased retrocardiac lucency

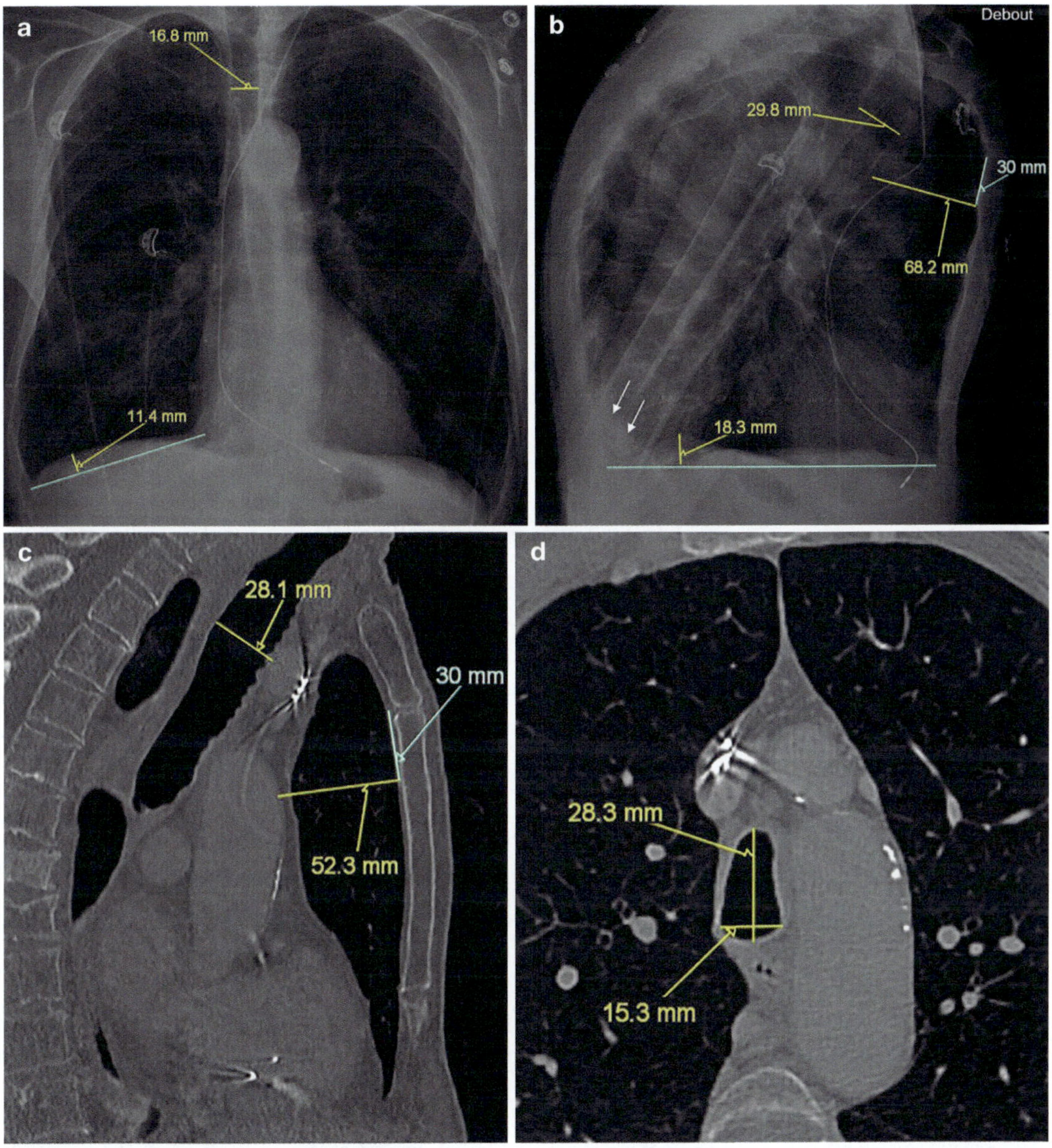

Fig. 23 Signs of pulmonary hyperinflation. In this 65-year-old patient with a history of COPD, frontal and lateral plain films (**a**, **b**) show a "barrel chest," flattening of the diaphragm, widening of the retrosternal space, and a "saber-sheath trachea" (coronal/sagittal diameter ratio = 0.56). Note that the arms backward (**b**) make it difficult to measure the trachea as the cortices of the humerus are parallel to the tracheal borders. Corresponding CT slices (**c**, **d**) confirm the signs of hyperinflation. The difference in size of the retrosternal space between X-ray and CT may be due to a different level of inspiration and positioning

- Presence of air under the heart
- Loss of vascular density within lungs (i.e., lung hyperlucency)
- Air trapping: diaphragmatic course less than 3 cm when comparing radiographs taken in maximal inspiration and expiration
- Comments:
  - Expiration X-ray cannot be however recommended for this research.
  - Physiological evaluation of diaphragm function currently relies on US or MRI.

7 Thoracic Vessels

The analysis of intrathoracic vessels is nowadays essentially visual, with the measurements being carried out on CT or MRI.

7.1 Arch of the Azygos Vein

The arch of the azygos vein can be seen on most plain PA views.

Measurement: On an upright frontal view, it appears as an oval opacity along the right side of the mediastinum, lateral to the angle between the trachea and the right main bronchus. In the common variant azygos lobe, the azygos vein is located in the azygos fissure, above its usual paratracheal course (Fig. 24).

Threshold values: The upper limit value is **7 mm** according to some authors (Heitzman 1973) but could be as high as **10 mm** according to some others (Felson 1973).

Comments: Enlargement of the azygos vein may be related to azygos continuation of the inferior vena cava, superior or inferior vena cava obstruction, congestive heart failure, portal hypertension, pregnancy, etc.

7.2 Aortic Nipple

An aortic nipple could be seen in up to 10% of frontal chest view. It corresponds to the arch of the left superior intercostal vein when lying along the aortic knob, slightly lower than its normal location.

Measurement: On a frontal PA view, it appears as small nodule or « nipple », adjacent to the superior or lateral margin of the aortic knob (Fig. 25).

Threshold values: The upper limit value is **4.5 mm** (McDonald et al. 1970).

Comments: Beyond this threshold, obstruction of the superior vena cava should be suspected,

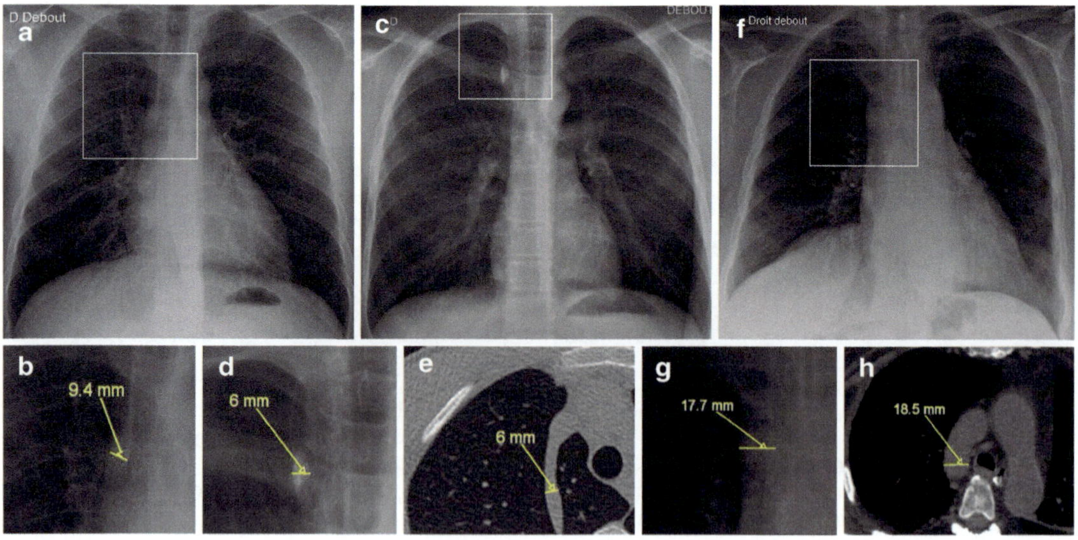

Fig. 24 Arch of the azygos vein. (**a**, **b**) Normal arch of azygos vein in a healthy 26-year-old man. (**c**–**e**) Normal diameter of azygos vein within an azygos fissure delimitating an azygos lobe in a healthy 23-year-old man. (**f**–**h**) Enlargement of the arch of the azygos vein in a 78-year-old woman with an azygos continuation of the inferior vena cava

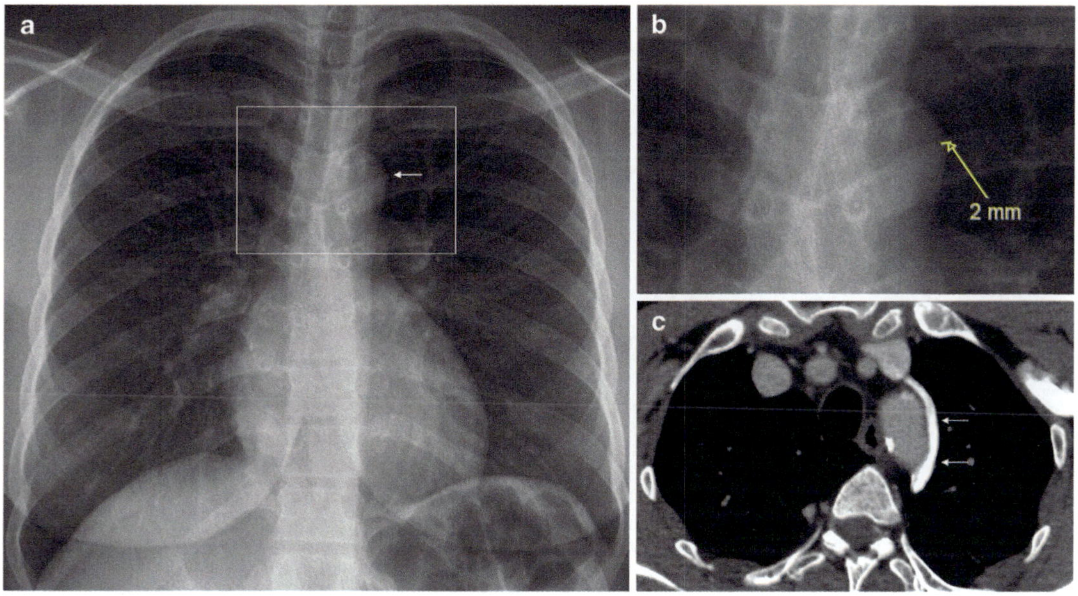

Fig. 25 Aortic nipple. (**a**, **b**) Chest radiograph in a 28-year-old healthy woman showing a small nodular opacity adjacent to the lateral border of the aortic knob (arrow). (**c**) Chest CT scan with IV contrast showing a non-dilated left arch of the superior intercostal vein (arrows)

with the dilated left superior intercostal vein serving as a collateral pathway.

7.3 Right Interlobar Pulmonary Artery

Measurements of pulmonary artery diameters on plain radiographs have become rarely performed, but it is still important to recognize a hilar enlargement and to try to distinguish between vascular and nodal origin. The right interlobar pulmonary artery is the most easily recognized.

Measurement: On frontal view, the interlobar pulmonary artery runs downwards, parallel and lateral to the lucency of the bronchus intermedius (Fig. 26).

Threshold values: The upper limit value is **17 mm** in men and **15 mm** in women (Webb and Higgins 2010; Chang 1962).

Comments: Enlargement may be related to pulmonary hypertension (Fig. 27), acute massive pulmonary embolism, and congenital heart disease.

7.4 Left Pulmonary Artery

The left pulmonary artery may occasionally be visible on a frontal view (Fig. 26) but would be easier to measure on a lateral view.

Measurement: On a lateral view, the left pulmonary artery appears as a curved opacity above the left main bronchus before continuing downward as the left interlobar artery (Fig. 28). However, it may be difficult to identify.

Threshold values: The upper limit value is **18 mm** (Reed 2010).

Comments: Causes of enlargement are the same as those mentioned above.

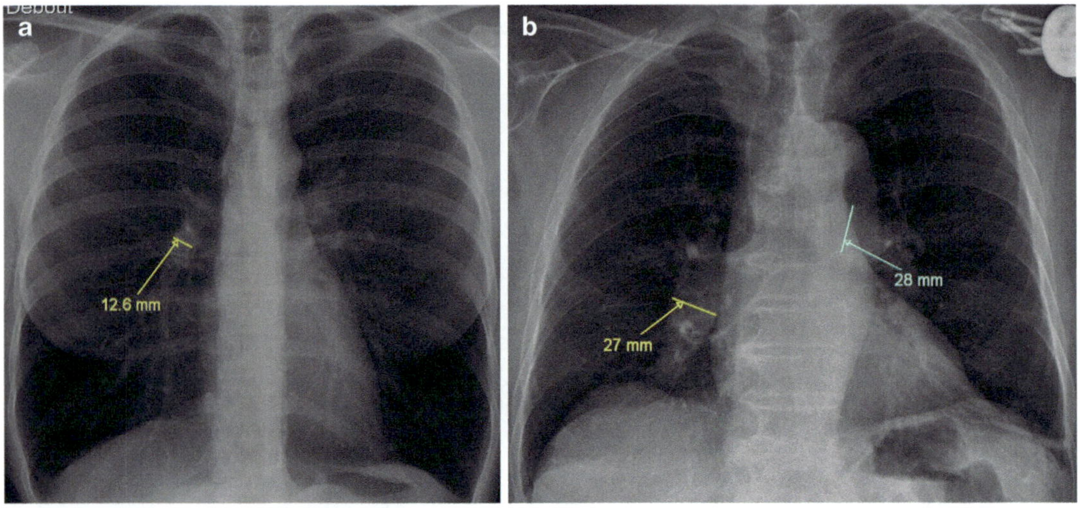

Fig. 26 Normal and enlarged right interlobar pulmonary artery. (**a**) Normal diameter of the right interlobar artery in a 36-year-old woman with no history of cardiopulmonary disease. (**b**) Enlargement of the right interlobar pulmonary artery in an 82-year-old man with chronic thromboembolic pulmonary hypertension. The left pulmonary artery is also measurable on this frontal view

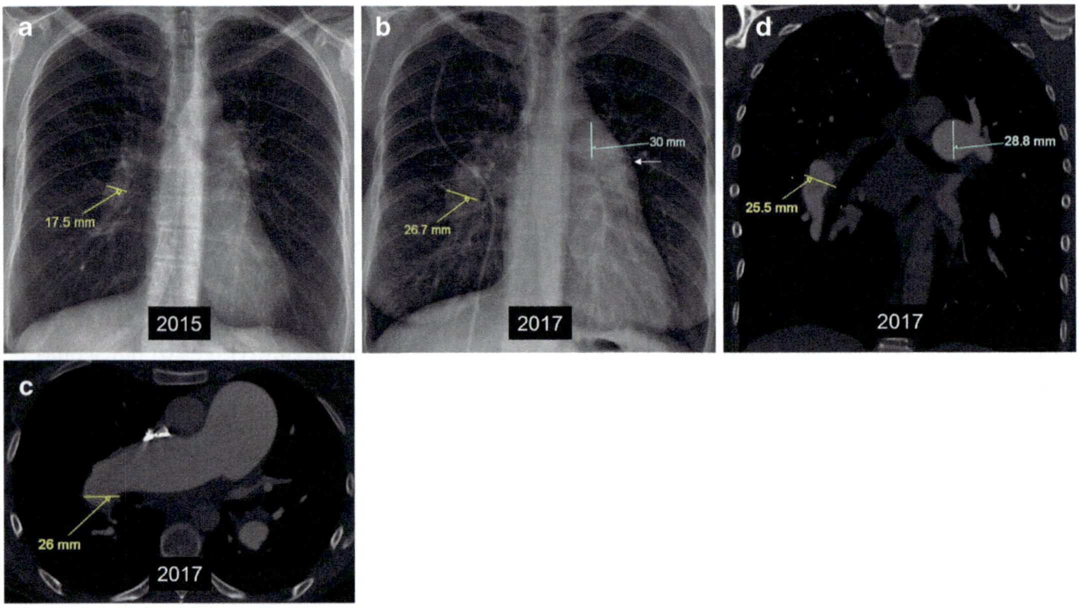

Fig. 27 Pulmonary hypertension. Evolution of the diameter of the right interlobar pulmonary artery in a 46-year-old woman diagnosed with pulmonary hypertension secondary to capillary hemangiomatosis. Frontal chest X-rays taken 2 years apart (**a**, **b**) show increase over time of the diameter of the right interlobar artery. In 2017, the left pulmonary artery is also measurable above the left main bronchus, and the convexity of the middle portion of the left mediastinal border is more pronounced due to pulmonary trunk dilation (arrow). CT angiography performed in 2017 (**c**, **d**) confirms the dilation of the pulmonary arteries

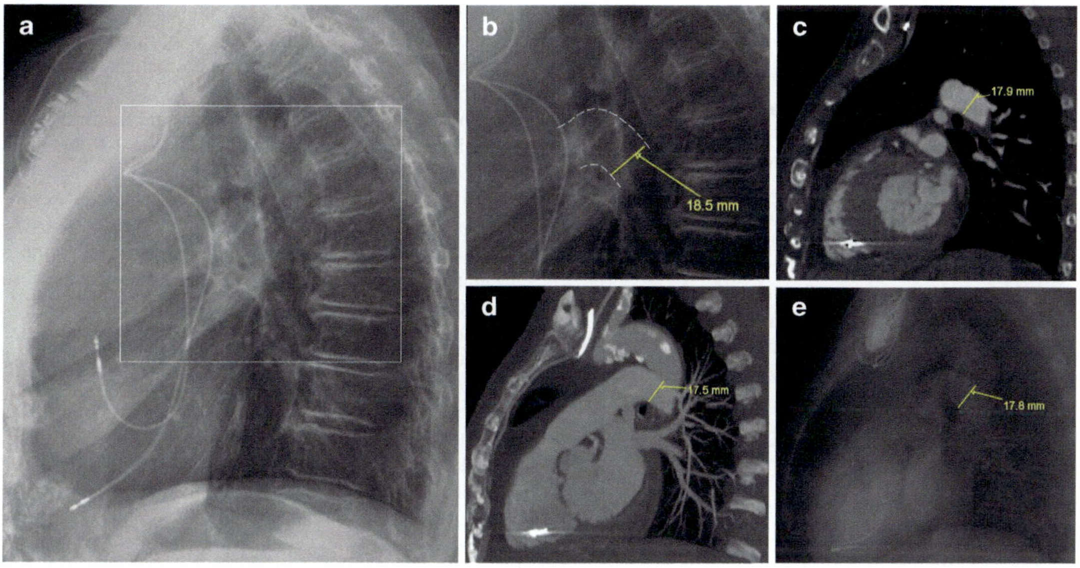

Fig. 28 Left main pulmonary artery. Lateral chest X-ray (**a**, **b**) and sagittal CT views (**c**–**e**) in an 86-year-old woman with a history of heart rhythm disorders but no hemodynamic evidence of pulmonary hypertension. The sagittal reformats in 20 mm thick MIP (**d**) and 150 mm thick average MPR (**e**) provide insight into the radiographic appearance of the left pulmonary artery

8 Conclusion

This chapter is an opportunity to take a trip down memory lane, and it is quite fascinating to look back at the amount and the accuracy of measurements that had been derived from chest X-rays, especially since most of them had their diagnostic value confirmed later on with CT. After reviewing this catalog, it appears that most of these measurements can still be useful. However, all measurements, particularly those in absolute value, should be considered with caution and interpreted according to subjects' age, sex, BMI, BSA, as well as technical parameters.

It should be remembered that measurements are necessary but not sufficient to properly read a chest X-ray. Taking measures can be reassuring since it is a mechanical and often easy task, but it is essential not to lose sight of the main objective, which is the detection of abnormal opacities/lucencies and their interpretation. Currently, plain chest X-ray is mainly used as a screening tool and is rarely conclusive on its own. Thus, any abnormal measurement on chest X-ray should be confirmed by a cross-sectional imaging technique, most often chest CT, or transthoracic echocardiogram for cardiac measurements.

Disclaimer All measurements in this book have been obtained from peer-reviewed papers and guidelines from professional organizations, unless explicitly stated otherwise. While the authors, editors, and publisher have gone through a rigorous process to establish their correct reproduction from the original source, each measurement must be interpreted in the correct clinical context, this along with an accurate way of measurement, and taking into account all technical variables, this including follow-up exams with various equipment or software. Neither the authors, the editors, nor the publisher can accept any legal responsibility for any improper application or interpretation of these measurements as well as their potential consequences.

References

Alavi SM, Keats TE, O'Brian WM (1970) The angle of tracheal bifurcation: its normal mensuration. AJR Am J Roentgenol 8:546–549

Bradley AJ, Carrington BM, Lawrance JA, Ryder WD, Radford JA (1999) Assessment and significance of mediastinal bulk in Hodgkin's disease: comparison between computed tomography and chest radiography. J Clin Oncol 17:2493–2498

Brakohiapa EKK, Botwe BO, Sarkodie BD, Ofori EK, Coleman J (2017) Radiographic determination of cardiomegaly using cardiothoracic ratio and transverse cardiac diameter: can one size fit all? Part one. Pan Afr Med J 27:201

Brant WE, Helms C (2012) Fundamentals of diagnostic radiology. Lippincott Williams & Wilkins. ISBN: 1608319113

Breatnach E, Abbott GC, Fraser RG (1984) Dimensions of the normal human trachea. AJR Am J Roentgenol 142:903–906

Chang CH (1962) The normal roentgenographic measurement of the right descending pulmonary artery in 1,085 cases. Am J Roentgenol Radium Ther Nucl Med 87:929–935

Chen JT, Putman CE, Hedlund LW, Dahmash NS, Roberts L (1982) Widening of the subcarinal angle by pericardial effusion. AJR Am J Roentgenol 139:883–887

Ciccarese F, Poerio A, Stagni S, Attinà D, Fasano L, Carbonara P, Bacchi Reggiani ML, Zompatori M (2014) Saber-sheath trachea as a marker of severe airflow obstruction in chronic obstructive pulmonary disease. Radiol Med 119:90–96

Collins J, Stern EJ (2008) Chest radiology, the essentials. Wolters Kluwer Health, Lippincott Williams & Wilkins. ISBN: 0781763142

Danzer CS (1919) The cardiothoracic ratio. Am J Med Sci 157:513–554

Edwards DK, Higgins CB, Gilpin EA (1981) The cardiothoracic ratio in newborn infants. AJR Am J Roentgenol 136:907–913

Fabre C, Proisy M, Chapuis C, Jouneau S, Lentz PA, Meunier C, Mahé G, Lederlin M (2018) Radiology residents' skill level in chest X-ray reading. Diagn Interv Imaging 99:361–370

Felson B (1973) Fundamentals of chest roentgenology. Saunders. ISBN: 9780721635910

Franquet T, Erasmus JJ, Giménez A, Rossi S, Prats R (2002) The retrotracheal space: normal anatomic and pathologic appearances. Radiographics 22(Spec No):S231–S246

Freeman V, Mutatiri C, Pretorius M, Doubell A (2003) Evaluation of left ventricular enlargement in the lateral position of the chest using the Hoffman and Rigler sign. Cardiovasc J S Afr 14:134–137

Gibbs JM, Chandrasekhar CA, Ferguson EC, Oldham SA (2007) Lines and stripes: where did they go? From conventional radiography to CT. Radiographics 27:33–48

Greene R, Lechner GL (1975) "Saber-sheath" trachea: a clinical and functional study of marked coronal narrowing of the intrathoracic trachea. Radiology 115:265–268

Haskin PH, Goodman LR (1982) Normal tracheal bifurcation angle: a reassessment. AJR Am J Roentgenol 139:879–882

Heitzman ER (1973) Radiologic appearance of the azygos vein in cardiovascular disease. Circulation 47:628–634

Hoffman R, Rigler L (1965) Evaluation of the left ventricular enlargement in the lateral projection of the chest. Radiology 85:93–100

Kabala JE, Wilde P (1987) The measurement of heart size in the antero-posterior chest radiograph. Br J Radiol 60:981–986

Kearney MT, Fox KA, Lee AJ, Prescott RJ, Shah AM, Batin PD, Baig W, Lindsay S, Callahan TS, Shell WE, Eckberg DL, Zaman AG, Williams S, Neilson JM, Nolan J (2002) Predicting death due to progressive heart failure in patients with mild-to-moderate chronic heart failure. J Am Coll Cardiol 40:1801–1808

Lister TA, Crowther D, Sutcliffe SB, Glatstein E, Canellos GP, Young RC, Rosenberg SA, Coltman CA, Tubiana M (1989) Report of a committee convened to discuss the evaluation and staging of patients with Hodgkin's disease: Cotswolds meeting. J Clin Oncol 7:1630–1636

Marano R, Liguori C, Savino G, Merlino B, Natale L, Bonomo L (2011) Cardiac silhouette findings and mediastinal lines and stripes: radiograph and CT scan correlation. Chest 139:1186–1196

Maresh MM, Washburn AH (1938) Size of the heart in healthy children. Am J Dis Child 56:33–60

McDonald CJ, Castellino RA, Blank N (1970) The aortic "nipple". The left superior intercostal vein. Radiology 96:533–536

Milne EN, Pistolesi M, Miniati M, Giuntini C (1984) The vascular pedicle of the heart and the vena azygos. Part I: The normal subject. Radiology 152(1):1–8

Milne EN, Pistolesi M, Miniati M, Giuntini C (1985) The radiologic distinction of cardiogenic and noncardiogenic edema. AJR Am J Roentgenol 144(5):879–894

Milne ENC, Burnett K, Aufrichtig D, McMillan J, Imray TJ (1988) Assessment of cardiac size on portable chest films. J Thorac Imaging 3:64–72

Miwa K, Fujita M (2008) Small heart syndrome in patients with chronic fatigue syndrome. Clin Cardiol 31:328–333

Morales MA, Prediletto R, Rossi G, Catapano G, Lombardi M, Rovai D (2012) Routine chest X-ray: still valuable for the assessment of left ventricular size and function in the era of super machines? J Clin Imaging Sci 2:25

Murray JG, Brown AL, Anagnostou EA, Senior R (1995) Widening of the tracheal bifurcation on chest radiographs: value as a sign of left atrial enlargement. AJR Am J Roentgenol 164:1089–1092

Petersen JA (1960) Recognition of infrapulmonary pleural effusion. Radiology 74:34–41

Pfaffenberger S, Bartko P, Graf A, Pernicka E, Babayev J, Lolic E, Bonderman D, Baumgartner H, Maurer G, Mascherbauer J (2013) Size matters! Impact of age, sex, height, and weight on the normal heart size. Circ Cardiovasc Imaging 6:1073–1079

Reed JC (2010) Chest radiology plain film patterns and differential diagnoses. Mosby. E-Book

Simkus P, Gutierrez Gimeno M, Banisauskaite A, Noreikaite J, McCreavy D, Penha D, Arzanauskaite M (2021) Limitations of cardiothoracic ratio derived from chest radiographs to predict real heart size: comparison with magnetic resonance imaging. Insights Imaging 12:158

Simon G (1971) Principles of chest X-ray diagnosis, 3rd edn. Butterworths, London

Simon G, Pride NB, Jones NL, Raimondi AC (1973) Relation between abnormalities in the chest radiograph and changes in pulmonary function in chronic bronchitis and emphysema. Thorax 28:15–23

Taskin V, Bates MC, Chillag SA (1991) Tracheal carinal angle and left atrial size. Arch Intern Med 151:307–308

Thurlbeck WM, Simon G (1978) Radiographic appearance of the chest in emphysema. AJR Am J Roentgenol 130:429–440

Torres FS, Eifer DA, Sanchez Tijmes F, Nguyen ET, Hanneman K (2021) Diagnostic performance of chest radiography measurements for the assessment of cardiac chamber enlargement. CMAJ 193:E1683–E1692

Truszkiewicz K, Poręba R, Gać P (2021) Radiological cardiothoracic ratio in evidence-based medicine. J Clin Med 10:2016

United Nations Scientific Committee on the Effects of Atomic Radiation (2008) Sources and Effects of ionizing radiation. 2008 Report to the General Assembly, with scientific annexes, vol I. United Nations, New York

Webb WR, Higgins CB (2010) Thoracic imaging. Lippincott Williams & Wilkins. ISBN: 1605479764

Whitten C, Khan S, Munneke G, Grubnic S (2007) A diagnostic approach to mediastinal abnormalities. Radiographics 27:657–671

Wigh RE (1978) On defining microcardia: application in pulmonary emphysema. South Med J 71:150–154

Xu Y, Yamashiro T, Moriya H, Tsubakimoto M, Tsuchiya N, Nagatani Y, Matsuoka S, Murayama S (2017) Hyperinflated lungs compress the heart during expiration in COPD patients: a new finding on dynamic-ventilation computed tomography. Int J Chron Obstruct Pulmon Dis 12:3123–3131

Yamazaki T, Suzuki, Shimamoto R, Tsuji T, Nakajima T, Nagai R, Komatsu S, Otomo K, Toyo-Oka T, Omata M (2002) Fluctuation of cardiac size on radiographs during a cardiac cycle: re-examination with magnetic resonance imaging. Radiography 8:181–187

Pulmonary Nodule

Guillaume Chassagnon and Marie-Pierre Revel

Contents

G. Chassagnon (✉) · M.-P. Revel
Radiology Department, Hôpital Cochin,
AP-HP. Centre Université Paris Cité, Paris, France
e-mail: guillaume.chassagnon@aphp.fr

Abstract

This chapter will review the different methods of measuring lung nodules, how these measurements are incorporated into malignancy risk assessment and management, and management strategies for pulmonary nodules, whether discovered incidentally or as part of lung cancer screening. Both manual and automated methods for measuring nodule size will be described. The advantages of automated methods, such as greater reproducibility and the ability to calculate volume doubling time, will be discussed, as will their limitations. The differences between solid and subsolid nodules will be presented, with particular emphasis on the differentiation between pure and partially ground glass nodules and the impact of this differentiation on size measurement. Density measurements and morphological criteria suggesting benignity or malignancy will also be reviewed.

Abbreviations

AAH	Atypical adenomatous hyperplasia
AIS	Adenocarcinoma in situ
BTS	British Thoracic Society
CT	Computed tomography
GGNs	Ground-glass nodules

Med Radiol Diagn Imaging (2026)

https://doi.org/10.1007/174_2025_604,
Published Online: 26 September 2025

GGO	Ground glass opacity
HU	Hounsfield units
Lung-RADS	Lung CT Screening Reporting and Data System
MIA	Minimally invasive adenocarcinoma
PET	Positron emission tomography
PFNs	Perifissural nodules
VDT	Volume doubling time

1 Introduction

Measurements play an essential role in the management of pulmonary nodules, as they are one of the main parameters for determining their diagnostic strategy. In this chapter, we will review the different methods of measurements, how to obtain and interpret them, and their role in the management of lung nodules when using CT.

2 Definitions

2.1 Nodule Versus Mass Versus Micronodule

By definition, a pulmonary nodule is a rounded, well- or poorly defined opacity measuring from 6 mm to 3 cm in diameter (Bankier et al. 2024). Nodules smaller than 6 mm are called micronodules, while lesions larger than 3 cm are called masses.

2.2 Subtypes of Nodules

Pulmonary nodules are subdivided into solid and subsolid nodules according to their attenuation (Fig. 1). The term *subsolid* refers to nodules showing, at least partially, a ground-glass opacity (GGO) component. Among subsolid nodules, a distinction is made between *pure ground-glass* nodules (GGNs) and *part-solid* GGNs comprising both a solid and a non-solid (GGO) component.

Histological studies have shown that 75% of persistent subsolid nodules correspond to pulmonary adenocarcinomas with lepidic growth (either adenocarcinoma in situ (AIS), minimally invasive adenocarcinoma (MIA), or invasive adenocarcinoma), and 6% correspond to atypical adenomatous hyperplasia (AAH), which is a premalignant lesion for lung adenocarcinoma (Kim et al. 2007). The proportion of cancer is therefore much higher for subsolid than for solid nodules, but the prognosis of subsolid cancer is better as the 5-year survival is near 100% for patients who have undergone surgical resection of an AIS or MIA (Naidich et al. 2013). In subsolid nodules seen in the spectrum of lung adenocarcinomas, the GGO component usually represents lepidic growth. Several studies have shown a close correlation between computed tomography (CT) and pathological findings in these lesions (Naidich et al. 2013). Pure GGNs generally correspond to premalignant lesions (most likely AAH when ≤5 mm and adenocarcinoma in situ when >5 mm) while partially solid GGNs generally correspond to malignant lesions (most likely MIA when the solid component is ≤5 mm and invasive adenocarcinoma when the solid component is >5 mm). It is therefore important to identify subsolid nodules and to distinguish between pure GGNs and part-solid GGNs.

Identification of the type of nodule (solid or subsolid) is not based on density measurements but on the visual identification of a solid component. Several studies have demonstrated poor agreement between radiologists in categorizing subsolid nodules as part-solid GGNs or pure GGNs. A criterion for improving inter-observer reproducibility is the detectability of a solid component on a modified mediastinal window setting (W:400/C:0 Hounsfield units (HU)). The use of this simple criterion considerably improves inter-observer reproducibility (*kappa* = 0.89 vs. 0.54) (Revel et al. 2018). Of note, when the solid component of a part-solid nodule is more than 80% of the nodule diameter, this nodule should be classified as solid (Yip et al. 2017).

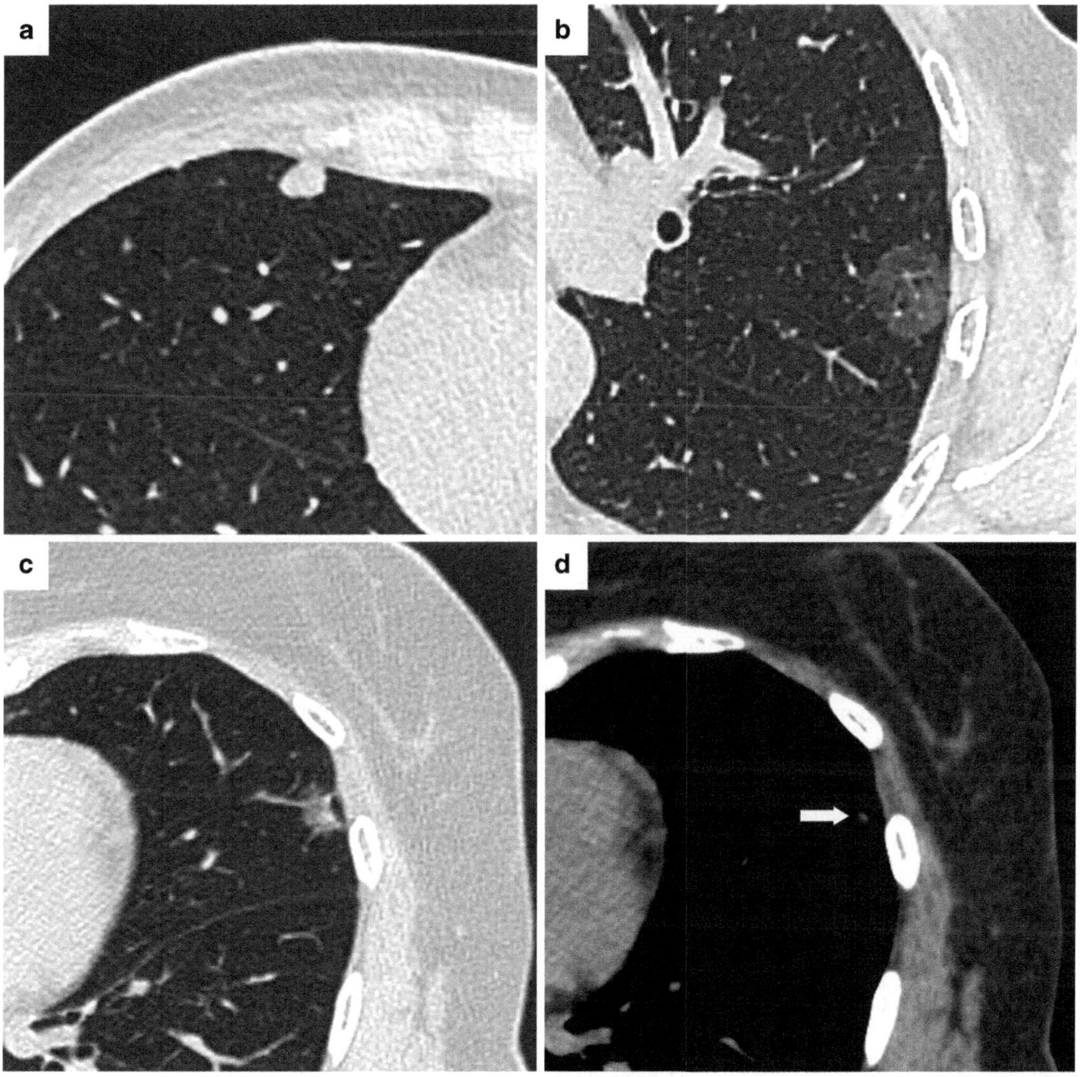

Fig. 1 Illustration of the different subtypes of lung nodules. Nodules can be either solid (**a**) or subsolid (**b–d**) when the latter shows, at least partially, a ground-glass opacity component. Subsolid nodules are divided into pure ground glass nodules (GGNs) when they only contain ground glass (**b**) or part-solid GGNs when they also contain a solid component (**c**, **d**). Identification of the solid component in the mediastinal window setting improves inter-observer reproducibility (arrow in **d**)

3 Measurements

In routine clinical practice, the two relevant measurements for the management of pulmonary nodules are their size and their attenuation. Size measurements can be made manually with electronic calipers (diameter measurements) or automatically/semi-automatically using dedicated software (diameter and volume measurements).

3.1 Diameter Measurement

Manual diameter measurements should be performed on a lung window setting (W:1600/C:−600 HU), ideally on images reconstructed using the lung kernel, which offers a better spatial resolution compared to the mediastinal one. It is highly recommended to zoom in on the nodule for more accurate measurement. Methods of diameter measurements vary according to nodule type.

- *For solid nodules*, the mean of the long- and short-axis diameters should be used for nodules below 10 mm, both of which should be obtained on the same transverse, coronal, or sagittal reconstructed image (Fig. 2). As an example, an oval nodule of 6 mm in major diameter and 4 mm in minor diameter has a mean diameter of (6 + 4)/2 = 5 mm. For nodules larger than 10 mm, both long- and short-axis dimensions should be recorded, as the long-axis dimension is used to determine the T factor in the TNM lung cancer staging (Bankier et al. 2017). The Fleischner society recommends using the mean diameter rounded to the nearest whole millimeter for subcentimeter nodules (e.g., mean diameter of 8.4 = 8 mm and 8.6 = 9 mm), because the mean of the long and short axes more accurately reflects the volume of the nodule (MacMahon et al. 2017).
- *For part-solid nodules*, the mean of the long- and short-axis diameters of the nodule, including the whole GGO and any cystic component, should be measured for nodules <10 mm and both long- and short-axis diameters should be recorded for larger nodules. If larger than 3 mm, the maximum diameter of the solid component should be measured (Fig. 3). While mediastinal window setting is useful for its identification, the solid component, however, must be measured on a lung window setting (Bankier et al. 2017).

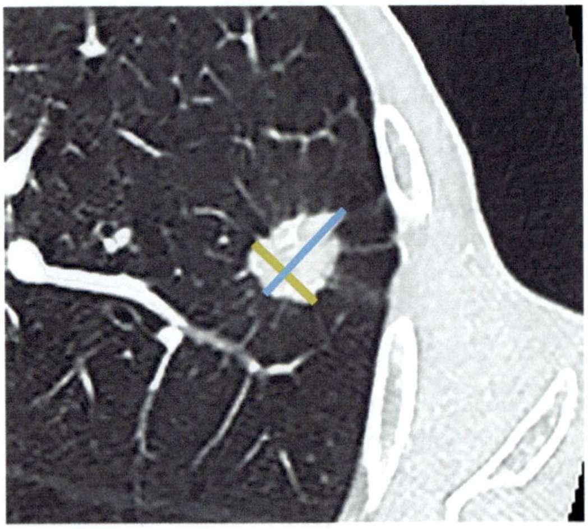

Fig. 2 Measuring the diameter of a solid nodule. Both long- (blue caliper) and short-axis (yellow caliper) diameters should be measured. The nodule size is the average of these two diameters for nodules smaller than 10 mm

Manual diameter measurements suffer from intra- and inter-reader variability. Revel et al. (2004) have shown that to be considered significant, an increase in the largest nodule diameter must be at least 1.73 mm when measurements are made by two different readers. Manual diameter measurements are especially known to be affected by irregular and spiculated margins, which increase inter-reader variability and cause substantial misclassification of nodule growth. Han et al. in a study on 25 nodules from the NELSON study, which were manually measured by 3 radiologists, showed that intra-reader variability of both spiculated nodules (±2.4 mm) and irregular nodules (±2.9 mm) exceeded the 1.5-mm nodule growth cut-off used in the Lung CT Screening Reporting and Data System (Lung-RADS) (Han et al. 2018).

3.2 Volumetric Measurement

Nodule volumetry is more effective than diameter measurement for the assessment of nodule growth, as it allows for the calculation of the volume doubling time (VDT) (Mehta et al. 2014). Doubling the volume of a nodule corresponds to a 26% increase in its diameter. The volume of a nodule can be estimated from its diameter when measured manually, using the following formula, which assumes that the nodule is spherical:

$$V = 1/6 \times \pi \times D^3$$

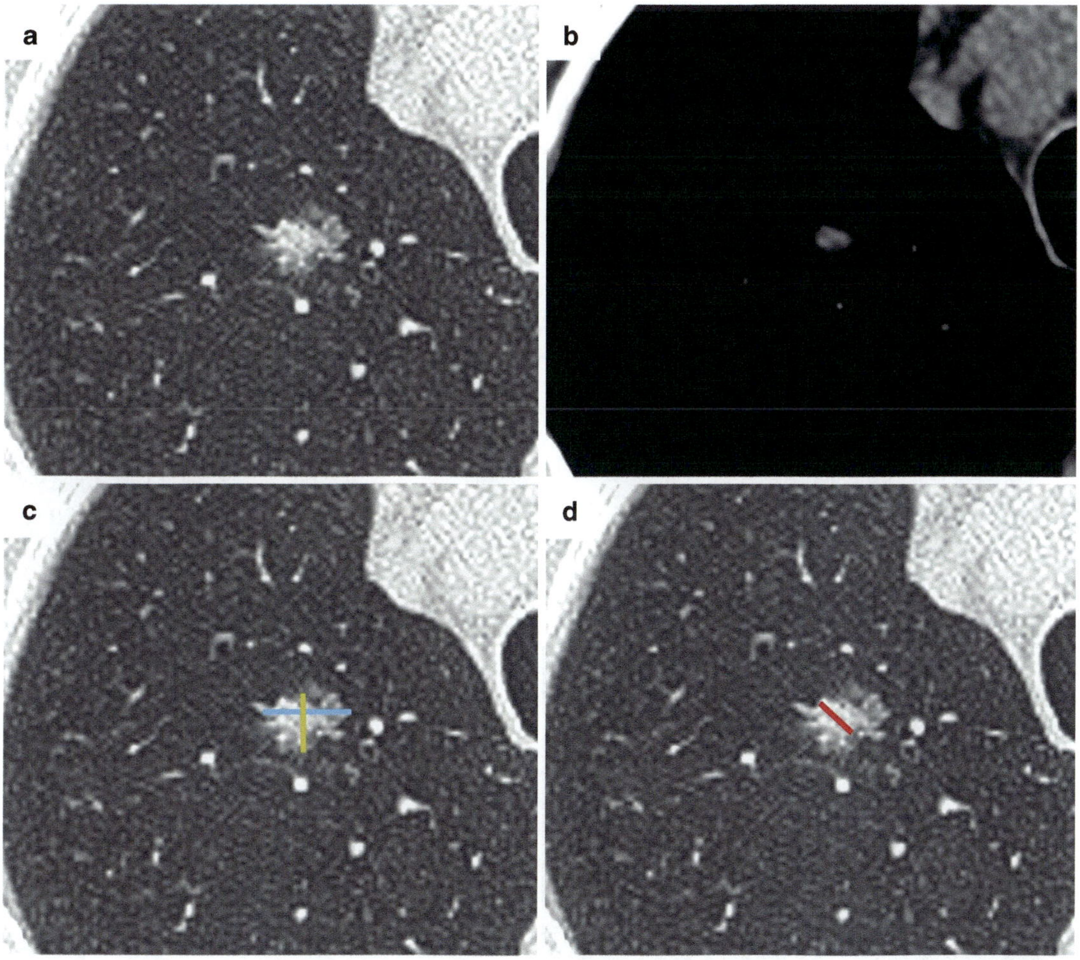

Fig. 3 Measuring the diameter of a part-solid nodule. The subsolid nodule of the right upper lobe (**a**) has a solid component, which is better seen in the mediastinal window setting (**b**). Both long- (blue caliper) and short-axis (yellow caliper) diameters should be measured (and averaged if <10 mm) for the whole nodule size (**c**), while only the long-axis diameter (red caliper) should be measured for the solid component (if >3 mm) (**d**). All measurements should be performed in the lung window setting (**c**, **d**)

V = volume, *D* = diameter

However, the actual volume of a nodule is more accurately obtained when using automated or semi-automated software: automated or semi-automated measurements have the advantage of being more reproducible than manual diameter measurements. However, they suffer from inter-scan variability, particularly related to the degree of inspiration (Devaraj et al. 2017). Studies that performed CT scans of patients twice on the same day found a similar 95% confidence interval for a relative difference of an order of 25% in volume between CT scans (Wormanns et al. 2004; Gietema et al. 2007). Volumetry is also dependent on the software used (Fig. 4). Peters et al. who evaluated the impact of volumetric variation between two software systems in a phantom study, found that 15% of the solid nodules were classified differently according to Lung-RADS between the two systems applied on the same images (Peters et al. 2023). The mean relative volume differences between the two systems were 1.3 ± 18.6% for solid nodules and −15.2 ± 23.5% for GGNs. Automatic volumetric

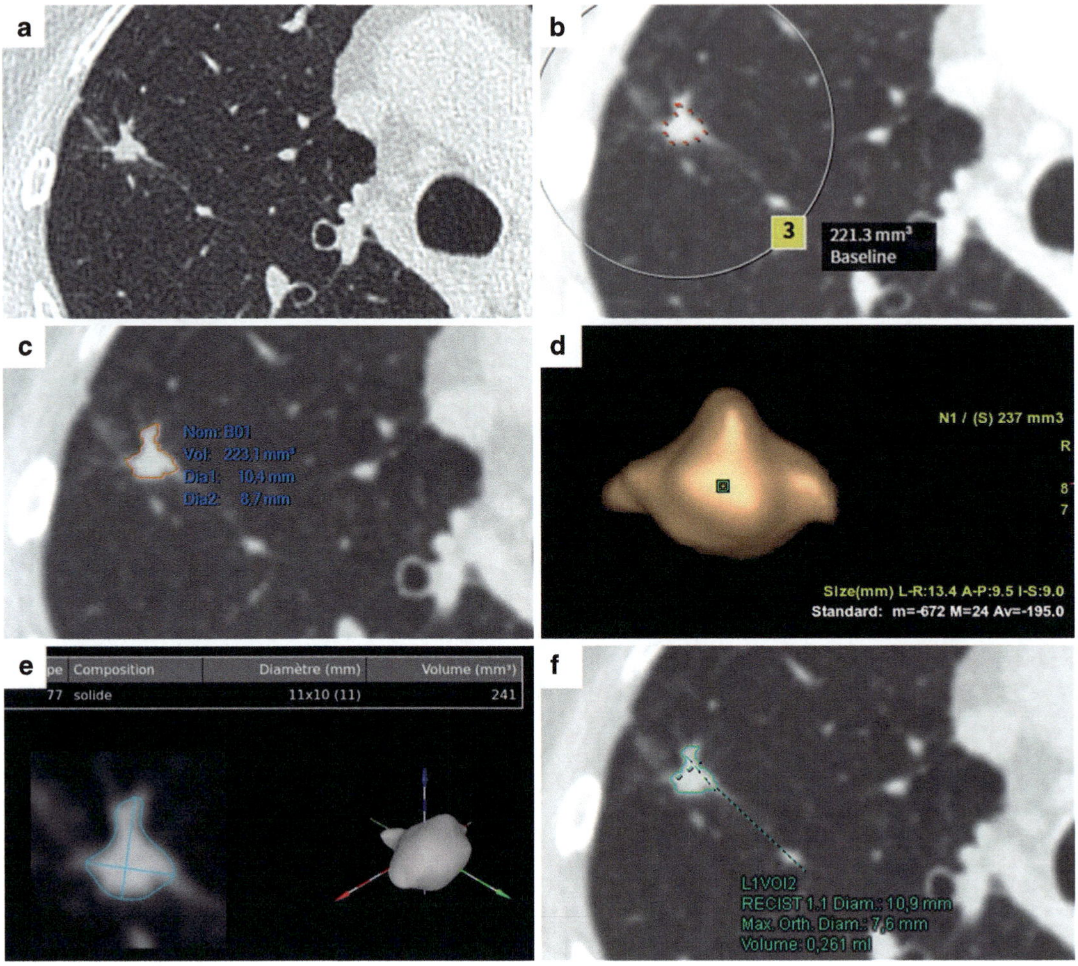

Fig. 4 Example of differences in nodule volumetry depending on the software used. Five software were used to assess the volume of this spiculated nodule located in the right upper lobe (**a**). Depending on the software, the volume ranged from 221 to 261 mm^3 (**b–f**), resulting in a relative difference of 18%

software has the advantage of offering perfect intrinsic reproducibility. On the other hand, semi-automatic software enables editing of nodule contours in the event of segmentation error at the expense of the risk of lower reproducibility. Due to size variations between various software, it is therefore important to always use the same software for volume comparisons on the same patient and to consider if there has been a manual editing or not.

It is important to note that when automated or semi-automated volumetric software is used, it must be applied to images reconstructed with the correct reconstruction kernel according to the manufacturer's recommendations (more often the mediastinal kernel).

3.3 Attenuation Measurement

Attenuation measurement can be useful in indicating the presence of fat (−40 to −120 HU), aeric content, or calcification within the nodule. Attenuation measurements must be made on images reconstructed with the mediastinal (soft) kernel and never by using a lung (edge-enhancing) filter. Importantly, caution is required when measuring attenuation values within a nodule, as partial volume with adjacent lung air can alter measurement and mimic fat density, and noise can also affect measurements. A small region of interest should be used, and one-pixel measurements (point value) should be avoided (Fig. 5). A large standard deviation should be taken as an indicator of poor measurement quality (Fig. 6). In doubtful cases, a close-up view using a smaller reconstructed FOV may be useful for more accurate evaluation of nodule densities.

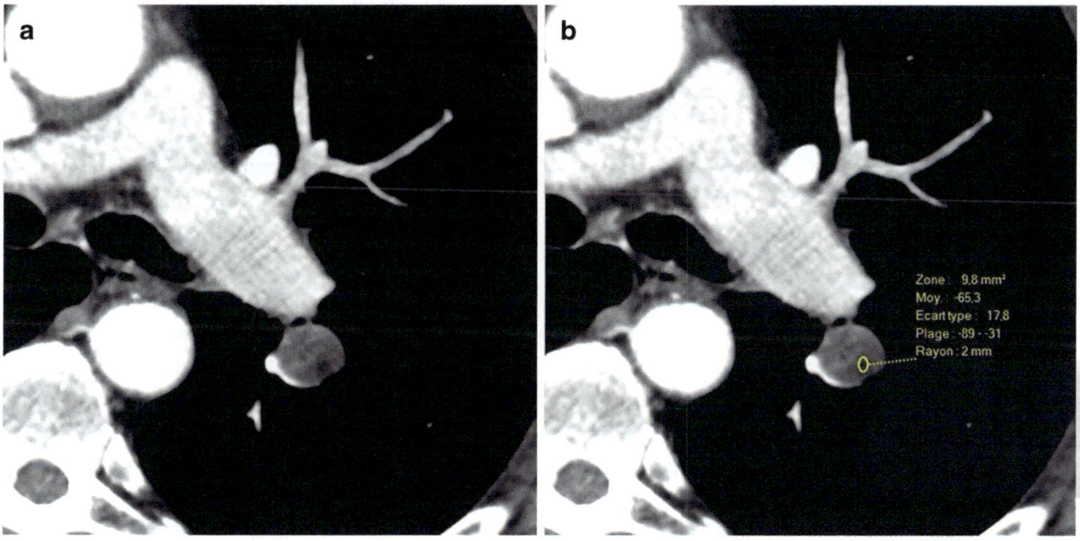

Fig. 5 Measuring the attenuation within a nodule. Attenuation measurement is needed to assess the presence of a fatty component (**a**). A region-of-interest should be drawn, avoiding overlap with the lung parenchyma (**b**). In this case, the attenuation is −65 HU with an acceptable standard deviation of 18 HU, assessing the presence of fat and enabling the diagnosis of pulmonary hamartoma

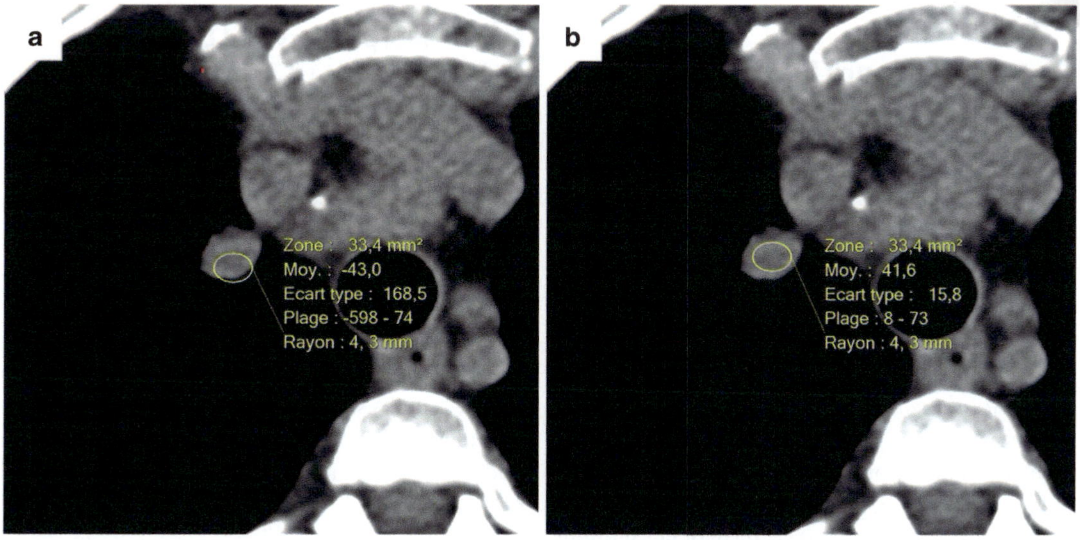

Fig. 6 Importance of standard deviation in assessing measurement quality. In **a**, the region of interest overlaps the lung parenchyma, resulting in an attenuation value of −43 Hounsfield Units (HU), but the standard deviation of 169 HU is a marker of poor measurement quality. In **b**, the region of interest is correctly drawn. The attenuation is then +42 HU with a low standard deviation (16 HU)

Attenuation of the whole nodule can also be used to calculate its mass. The concept of mass (nodule volume x nodule density) has been suggested to account for both the increase in size and density for subsolid nodules (De Hoop et al. 2012).

3.4 Other Nonquantitative Nodule Characteristics in Clinical Routine

Other characteristics are used routinely to characterize pulmonary nodules but are not measurable in clinical practice. These include the nodule's location, shape, and margin (well- or ill-defined, smooth, lobulated, or spiculated), as well as the presence of calcification. These characteristics are also used to assess the nodule's risk of malignancy.

Shape (such as sphericity index) and texture parameters can be calculated and are used in radiomic signatures to predict the risk of malignancy, the histological subtype, or the response to treatment (Beig et al. 2019; Sun et al. 2020). However, prospective validation of these approaches is still lacking and prevents their use in clinical practice.

4 Malignancy Risk Assessment

4.1 Criteria Suggesting Malignancy

4.1.1 Size

The risk of malignancy for solid nodules strongly depends on their size, which explains why decision criteria for nodule follow-up are mainly based on this criterion.

For *solid nodules*, nodules smaller than 6 mm have a risk of malignancy of less than 1%, even in high-risk populations from lung cancer screening programs (Horeweg et al. 2014; McWilliams et al. 2013; Swensen 1997). In patients without history of malignant disease, this has led the Fleischner Society to recommend no follow-up for nodules smaller than 6 mm except in cases of suspicious morphology or upper lobe location, whereby an optional 12-month follow-up may be proposed (MacMahon et al. 2017). Nodules measuring 8 mm have a risk of malignancy of around 3%, and thus nodules ≥8 mm should be investigated more proactively, either by a follow-up CT scan at 3 months, a positron emission tomography (PET) scan, or a biopsy (MacMahon et al. 2017). The subsequent approach of management to adopt depends on the morphology and location of the nodule, which may influence the probability of malignancy.

In *pure GGNs*, nodule size also correlates with risk of malignancy. Smaller lesions are thought to correspond to preinvasive lesions (AAH and AIS), with the majority of pure GGNs ≤5 mm being AAH (Lee and Lee 2011). Several studies have shown that pure GGNs ≥10 mm have a significantly higher risk to be invasive adenocarcinoma compared to those <10 mm (Lee et al. 2019a; AlShammari et al. 2024).

In *part-solid GGNs*, global lesion size and solid component size are associated with lesion invasiveness (Aherne et al. 2018).

4.1.2 Morphology and Location

Data from the first CT screening of the Pan-Canadian Early Detection of Lung Cancer Study (PanCan) were used to determine factors that could be predictive of the probability of malignancy of lung nodules. These data were used to build what is known as the Brock model (McWilliams et al. 2013). Along with larger nodule size, the nodule characteristics that are predictive of cancer in the Brock model include spiculated margins, part-solid GGN, low nodule count, emphysema, and upper lobe location. Spiculated margins and upper lobe location had odds ratios around 2, whereas emphysema and part-solid GGN had odds ratio around 1.4 (Table 1).

Other morphological characteristics are associated with malignancy, including a complex shape for solid nodules or a round shape for subsolid nodules, lobulated margins, pleural retraction, air bronchograms, and bubble-like lucencies (Snoeckx et al. 2018). Additionally, the presence of pulmonary fibrosis and family history of cancer are also associated with an increased risk of malignancy.

Table 1 Variables included in the Brock Model (McWilliams et al. 2013)

	Variables
Patients characteristics	Age Sex Family history of lung cancer Emphysema
Nodules characteristics	Nodule size Nodule type (non-solid/subsolid/solid) Nodule located in an upper lobe Number of nodules Spiculation

4.1.3 Atypical Pulmonary Cysts

Atypical lung cysts may correspond to cystic lung cancer or precursors of cystic lung cancer. Atypical pulmonary cysts include thick-walled unilocular cysts (>2 mm wall thickness) and multilocular cysts (Fig. 7). These lesions are now included in the 2022 update of Lung-RADS (Christensen et al. 2024), which recommends 3- to 6-month follow-up or referral for further evaluation based on their morphology and evolution (Table 2).

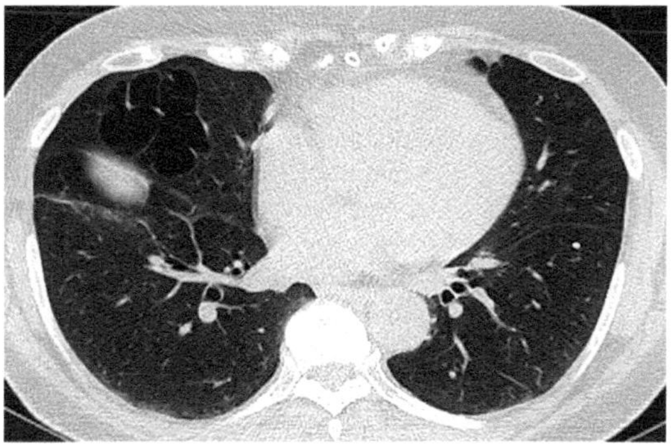

Fig. 7 Example of a multilocular cyst of the right middle lobe. The lesion was resected and corresponded to pulmonary adenocarcinoma

Table 2 Lung-RADS v2022

Lung-RADS	Findings	Management
0 *(Incomplete)*	Findings suggesting inflammatory or infectious lesion	1–3 month LDCT
	Incomplete CT examination or prior CT study existing but not being available for comparison	Comparison to prior CT examination
1 *(Negative)*	**No lung nodule**	12-month screening LDCT
	Lung nodule(s) with benign features: Complete / Central / Popcorn / Concentric ring calcification **Or:** fat-containing nodules	
2 *(Benign)*	**Juxtapleural nodule(s):** Solid nodule, measuring <10 mm in mean diameter, with smooth margin, and oval, lentiform, or triangular shape.	12-month screening LDCT
	Solid nodule(s): <6 mm (<113 mm^3) at baseline New nodule <4 mm (<34 mm^3)	
	Part-solid nodule(s): <6 mm total mean diameter (<113 mm^3) at baseline	
	Ground glass nodule(s): <30 mm (<14,137 mm^3) at baseline, new or growing ≥30 mm (≥14,137 mm^3) and unchanged or slowly growing	
	Airway nodule(s): Subsegmental airway nodule at baseline, new, or stable	
	Other: Lung-RADS 3 nodules that are stable or decreased at 6 months Lung-RADS 3 or 4B lesion that resolve on follow-up Lung-RADS 4B lesion that has a benign diagnosis on diagnostic work-up	

(continued)

Table 2 (continued)

Lung-RADS	Findings	Management
3 *(Probably benign)*	**Solid nodule(s):** ≥6 to 8 mm (≥113 mm^3 to <268 mm^3) at baseline New nodule between 4 mm and 6 mm (≥34 mm^3 to <113 mm^3)	6-month LDCT
	Subsolid nodule(s): ≥6 mm (≥113 mm^3) total diameter with solid component <6 mm (<113 mm^3) **Or:** new nodule measuring <6 mm in total diameter (<113 mm^3)	
	Ground glass nodule(s): ≥30 mm (at baseline or new)	
	Atypical pulmonary cyst: Atypical thick-walled lung cyst with growing cystic component (mean diameter)	
	Other: Category 4A lesion that is stable or decreased in size at 3-month follow-up (excluding airway nodules)	
4A *(Supicious)*	**Solid nodule(s):** ≥8 mm to <15 mm (≥268 mm^3 to <1717 mm^3) at baseline **Or:** growing nodule(s) <8 mm (<268 mm^3) **Or:** new nodule ≥6 mm to <8 mm (≥113 mm^3 to <268 mm^3)	**3-month LDCT** *PET-CT may be considered if there is a 8 mm (268 mm^3) solid nodule or solid component*
	Part-solid nodule(s): ≥6 mm (≥113 mm^3) total diameter with solid component ≥6 mm to <8 mm (≥113 mm^3 to <268 mm^3) **Or:** new or growing <4 mm solid component (<34 mm^3)	
	Atypical pulmonary cyst: Thick-walled cyst **Or:** multilocular cyst at baseline **Or:** thin- or thick-walled cyst that becomes multilocular	
	Airway nodules: Endotracheal or endobronchial nodule at baseline	
4B *(Very suspicious)*	**Solid nodule(s):** ≥15 mm (≥1767 mm^3) at baseline **Or:** New or growing, and ≥8 mm (268 mm^3)	**PET-CT** *(possible if there is a solid component ≥8 mm),* **biopsy,** and/or **referral for further clinical evaluation**
	Part-solid nodule(s): Solid component 8 mm (268 mm^3) **Or:** New or growing ≥4 mm (34 mm^3) solid component	
	Atypical pulmonary cyst: Thick-walled cyst with growing wall thickness/nodularity **Or:** growing multilocular cyst **Or:** multilocular cyst with increased loculation or new/increased opacity (nodular, ground glass, or consolidation)	
	Airway nodules: Endotracheal or endobronchial nodule that are stable or growing at 3-month follow-up	**Referral for further clinical evaluation**
4X *(Very suspicious)*	Category 3 or 4 nodules with additional features or imaging findings that increase the suspicion of malignancy, including: Spiculation Ground glass nodule(s) that double in size in 1 year Enlarged regional lymph nodes Frank metastatic disease	**PET-CT** *(possible if there is a solid component ≥8 mm),* **biopsy,** and/or **referral for further clinical evaluation**

4.2 Criteria Suggesting Benignity

Some nodule characteristics can also be used to identify benign nodules, which therefore do not require further investigation or follow-up. These are the features suggestive of intrapulmonary lymph nodes, hamartomas, and calcified granulomas.

4.2.1 Intrapulmonary Lymph Nodes

Intrapulmonary lymph nodes represent 1–66% of all lung nodules, according to the literature (Schreuder et al. 2020). These nodules are often perifissural and have been shown to never be malignant (De Hoop et al. 2012; Ahn et al. 2010). In the literature, the term *perifissural nodules* (PFNs) has been used to describe intrapulmonary lymph nodes because, in most cases, their nodal origin was not confirmed by histology. Whereas benign, they can, however, show growth rates in the range of malignant nodules (De Hoop et al. 2012). According to the criteria proposed by Schreuder et al., PFNs are defined as non-calcified, solid, well-circumscribed, smoothly marginated nodules with oval, lentiform, or polygonal shapes. PFNs are often attached to veins but not arteries (Barnett et al. 2019). PFNs must be either in contact with a major, minor, or accessory fissure or within 15 mm from the visceral pleura and located in the lower lobes, middle lobe, or lingula (Schreuder et al. 2020). They usually measure 12 mm or less (Schreuder et al. 2020). A localization above the level of the carina should be considered as an exclusion criterion (Schreuder et al. 2018).

4.2.2 Fatty Component

A fatty component within a well-circumscribed nodule is suggestive of benignity. Fat-containing nodules are most often pulmonary hamartomas. Endobronchial lipomas can also be seen and appear to be entirely fatty. Endobronchial lesions that are not entirely fatty may exceptionally correspond to a liposarcoma, in which case the diagnosis is based on bronchoscopy (Martinez Trevino et al. n.d.).

Pulmonary hamartomas are the most frequent benign tumors of the lung after intrapulmonary lymph nodes and account for approximately 6–8% of solitary pulmonary nodules (Siegelman et al. 1986). They present as well-circumscribed lesions with either smooth or lobulated margins. The presence of focal areas of fat within the nodule is suggestive of the diagnosis. Siegelman et al. defined fat content as the measurement of a mean attenuation value between −40 and −120 HU when using a region of interest (ROI) of at least 8 voxels (Siegelman et al. 1986). Fat is identified in up to 50% of hamartomas on CT, meaning that the absence of detectable fat component on CT does not rule out this diagnosis (Siegelman et al. 1986). Popcorn-like or central calcifications are seen in about 15–30% of the cases.

4.2.3 Calcifications

Benign calcifications include complete, central, laminated, or popcorn-like calcifications (Webb 1990). This is in contrast with eccentric calcifications that can be seen in malignant lesions. Popcorn-like calcifications are usually seen in hamartomas, whilst complete, central, and laminated calcifications are seen in granulomas. The most frequent causes of calcified granulomas include sequelae of tuberculosis or histoplasmosis. However, calcified/ossified metastases originating in particular from osteogenic sarcoma or chondrosarcoma can mimic benign calcifications.

5 Management Strategies

The choice of the management strategy depends on nodule type, its size, and the context in which it is discovered. For example, Lung-RADS can only be used in the context of a lung cancer screening program (Christensen et al. 2024). In all strategies, however, nodule measurement plays an essential role. Some recommendations are based on diameter assessment, others on volumetric assessment. Recommendations using a volumetric approach are based on the calculation of VDT according to the following formula (Fig. 6):

$$\mathrm{VDT} = \left[\ln 2 \times \Delta T\right] / \left[\ln\left(X2 / X1\right)\right]$$

$X2$ and $X1$ are the final and initial nodule volumes

ΔT is the number of days between the two scans

In the NELSON study, the cut-off value of VDT for differentiating malignant from benign pulmonary nodules was set at 400 days, and nodules with a VDT between 400 and 600 days at the second-round CT were considered indeterminate, requiring an additional 1-year follow-up CT (van Klaveren et al. 2009). These cut-off values were subsequently adopted by the British Thoracic Society (BTS) guidelines (Baldwin and Callister 2015). Lung cancers with the shortest volume doubling time are small cell carcinomas with a VDT of around 86 days (Arai et al. 1994), VDT of squamous cell carcinomas is around 122 days (Takashima et al. 2003), and VDT of adenocarcinoma ranges from 229 days for the solid or micropapillary subtypes to 647 days for the lepidic subtype (Park et al. 2020). Consistently, mean VDT of malignant lesions is 149 days for solid nodules, 457 days for part-solid nodules, and 813 days for pure GGNs (Hasegawa et al. 2000). It must be kept in mind that carcinoid tumors may have long doubling times largely exceeding 600 days, with overlapping VDT values compared to those of hamartomas (Ryan and Hammer 2023). Conversely, very short volume doubling times are not consistent with primary malignant lesions. In solid nodules, volume doubling times of less than 20–30 days are usually associated with inflammatory or infectious causes (Martin et al. 2017).

In general, when monitoring a nodule, it is important to compare the new CT scan not only with the most recent CT scan but also with the earliest available CT scan. This is particularly true for subsolid nodules, which can represent slow-growing lung cancers.

5.1 Incidentally Detected Lung Nodules

Outside the context of lung cancer screening, the most widely used recommendations are those of the Fleischner Society (Figs. 8 and 9) and of the BTS (MacMahon et al. 2017; Baldwin and Callister 2015) (Figs. 10 and 11). Both propose a

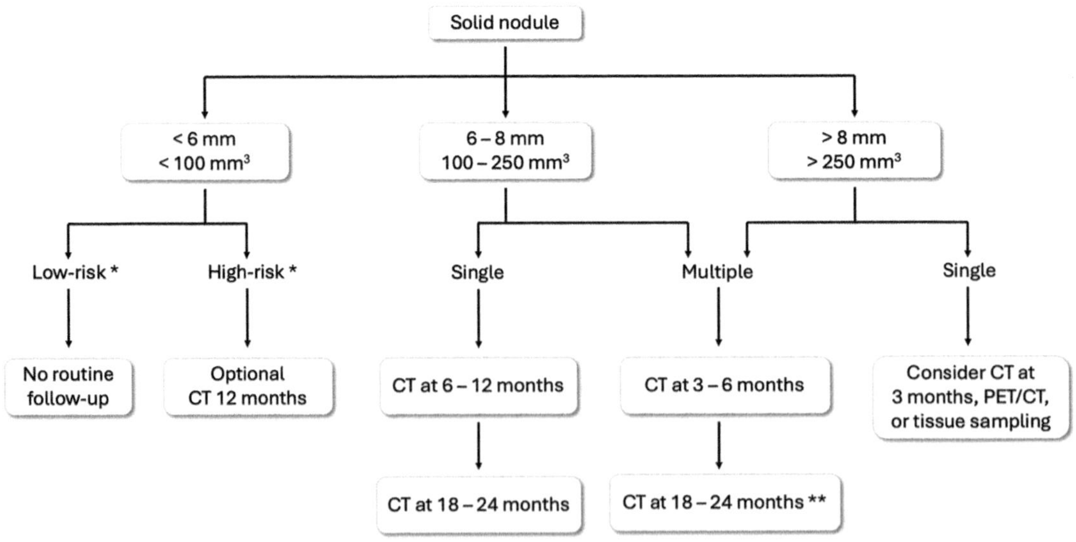

Fig. 8 Recommendations of the Fleischner society for the management of solid nodules. (Adapted from MacMahon et al. (2017)). Note: * High-risk factors include older age, heavy smoking, irregular or spiculated margins, and upper lobe location. ** Optional if low-risk

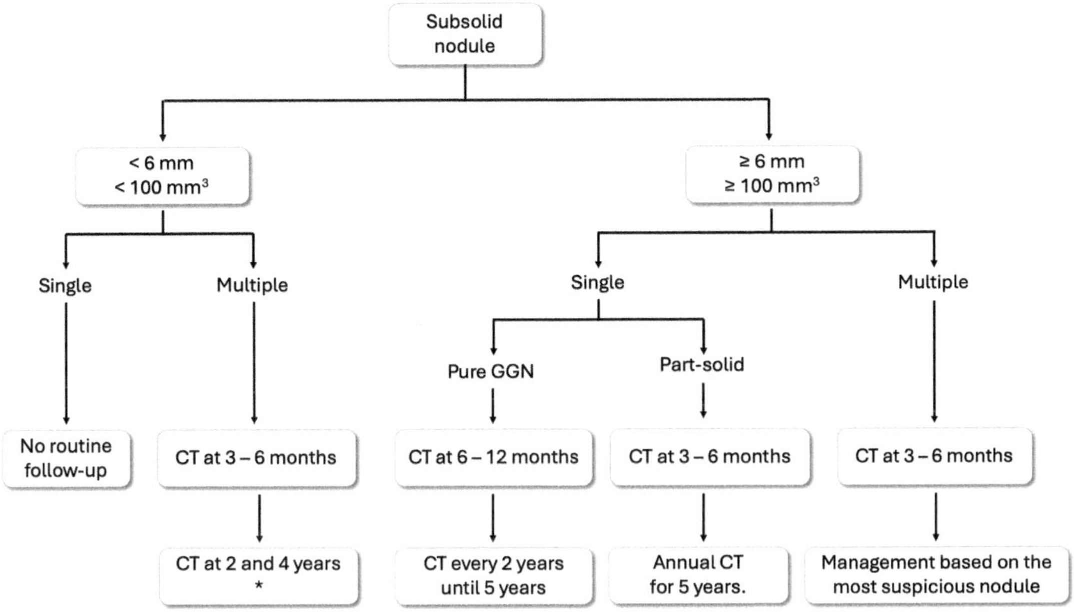

Fig. 9 Guidelines of the Fleischner society for the management of subsolid nodules. Adapted from Bankier et al. (2017). *Note*: * Optional; *GGN = ground glass nodule*

different strategy for solid and subsolid nodules and exclude nodules with clear features of benignity. The guidelines of the BTS are more complex but favor volumetry instead of diameter and are the only guidelines that provide a clear definition of nodule growth. However, this applies only for solid nodules. According to BTS guidelines, a VDT ≤400 days for solid nodules at 3 months is considered suspicious for malignancy and requires a specific management. At 1 year, only a VDT >600 days rules out malignancy, and a nodule showing a VDT between 400 and 600 days should be biopsied or followed up. As mentioned above, cautious remains to be maintained regarding carcinoid tumors. When comparison is based on diameter, growth should be reported if the change in measured diameter is at least of 2 mm (Bankier et al. 2017).

5.1.1 Solid Nodules

For small nodules (<5 mm or <80 mm^3 according to the BTS or <6 mm or <100 mm^3 according to the Fleischner Society guidelines), no follow-up is recommended except for high-risk nodules for which the Fleischner Society recommends an optional follow-up at 12 months. High-risk factors include older age, heavy smoking, irregular or spiculated margins, and upper lobe location.

For intermediate-size nodules (5–8 mm or 80–300 mm^3 according to the BTS or 6–8 mm or 100–250 mm^3 according to the Fleischner Society guidelines), a first follow-up CT scan is recommended at 3 or 6–12 months (3–6 months in the case of multiple nodules), respectively. If the nodule is stable on the first follow-up CT, the next follow-up CT is recommended at 18–24 months by the Fleischner Society, while according to the BTS guidelines, follow-up can be discontinued at 12 months in case of volume stability at 3 and 12 months or for nodules with VDT ≥400 days at 3 months and >600 days at 1 year.

For larger nodules (≥8 mm or ≥300 mm^3 according to the BTS or ≥8 mm or >250 mm^3 according to the Fleischner Society guidelines), there are various options, including 3-month follow-up, PET-CT, or tissue sampling. According to the Fleischner Society guidelines, the choice is guided by the nodule morphology, whereas in the BTS guidelines, the choice depends on the Brock model (Table 1) (McWilliams et al. 2013).

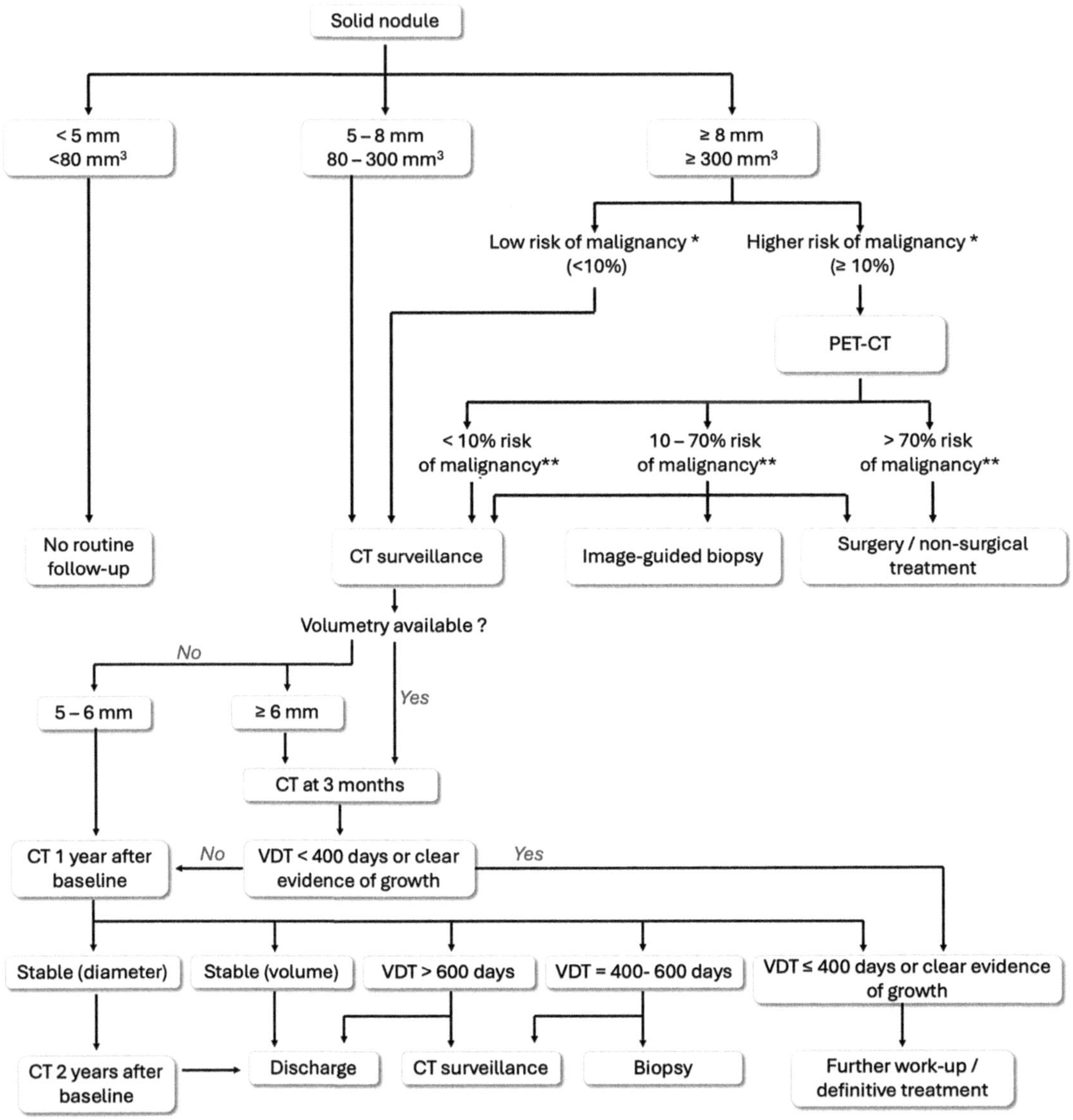

Fig. 10 Guidelines of the British Thoracic Society for the management of solid nodules. (Adapted from Baldwin and Callister (2015)). *Note:* * Using Brock Model. ** Using Herder model. *VDT = volume doubling time*

5.1.2 Subsolid Nodules

Both BTS and Fleischner Society guidelines agree that follow-up is not recommended for small subsolid nodules (<5 mm according to the BTS or <6 mm according to the Fleischner Society guidelines), except in cases of multiple subsolid nodules, for which the Fleischner Society recommends to consider CT follow-up at 3–6 months, 2 years, and 4 years.

For larger subsolid nodules (≥5 mm according to the BTS or ≥6 mm according to Fleischner Society guidelines), only the Fleischner guidelines differentiate between pure GGNs and part-solid GGNs. In BTS guidelines, all nodules should be re-evaluated at 3 months, whereas according to the Fleischner guidelines, pure GGNs should be re-evaluated at 6–12 months and part-solid GGNs at 3 months. The major

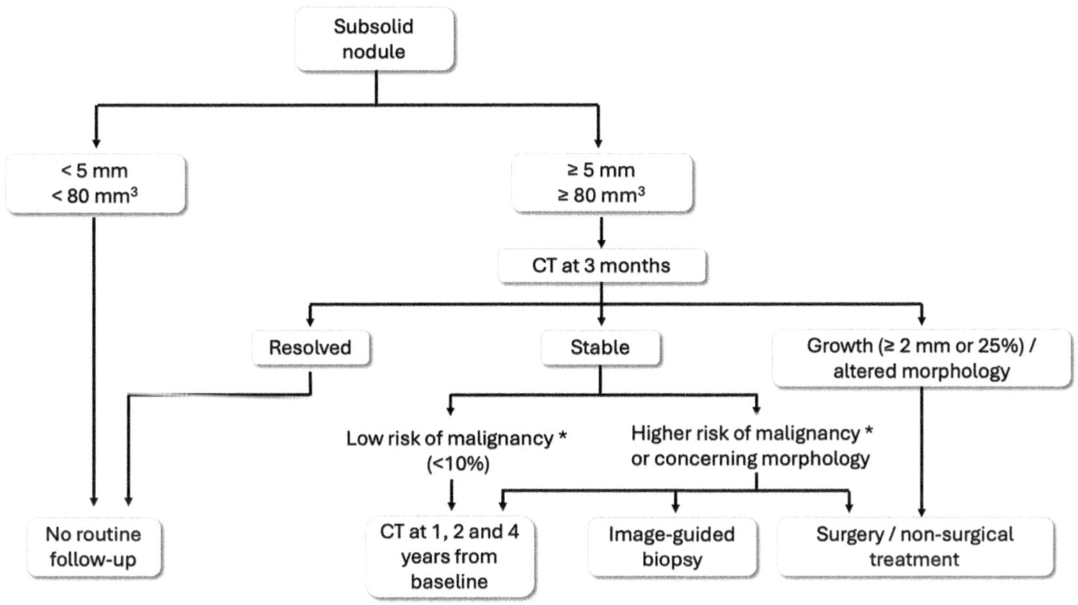

Fig. 11 Guidelines of the British Thoracic Society for the management of subsolid nodules. (Adapted from Baldwin and Callister (2015)). *Note: * Using Brock Model VDT = volume doubling time*

interest at this stage is to evaluate the persistence or not of the subsolid nodules. As a recall, around 60% of them will disappear, owing to their inflammatory or infectious nature. In both cases, the criteria for further workup or resection are an increase in size ≥2 mm or in attenuation (Azour et al. 2021), the appearance or increase in size of a solid component ≥2 mm, the presence of suspicious morphological criteria (lobulated margins or cystic components), or a solid component ≥8 mm (only for the Fleischner guidelines). Subsolid nodule follow-up lasts longer than for solid nodules (4 and 5 years according to BTS and Fleischner guidelines, respectively). The interest of follow-up greater than 5 years has also been discussed (Lee et al. 2019b; Herskovitz et al. 2022).

For pure GGNs, it is important to note that in the Multicentric Italian Lung Detection (MILD) study, the progression rate of these nodules towards clinically relevant disease was extremely low, which supports an active surveillance attitude instead of surgical resection (Silva et al. 2012).

To note, in all cases, a careful reading should look at new solid nodules that may have a more aggressive course than the subsolid one followed (Schreuder et al. 2021).

5.1.3 Atypical Pulmonary Cysts

Atypical lung cysts are not included in the Fleischner Society and BTS recommendations. However, Lung-RADS v2022, which applies to lung screening, recommends a 3-month follow-up (Christensen et al. 2024). If a comparison with the previous examination is available, a 6-month follow-up is recommended if the cystic component is growing, and a 3-month follow-up is recommended if a thick-walled unilocular cyst becomes multilocular. Further referral for clinical evaluation, PET-CT, or biopsy is recommended if the wall thickness or nodularity increases, if the size or loculation of a multilocular cyst increases, or if a nodular, ground glass, or consolidation component increases in size or density. These recommendations do not apply to thin-walled cysts (wall thickness <2 mm) and diffuse cystic lung disease.

5.2 Lung Cancer Screening

The management strategies adopted in lung cancer screening programs are inspired by the two major clinical trials that demonstrated the efficacy of screening: National Lung Cancer Screening (NLST) and Nelson. The main difference between these strategies and the guidelines for incidentally detected nodules is that a follow-up at 1 or 2 years will be systematically performed as part of the screening, whereas this is not the case outside this context. Their aim is therefore to identify nodules requiring management within this timeframe. The Lung-RADS recommendation by the American College of Radiology was updated in 2022 (Lung-RADS v2022) (Christensen et al. 2024). Compared to its previous version 1.1, Lung-RADS v2022 now includes, in addition to cystic lesions, nodule volumetry, which should be used by default nowadays. Lung-RADS v2022 is presented in Table 2.

6 Conclusion

In conclusion, measurements play a pivotal role in the management of pulmonary nodules, as the management strategy largely depends on size. Volumetric measurements should be preferred whenever possible, especially for solid nodules, as they allow a more accurate assessment of growth. It is important to bear in mind, however, that volumetric measurements are in particular software-dependent, and, in addition to similar acquisition CT conditions, it is imperative to use the same software for consecutive measurements in the same patient.

Disclaimer All measurements in this book have been obtained from peer-reviewed papers and guidelines from professional organizations, unless explicitly stated otherwise. While the authors, editors, and publisher have gone through a rigorous process to establish their correct reproduction from the original source, each measurement must be interpreted in the correct clinical context, this along with an accurate way of measurement, and taking into account all technical variables, this including follow-up exams with various equipment or software. Neither the authors, the editors, nor the publisher can accept any legal responsibility for any improper application or interpretation of these measurements as well as their potential consequences.

References

Aherne EA, Plodkowski AJ, Montecalvo J, Hayan S, Zheng J, Capanu M et al (2018) What CT characteristics of lepidic predominant pattern lung adenocarcinomas correlate with invasiveness on pathology? Lung Cancer 118:83–89. https://doi.org/10.1016/j.lungcan.2018.01.013

Ahn MI, Gleeson TG, Chan IH, McWilliams AM, MacDonald SL, Lam S et al (2010) Perifissural nodules seen at CT screening for lung cancer. Radiology 254:949–956. https://doi.org/10.1148/radiol.09090031

AlShammari A, Patel A, Boyle M, Proli C, Gallesio JA, Wali A et al (2024) Prevalence of invasive lung cancer in pure ground glass nodules less than 30 mm: a systematic review. Eur J Cancer 213:115116. https://doi.org/10.1016/j.ejca.2024.115116

Arai T, Kuroishi T, Saito Y, Kurita Y, Naruke T, Kaneko M (1994) Tumor doubling time and prognosis in lung cancer patients: evaluation from chest films and clinical follow-up study. Japanese Lung Cancer Screening Research Group. Jpn J Clin Oncol 24:199–204

Azour L, Ko JP, Naidich DP, Moore WH (2021) Shades of gray: subsolid nodule considerations and management. Chest 159:2072–2089. https://doi.org/10.1016/j.chest.2020.09.252

Baldwin DR, Callister ME (2015) The British Thoracic Society guidelines on the investigation and management of pulmonary nodules. Thorax 70:794–798. https://doi.org/10.1136/thoraxjnl-2015-207221

Bankier AA, MacMahon H, Goo JM, Rubin GD, Schaefer-Prokop CM, Naidich DP (2017) Recommendations for measuring pulmonary nodules at CT: a statement from the Fleischner Society. Radiology 285:584–600. https://doi.org/10.1148/radiol.2017162894

Bankier AA, MacMahon H, Colby T, Gevenois PA, Goo JM, Leung ANC et al (2024) Fleischner Society: glossary of terms for thoracic imaging. Radiology 310:e232558. https://doi.org/10.1148/radiol.232558

Barnett J, Pulzato I, Wilson R, Padley S, Nicholson AG, Devaraj A (2019) Perinodular vascularity distinguishes benign intrapulmonary lymph nodes from lung cancer on computed tomography. J Thorac Imaging 34:326–328. https://doi.org/10.1097/RTI.0000000000000394

Beig N, Khorrami M, Alilou M, Prasanna P, Braman N, Orooji M et al (2019) Perinodular and intranodular radiomic features on lung CT images distinguish adenocarcinomas from granulomas. Radiology 290:783–792. https://doi.org/10.1148/radiol.2018180910

Christensen J, Prosper AE, Wu CC, Chung J, Lee E, Elicker B et al (2024) ACR lung-RADS v2022:

assessment categories and management recommendations. Chest 165:738–753. https://doi.org/10.1016/j.chest.2023.10.028

De Hoop B, Van Ginneken B, Gietema H, Prokop M (2012) Pulmonary perifissural nodules on CT scans: rapid growth is not a predictor of malignancy. Radiology 265:611–616. https://doi.org/10.1148/radiol.12112351

Devaraj A, Van Ginneken B, Nair A, Baldwin D (2017) Use of volumetry for lung nodule management: theory and practice. Radiology 284:630–644. https://doi.org/10.1148/radiol.2017151022

Gietema HA, Schaefer-Prokop CM, Mali WPTM, Groenewegen G, Prokop M (2007) Pulmonary nodules: interscan variability of semiautomated volume measurements with multisection CT—influence of inspiration level, nodule size, and segmentation performance. Radiology 245:888–894. https://doi.org/10.1148/radiol.2452061054

Han D, Heuvelmans MA, Vliegenthart R, Rook M, Dorrius MD, De Jonge GJ et al (2018) Influence of lung nodule margin on volume- and diameter-based reader variability in CT lung cancer screening. Br J Radiol 91:20170405. https://doi.org/10.1259/bjr.20170405

Hasegawa M, Sone S, Takashima S, Li F, Yang ZG, Maruyama Y et al (2000) Growth rate of small lung cancers detected on mass CT screening. Br J Radiol 73:1252–1259. https://doi.org/10.1259/bjr.73.876.11205667

Herskovitz E, Solomides C, Barta J, Evans N, Kane G (2022) Detection of lung carcinoma arising from ground glass opacities (GGO) after 5 years – a retrospective review. Respir Med 196:106803. https://doi.org/10.1016/j.rmed.2022.106803

Horeweg N, van Rosmalen J, Heuvelmans MA, van der Aalst CM, Vliegenthart R, Scholten ET et al (2014) Lung cancer probability in patients with CT-detected pulmonary nodules: a prespecified analysis of data from the NELSON trial of low-dose CT screening. Lancet Oncol 15:1332–1341. https://doi.org/10.1016/S1470-2045(14)70389-4

Kim HY, Shim YM, Lee KS, Han J, Yi CA, Kim YK (2007) Persistent pulmonary nodular ground-glass opacity at thin-section CT: histopathologic comparisons. Radiology 245:267–275. https://doi.org/10.1148/radiol.2451061682

Lee HY, Lee KS (2011) Ground-glass opacity nodules: histopathology, imaging evaluation, and clinical implications. J Thorac Imaging 26:106–118. https://doi.org/10.1097/RTI.0b013e3181fbaa64

Lee GD, Park CH, Park HS, Byun MK, Lee IJ, Kim TH et al (2019a) Lung adenocarcinoma invasiveness risk in pure ground-glass opacity lung nodules smaller than 2 cm. Thorac Cardiovasc Surg 67:321–328. https://doi.org/10.1055/s-0037-1612615

Lee HW, Jin K-N, Lee J-K, Kim DK, Chung HS, Heo EY et al (2019b) Long-term follow-up of ground-glass nodules after 5 years of stability. J Thorac Oncol 14:1370–1377. https://doi.org/10.1016/j.jtho.2019.05.005

MacMahon H, Naidich DP, Goo JM, Lee KS, Leung ANC, Mayo JR et al (2017) Guidelines for management of incidental pulmonary nodules detected on CT images: from the Fleischner Society 2017. Radiology:161659. https://doi.org/10.1148/radiol.2017161659

Martin MD, Kanne JP, Broderick LS, Kazerooni EA, Meyer CA (2017) Lung-RADS: pushing the limits. Radiographics 37:1975–1993. https://doi.org/10.1148/rg.2017170051

Martinez Trevino EF, Sohail M, Mijares-Rojas IA, Qaddorah S, Levenson A (n.d.) Endobronchial obstruction: a case of well-differentiated liposarcoma. Cureus 16:e57731. https://doi.org/10.7759/cureus.57731

McWilliams A, Tammemagi MC, Mayo JR, Roberts H, Liu G, Soghrati K et al (2013) Probability of cancer in pulmonary nodules detected on first screening CT. N Engl J Med 369:910–919. https://doi.org/10.1056/NEJMoa1214726

Mehta HJ, Ravenel JG, Shaftman SR, Tanner NT, Paoletti L, Taylor KK et al (2014) The utility of nodule volume in the context of malignancy prediction for small pulmonary nodules. Chest 145:464–472. https://doi.org/10.1378/chest.13-0708

Naidich DP, Bankier AA, MacMahon H, Schaefer-Prokop CM, Pistolesi M, Goo JM et al (2013) Recommendations for the management of subsolid pulmonary nodules detected at CT: a statement from the Fleischner Society. Radiology 266:304–317. https://doi.org/10.1148/radiol.12120628

Park S, Lee SM, Kim S, Lee J-G, Choi S, Do K-H et al (2020) Volume doubling times of lung adenocarcinomas: correlation with predominant histologic subtypes and prognosis. Radiology 295:703–712. https://doi.org/10.1148/radiol.2020191835

Peters AA, Christe A, Von Stackelberg O, Pohl M, Kauczor H-U, Heußel CP et al (2023) "Will I change nodule management recommendations if I change my CAD system?"—impact of volumetric deviation between different CAD systems on lesion management. Eur Radiol. https://doi.org/10.1007/s00330-023-09525-z

Revel M-P, Bissery A, Bienvenu M, Aycard L, Lefort C, Frija G (2004) Are two-dimensional CT measurements of small noncalcified pulmonary nodules reliable? Radiology 231:453–458. https://doi.org/10.1148/radiol.2312030167

Revel M-P, Mannes I, Benzakoun J, Guinet C, Léger T, Grenier P et al (2018) Subsolid lung nodule classification: a CT criterion for improving interobserver agreement. Radiology 286:316–325. https://doi.org/10.1148/radiol.2017170044

Ryan JW, Hammer MM (2023) Growth rates of pulmonary carcinoid tumors and hamartomas. J Comput Assist Tomogr 47:396–401. https://doi.org/10.1097/RCT.0000000000001413

Schreuder A, van Ginneken B, Scholten ET, Jacobs C, Prokop M, Sverzellati N et al (2018) Classification of CT pulmonary opacities as perifissural nodules: reader variability. Radiology 288:867–875. https://doi.org/10.1148/radiol.2018172771

Schreuder A, Jacobs C, Scholten ET, van Ginneken B, Schaefer-Prokop CM, Prokop M (2020) Typical CT features of intrapulmonary lymph nodes: a review. Radiol: Cardiothorac Imaging 2:e190159. https://doi.org/10.1148/ryct.2020190159

Schreuder A, Prokop M, Scholten ET, Mets OM, Chung K, Mohamed Hoesein FAA et al (2021) CT-detected subsolid nodules: a predictor of lung cancer development at another location? Cancers (Basel) 13:2812. https://doi.org/10.3390/cancers13112812

Siegelman SS, Khouri NF, Scott WW, Leo FP, Hamper UM, Fishman EK et al (1986) Pulmonary hamartoma: CT findings. Radiology 160:313–317. https://doi.org/10.1148/radiology.160.2.3726106

Silva M, Sverzellati N, Manna C, Negrini G, Marchianò A, Zompatori M et al (2012) Long-term surveillance of ground-glass nodules: evidence from the MILD trial. J Thorac Oncol 7:1541–1546. https://doi.org/10.1097/JTO.0b013e3182641bba

Snoeckx A, Reyntiens P, Desbuquoit D, Spinhoven MJ, Van Schil PE, Van Meerbeeck JP et al (2018) Evaluation of the solitary pulmonary nodule: size matters, but do not ignore the power of morphology. Insights Imaging 9:73–86. https://doi.org/10.1007/s13244-017-0581-2

Sun Y, Li C, Jin L, Gao P, Zhao W, Ma W et al (2020) Radiomics for lung adenocarcinoma manifesting as pure ground-glass nodules: invasive prediction. Eur Radiol 30:3650–3659. https://doi.org/10.1007/s00330-020-06776-y

Swensen SJ (1997) The probability of malignancy in solitary pulmonary nodules. Application to small radiologically indeterminate nodules. Arch Intern Med 157:849–855. https://doi.org/10.1001/archinte.157.8.849

Takashima S, Sone S, Li F, Maruyama Y, Hasegawa M, Kadoya M (2003) Indeterminate solitary pulmonary nodules revealed at population-based CT screening of the lung: using first follow-up diagnostic CT to differentiate benign and malignant lesions. AJR Am J Roentgenol 180:1255–1263. https://doi.org/10.2214/ajr.180.5.1801255

van Klaveren RJ, Prokop M, Nackaerts K (2009) Management of lung nodules detected by volume CT scanning. N Engl J Med 361(23):2221–2229

Webb WR (1990) Radiologic evaluation of the solitary pulmonary nodule. AJR Am J Roentgenol 154:701–708. https://doi.org/10.2214/ajr.154.4.2107661

Wormanns D, Beyer F, Diederich S, Ludwig K, Heindel W (2004) Diagnostic performance of a commercially available computer-aided diagnosis system for automatic detection of pulmonary nodules: comparison with single and double reading. Rofo 176:953–958. https://doi.org/10.1055/s-2004-813251

Yip R, Henschke CI, Xu DM, Li K, Jirapatnakul A, Yankelevitz DF (2017) Lung cancers manifesting as part-solid nodules in the national lung screening trial. Am J Roentgenol 208:1011–1021. https://doi.org/10.2214/AJR.16.16930

Follow Up After Chemo/Immunotherapy

Caroline Caramella

Contents

C. Caramella (✉)
Department of Radiology, Hôpitaux Paris Saint-Joseph et Marie Lannelongue, International Center for Thoracic Cancers, Le Plessis Robinson, France

Laboratoire d'Imagerie Biomédicale Multimodale Paris-Saclay, BIOMAPS, UMR 1281, Université Paris-Saclay, Inserm, CNRS, CEA, Villejuif, France
e-mail: ca.caramella@ghpsj.fr

Abstract

Imaging plays a central role in the follow-up of patients under systemic treatment for advanced or metastatic cancers, both in clinical trials and in routine. Indeed, measurements of tumoral lesions have always been used to monitor treatment efficacy: Before imaging, clinical examination was requested, and the reliability and reproducibility of tumor evaluation were already questioned. In 1981, the World Health Organization (WHO) published recommendations for "reporting results in cancer treatment": The goal of this publication was "to make it possible for investigators to compare validly their results with those of others." These first recommendations paved the way to tumor evaluation with imaging. Nowadays, its use in cancer patient monitoring is mandatory in clinical trials with the adoption of Response Evaluation Criteria in Solid Tumors (RECIST) that were proposed by an international academic working group and largely accepted in the oncologic community. Nevertheless, due to the rapidly evolving landscape of anticancer therapies targeting different tumor components, RECIST criteria are sometimes insufficient for treatment assessment, and other criteria can be used. This chapter aims at describing the principles of tumor evaluation on imaging.

Med Radiol Diagn Imaging (2026)

https://doi.org/10.1007/174_2025_603,
Published Online: 24 August 2025

Abbreviations

CR	Complete response
CT	Computed tomography
CTLA4	Cytotoxic-T-lymphocyte-antigen 4 protein
DFS	Disease-free survival
EFS	Event-free survival
EMA	European Medical Agency
EORTC	European Organization for Research and Treatment of Cancer
FDA	Food and Drug Administration (US)
iCPD	Immune confirmed progressive disease
iRECIST	Immune-RECIST
iUPD	Immune unconfirmed progressive disease
MRI	Magnetic resonance imaging
NCI	National Cancer Institute (US)
NCIC	National Cancer Institute of Canada
ORR	Overall response rate
OS	Overall survival
PD	Progressive disease
PD1	Programmed cell death protein 1
PDL1	Programmed cell death-Ligand 1
PET-CT	Positron emission tomography coupled with computed tomography
PFS	Progression free survival
PR	Partial response
RECIST	Response Evaluation Criteria in Solid Tumors
SD	Stable disease
TFF	Time to treatment failure
TGR	Tumor growth rate
WB-MRI	Whole body magnetic resonance imaging
WHO	World Health Organization

1 Tumor Evaluation in Cancer Trials: History

Measurements of tumoral nodules or masses have always been used to monitor treatment efficacy: Before the advent of imaging, tumor evolution was based on clinical examination, and the reliability and reproducibility of tumor evaluation were already questioned (Moertel and Hanley 1976). In 1981, the World Health Organization (WHO) published recommendations for "reporting results in cancer treatment": The goal of this publication was "to make it possible for investigators to compare validly their results with those of others." This was the first introduction of imaging (either chest X-ray or CT) for this topic. They proposed to define tumor response when a decrease of at least 50% of the bidimensional measurable tumoral burden was achieved and progression when an increase of at least 25% was observed (Miller et al. 1981).

These first recommendations paved the way to tumor evaluation in imaging. As expected, imaging became widely available; its use in cancer patient monitoring became mandatory in clinical trials. Subsequently, the need for more precise guidelines (i.e., the definition of a measurable nodule, the number of nodules and technical issues) led to the publication of the RECIST (Response Evaluation Criteria in Solid Tumors) by a working group of European, Canadian and American organizations (EORTC, NCI, NCIC) in 2000 (Therasse et al. 2000). Although the oncologic community quickly adopted these criteria, many practical issues remained, and the same organization published a new version (RECIST v1.1) in 2009 (Eisenhauer et al. 2009). These RECIST 1.1 guidelines are still the reference standard for evaluating the effectiveness of solid tumor treatment in current clinical trials. The Food and Drug Administration (FDA) guidance for industry specified that "if available, standardized criteria should be used to ascertain response. A variety of response criteria have been considered appropriate (e.g., revised RECIST guideline (version 1.1)). The response criteria should be predefined in the protocol before the start of the study." (Clinical Trial 2018) The European Medical Agency (EMA) also recommended that overall response rate should be documented according to international standards (e.g., RECIST, volumetric RECIST or WHO criteria (ema.europa.eu)).

2 New Drug Development, an Overview

The development of novel anticancer therapies is a real challenge. Each new molecule that has shown a potential interest for cancer patients after preclinical testing needs to be tested through a complex pipeline of three phases of trials before it might be validated and endorsed for clinical prescription. According to the EMA guideline, phases I and II are exploratory studies, and phase III constitutes the confirmatory trials (Guideline on the evaluation of anticancer medicinal products in man EMA/CHMP/205/95 Rev. 6).

Briefly, phase I studies are proposed to patients who will receive for the "first-in-human" time the new treatment. The main objective is to define dose-limiting toxicities with a dose-escalation method in order to determine the optimal therapeutic dosage. Phase II studies may investigate single-agent activity in a variety of tumor types, or in a selected tumor type, or investigate the activity and feasibility of combination or multimodality regimens. Finally, phase III trials compare the activity of the new treatment with the reference therapy, generally with a randomized and blinded design.

In comparative studies, the effectiveness of the new drug will be generally based on survival: Basically, if the group of randomized patients who received the new treatment has a statistically significant better survival than the group receiving standard of care, then the drug will become a good candidate for final approval. More and more, trials also take care of toxicity and quality of life of patients.

2.1 How Is Survival Evaluated? Endpoints in Cancer Treatments

There are two main endpoints, namely overall survival (OS) and progression-free survival (PFS). Nevertheless, many others can be defined, such as EFS (event-free survival), DFS (disease-free survival), ORR (overall response rate) or TFF (time to treatment failure).

OS is the time interval from randomization to death (from any cause) of the patients. It can be easily measured and is objective. For patients who will live longer, the assessment of OS increases the length of the trial, thus delaying the potential clinical availability of a new effective treatment. For this reason, PFS is of interest. It is defined as the time from randomization to objective tumor progression or death. If the new treatment allows a delay in the time to progression, then it may be assumed that it will translate into a better OS, although this remains controversial (Fleming et al. 2009). That said, the precise definition of "progression" constitutes a real challenge. New cancer treatment development is a very competitive and costly field, while many cancer patients are hoping for new effective drugs.

2.2 How to Evaluate the Treatment, What Is a Progression?

Clinical symptoms of progression are systematically reported in clinical trials. However, they are difficult to assess and subjective. For this reason, the need for an objective definition of progression has led to the development of "biomarkers," mainly based on imaging. Imaging allows for an objective capture of tumor size, and the modification of this parameter is recognized as a good biomarker for response evaluation.

2.2.1 The WHO Criteria

Although the WHO criteria (Miller et al. 1981; Haanen and Robert 2015) were published in 1981, they are still recommended for cancer evaluation, mainly in lymphoma. According to the reference paper, disease should be described as "measurable, bidimensional (2D); measurable, unidimensional or non-measurable but evaluable." They were published at a time when CT was not widely available, but it was the first introduction of imaging in this topic, which explains that some of the recommendations are not considered anymore: e.g., "mediastinal and hilar involvement may be measured (…) by subtract-

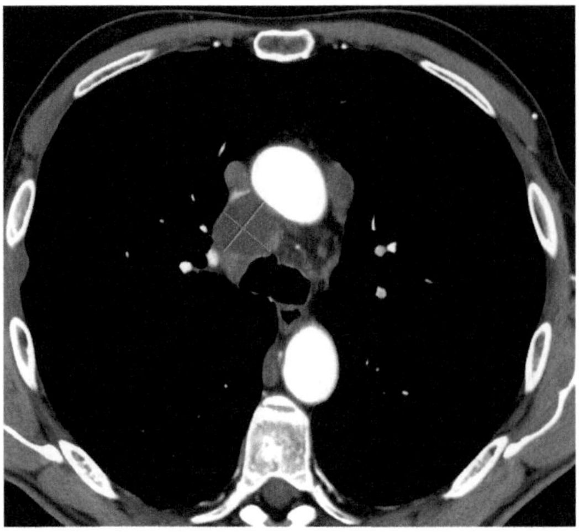

Fig. 1 According to WHO recommendation, in this patient with lymphoma, the paratracheal adenomegaly must be measured as the product of the longest diameter by the largest perpendicular diameter

ing the normal mediastinal or hilar width on the pre-involvement X-ray from the on-study width."

In current clinical trials, with the use of CT, the WHO guidelines specify the 2D assessment of tumoral nodules/lymph nodes as "determined by multiplying the longest diameter by the largest perpendicular diameter" and reported as a surface area (Fig. 1).

Progressive disease (PD) is defined as a "25% or more increase in the size of one or more measurable lesions or the appearance of new lesion(s)." In parallel, partial response (PR) is defined as a "50% or more decrease in total tumor load of the lesions (i.e., the sum of the surface area if multiple lesions are measured), without new lesion or progression of any lesion." In between, evaluation is considered as "no change."

2.2.2 The RECIST 1.1

The RECIST 1.1 criteria are the reference standard for evaluating the efficacy of solid tumor treatment in clinical trials (Eisenhauer et al. 2009). They are cited in the FDA guidance for industry, although they specify that "the response criteria should be predefined in the protocol before the start of the study."

In the following subchapter, we will overview the RECIST 1.1: definition of baseline, Nadir, target lesions, nontarget lesions, considerations about target measurability, especially in bone lesions, detection of new lesions and response evaluation. Thereafter, we will give a brief summary of the main differences with the previous 1.0 version.

2.2.2.1 Definition of Baseline and Nadir

The baseline examination is the first reference exam on which target lesion(s) and nontarget lesion(s) are defined. Theoretically, the treatment begins shortly after the baseline examination.

The Nadir is the examination on which the best response is observed compared to baseline. Consecutively, the Nadir can change during follow-up. The knowledge of Nadir is crucial to assess a progression, which may happen after a period of response (i.e., relapse). An illustration is given in Fig. 2.

2.2.2.2 Definition of Target Lesion

A target lesion is a nodule that is selected at baseline (i.e., imaging that is performed right before the initiation of a new treatment) with the following requirements: A nodule that is certainly tumoral can be accurately measured in at least one dimension and is ≥10 mm.

RECIST 1.1 gave an additional requirement for lymph nodes. Indeed, non-pathological lymph node can have a long axis of more than 10 mm. Moreover, the long axis of a node may change in orientation with time and therefore does not ensure an accurate measurement, conversely to the short axis. For these reasons, lymph nodes should be measured in their short axis (i.e., the largest perpendicular diameter to the longest diameter), with a size ≥15 mm to be considered as a target lesion (Fig. 3). To note, smaller nodes may be malignant and are a known limit of RECIST 1.1 criteria. These small nodes are best depicted by PET-CT. The latter point will be discussed in the dedicated chapter.

In RECIST 1.1, 5 target lesions may be selected with a maximum of 2 per organ. The sum of the size of the target lesion(s) defines the overall tumor burden, to which subsequent measurements will be compared. The percentage of change in the sum of target lesion(s) will be key

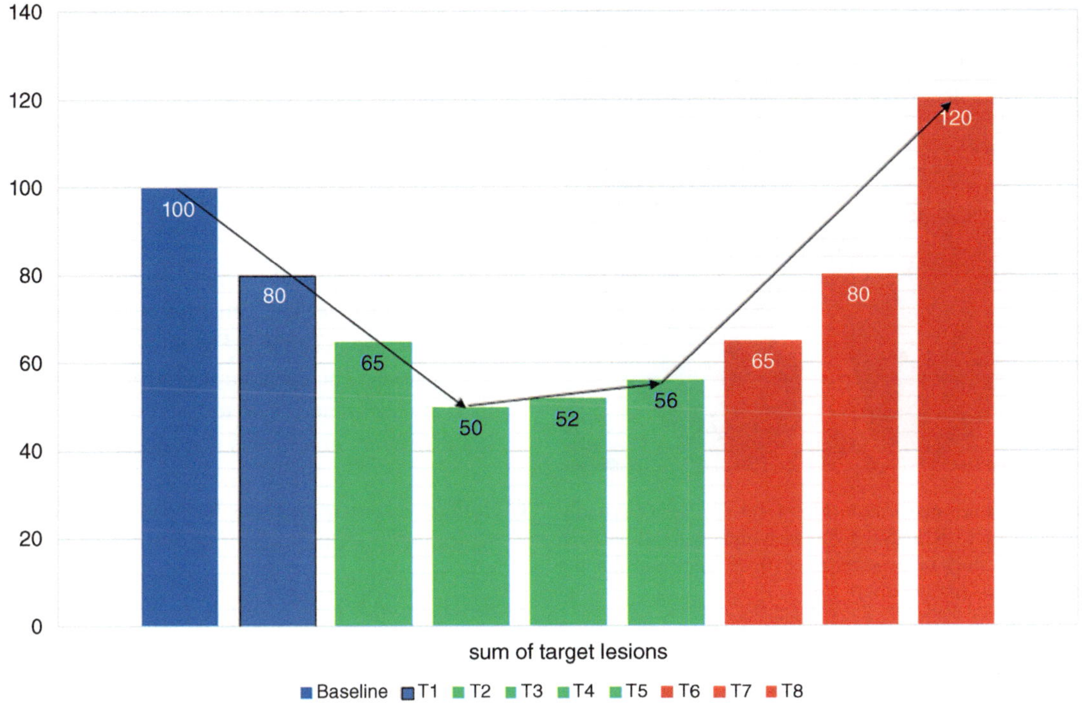

Fig. 2 In this example, at Baseline, the sum of target lesions is 100 mm. Assuming there is no nontarget lesion and there will be no new lesion during follow-up
At T1, the sum of target lesions is 80. The conclusion will then be stable disease (−20%) compared to baseline. This evaluation T1 then becomes the Nadir (best observed response so far)
At T2, the sum of target lesions is 65 mm. The conclusion will then be partial response (−35%) compared to baseline. This evaluation T2 then becomes the new Nadir (best observed response so far)
At T3, the sum of target lesions is 50 mm. The conclusion will then be partial response (−50%) compared to baseline. This evaluation T3 then becomes once again the new Nadir (best observed response so far)
At T4, the sum of target lesions is 52 mm. The conclusion will then be partial response (−48%) compared to baseline, no progression compared to Nadir (+4%) (T3)
At T5, the sum of target lesions is 56 mm. The conclusion will then be partial response (−44%), compared to baseline, no progression compared to Nadir (+12%) (T3)
At T6, the sum of target lesions is 65 mm. The conclusion will then be progressive disease compared to Nadir (T3) because of the increase in the sum of target lesions of 30% (more than 20%)
T7 and T8 are an illustration of the potential continued growth of the disease if the progression was not depicted at T6

for the final evaluation. The same target lesion(s) and method of evaluation must be used at each time point. The number of targets to be considered will be described later.

The choice of target lesion(s) depends on their size (those with the longest diameter with no upper limit) and their suitability for accurate repeated measurements. CT and MRI are the best currently available and most reproducible methods for morphological assessment. For skin lesions, documentation by color photography including a ruler is required. Chest X-ray is acceptable only for lesions that are clearly defined and surrounded by aerated lung. Ultrasound should not be used to measure tumor lesions.

2.2.2.3 Definition of Nontarget Lesion

A nontarget lesion is defined as a certainly tumoral lesion that cannot be selected as a target lesion either because the lesion has a size <1 cm, or because the lesion is not measurable, such as effusion or lymphangitic carcinomatosis. In RECIST 1.1 guidelines, lymph nodes that have a short axis ≥10 and <14 mm are considered non-

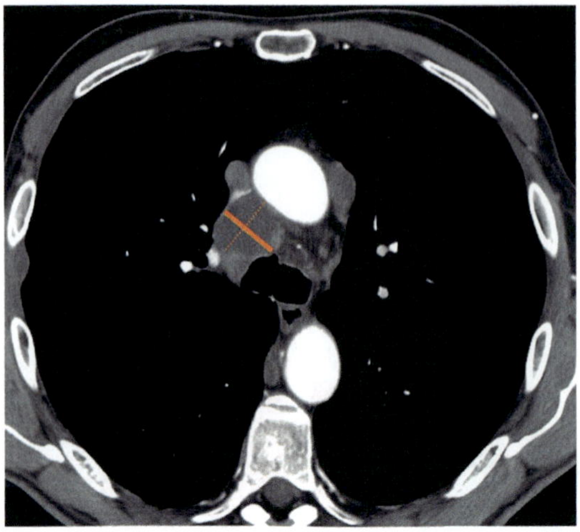

Fig. 3 Same image as in Fig. 1 for the WHO criteria. According to RECIST 1.1, the lymph node should be measured only in its short axis (thick line) and not the longest axis (dotted line)

target lesions. During follow-up, nontarget lesions will be assessed qualitatively as a unique entity, and the response will be defined as complete response, persistent, or unequivocal progression. An unequivocal progression is defined as "an overall level of substantial worsening in nontarget disease that is of a magnitude that, even in the presence of stable disease or partial response in target lesions, the treating physician would feel it important to change therapy" (Eisenhauer et al. 2009).

2.2.2.4 Other Considerations Regarding Lesion Measurability

Bone lesions are considered as nontarget lesions unless they are lytic and have an "identifiable soft tissue component" that can be measured and considered as a target lesion (i.e., ≥10 mm). Lesions located in previously irradiated areas or other focal therapies are not considered as target lesions unless they have demonstrated progression (Eisenhauer et al. 2009).

Of note, lesions that have been treated by focal therapy (stereotactic radiotherapy or thermal ablation) may not be considered as target lesions. Indeed, a successful focal treatment may result in a lesion larger than the primary target. Thus, they must not be selected as target lesions unless there is evidence of local recurrence.

2.2.2.5 Definition of New Lesion

New lesions are only assessed during follow-up examinations. They are defined as definitely tumoral lesions that were not present at baseline.

2.2.2.6 Evaluation of Target Lesions, Nontarget Lesions and New Lesions (Table 1, Fig. 2)

Target Lesions: The same target lesions that were defined at baseline must be measured.

Four different conditions may occur:

Complete response (CR) is the complete disappearance of all target lesions and all nontarget lesions, and no new lesion is detected.

Partial response (PR) is defined as ≥30% decrease in the sum of the diameters of target lesions, while nontarget lesions are not unequivocally progressive and there is no new lesion. A PR is also achieved in case of a complete response of target lesion, while non target lesions did not all disappear in the absence of any new lesion.

A special consideration must be given to response in lymph nodes that have been chosen as target lesions. They are considered in CR as soon as their short axis is <10 mm (even though their size has still to be recorded in the sum of the measurements of target lesions) (Fig. 4).

Progressive disease (PD) is defined as a ≥20% increase in the sum of the diameters of target lesions and/or the unequivocal progression of nontarget lesions and/or the appearance of new lesion(s) (Fig. 5).

Stable disease (SD) is defined as a change in the sum of the diameter of target lesions that is neither sufficient to qualify for PR nor PD.

2.2.2.7 Differences Between RECIST 1.0 and RECIST 1.1

Although nowadays, the great majority of trials using RECIST criteria are based on its 1.1 version, a reminder of the main differences between the first version and the latter is given in the

Table 1 RECIST 1.1 assessment of target lesion(s), nontarget lesion(s) and new lesion(s) and their corresponding final conclusion

Target lesion(s) assessment	Nontarget lesion(s) assessment	New lesion(s)	Conclusion of the evaluation
Complete Response	Complete Response	No	Complete Response
Complete Response	No complete response and no progression	No	Partial Response
Partial Response (regression >30%)	No complete response and no progression	No	Partial Response
Stable Disease (between −30% and +20%)	No complete response and no progression	No	Stable Disease
Progressive disease (progression >20%)	Whatever	Whatever	Progressive Disease
Whatever	Unequivocal progression	Whatever	Progressive Disease
Whatever	Whatever	Yes	Progressive Disease

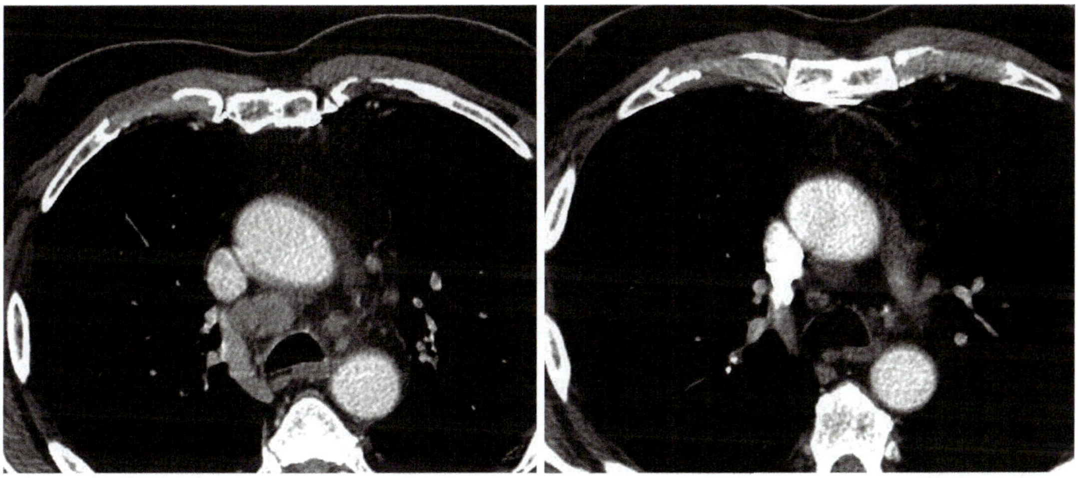

Fig. 4 On the left, a pathological mediastinal lymph node (short axis of 15 mm) at baseline is shown in station R4. On the right, after chemotherapy, the size of the lymph node becomes lower than 10 mm (in this case, around 5 mm). This lymph node is considered in complete response even though its size is still measurable and should be reported in the sum of target lesions

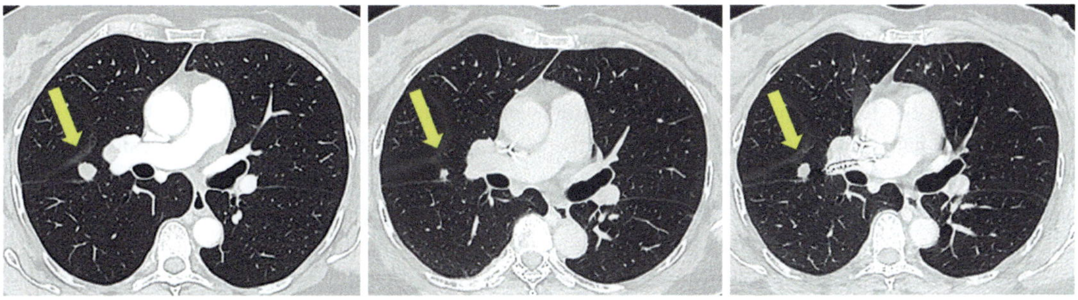

Fig. 5 Three consecutive images in a patient with metastatic lung cancer. On the left baseline evaluation shows a 14 mm right upper lobe nodule, which is selected as target lesion. In the middle, the first evaluation shows a decrease in the nodule size (5 mm). On the right, a subsequent evaluation shows a progression in the size of the nodule (12 mm)

RECIST 1.1 paper (Therasse et al. 2000; Eisenhauer et al. 2009). The main differences are the number of target lesions that can be selected (up to 10 in RECIST 1.0 with a maximum of 5 lesions per organ and only up to 5 in the 1.1 version with a maximum of 2 per organ) and the clarification in the management of lymph nodes.

3 Other Criteria

The development of new therapeutic agents in oncology, with different mechanisms of action, led to the ascertainment of new tumoral behavior under treatment and the need to adapt tumor evaluation by imaging, accordingly. Many new "criteria" were then proposed, for example CHOI criteria for the assessment of gastrointestinal stromal tumors (GIST) receiving imatinib, or EASL (European Association for the Study of the Liver) criteria for the assessment of hepatocarcinomas.

However, as of today, the FDA authorities don't directly recognize any of them. Their use must be justified in clinical trial files, and their results are reported in a separate chapter of the results of clinical trials.

More recently, a new family of drugs has been discovered and has rapidly gained a major place in the treatment of several types of cancers: checkpoint inhibitors (generally referred to as "immunotherapy").

3.1 Immunotherapy

Immunotherapy is a general term describing the compounds that would treat diseases by stimulating the immune response. A lot of research has been done in this field of oncology, but a major breakthrough happened in the late 2000s with the discovery and use of monoclonal antibodies targeting "immune check points inhibitors," i.e., the relationship between T-cells and tumor cells.

The first targeted cancer for immunotherapy was metastatic melanoma. Anti-CTLA4 and anti-PD1/PDL-1 treatment successively showed an improvement in the survival of these patients (Haanen and Robert 2015). Thereafter, many new cancer types and new molecules were (and are still) pushed under trials. Although the main characteristic of immune response remains a decrease of the tumor burden, new response patterns were also observed.

Pseudo-progression is defined as an initial increase of the tumor burden, followed by a decrease. This phenomenon resulting from massive influx of lymphocytes in the tumor was described in the first trials involving melanoma patients in up to 10% of cases. Following this observation, new guidelines were proposed: the main rule was to continue treatment with immunotherapy for 4–8 more weeks despite RECIST 1.1 evaluation showing progression on imaging (Wolchok et al. 2009). A subsequent CT has then to be obtained, and the results of this evaluation would give the final response: persistent disease progression or improvement. The first and complex criteria dedicated to immunotherapy (irRC for immune-related Response Criteria) were released in 2009, at the time RECIST 1.0 criteria were being revised in their new version 1.1 (Wolchok et al. 2009). Those criteria were never really adopted by the oncologic community.

As immunotherapy deployment went very fast for the treatment of various tumor types, such as non-small cell lung cancer, similar cases of pseudo-progression were also observed for various cancers, and new guidelines were needed (Tazdait et al. 2018; Wang et al. 2017). RECIST 1.1 criteria were therefore adapted for the management of potential pseudo-progression under immunotherapy and named iRECIST criteria (for immune-RECIST) (Seymour et al. 2017).

iRECIST guidelines differ from RECIST 1.1 only in the case of lesion progression, meaning that there is no change in the evaluation of patients at baseline and during follow-up in the case of SD, PR or CR. In case of lesion progression according to RECIST 1.1 criteria (i.e., ≥20% increase in the sum of the size of target lesions and/or the unequivocal progression of nontarget lesions and/or the appearance of new lesion(s)), the conclusion should constantly be *iUPD* for "immune-unconfirmed Progressive Disease." In case of any new lesion, their size and location have to be recorded apart: they have to be assessed as "new target lesion" or "new nontarget lesion," respectively, according to the definition of target and nontarget lesions as per RECIST 1.1. This new status *iUPD* automatically implies that the treatment might be pursued unless the clinical state of the patient is too deteriorated. A new evaluation on imaging is then recommended at least 4 weeks and no more than 8 weeks later. On this subsequent examination, the goal is to differentiate a transient pseudo-progression from a "true" progression by identifying anything that is worse than on the previous examination (namely imaging of the iuPD) among:

- ≥5 mm increase in the sum of the diameters of target lesion(s)
- and/or ≥5 mm increase in the sum of the diameters of previous new target lesion(s)
- and/or the worsening of nontarget lesion(s)
- and/or the emergence of new lesion

If one or more of those criteria is/are present, then the true progression is confirmed, and the status becomes *iCPD* for "immune-confirmed progressive disease."

On the other hand, if none of the above is observed, then the evaluation will be compared back to baseline (before the introduction of immunotherapy). There will be four possible conditions:

- All target lesion(s), nontarget lesion(s) and new lesion(s) have disappeared: then the conclusion is CR. By convention, an "i" should be placed before CR to acknowledge the previous unconfirmed progression = *iCR* for iComplete Response
- The sum of the diameters of target lesion(s) is ≥−30% compared to baseline, there is no increase of nontarget lesion(s), no increase of new lesion(s), no new lesion: the conclusion would then be *iPR* for iPartial Response
- The sum of the diameter of target lesion(s) is comprised between −30% and +20% compared to baseline, then the conclusion indicates *iSD* for iStable Disease
- Finally, the situation where the disease is not worse than during the previous iUPD evaluation but has not improved over the extent of iSD, then the conclusion would be iUPD again. This status authorizes the pursuit of the treatment.

These conditions are illustrated in Fig. 6. The great majority of iUPD are observed early (first or second evaluation) after administration of immunotherapy. However, iRECIST guidelines specify that any progression arising at any time of the treatment could be assessed as iuPD, despite late pseudo-progressions being uncommon (Seymour et al. 2017) (Fig. 6).

3.2 Density-Based Criteria: CHOI Criteria

CHOI criteria are mainly validated in gastrointestinal stromal tumor (GIST) treated with imatinib (a tyrosine-kinase inhibitor) (Fig. 7). The mechanism of action of this molecule targets the vascularity and induces some "necrosis," which translates into a decrease in CT density of the lesion before any significant decrease in size is seen and sometimes even leads to an apparent increase in the tumor size (Choi et al. 2004). The region of interest must be drawn on the whole metastasis. New criteria adapted for GIST under imatinib were then proposed, combining changes in size and tumor density on contrast-enhanced CT to determine tumor response. A better correlation with survival rates is observed when using these criteria compared to RECIST ones (Choi et al. 2004).

Partial response (PR) is defined as a decrease of ≥10% in the sum of the diameters of up to 5 target lesions or a decrease of ≥15% in tumor density measured in Hounsfield Units of target lesions.

Progressive disease (PD) is defined as a ≥10% increase in size of the sum of the diameters of up to 5 target lesions and not meeting the PR criteria for tumor density.

Stable Disease (SD) is declared if none of the above criteria is seen.

Following the CHOI criteria publication, several other teams tried to apply this new concept of evaluating not only the size but also the density of lesions under treatment (Lucidarme et al. 2019; van der Veldt et al. 2010).

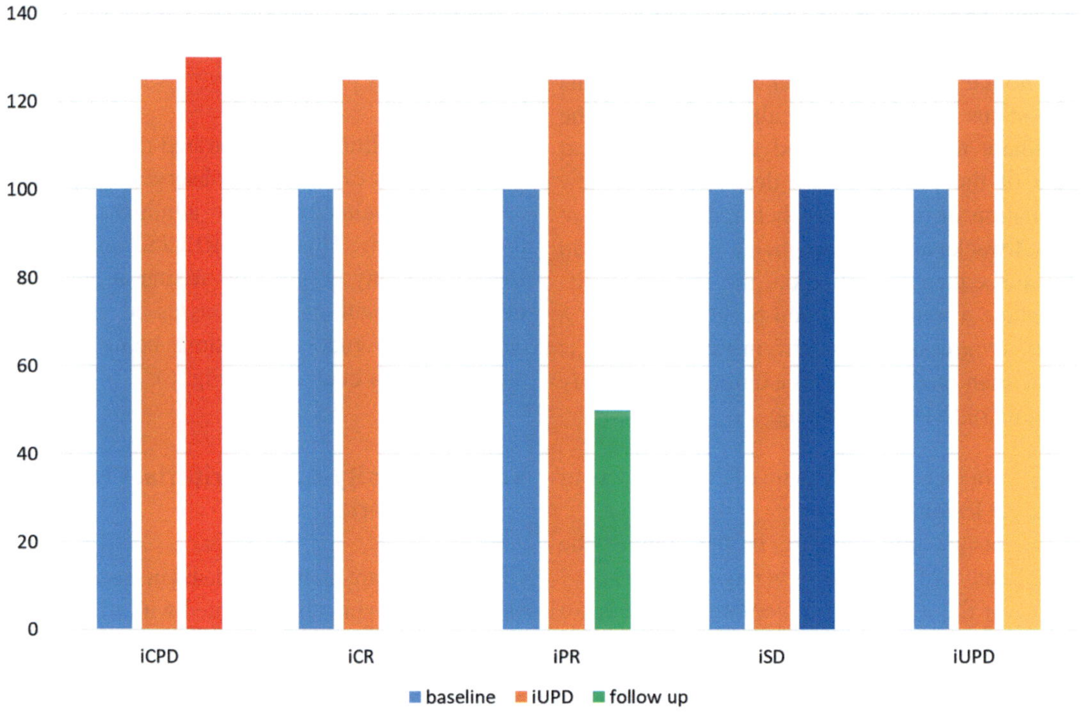

Fig. 6 Illustration of the different conditions encountered after iUPD. The first blue bars are the sum of target lesions at baseline (100). The orange bars represent an iUPD due to the increase of the sum of target lesions (125, i.e., +25%). The next bars represent five different conditions. The red bar illustrates the case of iCPD because the sum of target lesions increases by +5 mm. In case of complete disappearance of target lesions, the response will be iCR. The green bar illustrates the case of iPR, because the sum of target lesions decreases to 50 (which is better than the −30% compared to baseline). The dark blue bar illustrates the case of iSD, because the sum of target lesions decreases to 100 (which is comprised between +20% and −30% compared to baseline). The yellow bar illustrates the case of iUPD again, because the sum of target lesions did not increase compared to iUPD (there are no criteria to declare iCPD), and the sum of target lesions is still more than +20% compared to baseline

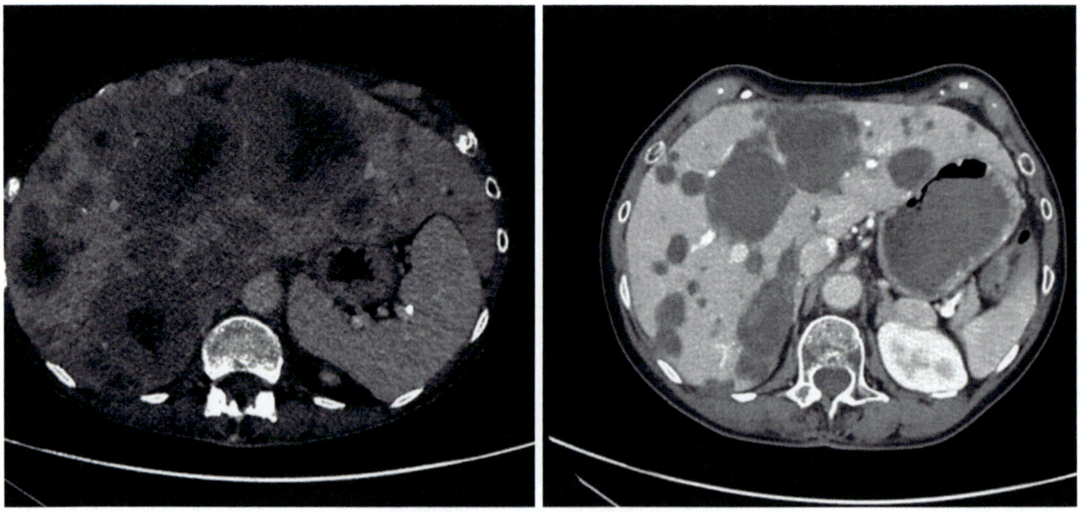

Fig. 7 Illustrates the appearance of liver metastases under an antiangiogenic compound: both the density of lesions and their size decreased

3.3 Mesothelioma

The behavior of tumoral extension in malignant mesothelioma is a challenge for tumor evaluation. The thickening of pleura, including fissures, is typically improper for RECIST criteria. Thus, new criteria called "modified RECIST" were proposed in 2004 and amended for more precise measurements in 2018 (Byrne and Nowak 2004; Armato and Nowak 2018). Of note, these modified RECIST criteria for mesothelioma are different than those used for the homonymous "mRECIST" criteria developed for the evaluation of hepatocarcinoma.

First, up to three different sections (on axial plane) are selected. These three sections must be more than 1 cm apart from each other (Fig. 8). Then, these sections must be identified in terms of specific anatomic landmarks (for example, carina, aortic arch, ...). Finally, one or two measurement(s) of the thickness of the pleura perpendicular to the chest wall or mediastinum at each level are reported. Of note, all selected sites must meet the criterion for minimally measurable disease, which is 7 mm and not 10 mm as per RECIST 1.1. Pleural effusion should never be included in measurements. The sum of these (up to) six measurements is considered as one target lesion. Any other tumoral lesion (lymph node(s), distant metastasis) is selected and measured as per RECIST 1.1 criteria.

During follow-up, measurements must be performed on the same areas of pleural thickening. If the thickening decreases but is persistent and is no more precisely measurable, the RECIST 1.1 rule of "too small to measure" is applied with a reporting of 2 mm (and not 5 mm as per RECIST 1.1).

3.4 Tumor Growth Rate

RECIST 1.1 criteria don't consider the kinetics of tumor growth. The baseline examination is the reference for tumor response, completely ignoring the type of tumoral behavior that existed beforehand. However, in experimental drug evaluation, it would be of interest to consider a relative decrease in tumor growth attributed to the new drug, despite a "poor" response according to

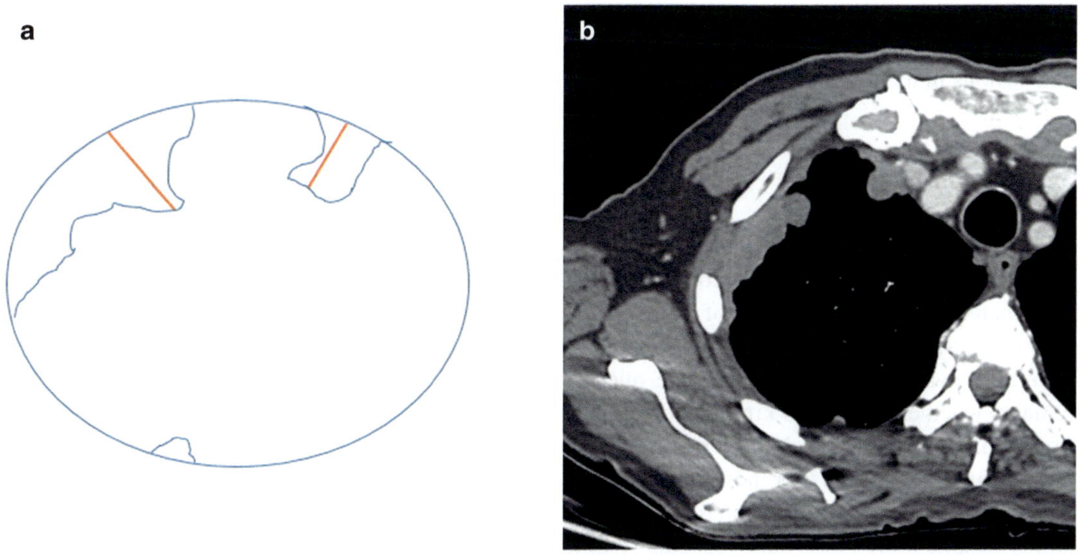

Fig. 8 (**a**) Drawing showing the method for measurement of pleural thickening done by drawing a line perpendicular to the pleura surface at the level of the greatest thickening; (**b**) Axial slice focused on the right upper area showing a selected level at the level of supra-aortic vessels

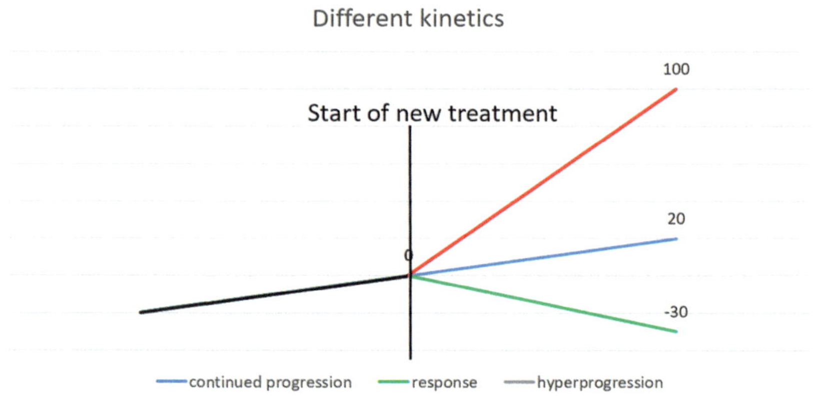

Fig. 9 Tumor Growth Rate illustration: Before the start of the new treatment, a degree of increase in tumor volume is observed. The effect of new treatment is illustrated as three different kinetics of the tumor volume: in green, a decrease (= response to treatment); in blue, a continued linear progression; and in red, an accelerated progression

RECIST criteria. For example, if the growth of the tumor was +80% before the initiation of treatment and is reduced to a rate +30% under treatment, this would indeed suggest an anti-tumoral effect of the drug (Ferté et al. 2014).

In order to consider account kinetics, *TGR* (tumor growth rate) has been proposed, considering the interval time (in days) between the successive evaluations and the size of the same target lesions before experimental treatment is introduced and then under treatment. This criterion, however, does not consider the occurrence of new lesions in the evaluation (Fig. 9).

3.5 Volumetry

RECIST 1.1 is based on the measurement of a single diameter, assuming that lesions are spherical. Thanks to the development of more precise CT devices, 3D segmentation of lesions is becoming available and accurate. The question remains whether or not this kind of implementation would give better results in terms of cohorts of patients' evaluation. For now, in metastatic patients, results show a lower interobserver variability despite more constraints (especially time-consuming) (Rothe et al. 2013; Fournier et al. 2021). There are currently not recommended in clinical routine.

3.6 MRI

Currently, MRI is not recommended in routine for lung cancer or any other thoracic cancer patients. In some specific cases, a thoracic MRI can be proposed in the initial work-up (superior sulcus tumors, especially in a paravertebral location and thymic malignancies) (Mihoubi Bouvier et al. 2021; Park et al. 2021). Although bone MRI has added value over CT scan, there are currently no recommendation for the use of serial bone MRI for the evaluation of bone metastasis response to treatment. The role of whole-body MRI (WB-MRI) has been evaluated in comparison to PET-CT for staging of lung cancer in a recent meta-analysis in 2020: WB-MRI showed the same diagnostic performances for the detection of metastasis (Machado Medeiros et al. 2020). Although MRI offers a radiation-free alternative, this modality is not currently recommended, neither for staging nor for treatment evaluation, in particular considering its low availability.

4 Perspectives and Conclusion

RECIST 1.1 criteria are widely used for the evaluation of tumor response in clinical trials. They offer the opportunity to identify responders versus non-responders on a population level, and they are validated by large retrospective analyses (Willemink et al. 2018; McCollough et al. 2015). Their limits are now well known, especially regarding the specificity of responses of some anti-tumoral agents. On a patient's level, RECIST 1.1 evaluation should be only one of the parameters that clinicians have to consider when deciding whether or not a treatment should be dismissed. Radiologists should use them in clinical routine, and this therefore could be considered a win-win: standardized reporting is helpful for both the radiologist and the clinician, and ultimately for the patient.

The development of advanced CT techniques such as dual-energy CT and, more recently, photon-counting CT gives hope to a better characterization of cancer nodules (Willemink et al. 2018). They allow the "material decomposition" of tissue by generating material- and iodine-specific maps, thus leading to a more precise analysis of tumor tissue. Several studies tested its accuracy in the characterization of suspicious lung nodules or mediastinal lymph nodes (Dewaguet et al. 2022; Nagano et al. 2022). Dual-energy CT images may offer access to the quantification of iodine concentration that in turn may allow quantitative comparison of tumoral versus non-tumoral structures, including necrotic content. Their routine applications are not yet validated.

Software that could automatically detect nodules and/or could subsequently retrieve the same nodules on the previous examinations and measure their size during a longitudinal follow-up is already available on the market. They offer a dedicated environment for oncologic imaging examination, with semi-automatic registration of target lesions and nontarget lesions and, most of the time, a dedicated "Case Report Form" (CRF). They are dedicated for clinical trial reviewers and are not yet displayed for clinical routine. Cautious verification remains required in all cases to avoid misregistration of lesions, especially lung nodules.

The promises of artificial intelligence applied to oncologic evaluation are still pending. However, one could dream of the day the radiologist would be really assisted by intelligent software enabling the immediate and automatic detection of true tumoral lesions within the 3000 images of a thoraco-abdomino-pelvic CT scan, while non-tumoral, infectious or inflammatory abnormalities would be correctly extracted. This could be facilitated if this software were able to retrieve relevant clinical information out of the medical file of a patient.

References

Armato SG, Nowak AK (2018) Revised modified response evaluation criteria in solid tumors for assessment of response in malignant pleural mesothelioma (version 1.1). J Thorac Oncol 13(7):1012–1021. https://doi.org/10.1016/j.jtho.2018.04.034

Byrne MJ, Nowak AK (2004) Modified RECIST criteria for assessment of response in malignant pleural mesothelioma. Ann Oncol 15(2):257–260. https://doi.org/10.1093/annonc/mdh059

Choi H, Charnsangavej C, de Castro FS et al (2004) CT evaluation of the response of gastrointestinal stromal tumors after imatinib mesylate treatment: a quantitative analysis correlated with FDG PET findings. AJR Am J Roentgenol 183(6):1619–1628. https://doi.org/10.2214/ajr.183.6.01831619

Clinical trial endpoints for the approval of cancer drugs and biologics. Published online 2018:19

Dewaguet J, Copin MC, Duhamel A et al (2022) Dual-energy CT perfusion of invasive tumor front in non-small cell lung cancers. Radiology 302(2):448–456. https://doi.org/10.1148/radiol.2021210600

Eisenhauer EA, Therasse P, Bogaerts J et al (2009) New response evaluation criteria in solid tumours: revised RECIST guideline (version 1.1). Eur J Cancer 45(2):228–247. https://doi.org/10.1016/j.ejca.2008.10.026

Ferté C, Fernandez M, Hollebecque A et al (2014) Tumor growth rate is an early indicator of antitumor drug activity in phase I clinical trials. Clin Cancer Res 20(1):246–252. https://doi.org/10.1158/1078-0432.CCR-13-2098

Fleming TR, Rothmann MD, Lu HL (2009) Issues in using progression-free survival when evaluating oncology products. J Clin Oncol 27(17):2874–2880. https://doi.org/10.1200/JCO.2008.20.4107

Fournier L, de Geus-Oei LF, Regge D et al (2021) Twenty years on: RECIST as a biomarker of response in solid tumours an EORTC Imaging Group – ESOI joint paper. Front Oncol 11:800547. https://doi.org/10.3389/fonc.2021.800547

Haanen JBAG, Robert C (2015) Immune checkpoint inhibitors. Prog Tumor Res 42:55–66. https://doi.org/10.1159/000437178

Lucidarme O, Wagner M, Gillard P et al (2019) RECIST and CHOI criteria in the evaluation of tumor response in patients with metastatic colorectal cancer treated with regorafenib, a prospective multicenter study. Cancer Imaging 19(1):85. https://doi.org/10.1186/s40644-019-0271-z

Machado Medeiros T, Altmayer S, Watte G et al (2020) 18F-FDG PET/CT and whole-body MRI diagnostic performance in M staging for non-small cell lung cancer: a systematic review and meta-analysis. Eur Radiol 30(7):3641–3649. https://doi.org/10.1007/s00330-020-06703-1

McCollough CH, Leng S, Yu L, Fletcher JG (2015) Dual- and multi-energy CT: principles, technical approaches, and clinical applications. Radiology 276(3):637–653. https://doi.org/10.1148/radiol.2015142631

Mihoubi Bouvier F, Thomas De Montpréville V, Besse B et al (2021) Can MRI differentiate surrounding vertebral invasion from reactive inflammatory changes in superior sulcus tumor? Eur Radiol 31(12):8991–8999. https://doi.org/10.1007/s00330-021-08001-w

Miller AB, Hoogstraten B, Staquet M, Winkler A (1981) Reporting results of cancer treatment. Cancer 47(1):207–214. https://doi.org/10.1002/1097-0142(19810101)47:1<207::aid-cncr2820470134>3.0.co;2-6

Moertel CG, Hanley JA (1976) The effect of measuring error on the results of therapeutic trials in advanced cancer. Cancer 38(1):388–394. https://doi.org/10.1002/1097-0142(197607)38:1<388::aid-cncr2820380156>3.0.co;2-a

Nagano H, Takumi K, Nakajo M et al (2022) Dual-energy CT-derived electron density for diagnosing metastatic mediastinal lymph nodes in non-small cell lung cancer: comparison with conventional CT and FDG PET/CT findings. AJR Am J Roentgenol 218(1):66–74. https://doi.org/10.2214/AJR.21.26208

Park JW, Jeong WG, Lee JE et al (2021) Pictorial review of mediastinal masses with an emphasis on magnetic resonance imaging. Korean J Radiol 22(1):139–154. https://doi.org/10.3348/kjr.2019.0897

Rothe JH, Grieser C, Lehmkuhl L et al (2013) Size determination and response assessment of liver metastases with computed tomography—comparison of RECIST and volumetric algorithms. Eur J Radiol 82(11):1831–1839. https://doi.org/10.1016/j.ejrad.2012.05.018

Seymour L, Bogaerts J, Perrone A et al (2017) iRECIST: guidelines for response criteria for use in trials testing immunotherapeutics. Lancet Oncol 18(3):e143–e152. https://doi.org/10.1016/S1470-2045(17)30074-8

Tazdait M, Mezquita L, Lahmar J et al (2018) Patterns of responses in metastatic NSCLC during PD-1 or PDL-1 inhibitor therapy: comparison of RECIST 1.1, irRECIST and iRECIST criteria. Eur J Cancer 88:38–47. https://doi.org/10.1016/j.ejca.2017.10.017

Therasse P, Arbuck SG, Eisenhauer EA et al (2000) New guidelines to evaluate the response to treatment in solid tumors. European Organization for Research and Treatment of Cancer, National Cancer Institute of the United States, National Cancer Institute of Canada. J Natl Cancer Inst 92(3):205–216. https://doi.org/10.1093/jnci/92.3.205

van der Veldt AAM, Meijerink MR, van den Eertwegh AJM, Haanen JBAG, Boven E (2010) Choi response criteria for early prediction of clinical outcome in patients with metastatic renal cell cancer treated with sunitinib. Br J Cancer 102(5):803–809. https://doi.org/10.1038/sj.bjc.6605567

Wang GX, Kurra V, Gainor JF et al (2017) Immune checkpoint inhibitor cancer therapy: spectrum of imaging findings. Radiographics 37(7):2132–2144. https://doi.org/10.1148/rg.2017170085

Willemink MJ, Persson M, Pourmorteza A, Pelc NJ, Fleischmann D (2018) Photon-counting CT: technical principles and clinical prospects. Radiology 289(2):293–312. https://doi.org/10.1148/radiol.2018172656

Wolchok JD, Hoos A, O'Day S et al (2009) Guidelines for the evaluation of immune therapy activity in solid tumors: immune-related response criteria. Clin Cancer Res 15(23):7412–7420. https://doi.org/10.1158/1078-0432.CCR-09-1624

Follow-Up After Radiation Therapy

Cecilia Strappa, Giuseppe Cicchetti, Antonella Martino, Francesco Scrocca, Annemilia del Ciello, Lucio Calandriello, Alessandra Farchione, Mariangela Massaccesi, and Anna Rita Larici

Contents

C. Strappa (✉) · G. Cicchetti · A. del Ciello · L. Calandriello · A. Farchione
Advanced Radiology Center, Department of Diagnostic Imaging and Oncological Radiotherapy, Fondazione Policlinico Universitario "A. Gemelli" IRCCS, Rome, Italy
e-mail: cecilia.strappa@guest.policlinicogemelli.it; giuseppe.cicchetti@policlinicogemelli.it; annemilia.delciello@policlinicogemelli.it; lucio.calandriello@policlinicogemelli.it; alessandra.farchione@policlinicogemelli.it

A. Martino · M. Massaccesi
Radiation Oncology, Department of Diagnostic Imaging and Oncological Radiotherapy, Fondazione Policlinico Universitario "A. Gemelli" IRCCS, Rome, Italy
e-mail: antonella.martino@policlinicogemelli.it; mariangela.massaccesi@policlinicogemelli.it

F. Scrocca
Section of Radiology, Department of Radiological and Hematological Sciences, Università Cattolica del Sacro Cuore, Rome, Italy
e-mail: francesco.scrocca01@icatt.it

A. R. Larici
Advanced Radiology Center, Department of Diagnostic Imaging and Oncological Radiotherapy, Fondazione Policlinico Universitario "A. Gemelli" IRCCS, Rome, Italy

Section of Radiology, Department of Radiological and Hematological Sciences, Università Cattolica del Sacro Cuore, Rome, Italy
e-mail: annarita.larici@unicatt.it

Med Radiol Diagn Imaging (2026)
https://doi.org/10.1007/174_2025_622,
Published Online: 26 September 2025

Abstract

Lung toxicity following radiation therapy (RT) for thoracic neoplasms shows a wide range of severity, with different temporal occurrence and evolution on computed tomography (CT) according to the fractionation scheme. Radiation-induced lung injury (RILI) may appear early or later after treatment completion and may increase over time or tend to resolve or stabilize. RILI in lung neoplasms is often indistinguishable from the treated lesion, thus preventing the application of size-based criteria to assess treatment response and local recurrence.

In this chapter, we will focus on RT techniques and applications in lung neoplasms and lung toxicity, described in terms of risk factors, CT characteristics, and clinical-radiological grading scales. Differential diagnoses and issues related to the prompt recognition of local recurrence will be discussed. Finally, the applications of RT in other thoracic neoplasms and radiation-induced toxicities in thoracic structures other than the lungs will be briefly outlined.

Abbreviations

ADC	Apparent diffusion coefficient
ADL	Activities of daily living
CAD	Coronary artery disease
COPD	Chronic obstructive pulmonary disease
CRT	Conformal radiation therapy
CT	Computed tomography
CTCAE	Common Terminology Criteria for Adverse Events
EGJ	Esophagogastric junction
FDG-PET/CT	Fluorodeoxyglucose-positron emission tomography/computed tomography
FEV1	Forced expiratory volume in 1 s
GLCM	Gray level co-occurrence matrix
Gy	Gray
HU	Hounsfield units
IGRT	Image-guided radiotherapy
IMRT	Intensity-modulated radiation therapy
LENT/SOMA	Late Effects of Normal Tissue—Subjective, Objective, Management and Analytic scale
MLD	Mean lung dose
MRI	Magnetic resonance imaging
NSCLC	Non-small cell lung cancer
OAR	Organs at risk
OR	Odds ratio
PTV	Planning target volume
RECIST	Response Evaluation Criteria In Solid Tumor
RILI	Radiation-induced lung injury
RT	Radiation therapy
RTOG/EORTC	Radiation Therapy Oncology Group/European Organization for Research and Treatment of Cancer
SABR	Stereotactic ablative radiation therapy
SBRT	Stereotactic body radiation therapy
SCLC	Small cell lung cancer
SWOG	Southwest Oncology Group
VMAT	Volumetric-modulated arc therapy

1 Introduction

Radiation therapy (RT) is one of the mainstays in the treatment of lung malignancies, with potential role in all stages of primary pulmonary neoplasms as well as in oligometastatic lung disease (National Comprehensive Cancer Network 2025a, b; Palma et al. 2020). RT also represents a valuable treatment option for mediastinal lymph node involvement in lung cancer and other solid tumor (Cozzi et al. 2022). Furthermore, RT is a treatment option in case of less frequent thoracic neoplasms, such as pleural mesothelioma, esophageal cancer, thymic tumors, and lymphoma (Pleural 2023; Hang et al. 2024; Kristina Gregory et al. 2023; Lymphoma 2024).

Although advancements in RT delivery technique, imaging guidance, and motion management have led to increasingly accurate dose administration, lung toxicity remains a challenge. Lung toxicity may have a wide range of clinical manifestations from asymptomatic to life-threatening conditions, and radiological abnormalities, in terms of entity, extent, and time of appearance (early and late phases) (Konkol et al. 2022).

The most widely used grading systems in clinical practice for lung toxicity assessment, such as the Common Terminology Criteria for Adverse Events (CTCAE) (Cancer Institute N 2017) and the Radiation Therapy Oncology Group/European Organization for Research and Treatment of Cancer (RTOG/EORTC) (Cox et al. 1995; Rubin et al. 1995), are mainly based on clinical presentation, even though symptoms may be absent despite extensive radiological changes.

In this chapter, we will present an overview of RT techniques used in thoracic neoplasms and radiation-induced lung injury (RILI) resulting from the treatment of lung neoplasms and its risk factors. The computed tomography (CT) appearance and physiological evolution of RILI according to the time of occurrence will be extensively reported, and the grading systems for RILI severity assessment will be outlined, emphasizing the importance of having tools for a standardized evaluation of RILI on CT. Finally, the applications of RT on other thoracic neoplasms will be briefly illustrated, including pleural and mediastinal tumors.

2 Radiotherapy Techniques and Applications in Lung Neoplasms

Over the years, advances in RT techniques and in image-guided radiotherapy (IGRT) have led to an increasingly accurate dose delivery to the tumoral target, while progressively minimizing dose to the surrounding organs at risk (OAR); therefore, RT has been increasingly employed, with fast-growing expansion of its applications. Early RT relied on bidimensional (2D) imaging (chest X-ray) and was based on a reduced number of square or rectangular beams, resulting in the inclusion of large healthy tissues within the radiation field. The groundbreaking advent of CT allowed the introduction of tridimensional (3D) treatment planning, which enabled the development of 3D conformal RT (CRT). In fact, through increased awareness of dose distribution and use of multiple beams with multileaf collimators, more conformal doses could be administered, ensuring sparing the OAR. Further refinements in dose delivery included the intensity-modulated radiation therapy (IMRT), which enabled the generation of nonuniform intensity radiation beams to better sculpt the dose, and, subsequently, the volumetric-modulated arc therapy (VMAT), which permitted faster and even more accurate dose distribution through the continuous delivery of modulated doses during rotation (Belderbos and Sonke 2009; Rammohan et al. 2022; Hall et al. 2022) (Fig. 1).

Such advancements in RT delivery would not have been achieved without concurrent evolution of IGRT. Advances in on-board imaging modalities, from initial 2D imaging to four-dimensional (4D) imaging, mainly including CT and more recently magnetic resonance imaging (MRI), have allowed an increasingly better visualization of both target and OAR, not only during the treatment planning but also during the treatment fraction. As a result, the planning target volume (PTV) margins have been progressively reduced, enabling dose administration in an increasingly safe manner (Zou et al. 2018; Herrmann et al. 2019).

Improved target and OAR visualization, coupled with accurate dose delivery, have led to development and rapid widespread of stereotactic body radiation therapy (SBRT), also called stereotactic ablative radiation therapy (SABR), which permits the administration of ablative doses to small-size targets (generally up to 5 cm in size) in fewer fractions compared to conventional fractionated RT (National Comprehensive Cancer Network 2025a, b; Finazzi et al. 2021).

Due to improved outcomes compared to conventionally fractionated RT (Ball et al. 2019; Li et al. 2020) and good tolerability even in case of

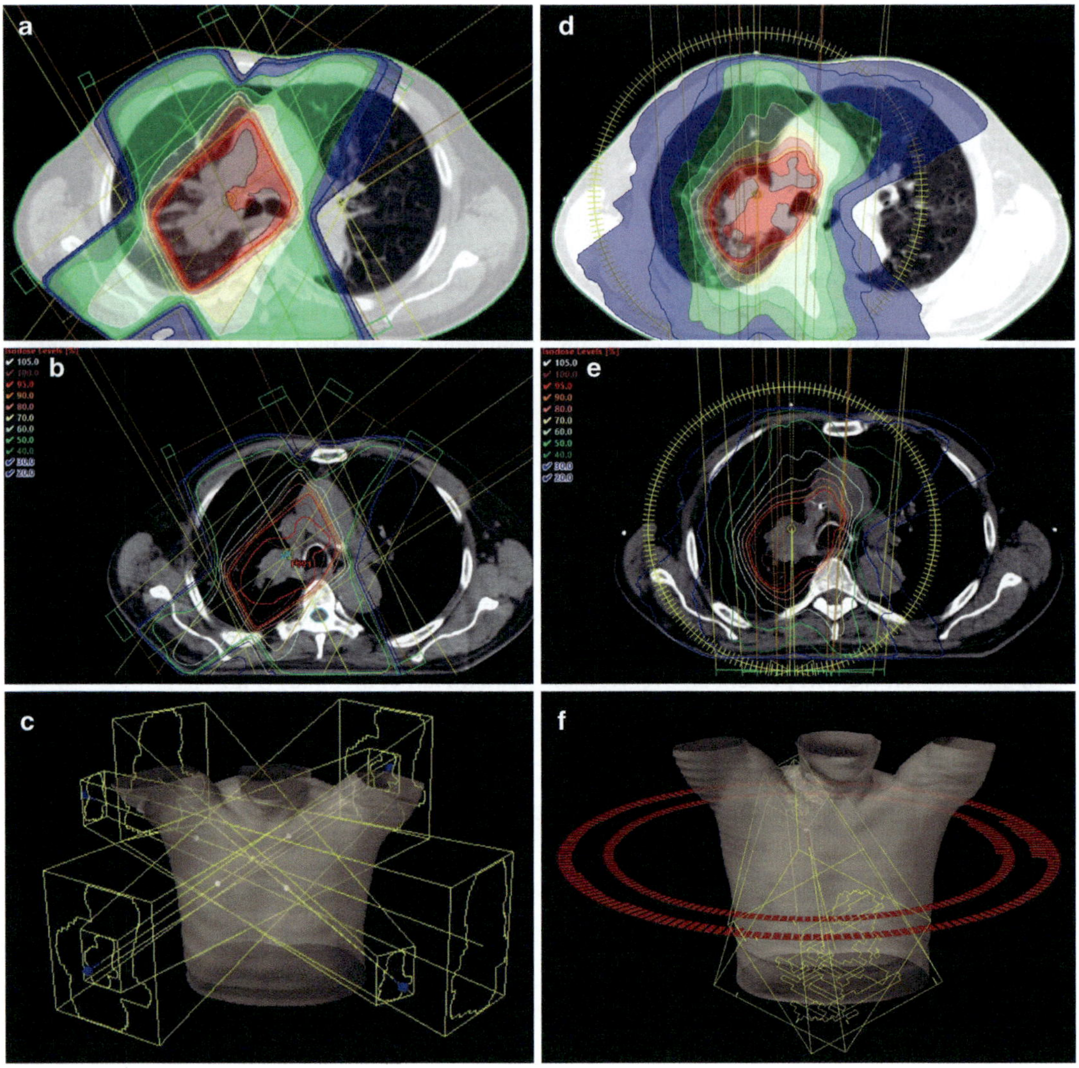

Fig. 1 Comparison of different radiotherapy techniques. 3D-conformal radiotherapy (3D-CRT) (**a–c**) and volumetric-modulated arc therapy (VMAT) (**d–f**) of a right upper lobe non-small cell lung cancer (NSCLC) (same patient, different treatments). Dose color wash (**a**, **d**) and corresponding isodose levels (**b**, **e**) ranging from 100% to 20%, focused on the target region. 3D anatomical renderings for both 3D-CRT (**c**) and VMAT (**f**) techniques, demonstrating the geometrical configuration of beam angles and radiation delivery mechanisms. VMAT treatment plan shows a more conformal and precise dose distribution on the target region in order to spare surrounding tissues

coexisting comorbidities (Guckenberger et al. 2017), SBRT has become the treatment of choice in patients with early-stage non-small cell lung cancer (NSCLC) who are medically inoperable or when surgical treatment is declined (National Comprehensive Cancer Network 2025a). Similarly, in patients with local or locoregional recurrence from NSCLC, if surgery is not feasible, SBRT may effectively be employed as salvage therapy, even after previous RT (Brooks et al. 2018). SBRT followed by systemic therapy is also a guideline-recommended option for patients with limited stage small cell lung cancer (SCLC), who are unfit or unwilling to undergo surgery (National Comprehensive Cancer Network 2025b). Furthermore, growing evidence favors the role of SBRT in oligometastatic diseases from both primary lung cancer (National Comprehensive Cancer Network 2025a) and extrapulmonary malignancies (Palma et al. 2020; Ricco et al. 2017). With various fractionation schemes and possible combination with chemotherapy, RT is also indicated in the heterogeneous group of patients with locally advanced NSCLC (National Comprehensive Cancer Network 2025a; Finazzi et al. 2021). Finally, in both advanced/metastatic NSCLC and extensive stage SCLC, RT can be used for palliative purposes (National Comprehensive Cancer Network 2025a, b).

Mediastinal and hilar lymph nodes are elective sites for lung cancer spread and frequently included in the PTV. Alongside the well-established use of conventional fractionated RT, SBRT is increasingly employed in mediastinal and hilar lymph node metastases, with encouraging results in terms of local control and safety. The abovementioned technological advancements enabled its feasibility despite the very close proximity of lymph nodes to OAR, such as great vessels, heart, central airways, and esophagus. Comparable results have been observed even in the setting of mediastinal and hilar lymph node dissemination of other solid tumors (Cozzi et al. 2022).

3 Risk Factors for Lung Toxicity

Lung toxicity remains a challenge regardless of the abovementioned advancements in RT delivery techniques and imaging guidance.

Several risk factors for RILI development after treatment completion exist, which are related to treatment, tumor characteristics, and patient factors. The most robust evidence is related to dose and irradiated volume (Käsmann et al. 2020; Arroyo-Hernández et al. 2021) with the mean lung dose (MLD), representing the average dose received by the whole lung, and the V20, which is the lung volume delivered with at least 20 Gy. The concept of V20 is crucial especially in conventionally fractionated RT, in which a V20 =35–40% of the irradiated lung is currently recommended (National Comprehensive Cancer Network 2025a), while in SBRT, the volumes are lower, and the generally recommended V20 values are =10–15% (Diez et al. 2022).

V20 has been proved to be the only factor significantly related to the development of grade =2 pneumonitis in the study of Graham et al. (1999). The same study also showed that no grade =2 pneumonitis was observed at V20 <22%, while at values >32%, fatal pneumonitis may occur. Similar results in terms of correlation between V20 and development of symptomatic radiation pneumonitis have also been reported in subsequent studies (Palma et al. 2024).

Although MLD and V20 were found to be independently and positively correlated with the risk of radiation pneumonitis (Graham et al. 1999; Zhang et al. 2012), dose and volume are highly interconnected. Indeed, the dose at which lung changes appear is inversely correlated with the V20 (Aoki et al. 2004); in other words, the higher the V20, the lower the mean dose at which toxicity may appear. Nevertheless, in some cases, RILI appears disproportionated with respect to dose and irradiated volume, with manifestations often resolving without fibrotic changes in the late phase. These cases, accounting for approximately 10%, are referred to "sporadic radiation pneumonitis" (Konkol et al. 2022; Hanania et al. 2019).

In addition to dosimetric parameters, other treatment-related factors have a potential influence on lung toxicity, such as previous surgery, sequential and concurrent chemotherapy (including targeted therapy), and immunotherapy.

A few studies analyzed the role of previous surgery in the development of radiation pneumonitis in patients undergoing RT, even though results are controversial and somewhat questionable (Dang et al. 2014; Vogelius and Bentzen 2012). Several systemic therapeutic regimens commonly employed in lung cancer treatment may represent risk factors for lung toxicity (Thomas et al. 2000; Pellegrino et al. 2018; Tseng et al. 2022); as expected, their use in combination with RT has been related to an increased risk of development of pneumonitis (Zhang et al. 2012; Geng et al. 2021). Concerning chemotherapy, a meta-analysis conducted by Zhang et al. showed that patients receiving RT combined with chemotherapy were at higher risk of developing radiation pneumonitis than patients receiving RT alone (Zhang et al. 2012). Even though there are conflicting results regarding the impact of using concomitant rather than sequential chemoradiotherapy schedule on lung toxicity (Vogelius and Bentzen 2012; Aupérin et al. 2010), a consensus exists that some chemotherapeutic drugs are more likely to induce pulmonary toxicity, such as gemcitabine, taxanes, and bevacizumab (Bledsoe et al. 2017; Chen et al. 2023).

Due to the relatively recent introduction of immunotherapy among the therapeutic options for lung cancer treatment, robust data on its relationship with RILI are still limited. However, data seem to suggest an increase in rates of pneumonitis resulting from the addition of immunotherapy to RT (Geng et al. 2021; Liu et al. 2023; Anscher et al. 2022) or to chemoradiation therapy (Han et al. 2024), with variable grades of severity.

4 When: Time as Measurement of Toxicity

Since the first descriptions of lung toxicity resulting from RT of thoracic neoplasms, it has been reported that, after treatment completion, two distinct temporal phases of RILI could be identified: an early phase, named *radiation pneumonitis*, and a later phase, named *radiation fibrosis* (Davis et al. 1992). Even though a clear distinction between these two different phases according to a precise time cut-off has not yet been defined, it is generally agreed that the early phase of RILI occurs within the first 6 months after RT completion, while the *late phase* from 6 months onward. The last day of RT administration is considered as the *"reference point"* for the definition of the two following phases. Notably, *early* and *late phases* show a good correspondence with clinical, pathological, and radiological appearances; therefore, the last day of RT represents a benchmark for the correct dating and interpretation of any lung changes occurring after treatment (Ghaye et al. 2016; Choi et al. 2004). Despite the two conventionally described phases apply to all types of RT, lung toxicity may occur at different time points according to the fractionation scheme. Indeed, due to radiobiological reasons, the higher the radiation dose per fraction, the greater the likelihood of lung alterations appearing later (Linda et al. 2011). As a result, whereas RILI after conventional fractionated RT usually occurs after weeks from the reference point, RILI after SBRT appears at least 3 months after, with possible first manifestation at CT imaging even after 6–12 months (Febbo et al. 2018). Similarly, even the evolution of lung alterations at CT shows different durations. Indeed, while changes induced by conventional fractionated RT rarely continue to evolve after 2 years, conversely, SBRT-induced RILI may evolve far beyond 2 years after treatment completion, even up to 4–5 years from the reference point (Febbo et al. 2018).

4.1 Clinical Measurement

Clinical manifestation of radiation pneumonitis may range from radiological evidence of lung abnormalities without any symptoms to life-threatening conditions. During the early phase, symptoms include dyspnea of various grades, dry cough, fatigue, fever, and pleuritic pain, variably combined (Konkol et al. 2022). These symptoms are typically temporary and tend to resolve with treatment. In the late phase, radiation fibrosis showing limited extent at CT is usually asymptomatic, while extensive lung alterations can determine progressive dyspnea, pulmonary hypertension, up to the development of *cor pulmonale* (Konkol et al. 2022; Larici et al. 2011).

Although robust evidence regarding the treatment of pulmonary toxicity is still lacking, radiation pneumonitis is usually treated according to symptom severity, either with inhaled or systemic steroids, with azathioprine or cyclosporine A reserved in case of steroid resistance. However, steroids do not appear to be effective in either preventing or treating radiation fibrosis (Konkol et al. 2022; Arroyo-Hernández et al. 2021; Rahi et al. 2021).

4.2 Pathological Measurement

RILI evolves through successive stages, from radiation-induced lung cell injury, followed by an inflammatory response and a subsequent attempt of tissue healing, which may result in development of fibrotic changes (Hanania et al. 2019).

Despite variable subdivisions of RILI into stages, with different designations according to various authors (Konkol et al. 2022; Arroyo-Hernández et al. 2021; Hanania et al. 2019; Larici et al. 2011; Rahi et al. 2021), evidence reports the onset of the fibrotic phase at approximately 6 months after radiation exposure (Konkol et al. 2022; Arroyo-Hernández et al. 2021; Larici et al. 2011; Rahi et al. 2021).

The pathological evolution of RILI has been distinguished according to time into five stages: early phase, latent phase, exudative phase, intermediate phase, and fibrotic phase (Konkol et al. 2022; Arroyo-Hernández et al. 2021). The *early phase* (from hours to days after RT exposure) is characterized by alveolar and endothelial damage, with vascular congestion, edema, and inflammatory infiltrates. In the subsequent *latent phase* (1–3 weeks), epithelial and endothelial degenerative changes progress. The following *exudative phase* (3–12 weeks) is characterized by hyaline membrane formation, resulting from detached pneumocytes and a fibrin-rich alveolar exudate, and corresponds to the clinical radiation pneumonitis; during this phase, repair phenomena begin to take place. In the *intermediate phase* (3–6 months), hyaline membranes are dissolved, and tissue integrity is restored through the synthesis of collagen (Konkol et al. 2022; Arroyo-Hernández et al. 2021). Through not completely understood mechanisms, this healing process may trigger the development of *fibrosis,* which begins about 6 months after RT and may continue to evolve for years (Arroyo-Hernández et al. 2021; Rahi et al. 2021). This stage is characterized by pneumocytes and myofibroblast hyperplasia, as well as extensive collagen deposits in both the interstitium and the alveoli, resulting in alveolar collapse and lung volume reduction (Konkol et al. 2022; Arroyo-Hernández et al. 2021).

4.3 Radiological Measurement

Radiological changes are distinguished according to whether they occur within (*early phase*) or after 6 months (*late phase*) following RT treatment completion. This classification may apply to all RT techniques (3D-CRT, IMRT, VMAT), even though the time of RILI appearance varies according to the fractionation scheme. As stated above, in conventional RT, lung changes generally appear after 4 weeks from the reference point and tend to stabilize within 2 years (Febbo et al. 2018). Conversely, in SBRT, lung abnormalities may appear later than 3–6 months or more than 1 year after the end of treatment (Febbo et al. 2018). Moreover, RILI after SBRT tends to evolve longer, for more than 2 years, with a peak of severity usually between the first and second year after the reference point (Febbo et al. 2018; Dahele et al. 2011).

Undoubtedly, CT is the imaging modality of choice for RILI evaluation (Käsmann et al. 2020). On CT, early changes induced by RT consist of ground-glass abnormalities and consolidation of variable extent and combination, while late changes consist of fibrotic abnormalities (Fig. 2). Although early changes may directly evolve into late abnormalities, especially in cases of severe injury, the two phases may also occur independently. Indeed, early alterations may resolve within 6 months without any radiological sequelae, while fibrosis may be observed on imaging without prior signs of radiation pneumonitis (Ghaye et al. 2016; Larici et al. 2011).

Among the various factors affecting morphological aspect and extent of RILI on CT, the RT technique assumes a crucial role. Early descriptions of RILI resulting from the treatment of thoracic neoplasms were based on *2D-RT* (Libshitz and Shuman 1984). Due to the limited number of beams and their non-conformal shape, these changes tended to be relatively extensive,

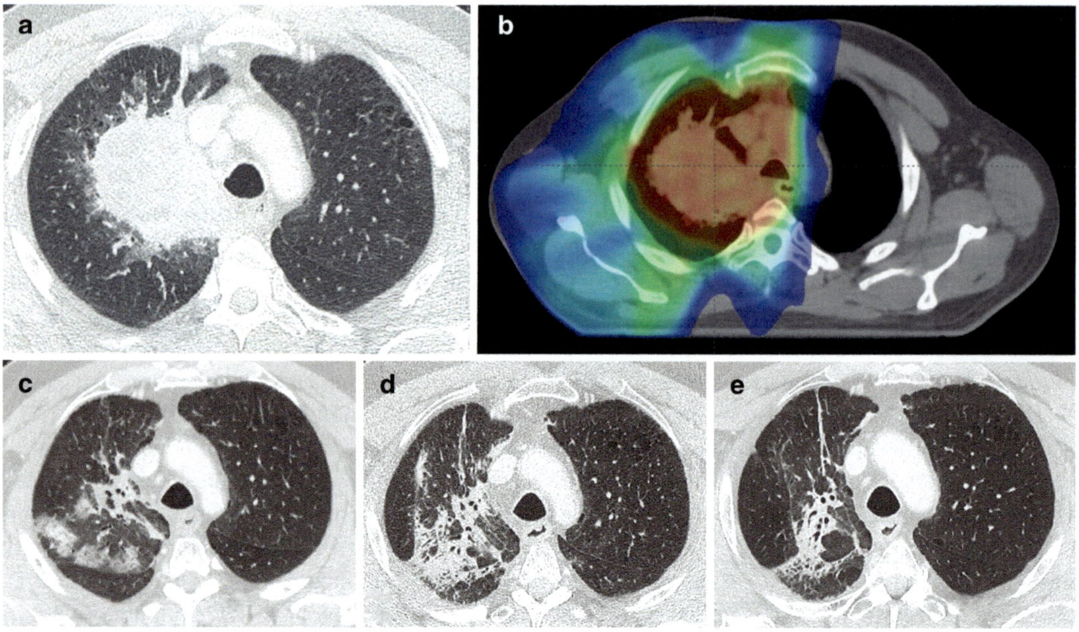

Fig. 2 Computed tomography (CT) abnormalities after volumetric-modulated arc therapy (VMAT) conventional radiation therapy (RT). CT axial image of a 55-year-old man with a right upper lobe non-small cell lung cancer (NSCLC) undergoing concomitant chemoradiation therapy (**a**). RT treatment plan showing dose distribution (**b**). CT axial images (**c**–**e**) showing radiation-induced lung injury (RILI) evolution from patchy consolidation observed 3 months after treatment completion (**c**) to the modified conventional pattern after 6 months (**d**); shrinkage of the consolidation was observed at 12 months, associated with mild parenchymal distortion and volume loss (**e**). Due to the involvement of less than four pulmonary segments, the RILI changes in both early (**c**) and late phase (**d**, **e**) can be classified as grade 1 according to the grading system proposed by Szejniuk et al. (2021)

usually corresponding to the radiation field edges (Larici et al. 2011), thus potentially involving a large lung volume.

The introduction of *3D-CRT* allowed a more limited RILI extent. Koenig et al. (2002) demonstrated that parenchymal lung changes induced by 3D-CRT in the early phase were limited to an area of 2 cm surrounding the tumor. They also distinguished late phase abnormalities into the following: *modified conventional*, defined as consolidation associated with volume loss and traction bronchiectasis, similar in shape to but less extensive than that induced by 2D-RT; *mass-like,* representing a consolidation with traction bronchiectasis in a 2 cm area around the tumor; *scar-like,* defined as a linear opacity of maximum 10 mm in thickness at the site of the previous tumor.

Due to the introduction and rapid spread of *SBRT*, several studies have dealt with the description of RILI induced by SBRT performed with different techniques (3D-CRT, IMRT, VMAT) (Dahele et al. 2011; Kimura et al. 2006; Trovo et al. 2010; Palma et al. 2011a). The RILI classification reported by Palma et al. (2011a) attempts to categorize the early phase alterations according to numerical cut-offs, rather than providing only a qualitative description of the abnormalities. Indeed, the authors distinguished early phase changes into *diffuse consolidation, patchy consolidation, diffuse ground-glass opacities,* and *patchy ground-glass opacities,* with the term "diffuse" applied to abnormalities at least 5 cm large in diameter or affecting more than 50% of the lung in the involved region, and the term "patchy" used to define alterations less than 5 cm in diameter and/or occupying less than 50% of the affected region.

Conversely, late SBRT-induced RILI usually follows Koenig et al. classification (Koenig et al. 2002) into *modified conventional pattern*, *mass-like fibrosis,* and *scar-like fibrosis*, as previously

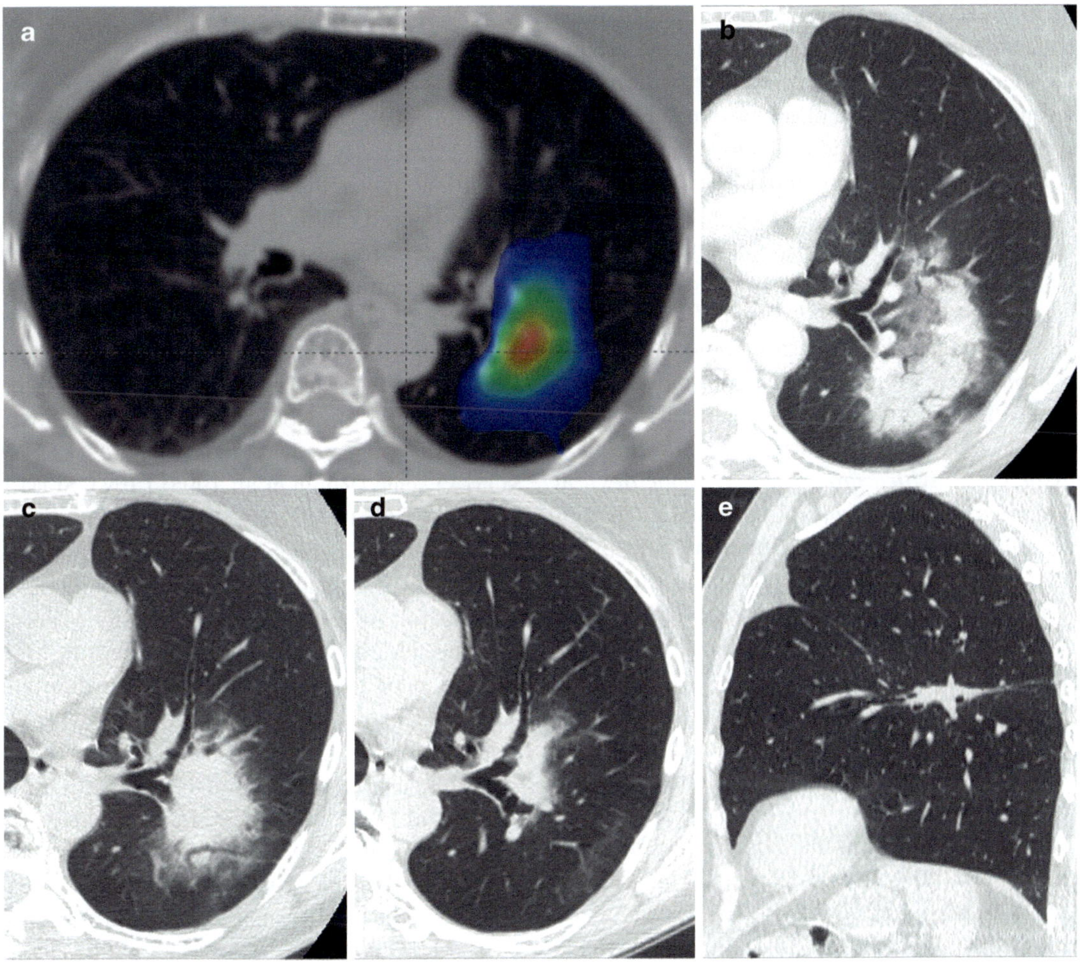

Fig. 3 **Temporal evolution of radiation-induced lung injury (RILI) after stereotactic body radiation therapy (SBRT).** Radiotherapy (RT) treatment plan (**a**) showing dose distribution in a 66-year-old woman with previous history of left upper lobectomy, affected by a left lower lobe lung adenocarcinoma, undergoing SBRT (50 Gy in 5 fractions to the 80% isodose line). CT axial image depicting a *diffuse consolidation* pattern (>5 cm, according to definition the definition by Palma et al. (2011a)) 3 months after treatment completion (**b**). CT axial image showing a *mass-like* pattern, observed 2 years after treatment completion (**c**). Axial and sagittal CT images (**d, e**) depicting the evolution into a *scar-like* pattern 3 years after RT. Sagittal reconstruction (**e**) better demonstrates the linear appearance of the consolidation compared to the axial image (**d**). RILI changes in late phase correspond to a grade 3 according to the grading system by Yamamoto et al. (2018) (diffuse radiographic changes <25% of lung volume)

mentioned. This classification also provides a qualitative definition of these alterations, without dimensional cut-offs. Particularly, the *modified conventional pattern* is defined as a consolidation associated with bronchiectasis and volume reduction, less extensive than conventional radiation fibrosis, possibly larger than the original lesion and associated with ground-glass abnormalities; the term *mass-like fibrosis* refers to a focal rounded consolidation larger than the original tumor; the *scar-like fibrosis* correspond to a linear opacity at the site of the treated lesion, associated with volume reduction (Dahele et al. 2011; Trovo et al. 2010; Huang et al. 2012; Chassagnon et al. 2020) (Fig. 3).

Al Umairi et al. (2022) analyzed the evolution of SBRT-induced RILI in 183 lung tumors, trying to define frequency, time of occurrence, and persistence over time. In their study, beyond the previously reported patterns, they also included the *nodule-like* pattern, defined as a rounded focal consolidation smaller than 3 cm in size around the treated lesion, and the *orbit-like pattern,* representing a nodule or a mass surrounded by a circumferential consolidative band with relatively normal lung parenchyma interposed. The authors reported a variety of CT patterns of RILI observed at different median time point after treatment completion, and in particular: *patchy/peribronchial consolidation, patchy ground-glass opacities,* and *nodule-like* pattern at 4 months; *diffuse consolidation* (homogeneous distribution in the areas of high radiation dose without areas of spared lung parenchyma) and *consolidation associated with ground-glass opacities* at 5 months; *diffuse ground-glass opacities* (homogeneous *ground-glass*) at 6 months; and *orbit-like pattern* and *mass-like pattern* at 8 months. After 12 months, the *modified conventional* and *scar-like patterns* were the most frequently observed RILI changes.

It is important to note that over time, each pattern may change, with the possibility of transformation of one pattern into another during follow-up (i.e., from the *orbit-like* to the *mass-like pattern,* and from the *mass-like* to the *scar-like* pattern) (Dahele et al. 2011; Al-Umairi et al. 2022). Furthermore, CT lung changes stabilized at a median time of 20 months, with a wide range of 8–62 months and with the *modified conventional pattern* being the most frequent at this stage (49%), followed by *scar-like* (23%) and *mass-like patterns* (12%), respectively (Al-Umairi et al. 2022). These results were consistent with other studies (Febbo et al. 2018; Dahele et al. 2011; Trovo et al. 2010).

5 How: Measurement of Toxicity Severity

Since the beginning of RT use in the treatment of thoracic neoplasms, lung toxicity has always been one of the major dose-limiting factors. The assessment of RILI severity relies on both clinical presentation and imaging findings (Käsmann et al. 2020).

5.1 Clinical Measurement of Toxicity Severity

The clinical presentation of lung toxicity variably ranges from asymptomatic to life-threatening conditions. Over the years, various scales have been proposed (Table 1) to establish a standardized system for classifying RILI that could be useful for clinical practice as well as for clinical trials (Trotti et al. 2003).

Among the proposed grading scales, the RTOG/EORTC criteria (Cox et al. 1995) and the Late Effects of Normal Tissue—Subjective, Objective, Management and Analytic (LENT/SOMA) scale (Rubin et al. 1995; LENT SOMA 1995) specifically classify the RT effects, while the Southwest Oncology Group (SWOG) (Green and Weiss 1992) and the Common Terminology Criteria for Adverse Events (CTCAE) (Cancer Institute N 2017) may be employed for the evaluation of toxicities deriving from different oncological treatments, including RT (Trotti et al. 2003).

In this section, we focus on the RTOG/EORTC (Cox et al. 1995) and the CTCAE (version 5) (Cancer Institute N 2017), which are the two grading systems most widely used in the clinical practice and trials (Käsmann et al. 2020).

The RTOG/EORTC (Cox et al. 1995) classifies RILI into *acute* and *late* effects, with acute criteria applicable from the day 1 of therapy until day 90, and late criteria from day 90 onward. Acute lung toxicity and late lung toxicity are graded on a five-point scale (0–4) and six-point scale (0–5), respectively, with increasing severity (Table 1). For both acute lung toxicity and late lung toxicity, grade 4 indicates a condition of severe respiratory insufficiency or requiring continuous oxygen/assisted ventilation, and grade 5 refers to death related to the adverse event(s). Acute lung toxicity from grade 0 to 3 is graded according to the symptom severity (cough and dyspnea) and the treatment required, with grade 3 classified also on radiological evidence of pneumonitis. Late lung toxicity is graded according to the severity of both symptoms and radiographic appearance.

Table 1 Clinical grading systems for lung toxicity

Scale	Grade 0	Grade 1	Grade 2	Grade 3	Grade 4	Grade 5
Pneumonitis						
CTCAE v5.0 (Cancer Institute N 2017)	–	Asymptomatic; clinical or diagnostic observations only; intervention not indicated	Symptomatic; medical intervention indicated; limiting instrumental ADL	Severe symptoms; limiting self-care ADL; oxygen indicated	Life-threatening respiratory compromise; urgent intervention indicated (e.g., tracheotomy or intubation)	Death
RTOG/ EORTC (Cox et al. 1995)	No change	Mild symptoms of dry cough or dyspnea on exertion	Persistent cough requiring narcotic, antitussive, agents/dyspnea with minimal effort but not at rest	Severe cough unresponsive to narcotic antitussive agent or dyspnea at rest/clinical or radiological evidence of acute pneumonitis/intermittent oxygen or steroids may be required	Severe respiratory insufficiency/ continuous oxygen or assisted ventilation	Not reported[a]
Fibrosis						
CTCAE v5.0 (Cancer Institute N 2017)	–	Radiologic pulmonary fibrosis <25% of lung volume associated with hypoxia	Evidence of pulmonary hypertension; radiographic pulmonary fibrosis 25–50% associated with hypoxia	Severe hypoxia; evidence of right-sided heart failure; radiographic pulmonary fibrosis >50–75%	Life-threatening consequences (e.g., hemodynamic/pulmonary complications); intubation with ventilatory support indicated; radiographic pulmonary fibrosis >75% with severe honeycombing	Death
RTOG/ EORTC[a] (Cox et al. 1995)	None	Asymptomatic or mild symptoms (dry cough); slight radiographic appearances	Moderate symptomatic fibrosis or pneumonitis (severe cough); low-grade fever; patchy radiographic appearances	Severe symptomatic fibrosis or pneumonitis; dense radiographic changes	Severe respiratory insufficiency/ continuous O_2/assisted ventilation	Death

CTCAE common terminology criteria for adverse events, *ADL* activities of daily living, *RTOG* radiation therapy oncology group, *EORTC* European Organization for Research and Treatment of Cancer

[a]Toxicity causing death is always graded as 5

In the effort to establish a common terminology and grading scale applicable to lung toxicity related to different oncological treatments, including RT, version 3 of CTCAE was released (Trotti et al. 2003), with subsequent updates till version 5 in 2017 (Cancer Institute N 2017). In this scale, pneumonitis is graded according to the severity of symptoms and limitation in activities of daily living (ADL), and appropriate treatment is provided for each grade. Conversely, pulmonary fibrosis is classified according to the percentage of the affected lung volume calculated at CT and the presence of hypoxia and hemodynamic consequences, with treatment indications only for grade 4 toxicity. Of note, in the evaluation of SBRT-induced fibrosis, the CTCAE fibrosis scale is not appropriate (Yamamoto et al. 2018), as SBRT-induced fibrotic changes tend to develop in the lung parenchyma immediately surrounding the treated lesion, without involving large amounts of lung volume. For this reason, volume percentages of fibrotic changes considered in the CTCAE grading scale are too high for SBRT.

The abovementioned scales are mainly based on symptom severity rather than radiological appearance, and symptoms may not correlate with the radiological extent of RILI (Deng et al. 2017). It may occur that patients showing extensive lung changes are paucisymptomatic and, therefore, classified as having grade 2 RILI. In terms of RILI grading, due to refinements in RT techniques, the occurrence of grade =2 radiation pneumonitis has progressively decreased from 30–47% with 2D-RT, to 30–35% with 3D-RT, to 29–32% with IMRT, to 24–29% with the more recent VMAT and even to less than 5% with proton therapy (Käsmann et al. 2020), with a reported incidence of 9.1% in case of SBRT (Zhang et al. 2022).

5.2 Radiological Measurement of Lung Toxicity

Several studies have proposed various RILI grading systems entirely based on CT imaging appearance (Palma et al. 2011a; Yamamoto et al. 2018; Geara et al. 1998; Jenkins and Welsh 2011; Kouloulias et al. 2013; Moran et al. 2017; Bernchou et al. 2017; Szejniuk et al. 2021) (Table 2), trying to identify correlations with predictive clinical and treatment data (Palma et al. 2011a; Yamamoto et al. 2018; Geara et al. 1998; Jenkins and Welsh 2011; Kouloulias et al. 2013; Bernchou et al. 2017; Szejniuk et al. 2021). Some classification systems are based on a qualitative description of lung abnormalities (Palma et al. 2011a; Geara et al. 1998; Jenkins and Welsh 2011; Kouloulias et al. 2013; Moran et al. 2017), while others define RILI extent using the affected lung volume or the number of affected segments (Yamamoto et al. 2018; Bernchou et al. 2017; Szejniuk et al. 2021).

The studies providing a qualitative description of RILI mainly rely on density of the lung abnormalities and their extent, according to a visual assessment. Correlations have been found between alteration severity and treatment-related factors (dosimetric parameters, fractionation scheme) (Palma et al. 2011a; Geara et al. 1998; Jenkins and Welsh 2011; Kouloulias et al. 2013), as well as between radiological changes and symptoms of radiation pneumonitis occurrence (Jenkins and Welsh 2011) or forced expiratory volume in 1 s (FEV1) reduction (Kouloulias et al. 2013). A classification system based on RILI qualitative description, adapted from Palma et al. (2011a), is also reported in the study by Moran et al. (2017), with the aim of exploring the potential of radiomics features to distinguish moderate/severe from none/light categories.

Other studies have addressed the issue of establishing a more objective method to assess RILI on CT imaging. Bernchou et al. (2017) evaluated CT scans performed within 6 months from RT initiation in 220 patients with NSCLC and categorized RILI into interstitial changes, ground-glass opacities, and patchy or confluent consolidations, establishing for each category a grading system based on the relative volume of lung affected by radiation injury with respect to the whole-lung volume. According to their analysis, a higher degree of lung injury was found to be associated with a longer time between the start of RT and follow-up, as well as with most of the dose metrics (Bernchou et al. 2017).

Table 2 Computed tomography (CT) radiotherapy-induced lung injury (RILI) grading systems

Authors	RT type	Grade 0	Grade 1	Grade 2	Grade 3	Grade 4	Grade 5
Jenkins and Welsh (2011)	3D-CRT; 54 Gy in 36 fr	No change	Slight homogeneous increase in density (e.g., ground-glass appearance)	Patchy or multifocal consolidation that does not conform to the irradiated area	Severe confluent consolidation that conforms to the shape of the irradiated area but does not uniformly involve it	–	–
Kouloulias et al. (2013)	3D-CRT; 60–66 Gy in 30–33 fr	No findings	Ground-glass opacities without fuzziness of underlying pulmonary vessels	Findings variable from ground-glass opacities, extending beyond the radiation field to consolidation	Clear focal consolidation ± elements of fibrosis	Dense consolidation, cicatricial atelectasis, air bronchogram and bronchial extension (traction bronchiectasis), significant pulmonary volume loss, and pleural thickening	–
Moran et al. (2017)	3D-CRT, IMRT, VMAT; 50–60 Gy in 3–5 fr	No significant change	Mild change felt to be of little clinical importance	Moderate change commonly seen with SBRT	Severe change more extensive than would be expected following SBRT	–	–
Bernchou et al. (2017)	IMRT, VMAT; 60–66 Gy in 30–33 fr	No injury	A fraction of lung affected in the range 0–0.05	A fraction of lung affected in the range 0.05–0.1	A fraction of lung affected above 0.1	–	–
Yamamoto et al. (2018)	3D-CRT; 40/48 Gy in 4 fr	None	Slight radiographic appearance	Patchy radiographic appearance	Diffuse radiographic changes <25% of lung volume	Diffuse radiographic changes =25% of lung volume	Death
Szejniuk et al. (2021)	3D-CRT or IMRT; 60–66 Gy in 30–33 fr	No RILI	*At least one of the following items:* Ground-glass opacities; Consolidation (nodular, patchy or confluent); Volume loss; Pleural thickening; Interstitial changes; Fibrosis ***In <4 segments*** *± ipsilateral pleural effusion* ***<1 cm***	*At least one of the following items:* Ground-glass opacities; Consolidation (nodular, patchy or confluent); Volume loss; Pleural thickening; Interstitial changes; Fibrosis ***In 4–5 segments*** *± ipsilateral pleural effusion* ***1–2 cm***	*At least one of the following items:* Ground-glass opacities; Consolidation (nodular, patchy, or confluent); Volume loss; Pleural thickening; Interstitial changes; Fibrosis ***In >5 segments*** *± ipsilateral pleural effusion* ***>2 cm***	–	–

RT radiation therapy, *3D-CRT* three-dimensional conformal radiation therapy, *Gy* gray, *fr* fractions, *IMRT* intensity-modulated radiation therapy, *VMAT* volumetric-modulated arc therapy

Yamamoto et al. (2018) proposed a 5-point severity grading system for late SBRT-induced injuries, reporting a qualitative description of CT alterations adapted from the *Modified RTOG/EORTC Late Radiation Morbidity Scoring Schema,* introducing a percentage volume cut-off (derived from the CTCAE scale of pulmonary fibrosis) to distinguish among grades 3 and 4. Age, oxygen requirement, and interstitial changes resulted to be significant predictors of grades =2 alterations, with a good interobserver agreement for the grading system application (quadratic weighted kappa = 0.66; 95% CI: 0.23–1.00) (Yamamoto et al. 2018).

Another method proposed for the quantitative estimation of radiological RILI distinguished different grades according to the number of affected lung segments, showing a high interobserver reproducibility (Kendall's W coefficient of concordance = 0.80, $p < 0.01$) and a significant association between grades 2 and 3 and the development of symptomatic radiation pneumonitis (Szejniuk et al. 2021).

In the effort to find a tool allowing a more objective and quantitative assessment of RILI, several studies explored the potential role of variation in Hounsfield Units (HU) between pre-treatment and post-treatment CT scans, also trying to find correlation with dosimetric or baseline imaging-based parameters and clinical symptoms (Palma et al. 2011b, c; Bernchou et al. 2013; Ma et al. 2010; Defraene et al. 2015; Schröder et al. 2019; Al Feghali et al. 2020). The dose-dependent increase in lung density is well established (Bernchou et al. 2013; Ma et al. 2010; Defraene et al. 2015; Schröder et al. 2019); in addition, a significant correlation with the time elapsed since RT treatment has been described, with an increase in lung density in the first 6 months and a subsequent plateau at approximately 6–12 months (Ma et al. 2010), consistent with the conventional subdivision into radiation pneumonitis and fibrosis (Bernchou et al. 2013; Ma et al. 2010). A positive correlation between HU variation in the peritumoral region and radiation pneumonitis grade according to the CTCAE grading scale was also observed (Al Feghali et al. 2020). However, variation in HU may result from several other causes, either related to different pathological processes, including tumor recurrence, atelectasis, infectious, and drug-induced pneumonitis, or to technical factors, such as contrast medium administration (Chandy et al. 2022).

To overcome these limitations, a more complex model to classify RILI at a voxel level has been proposed (Chandy et al. 2022), which distinguished five different classes of lung parenchymal textures according to the density, ranging from *normal/emphysematous lung* to *homogeneously dense lung tissue.* A deep-learning algorithm analyzed the changes in the relative volume of each class from the pre-RT CT to the various follow-up time points up to 24 months, providing interesting insights in the evolution over time of RILI, particularly demonstrating different trends in the prevalence of each category during follow-up. Moreover, a mild-to-moderate correlation between volume changes of different classes and dosimetric parameters was determined, as well as a correlation, albeit weak, with spirometric parameters and dyspnea score (Chandy et al. 2022).

Lastly, Huang et al. (2023) proposed a simpler and easily applicable quantitative model based on the relative volume of RILI, correlating the affected volume and the severity symptoms, as defined by the CTCAE grading scale, determining a volume cut-off of 4.79% for the onset of symptoms. Furthermore, the correlation between isodose lines and development of RILI was observed by superimposing the dose curves of the treatment planning CT on the RILI changes in the posttreatment CT (Figs. 4 and 5). This study demonstrated that =80% of RILI grade 1 or 2 occurred within the 26 Gy isodose (Huang et al. 2023).

The potential of radiomics has been explored to find higher-order features with respect to density that could be applied to the evaluation of RILI (Moran et al. 2017; Cunliffe et al. 2015). Moran et al. (2017) observed the potential of radiomics features in distinguishing the severity of SBRT-induced lung injury in patients with stage I NSCLC (none/mild vs. moderate/severe); in addition, a significant dose-response relation-

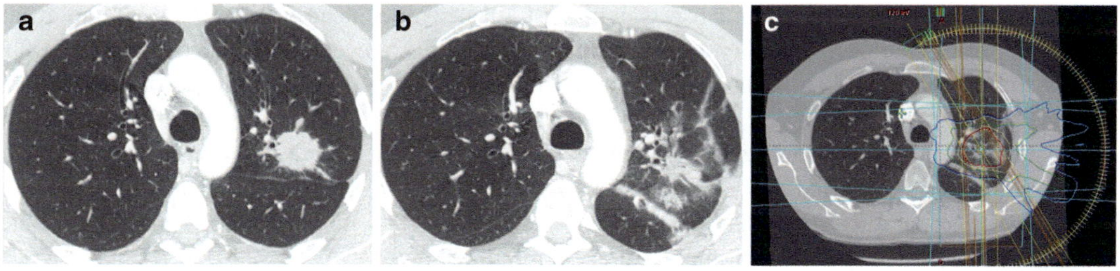

Fig. 4 Superposition of the isodose lines of a stereotactic body radiation therapy (SBRT) treatment plan for lung metastasis on the post-radiotherapy CT scan. Axial CT image demonstrating a 3.0 cm lung nodule of the left upper lobe (**a**) treated with SBRT-volumetric-modulated arc therapy (VMAT), in a patient with oligoprogressive gastric cancer. Axial CT image of RILI at 3 months after treatment completion, showing the *orbit-like* pattern (**b**). SBRT treatment plan (50 Gy in 5 fractions to the 80% isodose line) with isodose lines superimposed on the follow-up CT scan performed 3 months after radiotherapy (**c**), highlighting the posttreatment parenchymal changes within the treated volume. The superimposed isodose lines visually indicate the lesion shrinkage in the region within the inner isodose (*red line*, corresponding to the region receiving the highest dose) and slight radiation-induced abnormalities in the peripheral regions delineated by the isodose lines corresponding to lower doses (approximately within the *blue line*, corresponding to 20 Gy). *Isodose color legend: red = 50 Gy (80% isodose); yellow = 40 Gy; green = 30 Gy; blue = 20 Gy*

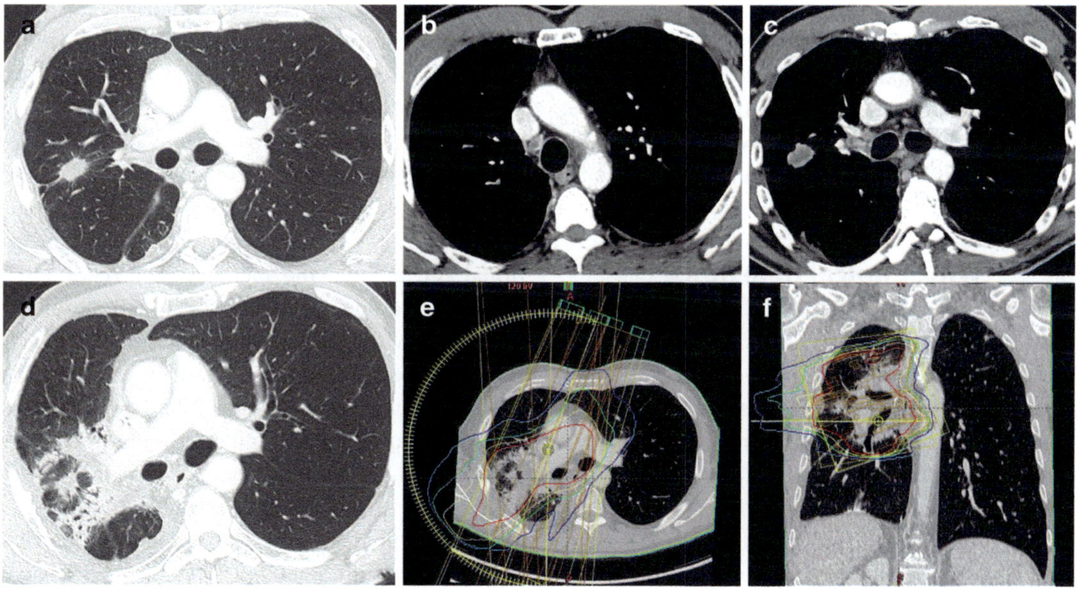

Fig. 5 Radiation therapy (RT) with volumetric-modulated arc therapy (VMAT) for stage III non-small cell lung cancer (NSCLC), with superposition of isodose lines on the post-RT CT scan. Axial CT images in the lung window setting (**a**) and mediastinal window setting (**b**, **c**) demonstrating a 2.3 cm adenocarcinoma of the right upper lobe with ipsilateral mediastinal and hilar lymphadenopathies (stage IIIa). Axial CT image depicting the radiotherapy-induced lung injury (RILI) at 3 months after treatment completion (60 Gy in 30 fractions) (**d**), which shows a reduction in size of the treated lesion with a surrounding consolidation and an interposed area of spared lung parenchyma (*orbit-like* pattern). The isodose lines superimposed on the follow-up CT scan in both the axial plane (**e**) and coronal plane (**f**) help visualize the correlation between the delivered radiation dose and the post-treatment parenchymal changes within the treated lung volume, with high-dose areas confined to the tumor and resulting in more significant RILI changes. *Isodose color legend: red = 50 Gy (80% isodose); yellow = 40 Gy; green = 30 Gy; blue = 20 Gy*

ship at 3 and 6 months after treatment was demonstrated for changes in first-order and higher-order (gray level co-occurrence matrix; GLCM) features.

Despite the several proposed radiological RILI grading systems, based on both qualitative and quantitative parameters, to date, a validated grading scale easily applicable in clinical practice is still lacking. Finding a radiological grading system with a good correlation with both treatment parameters and clinical symptoms remains an urgent need. Since qualitative parameters for assessing RILI are affected by interindividual variability and poor standardization, a grading system based on quantitative tools would be preferable. Among the various investigated options, the HU employment is affected by several limitations, and radiomics—though promising—still represents a field of research. In this context, a grading system based on isodose lines (Huang et al. 2023) could represent a readily applicable method, useful for radiation oncologists. The correspondence between an isodose line and lung toxicity may have major implications in terms of treatment planning.

6 Why: Clinical Relevance of Lung Toxicity

The proper recognition of RILI and its distinction from other chest disease that may occur in patients undergoing RT for thoracic neoplasms is of paramount importance for patient management. The main differential diagnoses include local recurrence, infectious disease, lymphangitic carcinomatosis, organizing pneumonia, and radiation recall pneumonitis (Larici et al. 2011; Jo et al. 2024). The accurate evaluation of imaging findings, taking into consideration the time of RILI occurrence with respect to the reference point (last day of RT administration) and clinical-laboratory data, contributes to the correct diagnosis.

Local recurrence The local recurrence rate after conventional RT in stage I NSCLC varied between 6.4% and 70% according to different studies, with a mean value of 40% (Qiao et al. 2003), while a recent systematic review on SBRT reports a rate of local recurrence of 13% over a median follow-up of about 24 months for both NSCLC and lung metastases (Lee et al. 2022). It is worth noting that local recurrence is more likely to occur within the first 24 months after the reference point.

The correct and prompt recognition of recurrence is of paramount importance to enable salvage therapy (National Comprehensive Cancer Network 2025a). Indeed, comparable outcome in terms of overall survival have been reported between patients undergoing salvage therapy after initial SBRT and patients without local recurrence (Brooks et al. 2018). Furthermore, growing evidence supports the safety and efficacy of reirradiation with SBRT (Kinj et al. 2021; Kennedy et al. 2020). On the contrary, misdiagnosis of recurrence may result in performing invasive procedures and even unnecessary treatments.

CT findings suggestive of local recurrence after RT treatment mimic the appearance of the primary neoplasm. Commonly reported CT findings suggestive of local recurrence after conventional RT include the increase in size of RILI changes, the development of a soft tissue growing mass, with convex or lobulated margins and inhomogeneous contrast enhancement, and the obstruction of the bronchial dilation within the fibrotic area (loss of air bronchogram) (Larici et al. 2011; Libshitz and Sheppard 1999; Benveniste et al. 2013) (Fig. 6). Although less frequent, the distinction of CT signs of RILI post-SBRT from local recurrence represents a challenge, due to the CT morphological appearance of SBRT-induced RILI and its potential evolution for even more than 2 years, up to a maximum of 5 years (Febbo et al. 2018).

Despite the widespread use of Response Evaluation Criteria In Solid Tumour (RECIST) 1.1 (Eisenhauer et al. 2009) in clinical practice, an International Delphi Consensus study stated their insufficiency in diagnosing recurrence after SBRT at CT imaging (Nguyen et al. 2018). In fact, the presence of fibrosis in the high-dose

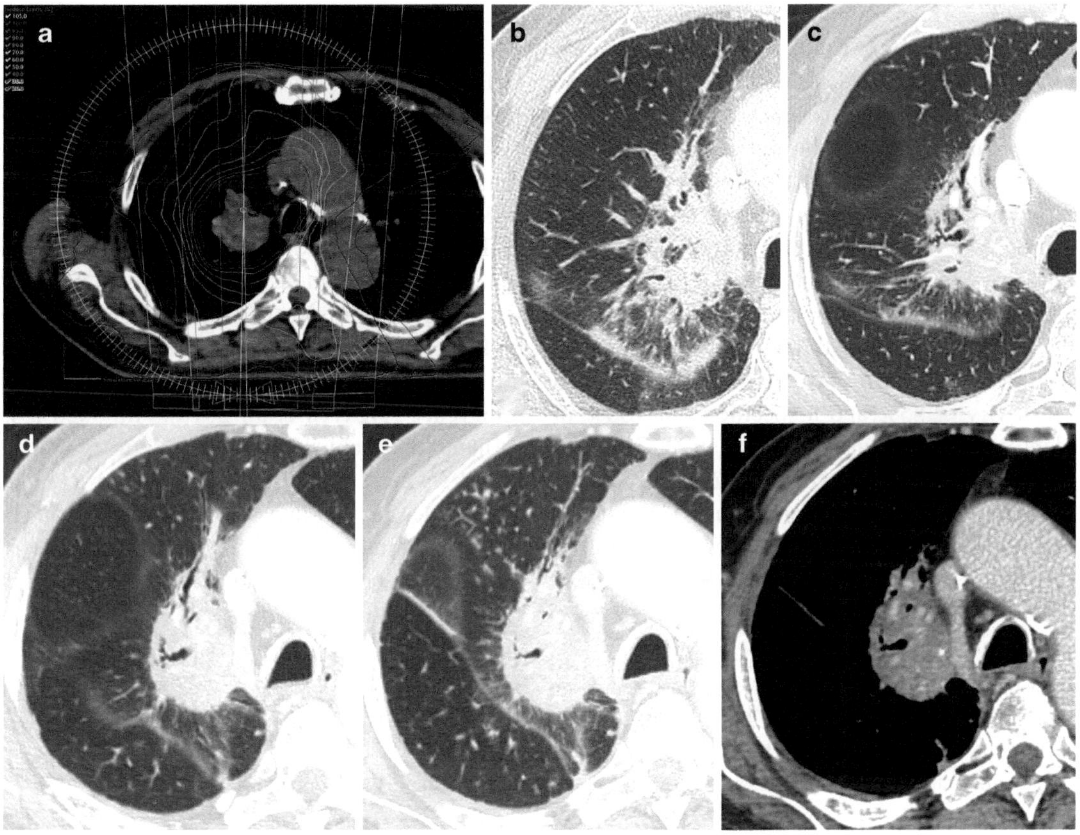

Fig. 6 Computed tomography (CT) findings suggestive of local recurrence after conventional radiotherapy (RT) with volumetric-modulated arc therapy (VMAT). RT treatment plan with dose distribution (**a**) in a 78-year-old man affected by right upper lobe squamous cell carcinoma, undergoing concomitant chemoradiation therapy. Axial CT images (**b**–**f**) showing the evolution of the treated lesion and the radiotherapy-induced lung injury (RILI) at 6 months (**b**), 12 months (**c**), 18 months (**d**), and 24 months (**e**, **f**) after RT completion, respectively. The serial images demonstrated the presence of multiple red flags for local recurrence, namely, the sustained growth over multiple scans, the mass-like/spherical appearance, the development of bulging margins (**d**, **e**), and an inhomogeneous contrast enhancement (**f**). Moreover, a progressive bronchial narrowing and obliteration is clearly evident, with development of post-obstructive airway inflammation in the downstream right upper lobe parenchyma (**e**)

region may hinder SBRT local response assessment (Senan et al. 2011). In addition, other limitations in using RECIST criteria in the follow-up are the following: the definition of a lesion <10 mm as non-measurable, while SBRT is mainly indicated in the treatment of small lesions; the indication to measure the longest diameter of a lesion at CT in the axial plane, while recurrence often involves limited or peripheral portion of the irradiated lung area resulting, for example, in cranio-caudal growth; and the difficulty and variability in measuring nonspherical lesions (Mattonen et al. 2016a). Therefore, the same Consensus suggests using a formal scoring system to classify the risk of local recurrence after SBRT, based on previously published CT high-risk features, as infiltration of adjacent organs/structures, sustained growth over serial scans, bulging margins, mass-like growth, predominantly spherical growth, cranio-caudal growth, and air space obliteration/loss of air bronchograms (Nguyen et al. 2018).

High-risk features were categorized by Huang et al. (2012) and subsequently broadened and validated (Lee et al. 2022; Huang et al. 2013). The high-risk features and their definitions (Lee et al. 2022; Huang et al. 2013; Peulen et al. 2016; Ronden et al. 2018; Kato et al. 2010; Halpenny et al. 2015) are listed in Table 3. Two of these features, namely, the bulging margins and the cranio-caudal growth, showed a relatively good performance according to a systematic review of 32 studies, with sensitivity and specificity of 72% and 84% for bulging margins and 87% and 81% for cranio-caudal growth, respectively (Lee et al. 2022). In the multicenter study, Peulen et al. used the cranio-caudal growth and the bulging margin features to develop a simplified model, reaching a sensitivity of 85% and a specificity of 100% in identifying local recurrence, with an AUC of 0.96 (95% CI 0.9–1.0) (Peulen et al. 2016). Nonetheless, the best performing CT feature turned out to be the presence of an enlarging opacity in the lung abnormalities after SBRT from 12 months onward, with a sensitivity of 94% and a specificity of 82%. This feature singularly showed a performance comparable to that observed in the presence of =3 of any other high-risk CT features considered (Lee et al. 2022), thus highlighting the importance of serial imaging evaluation to assess the lesion growth.

Fluorodeoxyglucose-positron emission tomography/computed tomography (FDG-PET/CT) may play a role in identifying recurrence and, according to the Delphi Consensus, its use is strongly recommended in cases of suspected recurrence (Nguyen et al. 2018). Although it is difficult to establish a consensus on SUVmax cut-offs, Lee et al. suggested that a relative reduction of SUVmax from baseline of less than 5% in the first 12 months post-SBRT is predictive of local recurrence, while a SUVmax >5 or 4.5 in

Table 3 High-risk features of local recurrence after stereotactic body radiation therapy (SBRT) in lung neoplasms (Lee et al. 2022) and their definitions (Huang et al. 2013; Peulen et al. 2016; Ronden et al. 2018; Kato et al. 2010; Halpenny et al. 2015)

Feature	Definition
Enlargement after 12 months	Increase in size in the axial plane of the lung abnormalities from 12 months onwards. (Peulen et al. 2016)
Cranio-caudal growth	Longitudinal growth of lung abnormalities of =5 mm or =20% in dimension. (Huang et al. 2013)
Bulging margin	Development or persistence of a convexity in the treated lesion in place of a previous straight or concave margin. (Ronden et al. 2018)
Linear margin disappearance	The former straight edge of the treated area is replaced by a convex margin. (Ronden et al. 2018)
Loss of air bronchogram	Reduction in caliber or disappearance of previously air-filled bronchi within a consolidation. (Ronden et al. 2018)
Enlarging opacity at primary site	Enlargement of the area of increased lung parenchymal density within the radiation field. (Ronden et al. 2018)
New or enlarging unilateral/ipsilateral pleural effusion	Occurrence or increase of pleural effusion in the side of the treated lesion. (Kato et al. 2010)
Sequential enlargement	A consolidation that progressively increases in size during follow-up CT scans. (Ronden et al. 2018)
New mass	Appearance or persistence of a lung lesion within 2 cm of the SBRT field, but distinct from the treated lesion. (Halpenny et al. 2015)
Density increase	Increase in CT attenuation of the treated lesion since the last follow-up. (Halpenny et al. 2015)
Appearance of lymph node enlargement	Occurrence of hilar or mediastinal lymph nodes with short axis >10 mm on serial CT scans. (Kato et al. 2010)
Inhomogeneity of contrast enhancement	Appearance of area of contrast enhancement within the typically hypodense treated lesion.
Appearance of angiogram sign	Branched linear structure within the lung abnormality that enhances after contrast administration, reproducing the normal vascularization of the area. (Kato et al. 2010)
Relative growth	Volume of the treated lesion compared to the volume of the primary tumor. (Peulen et al. 2016)

combination with qualitative features (i.e., a mass-like uptake visually higher than the blood pool taken as reference) is predictive of local recurrence after 12 months (Lee et al. 2022). Nevertheless, due to the lack of robust evidence on reliability of CT features alone in the first 12 months post-SBRT rather than after 12 months, the combined use of CT and PET/CT is advised to increase the likelihood of a correct identification of local recurrence (Lee et al. 2022).

Other tools are currently under investigation to address this issue, including magnetic resonance imaging (MRI) and radiomics. Studies exploring the role of MRI found that the apparent diffusion coefficient (ADC) showed good potential in identifying local recurrence (Sampath et al. 2019; Munoz-Schuffenegger et al. 2019; Kirshenboim et al. 2023). In particular, two prospective studies agreed that ADC values appeared to be lower in local recurrence than in relapse-free cases (Munoz-Schuffenegger et al. 2019; Kirshenboim et al. 2023), with values of 1.08×10^{-3} mm^2/s (interquartile range $1.00–1.19 \times 10^{-3}$ mm^2/s) vs. 1.60×10^{-3} mm^2/s (interquartile range $1.38–1.99 \times 10^{-3}$ mm^2/s) in the study by (Kirshenboim et al. 2023). Despite being limited so far to the field of research, radiomics has also shown promising results in both identification and prediction of recurrence (Mattonen et al. 2014, 2016b).

Infectious diseases The occurrence of areas of increased parenchymal density less than 4 weeks after the reference point or even before the radiation treatment termination may be suggestive of infection, even in case of slight or absent symptoms and laboratory testing, as RILI has generally not yet evident at this time (Toussie et al. 2024). Moreover, abnormalities suggestive of infection are more likely to occur outside the radiation field or bilaterally and tend to respect lung anatomic boundaries. Possibly associated ancillary findings, including centrilobular micronodules with or without a tree-in-bud pattern, cavitation, and mucoid impaction, may help the diagnosis of infection. Likewise, an infectious disease may also overlap with the physiological evolution of RILI, especially in patients with chronic obstructive pulmonary disease (COPD); in this case, the sudden onset of pulmonary abnormalities superimposed on the typically indolent course of RILI may suggest the correct diagnosis (Larici et al. 2011; Toussie et al. 2024).

Lymphangitic carcinomatosis Lymphangitic carcinomatosis may be found in lung neoplasms, especially NSCLC. It is characterized by distinctive CT findings, including smooth or nodular thickening of the interlobular septa and thickening of peribronchovascular interstitium (Desai et al. 2024). These abnormalities are often located outside the radiation portal and can be found even in both lungs (Larici et al. 2011). The association with pleural effusion and hilar or mediastinal nodal enlargement may guide the diagnosis.

Organizing pneumonia Apart from representing an adverse effect of systemic therapies, especially following immunotherapy, organizing pneumonia may occur after RT treatment. It may appear 6–18 months after SBRT, with a reported incidence of up to 4% after 1 year and 8% after 2 years and consists of patchy consolidations or ground-glass opacities arising outside the radiation field, with peripheral and peribronchovascular distribution and migratory behavior. These abnormalities may improve rapidly upon steroid therapy, although they often relapse with steroid withdrawal or tapering (Ochiai et al. 2015; Murai et al. 2012).

Radiation recall pneumonitis Radiation recall pneumonitis consists of ground-glass areas and/or consolidation occurring in the lung regions included in the radiation field, triggered by the administration of chemotherapy, targeted therapy or, more commonly, immunotherapy. This abnormality may develop months to years after RT completion and usually resolves quickly after steroid therapy, without residual alterations (Jo et al. 2024).

Radiation-induced neoplasms Patients who received RT to the chest are at risk of developing radiation-induced cancers, including sarcomas, breast cancer, lung cancer, esophageal cancer, and pleural mesothelioma (Benveniste et al. 2019). Particularly, studies conducted on patients undergoing RT for breast cancer have shown an increased risk of developing a second tumor compared to non-irradiated subjects (Grantzau and Overgaard 2016; Xia et al. 2022; Wennstig et al. 2021), with an estimated risk of developing second non-breast cancer of 23% (vs. 8%) (Grantzau and Overgaard 2016). This risk gradually increases over time, peaking at =10–15 years after diagnosis of the primary tumor (Grantzau and Overgaard 2016; Wennstig et al. 2021). Concerning radiation-induced lung cancer, a meta-analysis conducted on 113,516 irradiated and 203,957 non-irradiated breast cancer patients demonstrated that the standardized incidence ratio was of 1.21 at =5 years, 1.58 at =10 years, and 1.91 at =15 years, respectively (Grantzau and Overgaard 2016).

At imaging, the suspicion of radiation-induced lung cancer should arise when a newly appearing opacity is observed within or at the edge of the previous radiation field (Benveniste et al. 2019).

7 Other Thoracic RT Applications: Pleura and Mediastinum

Pleura The management of *pleural mesothelioma* is generally multimodal, and RT can be used in different settings. Particularly, in patients with resectable pleural mesothelioma undergoing extrapleural pneumonectomy, adjuvant RT can be recommended in case of good performance status in order to improve local control. RT may be applied also as an effective palliative treatment for chest pain relief, bronchial or esophageal obstruction, and other symptomatic sites. The use of IMRT is the preferred choice based on comprehensive consideration of target coverage and clinically relevant OAR tolerance (such as the contralateral lung) (Pleural 2023). Moreover, RT can be also used, with both curative and palliative intent, in the treatment of pleural metastasis, from either lung cancer or other thoracic and extra-thoracic malignancies, particularly in case of thoracic wall infiltration (Shepherd and Rimner 2022).

Esophagus RT is a fundamental part of treatment for esophageal and esophagogastric junction (EGJ) cancers as it is applied in preoperative, postoperative, or palliative settings. Treatment recommendations depend on the location of the bulk tumor and different guidelines are applied according to the tumor site, especially for EGJ lesions (Hang et al. 2024).

Thymus RT is an essential part of the multidisciplinary management of thymoma or thymic carcinoma. Definitive RT is indicated for patients with unresectable tumor or if disease progresses on induction systemic treatment. RT can be also recommended in patients with incompletely resected invasive tumor, or as adjuvant treatment after systemic therapy and surgery in patients with locally advanced disease (Kristina Gregory et al. 2023), as well as, in case of pleural metastases either to palliate symptoms or to maximize disease control, particularly in patients with limited sites of diseases (Shepherd and Rimner 2022; Pasquini 2021).

Lymphoma RT has an important role in the treatment of Hodgkin lymphoma, either alone or in combination with chemotherapy (Balosso et al. 2022). Hematological malignancies are usually treated with much lower RT doses than epithelial or mesenchymal tumors, with generally more favorable long-term outcomes (Lymphoma 2024).

7.1 Toxicity

RILI represents one of the major dose-limiting factors not only after treatment of lung cancer but also after RT for pleural and mediastinal tumors. Toxicity is sustained by the same pathogenetic mechanisms of RILI induced by lung cancer RT and follows the same conventional classification, distinguishing lung abnormalities appearing within the first 6 months (*early phase*) and 6 months onward (*late phase*) after the reference point, as defined above (Hanania et al. 2019; Käsmann et al. 2020). Furthermore, in addition to lung toxicity, RT treatment of both lung cancer and other thoracic neoplasms may induce complications also in other thoracic structures (Febbo et al. 2018; Benveniste et al. 2019) (Table 4).

The most important risk factors for toxicity are dose-volume metrics (e.g., MLD). Nevertheless, other treatment (especially concomitant chemotherapy and immunotherapy) and patient-related factors (age, comorbidities, smoking history, etc.) may contribute to the development of toxicity in the lungs and in other thoracic organs (Hang et al. 2024; Lymphoma 2024; Pozzessere et al. 2020, 2021).

Similar to lung cancers, RT of other thoracic malignancies requires careful definition of the target volumes while designing treatment plans; particularly, uncertainties from variations in respiratory motion should be considered. Moreover, in this setting, treatment planning is essential to reduce RT doses to OAR other than the lungs, and limiting as much as possible the radiation dose to susceptible organs is fundamental (i.e., esophagus, heart) (Hang et al. 2024). In addition, particularly when dealing with the treatment of young patients, attention should be paid to the potential development of secondary malignancies (Balosso et al. 2022).

Among the complications of thoracic RT, those affecting the heart and great vessels are of relevance due to their impact on mortality (Benveniste et al. 2019; Ramin et al. 2021). Radiation-induced cardiovascular injury may affect different structures, including the pericardium, atria and ventricles, valves, coronary arteries, superior vena cava, aorta, and pulmonary arteries (Bergom et al. 2021). The most common

Table 4 Radiotherapy-induced toxicities after radiation therapy (RT) for thoracic neoplasms other than lung cancer (Febbo et al. 2018; Benveniste et al. 2019)

Site	Early toxicity	Late toxicity
Airway	Airway wall thickening, with or without narrowing	Trachea or bronchus focal stricture Tracheoesophageal fistula
Pleura	Pleural effusion	Smooth pleural thickening
Heart	–	*Direct*: coronary artery disease, myocardial fibrosis, valvular fibrosis, and calcification *Indirect*: pulmonary hypertension and right ventricular alterations secondary to radiation fibrosis
Pericardium	Acute pericarditis	Chronic pericarditis up to constrictive pericarditis
Great vessels	Aorta wall thickening Aortic dissection Aortic rupture Aneurysm Hemoptysis	Calcifications of vessel walls Vascular occlusion Pseudoaneurysms
Lymph nodes	–	Mediastinal lymph node calcifications Fibrotic mass
Esophagus	Circumferential wall thickening, with or without narrowing Perforation Fistula	Stricture Chronic ulceration Perforation Fistula
Thymus	Cysts	–
Bones	Bone edema Osteopenia	Fractures Osteochondromas Osteoradionecrosis
Miscellaneous	–	Second malignancies: Sarcoma Lung cancer Bone tumor Pleural mesothelioma Esophageal cancer

radiation-induced cardiovascular complication is coronary artery disease (CAD), which can occur in up to 85% of cases, followed by pericardial disease (6%–30%), cardiomyopathy (up to 10%), and conduction system abnormalities (up to 5%). The incidence of valvular heart disease varies according to the type of alteration, with regurgitation being more frequent in the early phase while stenosis later, and according to side, with left valves more frequently affected than right valves (Chang et al. 2017). In the acute phase, complications are related to radiation-induced inflammation, while those occurring later are related to fibrotic modification of the involved structures (Narowska et al. 2023). Indeed, acute pericarditis may develop within days to months after RT; conversely, CAD and valvular heart disease tend to occur 5–10 years after (Chang et al. 2017), with a risk of developing any cardiovascular disease that may persist up to 47 years after RT (Van Nimwegen et al. 2015). Since many diseases may remain asymptomatic for long, imaging plays a key role in their identification before symptoms occur (Walker et al. 2013).

Pericarditis is characterized by pericardial effusion associated with pericardial thickening. Unless the effusion is large enough to cause tamponade, the clinical manifestation of acute pericarditis may range from asymptomatic to self-limiting symptoms, with only a few patients developing chronic pericarditis (Benveniste et al. 2019). In 20% of chronic cases, constrictive pericarditis may occur (Narowska et al. 2023), manifesting with pericardial thickening and calcifications, dilation of systemic veins, and flattening or diastolic bouncing of the interventricular septum (Benveniste et al. 2019).

Endothelial damage and inflammation induced by RT also lead to the formation of atherosclerotic plaques in the coronary arteries with a pathogenesis like CAD in the general population; however, in radiation-induced CAD, in addition to intimal plaque, a thinning of the medial vessel wall and adventitial fibrosis occur. CT is useful to evaluate and quantify coronary artery calcification and can be used to perform coronary angiography (Benveniste et al. 2019; Narowska et al. 2023; Walker et al. 2013).

8 Conclusions

The use of RT has become a cornerstone in the treatment of lung neoplasms and other thoracic malignancies, although toxicity still represents one of the major dose-limiting factors. The knowledge of CT appearance and the evolution over time of physiologic lung changes due to RILI is pivotal to assess toxicity severity and differentiate it from local recurrence and other potential coexisting lung diseases. Several radiological classification systems have been proposed for RILI assessment, even though with current limitations. Qualitative parameters are subject to interindividual variability and are poorly standardized, while quantitative parameters often rely on complex tools and are still a field of research. In terms of future perspectives, development and implementation of easily applicable grading system based on both clinical and radiological features would greatly assist in maximizing RT effectiveness while minimizing adverse effects.

References

Al Feghali KA, Wu Q (Charles), Devpura S, Liu C, Ghanem AI, Wen N (Winston) et al (2020) Correlation of normal lung density changes with dose after stereotactic body radiotherapy (SBRT) for early stage lung cancer. Clin Transl Radiat Oncol [Internet] 22:1. Available from: https://pubmed.ncbi.nlm.nih.gov/32140574/

Al-Umairi R, Tarique U, Moineddin R, Jimenez-Juan L, Kha LC, Cheung P et al (2022) CT patterns and serial CT changes in lung cancer patients post stereotactic body radiotherapy (SBRT). Cancer Imaging [Internet] 22(1):15. Available from: https://pubmed.ncbi.nlm.nih.gov/36114585/

Anscher MS, Arora S, Weinstock C, Amatya A, Bandaru P, Tang C et al (2022) Association of radiation therapy with risk of adverse events in patients receiving immunotherapy: a pooled analysis of trials in the US Food and Drug Administration database. JAMA Oncol [Internet] 8(2):232–240. Available from: https://mdanderson.elsevierpure.com/en/publications/association-of-radiation-therapy-with-risk-of-adverse-events-in-p

Aoki T, Nagata Y, Negoro Y, Takayama K, Mizowaki T, Kokubo M et al (2004) Evaluation of lung injury after three-dimensional conformal stereotactic radiation therapy for solitary lung tumors: CT appearance. Radiology [Internet] 230(1):101–108. Available from: https://pubmed.ncbi.nlm.nih.gov/14645881/

Arroyo-Hernández M, Maldonado F, Lozano-Ruiz F, Muñoz-Montaño W, Nuñez-Baez M, Arrieta O (2021) Radiation-induced lung injury: current evidence. BMC Pulm Med [Internet] 21(1). Available from: https://pubmed.ncbi.nlm.nih.gov/33407290/

Aupérin A, Le Péchoux C, Rolland E, Curran WJ, Furuse K, Fournel P et al (2010) Meta-analysis of concomitant versus sequential radiochemotherapy in locally advanced non-small-cell lung cancer. J Clin Oncol [Internet] 28(13):2181–2190. Available from: https://pubmed.ncbi.nlm.nih.gov/20351327/

Ball D, Mai GT, Vinod S, Babington S, Ruben J, Kron T et al (2019) Stereotactic ablative radiotherapy versus standard radiotherapy in stage 1 non-small-cell lung cancer (TROG 09.02 CHISEL): a phase 3, open-label, randomised controlled trial. Lancet Oncol [Internet] 20(4):494–503. Available from: https://pubmed.ncbi.nlm.nih.gov/30770291/

Balosso J, Missohou F, Antoni D, Hennequin C, Mahé MA, Simon L et al (2022) Radiotherapy of lymphomas. Cancer Radiother [Internet] 26(1–2):388–396. Available from: https://pubmed.ncbi.nlm.nih.gov/34953716/

Belderbos J, Sonke JJ (2009) State-of-the-art lung cancer radiation therapy. Expert Rev Anticancer Ther [Internet] 9(10):1353–1363. Available from: https://pubmed.ncbi.nlm.nih.gov/19827995/

Benveniste MFK, Welsh J, Godoy MCB, Betancourt SL, Mawlawi OR, Munden RF (2013) New era of radiotherapy: an update in radiation-induced lung disease. Clin Radiol [Internet] 68(6). Available from: https://pubmed.ncbi.nlm.nih.gov/23473474/

Benveniste MF, Gomez D, Carter BW, Betancourt Cuellar SL, Shroff GS, Benveniste APA et al (2019) Recognizing radiation therapy-related complications in the chest. Radiographics [Internet] 39(2):344–366. Available from: https://pubmed.ncbi.nlm.nih.gov/30844346/

Bergom C, Bradley JA, Ng AK, Samson P, Robinson C, Lopez-Mattei J et al (2021) Past, present, and future of radiation-induced cardiotoxicity: refinements in targeting, surveillance, and risk stratification. JACC CardioOncol [Internet] 3(3):343–359. Available from: https://pubmed.ncbi.nlm.nih.gov/34604796/

Bernchou U, Schytte T, Bertelsen A, Bentzen SM, Hansen O, Brink C (2013) Time evolution of regional CT density changes in normal lung after IMRT for NSCLC. Radiother Oncol [Internet] 109(1):89–94. Available from: https://pubmed.ncbi.nlm.nih.gov/24060177/

Bernchou U, Christiansen RL, Asmussen JT, Schytte T, Hansen O, Brink C (2017) Extent and computed tomography appearance of early radiation induced lung injury for non-small cell lung cancer. Radiother Oncol [Internet] 123(1):93–98. Available from: https://pubmed.ncbi.nlm.nih.gov/28259449/

Bledsoe TJ, Nath SK, Decker RH (2017) Radiation pneumonitis. Clin Chest Med [Internet] 38(2):201–208. Available from: https://pubmed.ncbi.nlm.nih.gov/28477633/

Brooks ED, Sun B, Feng L, Verma V, Zhao L, Gomez DR et al (2018) Association of long-term outcomes and survival with multidisciplinary salvage treatment for local and regional recurrence after stereotactic ablative radiotherapy for early-stage lung cancer. JAMA Netw Open [Internet] 1(4). Available from: https://pubmed.ncbi.nlm.nih.gov/30646121/

Cancer Institute N (2017) Common terminology criteria for adverse events (CTCAE) common terminology criteria for adverse events (CTCAE) v5.0. Available from: https://www.meddra.org/

Chandy E, Szmul A, Stavropoulou A, Jacob J, Veiga C, Landau D et al (2022) Quantitative analysis of radiation-associated parenchymal lung change. Cancers (Basel) [Internet] 14(4). Available from: https://pubmed.ncbi.nlm.nih.gov/35205693/

Chang HM, Okwuosa TM, Scarabelli T, Moudgil R, Yeh ETH (2017) Cardiovascular complications of cancer therapy: best practices in diagnosis, prevention, and management: part 2. J Am Coll Cardiol [Internet] 70(20):2552–2565. Available from: https://pubmed.ncbi.nlm.nih.gov/29145955/

Chassagnon G, Martini K, Giraud P, Revel MP (2020) Radiological assessment after stereotactic body radiation of lung tumours. Cancer Radiother [Internet] 24(5):379–387. Available from: https://pubmed.ncbi.nlm.nih.gov/32534799/

Chen F, Niu J, Wang M, Zhu H, Guo Z (2023) Re-evaluating the risk factors for radiation pneumonitis in the era of immunotherapy. J Transl Med [Internet] 21(1). Available from: https://pubmed.ncbi.nlm.nih.gov/37287014/

Choi YW, Munden RF, Erasmus JJ, Park KJ, Chung WK, Jeon SC et al (2004) Effects of radiation therapy on the lung: radiologic appearances and differential diagnosis. Radiographics [Internet] 24(4):985–997. Available from: https://pubmed.ncbi.nlm.nih.gov/15256622/

Cox JD, Stetz JA, Pajak TF (1995) Toxicity criteria of the Radiation Therapy Oncology Group (RTOG) and the European Organization for Research and Treatment of Cancer (EORTC). Int J Radiat Oncol Biol Phys

[Internet] 31(5):1341–1346. Available from: https://pubmed.ncbi.nlm.nih.gov/7713792/

Cozzi S, Alì E, Bardoscia L, Najafi M, Botti A, Blandino G et al (2022) Stereotactic body radiation therapy (SBRT) for oligorecurrent/oligoprogressive mediastinal and hilar lymph node metastasis: a systematic review. Cancers (Basel) [Internet] 14(11):2680. Available from: https://pubmed.ncbi.nlm.nih.gov/35681659/

Cunliffe A, Armato SG, Castillo R, Pham N, Guerrero T, Al-Hallaq HA (2015) Lung texture in serial thoracic computed tomography scans: correlation of radiomics-based features with radiation therapy dose and radiation pneumonitis development. Int J Radiat Oncol Biol Phys [Internet] 91(5):1048. Available from: https://pubmed.ncbi.nlm.nih.gov/25670540/

Dahele M, Palma D, Lagerwaard F, Slotman B, Senan S (2011) Radiological changes after stereotactic radiotherapy for stage I lung cancer. J Thorac Oncol [Internet] 6(7):()1–()8. Available from: https://pubmed.ncbi.nlm.nih.gov/21623237/

Dang J, Li G, Zang S, Zhang S, Yao L (2014) Comparison of risk and predictors for early radiation pneumonitis in patients with locally advanced non-small cell lung cancer treated with radiotherapy with or without surgery. Lung Cancer [Internet] 86(3):329–333. Available from: https://pubmed.ncbi.nlm.nih.gov/25454199/

Davis SD, Yankelevitz DF, Henschke CI (1992) Radiation effects on the lung: clinical features, pathology, and imaging findings. AJR Am J Roentgenol [Internet] 159(6):1157–1164. Available from: https://pubmed.ncbi.nlm.nih.gov/1442375/

Defraene G, Van Elmpt W, Crijns W, Slagmolen P, De Ruysscher D (2015) CT characteristics allow identification of patient-specific susceptibility for radiation-induced lung damage. Radiother Oncol [Internet] 117(1):29–35. Available from: https://pubmed.ncbi.nlm.nih.gov/26255763/

Deng G, Liang N, Xie J, Luo H, Qiao L, Zhang J et al (2017) Pulmonary toxicity generated from radiotherapeutic treatment of thoracic malignancies. Oncol Lett [Internet] 14(1):501. Available from: https://pubmed.ncbi.nlm.nih.gov/28693198/

Desai S, Lynch D, Elicker BM, Devaraj A, Sverzellati N. Webb, Müller and Naidich's high-resolution CT of ... [Internet]. [cited 2024 Oct 1]. Available from: https://shop.lww.com/Webb%2D%2DM-ller-and-Naidich-s-High-Resolution-CT-of-the-Lung/p/9781975144432

Diez P, Hanna GG, Aitken KL, van As N, Carver A, Colaco RJ et al (2022) UK 2022 consensus on normal tissue dose-volume constraints for oligometastatic, primary lung and hepatocellular carcinoma stereotactic ablative radiotherapy. Clin Oncol (R Coll Radiol) [Internet] 34(5):288–300. Available from: https://pubmed.ncbi.nlm.nih.gov/35272913/

Eisenhauer EA, Therasse P, Bogaerts J, Schwartz LH, Sargent D, Ford R et al (2009) New response evaluation criteria in solid tumours: revised RECIST guideline (version 1.1). Eur J Cancer [Internet] 45(2):228–247. Available from: https://pubmed.ncbi.nlm.nih.gov/19097774/

Febbo JA, Gaddikeri RS, Shah PN (2018) Stereotactic body radiation therapy for early-stage non-small cell lung cancer: a primer for radiologists. Radiographics [Internet] 38(5):1312–1336. Available from: https://pubmed.ncbi.nlm.nih.gov/30074857/

Finazzi T, Schneiders FL, Senan S (2021) Developments in radiation techniques for thoracic malignancies. Eur Respir Rev [Internet] 30(160). Available from: https://pubmed.ncbi.nlm.nih.gov/33952599/

Geara FB, Komaki R, Tucker SL, Travis EL, Cox JD (1998) Factors influencing the development of lung fibrosis after chemoradiation for small cell carcinoma of the lung: evidence for inherent interindividual variation. Int J Radiat Oncol Biol Phys [Internet] 41(2):279–286. Available from: https://pubmed.ncbi.nlm.nih.gov/9607342/

Geng Y, Zhang Q, Feng S, Li C, Wang L, Zhao X et al (2021) Safety and efficacy of PD-1/PD-L1 inhibitors combined with radiotherapy in patients with non-small-cell lung cancer: a systematic review and meta-analysis. Cancer Med [Internet] 10(4):1222–1239. Available from: https://pubmed.ncbi.nlm.nih.gov/33465302/

Ghaye B, Wanet M, El Hajjam M (2016) Imaging after radiation therapy of thoracic tumors. Diagn Interv Imaging [Internet] 97(10):1037–1052. Available from: https://pubmed.ncbi.nlm.nih.gov/27567554/

Graham MV, Purdy JA, Emami B, Harms W, Bosch W, Lockett MA et al (1999) Clinical dose-volume histogram analysis for pneumonitis after 3D treatment for non-small cell lung cancer (NSCLC). Int J Radiat Oncol Biol Phys [Internet] 45(2):323–329. Available from: https://pubmed.ncbi.nlm.nih.gov/10487552/

Grantzau T, Overgaard J (2016) Risk of second non-breast cancer among patients treated with and without postoperative radiotherapy for primary breast cancer: a systematic review and meta-analysis of population-based studies including 522,739 patients. Radiother Oncol [Internet] 121(3):402–413. Available from: https://pubmed.ncbi.nlm.nih.gov/27639892/

Green S, Weiss GR (1992) Southwest Oncology Group standard response criteria, endpoint definitions and toxicity criteria. Invest New Drugs [Internet] 10(4):239–253. Available from: https://pubmed.ncbi.nlm.nih.gov/1487397/

Guckenberger M, Andratschke N, Dieckmann K, Hoogeman MS, Hoyer M, Hurkmans C et al (2017) ESTRO ACROP consensus guideline on implementation and practice of stereotactic body radiotherapy for peripherally located early stage non-small cell lung cancer. Radiother Oncol [Internet] 124(1):11–17. Available from: https://pubmed.ncbi.nlm.nih.gov/28687397/

Hall WA, Paulson E, Li XA, Erickson B, Schultz C, Tree A et al (2022) Magnetic resonance linear accelerator technology and adaptive radiation therapy: an overview for clinicians. CA Cancer J Clin [Internet]

72(1):34–56. Available from: https://pubmed.ncbi.nlm.nih.gov/34792808/

Halpenny D, Ridge CA, Hayes S, Zheng J, Moskowitz CS, Rimner A et al (2015) Computed tomographic features predictive of local recurrence in patients with early stage lung cancer treated with stereotactic body radiation therapy. Clin Imaging [Internet] 39(2):254–258. Available from: https://pubmed.ncbi.nlm.nih.gov/25571791/

Han C, Qiu J, Bai L, Liu T, Chen J, Wang H et al (2024) Pneumonitis risk after chemoradiotherapy with and without immunotherapy in patients with locally advanced non-small cell lung cancer: a systematic review and meta-analysis. Int J Radiat Oncol Biol Phys [Internet] 119(4):1179–1207. Available from: https://pubmed.ncbi.nlm.nih.gov/38360117/

Hanania AN, Mainwaring W, Ghebre YT, Hanania NA, Ludwig M (2019) Radiation-induced lung injury: assessment and management. Chest [Internet] 156(1):150–162. Available from: https://pubmed.ncbi.nlm.nih.gov/30998908/

Hang L, McMillian N, MaryElizabeth Stein M, Ajani JA, D TA, Chair V et al (2024) NCCN guidelines version 3.2024 esophageal and esophagogastric junction cancers continue NCCN [Internet]. Available from: https://www.nccn.org/home/

Herrmann H, Seppenwoolde Y, Georg D, Widder J (2019) Image guidance: past and future of radiotherapy. Radiologe [Internet] 59(Suppl 1):21–27. Available from: https://pubmed.ncbi.nlm.nih.gov/31346650/

Huang K, Dahele M, Senan S, Guckenberger M, Rodrigues GB, Ward A et al (2012) Radiographic changes after lung stereotactic ablative radiotherapy (SABR)—can we distinguish recurrence from fibrosis? A systematic review of the literature. Radiother Oncol [Internet] 102(3):335–342. Available from: https://pubmed.ncbi.nlm.nih.gov/22305958/

Huang K, Senthi S, Palma DA, Spoelstra FOB, Warner A, Slotman BJ et al (2013) High-risk CT features for detection of local recurrence after stereotactic ablative radiotherapy for lung cancer. Radiother Oncol [Internet] 109(1):51–57. Available from: https://pubmed.ncbi.nlm.nih.gov/23953413/

Huang JW, Lin YH, Chang GC, Chen JJW (2023) A novel tool to evaluate and quantify radiation pneumonitis: a retrospective analysis of correlation of dosimetric parameters with volume of pneumonia patch. Front Oncol [Internet] 13. Available from: https://pubmed.ncbi.nlm.nih.gov/36994217/

Jenkins P, Welsh A (2011) Computed tomography appearance of early radiation injury to the lung: correlation with clinical and dosimetric factors. Int J Radiat Oncol Biol Phys [Internet] 81(1):97–103. Available from: https://pubmed.ncbi.nlm.nih.gov/21543163/

Jo NC, Shroff GS, Ahuja J, Agrawal R, Price MC, Wu CC (2024) Radiation recall pneumonitis: imaging appearance and differential considerations. Korean J Radiol [Internet] 25(9):843–850. Available from: https://pubmed.ncbi.nlm.nih.gov/39197829/

Käsmann L, Dietrich A, Staab-Weijnitz CA, Manapov F, Behr J, Rimner A et al (2020) Radiation-induced lung toxicity – cellular and molecular mechanisms of pathogenesis, management, and literature review. Radiat Oncol [Internet] 15(1):214. Available from: https://pubmed.ncbi.nlm.nih.gov/32912295/; https://pmc.ncbi.nlm.nih.gov/articles/PMC7488099/

Kato S, Nambu A, Onishi H, Saito A, Kuriyama K, Komiyama T et al (2010) Computed tomography appearances of local recurrence after stereotactic body radiation therapy for stage I non-small-cell lung carcinoma. Jpn J Radiol [Internet] 28(4):259–265. Available from: https://pubmed.ncbi.nlm.nih.gov/20512542/

Kennedy WR, Gabani P, Nikitas J, Robinson CG, Bradley JD, Roach MC (2020) Repeat stereotactic body radiation therapy (SBRT) for salvage of isolated local recurrence after definitive lung SBRT. Radiother Oncol [Internet] 142:230–235. Available from: https://pubmed.ncbi.nlm.nih.gov/31481272/

Kimura T, Matsuura K, Murakami Y, Hashimoto Y, Kenjo M, Kaneyasu Y et al (2006) CT appearance of radiation injury of the lung and clinical symptoms after stereotactic body radiation therapy (SBRT) for lung cancers: are patients with pulmonary emphysema also candidates for SBRT for lung cancers? Int J Radiat Oncol Biol Phys [Internet] 66(2):483–491. Available from: https://pubmed.ncbi.nlm.nih.gov/16904838/

Kinj R, Casutt A, Bennassi A, Bouchaab H, Vallet V, Lovis A et al (2021) Stereotactic lung reirradiation for local relapse: a case series. Clin Transl Radiat Oncol [Internet] 28:85. Available from: https://pubmed.ncbi.nlm.nih.gov/33912693/

Kirshenboim Z, Dan Lantsman C, Appel S, Klug M, Onn A, Truong MT et al (2023) Magnetic resonance imaging for prospective assessment of local recurrence of non-small cell lung cancer after stereotactic body radiation therapy. Lung Cancer [Internet] 182:107265. Available from: https://pubmed.ncbi.nlm.nih.gov/37327593/

Koenig TR, Munden RF, Erasmus JJ, Sabloff BS, Gladish GW, Komaki R et al (2002) Radiation injury of the lung after three-dimensional conformal radiation therapy. AJR Am J Roentgenol [Internet] 178(6):1383–1388. Available from: https://pubmed.ncbi.nlm.nih.gov/12034601/

Konkol M, Sniatala P, Milecki P (2022) Radiation-induced lung injury — what do we know in the era of modern radiotherapy? Rep Pract Oncol Radiother [Internet] 27(3):552. Available from: https://pubmed.ncbi.nlm.nih.gov/36186693/

Kouloulias V, Zygogianni A, Efstathopoulos E, Victoria O, Christos A, Pantelis K et al (2013) Suggestion for a new grading scale for radiation induced pneumonitis based on radiological findings of computerized tomography: correlation with clinical and radiotherapeutic parameters in lung cancer patients. Asian Pac J Cancer Prev [Internet] 14(5):2717–2722. Available from: https://pubmed.ncbi.nlm.nih.gov/23803021/

Kristina Gregory N, Lisa Hang M, Riely GJ, Aisner DL, Akerley W; Hutchinson Cancer Center F et al (2023) NCCN guidelines version 1.2024 thymomas and thymic carcinomas continue NCCN guidelines panel disclosures [Internet]. Available from: https://www.nccn.org/home/member

Larici AR, del Ciello A, Maggi F, Santoro SI, Meduri B, Valentini V et al (2011) Lung abnormalities at multimodality imaging after radiation therapy for non-small cell lung cancer. Radiographics [Internet] 31(3):771–789. Available from: https://pubmed.ncbi.nlm.nih.gov/21571656/

Lee K, Le T, Hau E, Hanna GG, Gee H, Vinod S et al (2022) A systematic review into the radiologic features predicting local recurrence after stereotactic ablative body radiotherapy (SABR) in patients with non-small cell lung cancer (NSCLC). Int J Radiat Oncol Biol Phys [Internet] 113(1):40–59. Available from: https://pubmed.ncbi.nlm.nih.gov/34879247/

LENT SOMA scales for all anatomic sites. Int J Radiat Oncol Biol Phys [Internet]. 1995;31(5):1049–1091. Available from: https://pubmed.ncbi.nlm.nih.gov/7713776/

Li C, Wang L, Wu Q, Zhao J, Yi F, Xu J et al (2020) A meta-analysis comparing stereotactic body radiotherapy vs conventional radiotherapy in inoperable stage I non-small cell lung cancer. Medicine [Internet] 99(34):E21715. Available from: https://pubmed.ncbi.nlm.nih.gov/32846789/

Libshitz HI, Sheppard DG (1999) Filling in of radiation therapy-induced bronchiectatic change: a reliable sign of locally recurrent lung cancer. Radiology [Internet] 210(1):25–27. Available from: https://pubmed.ncbi.nlm.nih.gov/9885581/

Libshitz HI, Shuman LS (1984) Radiation-induced pulmonary change: CT findings. J Comput Assist Tomogr [Internet] 8(1):15–19. Available from: https://pubmed.ncbi.nlm.nih.gov/6690504/

Linda A, Trovo M, Bradley JD (2011) Radiation injury of the lung after stereotactic body radiation therapy (SBRT) for lung cancer: a timeline and pattern of CT changes. Eur J Radiol [Internet] 79(1):147–154. Available from: https://pubmed.ncbi.nlm.nih.gov/19954913/

Liu Z, Xu T, Chang P, Fu W, Wei J, Xia C et al (2023) Efficacy and safety of immune checkpoint inhibitors with or without radiotherapy in metastatic non-small cell lung cancer: a systematic review and meta-analysis. Front Pharmacol 14:1064227

Lymphoma H (2024) NCCN clinical practice guidelines in oncology (NCCN guidelines®). NCCN.org. NCCN guidelines for patients®. Available from: www.nccn.org/patients

Ma J, Zhang J, Zhou S, Hubbs JL, Foltz RJ, Hollis DR et al (2010) Regional lung density changes after radiation therapy for tumors in and around thorax. Int J Radiat Oncol Biol Phys [Internet] 76(1):116–122. Available from: https://pubmed.ncbi.nlm.nih.gov/19406588/

Mattonen SA, Palma DA, Haasbeek CJA, Senan S, Ward AD (2014) Early prediction of tumor recurrence based on CT texture changes after stereotactic ablative radiotherapy (SABR) for lung cancer. Med Phys [Internet] 41(3):033502. Available from: https://researchinformation.amsterdamumc.org/en/publications/early-prediction-of-tumor-recurrence-based-on-ct-texture-changes-

Mattonen SA, Ward AD, Palma DA (2016a) Pulmonary imaging after stereotactic radiotherapy—does RECIST still apply? Br J Radiol [Internet] 89(1065). Available from: https://pubmed.ncbi.nlm.nih.gov/27245137/

Mattonen SA, Palma DA, Johnson C, Louie AV, Landis M, Rodrigues G et al (2016b) Detection of local cancer recurrence after stereotactic ablative radiation therapy for lung cancer: physician performance versus radiomic assessment. Int J Radiat Oncol Biol Phys [Internet] 94(5):1121–1128. Available from: https://pubmed.ncbi.nlm.nih.gov/26907916/

Moran A, Daly ME, Yip SSF, Yamamoto T (2017) Radiomics-based assessment of radiation-induced lung injury after stereotactic body radiotherapy. Clin Lung Cancer [Internet] 18(6):e425–e431. Available from: https://pubmed.ncbi.nlm.nih.gov/28623121/

Munoz-Schuffenegger P, Kandel S, Alibhai Z, Hope A, Bezjak A, Sun A et al (2019) A prospective study of magnetic resonance imaging assessment of post-radiation changes following stereotactic body radiation therapy for non-small cell lung cancer. Clin Oncol (R Coll Radiol) [Internet] 31(10):720–727. Available from: https://pubmed.ncbi.nlm.nih.gov/31176537/

Murai T, Shibamoto Y, Nishiyama T, Baba F, Miyakawa A, Ayakawa S et al (2012) Organizing pneumonia after stereotactic ablative radiotherapy of the lung. Radiat Oncol [Internet] 7(1):1–7. Available from: https://ro-journal.biomedcentral.com/articles/10.1186/1748-717X-7-123

Narowska G, Gandhi S, Tzeng A, Hamad EA (2023) Cardiovascular toxicities of radiation therapy and recommended screening and surveillance. J Cardiovasc Dev Dis [Internet] 10(11). Available from: https://pubmed.ncbi.nlm.nih.gov/37998505/

National Comprehensive Cancer Network (2025a) Non-small cell lung cancer (version 3.2025). https://www.nccn.org/professionals/physician_gls/pdf/nscl.pdf

National Comprehensive Cancer Network (2025b) Small cell lung cancer (version 4.2025). https://www.nccn.org/professionals/physician_gls/pdf/sclc.pdf

Nguyen TK, Senan S, Bradley JD, Franks K, Giuliani M, Guckenberger M et al (2018) Optimal imaging surveillance after stereotactic ablative radiation therapy for early-stage non-small cell lung cancer: findings of an International Delphi Consensus Study. Pract Radiat Oncol [Internet] 8(2):e71–e78. Available from: https://pubmed.ncbi.nlm.nih.gov/29291965/

Ochiai S, Nomoto Y, Yamashita Y, Murashima S, Hasegawa D, Kurobe Y et al (2015) Radiation-induced organizing pneumonia after stereotactic body radiotherapy for lung tumor. J Radiat Res [Internet] 56(6):904. Available from: https://pmc.ncbi.nlm.nih.gov/articles/PMC4628220/

Palma DA, Senan S, Haasbeek CJA, Verbakel WFAR, Vincent A, Lagerwaard F (2011a) Radiological and clinical pneumonitis after stereotactic lung radiotherapy: a matched analysis of three-dimensional conformal and volumetric-modulated arc therapy techniques. Int J Radiat Oncol Biol Phys [Internet] 80(2):506–513. Available from: https://pubmed.ncbi.nlm.nih.gov/20584582/

Palma DA, Van Sörnsen De Koste J, WFAR V, Vincent A, Senan S (2011b) Lung density changes after stereotactic radiotherapy: a quantitative analysis in 50 patients. Int J Radiat Oncol Biol Phys [Internet] 81(4):974–978. Available from: https://pubmed.ncbi.nlm.nih.gov/20932655/

Palma DA, Van Sörnsen De Koste JR, Verbakel WFAR, Senan S (2011c) A new approach to quantifying lung damage after stereotactic body radiation therapy. Acta Oncol [Internet] 50(4):509–517. Available from: https://pubmed.ncbi.nlm.nih.gov/21174519/

Palma DA, Olson R, Harrow S, Gaede S, Louie AV, Haasbeek C et al (2020) Stereotactic ablative radiotherapy for the comprehensive treatment of oligometastatic cancers: long-term results of the SABR-COMET phase II randomized trial. J Clin Oncol [Internet] 38(25):2830–2838. Available from: https://pubmed.ncbi.nlm.nih.gov/32484754/

Palma DA, Senan S, Tsujino K, Barriger RB, Rengan R, Moreno M et al (2024) Predicting radiation pneumonitis after chemoradiation therapy for lung cancer: an international individual patient data meta-analysis. Int J Radiat Oncol Biol Phys [Internet] 85(2):444–450. Available from: https://www.iris.unicampus.it/handle/20.500.12610/12477

Pasquini G, Menichelli C, Pastore G, Casamassima F, Fabrini MG, Cappelli S et al (2021) Stereotactic body radiation therapy for the treatment of pleural metastases in patients with thymoma: a retrospective review of 22 patients. J Thorac Dis [Internet] 13(11):6373–6380. Available from: https://pubmed.ncbi.nlm.nih.gov/34992817/

Pellegrino B, Facchinetti F, Bordi P, Silva M, Gnetti L, Tiseo M (2018) Lung toxicity in non-small-cell lung cancer patients exposed to ALK inhibitors: report of a peculiar case and systematic review of the literature. Clin Lung Cancer [Internet] 19(2):e151–e161. Available from: https://pubmed.ncbi.nlm.nih.gov/29174221/

Peulen H, Mantel F, Guckenberger M, Belderbos J, Werner-Wasik M, Hope A et al (2016) Validation of high-risk computed tomography features for detection of local recurrence after stereotactic body radiation therapy for early-stage non-small cell lung cancer. Int J Radiat Oncol Biol Phys [Internet] 96(1):134–141. Available from: https://pubmed.ncbi.nlm.nih.gov/27325481/

Pleural M: NCCN clinical practice guidelines in oncology (NCCN Guidelines®). NCCN.org. NCCN guidelines for patients®. Available at www.nccn.org/patients [Internet]. 2023. Available from: www.nccn.org/patients

Pozzessere C, Bouchaab H, Jumeau R, Letovanec I, Daccord C, Bourhis J et al (2020) Relationship between pneumonitis induced by immune checkpoint inhibitors and the underlying parenchymal status: a retrospective study. ERJ Open Res [Internet] 6(1):00165-2019. Available from: https://pubmed.ncbi.nlm.nih.gov/32201690/

Pozzessere C, Lazor R, Jumeau R, Peters S, Prior JO, Beigelman-Aubry C (2021) Imaging features of pulmonary immune-related adverse events. J Thorac Oncol [Internet] 16(9):1449–1460. Available from: https://pubmed.ncbi.nlm.nih.gov/34087477/

Qiao X, Tullgren O, Lax I, Sirzén F, Lewensohn R (2003) The role of radiotherapy in treatment of stage I non-small cell lung cancer. Lung Cancer [Internet] 41(1):1–11. Available from: https://pubmed.ncbi.nlm.nih.gov/12826306/

Rahi MS, Parekh J, Pednekar P, Parmar G, Abraham S, Nasir S et al (2021) Radiation-induced lung injury-current perspectives and management. Clin Pract [Internet] 11(3):410–429. Available from: https://pubmed.ncbi.nlm.nih.gov/34287252/

Ramin C, Schaeffer ML, Zheng Z, Connor AE, Hoffman-Bolton J, Lau B et al (2021) All-cause and cardiovascular disease mortality among breast cancer survivors in CLUE II, a long-standing community-based cohort. J Natl Cancer Inst [Internet] 113(2):137–145. Available from: https://pubmed.ncbi.nlm.nih.gov/32634223/

Rammohan N, Randall JW, Yadav P (2022) History of technological advancements towards MR-Linac: the future of image-guided radiotherapy. J Clin Med [Internet] 11(16). Available from: https://pubmed.ncbi.nlm.nih.gov/36012969/

Ricco A, Davis J, Rate W, Yang J, Perry D, Pablo J et al (2017) Lung metastases treated with stereotactic body radiotherapy: the RSSearch® Patient Registry's experience. Radiat Oncol [Internet] 12(1). Available from: https://pubmed.ncbi.nlm.nih.gov/28143558/

Ronden MI, Palma D, Slotman BJ, Senan S (2018) Brief report on radiological changes following stereotactic ablative radiotherapy (SABR) for early-stage lung tumors: a pictorial essay. J Thorac Oncol [Internet] 13(6):855–862. Available from: https://pubmed.ncbi.nlm.nih.gov/29518554/

Rubin P, Constine LS, Fajardo LF, Phillips TL, Wasserman TH (1995) RTOG Late Effects Working Group. Overview. Late Effects of Normal Tissues (LENT) scoring system. Int J Radiat Oncol Biol Phys [Internet] 31(5):1041–1042. Available from: https://pubmed.ncbi.nlm.nih.gov/7713774/

Sampath S, Rahmanuddin S, Sahoo P, Frankel P, Boswell S, Wong J et al (2019) Change in apparent diffusion coefficient is associated with local failure after stereotactic body radiation therapy for non-small cell lung cancer: a prospective clinical trial. Int J Radiat Oncol Biol Phys [Internet] 105(3):659–663. Available from: https://pubmed.ncbi.nlm.nih.gov/31271822/

Schröder C, Engenhart-Cabillic R, Kirschner S, Blank E, Buchali A (2019) Changes of lung parenchyma density following high dose radiation therapy for thoracic carcinomas – an automated analysis of follow up CT scans. Radiat Oncol [Internet] 14(1). Available from: https://pubmed.ncbi.nlm.nih.gov/31036015/

Senan S, Palma DA, Lagerwaard FJ (2011) Stereotactic ablative radiotherapy for stage I NSCLC: recent advances and controversies. J Thorac Dis [Internet] 3(3):189–196. Available from: https://pubmed.ncbi.nlm.nih.gov/22263087/

Shepherd AF, Rimner A (2022) Radiation strategy and techniques for metastatic pleural disease from thymic malignancies: extended abstract. Mediastinum [Internet] 6:27. Available from: https://pubmed.ncbi.nlm.nih.gov/36164364/

Szejniuk WM, Nielsen MS, Takács-Szabó Z, Pawlowski J, Al-Saadi SS, Maidas P et al (2021) High-dose thoracic radiation therapy for non-small cell lung cancer: a novel grading scale of radiation-induced lung injury for symptomatic radiation pneumonitis. Radiat Oncol [Internet] 16(1):131. Available from: https://pubmed.ncbi.nlm.nih.gov/34266462/

Thomas AL, Cox G, Sharma RA, Steward WP, Shields F, Jeyapalan K et al (2000) Gemcitabine and paclitaxel associated pneumonitis in non-small cell lung cancer: report of a phase I/II dose-escalating study. Eur J Cancer [Internet] 36(18):2329–2334. Available from: https://pubmed.ncbi.nlm.nih.gov/11094306/

Toussie D, Ginocchio LA, Cooper BT, Azour L, Moore WH, Villasana-Gomez G et al (2024) Radiation therapy for lung cancer: imaging appearances and pitfalls. Clin Chest Med [Internet] 45(2):339–356. Available from: https://pubmed.ncbi.nlm.nih.gov/38816092/

Trotti A, Colevas AD, Setser A, Rusch V, Jaques D, Budach V et al (2003) CTCAE v3.0: development of a comprehensive grading system for the adverse effects of cancer treatment. Semin Radiat Oncol [Internet] 13(3):176–181. Available from: https://pubmed.ncbi.nlm.nih.gov/12903007/

Trovo M, Linda A, El Naqa I, Javidan-Nejad C, Bradley J (2010) Early and late lung radiographic injury following stereotactic body radiation therapy (SBRT). Lung Cancer [Internet] 69(1):77–85. Available from: https://pubmed.ncbi.nlm.nih.gov/19910075/

Tseng SC, Lee HY, Nishino M (2022) Imaging of drug-related pneumonitis in oncology. Semin Respir Crit Care Med [Internet] 43(6):887–898. Available from: https://pubmed.ncbi.nlm.nih.gov/36307109/

Van Nimwegen FA, Schaapveld M, Janus CPM, Krol ADG, Petersen EJ, Raemaekers JMM et al (2015) Cardiovascular disease after Hodgkin lymphoma treatment: 40-year disease risk. JAMA Intern Med [Internet] 175(6):1007–1017. Available from: https://pubmed.ncbi.nlm.nih.gov/25915855/

Vogelius IR, Bentzen SM (2012) A literature-based meta-analysis of clinical risk factors for development of radiation induced pneumonitis. Acta Oncol [Internet] 51(8):975–983. Available from: https://pubmed.ncbi.nlm.nih.gov/22950387/

Walker CM, Saldaña DA, Gladish GW, Dicks DL, Kicska G, Mitsumori LM et al (2013) Cardiac complications of oncologic therapy. Radiographics [Internet] 33(6):1801–1815. Available from: https://pubmed.ncbi.nlm.nih.gov/24108563/

Wennstig AK, Wadsten C, Garmo H, Johansson M, Fredriksson I, Blomqvist C et al (2021) Risk of primary lung cancer after adjuvant radiotherapy in breast cancer-a large population-based study. NPJ Breast Cancer [Internet] 7(1). Available from: https://pubmed.ncbi.nlm.nih.gov/34075042/

Xia C, Qin L, Wang Y, Yao L, Shia B, Wu SY (2022) Risk factors and specific cancer types of second primary malignancies in patients with breast cancer receiving adjuvant radiotherapy: a case-control cohort study based on the SEER database. Am J Cancer Res [Internet] 12(6):2744. Available from: https://pmc.ncbi.nlm.nih.gov/articles/PMC9251704/

Yamamoto T, Kadoya N, Morishita Y, Sato Y, Matsushita H, Umezawa R et al (2018) Assessment and agreement of the CT appearance pattern and its severity grading of radiation-induced lung injury after stereotactic body radiotherapy for lung cancer. PLoS One [Internet] 13(10):e0204734. Available from: https://pubmed.ncbi.nlm.nih.gov/30286105/

Zhang XJ, Sun JG, Sun J, Ming H, Wang XX, Wu L et al (2012) Prediction of radiation pneumonitis in lung cancer patients: a systematic review. J Cancer Res Clin Oncol [Internet] 138(12):2103–2116. Available from: https://pubmed.ncbi.nlm.nih.gov/22842662/

Zhang R, Kang J, Ren S, Xing L, Xu Y (2022) Comparison of stereotactic body radiotherapy and radiofrequency ablation for early-stage non-small cell lung cancer: a systematic review and meta-analysis. Ann Transl Med [Internet] 10(2):104. Available from: https://pubmed.ncbi.nlm.nih.gov/35282118/

Zou W, Dong L, Kevin Teo BK (2018) Current state of image guidance in radiation oncology: implications for PTV margin expansion and adaptive therapy. Semin Radiat Oncol [Internet] 28(3):238–247. Available from: https://pubmed.ncbi.nlm.nih.gov/29933883/

Quantitative CT Imaging of Chronic Airway Diseases

Gael Dournes

Contents

G. Dournes (✉)
Université de Bordeaux, Centre de Recherche Cardio-Thoracique de Bordeaux, INSERM U1045, CIC 1401, Bordeaux, France

CHU de Bordeaux, Service d'Imagerie Cardiovasculaire et Thoracique, Service des Maladies Respiratoires, Service d'Exploration Fonctionnelle Respiratoire, Centre de référence pédiatrique de la mucoviscidose, CIC 1401, Pessac, France

Inserm, Centre de Recherche Cardio-Thoracique de Bordeaux, U1045, CIC 1401, Bordeaux, France
e-mail: gael.dournes@chu-bordeaux.fr

Abstract

Chronic airway diseases are associated with morphological changes involving all three parts of the lung, namely the bronchi, parenchyma and pulmonary vessels. In vivo imaging, with its ability to describe the different types of lung alterations and their regional distribution, can help to elucidate the relationship between lung structure and respiratory function. High-resolution computed tomography (CT) of the lung is the imaging modality of choice for assessing the pathological changes associated with airflow obstruction occurring in chronic airway diseases. Over the last few decades, numerous studies have demonstrated the role of CT as a morphological and functional method conducive to the phenotyping of airway diseases. This chapter aims to examine the data on CT imaging of airway diseases with a critical approach to recent data and to determine the extent to which CT could be integrated into the care of patients with this/these disease(s).

Abbreviations

ABPA	Allergic bronchopulmonary aspergillosis
AP/Ao	Ratio between pulmonary artery and aorta diameters

https://doi.org/10.1007/174_2025_606,

Published Online: 15 July 2025

BOS	Bronchiolitis obliterans syndrome
CF	Cystic fibrosis
COPD	Chronic obstructive pulmonary disease
CT	Computed tomography
fSAD	Functional small airway disease
FWHM	Full width at half maximum
GOLD	Global initiative for COPD
HAM	Hyperattenuated mucus
HU	Hounsfield Unit
IMIS	Inverted mucoid impaction signal
LA	Lumen area
LAV	Low attenuation volume
MinIP	Minimum intensity projection
MRI	Magnetic resonance imaging
NOVAA-CT	Normalized volume of airway abnormalities CT score
Pi10	Square root wall area of a hypothetical bronchus with an internal perimeter of 10 mm
PRM	Parametric response mapping
TA	Total area
TAC	Total airway count
WA	Wall area

1 Introduction

Chronic airway diseases such as chronic obstructive pulmonary disease (COPD), asthma or cystic fibrosis (CF) are leading causes of death worldwide (Stolz et al. 2022). These chronic airway diseases lead to functional obstruction, which is progressive and eventually irreversible. These diseases are associated with environmental factors such as allergens, viruses, bacteria, or toxins leading to an inflammatory response in genetically susceptible patients, the first of them being tobacco. Airway inflammation triggers chronic inflammation, leading to airway remodeling. In COPD, the epithelium displays mucous metaplasia, while inflammation is associated with loss of alveolar attachments, surrounded by peribronchial fibrosis. Destruction of alveolar wall leads to emphysema, which is a structural alteration seen in severe COPD. Computed tomography (CT) appears to be the major noninvasive tool to investigate structural components in vivo. Submillimetric acquisition can be obtained with an isotropic voxel over the whole lung volume, and automatic quantification measurements are achievable using commercially available software. CT also provides an accurate research tool, suitable to help understand the complex physiopathology underlying the disease, which is still not totally understood. Clinical, functional, and histological correlations with imaging have been reported. This article is focused on the most recent developments made in the last decade to quantify the lung alterations, besides visual analyses. Thus, we will review the quantitative possibilities offered by CT, their findings, their limits, and their perspectives.

2 Quantitative Measurement of the Trachea

The trachea corresponds to the initial part of the conductive airway tree, before subsequent division into bronchi at the level of the carina. The anterolateral part is mainly cartilaginous, and the posterior part is formed by a membrane. During expiration, the caliber of the trachea is reduced, and there is bulging of the posterior layer of the trachea.

To obtain reproducible assessment of tracheal dimensions, measurements should be performed 2 cm above the aortic arch. The normal tracheal shape is roughly circular in children and young adults and becomes more ovoid starting at 20 years old. In addition, tracheal dimensions are influenced by gender and age, but no relationship with height or weight was found in a study (Breatnach et al. 1984). Assuming a normative range that encompasses three SDs from the mean, the upper limits of normal for coronal (transversal) and sagittal (antero-posterior) diameters of the tracheal air column in men aged 20–79 are 25 and 27 mm, respectively; in women aged 20–79, they are 21 and 23 mm, respectively. The lower limit of normal for both dimensions is 13 mm in men and 10 mm in women (Breatnach et al. 1984).

Changes in tracheal dimensions occur in various conditions; for example, in full inspiration, there is dilation in tracheobronchomegaly (Celik et al. 2011) and tracheomalacia and narrowing in tracheobronchopathia osteochondroplastica, relapsing polychondritis (Borgia et al. 2018), fibrosing mediastinitis, rhinoscleroma, and "saber sheath" trachea (Greene and Lechner 1975). Saber-sheath trachea involves a coronal tracheal diameter less than two-thirds of the sagittal diameter, and it is strongly associated to COPD (Greene and Lechner 1975).

In COPD, it has been showed that the tracheal wall may be weakened by chronic inflammation. The main consequence is a tracheal collapse, which can be assessed by using paired inspiratory and expiratory CT acquisitions. For this, both acquisitions can be acquired during two independent static maneuvers. However, collapsibility of the trachea may be better assessed by acquisition during a dynamic expiratory maneuver by the patient (O'Donnell et al. 2014).

The threshold to acknowledge a tracheal collapse is often a reduction of 50% in tracheal lumen during expiration. Nevertheless, studies in healthy volunteers showed that this threshold is reached in a substantial number of healthy volunteers, probably because healthy subjects may be able to develop high intrathoracic pressure without any weakening of their tracheal layers. Therefore, an alternative threshold of 70% was also proposed, and the choice between 50% or 70% may be a compromise between sensitivity or specificity of detection (Boiselle et al. 2009).

In COPD, the clinical relevance of the measurement was studied, and reports from the COPDgene cohort demonstrated that tracheal collapse found on expiratory CT was a predictor of worse quality of life, independently from pulmonary function tests or emphysema (Bhatt et al. 2016).

3 Quantitative Measurement of Central Bronchi

3.1 Quantification of Airway Wall Remodeling

There is no standardized measurement of central airway wall thickness. Theoretical models to predict these dimensions have been proposed by Weibel et al.; however, human studies have shown that actual measurements of airway dimensions significantly differ from these theoretical models (Montaudon et al. 2007a). In addition, it has been shown that airway calibers may vary according to various factors, including prone or supine positioning or altitude (Kim et al. 1997). However, airway wall remodeling is a key component of airway diseases such as asthma, COPD, or cystic fibrosis. Two approaches have been proposed in the literature to enable semi-quantitative or quantitative evaluations of this important issue.

3.1.1 Visual Assessment

For visual analysis, scoring systems have been developed, although with various definitions, mainly in cystic fibrosis conditions. Brody et al. have proposed a threshold of one third of the diameter of the adjacent artery to consider airway wall thickening (Brody et al. 2006). Bhalla et al. are using a threshold of one time the adjacent artery dimension to consider a "peribronchial thickening", considering that, at CT, it is not possible to discriminate between bronchial walls and mucus plugging encroached to the bronchial wall (Bhalla et al. 1991) (Table 1). Rosenow et al. assume a pure subjective definition and accept a mixed evaluation of either an enlarged wall thickness or a higher wall attenuation (Rosenow et al. 2015). These visual analyses may appear imprecise or subjective. Nevertheless, they are still supported by compelling literature data demonstrating that these evaluations are related to the disease severity and can predict clinically important outcomes such as exacerbations (Calder et al. 2014). In addition, this visual analysis requires experienced readers.

Table 1 Bhalla score template

Category	Scores 0	1	2	3
Severity of bronchiectasis	Absent	Mild	Moderate	Severe
Peribronchial thickening	Absent	Mild	Moderate	Severe
The extent of bronchiectasis (no. of segments)	Absent	1–5	6–9	>9
Extent of mucus plugging (no. of segments)	Absent	1–5	6–9	>9
Sacculation or abscesses (no. of segments)	Absent	1–5	6–9	>9
Generation of bronchial divisions involved (bronchiectasis/plugging)	Absent	Up to 4th generation	Up to 5th generation	Up to 6th generation and distal
No. of bullae	Absent	Unilateral (not >4)	Bilateral (not >4)	>4
Emphysema (no. of segments)	Absent	1–5	>5	
Collapse/consolidation	Absent	Subsegmental	Segmental/ lobar	

Note: The template is adapted from Bhalla et al. (1991). The score is calculated as follows: Total Bhalla score = 25—(sum of scores)
When present, bronchiectasis and peribronchial thickening were assigned a severity score as follows:
Bronchiectasis severity: Absent (0), luminal diameter slightly greater than diameter of adjacent vessel (Mild (1)), luminal diameter 2–3× the adjacent vessel (Moderate (2)), luminal diameter > 3× the adjacent vessel (Severe (3))
Peribronchial thickening severity: Absent (0), wall thickness equal to the diameter of adjacent vessel (Mild (1)), wall thickness ≤ 2× the adjacent vessel (Moderate (2)), wall thickness > 2× the adjacent vessel (Severe (3))

3.1.2 Software Assessment

At quantitative analysis, the rationale of airway wall quantification using CT is the presence of an increased airway wall thickness in patients with chronic airway disease as compared with control subjects (Dournes et al. 2015). Several softwares have been reported, and the first step is to segment the bronchial volume, which is subsequently skeletonized to obtain a bronchial tree (Montaudon et al. 2007b; Brillet et al. 2007). Then, to prevent parallax errors, CT reformats orthogonal to the target bronchi main axis can be acquired, and geometrical information of the bronchial calibers can be obtained. The most common measurements are airway wall and lumen dimensions, including the wall area (WA) and the lumen area (LA). These softwares allow a fast and accurate postprocessing quantification, and this is relevant knowing the heterogeneity of alterations in chronic airway diseases such as asthma or COPD.

The most widely published measurements correspond to the 2D evaluations of airway cross-sectional areas, as a surrogate of airway wall and lumen remodeling. The airway intraluminal area (LA) and the total bronchial layer area (TA) are measured, in millimeters square. The wall area (WA) corresponds to the difference WA = TA − LA (Fig. 1). WA% represents WA normalized on TA, that is, WA% = (WA/TA) × 100. WA and LA are not independent from body height, so they may be normalized on body surface area to reduce interindividual variations.

Computational methods have been developed to allow automated segmentation of the wall contours of the bronchial tree. Briefly, among most of published applications, active energy-driven contours are a region-based active contour model to extract the local image information. The Full-Width-at-Half-Maximum (FWHM) principle is given by the difference between the two extreme values at which the wall attenuation is equal to half to its maximum (Fig. 1). The Laplacian-of-Gaussian algorithm is a function that combines a Laplace operator to detect edges as well as noise, and a convolution with a Gaussian kernel to smooth the image first. These algorithms have been used to segment airways wall contours, but none of them have demonstrated any superiority from each other. However, it has been showed

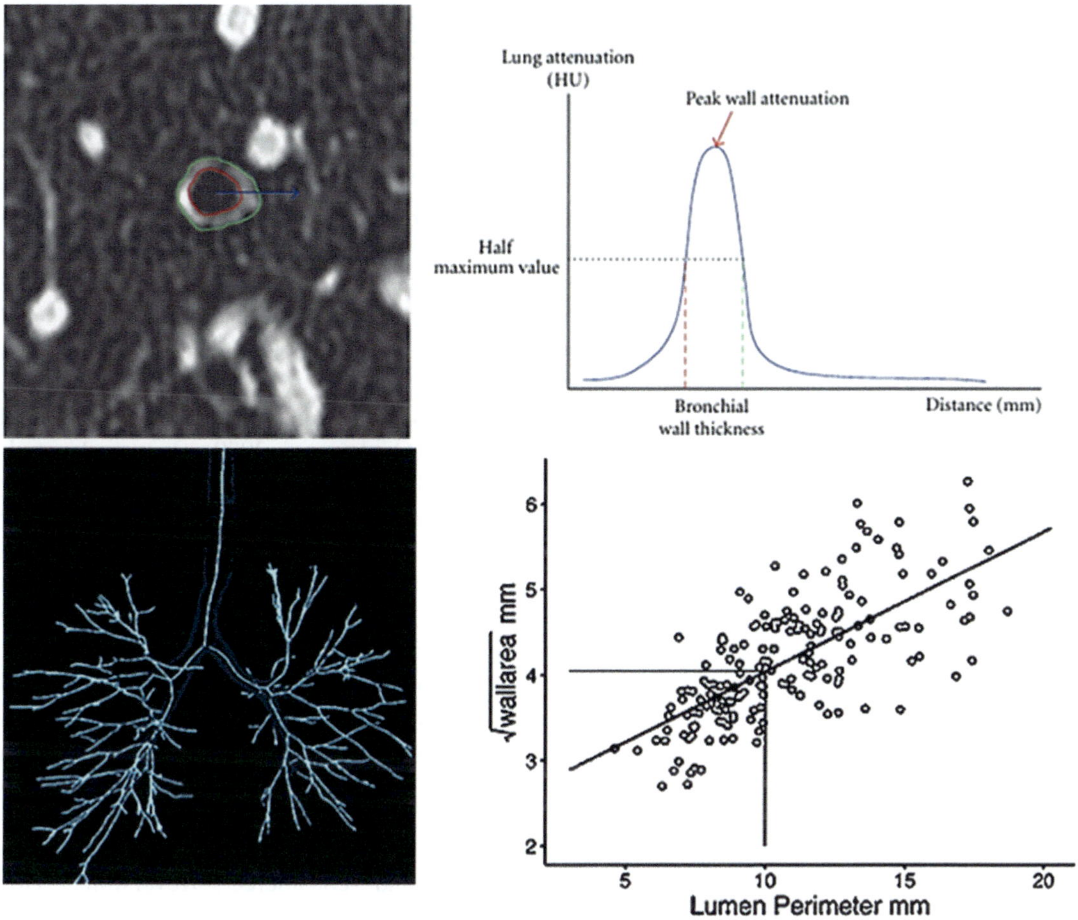

Fig. 1 Bronchial tree volume is automatically segmented using a homemade dedicated software (bottom left panel), extracted from a whole set of lung CT images. The skeleton of the bronchial tree is computed to obtain a simplified three-dimensional geometry of the bronchial tree. On top left panel, a thin-section CT image perpendicular to the third generation of the right segmental apical bronchus is displayed. Green line indicates the external wall contour, and red line the internal layer. On right panel, theorical single intensity curve (blue line) representing voxel attenuation variation along the blue line seen in left upper panel. One dimensional measurement of the bronchial wall thickness can be calculated with the Full Width at Half Maximum (FWHM) principle that is given by the difference between the two extreme values at which the mural attenuation is equal to half to its maximum (green and red dashed lines). Additionally, two-dimensional measurement of the wall area (WA), the lumen area (LA) or the percentage wall area (WA% = WA/LA * 100) can be calculated. On bottom right panel, scatterplot shows the square root of the wall area against the internal perimeter of the corresponding airway sections. The tangent drawn onto the y-axis corresponds to the airway with a 10-mm internal perimeter, representing the square root of a theoretical summary airway with an internal perimeter of 10 mm (i.e., Pi10). The regression line is used to calculate the PiSlope

that they are not interchangeable in longitudinal studies (Dournes and Laurent 2012).

The results are usually reported in the form of an average value of all measurements, which can also be decomposed regionally to provide the distribution across airway generations (Dettmer et al. 2023). It is also possible to integrate these measurements to calculate the Pi10 value, which is an estimated perimeter of a hypothetical "normalized" airway with an internal perimeter of 10 mm. It is derived from regression equations between the square root of airway WA and its internal perimeter (Kahnert et al. 2023) (Fig. 1). Recently, the slope of this regression has been proposed as a biomarker of airway remodeling and showed to correlate to clinical outcomes such as exacerbation or mortality in COPD (Bhatt et al. 2024) (Fig. 1).

3.1.3 Total Airway Count

Another interesting application is the total airway count (TAC). Indeed, the number of airways that can be segmented and skeletonized automatically in a CT bronchial volume is limited because of clinical features such as airway narrowing and mucus obstruction, or technical reasons such as air leakage, mainly because of surrounding emphysema. Kirby et al. (2021) showed that TAC was significantly associated with the disease severity status. For instance, TAC is reduced in patients with Global Initiative for Chronic Obstructive Lung Disease (GOLD) I and II COPD when compared with both never-smokers and smokers without COPD (Elbehairy et al. 2024).

3.1.4 Dysanapsis

In addition, dysanapsis, a mismatch between the airway tree caliber (*a*) and the lung size (*l*), can also be directly quantified using CT; lower *a/l* ratio values indicate smaller airway tree lumens relative to lung size and thus greater dysanapsis (Mochizuki et al. 2024). The concept of the disproportionate growth between lung size and airway caliber was termed "dysanaptic growth" by Green et al. in 1974 (Thompson 2017), who described the wide variations in maximum expiratory flows in normal subjects with similar lung size. They postulated that the differences in maximum expiratory flows observed were due to between-individual differences in airway caliber and geometry (caliber vs. length) and suggested that the proposed disconnect between lung size and airway size was indeed a normal variant and may have an embryological basis. This physiological variation was found to be clinically important. For instance, Forno et al. showed that airway dysanapsis is associated with asthma morbidity in obese children (Forno et al. 2017). In COPD, airway dysanapsis and emphysema were independently associated with pulmonary function test severity (Mochizuki et al. 2024).

3.2 Quantification of Lumen Caliber

3.2.1 Bronchial Dilation

Bronchiectasis is defined as abnormal dilation of the bronchi, usually due to chronic airway inflammation and/or infection (Fig. 2). Similarly to bronchial wall thickness, there is no standardized measurement to give a range of absolute measurement of normal airway lumen, and actual measurement significantly differs from theoretical models (Montaudon et al. 2007a). Also, bronchial dilatation may be associated with age (Copley et al. 2009). Conversely, studies from lung explants have showed that airway lumen and adjacent vessel diameters are closely related to each other. This is why the evaluation often relies on a relative comparison between airway lumen and the adjacent artery dimension.

Several concepts have recently been reported in literature. The Fleischner Society 2024 update of its Glossary of Thoracic CT Terms (Bankier et al. 2024) mentions discrimination between the terms "bronchiectasis" and "bronchial dilation," the former having to be proven chronic and considered irreversible. This implies that the glossary's authors acknowledge that there is now evidence that "bronchial dilation" can be potentially reversible, particularly when managed early. This was shown recently in a pediatric study, where around 80% of patients showed reversibility under treatment, with a majority of patients carrying post-infectious bronchial dilations (Mills et al. 2024). In another study comparing patients with and without reversibility of these dilations, David et al. showed that younger patients, with less severe cylindrical-type bronchial dilations, were those most likely to present reversibility (David et al. 2024).

It is notable that there are several possible definitions of bronchiectasis (Aliberti et al. 2022). In the absence of a standard measurement, dilation is judged relatively, in comparison with the adjacent vessel. A ratio between the lumen of the bronchus and the diameter of the adjacent pulmonary artery (including its walls) that is

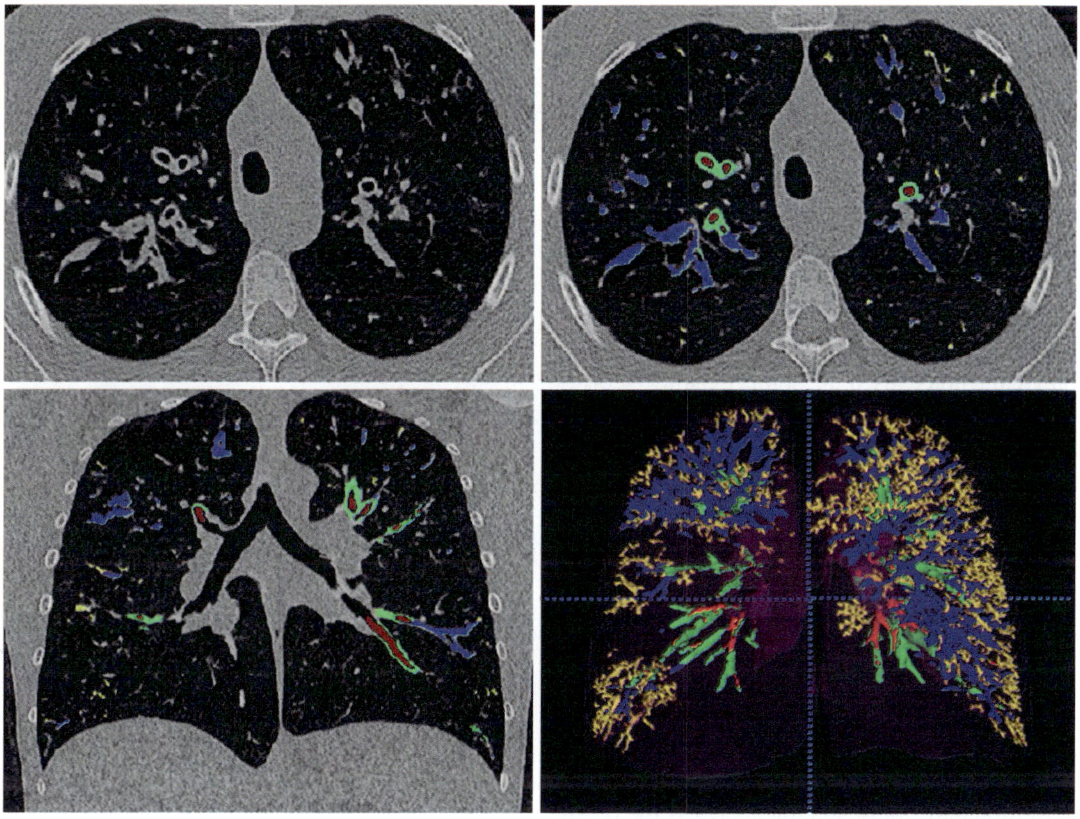

Fig. 2 CT scan in a cystic fibrosis patient with native axial reformation (top left panel). After segmentation by a dedicated deep learning algorithm, five structural alterations are labeled (top right panel): bronchiectasis (red color), peribronchial thickening (green color), bronchial mucus (blue color), bronchiolar mucus (yellow color). A coronal reformation (bottom left panel) and a volume rendering of the full airway tree alterations (bottom right panel) are displayed allowing the calculation of normalized volume of airway abnormalities at CT (NOVAA-CT) as a 3-D holistic quantitative outcome

greater than 1:1 is the most commonly accepted and used in the literature (Meerburg et al. 2020). However, a group of experts has proposed that a ratio greater than 1.5:1 may be used in the specific context of a clinical trial (Aliberti et al. 2022). In this context, the rationale for a higher threshold was to increase the probability of recruiting patients presenting with this abnormality on imaging and with clinical symptoms. However, with a view to using an imaging biomarker, it can be argued that such a high threshold is not suitable to reflect the totality of possible impairments, particularly if the aim is to quantify reversibility of bronchial dilation under the effect of a given therapy in patients who have become precisely asymptomatic as a result of effective treatment (Mills et al. 2024; David et al. 2024; Hadj Bouzid et al. 2025).

Conversely, in children, an airway-artery ratio of 0.8:1 has been proposed (Chang et al. 2021). The rationale is to consider early modifications for allowing early therapeutic management. However, literature is currently lacking, for instance, to assess the visual reproducibility of this evaluation (a ratio between 0.7:1 and 0.9:1, for instance), as compared to a simple 1:1 comparison. In addition, in a recent study, no significant difference in sensitivity analyses was found between measurements of bronchiectasis made with a 0.8:1 ratio or a 1:1 ratio. It is also unclear at which age this 0.8:1 may be considered, fromv infants, preschool children, children, and teenagers.

Moreover, there is no consensus on whether to use the external or internal contour to define a bronchial dilatation. The impact of this choice is consequential, as the underlying abnormalities differ. Indeed, by using the external contour of the bronchi, the term "bronchiectasis" includes parietal thickening and bronchoceles in the definition. This synthetic approach is the methodological choice used in some existing scoring systems, such as a visual MR score (Eichinger et al. 2012) or manual CT score (Rosenow et al. 2015). Conversely, a definition based on the inner lumen will consider these alterations as independent but may be biased when mucus clinging to the walls would partially reduce the bronchial lumen (Aliberti et al. 2022). The second analytic approach is considered in scoring systems such as NOVAA-CT (Dournes et al. 2022).

Because the outer bronchus includes both lumen and wall components in the definition of "bronchiectasis," it can be discussed that this definition may not be suitable to assess the recent finding of bronchiectasis reversibility (Mills et al. 2024; David et al. 2024; Bugenhagen et al. 2024; Cazier et al. 2024). Indeed, the reduction in bronchial caliber, with this synthetic approach, may refer to either the reduction in wall thickening and/or lumen variation indiscriminately (McNally et al. 2023).

Automated 2D methods have been reported to describe the degree of bronchial dilation, with or without the aid of artificial intelligence (Dournes et al. 2022; Lv et al. 2023). Among these latter methods, the NOVAA-CT (Normalized Volume of Airway Abnormalities at CT) score has recently been established in cystic fibrosis and quantifies this phenomenon in 3D, thus including both the degree of dilation and the spatial extent of this involvement (Hadj Bouzid et al. 2025) (Fig. 2).

3.2.2 Bronchial Narrowing

Recently, an alternative and opposite concept has emerged, which is airway lumen narrowing instead of airway lumen dilation (Bodduluri et al. 2024). As compared to dysanapsis, which is the measurement of an overall bronchial tree volume, airway narrowing may be assessed by using the calculation of a "T-slope," which corresponds to a measurement of airway tapering of bronchi across several generations. This measurement appeared to demonstrate a higher slope toward airway narrowing of the more distal airways in COPD.

3.3 Quantification of Bronchial Mucus

The importance of mucoid impactions in chronic airway diseases has recently been highlighted. Indeed, it is notable that in the scientific literature on visual or quantitative CT, the assessment of mucoid plugs has only been very recently reported.

In COPD, the majority of these mucoid plugs are generally located in the distal airways, and the current accuracy of CT scans does not allow discrimination of parietal bronchial thickening and mucoid impaction in these small airways due to a lack of spatial resolution (Hogg et al. 2004). In contrast to particular conditions such as cystic fibrosis, mucoid impactions in medium-sized airways are therefore relatively uncommon in the central airways of stable post-smoking COPD or asthma patients.

Nevertheless, it has been shown that the presence of just three lung segments (out of a total of 20) showing mucus plugs within medium-sized airways is associated with a greater risk of mortality and exacerbations compared with patients without mucus plugs (Diaz et al. 2023). A low number of mucoid impactions does not therefore indicate a low risk, and their detection therefore seems relevant. The visual scores proposed for this purpose are simple: they count the number of segments in which at least one mucous plug is visible within medium-sized airways. This visual score can vary from 0 to 20, with a risk of complications/mortality starting at just 3 (Diaz et al. 2023).

Software methods have also been developed, either specifically dedicated to the description of this anomaly or associated with a more global quantitative score, namely the NOVAA-CT score mentioned above (Fig. 2). This "holistic" approach differs from "hierarchical" approaches in that the former allows us to assess the current value of all structural alterations at voxel level. Conversely, "hierarchical" approaches, in which alterations are scored in order of priority, allow only a total score and the component of highest importance to be assessed longitudinally; to note existing hierarchical scores, do not allow reliable mucus assessment.

Another interest of analyzing mucoid impactions lies not only in their detection or extent but also in their characterization. In particular, the presence of hyperattenuated mucus (HAM) is recognized as a diagnostic marker of allergic bronchopulmonary aspergillosis (ABPA) (Agarwal et al. 2024). Several comments can be made on this subject. Indeed, the ISHAM group recently updated their diagnostic criteria for ABPA in 2024. Whereas, in their 2013 version, the predisposing conditions for ABPA were asthma and cystic fibrosis (Agarwal et al. 2013), the revised version of ISHAM in 2024 considers that COPD and any condition associated with bronchiectasis are also one of these predisposing conditions (Agarwal et al. 2024). On the other hand, these authors considered that HAM can be seen as pathognomonic of ABPA and allows, according to them, confirmation of ABPA in the absence of a complete picture based on other clinical, biological or immunological criteria. Given the importance of this criterion, defining HAM as mucous plugging showing greater attenuation than the adjacent paraspinal muscle is debatable. Indeed, in COPD, for example, it is known that sarcopenia or fatty muscle remodeling can lead to a drop in muscle density, and therefore a risk of false-positive HAM, based on this relative criterion (Mills et al. 2024). No threshold in HU was specified for this relative increase in density. In addition, the CT parameters recommended for this assessment mention a CT dose of between 3 and 7 milliSieverts (Agarwal et al. 2024). However, current CT scans are often performed at ultra-low doses, <1 mSv. The applicability of a definite diagnosis of ABPA on the basis of an attenuation greater than that of a muscle therefore deserves caution and attention. Note also that HAM are not mandatory for the diagnosis of ABPA and that high attenuation artefacts in the area of the lingula may result in false positive results. A possible alternative is MRI, which can also be used to characterize the lesion signal, in the form of mucoid impaction signal inversion or IMIS (Dournes et al. 2017, 2021). Inverted mucoid impaction signal (IMIS) is the MR equivalent of HAM at CT, with the particularity of not being dependent on a threshold or an assessment relative to a muscle, and thus freeing itself from the diagnostic thresholding problem at CT. However, MRI may lack accessibility and is more expensive than CT, so it cannot be recommended on a large scale in healthcare, outside specific contexts such as cystic fibrosis for which lung MRI using a combination of T1-weighted and T2-weighted sequences is already part of routine care (Dournes et al. 2021; Hatabu et al. 2020).

From a practical point of view, mucoid impactions are well visualized on lung CT reconstruction in "hard" or "parenchymal" filter and sensitized by maximum intensity projection (MIP) reconstruction, while mucus density analysis should be performed on "soft" or "standard" filter reconstruction.

4 Quantification of Small Airways

The small airways, defined as those having a diameter inferior to 2 mm, are considered as the main site of increased resistance and airflow obstruction prior to emphysematous destruction of the alveolar wall. HRCT allows a direct visualization of about 10–13 bronchial generations, while the human airway tree is composed of 25 generations, meaning that only less than half of airways are directly assessable using CT. Moreover, Tanabe et al. reported that the bronchial volumes measured in the right upper and middle lobes of adult COPD patients using dedicated CT software ranged approximately between 9 and 20 ml, therefore corresponding to a mean of 0.5% of the lung volume only (Tanabe et al. 2019). Indeed, small conductive and distal airways are beyond the spatial resolution of CT. Intralobular structures are also not clearly visible, such as alveolar membranes, capillaries, or interstitial tissue. However, lung parenchyma density is a consequence of the X-ray attenuation by these lung structures, and any change in either of these structures may alter its density.

Areas of air trapping are well-known manifestations of small airway involvement, although they suffer from poor reproducibility in their visual detection and characterization of their extent (O'Donnell et al. 2004). From a practical standpoint, the analysis of small airway involvement calls for a complementary acquisition during expiration, with analysis of attenuation variations in the lung parenchyma sensitized by using minimum intensity projection (MinIP) reconstructions from "soft" or "standard" filter reconstructions. Areas of air trapping are generally depicted by a less-than-normal increase in attenuation areas on expiratory CT. However, some extent of lobular or areas of air-trapping have also been reported in healthy non-smoking subjects (Galbán et al. 2012) and the elderly. In Bronchiolitis Obliterans Syndrome (BOS) in heart-lung transplant recipients, a visual threshold of 32% in air trapping extent has been proposed to distinguish between patients with and without BOS (Bankier et al. 2001). Moreover, diffuse air trapping can be extremely difficult to assess visually.

Methods for quantifying small airway dysfunction have been proposed with relative success in defining and characterizing COPD or asthma patients. These methods use either expiratory CT images to calculate lung volume with an attenuation value of less than −856 HU (Matsuoka et al. 2008), or paired expiratory and inspiratory CT images to calculate the ratio of mean lung density in Hounsfield Units (HU) (Fig. 3). Voxel-by-voxel comparison of recorded and paired expiratory and inspiratory CT images has also been used to quantify so-called functional small airway disease (fSAD) using the parametric response mapping (PRM) technique (Galbán et al. 2012). Another approach using the registration of inspiratory and expiratory CT images has been developed to quantify the Jacobian determinant and the anisotropic deformation index as a surrogate for the biomechanical properties of the lung (Bodduluri et al. 2017). However, none of these methods has shown superiority over the others, and the lack of consensus in their use precludes any comparison between cohorts.

Studies on the prognostic value of these measurements/quantifications have also been carried out in terms of predicting exacerbations, mortality (Johannessen et al. 2013) or association with a genetic risk score (Oelsner et al. 2019).

Nevertheless, such quantitative methods are based on the detection and measurement of hypoattenuated areas due to expiratory air trapping or obliterative bronchiolitis. Alternatively, cellular or proliferative bronchiolitis can manifest as an abnormal increase in attenuation and visibility of small airways because of the thickening of their walls and/or mucus filling of their lumen. Visually, the branching appearance of the small airways is called the "tree-in-bud" or "mimosa flower" pattern. Recent studies have shown that AI enables quantitative segmentation of this pattern with a calculation of their volume (Dournes et al. 2022) (Fig. 2). Despite some underestimation of the bronchiolar impaction extent as compared to manual ground truth, the quantitative evaluation was demonstrated valid to correlate to the disease severity status in patients with cystic fibrosis and to demonstrate a reduction in patients with effective treatments (Hadj Bouzid et al. 2025; Dournes et al. 2022). This recent application may typically highlight the novel possibilities of AI for local detection and extracting local features, with precision down to millimetric small structures, that non-AI methods did not reach in the past literature.

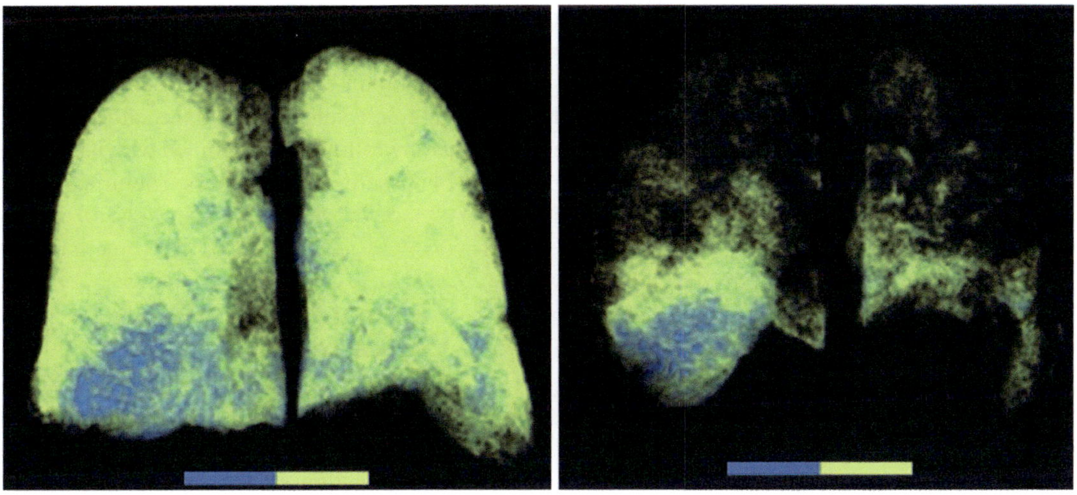

Fig. 3 Coronal views of lung attenuation volume samples computed using the density mask technique to extract voxels below −856 HU. Green areas are representative of voxels between −950 HU and −856 HU, and blue areas between −1000 and −950 HU. Images were acquired in inspiration (left panel) and in expiration (right panel) in a patient with chronic obstructive airway disease

4.1 Quantitative Assessment of Emphysema

Quantitative measurement of emphysema is developed in a dedicated chapter of this book. Some peculiar points will be described in this chapter.

Visual scoring systems were originally used to assess emphysema in COPD patients (COPDGene CT Workshop Group et al. 2012). This visual assessment showed significant correlations with obstructive EFR parameters. In addition, visual classification of emphysema pattern (centrilobular, panlobular, paraseptal) proved to be an independent predictor of mortality. However, visual analyses come up against several pitfalls. For example, it has been shown that reading CT scans in axial slices fails to assess a key marker in emphysema imaging, namely the flattening of the diaphragmatic cupolas. This flattening cannot be correctly seen on axial sections, and it is therefore important, during a COPD imaging workup, to use multiplanar sagittal reconstructions (Hightower et al. 2016), which amounts in a way to complement thin-section CT analysis with semiology derived from that of standard chest X-ray.

The second pitfall is that not all emphysema is visible to the naked eye. This is the case, for example, when the enlargement or destruction only affects the distal compartment such as the alveolar walls, below the resolution of any clinical imaging modality, and the density reduction is diffuse and homogeneous in the image, particularly in panlobular emphysema. Thus, intra- and extra-observer variability has led to automated quantification techniques (Gevenois et al. 1995; Lynch et al. 2015). Indeed, it has been shown that the reproducibility of visual assessment of the extent of emphysema is only moderate. Furthermore, this assessment can be compromised when CT attenuation lowering, secondary to lung parenchyma destruction, is homogeneous and diffuse, resulting in a lack of visual detection. The density mask technique with empirically determined thresholds or percentile points has been widely used to quantify emphysema and has shown significant correlations with histology.

Areas of low relative attenuation volume on inspiratory CT scans and "soft" or "standard" filter reconstruction, corresponding to LAA% or LAV% (= "low attenuation area" or "low attenuation volume") below a threshold of −950 HU or the 15th percentile of the cumulative lung density histogram can provide reproducible measurements and important functional information in COPD patients. An LAV% threshold of 5% has been proposed in the COPDGene study, or 6% by the Fleischner Society, in order to consider this quantitative measure as significant.

There are several points to discuss here. It is important to consider that the thresholds of 5% or 6% correspond to a percentage of voxels. Because of the millimetric spatial resolution of CT scans, a lung volume contains several million voxels, and so the 5% and 6% figures are not trivial but correspond to a very large number of voxels, whereas a 1% difference corresponds to a significant difference. It can be argued that small patches of incipient paraseptal or centro-lobular emphysema are common, without the LAV% exceeding 6%. Conversely, pan-lobular emphysema can be unmasked using this technique, particularly when the contrast variation is not perceptible to the naked eye. These thresholds should therefore be considered more specific than sensitive. Conversely, it is also true that bronchiectasis, honeycomb or any other intrapulmonary cavitary image may falsely increase this value. Thus, the main interest is to have a reproducible and reliable quantification of the extent of areas of "excess air," including emphysema, rather than to have a diagnostic criterion (Dournes et al. 2024).

As a biomarker, we consider that this measurement, while not without limitations, is in all cases more robust and reproducible over time than visual analyses for quantifying the extent of damage, while their practical implementation is now very straightforward. Moreover, reconstructions made on standard kernels have been shown to be similar between different machines from different manufacturers (Mackin et al. 2019). Clinical validation of this measurement is also widely supported by numerous articles in the literature.

The regional distribution of emphysema enabled by this quantification can also help in the pre-implantation assessment of endobronchial valves in emphysema reduction treatment and in post-therapy follow-up, combined with an assessment of fissure completeness (Sciurba et al. 2010).

5 Pulmonary Vessels Assessment

Pulmonary vascular changes have been described in the pathophysiology of chronic airway diseases. The reduction of distal vessels and endothelial dysfunction in response to hypoxic vasoconstriction are thought to be linked to inflammation in smokers and COPD patients. The main pulmonary artery to aorta ratio (PA/Ao) is a very simple measurement of large vessels, performed on any axial CT image showing the main pulmonary artery and ascending aorta side by side. This index was initially used to assess pulmonary arterial pressure (PAP) (Estépar et al. 2013). This ratio has been associated with an increased risk of COPD exacerbations and mortality (Coste et al. 2019; Terzikhan et al. 2017).

Pulmonary hypertension (PH) may causally be linked to COPD. Earlier studies suggested that PH was due to emphysematous destruction of the lung. However, recent studies do not support this hypothesis (Dournes et al. 2015). Pulmonary vascular changes can also be investigated in the small intrapulmonary vessels. Various methods using 2D or 3D images have been proposed for measuring the surface area of small vessels, the easiest to apply not seeking to separate arteries and veins. Quantification of small pulmonary vessels in mild-to-moderate PH secondary to COPD has shown a negative correlation with mean PAP (Matsuoka et al. 2010; Coste et al. 2016) (Fig. 4). Higher artery and vein volumes have also been shown to relate to mortality in current and former smokers (Kwee et al. 2024).

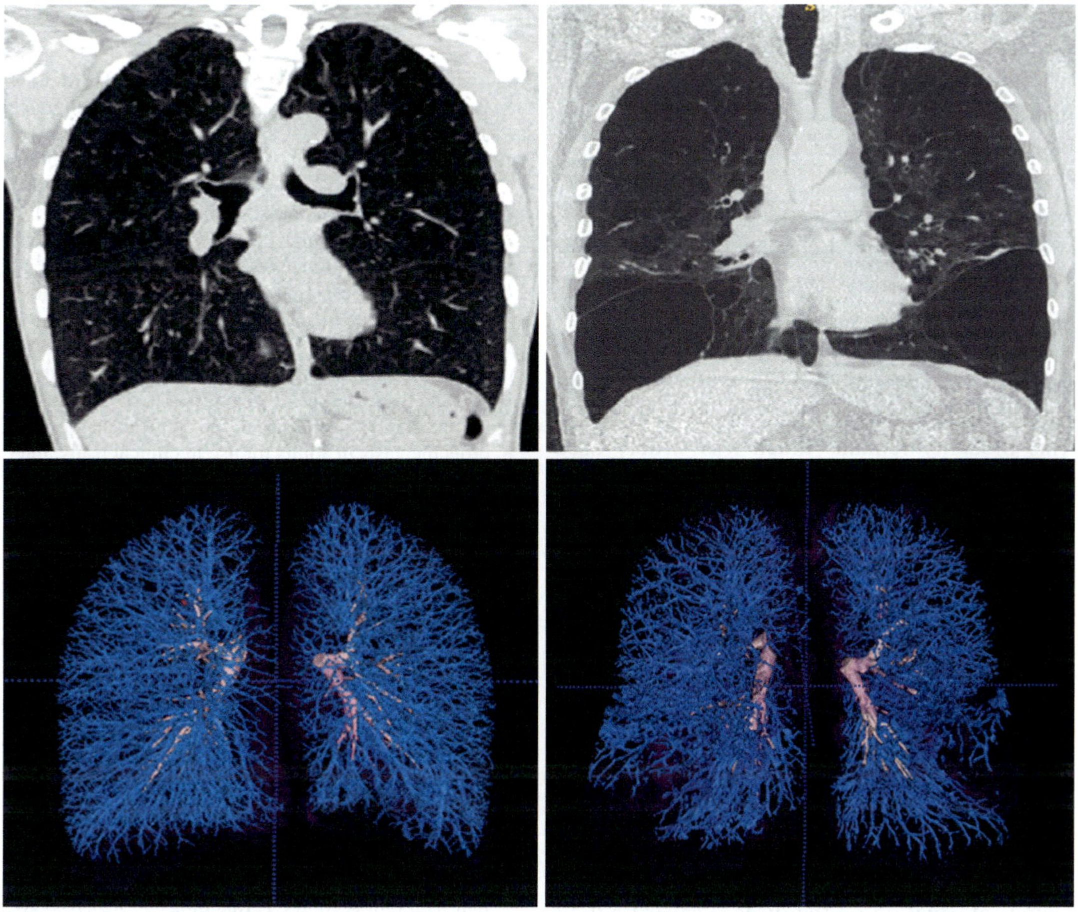

Fig. 4 Vascular tree segmentations in patients with chronic obstructive pulmonary disease (COPD) without (left panels) and with (right panel) emphysematous destruction of the lung. Coronal reformations of the native CT scans are displayed on top panels, and volume rendering of their bronchial tree volume (pink labels) and vascular tree volumes (blue labels) are displayed on bottom panels. Note the reduction of the vascular tree volume in the COPD patients with severe emphysema

6 Perspectives/Conclusion

Strong efforts have been made during the last decade to assess CT as a research tool to better understand COPD. The major advantage of quantitative tools is their reproducibility compared to subjective visual analysis. They also allow to investigate the complexity and diversity of these disorders with an increased precision.

However, several caveats remain. Although CT quantitative measurements of emphysema are fast, reproducible, and simple to implement in a clinical context, most of quantitative measurements of airway remodeling are still time-consuming and the associated literature appears heterogeneous.

AI should bring greater precision, with recent possibilities for automatically detecting and quantifying anomalies such as bronchiectasis, parietal thickening or mucoid impactions (Dournes et al. 2022; Diaz et al. 2023; Díaz et al. 2023). AI could thus enable measurements of airway caliber or small intra-pulmonary vessels to be considered for routine use, which tediousness and lack of reproducibility have so far prevented from achieving consensual use outside research.

The photon-counting scanner is expected to improve the spatial resolution of imaging, with the potential for better tissue characterization (Fletcher et al. 2024).

Pulmonary MRI has also seen major advances, such as compartmental characterization of damage (Mummy et al. 2021), ultra-short echo time imaging (Dournes et al. 2021; Hatabu et al. 2020), hybrid CT-MRI imaging (Longuefosse et al. 2023), and the possibility of assessing bronchial parietal inflammation (Benlala et al. 2020). This modality remains much less widely used than CT, however, and a dedicated literature review has not been included in our manuscript, due to the richness and diversity of this theme.

To conclude, CT remains the major modality as it is a rich and opportunistic tool to investigate chronic airway diseases in vivo. CT possibilities to quantify airway wall and lung parenchyma involvement are multiple, showing clinically relevant correlations with functional and pathological outcomes. Research applications are possible, and, in expert centers, translation to clinical routine is applicable (Dournes et al. 2024) to provide reproducible and automated information on the disease severity, their spatial distribution and longitudinal variations, in a novel era of emerging therapies. Target interventions toward bronchial, parenchymal or vascular compartments of the lungs are currently being evaluated and may underscore the need for precision medicine and patient phenotyping in the years to come.

Disclaimer All measurements in this book have been obtained from peer-reviewed papers and guidelines from professional organizations, unless explicitly stated otherwise. While the authors, editors, and publisher have gone through a rigorous process to establish their correct reproduction from the original source, each measurement must be interpreted in the correct clinical context, this along with an accurate way of measurement, and taking into account all technical variables, this including follow-up exams with various equipment or software. Neither the authors, the editors, nor the publisher can accept any legal responsibility for any improper application or interpretation of these measurements as well as their potential consequences.

References

Agarwal R, Chakrabarti A, Shah A, Gupta D, Meis JF, Guleria R et al (2013) Allergic bronchopulmonary aspergillosis: review of literature and proposal of new diagnostic and classification criteria. Clin Exp Allergy 43(8):850–873

Agarwal R, Singh Sehgal I, Muthu V, Denning DW, Chakrabarti A, Soundappan K et al (2024) Revised clinical practice guidelines for diagnosing, classifying, and treating allergic bronchopulmonary aspergillosis/mycoses: a Delphi statement from the ISHAM-ABPA working group. Eur Respir J 63:2400061

Aliberti S, Goeminne PC, O'Donnell AE, Aksamit TR, Al-Jahdali H, Barker AF et al (2022) Criteria and definitions for the radiological and clinical diagnosis of bronchiectasis in adults for use in clinical trials: international consensus recommendations. Lancet Respir Med 10(3):298–306

Bankier AA, Van Muylem A, Knoop C, Estenne M, Gevenois PA (2001) Bronchiolitis obliterans syndrome in heart-lung transplant recipients: diagnosis with expiratory CT. Radiology 218(2):533–539

Bankier AA, MacMahon H, Colby T, Gevenois PA, Goo JM, Leung ANC et al (2024) Fleischner Society: glossary of terms for thoracic imaging. Radiology 310(2):e232558

Benlala I, Hocke F, Macey J, Bui S, Berger P, Laurent F et al (2020) Quantification of MRI T2-weighted high signal volume in cystic fibrosis: a pilot study. Radiology 294(1):186–196

Bhalla M, Turcios N, Aponte V, Jenkins M, Leitman BS, McCauley DI et al (1991) Cystic fibrosis: scoring system with thin-section CT. Radiology 179(3):783–788

Bhatt SP, Terry NLJ, Nath H, Zach JA, Tschirren J, Bolding MS et al (2016) Association between expiratory central airway collapse and respiratory outcomes among smokers. JAMA 315(5):498–505

Bhatt SP, Nakhmani A, Sthanam V, Kizhakke Puliyakote A, Reinhardt JM, Bodduluri S (2024) PiSlope: a new CT metric for quantifying airway remodeling in chronic obstructive pulmonary disease. Radiology 313(2):e240717

Bodduluri S, Bhatt SP, Hoffman EA, Newell JD, Martinez CH, Dransfield MT et al (2017) Biomechanical CT metrics are associated with patient outcomes in COPD. Thorax 72(5):409–414

Bodduluri S, Nakhmani A, Kizhakke Puliyakote AS, Reinhardt JM, Dransfield MT, Bhatt SP (2024) Airway tapering in COPD. Eur Respir J 64(6):2400191

Boiselle PM, O'Donnell CR, Bankier AA, Ernst A, Millet ME, Potemkin A et al (2009) Tracheal collapsibility in healthy volunteers during forced expiration: assessment with multidetector CT. Radiology 252(1):255–262

Borgia F, Giuffrida R, Guarneri F, Cannavò SP (2018) Relapsing polychondritis: an updated review. Biomedicines 6(3):84

Breatnach E, Abbott GC, Fraser RG (1984) Dimensions of the normal human trachea. AJR Am J Roentgenol 142(5):903–906

Brillet PY, Fetita CI, Beigelman-Aubry C, Saragaglia A, Perchet D, Preteux F et al (2007) Quantification of bronchial dimensions at MDCT using dedicated software. Eur Radiol 17(6):1483–1489

Brody AS, Kosorok MR, Li Z, Broderick LS, Foster JL, Laxova A et al (2006) Reproducibility of a scoring system for computed tomography scanning in cystic fibrosis. J Thorac Imaging 21(1):14–21

Bugenhagen SM, Grant JCE, Rosenbluth DB, Bhalla S (2024) Update on the role of chest imaging in cystic fibrosis. Radiographics 44(9):e240008

Calder AD, Bush A, Brody AS, Owens CM (2014) Scoring of chest CT in children with cystic fibrosis: state of the art. Pediatr Radiol 44(12):1496–1506

Cazier P, Chassagnon G, Dhote T, Da Silva J, Kanaan R, Honore I et al (2024) Reversal of cylindrical bronchial dilatations in a subset of adults with cystic fibrosis treated with elexacaftor-tezacaftor-ivacaftor. Eur Respir J 63:2301794

Celik B, Bilgin S, Yuksel C (2011) Mounier-Kuhn syndrome: a rare cause of bronchial dilation. Tex Heart Inst J 38(2):194–196

Chang AB, Fortescue R, Grimwood K, Alexopoulou E, Bell L, Boyd J et al (2021) European Respiratory Society guidelines for the management of children and adolescents with bronchiectasis. Eur Respir J 58(2):2002990

COPDGene CT Workshop Group, Barr RG, Berkowitz EA, Bigazzi F, Bode F, Bon J et al (2012) A combined pulmonary-radiology workshop for visual evaluation of COPD: study design, chest CT findings and concordance with quantitative evaluation. COPD 9(2):151–159

Copley SJ, Wells AU, Hawtin KE, Gibson DJ, Hodson JM, Jacques AET et al (2009) Lung morphology in the elderly: comparative CT study of subjects over 75 years old versus those under 55 years old. Radiology 251(2):566–573

Coste F, Dournes G, Dromer C, Blanchard E, Freund-Michel V, Girodet PO et al (2016) CT evaluation of small pulmonary vessels area in patients with COPD with severe pulmonary hypertension. Thorax 71(9):830–837

Coste F, Benlala I, Dournes G, Dromer C, Blanchard E, Girodet PO et al (2019) Quantitative CT assessment of bronchial and vascular alterations in severe precapillary pulmonary hypertension. Int J Chron Obstruct Pulmon Dis 14:381–389

David M, Benlala I, Bui S, Benkert T, Berger P, Laurent F et al (2024) Longitudinal evaluation of bronchial changes in cystic fibrosis patients undergoing elexacaftor/tezacaftor/ivacaftor therapy using lung MRI with ultrashort echo-times. J Magn Reson Imaging 60(1):116–124

Dettmer S, Weinheimer O, Sauer-Heilborn A, Lammers O, Wielpütz MO, Fuge J et al (2023) Qualitative and quantitative evaluation of computed tomography changes in adults with cystic fibrosis treated with elexacaftor-tezacaftor-ivacaftor: a retrospective observational study. Front Pharmacol 14:1245885

Diaz AA, Orejas JL, Grumley S, Nath HP, Wang W, Dolliver WR et al (2023) Airway-occluding mucus plugs and mortality in patients with chronic obstructive pulmonary disease. JAMA 329:e232065

Díaz AA, Nardelli P, Wang W, San José Estépar R, Yen A, Kligerman S et al (2023) Artificial intelligence-based CT assessment of bronchiectasis: the COPDGene study. Radiology 307(1):e221109

Dournes G, Laurent F (2012) Airway remodelling in asthma and COPD: findings, similarities, and differences using quantitative CT. Pulm Med 2012:670414

Dournes G, Laurent F, Coste F, Dromer C, Blanchard E, Picard F et al (2015) Computed tomographic measurement of airway remodeling and emphysema in advanced chronic obstructive pulmonary disease. Correlation with pulmonary hypertension. Am J Respir Crit Care Med 191(1):63–70

Dournes G, Berger P, Refait J, Macey J, Bui S, Delhaes L et al (2017) Allergic bronchopulmonary aspergillosis in cystic fibrosis: MR imaging of airway mucus contrasts as a tool for diagnosis. Radiology 285(1):261–269

Dournes G, Walkup LL, Benlala I, Willmering MM, Macey J, Bui S et al (2021) The clinical use of lung MRI in cystic fibrosis: what, now, how? Chest 159(6):2205–2217

Dournes G, Hall CS, Willmering MM, Brody AS, Macey J, Bui S et al (2022) Artificial intelligence in computed tomography for quantifying lung changes in the era of CFTR modulators. Eur Respir J 59(3):2100844

Dournes G, Zysman M, Benlala I, Berger P (2024) CT imaging of chronic obstructive pulmonary disease: what aspects and what role? Rev Mal Respir 41(10):738–750

Eichinger M, Optazaite DE, Kopp-Schneider A, Hintze C, Biederer J, Niemann A et al (2012) Morphologic and functional scoring of cystic fibrosis lung disease using MRI. Eur J Radiol 81(6):1321–1329

Elbehairy AF, Marshall H, Naish JH, Wild JM, Parraga G, Horsley A et al (2024) Advances in COPD imaging using CT and MRI: linkage with lung physiology and clinical outcomes. Eur Respir J 63(5):2301010

Estépar RSJ, Kinney GL, Black-Shinn JL, Bowler RP, Kindlmann GL, Ross JC et al (2013) Computed tomographic measures of pulmonary vascular morphology in smokers and their clinical implications. Am J Respir Crit Care Med 188(2):231–239

Fletcher JG, Inoue A, Bratt A, Horst KK, Koo CW, Rajiah PS et al (2024) Photon-counting CT in thoracic imaging: early clinical evidence and incorporation into clinical practice. Radiology 310(3):e231986

Forno E, Weiner DJ, Mullen J, Sawicki G, Kurland G, Han YY et al (2017) Obesity and airway dysanapsis in children with and without asthma. Am J Respir Crit Care Med 195(3):314–323

Galbán CJ, Han MK, Boes JL, Chughtai KA, Meyer CR, Johnson TD et al (2012) Computed tomography-based

biomarker provides unique signature for diagnosis of COPD phenotypes and disease progression. Nat Med 18(11):1711–1715
Gevenois PA, de Maertelaer V, De Vuyst P, Zanen J, Yernault JC (1995) Comparison of computed density and macroscopic morphometry in pulmonary emphysema. Am J Respir Crit Care Med 152(2):653–657
Greene R, Lechner GL (1975) "Saber-Sheath" Trachea: a clinical and functional study of marked coronal narrowing of the intrathoracic trachea. Radiology 115(2):265–268
Hadj Bouzid AI, Bui S, Benlala I, Berger P, Hutt A, Liberge R et al (2025) Artificial intelligence-driven volumetric CT outcome score in cystic fibrosis: longitudinal and multicenter validation with/without modulators treatment. Eur Radiol 35(2):815–827
Hatabu H, Ohno Y, Gefter WB, Parraga G, Madore B, Lee KS et al (2020) Expanding applications of pulmonary MRI in the clinical evaluation of lung disorders: Fleischner society position paper. Radiology 297(2):286–301
Hightower JS, Amadi C, Den E, Schmitt JE, Shah RM, Miller WT (2016) Back to the future: sagittal CT in the evaluation of COPD. Eur Radiol 26(8):2730–2739
Hogg JC, Chu F, Utokaparch S, Woods R, Elliott WM, Buzatu L et al (2004) The nature of small-airway obstruction in chronic obstructive pulmonary disease. N Engl J Med 350(26):2645–2653
Johannessen A, Skorge TD, Bottai M, Grydeland TB, Nilsen RM, Coxson H et al (2013) Mortality by level of emphysema and airway wall thickness. Am J Respir Crit Care Med 187(6):602–608
Kahnert K, Jörres RA, Kauczor HU, Alter P, Trudzinski FC, Herth F et al (2023) Standardized airway wall thickness Pi10 from routine CT scans of COPD patients as imaging biomarker for disease severity, lung function decline, and mortality. Ther Adv Respir Dis 17:17534666221148663
Kim JS, Müller NL, Park CS, Lynch DA, Newman LS, Grenier P et al (1997) Bronchoarterial ratio on thin section CT: comparison between high altitude and sea level. J Comput Assist Tomogr 21(2):306–311
Kirby M, Smith BM, Tanabe N, Hogg JC, Coxson HO, Sin DD et al (2021) Computed tomography total airway count predicts progression to COPD in at-risk smokers. ERJ Open Res 7(4):00307–02021
Kwee AKAL, Andrinopoulou ER, van der Veer T, Gallardo-Estrella L, Charbonnier JP, Humphries SM et al (2024) Higher small pulmonary artery and vein volume on computed tomography is associated with mortality in current and former smokers. EBioMedicine 108:105366
Longuefosse A, Raoult J, Benlala I, Denis de Senneville B, Benkert T, Macey J et al (2023) Generating high-resolution synthetic ct from lung mri with ultrashort echo times: initial evaluation in cystic fibrosis. Radiology 308(1):e230052
Lv Q, Gallardo-Estrella L, Andrinopoulou ER, Chen Y, Charbonnier JP, Sandvik RM et al (2023) Automatic analysis of bronchus-artery dimensions to diagnose and monitor airways disease in cystic fibrosis. Thorax 79(1):13–22
Lynch DA, Austin JHM, Hogg JC, Grenier PA, Kauczor HU, Bankier AA et al (2015) CT-definable subtypes of chronic obstructive pulmonary disease: a statement of the Fleischner Society. Radiology 277(1):192–205
Mackin D, Ger R, Gay S, Dodge C, Zhang L, Yang J et al (2019) Matching and homogenizing convolution kernels for quantitative studies in computed tomography. Investig Radiol 54(5):288–295
Matsuoka S, Kurihara Y, Yagihashi K, Hoshino M, Watanabe N, Nakajima Y (2008) Quantitative assessment of air trapping in chronic obstructive pulmonary disease using inspiratory and expiratory volumetric MDCT. AJR Am J Roentgenol 190(3):762–769
Matsuoka S, Washko GR, Yamashiro T, Estepar RSJ, Diaz A, Silverman EK et al (2010) Pulmonary hypertension and computed tomography measurement of small pulmonary vessels in severe emphysema. Am J Respir Crit Care Med 181(3):218–225
McNally P, Lester K, Stone G, Elnazir B, Williamson M, Cox D et al (2023) Improvement in lung clearance index and chest CT scores with elexacaftor/tezacaftor/ivacaftor treatment in people with cystic fibrosis aged 12 years and older – the RECOVER Study. Am J Respir Crit Care Med 208(9):917–929
Meerburg JJ, Veerman GDM, Aliberti S, Tiddens HAWM (2020) Diagnosis and quantification of bronchiectasis using computed tomography or magnetic resonance imaging: a systematic review. Respir Med 170:105954
Mills DR, Masters IB, Yerkovich ST, McEniery J, Kapur N, Chang AB et al (2024) Radiographic outcomes in pediatric bronchiectasis and factors associated with reversibility. Am J Respir Crit Care Med 210(1):97–107
Mochizuki F, Tanabe N, Shimada T, Iijima H, Sakamoto R, Shiraishi Y et al (2024) Centrilobular emphysema and airway dysanapsis: factors associated with low respiratory function in younger smokers. ERJ Open Res 10(2):00695–02023
Montaudon M, Desbarats P, Berger P, de Dietrich G, Marthan R, Laurent F (2007a) Assessment of bronchial wall thickness and lumen diameter in human adults using multi-detector computed tomography: comparison with theoretical models. J Anat 211(5):579–588
Montaudon M, Berger P, Cangini-Sacher A, de Dietrich G, Tunon-de-Lara JM, Marthan R et al (2007b) Bronchial measurement with three-dimensional quantitative thin-section CT in patients with cystic fibrosis. Radiology 242(2):573–581
Mummy DG, Bier EA, Wang Z, Korzekwinski J, Morrison L, Barkauskas C et al (2021) Hyperpolarized 129Xe MRI and spectroscopy of gas-exchange abnormalities in nonspecific interstitial pneumonia. Radiology 301(1):211–220
O'Donnell RA, Peebles C, Ward JA, Daraker A, Angco G, Broberg P et al (2004) Relationship between peripheral airway dysfunction, airway obstruction, and neutrophilic inflammation in COPD. Thorax 59(10):837–842

O'Donnell CR, Bankier AA, O'Donnell DH, Loring SH, Boiselle PM (2014) Static end-expiratory and dynamic forced expiratory tracheal collapse in COPD. Clin Radiol 69(4):357–362

Oelsner EC, Ortega VE, Smith BM, Nguyen JN, Manichaikul AW, Hoffman EA et al (2019) A genetic risk score associated with chronic obstructive pulmonary disease susceptibility and lung structure on computed tomography. Am J Respir Crit Care Med 200(6):721–731

Rosenow T, Oudraad MCJ, Murray CP, Turkovic L, Kuo W, de Bruijne M et al (2015) PRAGMA-CF. a quantitative structural lung disease computed tomography outcome in young children with cystic fibrosis. Am J Respir Crit Care Med 191(10):1158–1165

Sciurba FC, Ernst A, Herth FJF, Strange C, Criner GJ, Marquette CH et al (2010) A randomized study of endobronchial valves for advanced emphysema. N Engl J Med 363(13):1233–1244

Stolz D, Mkorombindo T, Schumann DM, Agusti A, Ash SY, Bafadhel M et al (2022) Towards the elimination of chronic obstructive pulmonary disease: a Lancet Commission. Lancet 400(10356):921–972

Tanabe N, Sato S, Oguma T, Shima H, Sato A, Muro S et al (2019) Associations of airway tree to lung volume ratio on computed tomography with lung function and symptoms in chronic obstructive pulmonary disease. Respir Res 20(1):77

Terzikhan N, Bos D, Lahousse L, Wolff L, Verhamme KMC, Leening MJG et al (2017) Pulmonary artery to aorta ratio and risk of all-cause mortality in the general population: the Rotterdam Study. Eur Respir J 49(6):1602168

Thompson BR (2017) Dysanapsis-once believed to be a physiological curiosity-is now clinically important. Am J Respir Crit Care Med 195(3):277–278

Lung Volume, Emphysema, and Air Trapping

Constance de Margerie-Mellon and Alexander A. Bankier

Contents

C. de Margerie-Mellon (✉)
Université Paris Cité, AP-HP, Hôpital Saint-Louis, Paris, France

Department of Radiology, PARCC UMRS 970, INSERM, Paris, France
e-mail: constance.de-margerie@aphp.fr

A. A. Bankier
Department of Radiology, University of Massachusetts Memorial Health and University of Massachusetts Chan Medical School, Worcester, MA, USA
e-mail: alexander.bankier@umassmemorial.org

Abstract

In the framework of evidence-based medicine, quantitative biomarkers are needed to adequately diagnose disease, predict prognosis, and assess the effects of therapy. Among others, respiratory conditions such as COPD or asthma are common chronic diseases that place an important burden on healthcare costs. Reliable measurements of respiratory parameters that are altered in these diseases could contribute to standardizing and rationalizing their management and potentially decreasing the associated expenses. Quantitative measurements of lung volumes, emphysema, and air trapping are now achievable in routine practice through imaging. The aim of this chapter is to review the pathophysiological basis of these respiratory parameters, the principles on which their measurements rely, the technical requirements for adequate quantitative assessments, and the interpretation of the measurement results.

Abbreviations

$\%LAA_{-950}$	Percentage of low attenuation areas below −950 HU
$\%LAA_{-856expi}$	Percentage of low attenuation areas below −856 HU on expiratory CT
ADC	Apparent diffusion coefficient

Med Radiol Diagn Imaging (2026)
https://doi.org/10.1007/174_2024_523,
Published Online: 13 February 2025

CTLV	Computed tomography lung volumetry
E/I-ratio$_{MLD}$	Expiratory to inspiratory ratio of mean lung density
FEV$_1$	Forced expiratory volume at the first second
LAA	Low attenuation areas
MLD	Mean lung density
Perc15	15th percentile point of the attenuation curve
PFT	Pulmonary function test
PRM	Parametric response mapping
QIBA	Quantitative Imaging Biomarker Alliance
RVC$_{-860\ to\ -950}$	Relative inspiratory to expiratory volume change of voxels with attenuation values between −860 and −950 HU
SAD	Small airway disease
TLC	Total lung capacity

1 Lung Volumes

1.1 Definition and Clinical Importance

Lung volume refers to the volume of gas in the lungs at a given time during the respiratory cycle. Inspired and expired lung volumes are easily measured by spirometry. Measurements of absolute lung volumes are technically more challenging (Wanger et al. 2005). Absolute lung volumes are the total lung capacity (TLC)—which represents the maximum volume of gas the lungs can accommodate—and its components, the residual volume and the vital capacity (Tseng et al. 2017). TLC can be altered in various respiratory conditions: it is reduced in restrictive lung disease, whereas it may be increased in disease as emphysema and asthma. TLC can be measured through several methods: body plethysmography, nitrogen washout, gas dilution (these three methods can be considered as part of pulmonary function tests (PFTs)), or imaging (Wanger et al. 2005).

As compared to PFTs, imaging, notably with CT, has the major advantage of being able to measure each lung and each lobe separately, thanks to the fissures that represent anatomic boundaries between lobes. In patients with emphysema for instance, precise lobe volumetry is helpful before lung volume reduction surgery or implementation of an endobronchial valve or coil and if required after the procedure (Tenda et al. 2019; Becker et al. 1998). Additionally, CT scanners are usually widely accessible, whereas nitrogen washout and gas dilution methods require specific equipment that is not as widespread. However, contrary to PFT-derived lung volumes, measuring lung volumes through CT implies the delivery of ionizing radiation. Nevertheless, if a patient needs a chest CT for diagnostic purposes, measurement of lung volume can be a useful adjunct without additional radiation or cost (Ruppel 2012).

1.2 Lung Volumetry with Radiograph

Initially, measurements of lung volumes with imaging were based on chest radiographs (Barnhard et al. 1960; Pierce et al. 1979). These measurements were inherently limited by the two-dimensional nature of conventional radiographs, and large differences between plethysmographic and radiographic TLCs have been reported (Rodenstein et al. 1985). For this reason, and because of the development of CT lung volumetry (CTLV), radiographic measurements of TLC are no longer performed.

1.3 Lung Volumetry with CT

Thanks to a fast image acquisition, a detailed anatomical depiction, and a wide availability, CT is the modality of choice for the morphological assessment of the lung parenchyma. CT is also an accurate tool for the measurement of functional data such as absolute lung volumes (Wanger et al. 2005; O'Donnell et al. 2010).

1.3.1 Principle

1.3.1.1 Total Lung Volumetry

TLC is a parameter that can be extracted from a chest CT examination. TLC simply corresponds to the volume of gas contained in the lungs at full inspiration.

In its early age, CTLV involved a manual delineation of the lung parenchyma on a stack of 2D sections, a multiplication by the section thickness, and a sum of the individual section volumes to obtain the TLC (Schlesinger et al. 1995; Wandtke et al. 1986).

The development of spiral CT and quantification software introduced a quicker and more accurate method based on an automated identification of voxels containing lung parenchyma. These voxels are segmented from the chest wall and mediastinum, are quantified, and are subsequently translated into lung volumes (Kauczor et al. 1996, 1998).

1.3.1.2 Individual Lobe Volumetry

A major strength of CTLV is its ability to provide data per lung and per lobe, in addition to TLC.

The segmentation of pulmonary lobes relies on the accurate identification of lung fissures. This task can be challenging: in patients with lung disease, the lobes can lose their normal shape, and the fissures become difficult to identify. Moreover, lung fissures can be incomplete, even in patients with normal lung parenchyma (Guelsuen et al. 2006).

There are now several different lung segmentation methods in order to avoid an entirely manual delineation of pulmonary lobes that would be extremely time consuming (Hu et al. 2001). These methods are usually semiautomated: the software provides an initial output, which can be easily manually corrected if needed. Whatever the chosen method, the first fundamental step is to identify the fissures (Tenda et al. 2019). The second step involves the generation of complete fissure planes and the separation of the different individual lobes. Most methods use the pulmonary airway and vascular trees to guide the subdivision of the lungs into lobes (Lassen et al. 2013; Palagyi et al. 2006; Tschirren et al. 2005). The software then provides a volume measurement per lung and per lobe. An example is provided in Fig. 1.

1.3.2 Comparison to PFTs

Direct comparison of volumes measured through PFTs and through CT is subject to two limitations. First, lung volumes measured on CT include not only the gas lung volume (as in PFTs) but also lung tissue volume. Second, CTLV is performed in the supine position, whereas PFTs are performed in the sitting position. The elevation of the diaphragm in supine position induced by a raised intra-abdominal pressure may underestimate the actual lung volumes (Vilke et al. 2000). In a recent study using a CT scanner prototype that allows acquisition in the upright positions, correlation between total lung volume on inspiratory CT and total lung capacity on PFTs was higher for upright CT than for supine CT (Yamada et al. 2020).

Lung volumes measured with PFTs and with CT therefore represent two different parameters. However, TLC calculated from CTs has been shown to be highly correlated with plethysmographic measurements of TLC (Kauczor et al. 1998; Nemec et al. 2015; Iwano et al. 2009; Brown et al. 1999, 2010). A recent study suggests that CT TLC may substitute for plethysmographic TLC when plethysmography is difficult to perform or not available (Matsumoto et al. 2017).

1.3.3 Source of Variations

1.3.3.1 Confounding Factors

For comparisons of CT-derived lung volumes, either in cross-sectional studies or in longitudinal assessments, several potential intrinsic and extrinsic confounding factors have to be considered.

Intrinsic Factors

The measurement of lung volumes is obviously influenced by the degree of inspiration. For TLC assessment, CT acquisition should be performed at full inspiration. The inability to follow the respiratory instructions may result in non-reliable measurements and limited longitudinal reproducibility. Nevertheless, spirometric monitoring dur-

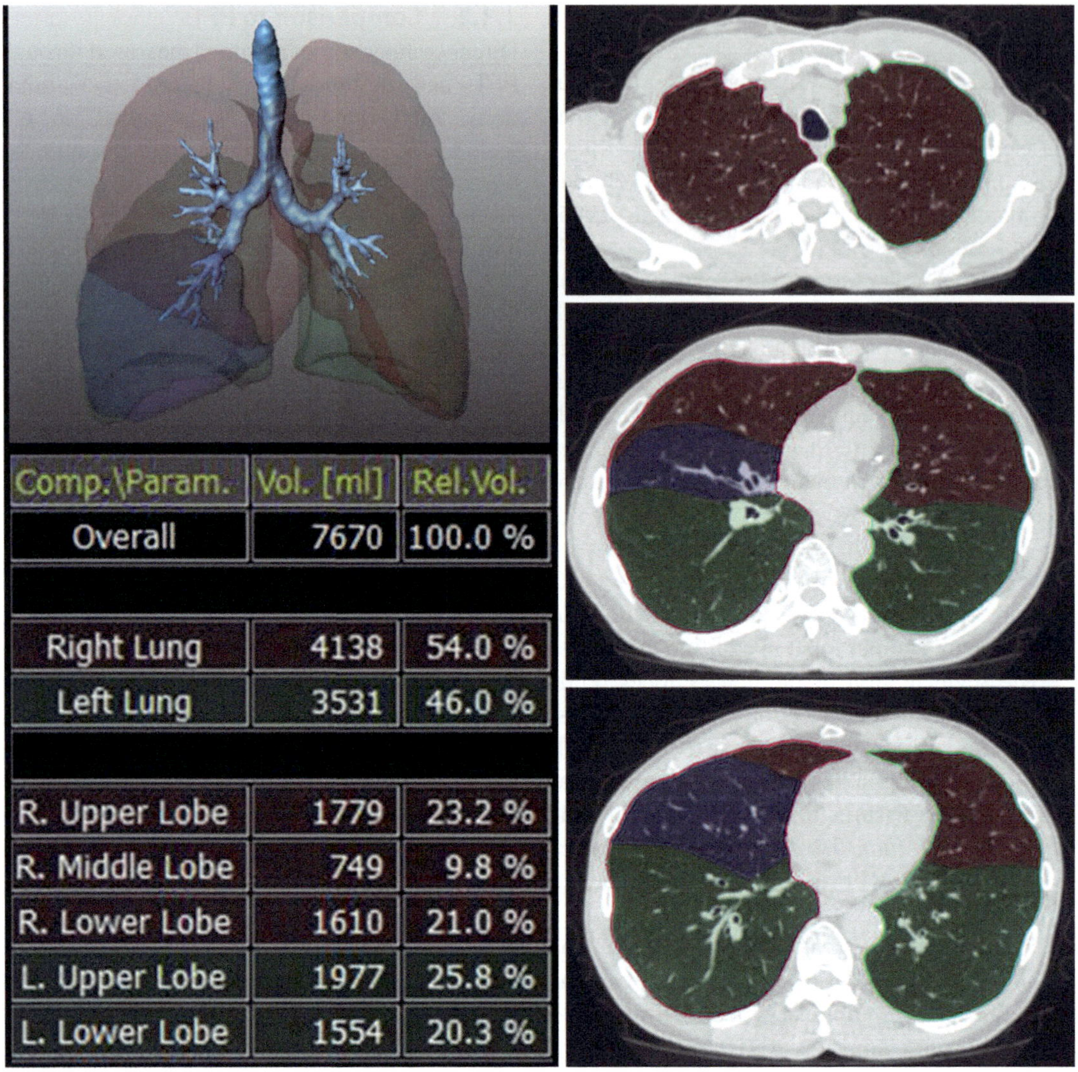

Fig. 1 Individual lobe volumetry (performed with PULMO3D, MeVis Medical Solutions, Bremen, Germany). Upper lobes are colored in red, lower lobes in green, and right middle lobe in blue. *Vol.* volume, *Rel. Vol.* relative volume

ing the acquisition is probably not necessary, when considering the high reproducibility of volume measured on longitudinal CTs with straightforward breathing instructions (Brown et al. 2010; Gierada et al. 2001; Shin et al. 2017).

Extrinsic Factors

The impact of the variation of acquisition and reconstruction parameters such as tube voltage, tube current, kernel, or section thickness on CTLV have not been precisely studied. However, because the lung segmentation is the first step of CTLV, and because this segmentation relies on attenuation values that can be influenced by these acquisition and reconstructions parameters, it is probably reasonable to keep identical protocols when performing serial measurements of lung volume on CT.

On the post-processing side, lung volumetric differences resulting from the use of different software packages have been proven to be small (Nemec et al. 2015), and, as a consequence, agreement was high. Of note, the strength of this agreement decreased with decreasing lung volumes especially for the assessment of functional residual capacity on expiratory acquisitions. The authors explained this observation by suggesting that the lower natural contrast between the lung parenchyma and the chest wall at smaller lung volumes could limit the ability of the segmentation software to differentiate between those structures on expiratory CT images.

1.3.3.2 Inter- and Intraobserver Reproducibility

Inter- and intraobserver reproducibility of CT lung volume measurements is high (Molinari et al. 2010, 2013). In one study, reproducibility was higher for total lung volumes than for lobar volumes: inter- and intraobserver variability was ±3.4% for total volume, while it could increase to 10.6% (intra) and 98.3% (inter) for lobar volumes (Molinari et al. 2010). This could be explained by the larger impact of manual corrections for the lobe segmentation, as compared to the corrections performed for the total lung segmentation. For lobar volumes, the reproducibility is probably additionally influenced by the considered lobe: one study demonstrated a lower reproducibility of volume measurements of the right upper lobe and the right middle lobe, as compared to the other lobes (Revel et al. 2008). This may be secondary to difficulties in the identification of the right minor fissure, due especially to its frequent incompleteness. In the latter case, the fissure location has to be determined by the radiologist which may be an undeniable source of variability. Automated and semiautomated approaches for the measurement of lobe volumes seem to have similar reproducibility (Revel et al. 2008), whereas entirely manual segmentation has a larger inter- and intraobserver variability (Molinari et al. 2013).

1.3.4 CTLV in Routine Practice

Recommended protocols for CT quantitative assessment of lung volume are suggested in Table 1. These parameters are valid for lung volumetry, but also for the measurement of emphysema and air trapping. They are derived from the CT protocol used in the COPDGene study (Regan et al. 2010) and from recommendations of the Quantitative Imaging Biomarkers Alliance (QIBA) regarding lung densitometry (Kay et al.

Table 1 Recommended CT parameters for quantitative assessment of lung volume, emphysema, and air trapping

	Parameters used in the COPDGene study	Parameters recommended by the QIBA
Contrast media	None	None
Tube potential (kVp)	120	Not reported
Tube current (mAs)		Use of automatic exposure control to meet $CTDI_{vol}$ requirement
– Inspiratory acquisition	<200	
– Expiratory acquisition (air trapping assessment)	<50	
$CTDI_{vol}$	Not reported	≤3 mGy (medium-sized subject, <75 kg) for inspiratory acquisition Not reported for expiratory acquisitions
Pitch	0.9–1.1	Chosen so to allow the completion of the scan in a single breath hold
Scan duration	Not reported	≤10 s (table speed ≥4 cm/s)
Detector configuration (mm)	16–128 × 0.6–0.75	>16 × ≤1
Reconstructed section thickness (mm)	0.625–1	≤1[a]
Reconstruction algorithms	High-resolution (visual assessment) Standard (quantitative assessment)	Not reported

Adapted from Litmanovich et al. (2014) and Quantitative Imaging Biomarkers Alliance (2019)

[a] In clinical practice, slices ≤1.5 mm are acceptable

2019). Data on ultralow-dose protocols for lung volume measurement are scarce; it is therefore not possible to recommend them in this framework. Dose reduction could limit fissure visibility, resulting in possibly more challenging measurement of lobar volumes (de Margerie-Mellon et al. 2016). However, deep learning-based segmentation algorithms and photon counting detectors may overcome these difficulties in the near future (Graafen et al. 2022; Zhang et al. 2021). Of note, lung volume assessment is seldom a clinical indication to perform chest CT and is rather a side measurement on an examination performed for another clinical indication, this indication being the main driver of the protocol choice.

For the assessment of lung volumes, an adequate full inspiration from the patient is of paramount importance. This should be obtained through appropriate breathing instructions and a practice breathing session by the CT technologist prior to the acquisition. Spirometric monitoring is not feasible in most centers and is probably not necessary as long as the patient's training is appropriate (Brown et al. 2010; Gierada et al. 2001; Shin et al. 2017). The completion of a full inspiration should be verified after the CT acquisition: when the lung is at its maximal volume, the trachea has a circular configuration, and peripheral vessels are thin and stretched with sparing of the immediate subpleural space, notably in the lung bases; the azygoesophageal recess is deployed, and the interlobar fissures are straight (Bankier et al. 2008). If these criteria are not met, TLC is likely to be underestimated.

Once the quality of the CT images has been verified, the lung volumetry software can be launched on the series reconstructed with the soft tissue kernel. The lung segmentation process can be automated or semiautomated; in both cases, the segmentation output provided by the software needs to be checked and corrected if necessary. Most lung volumetry software also include lung densitometry. Some of them are listed later in Sect. 2, Table 3.

Importantly, in the case of cross-sectional and longitudinal studies, the CT scanner, the acquisition protocol, the reconstruction parameters, and the post-processing software should be kept identical in order to limit the influence of confounding factors on volume measurements. In clinical practice, following these recommendations may be challenging, considering the fact that dose reduction approach, as well as reconstruction algorithms and post-processing software, is continuously updated.

Data about normal values for CTLV are scarce, and, as PFTs, are likely to vary according to age, sex, race/ethnicity, and height. Zach et al. studied the chest CT examinations of 92 healthy nonsmokers (within the COPDGene project) (Zach et al. 2012). Results are reported in Table 2.

1.4 Lung Volumetry with MR

Compared to CT, lung MR has the advantage of being radiation-free. Volumetric anatomic sequences are now available and could, theoretically, be used for volumetry (Johnson et al. 2013). However, due to its limited availability, the scan duration, and its high cost, lung MR volumetry is not, to date, be routinely performed.

1.5 Future Research Directions

Several research directions exist in the field of CTLV. First, the development of more accurate and entirely automatic processes for lobar segmentation that could uniformly be applied to healthy and non-healthy lungs would be useful (Mansoor et al. 2015). It would limit the need for manual corrections (and the additional time bur-

Table 2 Mean lung volume (*L*) in 92 healthy nonsmoker subjects

	Total lung	Right upper lobe[a]	Right middle lobe[a]	Right lower lobe[a]	Left upper lobe[a]	Left lower lobe[a]
Male	6.81	1.02	0.46	1.43	1.25	1.29
Female	4.83					

From Zach et al. (2012)

[a] Denotes average values for women ($n = 63$) and men ($n = 29$)

Table 3 List of lung densitometry software (alphabetic order) used in selected published studies for this chapter, some of them performed with previous versions of the cited software

Name of the software	Company/owner	Availability	References
Chest Imaging Platform in 3D SLICER	Brigham and Women's Hospital, Boston, MA, USA	Open-source	Gierada et al. (2011)
CALIPER (Computer-Aided Lung Informatics for Pathology Evaluation and Ratings)	Mayo Clinic, Rochester, MN, USA	Research	Matsumoto et al. (2017)
CT Lung Density Analysis in Vitrea software	Vital Images, Minnesota, MN, USA	Commercial	Haas et al. (2014)
Lung Density Analysis	Imbio, Minneapolis, MN, USA	Commercial	Vehar et al. (2019)
LungPrint	VIDA Diagnostics Inc., Coralville, IO, USA	Commercial	Nemec et al. (2015), Schroeder et al. (2013), Sieren et al. (2016)
Lung Segmentation in Aquarius iNtuition	TeraRecon, Foster City, California, USA	Commercial	Shin et al. (2017), Wielputz et al. (2014)
Myrian XP Lung	Intrasense, Paris, France	Commercial	Baumueller et al. (2016), Cheng et al. (2015)
Osirix MD	Pixmeo, Geneva, Switzerland	Commercial	Nemec et al. (2015)
PULMO3D	MeVis Medical Solutions, Bremen, Germany	Commercial	Nemec et al. (2015), Molinari et al. (2013)
Syngo Pulmo CT	Siemens Healthcare, Erlangen, Germany	Commercial	Lim et al. (2016), Wielputz et al. (2014)
YACTA (Yet another CT analyzer)	University Hospital of Heidelberg, Germany	Research	Lim et al. (2016), Wielputz et al. (2013, 2014), Heussel et al. (2009)

den for the radiologist) and could increase the reproducibility of the measurements. Second, the exact role of CTLV as compared to lung volume measured with PFTs has yet to be determined. To date, there are no recommendations about the use of CT-derived lung volume values. The actual contribution of lobar volumes measured on CT for clinical practice, notably, is still unknown. Finally, large datasets of normal and abnormal CTLV values are currently lacking, and studies of large, representative cohorts are needed in order to provide reliable references.

2 Emphysema

2.1 Definition and Clinical Importance

Emphysema is defined as a "condition of the lung characterized by abnormal, permanent enlargement of airspaces distal to the terminal bronchiole, accompanied by the destruction of their walls, and without obvious fibrosis" (Snider et al. 1985). Emphysema is one phenotype of COPD, resulting in increased lung compliance, and is mainly caused by tobacco smoke. Other causes include deficiency of alpha-1-antitrypsin, exposure to biomass smoke, and other air pollutants (Labaki et al. 2019; Barnes et al. 2015; Hu et al. 2010).

Emphysema is a pathological diagnosis. Consequently, emphysema diagnosis is mainly indirect during life, often based on imaging. Of note, any new CT technique used to quantify noninvasive emphysema should theoretically be compared to pathology for actual validation (Gevenois et al. 1995, 1996a).

In COPD, the phenotyping effort primarily aims at classifying the leading pathophysiological component as either emphysema or airway inflammation/remodeling. Traditionally, forced expiratory volume in one second (FEV_1) has been used to measure the baseline severity and progression of emphysema, but destructive changes in lung parenchyma often precede decreases in forced expiratory volume by several years (Gurney et al. 1992). These changes can be directly visualized on imaging. CT quantification of emphysema can therefore be a valuable addition to PFTs in the assessment of COPD patients. The relationship between CT-quantified emphysema and clinical parameters has been widely studied, and it has been proven that CT-derived parameters of emphysema are associated with lung function, lung function decline, and mortality (Kinsella et al. 1990; Arakawa et al. 2001; Mohamed Hoesein et al. 2011; Smith et al. 2014; Lynch et al. 2018).

Quantifying emphysema is a critical challenge to assess the natural history of the disease, its extent, and its evolution after specific treatments. As a key strength, CT allows not only an overall quantification of emphysema but also a lobar quantification that can be useful before and after lung volume reduction surgery and implantation of bronchial valves (Schroeder et al. 2013; Brown et al. 2012). At a broader scale, quantification of emphysema could be performed in all patients undergoing chest CT for lung cancer screening. By assessing the extent of emphysema, and monitoring its evolution, a more comprehensive assessment of patients with tobacco smoke exposure could be provided through lung cancer screening programs, and the cost-effectiveness of screening could thus be increased (Kumar et al. 2018).

2.2 Quantification with Radiograph

Chest radiograph can identify the presence of bullae or indirect signs of emphysema such as the reduction of the peripheral vasculature and overinflation (Miniati et al. 2008) as well as flattening of the diaphragms. In one study, a radiograph-based score of emphysema correlated with functional indices of airflow obstruction, overinflation, and impaired lung diffusing capacity in a way comparable to that obtained by using qualitative and quantitative CT data (Miniati et al. 1995). Nevertheless, chest radiograph does not allow any objective quantification of emphysema, limiting its use for this specific task with a less sensitivity than that of chest CT.

2.3 Quantification with CT

CT is currently the most widely available imaging technique for the in vivo measurement of emphysema. Measurement of emphysema can be performed in combination with airway measurements, leading to a comprehensive, quantitative assessment of the COPD phenotype. Emphysema quantification with CT, by visual scales or through objective methods, has been largely studied and will be detailed in this section. Functional evaluation of lung ventilation with CT, after inhalation of xenon gas, has also been investigated in patients with emphysema (Kong et al. 2014; Sugino et al. 2017; Lee et al. 2017). However, this technique is only used in research, and no quantification tool has been validated to date; therefore, the topic will not be discussed in this chapter.

On CT, emphysema is characterized by areas of decreased attenuation. Several anatomic subtypes of emphysema have been described, based on the disease distribution within secondary pulmonary lobules and cranio-caudal distribution at the lung level, with likely different underlying pathophysiology (Kim et al. 1991).

2.3.1 Morphological Subtypes of Emphysema

The three following subtypes of emphysema are commonly accepted subtypes (Smith et al. 2014; Thurlbeck and Muller 1994; Stern and Frank 1994; Snider et al. 1985; Takahashi et al. 2008; Wright and Churg 2006). Examples are shown in Fig. 2.

Centrilobular emphysema, the most common subtype, corresponds to an abnormal enlargement of airspaces centered on the respiratory bronchiole with coalescence of destroyed lobules in severe cases. On CT, it is defined by centrilobular areas of decreased attenuation, usually without visible walls, of nonuniform distribution

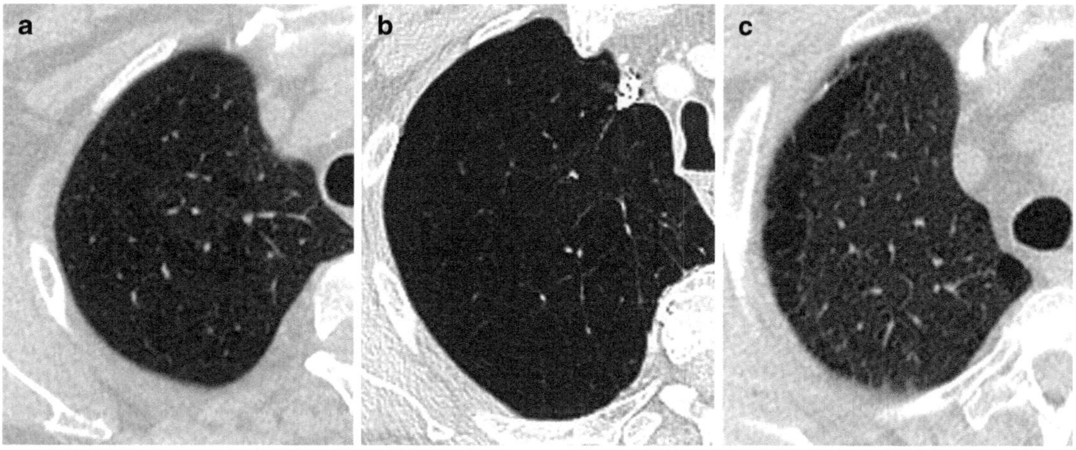

Fig. 2 Three emphysema subtypes on chest CT (right upper lobes of three distinct patients). (**a**) Centrilobular emphysema, (**b**) panlobular emphysema, and (**c**) paraseptal emphysema

and predominantly located in upper lung zones (Hansell et al. 2008).

Panlobular emphysema is characterized by a uniform overdistension and destruction of airspaces from the respiratory bronchioles to the alveoli. On CT, it appears as a generalized effacement of the lung parenchyma with a decrease in the caliber of blood vessels in the affected lung (Hansell et al. 2008). The decrease in lung attenuation is usually more homogeneous than in centrilobular emphysema.

Paraseptal (or distal acinar) emphysema is described as an enlarged airspace at the periphery of acini, commonly occurring adjacent to pleural spaces or interstitial interfaces. This subtype is often associated with other emphysema subtypes but may also occur as an isolated finding. On CT, paraseptal emphysema appears as single or multiple cyst-like lucencies or bullae in subpleural locations (Hansell et al. 2008).

Of note, CT-based automated methods for emphysema quantification do not allow the distinction between the different morphological subtypes of emphysema. The densitometry software will provide a global assessment for all areas with decreased attenuation.

2.3.2 Subjective Quantification (Visual Scale)

Subjective quantification (visual semiquantitative analysis) was the first method used to assess the severity of emphysema before the wide availability of automated analysis.

2.3.2.1 Available Scales

Semiquantitative Scale (4- or 5-Point Scale)

Goddard et al. described in 1982 the first visual scoring method. For each lung region, a score of 0 represented no abnormality, 1 was assigned if less than 25% of the parenchyma showed emphysema, 2 was assigned if 25–50% of the parenchyma showed emphysema, 3 was assigned if 50–75% of the parenchyma showed emphysema, and 4 was assigned if more than 75% of the parenchyma showed emphysema (Goddard et al. 1982). In the initial scoring system, emphysema was assessed in right lung and left lung on eight sections, leading to a maximum score of 64 ($8 \times 2 \times 4$).

Several authors have used this score, assessing a variable number of CT sections or lung regions for a complete scoring (Bankier et al. 1999; Cavigli et al. 2009; COPDGene CT Workshop Group et al. 2012; Stavngaard et al. 2006; Wille et al. 2014; Mascalchi et al. 2012; Koyama et al. 2010). In some studies, an additional category for a lung region showing less than 5% of emphysema was created, in order to isolate patients with very limited emphysema, including one study performed among patients from the COPDGene cohort (COPDGene CT Workshop Group et al. 2012).

Fleischner Society Scale

The Fleischner Society proposed an alternate classification in 2015 (Lynch et al. 2015). This scoring method is both semiquantitative and qualitative. It distinguishes centrilobular emphysema (CLE), paraseptal emphysema (PSE), and panlobular emphysema (only used for emphysema induced by a deficiency of alpha-1-antitrypsin, a lower lobe predominant pattern involving generalized destruction of all acini more or less equally).

CLE is graded as follows:

- Trace CLE: minimal centrilobular lucencies, involving less than 0.5% of a lung zone
- Mild CLE: scattered centrilobular lucencies, involving 0.5–5.0% of a lung zone
- Moderate CLE: many well-defined centrilobular lucencies, involving more than 5% of any lung zone
- Confluent emphysema: coalescent centrilobular or lobular lucencies without extensive hyperexpansion of secondary pulmonary lobules or distortion of pulmonary architecture
- Advanced destructive emphysema: panlobular lucencies with hyperexpansion of secondary pulmonary lobules or distortion of pulmonary architecture

PSE is graded as either mild (small (≤1 cm) well-demarcated rounded juxtapleural lucencies, aligned in a row along a pleural margin) or substantial (mainly large (>1 cm) juxtapleural cyst-like lucencies or bullae involving more than the lung apices, aligned in a row along a pleural margin).

This scoring method was then used in a recent large study based on the COPDGene cohort (Lynch et al. 2018).

2.3.2.2 Comparison to Clinical Data and Reproducibility

Comparison to Quantitative CT Measurements, Pathological and Clinical Data

The major strengths of visual analysis of emphysema are (1) the limited influence of image noise on the assessment and (2) the ability to detect even a small amount of parenchymal destruction, as compared to quantitative measurements. Visual analysis has also several weaknesses: it is reader dependent, time consuming, and usually performed on a limited number of sections, whereas the quantitative analysis offers an assessment of the entire lung parenchyma. As referenced to histology, Bankier et al. showed that the visual, semiquantitative scale had a tendency to overestimate the extent of emphysema and showed less agreement with macroscopic assessment of emphysema than the objective CT quantification (Bankier et al. 1999). In a study by Cavigli et al., the visual, semiquantitative assessment showed a weaker correlation to the DLCO, as compared to objective CT quantification (Cavigli et al. 2009). However, in a more recent study based on the Fleischner Society scale, Lynch et al. found that the visual analysis of emphysema patterns was an independent predictor of mortality (Lynch et al. 2018).

Interobserver Reproducibility

The limited interobserver reproducibility of the visual scale is one of its main important drawbacks. Regarding the original 4-point scale (or modified 5-point scale) designed by Goddard et al., a slight to moderate agreement has been described (Bankier et al. 1999; Cavigli et al. 2009; COPDGene CT Workshop Group et al. 2012; Mascalchi et al. 2012). Yet, in one recent study, the Fleischner grading system (Table 3) has shown better results, with weighted kappa values ranging from 0.71 to 0.80 among observers (Lynch et al. 2018). As a consequence, this grading system can be considered as reliable and be used for the assessment of emphysema morphological subtypes, complementary to objective quantification.

2.3.3 Objective Quantification

2.3.3.1 Origin

In order to objectively quantify the extent of emphysema, and to overcome the subjectivity and the limited reproducibility of visual scales, several methods based on CT attenuation values have been developed and validated against histopathological quantification of emphysema, which represents the ground truth.

CT has been initially developed as a measurement tool, and lung CT is an actual map of attenuation of the parenchyma. For this reason, it seems suited to the quantitative assessment of emphysema.

Three methods can be distinguished. The first method simply relies on the measurement of mean lung CT attenuation (often called mean lung density), which would be lowered in cases of emphysema. The two other methods are based on the distribution of lung attenuation values through the lung parenchyma. One is based on an absolute threshold of CT attenuation value. All lung areas presenting with attenuation lower than this threshold are considered as emphysema. Another approach relies on an analysis of the histogram of CT attenuation values. The degree of emphysema is quantified by a preselected given percentile (named *X*th percentile) point of the lung attenuation histogram derived from CT. This corresponds of the *X*% of voxels below this threshold. The approach of both methods is shown in Fig. 3.

In the earliest investigations, single-section analysis of CT attenuation values of the lung was applied; then the analysis shifted to multiple section levels and to volume assessment. The analysis is now performed on volumetric scans, using an algorithm that first segments the lung from the chest wall and the mediastinum, and traces its borders after removal of central pulmonary blood vessels and airways, as for lung volumetry. The software then calculates the proportion of pixels below a threshold value, extracts an attenuation histogram of the parenchyma, and computes the mean lung CT attenuation.

The first quantitative radiology-pathology correlation was presented by Hayhurst et al. (1984); the authors showed that emphysematous lung had lower CT attenuation values as compared to normal parenchyma (Hayhurst et al. 1984). Subsequent studies, based on histological evidence of emphysema, have discussed the most appropriate HU threshold or percentile to quantify emphysema on CT (Gevenois et al. 1995, 1996a; Gould et al. 1988; Muller et al. 1988; Madani et al. 2007).

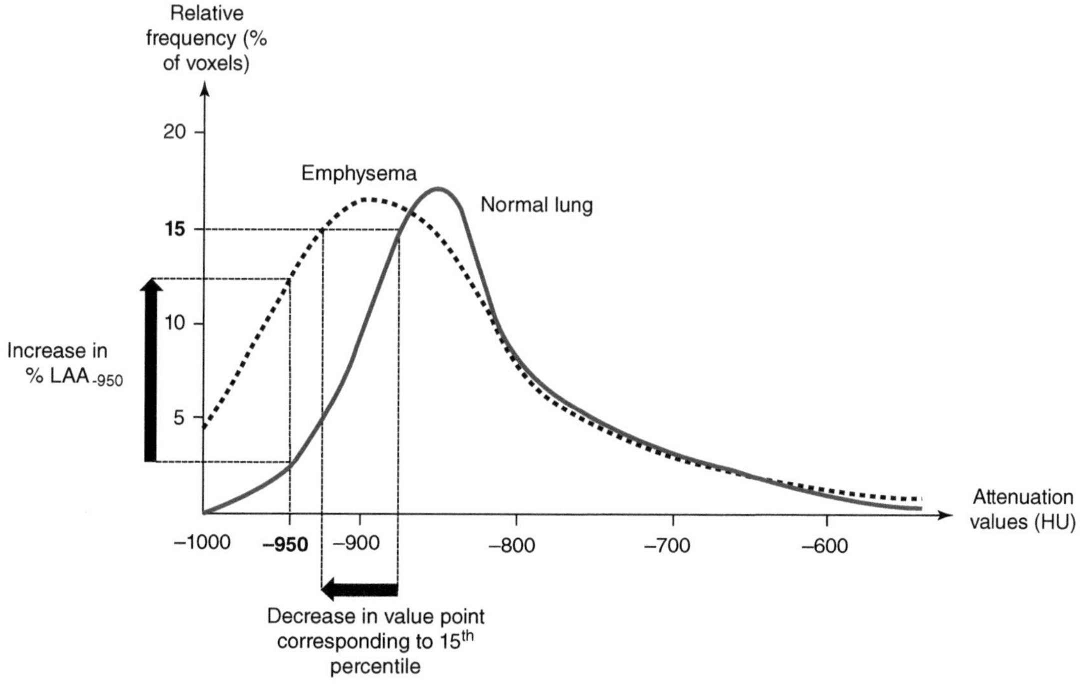

Fig. 3 Threshold and percentile methods. For this example, the threshold method is based on a −950 HU threshold and the percentile method on the 15th percentile point. If emphysema is present (dashed curve), the relative frequency of voxels below the predefined threshold (−950 HU usually) will increase, whereas the point representing the 15th percentile of the attenuation curve will decrease (displaced on the left of the curve)

For the threshold method, the most commonly accepted value today is −950 HU. This threshold comes from two studies from Gevenois et al. (1995, 1996a) who compared noncontiguous 1-mm-thick HRCT data obtained from several attenuation thresholds to the microscopic and macroscopic extent of emphysema on resected lungs. They found that the only threshold for which there was no statistically significant difference between the CT and the morphometric data was −950 HU. A few years later, Madani et al. repeated the experiment using volumetric chest CT acquisitions instead of sequential thin-section CT sections and identified −960 HU as the best reflection of the extent of emphysema as compared to microscopic and macroscopic measurements (Madani et al. 2008).

Regarding the percentile method, Gould et al. showed that the lowest fifth percentile of the histogram of attenuation values was significantly correlated with the extent of microscopic emphysema (Gould et al. 1988). Later, Madani et al. found that the first percentile was the parameter with the strongest correlation to microscopic and macroscopic histological measurements (Madani et al. 2006, 2007). In more recent studies, the 15th percentile point (Perc15) was used predominantly and shown to be reliable in longitudinal measurements of emphysema (Mohamed Hoesein et al. 2011; Dirksen et al. 1999, 2009; Shaker et al. 2009; Parr et al. 2006).

Finally, mean lung density (MLD) has been reported in several emphysema-centered studies and has been shown to be correlated to various PFT parameters (Giuntini et al. 2007; Lee et al. 2008; Camiciottoli et al. 2006; Sverzellati et al. 2013). Still, this CT-based emphysema parameter lacks histological validation and is less frequently used compared to the thresholds and the percentile methods.

2.3.3.2 Source of Variations

Confounding Factors

Objective quantitative measurements have been proven to be accurate by comparison to microscopic and macroscopic pathological measurements. However, it is important to keep in mind that they are prone to be influenced by numerous clinical and technical parameters.

Intrinsic Factors

CT measurements of emphysema vary with lung volume. Gevenois et al. identified a statistically significant correlation between TLC and both the relative area of pixels <−950 HU and MLD (Gevenois et al. 1996b), suggesting that normal densitometric values should be established as a function of body length and age, as both factors influence TLC. Madani et al. found that submaximal inspiration induces underestimation of pulmonary emphysema (Madani et al. 2010), and Nemec et al. confirmed that MLD increases with decreasing volumes (Nemec et al. 2015). Still, Gierada et al. demonstrated that spirometric control of lung volume does not significantly improve the repeatability of quantitative measurement of emphysema (Gierada et al. 2001). Nevertheless, in the longitudinal evaluation of emphysema, a correction for lung volume can be used and has been proven to substantially reduce the interscan variability (Bakker et al. 2005; Stoel et al. 2008; Staring et al. 2014).

CT lung densitometry is also influenced by gender (Walsdorff et al. 2016). Moreover, there is a distal airspace enlargement that increases with age, resulting in "pseudo-emphysema" in elderly patients (Fukuchi 2009).

Another factor to take into account is the smoking status of the patient. Interestingly, CT-quantified emphysema tends to increase after a recent smoking cessation (Shaker et al. 2011; Ashraf et al. 2011). A likely explanation for this phenomenon is that smokers have an increased number of inflammatory cells in the lung that partly offset the decrease of lung attenuation induced by emphysema (Karimi et al. 2014). Once the patient stops smoking, these inflammatory cells disappear and, as a consequence, the lung attenuation tends to decrease.

Extrinsic Factors

All other factors kept constant, variability can be induced by the CT scan itself, mainly as the result of differences in measured air attenuation (Bakker et al. 2005). Regular scanner calibration with standardized CT phantoms is necessary to ensure the accuracy of CT numbers and is of paramount importance in multicenter studies (Parr et al. 2004).

Tube current has been shown to substantially influence emphysema quantification. In a study simulating fixed low mAs settings with filtered back reconstruction, Zaporozhan et al. showed that settings below 50 mAs alter quantitative emphysema measurements as compared to the original protocol at 150 mAs (Zaporozhan et al. 2006). Madani et al. showed that lowering the tube current from 120 to 20 mAs affects the relative area of pixels <−950 and <−960 HU. However, there was no effect on the first percentile of the histogram (Madani et al. 2007).

Section thickness has a statistically significant effect on the relative area of pixels <−950 and <−960 HU and on MLD (Madani et al. 2007; Gierada et al. 2010). The CT reconstruction kernel may also strongly affect the lung densitometry, notably high-frequency kernels, as compared to standard ones (Boedeker et al. 2004). Increasing the section thickness and decreasing the kernel sharpness reduce the image noise and modify the attenuation histogram, resulting in lower measurements of emphysema percentage. On the contrary, decreasing the section thickness and increasing the kernel sharpness tend to increase the percentage of measured emphysema (Gierada et al. 2010; Hochhegger et al. 2010, 2011).

Additionally, it has been proven in several studies that iterative reconstruction algorithms significantly influence CT quantitative measurement of emphysema (Mets et al. 2012a; Choo et al. 2014; Martin et al. 2017; den Harder et al. 2018). Iterative reconstruction reduces the image noise but may also degrade the low-contrast resolution (McCollough et al. 2015), by smoothening the abrupt transitions between different attenuations. As a consequence, lower threshold and percentile-based measurements of emphysema have been reported when using iterative reconstruction as compared to filtered back projection (Mets et al. 2012a; Choo et al. 2014; Martin et al. 2017). Interestingly, MLD measurements of emphysema seem unaffected by the reconstruction algorithm (Mets et al. 2012a; Choo et al. 2014; Martin et al. 2017). This may be due to the fact that iterative reconstruction mainly affects the extreme values of the attenuation histogram, without modifying MLD (Mets et al. 2012a). More recently, a study showed significantly different emphysema volumes (using threshold-based measurement) of deep learning reconstructions as compared to iterative and filtered back projection algorithms (Ferri et al. 2022).

Finally, the software used to automatically quantify the emphysema can also induce substantial variability, notably for lobe-wise analysis (Heussel et al. 2006; Lim et al. 2016; Wielputz et al. 2014). Variability in the lobe segmentation output would inevitably result in variability in lobe densitometric analysis.

Inter- and Intraobserver Reproducibility

Bakker et al. showed a very high inter- and intraobserver reproducibility for Perc15 in total lung measurement of emphysema (Bakker et al. 2005). As expected, lobe-wise measurement of emphysema showed higher variability, because it relies first on the segmentation of the different lung lobes. As described above, this task can be challenging (Molinari et al. 2010, 2013).

2.3.4 Quantitative Measurements of Emphysema in Clinical Practice

2.3.4.1 Technical Requirement for Quantitative Measurement of Emphysema

Technical requirements for emphysema quantification on chest CT are similar to those described for lung volumetry and detailed in Table 2. Contrast material may influence the attenuation measurements; therefore, nonenhanced CT acquisition should be used. An adequate full inspiration should be obtained for the image acquisition, after appropriate training. Of note, recommendations on radiation dose are limited to an upper threshold of 3 mGy for CTDIvol, and no lower threshold is provided. In the framework of lung cancer screening, where emphysema identification jointly to lung nodule detection is relevant, chest CTs are performed at low dose levels that vary according to protocols but with CTDIvol that can be well below 3 mGy. Based on the bioMILD trial population, a recent work has shown that emphysema quantification on low-dose screening CTs was feasible and that %LAA_{-950} was correlated to all-cause mortality and airflow obstruction (Balbi et al. 2023). However, the minimal radiation dose for adequate emphysema detection is still unknown.

A first visual inspection on images reconstructed with the lung kernel should be done before any quantitative measurement, to check the quality of the image acquisition and to visually assess the presence and extent of emphysema. Quantitative measurements will be performed on images reconstructed with the standard (soft tissue) kernel to limit the noise. Most software combines CT lung volumetry and CT emphysema measurements; therefore, an emphysema measurement is usually possible for the whole lung, for the separated right and left lungs, and for each individual lobe. Lobar measurement of emphysema may be useful to provide an objective measurement of emphysema distribution heterogeneity before a potential endobronchial lung volume reduction (Sciurba et al. 2010). As for lobe volumetry, the adequate segmentation of the lung should be verified before proceeding to the quantitative analysis. A list of some selected lung densitometry software is presented in Table 3, and an example is provided in Fig. 4.

As described above, there are multiple sources of variations in attenuation measurements on CT scan (Table 4). For this reason, comparison of quantitative measures should ideally only be done on CT examinations performed with the same technique (same breathing instructions, CT scan, acquisition, and reconstruction parameters)

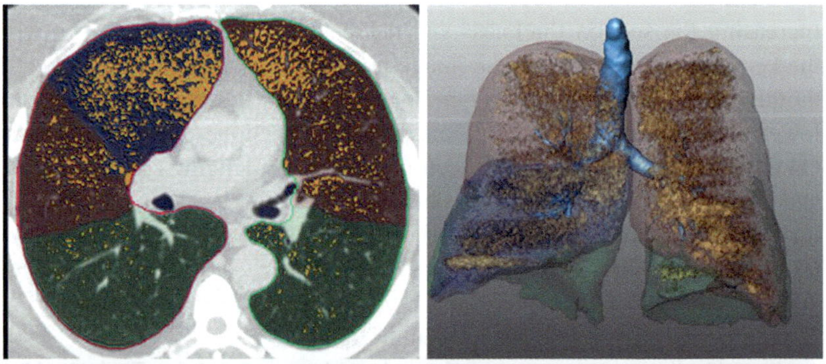

Comp.\Param.	Vol. [ml]	Rel.Vol.	MLD [HU]	P15 (HU)	LAV
Overall	7670	100.0 %	-866	-941	8.6 %
Right Lung	4138	54.0 %	-864	-939	8.1 %
Left Lung	3531	46.0 %	-869	-942	9.1 %
R. Upper Lobe	1779	23.2 %	-872	-940	8.2 %
R. Middle Lobe	749	9.8 %	-891	-954	18.3 %
R. Lower Lobe	1610	21.0 %	-842	-923	3.3 %
L. Upper Lobe	1977	25.8 %	-880	-947	12.1 %
L. Lower Lobe	1554	20.3 %	-855	-933	5.4 %

Fig. 4 Quantitative measurement of emphysema (performed with PULMO3D, MeVis Medical Solutions, Bremen, Germany). *MLD* mean lung density, *P15* 15th percentile point, *LAV* low-attenuation value areas (<−950 HU). The yellow areas represent the voxels with an attenuation value <−950 HU

Table 4 Source of variations in quantitative measurement of emphysema and suggestions for limiting their influence

Levels	Parameters	Comments
Patient	Lung volume at acquisition	Breathing practice session with standardized instruction in order to obtain an adequate full inspiration For longitudinal studies, consider lung volume adjustment
	Smoking status	For longitudinal studies: take into consideration a recent smoking cessation
CT technique	CT scan	Regular air and phantom calibrations For cross-sectional and longitudinal studies, use the same CT scan
	Tube voltage and tube current	For cross-sectional and longitudinal studies, keep the acquisition parameters constant
	Reconstruction algorithm	For cross-sectional and longitudinal studies, keep the reconstruction algorithm constant
	Reconstruction kernel	Use high-frequency (lung) kernel for lung visual assessment Use standard (soft tissue) kernel for quantitative analysis For cross-sectional and longitudinal studies, keep the kernel constant
Quantitative analysis	Analysis software	For cross-sectional and longitudinal studies, keep the same software

and analyzed with the same software. Additionally, air and phantom calibration should be done on a quarterly basis (Quantitative Imaging Biomarkers Alliance 2019). For longitudinal assessment of patients, lung volume adjustment should be considered if there is more than a 10% variation in TLC measured on CT (Quantitative Imaging Biomarkers Alliance 2019). The volume adjustment can be performed using a simple equation that assumes a proportional inverse relationship between lung volume and lung density. More complicated models include linear mixed-effects models (Stoel et al. 2008). However, to date, there is no recommended method to perform this volume adjustment (Quantitative Imaging Biomarkers Alliance 2019). Regarding other sources of variations, a recent study performed in patients from the COPDGene cohort showed that volume, noise, and interscanner bias for lung density change estimation over time could be corrected simultaneously, improving repeatability analyses and agreeing with visual readings (Vegas Sanchez-Ferrero et al. 2024). The authors applied an analytic technique to modify the paired baseline lung attenuation histogram to match the acquisition conditions of the follow-up scan, allowing to overcome the impact of the above-cited confounders. Such methods are not yet, however, available for clinical practice.

2.3.4.2 Thresholds and Normal Values in Clinical Practice

The relative lung area occupied by pixels with attenuation values lower than −950 HU on an inspiratory chest CT is now the parameter most commonly used in clinical practice and in scientific studies for the measurement of emphysema (Wang et al. 2013). This parameter is calculated by dividing the volume of lung pixels <−950 HU by the total volume of lung pixels. This parameter is often named $\%LAA_{-950}$, LAA standing for low-attenuation areas. When using the percentile method, it is usually the 15th percentile point of the attenuation curve (Perc15) that is mostly used (Dirksen 2008; Crossley et al. 2018). Both $\%LAA_{-950}$ and Perc15 have been identified by the QIBA as the key biomarkers for the assessment of emphysema (Quantitative Imaging Biomarkers Alliance 2019).

There are limited data for normal values of $\%LAA_{-950}$ and Perc15, which may vary according to intrinsic and extrinsic factors. Nevertheless, Table 5 summarizes values of these parameters reported in three studies performed on healthy subjects.

For longitudinal studies, the QIBA states that without lung volume adjustment, an increase in $\%LAA_{-950}$ of at least 3.7% or a decrease in Perc15 of at least 18 HU indicates an increase in the extent of emphysema, with 95% confidence

Table 5 Normal values for %LAA$_{-950}$, %LAA$_{-960}$, and 15th percentile of the attenuation curve

	Population	%LAA$_{-950}$	%LAA$_{-960}$	Perc15
Irion et al. (2009)	30 healthy young patients (male and female, age range 19–41 years old)	(Mean) 0.19%	Not recorded	Not recorded
Mets et al. (2012b)	70 young men (mean age 36 years old) with normal lung function	(Mean ± SD) 0.97 ± 1.1%	(Mean ± SD) 0.35 ± 0.33%	(Mean ± SD) −919 ± 13 HU
Zach et al. (2012)	92 healthy nonsmokers (male and female, mean age 63 years old)	(Mean ± SD) All: 2 ± 2.7% Male: 3.6 ± 3.2% Female: 1.3 ± 2%	Not recorded	Not recorded

(Quantitative Imaging Biomarkers Alliance 2019). The QIBA also mentions that with lung volume adjustment, a decrease in Perc15 of at least 11 HU is required for the detection of an increase in the extent of emphysema, with 95% confidence (Quantitative Imaging Biomarkers Alliance 2019). These statements are only valid if all technical requirements are met (including the stability of acquisition and reconstruction parameters).

2.4 Quantification with MRI

The low proton density and the magnetic susceptibility artifacts induced by the multiple air-lung tissue surfaces have initially limited the development of lung proton MRI. Yet, this radiation-free technique offers excellent soft tissue contrast and, thanks to recent technological improvements, is now able to generate anatomical and functional information about the lung pathophysiology.

Several MR techniques have proven to be useful in research settings for the assessment of emphysema and are described below. However, to date, there is no validated clinical application for MRI in the measurement of emphysema because of their limited availability, their technical requirements (notably for ventilation MRI), and their cost.

For morphological MR, ultrashort echo time sequences, that use radial k-space sampling to shorten the echo times well below 1 ms, have become available recently. MR with ultrashort echo time imaging may have the potential to assist detection of early and localized pathological destruction of lung tissue architecture observed in various pulmonary disorders such as emphysema (Togao et al. 2010). This sequence could quantitatively assess the loss of pulmonary function and help classify the clinical stage of COPD in smokers, similar to thin-section multidetector CT (Ohno et al. 2011).

Dynamic contrast-enhanced perfusion MR can also be useful in the context of COPD. In these patients, both airway obstruction (due to inflammation) and parenchymal destruction (due to emphysema) impair ventilation; as a consequence, a hypoxic vasoconstriction occurs. Additionally, parenchyma destruction occurs along with the destruction of the pulmonary vascular bed (Lee et al. 2013). Several studies have shown that the deterioration of perfusion parameters measured on CT was correlated with worsening of airflow limitation on PFTs and emphysema index on CT and that regional heterogeneity of emphysema on CT matches with the decreased perfusion on MR (Jang et al. 2008; Ley-Zaporozhan et al. 2007).

Finally, ventilation MR is also an interesting method to evaluate lung ventilation function without radiation. Ventilation MR is traditionally obtained either with the oxygen-enhanced technique or through the inhalation of hyperpolarized noble gas. Oxygen-enhanced MRI is a proton-based MR technique. Images are acquired before and after inhalation of 100%

oxygen by the patient. Oxygen molecules, which are paramagnetic substances, dissolve into the blood and produce a T1-shortening effect in the lungs. This shortening of the T1 relaxation time is proportional to the oxygen concentration in the inhaled gas and can be visualized as increased signal intensity on MRI (Ohno et al. 2001a). Several studies have shown that the intensity of oxygen-enhanced MRI is correlated to the DLCO in patients with emphysema (Ohno et al. 2001b, 2002). The alternative ventilation MR technique relies on the inhalation of hyperpolarized noble gas, either ^{3}He or ^{129}Xe. This technique uses the gas itself to visualize the airway and airspaces after inhalation of laser-polarized gas and can be used in functional imaging such as regional mapping of airflow in the lungs, measurement of diffusion in airspace, or measurement of regional oxygen concentration (Lee et al. 2013). The apparent diffusion coefficient (ADC) of hyperpolarized ^{3}He has been proven to be increased in patients with emphysema and correlated with PFT results, suggesting that the ADC of ^{3}He can provide quantitative information on the status of the pulmonary microstructure (Salerno et al. 2002; Ley et al. 2004). More recently, phase-revolved ventilation MRI, an innovative and cost-effective technique, has offered promising results for the assessment of the lung ventilation and perfusion (Klimes et al. 2024; Kaireit et al. 2021). This technique is based on a Fourier decomposition approach and does not require the use of any inhaled gas or contrast agent.

2.5 Future Research Directions

Because most CT acquisitions now fulfill the quality criteria for a reliable quantitative analysis, and because quantification software is now widespread, it is likely that automated quantification of emphysema will soon become a standard practice for all chest CT examinations where emphysema is diagnosed.

Nevertheless, the main challenge to be overcome for the quantitative measurement of emphysema (as, on a larger scale, for the quantitative imaging of COPD) is the comparability of various CT datasets, either for cross-sectional or for longitudinal studies. As described above, variability in emphysema measurements can appear at all levels (Table 4). Some confounding factors are relatively easy to avoid, by keeping the acquisition parameters constant and by using the same reconstruction kernel, given that there is no change in the CT scanner that is used for the examination. Other parameters are more challenging to control. It is well known that the use of iterative reconstruction can result in important differences in emphysema measurements (Mets et al. 2012a; Choo et al. 2014; Martin et al. 2017). Each vendor has his proprietary iterative reconstruction algorithm, whose details are not available to the public, and that is continually refined. The precise impact of these algorithms on quantitative measurements in the lung is not known, and no adjustment is therefore possible. Likewise, the exact influence of different densitometry software on emphysema quantification is difficult to predict, and thus, the comparability of results obtained with distinct programs is difficult to foresee. Future research should focus on quantifying the respective influence of each of these parameters and on developing detailed, standardized protocols that could be used across different CT vendors and densitometry software. The ultimate goal would be to normalize all results according to various parameters and vendors. The first step to achieve such goals would be to increase the transparency of CT image reconstruction and densitometry algorithms, which are currently "black boxes." Supporting these research directions and creating recommendations to reduce the variability across devices, sites, patients, and time are the aims of the QIBA, launched by the Radiological Society of North America in 2007 (Kay et al. 2019; Quantitative Imaging Biomarkers Alliance 2019).

3 Air Trapping

3.1 Definition and Clinical Importance

Air trapping in chest imaging refers to retention of air distal to a complete or partial airway obstruction. Air trapping is a hallmark of small airway disease (SAD) (defined as ≤2 mm in diameter), as the result of an airway obstruction (constrictive bronchiolitis, asthma, cystic fibrosis, hypersensitivity pneumonitis, …) or as the result of local abnormalities in pulmonary compliance (Arakawa and Webb 1998). In COPD, the airflow obstruction is secondary to an increase in the resistance of the small airways and/or to an increase in lung compliance caused by emphysematous lung destruction (Matsuoka et al. 2007).

As described above, small airways are a major site of pathology in various lung diseases (Cosio et al. 1978; McNulty and Usmani 2014). SAD may lead to reduction in airflow, increased airway resistance, gas trapping, and inhomogeneity of ventilation. These parameters are usually not easily accessible. The forced expiratory volume in 1 s (FEV_1), the spirometric parameter that is used in PFTs to assess airways, is widely available but mostly reflects the status of large airways. In small airway obstruction, a substantial amount of disease must accumulate before FEV_1 is decreased (McNulty and Usmani 2014). Plethysmographic parameters such as residual volume and airway resistance are more sensitive to early changes but lack specificity (McNulty and Usmani 2014). On the imaging side, small airway wall size is well beyond the spatial resolution of CT and MRI, but they can be assessed indirectly with air trapping and inhomogeneity of ventilation. Quantification of air trapping with CT is relatively simple to obtain after acquisition of end-expiration CT images, however at the cost of ionizing radiation to the patient. Nevertheless, CT measurement of air trapping has been proven to be well correlated to clinical diagnosis and prognostic categories in various diseases (Arakawa and Webb 1998; Leung et al. 1998; Goris et al. 2003; Busacker et al. 2009; Mets et al. 2013), and CT can be of important contribution for the assessment of SAD and complementary to the data provided by PFTs.

Of note, a limited amount of air trapping may sometimes be observed in individuals with normal lung function (Tanaka et al. 2003; Mastora et al. 2001). This amount may increase in elderly subjects, smokers, and subjects imaged in the prone position (Mastora et al. 2001; Bankier et al. 2010; Lee et al. 2000; Martinez et al. 2017).

3.2 Quantification with Radiograph

Chest X-ray has a very limited role in the quantification of air trapping. Only obstruction of the large airways (often secondary to the inhalation of a foreign body) resulting in the hyperinflation of one lung or one lobe can be visible on an expiration chest X-ray.

3.3 Quantification with CT

On CT, air trapping is diagnosed on end-expiration CT images when parenchymal areas fail to increase in attenuation and/or fail to decrease in volume (Hansell et al. 2008; Bankier et al. 2001). An example is provided in Fig. 5. Comparison between inspiratory and expiratory CT scans can be helpful when air trapping is subtle or diffuse (Hansell et al. 2008). To note, in some cases of severe constrictive bronchiolitis, no change may be observed between inspiratory and expiratory data due to the diffuse and severe involvement. In patients with severe emphysema, air trapping can be difficult to detect visually, as lung attenuation is already decreased because of the parenchymal destruction.

It is important to keep in mind that air trapping is an indirect radiological sign, which is the consequence of the disease (= trapped air distal to a diseased airway) but not the visualization of the diseased airway itself (which may exhibit features like centrilobular micronodules or tree-in-bud).

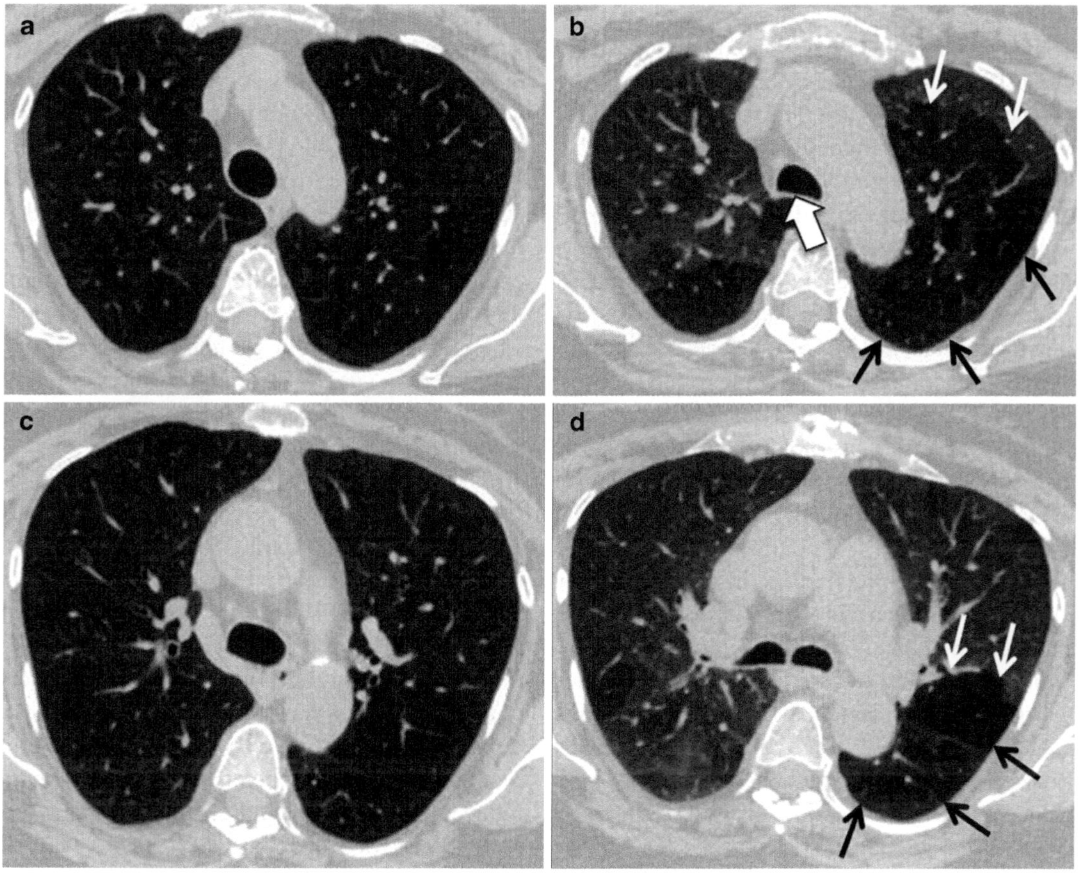

Fig. 5 Air trapping (four images from the same patient). (**a**, **c**) Inspiration CT images, (**b**, **d**) expiration CT images. On the expiration CT, the lung volume is decreased, and the posterior wall of the trachea is flattened (wide white arrow). Areas of air trapping appear as persistent low-attenuation areas (examples for the left lung are shown with white and black thin arrows)

3.3.1 Subjective Quantification

Before the widespread development of quantification software, semiquantitative scores have been used to assess the extent of air trapping. These 4- or 5-point scales harbor slight modifications from study to study (Arakawa and Webb 1998; Leung et al. 1998). To note, using minIP with a soft tissue kernel and increasing the contrast of the image with window/level adjustment may facilitate the visual detection of air trapping.

In three successive studies, Bankier et al. used the following scoring method: a score of 0 was assigned if there was no abnormality; 1, if less than 20%; 2, if 20–39%; 3, if 40–59%; 4, if 60–79%; or 5, if more than 80% showed air trapping (Bankier et al. 2001, 2003, 2007). These semiquantitative scores have been shown to be correlated to PFT values (Arakawa and Webb 1998; Hansell et al. 1997).

Of note, air trapping involving <25% of the cross-sectional area of the lung at a single scan level can be considered physiological (Lee et al. 2000; Webb et al. 1993), depending on the age and smoking history of the patient.

3.3.2 Objective Quantification

3.3.2.1 Quantification with Expiratory CT Alone

Similarly to emphysema, the most commonly used method to objectively quantify air trapping is threshold based. Air trapping is usually defined as the percentage of LAA ≤−856 HU on expiratory CT that can be named $\%LAA_{-856expi}$.

The selection of −856 HU as the threshold for air trapping on expiratory CT is based on the fact that −856 HU is the mean attenuation of normally inflated lung (≈6 mL air per gram of lung) on full inspiration (Newman et al. 1994). Therefore, in a normal lung, the attenuation on expiration should be higher than −856 HU (Schroeder et al. 2013). Of note, because air trapping is a functional parameter measured on expiratory CT, the above threshold has never been validated against a histological proof of airway disease. It is, indeed, not possible to reproduce the expiration phenomenon on lung histological samples.

Several studies focused on asthma and cystic fibrosis have shown that there is a strong relationship between quantitative measurements of expiratory air trapping and spirometric abnormalities (Goris et al. 2003; Busacker et al. 2009; Newman et al. 1994). These quantitative measurements also correlate strongly with physiologic measurements of airway obstruction in COPD (Schroeder et al. 2013; Lee et al. 2008; Matsuoka et al. 2008).

3.3.2.2 Quantification with Paired Inspiratory-Expiratory CTs

In patients with COPD, the presence of emphysema, defined as LAA ≤−950 HU on inspiratory CT, inevitably affects air trapping measurements, because air-trapped areas and emphysema areas will show similar low attenuation on expiratory CT. In order to avoid this pitfall, paired inspiratory and expiratory CTs are useful. Comparison between both set of images allows the distinction between permanent LAA (emphysema) and functional LAA that appear only on expiratory CT (air trapping).

Two different measures have been described in this context.

A simple measure is to compute the expiratory to inspiratory ratio of MLD (E/I-ratio$_{MLD}$) (Eda et al. 1997; Kubo et al. 1999). In case of air trapping, the absolute value of expiratory MLD decreases and the E/I-ratio$_{MLD}$ increases.

Another method has been described afterwards. Matsuoka et al. introduced the relative inspiratory to expiratory volume change (RVC) of voxels with attenuation values between −860 and −950 HU ($RVC_{-860\ to\ -950}$) (Matsuoka et al. 2007). For this measure, parenchymal volumes with attenuation values below −950 HU are excluded on inspiratory and expiratory CTs, to correct for emphysema. Next, the difference between expiratory and inspiratory relative lung volume below −860 HU in the resulting limited density range is computed. In case of air trapping, the expiratory relative lung volume below −860 HU increases, resulting in a higher $RVC_{-860\ to\ -950}$.

These two measures, E/I-ratio$_{MLD}$ and $RVC_{-860\ to\ -950}$, as well as the percentage of lung areas below −856 HU on expiratory CT ($\%LAA_{-856expi}$), have been compared by Mets et al. The authors showed that the E/I-ratio$_{MLD}$ was more suitable for detecting air trapping on low-dose screening CT than $RVC_{-860\ to\ -950}$ and $\%LAA_{-856expi}$ (Mets et al. 2012c). In a lung cancer screening cohort, air trapping assessed with the E/I-ratio$_{MLD}$ on low-dose CT was independently associated with reduced lung function and accelerated decline of FEV_1/FVC (Mets et al. 2013).

3.3.2.3 Quantification with Co-registered Inspiratory-Expiratory CTs

In 2012, Galban et al. developed the parameter response mapping (PRM) for the comprehensive assessment of COPD, including its air trapping component. Parametric response mapping is based on a voxel-by-voxel comparison of lung attenuation changes from digitally co-registered inspiratory and expiratory CT images (Galban et al. 2012). Each lung area on inspiratory CT is matched to the same area on expiratory CT, and the CT densities are compared. This technique automatically separates emphysema from air trapping and allows the distinction between different COPD phenotypes. Another major advantage is that it also provides detailed spatial information related to the disease distribution (Fig. 6). It may serve as a complementary readout to PFTs for more accurate diagnosis and treatment management.

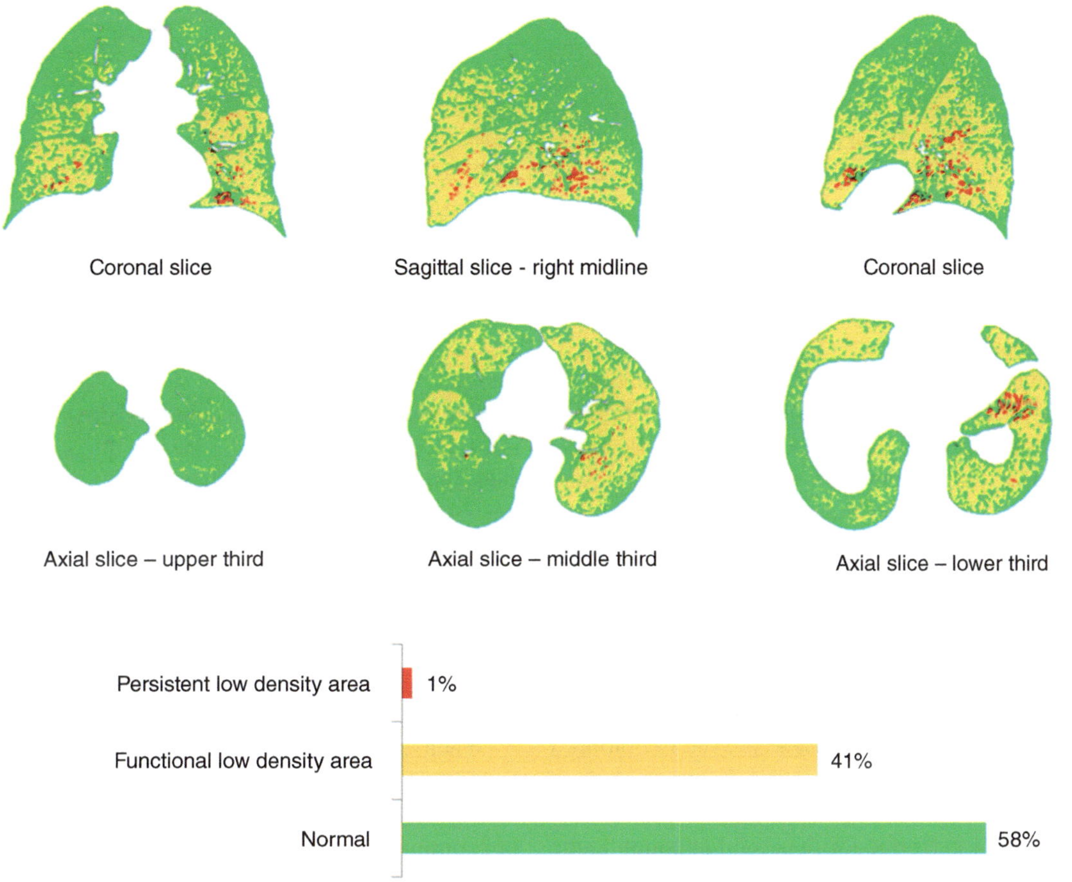

Fig. 6 Parametric response mapping (performed with Lung Density Analysis, Imbio, Minneapolis, MN, USA). Normal areas (voxels above −950 HU on inspiration images and above −856 HU on expiration images) are shown in green. Functional low-attenuation areas (voxels above −950 HU on inspiration images and below −856 HU on expiration images), or air trapping areas, are shown in yellow. Persistent low-attenuation areas (voxels below −950 HU on inspiration images and below −856 HU on expiration images), or emphysema areas, are shown in red

To date, PRM has been used in COPD to more precisely characterize the underlying disease phenotype (Boes et al. 2015). It has also been studied in bronchiolitis obliterans syndrome, where it was identified as a prognostic tool in transplant recipients with spirometric decline (Belloli et al. 2017; Galbán et al. 2014).

Registration-based algorithms are now commercially available in software packages for quantitative analysis of emphysema and SAD.

3.3.2.4 Confounding Factors

Intrinsic Factors

In a study analyzing participants from a lung cancer screening trial that were examined twice by CT within 3 months (with CT acquisition and reconstruction parameters kept constant), the authors showed that $\%LAA_{-856expi}$, and E/I-ratio$_{MLD}$ at a smaller extent, had important variations, even with reproducible breath holds and lung volume correction. Therefore, these quantitative measures of air trapping should be used cautiously for longitudinal assessment (Mets et al. 2012d). Regarding PRM, a study performed on 85 COPD patients showed that the limits of agreement between two sets of PRM values extracted from CTs performed 30 days apart could be wide, notably when no volume adjustment was performed (Hatt et al. 2017).

Extrinsic Factors

The impact of extrinsic factors on quantitative air trapping measurement has been less widely studied than on emphysema. However, because quantitative measurements of air trapping and emphysema both rely on CT attenuations, extrinsic factors that affect emphysema measurements are likely to affect air trapping measurements as well.

In a study centered on both emphysema and air trapping, Mets et al. demonstrated that the use of iterative reconstruction significantly influences $RVC_{-860\ \text{to}\ -950}$ and EXP_{-856}. Yet, E/I-ratio$_{MLD}$ was unaffected by this reconstruction method (Mets et al. 2012a). Quantitative CT of the lungs should be performed with careful attention to the CT protocol, notably when iterative reconstruction is introduced.

3.3.3 Quantitative Measurements of Air Trapping in Clinical Practice

Air trapping quantitative measurement requires data from a CT scan obtained at full inspiration and from a chest CT scan obtained at end expiration. For the expiratory acquisition, low-dose scanning is recommended (≤50 mAs, with automated dose modulation disabled). Other parameters are similar to the ones described in Table 2. As for inspiratory acquisition, appropriate coaching by the technologist and standardized breathing instructions are important to ensure that the patient expires to an appropriate level. A good understanding of these breathing instructions has to be verified before the acquisition of the images. Images obtained at end expiration will show a flattening of the posterior wall of the trachea and a decrease in bronchial diameters. In healthy individuals, there will also be a substantial decrease of the lung volume and an increase in lung attenuation.

Table 6 Normal values for %LAA$_{-856expi}$

	Population	%LAA$_{-856expi}$ (mean ± SD)	E/I-ratio$_{MLD}$ (mean ± SD)
Mets et al. (2012b)	70 young men (mean age 36 years old) with normal lung function	5.1 ± 8%	76.2 ± 7.3%
Zach et al. (2012)	92 healthy nonsmokers (male and female)	9.2 ± 6.8%	NA

As for attenuation measurements on inspiratory CT scans of healthy individuals, data on normal values of air trapping on expiratory CTs are scarce. Table 6 reports normal values for %LAA$_{-856expi}$ in two different studies performed on healthy subjects.

When using PRM, a certain amount of air trapping is also present in healthy individuals. In a study of 15 healthy volunteers, the mean extent of expiratory LAA was 20% (Silva et al. 2016).

3.4 Quantification of Air Trapping with Lung MRI

Morphologic MRI is not suited for the assessment of SAD; still, ventilation MRI allows for the assessment of distribution of ventilation and morphometry of the distal airways without exposure to ionizing radiation. Ventilation defects are present in asthma (Eda et al. 1997; Kubo et al. 1999), COPD (Mets et al. 2012c; Galban et al. 2012), and cystic fibrosis (Alam et al. 2023; Doellinger et al. 2024), resulting from airway narrowing or obstruction and uneven ventilation.

Nevertheless, as in emphysema, ventilation MRI is still limited to research applications, and its role in clinical management is unclear. Moreover, its limited availability and high cost do not allow its widespread diffusion for routine practice.

3.5 Future Research Directions

Two main challenges remain for quantitative measurement of air trapping on paired inspiratory/expiratory CT. The first concern is the important variability of longitudinal air trapping measurements. Additional research on the origins and solution for this issue is needed. As CT attenuation is related to lung volume, a difference in the expiration effort would certainly result in a change of parenchymal attenuation and, as a consequence, a change in air trapping quantification. Therefore, enhancing the standardization of respiratory training before image acquisition and volume adjustment for attenuation measurements are certainly part of the answer. Additionally, as for emphysema, various CT acquisition and reconstruction parameters may impact air trapping measurements. However, the effect of variation of each individual parameter is difficult to predict. In this regard, definitive technical recommendations from the QIBA Committee for lung attenuation are eagerly awaited (Kay et al. 2019).

Disclaimer All measurements in this book have been obtained from peer-reviewed papers and guidelines from professional organizations, unless explicitly stated otherwise. While the authors, editors, and publisher have gone through a rigorous process to establish their correct reproduction from the original source, each measurement must be interpreted in the correct clinical context, this along with an accurate way of measurement, and taking into account all technical variables, this including follow-up exams with various equipment or software. Neither the authors, the editors, nor the publisher can accept any legal responsibility for any improper application or interpretation of these measurements as well as their potential consequences.

References

Alam FS, Zanette B, Munidasa S, Braganza S, Li D, Woods JC, Ratjen F, Santyr G (2023) Intra- and inter-visit repeatability of (129) xenon multiple-breath washout MRI in children with stable cystic fibrosis lung disease. J Magn Reson Imaging 58:936–948

Arakawa H, Webb WR (1998) Air trapping on expiratory high-resolution CT scans in the absence of inspiratory scan abnormalities: correlation with pulmonary function tests and differential diagnosis. AJR Am J Roentgenol 170:1349–1353

Arakawa A, Yamashita Y, Nakayama Y, Kadota M, Korogi H, Kawano O, Matsumoto M, Takahashi M (2001) Assessment of lung volumes in pulmonary emphysema using multidetector helical CT: comparison with pulmonary function tests. Comput Med Imaging Graph 25:399–404

Ashraf H, Lo P, Shaker SB, de Bruijne M, Dirksen A, Tonnesen P, Dahlback M, Pedersen JH (2011) Short-term effect of changes in smoking behaviour on emphysema quantification by CT. Thorax 66:55–60

Bakker ME, Stolk J, Putter H, Shaker SB, Parr DG, Piitulainen E, Russi EW, Dirksen A, Stockley RA, Reiber JHC, Stoel BC (2005) Variability in densitometric assessment of pulmonary emphysema with computed tomography. Investig Radiol 40:777–783

Balbi M, Sabia F, Ledda RE, Milanese G, Ruggirello M, Silva M, Marchiano AV, Sverzellati N, Pastorino U (2023) Automated coronary artery calcium and quantitative emphysema in lung cancer screening: association with mortality, lung cancer incidence, and airflow obstruction. J Thorac Imaging 38:W52–W63

Bankier AA, De Maertelaer V, Keyzer C, Gevenois PA (1999) Pulmonary emphysema: subjective visual grading versus objective quantification with macroscopic morphometry and thin-section CT densitometry. Radiology 211:851–858

Bankier AA, Van Muylem A, Knoop C, Estenne M, Gevenois PA (2001) Bronchiolitis obliterans syndrome in heart-lung transplant recipients: diagnosis with expiratory CT. Radiology 218:533–539

Bankier AA, Van Muylem A, Scillia P, De Maertelaer V, Estenne M, Gevenois PA (2003) Air trapping in heart-lung transplant recipients: variability of anatomic distribution and extent at sequential expiratory thin-section CT. Radiology 229:737–742

Bankier AA, Schaefer-Prokop C, De Maertelaer V, Tack D, Jaksch P, Klepetko W, Gevenois PA (2007) Air trapping: comparison of standard-dose and simulated low-dose thin-section CT techniques. Radiology 242:898–906

Bankier AA, O'Donnell CR, Boiselle PM (2008) Quality initiatives. Respiratory instructions for CT examinations of the lungs: a hands-on guide. Radiographics 28:919–931

Bankier AA, Estenne M, Kienzl D, Muller-Mang C, Van Muylem A, Gevenois PA (2010) Gravitational gradients in expiratory computed tomography examinations of patients with small airways disease: effect of body position on extent of air trapping. J Thorac Imaging 25:311–319

Barnes PJ, Burney PGJ, Silverman EK, Celli BR, Vestbo J, Wedzicha JA, Wouters EFM (2015) Chronic obstructive pulmonary disease. Nat Rev Dis Primers 1:21

Barnhard HJ, Pierce JA, Joyce JW, Bates JH (1960) Roentgenographic determination of total lung capacity. A new method evaluated in health, emphysema and congestive heart failure. Am J Med 28:51–60

Baumueller S, Hilty R, Nguyen TD, Weder W, Alkadhi H, Frauenfelder T (2016) Influence of sinogram-affirmed iterative reconstruction on computed tomography-based lung volumetry and quantification of pulmonary emphysema. J Comput Assist Tomogr 40:96–101

Becker MD, Berkmen YM, Austin JHM, Mun IK, Romney BM, Rozenshtein A, Jellen PA, Yip CK, Thomashow B, Ginsburg ME (1998) Lung volumes before and after lung volume reduction surgery—quantitative CT analysis. Am J Respir Crit Care Med 157:1593–1599

Belloli EA, Degtiar I, Wang X, Yanik GA, Stuckey LJ, Verleden SE, Kazerooni EA, Ross BD, Murray S, Galbán CJ, Lama VN (2017) Parametric response mapping as an imaging biomarker in lung transplant recipients. Am J Respir Crit Care Med 195:942–952

Boedeker KL, McNitt-Gray MF, Rogers SR, Truong DA, Brown MS, Gjertson DW, Goldin JG (2004) Emphysema: effect of reconstruction algorithm on CT imaging measures. Radiology 232:295–301

Boes JL, Hoff BA, Bule M, Johnson TD, Rehemtulla A, Chamberlain R, Hoffman EA, Kazerooni EA, Martinez FJ, Han MK, Ross BD, Galban CJ (2015) Parametric response mapping monitors temporal changes on lung CT scans in the subpopulations and intermediate outcome measures in COPD Study (SPIROMICS). Acad Radiol 22:186–194

Brown MS, McNitt-Gray MF, Goldin JG, Greaser LE, Hayward UM, Sayre JW, Arid MK, Aberle DR (1999) Automated measurement of single and total lung volume from CT. J Comput Assist Tomogr 23:632–640

Brown MS, Kim HJ, Abtin F, Da Costa I, Pais R, Ahmad S, Angel E, Ni C, Kleerup EC, Gjertson DW, McNitt-Gray MF, Goldin JG (2010) Reproducibility of lung and lobar volume measurements using computed tomography. Acad Radiol 17:316–322

Brown MS, Kim HJ, Abtin FG, Strange C, Galperin-Aizenberg M, Pais R, Da Costa IG, Ordookhani A, Chong D, Ni C, McNitt-Gray MF, Tashkin DP, Goldin JG (2012) Emphysema lung lobe volume reduction: effects on the ipsilateral and contralateral lobes. Eur Radiol 22:1547–1555

Busacker A, Newell JD, Keefe T, Hoffman EA, Granroth JC, Castro M, Fain S, Wenzel S (2009) A multivariate analysis of risk factors for the air-trapping asthmatic phenotype as measured by quantitative CT analysis. Chest 135:48–56

Camiciottoli G, Bartolucci M, Maluccio NM, Moroni C, Mascalchi M, Giuntini C, Pistolesi M (2006) Spirometrically gated high-resolution CT findings in COPD: lung attenuation vs lung function and dyspnea severity. Chest 129:558–564

Cavigli E, Camiciottoli G, Diciotti S, Orlandi I, Spinelli C, Meoni E, Grassi L, Farfalla C, Pistolesi M, Falaschi F, Mascalchi M (2009) Whole-lung densitometry versus visual assessment of emphysema. Eur Radiol 19:1686–1692

Cheng T, Wan HY, Cheng QJ, Guo Y, Qian YR, Fan L, Feng Y, Song YY, Zhou M, Li QY, Shi GC, Huang SG (2015) Obvious emphysema on computed tomography during an acute exacerbation of chronic obstructive pulmonary disease predicts a poor prognosis. Intern Med J 45:517–526

Choo JY, Goo JM, Lee CH, Park CM, Park SJ, Shim M-S (2014) Quantitative analysis of emphysema and airway measurements according to iterative reconstruction algorithms: comparison of filtered back projection, adaptive statistical iterative reconstruction and model-based iterative reconstruction. Eur Radiol 24:799–806

COPDGene CT Workshop Group, Barr RG, Berkowitz EA, Bigazzi F, Bode F, Bon J, Bowler RP, Chiles C, Crapo JD, Criner GJ, Curtis JL, Dass C, Dirksen A, Dransfield MT, Edula G, Erikkson L, Friedlander A, Galperin-Aizenberg M, Gefter WB, Gierada DS, Grenier PA, Goldin J, Han MK, Hanania NA, Hansel NN, Jacobson FL, Kauczor HU, Kinnula VL, Lipson DA, Lynch DA, MacNee W, Make BJ, Mamary AJ, Mann H, Marchetti N, Mascalchi M, McLennan G, Murphy JR, Naidich D, Nath H, Newell JD Jr, Pistolesi M, Regan EA, Reilly JJ, Sandhaus R, Schroeder JD, Sciurba F, Shaker S, Sharafkhaneh A, Silverman EK, Steiner RM, Strange C, Sverzellati N, Tashjian JH, van Beek EJ, Washington L, Washko GR, Westney G, Wood SA, Woodruff PG (2012) A combined pulmonary-radiology workshop for visual evaluation of COPD: study design, chest CT findings and concordance with quantitative evaluation. COPD 9:151–159

Cosio M, Ghezzo H, Hogg JC, Corbin R, Loveland M, Dosman J, Macklem PT (1978) Relations between structural changes in small airways and pulmonary function tests. N Engl J Med 298:1277–1281

Crossley D, Renton M, Khan M, Low EV, Turner AM (2018) CT densitometry in emphysema: a systematic review of its clinical utility. Int J Chron Obstruct Pulmon Dis 13:547–563

de Margerie-Mellon C, de Bazelaire C, Montlahuc C, Lambert J, Martineau A, Coulon P, de Kerviler E, Beigelman C (2016) Reducing radiation dose at chest CT: comparison among model-based type iterative reconstruction, hybrid iterative reconstruction, and filtered back projection. Acad Radiol 23:1246–1254

den Harder AM, de Boer E, Lagerweij SJ, Boomsma MF, Schilham AMR, Willemink MJ, Milles J, Leiner T, Budde RPJ, de Jong PA (2018) Emphysema quantification using chest CT: influence of radiation dose reduction and reconstruction technique. Eur Radiol Exp 2:30–30

Dirksen A (2008) Monitoring the progress of emphysema by repeat computed tomography scans with focus on noise reduction. Proc Am Thorac Soc 5:925–928

Dirksen A, Dijkman JH, Madsen F, Stoel B, Hutchison DCS, Ulrik CS, Skovgaard LT, Kok-Jensen A, Rudolphus A, Seersholm N, Vrooman HA, Reiber JHC, Hansen NC, Heckscher T, Viskum K, Stolk J (1999) A randomized clinical trial of alpha(1)-antitrypsin augmentation therapy. Am J Respir Crit Care Med 160:1468–1472

Dirksen A, Piitulainen E, Parr DG, Deng C, Wencker M, Shaker SB, Stockley RA (2009) Exploring the role of CT densitometry: a randomised study of augmentation therapy in alpha(1)-antitrypsin deficiency. Eur Respir J 33:1345–1353

Doellinger F, Bauman G, Roehmel J, Stahl M, Posch H, Steffen IG, Pusterla O, Bieri O, Wielputz MO, Mall

MA (2024) Contrast agent-free functional magnetic resonance imaging with matrix pencil decomposition to quantify abnormalities in lung perfusion and ventilation in patients with cystic fibrosis. Front Med (Lausanne) 11:1349466

Eda S, Kubo K, Fujimoto K, Matsuzawa Y, Sekiguchi M, Sakai F (1997) The relations between expiratory chest CT using helical CT and pulmonary function tests in emphysema. Am J Respir Crit Care Med 155:1290–1294

Ferri F, Bouzerar R, Auquier M, Vial J, Renard C (2022) Pulmonary emphysema quantification at low dose chest CT using deep learning image reconstruction. Eur J Radiol 152:110338

Fukuchi Y (2009) The aging lung and chronic obstructive pulmonary disease: similarity and difference. Proc Am Thorac Soc 6:570–572

Galban CJ, Han MK, Boes JL, Chughtai KA, Meyer CR, Johnson TD, Galban S, Rehemtulla A, Kazerooni EA, Martinez FJ, Ross BD (2012) Computed tomography-based biomarker provides unique signature for diagnosis of COPD phenotypes and disease progression. Nat Med 18:1711–1715

Galbán CJ, Boes JL, Bule M, Kitko CL, Couriel DR, Johnson TD, Lama V, Telenga ED, van den Berge M, Rehemtulla A, Kazerooni EA, Ponkowski MJ, Ross BD, Yanik GA (2014) Parametric response mapping as an indicator of bronchiolitis obliterans syndrome after hematopoietic stem cell transplantation. Biol Blood Marrow Transplant 20:1592–1598

Gevenois PA, Demaertelaer V, Devuyst P, Zanen J, Yernault JC (1995) Comparision of computed density and macroscopic morphometry in pulmonary emphysema. Am J Respir Crit Care Med 152:653–657

Gevenois PA, DeVuyst P, deMaertelaer V, Zanen J, Jacobvitz D, Cosio MG, Yernault JC (1996a) Comparison of computed density and microscopic morphometry in pulmonary emphysema. Am J Respir Crit Care Med 154:187–192

Gevenois PA, Scillia P, deMaertelaer V, Michils A, DeVuyst P, Yernault JC (1996b) The effects of age, sex, lung size, and hyperinflation on CT lung densitometry. AJR Am J Roentgenol 167:1169–1173

Gierada DS, Yusen RD, Pilgram TK, Crouch L, Slone RM, Bae KT, Lefrak SS, Cooper JD (2001) Repeatability of quantitative CT indexes of emphysema in patients evaluated for lung volume reduction surgery. Radiology 220:448–454

Gierada DS, Bierhals AJ, Choong CK, Bartel ST, Ritter JH, Das NA, Hong C, Pilgram TK, Bae KT, Whiting BR, Woods JC, Hogg JC, Lutey BA, Battafarano RJ, Cooper JD, Meyers BF, Patterson GA (2010) Effects of CT section thickness and reconstruction kernel on emphysema quantification relationship to the magnitude of the CT emphysema index. Acad Radiol 17:146–156

Gierada DS, Guniganti P, Newman BJ, Dransfield MT, Kvale PA, Lynch DA, Pilgram TK (2011) Quantitative CT assessment of emphysema and airways in relation to lung cancer risk. Radiology 261:950–959

Giuntini C, Camiciottoli G, Maluccio NM, Mariani L, Lavorini F, Pistolesi M (2007) Chronic effort dyspnea explained by lung function tests and by HRCT and CRX radiographic patterns in COPD: a post-hoc analysis in 51 patients. COPD 4:169–176

Goddard PR, Nicholson EM, Laszlo G, Watt I (1982) Computed tomography in pulmonary emphysema. Clin Radiol 33:379–387

Goris ML, Zhu HYJ, Blankenberg F, Chan F, Robinson TE (2003) An automated approach to quantitative air trapping measurements in mild cystic fibrosis. Chest 123:1655–1663

Gould GA, Macnee W, McLean A, Warren PM, Redpath A, Best JJK, Lamb D, Flenley DC (1988) CT measurements of lung density in life can quantitate distal airspace enlargement: an essential defining feature of human emphysema. Am Rev Respir Dis 137:380–392

Graafen D, Emrich T, Halfmann MC, Mildenberger P, Duber C, Yang Y, Othman AE, O'Doherty J, Muller L, Kloeckner R (2022) Dose reduction and image quality in photon-counting detector high-resolution computed tomography of the chest: routine clinical data. J Thorac Imaging 37:315–322

Guelsuen M, Ariyuerek OM, Coemert RB, Karabulut N (2006) Variability of the pulmonary oblique fissures presented by high-resolution computed tomography. Surg Radiol Anat 28:293–299

Gurney JW, Jones KK, Robbins RA, Gossman GL, Nelson KJ, Daughton D, Spurzem JR, Rennard SI (1992) Regional distribution of emphysema: correlation of high-resolution CT with pulmonary function tests in unselected smokers. Radiology 183:457–463

Haas M, Hamm B, Niehues SM (2014) Automated lung volumetry from routine thoracic CT scans: how reliable is the result? Acad Radiol 21:633–638

Hansell DM, Rubens MB, Padley SP, Wells AU (1997) Obliterative bronchiolitis: individual CT signs of small airways disease and functional correlation. Radiology 203:721–726

Hansell DM, Bankier AA, MacMahon H, McLoud TC, Muller NL, Remy J (2008) Fleischner Society: glossary of terms for thoracic imaging. Radiology 246:697–722

Hatt CR, Fernandez-Baldera A, Hoffman EA, Martinez FJ, Galban CJ, Han MK, Investigators S (2017) Reproducibility of parametric response mapping at 30 days. Am J Respir Crit Care Med 195:2

Hayhurst MD, Flenley DC, McLean A, Wightman AJA, Macnee W, Wright D, Lamb D, Best J (1984) Diagnosis of pulmonary emphysema by computerized tomography. Lancet 2:320–322

Heussel CP, Achenbach T, Buschsieweke C, Kuhnigk J, Weinheimer O, Hammer G, Duber C, Kauczor HU (2006) Quantification of pulmonary emphysema in multislice-CT using different software tools. Rofo-Fortschritte Auf Dem Gebiet Der Rontgenstrahlen Und Der Bildgebenden Verfahren 178:987–998

Heussel CP, Herth FJF, Kappes J, Hantusch R, Hartlieb S, Weinheimer O, Kauczor HU, Eberhardt R (2009)

Fully automatic quantitative assessment of emphysema in computed tomography: comparison with pulmonary function testing and normal values. Eur Radiol 19:2391–2402
Hochhegger B, Irion KL, Marchiori E, Moreira JS (2010) Reconstruction algorithms and their influence in emphysema CT measurements. Acad Radiol 17:674–674
Hochhegger B, Irion KL, Marchiori E, Moreira JS (2011) Reconstruction algorithms influence the follow-up variability in the longitudinal CT emphysema index measurements. Korean J Radiol 12:169–175
Hu SY, Hoffman EA, Reinhardt JM (2001) Automatic lung segmentation for accurate quantitation of volumetric X-ray CT images. IEEE Trans Med Imaging 20:490–498
Hu GP, Zhou YM, Tian J, Yao WM, Li JG, Li B, Ran PX (2010) Risk of COPD from exposure to biomass smoke a meta-analysis. Chest 138:20–31
Irion KL, Marchiori E, Hochhegger B, da Silva Porto N, da Silva Moreira J, Anselmi CE, Holemans JA, Irion PO (2009) CT quantification of emphysema in young subjects with no recognizable chest disease. AJR Am J Roentgenol 192:W90–W96
Iwano S, Okada T, Satake H, Naganawa S (2009) 3D-CT volumetry of the lung using multidetector row CT: comparison with pulmonary function tests. Acad Radiol 16:250–256
Jang YM, Oh YM, Seo JB, Kim N, Chae EJ, Lee YK, Lee SD (2008) Quantitatively assessed dynamic contrast-enhanced magnetic resonance imaging in patients with chronic obstructive pulmonary disease: correlation of perfusion parameters with pulmonary function test and quantitative computed tomography. Investig Radiol 43:403–410
Johnson KM, Fain SB, Schiebler ML, Nagle S (2013) Optimized 3D ultrashort echo time pulmonary MRI. Magn Reson Med 70:1241–1250
Kaireit TF, Kern A, Voskrebenzev A, Pohler GH, Klimes F, Behrendt L, Gutberlet M, Moher-Alsady T, Dittrich AM, Wacker F, Hohlfeld J, Vogel-Claussen J (2021) Flow volume loop and regional ventilation assessment using phase-resolved functional lung (PREFUL) MRI: comparison with (129) xenon ventilation MRI and lung function testing. J Magn Reson Imaging 53:1092–1105
Karimi R, Tornling G, Forsslund H, Mikko M, Wheelock ÅM, Nyrén S, Sköld CM (2014) Lung density on high resolution computer tomography (HRCT) reflects degree of inflammation in smokers. Respir Res 15:23
Kauczor HU, Wolcke B, Fischer B, Mildenberger P, Lorenz J, Thelen M (1996) Three-dimensional helical CT of the tracheobronchial tree: evaluation of imaging protocols and assessment of suspected stenoses with bronchoscopic correlation. AJR Am J Roentgenol 167:419–424
Kauczor HU, Heussel CP, Fischer B, Klamm R, Mildenberger P, Thelen M (1998) Assessment of lung volumes using helical CT at inspiration and expiration: comparison with pulmonary function tests. AJR Am J Roentgenol 171:1091–1095
Kay FU, Oz OK, Abbara S, Mortani Barbosa EJ Jr, Agarwal PP, Rajiah P (2019) Translation of quantitative imaging biomarkers into clinical chest CT. Radiographics 39:957–976
Kim WD, Eidelman DH, Izquierdo JL, Ghezzo H, Saetta MP, Cosio MG (1991) Centrilobular and panlobular emphysema in smokers. Two distinct morphologic and functional entities. Am Rev Respir Dis 144:1385–1390
Kinsella M, Muller NL, Abboud RT, Morrison NJ, Dybuncio A (1990) Quantification of emphysema by computed tomography using a density mask program and correlation with pulmonary function tests. Chest 97:315–321
Klimes F, Voskrebenzev A, Wacker F, Vogel-Claussen J (2024) Three-dimensional phase resolved functional lung magnetic resonance imaging. J Vis Exp. https://doi.org/10.3791/66385
Kong X, Sheng HX, Lu GM, Meinel FG, Dyer KT, Schoepf UJ, Zhang LJ (2014) Xenon-enhanced dual-energy CT lung ventilation imaging: techniques and clinical applications. AJR Am J Roentgenol 202:309–317
Koyama H, Ohno Y, Yamazaki Y, Nogami M, Murase K, Onishi Y, Matsumoto K, Takenaka D, Sugimura K (2010) Quantitative and qualitative assessments of lung destruction and pulmonary functional loss from reduced-dose thin-section CT in pulmonary emphysema patients. Acad Radiol 17:163–168
Kubo K, Eda S, Yamamoto H, Fujimoto K, Matsuzawa Y, Maruyama Y, Hasegawa M, Sone S, Sakai F (1999) Expiratory and inspiratory chest computed tomography and pulmonary function tests in cigarette smokers. Eur Respir J 13:252–256
Kumar V, Cohen JT, van Klaveren D, Soeteman DI, Wong JB, Neumann PJ, Kent DM (2018) Risk-targeted lung cancer screening: a cost-effectiveness analysis. Ann Intern Med 168:161
Labaki WW, Kimmig LM, Mutlu GM, Han MK, Bhatt SP (2019) Update in chronic obstructive pulmonary disease 2018. Am J Respir Crit Care Med 199:1462–1470
Lassen B, van Rikxoort EM, Schmidt M, Kerkstra S, van Ginneken B, Kuhnigk J-M (2013) Automatic segmentation of the pulmonary lobes from chest CT scans based on fissures, vessels, and bronchi. IEEE Trans Med Imaging 32:210–222
Lee KW, Chung SY, Yang I, Lee Y, Ko EY, Park MJ (2000) Correlation of aging and smoking with air trapping at thin-section CT of the lung in asymptomatic subjects. Radiology 214:831–836
Lee YK, Oh YM, Lee JH, Kim EK, Lee JH, Kim N, Seo JB, Do Lee S, Grp KS (2008) Quantitative assessment of emphysema, air trapping, and airway thickening on computed tomography. Lung 186:157–165
Lee SM, Seo JB, Hwang HJ, Kim EY, Oh SY, Kim JE (2013) Thoracic magnetic resonance imaging for the evaluation of pulmonary emphysema. J Thorac Imaging 28:160–170
Lee SM, Seo JB, Hwang HJ, Kim N, Oh SY, Lee JS, Lee SW, Oh YM, Kim TH (2017) Assessment of regional

emphysema, air-trapping and Xenon-ventilation using dual-energy computed tomography in chronic obstructive pulmonary disease patients. Eur Radiol 27:2818–2827

Leung AN, Fisher K, Valentine V, Girgis RE, Berry GJ, Robbins RC, Theodore J (1998) Bronchiolitis obliterans after lung transplantation—detection using expiratory HRCT. Chest 113:365–370

Ley S, Zaporozhan J, Morbach A, Eberle B, Gast KK, Heussel CP, Biedermann A, Mayer E, Schmiedeskamp J, Stepniak A, Schreiber WG, Kauczor HU (2004) Functional evaluation of emphysema using diffusion-weighted (3)Helium-magnetic resonance imaging, high-resolution computed tomography, and lung function tests. Investig Radiol 39:427–434

Ley-Zaporozhan J, Ley S, Eberhardt R, Weinheimer O, Fink C, Puderbach M, Eichinger M, Herth F, Kauczor HU (2007) Assessment of the relationship between lung parenchymal destruction and impaired pulmonary perfusion on a lobar level in patients with emphysema. Eur J Radiol 63:76–83

Lim HJ, Weinheimer O, Wielputz MO, Dinkel J, Hielscher T, Gompelmann D, Kauczor HU, Heussel CP (2016) Fully automated pulmonary lobar segmentation: influence of different prototype software programs onto quantitative evaluation of chronic obstructive lung disease. PLoS One 11:15

Litmanovich DE, Hartwick K, Silva M, Bankier AA (2014) Multidetector computed tomographic imaging in chronic obstructive pulmonary disease: emphysema and airways assessment. Radiol Clin North Am 52:137–154

Lynch DA, Austin JH, Hogg JC, Grenier PA, Kauczor HU, Bankier AA, Barr RG, Colby TV, Galvin JR, Gevenois PA, Coxson HO, Hoffman EA, Newell JD Jr, Pistolesi M, Silverman EK, Crapo JD (2015) CT-definable subtypes of chronic obstructive pulmonary disease: a statement of the Fleischner Society. Radiology 277:192–205

Lynch DA, Moore CM, Wilson C, Nevrekar D, Jennermann T, Humphries SM, Austin JHM, Grenier PA, Kauczor HU, Han MLK, Regan EA, Make BJ, Bowler RR, Beaty TH, Curran-Everett D, Hokanson JE, Curtis JL, Silverman EK, Crapo JD, Genetic Epidemiology CC (2018) CT-based visual classification of emphysema: association with mortality in the COPDGene Study. Radiology 288:859–866

Madani A, Zanen J, de Maertelaer V, Gevenois PA (2006) Pulmonary emphysema: objective quantification at mufti-detector row CT—comparison with macroscopic and microscopic morphometry. Radiology 238:1036–1043

Madani A, De Maertelaer V, Zanen J, Gevenois PA (2007) Pulmonary emphysema: radiation dose and section thickness at multidetector CT quantification—comparison with macroscopic and microscopic morphometry. Radiology 243:250–257

Madani A, Van Muylem A, de Maertelaer V, Zanen J, Gevenois PA (2008) Pulmonary emphysema: size distribution of emphysematous spaces on multidetector CT images—comparison with macroscopic and microscopic morphometry. Radiology 248:1036–1041

Madani A, Van Muylem A, Gevenois PA (2010) Pulmonary emphysema: effect of lung volume on objective quantification at thin-section CT. Radiology 257:260–268

Mansoor A, Bagci U, Foster B, Xu ZY, Papadakis GZ, Folio LR, Udupa JK, Mollura DJ (2015) Segmentation and image analysis of abnormal lungs at CT: current approaches, challenges, and future trends. Radiographics 35:1056–1076

Martin SP, Gariani J, Hachulla AL, Botsikas D, Adler D, Karenovics W, Becker CD, Montet X (2017) Impact of iterative reconstructions on objective and subjective emphysema assessment with computed tomography: a prospective study. Eur Radiol 27:2950–2956

Martinez CH, Diaz AA, Meldrum C, Curtis JL, Cooper CB, Pirozzi C, Kanner RE, Paine R 3rd, Woodruff PG, Bleecker ER, Hansel NN, Barr RG, Marchetti N, Criner GJ, Kazerooni EA, Hoffman EA, Ross BD, Galban CJ, Cigolle CT, Martinez FJ, Han MK (2017) Age and small airway imaging abnormalities in subjects with and without airflow obstruction in SPIROMICS. Am J Respir Crit Care Med 195:464–472

Mascalchi M, Diciotti S, Sverzellati N, Camiciottoli G, Ciccotosto C, Falaschi F, Zompatori M (2012) Low agreement of visual rating for detailed quantification of pulmonary emphysema in whole-lung CT. Acta Radiol 53:53

Mastora I, Remy-Jardin M, Sobaszek A, Boulenguez C, Remy J, Edme JL (2001) Thin-section CT finding in 250 volunteers: assessment of the relationship of CT findings with smoking history and pulmonary function test results. Radiology 218:695–702

Matsumoto AJ, Bartholmai BJ, Wylam ME (2017) Comparison of total lung capacity determined by plethysmography with computed tomographic segmentation using CALIPER. J Thorac Imaging 32:101–106

Matsuoka S, Kurihara Y, Yagihashi K, Nakajima Y (2007) Quantitative assessment of peripheral airway obstruction on paired expiratory/inspiratory thin-section computed tomography in chronic obstructive pulmonary disease with emphysema. J Comput Assist Tomogr 31:384–389

Matsuoka S, Kurihara Y, Yagihashi K, Hoshino M, Watanabe N, Nakajima Y (2008) Quantitative assessment of air trapping in chronic obstructive pulmonary disease using inspiratory and expiratory volumetric MDCT. AJR Am J Roentgenol 190:762–769

McCollough CH, Yu LF, Kofler JM, Leng S, Zhang Y, Li ZB, Carter RE (2015) Degradation of CT low-contrast spatial resolution due to the use of iterative reconstruction and reduced dose levels. Radiology 276:499–506

McNulty W, Usmani OS (2014) Techniques of assessing small airways dysfunction. Eur Clin Respir J 1. https://doi.org/10.3402/ecrj.v1.25898

Mets OM, Willemink MJ, de Kort FPL, Mol CP, Leiner T, Oudkerk M, Prokop M, de Jong PA (2012a) The effect of iterative reconstruction on computed tomography

assessment of emphysema, air trapping and airway dimensions. Eur Radiol 22:2103–2109
Mets OM, van Hulst RA, Jacobs C, van Ginneken B, de Jong PA (2012b) Normal range of emphysema and air trapping on CT in young men. AJR Am J Roentgenol 199:336–340
Mets OM, Zanen P, Lammers JW, Isgum I, Gietema HA, van Ginneken B, Prokop M, de Jong PA (2012c) Early identification of small airways disease on lung cancer screening CT: comparison of current air trapping measures. Lung 190:629–633
Mets OM, Isgum I, Mol CP, Gietema HA, Zanen P, Prokop M, de Jong PA (2012d) Variation in quantitative CT air trapping in heavy smokers on repeat CT examinations. Eur Radiol 22:2710–2717
Mets OM, de Jong PA, van Ginneken B, Kruitwagen CL, Prokop M, Oudkerk M, Lammers JW, Zanen P (2013) CT air trapping is independently associated with lung function reduction over time. PLoS One 8:e61783
Miniati M, Filippi E, Falaschi F, Carrozzi L, Milne EN, Sostman HD, Pistolesi M (1995) Radiologic evaluation of emphysema in patients with chronic obstructive pulmonary disease. Chest radiography versus high resolution computed tomography. Am J Respir Crit Care Med 151:1359–1367
Miniati M, Monti S, Stolk J, Mirarchi G, Falaschi F, Rabinovich R, Canapini C, Roca J, Rabe KF (2008) Value of chest radiography in phenotyping chronic obstructive pulmonary disease. Eur Respir J 31:509–515
Mohamed Hoesein FA, de Hoop B, Zanen P, Gietema H, Kruitwagen CL, van Ginneken B, Isgum I, Mol C, van Klaveren RJ, Dijkstra AE, Groen HJ, Boezen HM, Postma DS, Prokop M, Lammers JW (2011) CT-quantified emphysema in male heavy smokers: association with lung function decline. Thorax 66:782–787
Molinari F, Amato M, Stefanetti M, Parapatt G, Macagnino A, Serricchio G, Pirronti T, Bonomo L (2010) Density-based MDCT quantification of lobar lung volumes: a study of inter- and intraobserver reproducibility. Radiol Med 115:516–525
Molinari F, Pirronti T, Sverzellati N, Diciotti S, Amato M, Paolantonio G, Gentile L, Parapatt GK, D'Argento F, Kuhnigk J-M (2013) Intra- and interoperator variability of lobar pulmonary volumes and emphysema scores in patients with chronic obstructive pulmonary disease and emphysema: comparison of manual and semi-automated segmentation techniques. Diagn Interv Radiol 19:279–285
Muller NL, Staples CA, Miller RR, Abboud RT (1988) Density mask: an objective method to quantitate emphysema using computed tomography. Chest 94:782–787
Nemec SF, Molinari F, Dufresne V, Gosset N, Silva M, Bankier AA (2015) Comparison of four software packages for CT lung volumetry in healthy individuals. Eur Radiol 25:1588–1597
Newman KB, Lynch DA, Newman LS, Ellegood D, Newell JD (1994) Quantitative computed-tomography detects air trapping due to asthma. Chest 106:105–109
O'Donnell CR, Bankier AA, Stiebellehner L, Reilly JJ, Brown R, Loring SH (2010) Comparison among different methods on measurement of total lung capacity in COPD response. Chest 138:459–460
Ohno Y, Chen Q, Hatabu H (2001a) Oxygen-enhanced magnetic resonance ventilation imaging of lung. Eur J Radiol 37:164–171
Ohno Y, Hatabu H, Takenaka D, Adachi S, Van Cauteren M, Sugimura K (2001b) Oxygen-enhanced MR ventilation imaging of the lung: preliminary clinical experience in 25 subjects. AJR Am J Roentgenol 177:185–194
Ohno Y, Hatabu H, Takenaka D, Van Cauteren M, Fujii M, Sugimura K (2002) Dynamic oxygen-enhanced MRI reflects diffusing capacity of the lung. Magn Reson Med 47:1139–1144
Ohno Y, Koyama H, Yoshikawa T, Matsumoto K, Takahashi M, Van Cauteren M, Sugimura K (2011) T2*measurements of 3-T MRI with ultrashort TEs: capabilities of pulmonary function assessment and clinical stage classification in smokers. AJR Am J Roentgenol 197:W279–W285
Palagyi K, Tschirren J, Hoffman EA, Sonka M (2006) Quantitative analysis of pulmonary airway tree structures. Comput Biol Med 36:974–996
Parr DG, Stoel BC, Stolk J, Nightingale PG, Stockley RA (2004) Influence of calibration on densitometric studies of emphysema progression using computed tomography. Am J Respir Crit Care Med 170:883–890
Parr DG, Stoel BC, Stolk J, Stockley RA (2006) Validation of computed tomographic lung densitometry for monitoring emphysema in alpha1-antitrypsin deficiency. Thorax 61:485–490
Pierce RJ, Brown DJ, Holmes M, Cumming G, Denison DM (1979) Estimation of lung volumes from chest radiographs using shape information. Thorax 34:726–734
Quantitative Imaging Biomarkers Alliance (2019) QIBA profile: computed tomography: lung densitometry
Regan EA, Hokanson JE, Murphy JR, Make B, Lynch DA, Beaty TH, Curran-Everett D, Silverman EK, Crapo JD (2010) Genetic epidemiology of COPD (COPDGene) study design. COPD 7:32–43
Revel M-P, Faivre J-B, Remy-Jardin M, Deken V, Duhamel A, Marquette C-H, Tacelli N, Bakai A-M, Remy J (2008) Automated lobar quantification of emphysema in patients with severe COPD. Eur Radiol 18:2723–2730
Rodenstein DO, Sopwith T, Denison DM, Stanescu DC (1985) Reevaluation of the radiographic method for measurement of total lung capacity. Bull Eur Physiopathol Respir 21:521–525
Ruppel GL (2012) What is the clinical value of lung volumes? Respir Care 57:26–38
Salerno M, de Lange EE, Altes TA, Truwit JD, Brookeman JR, Mugler JP 3rd. (2002) Emphysema: hyperpolarized helium 3 diffusion MR imaging of the lungs com-

pared with spirometric indexes—initial experience. Radiology 222:252–260
Schlesinger AE, White DK, Mallory GB, Hildeboldt CF, Huddleston CB (1995) Estimation of total lung capacity from chest radiography and chest CT in children: comparison with body plethysmography. AJR Am J Roentgenol 165:151–154
Schroeder JD, McKenzie AS, Zach JA, Wilson CG, Curran-Everett D, Stinson DS, Newell JD Jr, Lynch DA (2013) Relationships between airflow obstruction and quantitative CT measurements of emphysema, air trapping, and airways in subjects with and without chronic obstructive pulmonary disease. AJR Am J Roentgenol 201:W460–W470
Sciurba FC, Ernst A, Herth FJ, Strange C, Criner GJ, Marquette CH, Kovitz KL, Chiacchierini RP, Goldin J, McLennan G (2010) A randomized study of endobronchial valves for advanced emphysema. N Engl J Med 363:1233–1244
Shaker SB, Dirksen A, Ulrik CS, Hestad M, Stavngaard T, Laursen LC, Maltbaek N, Clementsen P, Skjaerbaek N, Nielsen L, Stoel B, Skovgaard LT, Tonnesen P (2009) The effect of inhaled corticosteroids on the development of emphysema in smokers assessed by annual computed tomography. COPD 6:104–111
Shaker SB, Stavngaard T, Laursen LC, Stoel BC, Dirksen A (2011) Rapid fall in lung density following smoking cessation in COPD. COPD 8:2–7
Shin JM, Kim TH, Haam S, Han K, Byun MK, Chang YS, Kim HJ, Park CH (2017) The repeatability of computed tomography lung volume measurements: comparisons in healthy subjects, patients with obstructive lung disease, and patients with restrictive lung disease. PLoS One 12:e0182849
Sieren JP, Newell JD Jr, Barr RG, Bleecker ER, Burnette N, Carretta EE, Couper D, Goldin J, Guo J, Han MK, Hansel NN, Kanner RE, Kazerooni EA, Martinez FJ, Rennard S, Woodruff PG, Hoffman EA (2016) SPIROMICS protocol for multicenter quantitative computed tomography to phenotype the lungs. Am J Respir Crit Care Med 194:794–806
Silva M, Nemec SF, Dufresne V, Occhipinti M, Heidinger BH, Chamberlain R, Bankier AA (2016) Normal spectrum of pulmonary parametric response map to differentiate lung collapsibility: distribution of densitometric classifications in healthy adult volunteers. Eur Radiol 26:3063–3070
Smith BM, Austin JHM, Newell JD Jr, D'Souza BM, Rozenshtein A, Hoffman EA, Ahmed F, Barr RG (2014) Pulmonary emphysema subtypes on computed tomography: the MESA COPD study. Am J Med 127:94.e7–94.23
Snider GL, Kleinerman JL, Thurlbeck WM, Bengali ZH (1985) The definition of emphysema—report of a National-Heart-Lung-and-Blood-Institute, Division of Lung-Diseases workshop. Am Rev Respir Dis 132:182–185
Staring M, Bakker ME, Stolk J, Shamonin DP, Reiber JHC, Stoel BC (2014) Towards local progression estimation of pulmonary emphysema using CT. Med Phys 41:13
Stavngaard T, Shaker SB, Bach KS, Stoel BC, Dirksen A (2006) Quantitative assessment of regional emphysema distribution in patients with chronic obstructive pulmonary disease (COPD). Acta Radiol 47:914–921
Stern EJ, Frank MS (1994) CT of the lung in patients with pulmonary emphysema: diagnosis, quantification, and correlation with pathological and physiological findings. AJR Am J Roentgenol 162:791–798
Stoel BC, Putter H, Bakker ME, Dirksen A, Stockley RA, Piitulainen E, Russi EW, Parr D, Shaker SB, Reiber JH, Stolk J (2008) Volume correction in computed tomography densitometry for follow-up studies on pulmonary emphysema. Proc Am Thorac Soc 5:919–924
Sugino K, Kobayashi M, Nakamura Y, Gocho K, Ishida F, Isobe K, Shiraga N, Homma S (2017) Xenon-enhanced dual-energy CT imaging in combined pulmonary fibrosis and emphysema. PLoS One 12:e0170289
Sverzellati N, Randi G, Spagnolo P, Marchiano A, Silva M, Kuhnigk JM, La Vecchia C, Zompatori M, Pastorino U (2013) Increased mean lung density: another independent predictor of lung cancer? Eur J Radiol 82:1325–1331
Takahashi M, Fukuoka J, Nitta N, Takazakura R, Nagatani Y, Murakami Y, Otani H, Murata K (2008) Imaging of pulmonary emphysema: a pictorial review. Int J Chron Obstruct Pulmon Dis 3:193–204
Tanaka N, Matsumoto T, Miura G, Emoto T, Matsunaga N, Ueda K, Lynch DA (2003) Air trapping at CT: high prevalence in asymptomatic subjects with normal pulmonary function. Radiology 227:776–785
Tenda ED, Ridge CA, Shen ML, Yang GZ, Shah PL (2019) Role of quantitative computed tomographic scan analysis in lung volume reduction for emphysema. Respiration 98:86–94
Thurlbeck WM, Muller NL (1994) Emphysema: definition, imaging and quantification. AJR Am J Roentgenol 163:1017–1025
Togao O, Tsuji R, Ohno Y, Dimitrov I, Takahashi M (2010) Ultrashort Echo Time (UTE) MRI of the lung: assessment of tissue density in the lung parenchyma. Magn Reson Med 64:1491–1498
Tschirren J, Hoffman EA, McLennan G, Sonka M (2005) Intrathoracic airway trees: segmentation and airway morphology analysis from low-dose CT scans. IEEE Trans Med Imaging 24:1529–1539
Tseng HJ, Henry TS, Veeraraghavan S, Mittal PK, Little BP (2017) Pulmonary function tests for the radiologist. Radiographics 37:1037–1058
Vegas Sanchez-Ferrero G, Diaz AA, Ash SY, Baraghoshi D, Strand M, Crapo JD, Silverman EK, Humphries SM, Washko GR, Lynch DA, San Jose Estepar R (2024) Quantification of emphysema progression at CT using simultaneous volume, noise, and bias lung density correction. Radiology 310:e231632
Vehar S, Kirupaharan P, Yadav R, Mazzone PJ, Choi H (2019) The association between emphysema detected

by lung density analysis and healthcare utilization in patients undergoing lung cancer screening. In: A24 COPD: therapy, imaging, and molecular markers. American Thoracic Society, p A1123

Vilke GM, Chan TC, Neuman T, Clausen JL (2000) Spirometry in normal subjects in sitting, prone, and supine positions. Respir Care 45:407–410

Walsdorff M, Van Muylem A, Gevenois PA (2016) Effect of total lung capacity and gender on CT densitometry indexes. Br J Radiol 89:20150631

Wandtke JC, Hyde RW, Fahey PJ, Utell MJ, Plewes DB, Goske MJ, Fischer HW (1986) Measurement of lung gas volume and regional density by computed tomography in dogs. Investig Radiol 21:108–117

Wang Z, Gu S, Leader JK, Kundu S, Tedrow JR, Sciurba FC, Gur D, Siegfried JM, Pu J (2013) Optimal threshold in CT quantification of emphysema. Eur Radiol 23:975–984

Wanger J, Clausen JL, Coates A, Pedersen OF, Brusasco V, Burgos F, Casaburi R, Crapo R, Enright P, van der Grinten CPM, Gustafsson P, Hankinson J, Jensen R, Johnson D, MacIntyre N, McKay R, Miller MR, Navajas D, Pellegrino R, Viegi G (2005) Standardisation of the measurement of lung volumes. Eur Respir J 26:511–522

Webb WR, Stern EJ, Kanth N, Gamsu G (1993) Dynamic pulmonary CT—findings in healthy adult men. Radiology 186:117–124

Wielputz MO, Eichinger M, Weinheimer O, Ley S, Mall MA, Wiebel M, Bischoff A, Kauczor HU, Heussel CP, Puderbach M (2013) Automatic airway analysis on multidetector computed tomography in cystic fibrosis: correlation with pulmonary function testing. J Thorac Imaging 28:104–113

Wielputz MO, Bardarova D, Weinheimer O, Kauczor HU, Eichinger M, Jobst BJ, Eberhardt R, Koenigkam-Santos M, Puderbach M, Heussel CP (2014) Variation of densitometry on computed tomography in COPD—influence of different software tools. PLoS One 9:e112898

Wille MM, Thomsen LH, Dirksen A, Petersen J, Pedersen JH, Shaker SB (2014) Emphysema progression is visually detectable in low-dose CT in continuous but not in former smokers. Eur Radiol 24:2692–2699

Wright JL, Churg A (2006) Advances in the pathology of COPD. Histopathology 49:1–9

Yamada Y, Yamada M, Chubachi S, Yokoyama Y, Matsuoka S, Tanabe A, Niijima Y, Murata M, Fukunaga K, Jinzaki M (2020) Comparison of inspiratory and expiratory lung and lobe volumes among supine, standing, and sitting positions using conventional and upright CT. Sci Rep 10:16203

Zach JA, Newell JD, Schroeder J, Murphy JR, Curran-Everett D, Hoffman EA, Westgate PM, Han MLK, Silverman EK, Crapo JD, Lynch DA, Investigators CO (2012) Quantitative computed tomography of the lungs and airways in healthy nonsmoking adults. Investig Radiol 47:596–602

Zaporozhan J, Ley S, Weinheimer O, Eberhardt R, Tsakiris I, Noshi Y, Herth F, Kauczor H-U (2006) Multi-detector CT of the chest: influence of dose onto quantitative evaluation of severe emphysema: a simulation study. J Comput Assist Tomogr 30:460–468

Zhang Z, Ren J, Tao X, Tang W, Zhao S, Zhou L, Huang Y, Wang J, Wu N (2021) Automatic segmentation of pulmonary lobes on low-dose computed tomography using deep learning. Ann Transl Med 9:291

Infiltrative Lung Disease

A. L. Brun and P. Y. Brillet

Contents

Abstract

Interstitial lung diseases (ILDs) encompass a large group of diseases with great variability in clinical severity and behavior. If computed tomography (CT) plays a key role in the detection and characterization of ILD, visual CT analysis is subjective and prone to inter- and intraobserver variability. Measurements in ILD may seem unrealistic as the disease may be diffuse, heterogeneous, and characterized by complex and sometimes subtle patterns. However, there has been growing interest in the recent years for the development of quantitative imaging biomarkers that could help the radiologist tracking disease progression and response to treatment.

This chapter will review the reasons why measurements in ILD are important, and the tools available for the radiologists, to address directly or indirectly the extent and severity of the disease.

Abbreviations

AI	Artificial intelligence
AMFM	Adaptive multiple feature method
CALIPER	Computer-Aided Lung Informatics for Pathology Evaluation and Rating
CNN	Convolutional neural network

A. L. Brun (✉)
Imaging Department, Foch Hospital, Suresnes, France
e-mail: al.brun@hopital-foch.com

P. Y. Brillet
Imaging Department, Avicenne Hospital, AP-HP, Bobigny, France

Med Radiol Diagn Imaging (2026)
https://doi.org/10.1007/174_2025_585,
Published Online: 28 May 2025

COVID-19	Coronavirus disease of 2019
DTA	Data-driven textural analysis
FVC	Forced vital capacity
GGO	Ground-glass opacities
GGR	GGO + reticulation
HAA	High attenuation areas
HP	Hypersensitivity pneumonitis
HRCT	High-resolution computed tomography
HU	Hounsfield Units
ILA	Interstitial lung abnormalities
ILD	Interstitial lung disease
IPF	Idiopathic pulmonary fibrosis
MDA-5	Melanoma differentiation-associated gene 5
mIP	Minimal intensity projection
MLD	Mean lung density
PVV	Pulmonary vessel volume
QCT	Quantitative CT
ROI	Regions of interest
TB	Traction bronchiectasis
TLC	Total lung capacity
UIP	Usual interstitial pneumonia

1 Introduction: Why

High-resolution computed tomography (HRCT) plays a key role in the diagnosis and assessment of interstitial lung diseases (ILDs). Computed tomography (CT) analysis in clinical practice is essentially qualitative, but data are increasingly being used to stage and quantify interstitial lesions.

The definition of interstitial lung abnormalities (ILAs) specifies a threshold of at least 5% of any lung zone to consider the diagnosis (Hatabu et al. 2020). An ILD extent of 10% is the most common cut-off threshold for inclusion in large clinical trials (Flaherty et al. 2019; Maher et al. 2020). Although arbitrary, these figures are meant to exclude minimal opacities and to conform to previous published literature.

Staging the severity of disease is also recognized as important to patients, as the extent of fibrosis on CT has been consistently linked to a worse prognosis, in idiopathic pulmonary fibrosis (IPF) (Lynch et al. 2005; Edey et al. 2011; Mogulkoc et al. 2001; Gay et al. 1998; Sumikawa et al. 2008), and other ILDs (Walsh et al. 2014; Ito et al. 2019).

In systemic sclerosis-associated ILD, Goh et al. developed a simple staging system for prediction of survival. Patients were categorized as having limited or extensive disease based on the extent of any features of ILD seen on HRCT (clearly <10% or clearly >30%, respectively), together with forced vital capacity (FVC) percent predicted in patients. For clinical practice, the optimal extent threshold was 20% ILD on HRCT and 70% of predicted values for FVC (Goh et al. 2008). Jacob et al. used the same composite staging system in rheumatoid arthritis associated ILD with a threshold of 25% to define the poor-outcome group (Jacob et al. 2019). In a study combining CT scoring and the GAP (gender, age, physiology) model in IPF patients, the worst prognosis was associated with more than 30% fibrosis (Ley et al. 2014).

Finally, tracking disease progression and response to therapy has become more and more important with the concept of progressive fibrosing ILD (George et al. 2020) and newly developed drug therapies. Criteria of disease progression as defined in the INBUILD trial include any increased (non-quantified) extent of fibrosis on chest HRCT, associated with relative 5–10% FVC decline or worsening respiratory symptoms (Flaherty et al. 2017, 2019). Visual assessment of disease extent and severity lacks sensitivity and is prone to inter- and intraobserver variability (Lynch et al. 2005). Computer-based methods for quantifying disease on HRCT (quantitative CT—QCT) can help solving these issues, by objectively assessing more subtle changes in nature or extent of disease. New emerging QCT tools can provide sensitive, objective, and reproducible measurement of disease extent and change over time (Wu et al. 2019). There is growing interest in the potential role of serial QCT as an effectiveness endpoint in clinical trials (Hansell et al. 2015).

2 How

2.1 Semiquantitative Visual Analysis

There is currently no standard method for scoring radiological extent or severity of ILD. Over the past two decades, multiple scoring methods have been used to characterize and quantify the disease, correlate with functional and clinical parameters, and assess disease progression and response to treatment. Most of these scoring systems combine an extent score and a texture (coarseness) score.

Semiquantitative visual estimation of the extent of disease can be reported literally by terms such as mild, moderate, and severe, or based on the total number of lobes or segments involved, or presented as an estimate of the percentage of lung affected (to the nearest 25%, 10%, or 5%). Rather than trying to display the total lung volume in 3D, it may be easier to work by sampling the levels of analysis (selected anatomical sections, lobes, and regions) (Fig. 1).

For textural score, different patterns associated with increasingly severe coarseness are being given increasingly high scores (ground-glass opacities (GGOs), reticulations, and honeycombing) (Assayag et al. 2012). Indeed, as the disease progresses, GGOs get being replaced with coarser interstitial reticulations associated with traction bronchiectasis and bronchiolectasis. Honeycombing also develops with time replacing reticulations and increasing number and size of cysts.

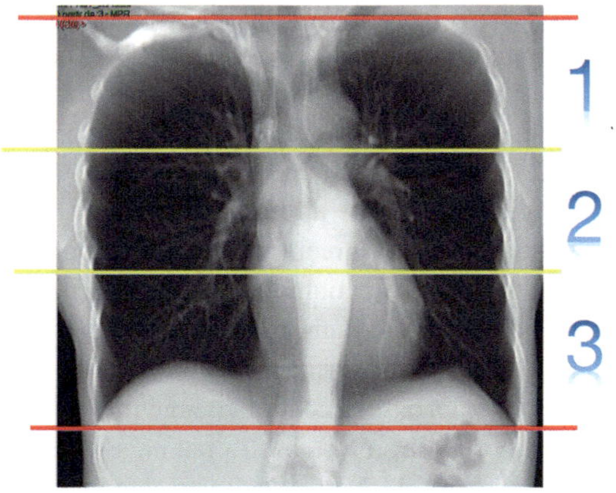

Fig. 1 Example of lung sampling for semiquantitative estimation of ILD. The lungs are divided in upper, mid, and lower zones based on the anatomical levels of the carina and inferior pulmonary veins. The extent of ILD can be estimated for each zone from 0% to 100% to the nearest 5%, 10%, or 25%. Total extent of fibrosis is obtained by the average of the 3 values

Most of these semiquantitative scoring systems are susceptible to observer bias, inter-reader, and intra-reader variability (Assayag et al. 2012). Furthermore, they may be too insensitive to display clinically relevant short-term changes (Flaherty et al. 2003a).

In contrast, QCT-derived measurements have outperformed visual CT assessment in predicting outcome in IPF and other fibrosing ILD (Jacob et al. 2016a, 2017a, b).

2.2 Technical Considerations

Measuring ILD on HRCT scans requires good and reproducible technical conditions. Volumetric acquisition with contiguous/overlapped thin sections is essential. For image reconstruction, a relatively "soft" kernel may be preferred to avoid excessive noise despite a lowering of the spatial resolution. Attention will be given to the position of the patient in case of isolated posterobasal opacities, as they can be related to gravitational changes. Additional prone imaging can be necessary to confirm or exclude limited / early interstitial changes in the dependent areas.

The quality of inspiration must be checked: sensibilizing and coaching the patient before the examination is crucial to get the maximal depth of inspiration. Radiologists should be aware that the injection of iodine contrast may be responsible for a slight increase in lung density, which may lead to false positive GGO. In clinical practice, the radiation dose can be relatively low, and dose modulation can be used. "Ultra-low dose" CT scans (<1 mSv) are however not recommended as they are responsible for increasing noise and loss of information (Fig. 2). For longitudinal follow-up, it is important to compare CT scans that are similar in terms of acquisition parameters including radiation dose, position, and depth of inspiration at all timepoints.

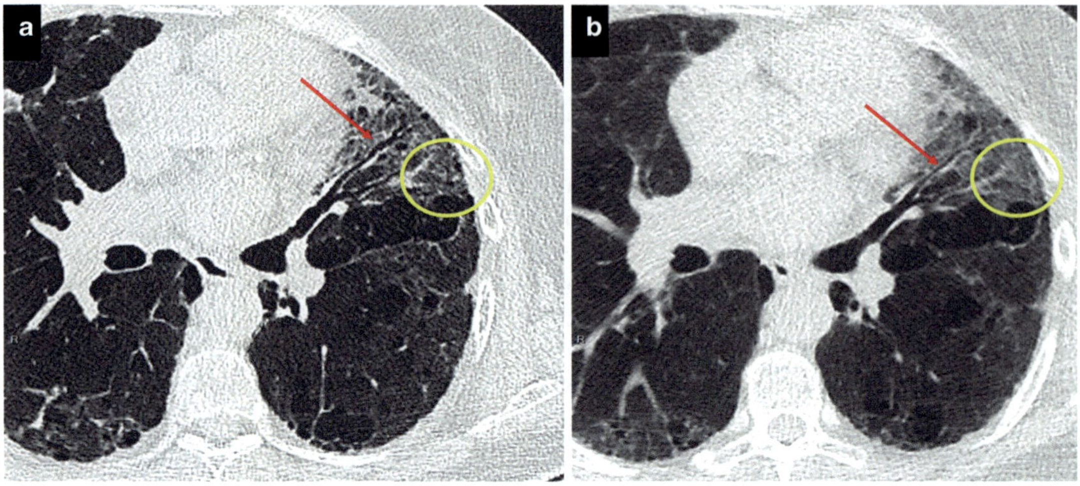

Fig. 2 Axial CT scan images in standard dose (**a**: DLP 150 mGy.cm) and ultra-low dose (**b**: DLP 10 mGy.cm). Note the effect of ultra-low dose on the detection of traction bronchiectasis (arrow) and reticulations (yellow circle) in the left upper lobe. Subtle findings of lung fibrosis may be blurred by excessive reduction of the dose

QCT scan requires even more restrictive parameters. Ideally, patients should be imaged using the same acquisition technique and the same CT scanner. Nevertheless, data concerning the reproducibility and robustness of computer-based programs according to various acquisition and reconstruction parameters are still missing. Iterative reconstruction techniques are not recommended in this area.

3 What?

This section will review the most relevant signs of ILD with their respective QCT-derived measurements.

3.1 Major CT Features of Fibrotic Diseases

HRCT features of fibrosis have been correlated to histological entities which are associated with clinical conditions and prognosis of patients. These phenotypes are well recognized in international consensus guidelines (Travis et al. 2013), and CT plays a key role in their identification. For example, subpleural and basal predominant honeycombing is highly suggestive of usual interstitial pneumonia (UIP), a pattern which is associated with IPF and a higher mortality (Kim et al. 2010; Flaherty et al. 2003b; Chiba et al. 2016).

3.1.1 Traction Bronchiectasis

The presence of traction bronchiectasis (TB) is usually a definite and strong feature of lung fibrosis, more sensitive and less prone to interobserver variation than honeycombing (Jacob et al. 2020). Large studies have shown that the severity of TB is strongly associated with survival (Edey et al. 2011; Walsh et al. 2014). In patients with ILA, the presence of TB is also associated with a poorer clinical outcome (Hata et al. 2022). The severity of TB can be appreciated visually, with good interobserver agreement. Applying the minimal intensity projection (mIP) post-processing technique on soft kernel images can be helpful in identifying TB and their progression over time (Fig. 3). Visual assessment of change in TB independently predicts mortality in patients with IPF showing marginal FVC declines (Jacob et al. 2020). In this way, a severity grade can be assigned for TB based on the average degree of airway dilation within areas of fibrosis as well as the extent of TB dilation within the lobe (final score 0 = none, 1 = mild, 2 = moderate, 3 = severe) (Jacob et al. 2016b) (Fig. 4).

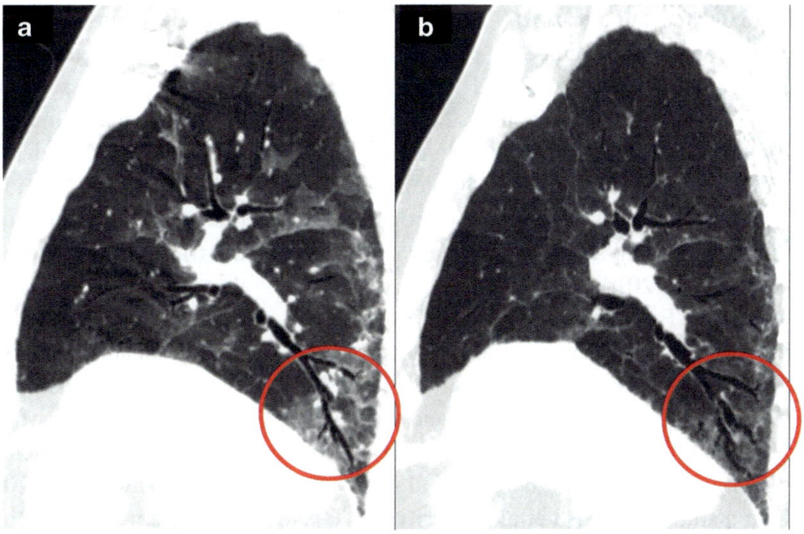

Fig. 3 Serial CT scan images in a 49-year-old patient with COVID-19 pneumonia (**a**: at discharge, **b**: 6 months after). Results are displayed in sagittal reconstructions, with a 3–4 mm mIP treatment applied on soft kernel images. Despite partial regression of ground-glass opacities and total ILD extent, there is clear worsening of traction bronchiectasis in the right lung base (red circles), suggestive of progressive fibrosis

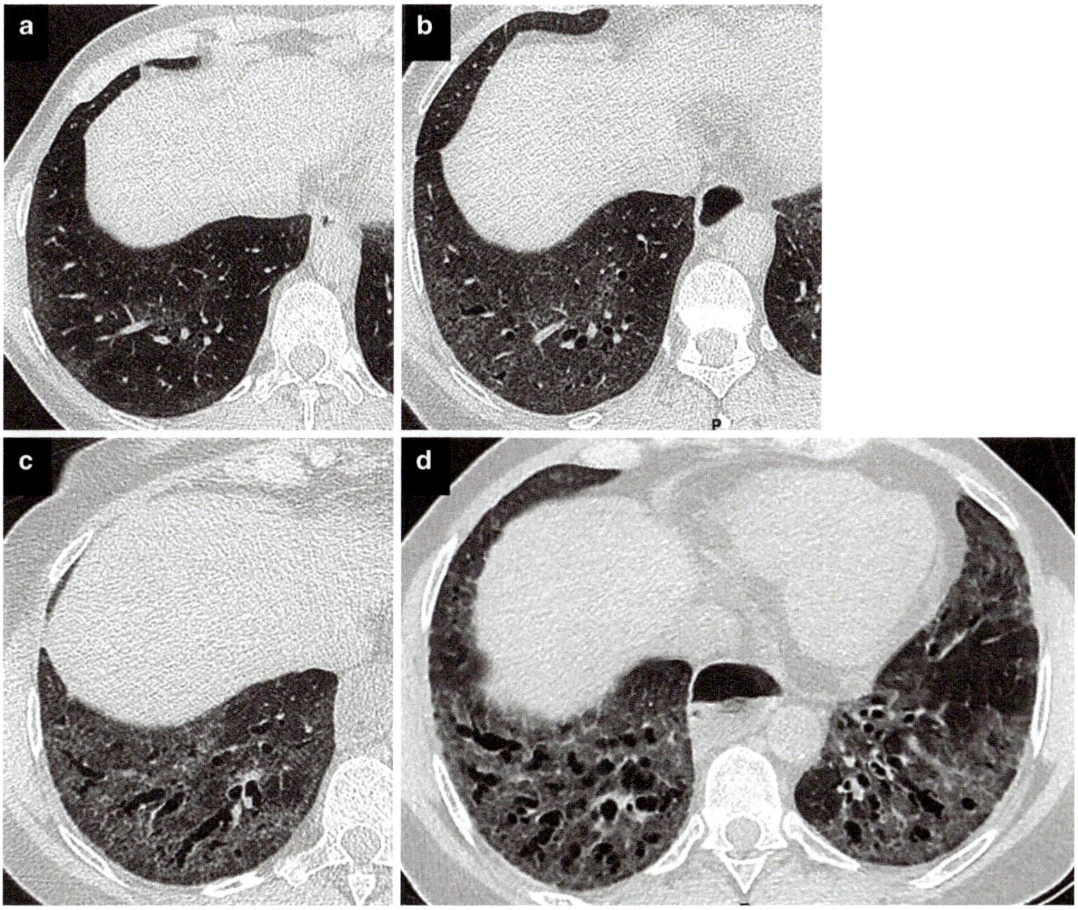

Fig. 4 A 32-year-old woman with systemic sclerosis. Serial CT scans (**a**–**d**) show the apparition (**b**) and progressive worsening (**c**, **d**) of traction bronchiectasis (arrows) and ground-glass opacities with reticulations within the lung bases, consistent with fibrotic nonspecific interstitial pneumonia. These bronchiectasis can be graded from mild to moderate and severe depending on their degree of dilation

3.1.2 Honeycombing

Honeycombing is defined by clustered cystic air spaces (usually between 3 and 10 mm in diameter, but occasionally as large as 2.5 cm) and represents end-stage lung fibrosis. Honeycombing is strongly associated with the pathological phenotype of UIP and has demonstrated prognostic significance in many studies over the past 15 years (Walsh et al. 2014; Wells et al. 1993; Sundaram et al. 2008; Fujimoto et al. 2012). However, identification of honeycombing at CT is subjective, and interobserver agreement is moderate at best, even among expert radiologists, and particularly in patients with emphysema (Lynch et al. 2005; Sundaram et al. 2008; Watadani et al. 2013).

In a study by Walsh et al., severity of TB and extent of honeycombing were strongly associated with mortality in connective tissue disease-associated ILD (Walsh et al. 2014). TB and honeycombing often spread when disease worsen, representing larger proportions of damaged lung, whereas other CT variables such as total ILD extent may underestimate disease progression because of lung shrinkage secondary to lung fibrosis.

3.2 Lung Density Analysis

3.2.1 Ground-Glass Opacities/Consolidation

Artificial intelligence (AI) algorithms trained to detect CT patterns commonly found in pneumonia, such as GGO and consolidation, in both lungs and/or lobe-wise, have been massively tested and validated during the COVID-19 pandemic. One of these solutions has more recently been applied to detect and quantify MDA5-associated ILD, with a percentage of consolidation significantly associated with overall survival (Yamaguchi et al. 2022).

3.2.2 High Attenuation Analysis

High attenuation areas (HAA) are defined as the percentage of lungs presenting CT attenuation values between −600 and −250 Hounsfield Units (HU). This quantitative value can be automatically obtained by software analysis on inspiratory CT scans. In patients not investigated for lung disease indications (i.e., cardiovascular screening), the presence of HAA is associated with a greater cumulative cigarette smoke exposure and a reduced FVC (Lederer et al. 2009), increased odds of identification of ILA, and increased all-cause mortality (Podolanczuk et al. 2016). In another study, Podolanczuk et al. found that higher HAA was associated in the general adult population, with increased odds of having an adjudicated ILD diagnosis, an increased rate of hospitalizations for respiratory or ILD causes, an increased rate of ILD death, and increased odds of subsequent self-reported dyspnea (Podolanczuk et al. 2017). This automated value could represent an index for preclinical ILD (Salisbury and Lynch 2017).

3.2.3 Histogram Kurtosis

The CT density histogram provides a distribution of HU for any single CT image or for the entire lung. The CT density histogram of normal lung tissue shows a peak at approximately −800 HU and is left-skewed. Kurtosis describes the sharpness of the histogram peak and is inversely proportional to the thickness of the two tails of the histogram. An increase in the amount of soft tissue, due to fibrosis, will increase mean lung density (MLD), decrease the histogram peak (kurtosis), and will skew the curve to the right (Hartley et al. 1994) (Fig. 5). Kurtosis and skewness are correlated with changes in FVC and survival in patients with IPF (Best et al. 2003, 2008). However, these global measurements can be confounded by other existing parenchymal changes such as air trapping (i.e., in hypersensitivity pneumonitis) or emphysema (i.e., in combined pulmonary fibrosis and emphysema syndrome).

3.3 Lung Volume

Pulmonary fibrosis is classically associated with shrinking and volume loss of the lungs. Volume loss can be appreciated on CT images by looking at the position of the fissures. Robbie et al. have recently evaluated 3 CT-derived manual measurements, namely, lung height,

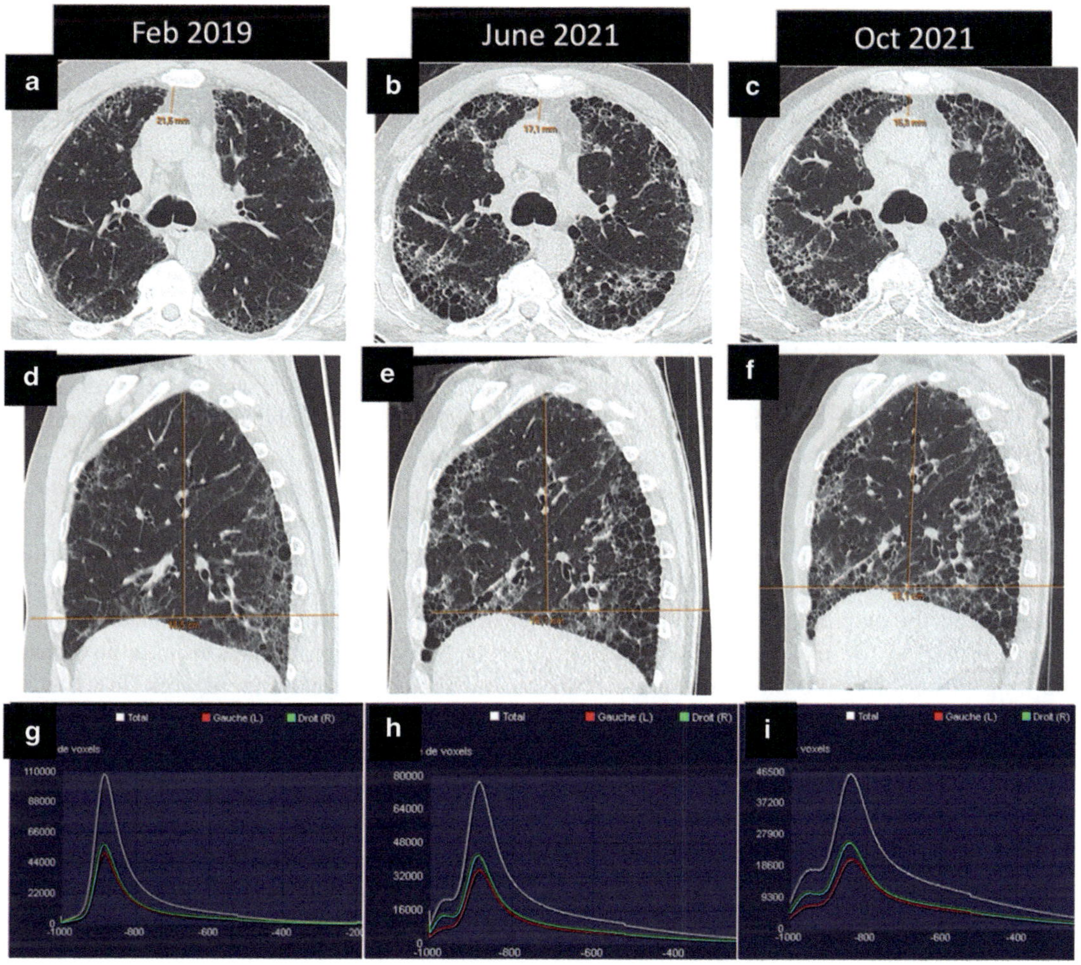

	Feb 2019	June 2021	Oct 2021
Total lung volume (ml)*	5099	4859	4750
Aorto-sternal distance (mm) (a, b, c)	21	17	15
Lung height (cm) (d, e, f)	18, 5	18, 1	18, 1
MLD (HU) (g, h, i) and kurtosis*	–780	–744	–702
Fissure retraction ratio	0,63	0,5	0,44

* Obtained par the CT Pulmo 3D software by *Syngo.via* (Siemens Healthineers®)

Fig. 5 Various CT measurements applied to serial CT scans in a 76-year-old patient diagnosed with IPF in February 2019 (**a**, **d**, **g**), June 2021 (**b**, **e**, **h**), and October 2021 (**c**, **f**, **i**). Aortosternal distance, lung height, and fissure retraction ratio have been calculated according to Robbie et al. (2019)

aortosternal distance, and oblique fissure retraction distance, and shown that these measurements were significantly related to percentage of predicted FVC, independently of fibrosis and emphysema (Robbie et al. 2019). In this study, lung height is corrected for body habitus. It is obtained by measuring the distance between the lung apex and diaphragmatic dome on sagittal reformation (at the mid clavicle landmark) and dividing the result by the sagittal height of the tallest vertebra in the lower thoracic spine (Fig. 5). Aortosternal distance represents the distance between the anterior aspect of the ascending aorta using the pulmonary trunk for anatomic landmark, and the posterior aspect of the sternum. The oblique fissure retraction distance is obtained by measuring for each lung the ratio between the distance from where the fissure meets the diaphragm to the retrosternum anteriorly and to the most posterior aspect of the lung posteriorly; the mean value for both lungs is then calculated (Fig. 5). Note that only serial changes were considered without definite threshold (Robbie et al. 2022).

Softwares dedicated to lung analysis can provide automatic segmentation of lungs and lung volume calculation (Fig. 5). There is a good correlation between CT-derived automated lung volume, FVC (Si-Mohamed et al. 2022), and total lung capacity (TLC) (Robbie et al. 2019; Si-Mohamed et al. 2022). In a retrospective study analyzing 4610 CT scans from 560 patients, Si-Mohamed et al. showed that median annual CT volume loss was significantly higher in patients with IPF than in patients with other fibrotic ILD. They proposed the measurement of lung volume as an alternative or a complementary biomarker to pulmonary function tests for the assessment of lung volume loss in ILD (Si-Mohamed et al. 2022).

3.4 Texture-Based Analysis and Machine Learning

This section will briefly present some of AI solutions dedicated to identification and quantification of ILD patterns.

3.4.1 The Adaptive Multiple Feature Method

The adaptive multiple feature method (AMFM) is a computer-based texture analysis tool designed to recognize and quantify HRCT patterns, including GGO, GGO + reticulation (GGR), honeycombing, and emphysema (Xu et al. 2006). An extended 3-D version has been used in a retrospective study to explore the association between AMFM regional analysis of the lungs and clinical outcomes in IPF patients. The authors demonstrated that both visual and AMFM extent of GGR at baseline predicted disease progression (Salisbury et al. 2017).

3.4.2 Data-Driven Textural Analysis

Data-driven textural analysis (DTA) is a learning program implemented as a simple convolutional neural network (CNN) that uses clustering analyses to find common features from large datasets of unlabeled images. The network is trained to discriminate fibrosis using radiologist-labeled regions of interest (ROI) demonstrating normal lung parenchyma and UIP patterns. A derived IPF index score can be calculated (fibrotic regions of interest (ROI)/total ROI) that has shown correlation with functional impairment at baseline (Humphries et al. 2017a), and longitudinally (Humphries et al. 2017b).

3.4.3 Computer-Aided Lung Informatics for Pathology Evaluation and Rating

Computer-Aided Lung Informatics for Pathology Evaluation and Rating (CALIPER) can identify and quantify normal lung + six specific parenchymal features of ILD (GGO, reticular density, honeycombing, and mild, moderate, or severe low attenuation areas) based on pathological validation (Zavaletta et al. 2007; Bartholmai et al. 2013). The technique is robust and reproducible (Raghunath et al. 2013; Maldonado et al. 2014). It has been successfully used to predict survival and FVC decline in IPF and non-IPF fibrosing lung diseases (Jacob et al. 2016b; Raghunath et al. 2013; Maldonado et al. 2014; Jacob et al. 2018).

In addition to lung parenchymal feature quantification, CALIPER provides automatic segmentation of the pulmonary vasculature. The sum of pulmonary vessel volume (PVV) may be a sign of vascular changes in ILD and has demonstrated prognostic value in two retrospective studies including patients with IPF, connective tissue disease-related ILD, HP, and unclassifiable ILD (Jacob et al. 2016a, 2017a; Maldonado et al. 2014; Silva et al. 2008).

3.5 Additional CT Features Associated to ILD

In most ILDs, some ancillary signs can be associated with pulmonary fibrosis and be quantified.

3.5.1 Air Trapping

Air trapping is seen on end-expiration CT scans as parenchymal areas with less than normal increase in attenuation and lack of volume reduction according to the Fleischner definition (Bankier et al. 2024). Air trapping related to small airway disease makes the diagnosis of fibrotic HP more likely than that of IPF, when extensive, but these descriptors do not state specific numerical values. The threshold of five or more lobules of mosaic attenuation in each of three or more lobes, bilaterally, has been proposed by Silva et al. (Silva et al. 2008) and was found to have the highest specificity for fibrotic HP and to help differentiate this disorder from IPF. However, a recent study demonstrated that air trapping is present in as much as 46% on expiratory CT in IPF patients (Barnett et al. 2019; Walsh and Richeldi 2019).

3.5.2 Extrapulmonary Findings

Extrapulmonary findings can be associated with ILD etiology (esophageal dilation in systemic sclerosis), prognosis (size of the pulmonary artery, lymph nodes), or reflect patient sarcopenia (muscle mass).

3.5.2.1 Esophagus

An increased esophageal diameter at CT is common in patients with systemic sclerosis (Perelas et al. 2020). It is due to dysmotility and is a key sign of the disease. Dilation is associated to esophageal reflux and increases the risk of death and faster disease progression. The largest distance (mm) between internal esophageal mucosal limits for three esophageal diameter measurements on supine axial CT images is most often considered, with various thresholds (9–15 mm) and various of levels of measurements (supra-aortic or infra-aortic arch). There is not clear mention in the literature on the height of the dilation to be considered (Takekoshi et al. 2015; Richardson et al. 2016; Pitrez et al. 2006; Winstone et al. 2018).

3.5.2.2 Pulmonary Artery

Pulmonary artery enlargement, in the context of ILD, may suggest pulmonary hypertension, a frequent complication of ILD (King and Shlobin 2020). A recent Position Paper from the Fleischner Society proposed to consider patients at high risk in case of values >30 mm for the diameter of the pulmonary artery and a ratio >0.9 for pulmonary to aorta ratio of the diameters (Remy-Jardin et al. 2021). Such a finding requires an additional cardiac workup.

3.5.2.3 Lymph Nodes

Finally, lymph node enlargement with a small diameter >10 mm is also a cause for concern in ILDs, as it can be associated with poor outcomes (Adegunsoye et al. 2019; Tyker et al. 2021; Walsh 2019). Lymph node enlargement remains however a poorly specific factor, as it can be occasionally seen in various other clinical conditions.

4 Perspectives

In clinical practice, quantitative imaging is widely used to evaluate the extent of ILD. Extensive versus limited fibrosis must be specified in the radiological report, and providing numerical value is also helpful as it allows to predict the prognosis of disease and to diagnose progression. Measurements are also helpful for the diagnosis of comorbidities, including pulmonary hypertension through enlargement of the pulmonary artery.

Regarding AI, things are going fast (Howell et al. 2024; Walsh et al. 2020), and the use of quantified imaging is now discussed as a meaningful endpoint in clinical trials (Raghu et al. 2024). Today, deep learning models are largely used in research to evaluate ILD and applications are numerous (Walsh et al. 2024). We have now data suggesting that the 4% change of extent between two acquisitions could be a threshold associated with a significant event (Kim et al. 2020; Humphries et al. 2018; Guerra et al. 2024). Nowadays, the trend is to dig deeper and develop biomarkers of bronchial (Cheung et al. 2023) and vascular remodeling (Devaraj et al. 2024; Harder et al. 2024; Jacob et al. 2018), which could be combined to the evaluation of ILD extent (Thillai et al. 2024). Finally, the future of quantitative imaging could also associate functional data, including functional respiratory imaging evaluating fluid dynamics in the airways (Clukers et al. 2018) or in the pulmonary arteries, or an evaluation of deformations of the fibrotic lungs based on elastic registration algorithm (Chassagnon et al. 2021). The future role of MRI for qualitative and quantitative assessment of ILD needs further evaluation (Lonzetti et al. 2019).

Disclaimer All measurements in this book have been obtained from peer-reviewed papers and guidelines from professional organizations, unless explicitly stated otherwise. While the authors, editors, and publisher have gone through a rigorous process to establish their correct reproduction from the original source, each measurement must be interpreted in the correct clinical context, this along with an accurate way of measurement, and taking into account all technical variables, this including follow-up exams with various equipment or software. Neither the authors, the editors, nor the publisher can accept any legal responsibility for any improper application or interpretation of these measurements as well as their potential consequences.

References

Adegunsoye A, Oldham JM, Bonham C et al (2019) Prognosticating outcomes in interstitial lung disease by mediastinal lymph node assessment. An observational cohort study with independent validation. Am J Respir Crit Care Med 199(6):747–759

Assayag D, Kaduri S, Hudson M, Hirsch A, Baron M (2012) High resolution computed tomography scoring systems for evaluating interstitial lung disease in systemic sclerosis patients. Rheumatology S1:003. https://doi.org/10.4172/2161-1149.S1-003

Bankier AA, MacMahon H, Colby T et al (2024) Fleischner society: glossary of terms for thoracic imaging. Radiology 310(2):e232558

Barnett J, Molyneaux PL, Rawal B et al (2019) Variable utility of mosaic attenuation to distinguish fibrotic hypersensitivity pneumonitis from idiopathic pulmonary fibrosis. Eur Respir J 54(1):1900531

Bartholmai BJ, Raghunath S, Karwoski RA et al (2013) Quantitative computed tomography imaging of interstitial lung diseases. J Thorac Imaging 28:298–307

Best AC, Lynch AM, Bozic CM, Miller D, Grunwald GK, Lynch DA (2003) Quantitative CT indexes in idiopathic pulmonary fibrosis: relationship with physiologic impairment. Radiology 228:407–414

Best AC, Meng J, Lynch AM, Bozic CM, Miller D, Grunwald GK, Lynch DA (2008) Idiopathic pulmonary fibrosis: physiologic tests, quantitative CT indexes, and CT visual scores as predictors of mortality. Radiology 246:935–940

Chassagnon G, Vakalopoulou M, Régent A et al (2021) Elastic registration-driven deep learning for longitudinal assessment of systemic sclerosis interstitial lung disease at CT. Radiology 298(1):189–198

Cheung WK, Pakzad A, Mogulkoc N et al (2023) Automated airway quantification associates with mortality in idiopathic pulmonary fibrosis. Eur Radiol 33(11):8228–8238

Chiba S, Tsuchiya K, Akashi T, Ishizuka M, Okamoto T, Furusawa H, Tateishi T, Kishino M, Miyazaki Y, Tateishi U, Takemura T, Inase N (2016) Chronic hypersensitivity pneumonitis with a usual interstitial pneumonia-like pattern: correlation between histopathologic and clinical findings. Chest 149:1473–1481

Clukers J, Lanclus M, Mignot B et al (2018) Quantitative CT analysis using functional imaging is superior in describing disease progression in idiopathic pulmonary fibrosis compared to forced vital capacity. Respir Res 19(1):213

Devaraj A, Ottink F, Rennison-Jones C et al (2024) e-lung computed tomography biomarker stratifies patients at risk of idiopathic pulmonary fibrosis progression in a 52-week clinical trial. Am J Respir Crit Care Med 209(9):1168–1169

Edey AJ, Devaraj AA, Barker RP, Nicholson AG, Wells AU, Hansell DM (2011) Fibrotic idiopathic interstitial pneumonias: HRCT findings that predict mortality. Eur Radiol 21:1586–1593

Flaherty KR, Mumford JA, Murray S, Kazerooni EA, Gross BH, Colby TV, Travis WD, Flint A, Toews GB, Lynch JP 3rd, Martinez FJ (2003a) Prognostic implications of physiologic and radiographic changes in idiopathic interstitial pneumonia. Am J Respir Crit Care Med 168:543–548

Flaherty KR, Thwaite EL, Kazerooni EA, Gross BH, Toews GB, Colby TV, Travis WD, Mumford JA,

Murray S, Flint A, Lynch JP 3rd, Martinez FJ (2003b) Radiological versus histological diagnosis in UIP and NSIP: survival implications. Thorax 58:143–148

Flaherty KR, Brown KK, Wells AU et al (2017) Design of the PF-ILD trial: a double-blind, randomised, placebo-controlled phase III trial of nintedanib in patients with progressive fibrosing interstitial lung disease. BMJ Open Respir Res 4:e000212

Flaherty KR, Wells AU, Cottin V, Devaraj A, Walsh SLF, Inoue Y, Richeldi L, Kolb M, Tetzlaff K, Stowasser S, Coeck C, Clerisme-Beaty E, Rosenstock B, Quaresma M, Haeufel T, Goeldner RG, Schlenker-Herceg R, Brown KK, INBUILD Trial Investigators (2019) Nintedanib in progressive fibrosing interstitial lung diseases. N Engl J Med 381(18):1718–1727

Fujimoto K, Taniguchi H, Johkoh T, Kondoh Y, Ichikado K, Sumikawa H, Ogura T, Kataoka K, Endo T, Kawaguchi A, Muller NL (2012) Acute exacerbation of idiopathic pulmonary fibrosis: high-resolution CT scores predict mortality. Eur Radiol 22:83–92

Gay SE, Kazerooni EA, Toews GB, Lynch JP 3rd, Gross BH, Cascade PN, Spizarny DL, Flint A, Schork MA, Whyte RI, Popovich J, Hyzy R, Martinez FJ (1998) Idiopathic pulmonary fibrosis: predicting response to therapy and survival. Am J Respir Crit Care Med 157:1063–1072

George PM, Spagnolo P, Kreuter M, Altinisik G, Bonifazi M, Martinez FJ, Molyneaux PL, Renzoni EA, Richeldi L, Tomassetti S, Valenzuela C, Vancheri C, Varone F, Cottin V, Costabel U, Erice ILD Working Group (2020) Progressive fibrosing interstitial lung disease: clinical uncertainties, consensus recommendations, and research priorities. Lancet Respir Med 8(9):925–934. https://doi.org/10.1016/S2213-2600(20)30355-6

Goh NS, Desai SR, Veeraraghavan S et al (2008) Interstitial lung disease in systemic sclerosis: a simple staging system. Am J Respir Crit Care Med 177:1248–1254

Guerra X, Rennotte S, Fetita C et al (2024) U-net convolutional neural network applied to progressive fibrotic interstitial lung disease: is progression at CT scan associated with a clinical outcome? Respir Med Res 85:101058

Hansell DM, Goldin JG, King TE et al (2015) CT staging and monitoring of fibrotic interstitial lung diseases in clinical practice and treatment trials: a Position Paper from the Fleischner Society. Lancet Respir Med 3:483–496

Harder EM, Abtin F, Nardelli P et al (2024) Pulmonary hypertension in idiopathic interstitial pneumonia is associated with small vessel pruning. Am J Respir Crit Care Med 209(9):1170–1173

Hartley PG, Galvin JR, Hunninghake GW et al (1994) High-resolution CT-derived measures of lung density are valid indexes of interstitial lung disease. J Appl Physiol 76:271–277

Hata A, Hino T, Putman RK, Yanagawa M, Hida T, Menon AA, Honda O, Yamada Y, Nishino M, Araki T, Valtchinov VI, Jinzaki M, Honda H, Ishigami K, Johkoh T, Tomiyama N, Christiani DC, Lynch DA, San José Estépar R, Washko GR, Cho MH, Silverman EK, Hunninghake GM, Hatabu H, COPDGene Investigators (2022) Traction bronchiectasis / bronchiolectasis on CT scans in relationship to clinical outcomes and mortality: the COPDGene Study. Radiology 304(3):694–701

Hatabu H, Hunninghake GM, Richeldi L et al (2020) Interstitial lung abnormalities detected incidentally on CT: a Position Paper from the Fleischner Society. Lancet Respir Med 8(7):726–737

Howell MD, Corrado GS, DeSalvo KB (2024) Three epochs of artificial intelligence in health care. JAMA 331(3):242–244

Humphries SM, Yagihashi K, Huckleberry J et al (2017a) Idiopathic pulmonary fibrosis: data-driven textural analysis of extent of fibrosis at baseline and 15-month follow-up. Radiology 285:270–278

Humphries SORT, Sundy JS, Zhang JJ, Gong Q, Bayly S, Sood R, Raghu G, Lynch DA (2017b) Change in CT-derived fibrosis score correlates with lung function progression in a clinical trial population with idiopathic pulmonary fibrosis. Am J Respir Crit Care Med 195:A6783

Humphries SM, Swigris JJ, Brown KK et al (2018) Quantitative high-resolution computed tomography fibrosis score: performance characteristics in idiopathic pulmonary fibrosis. Eur Respir J 52(3):1801384

Ito Y, Arita M, Kumagai S, Takei R, Noyama M, Tokioka F, Nishimura K, Koyama T, Tachibana H, Ishida T (2019) Radiological fibrosis score is strongly associated with worse survival in rheumatoid arthritis-related interstitial lung disease. Mod Rheumatol 29(1):98–104

Jacob J, Bartholmai BJ, Rajagopalan S et al (2016a) Evaluation of computer-based computer tomography stratification against outcome models in connective tissue disease-related interstitial lung disease: a patient outcome study. BMC Med 14:190

Jacob J, Bartholmai BJ, Rajagopalan S, Kokosi M, Nair A, Karwoski R et al (2016b) Automated quantitative computed tomography versus visual computed tomography scoring in idiopathic pulmonary fibrosis: validation against pulmonary function. J Thorac Imaging 31:304–311

Jacob J, Bartholmai BJ, Rajagopalan S et al (2017a) Mortality prediction in idiopathic pulmonary fibrosis: evaluation of computer-based CT analysis with conventional severity measures. Eur Respir J 49:16

Jacob J, Bartholmai BJ, Egashira R, Brun AL, Rajagopalan S, Karwoski R, Kokosi M, Hansell DM, Wells AU (2017b) Chronic hypersensitivity pneumonitis: identification of key prognostic determinants using automated CT analysis. BMC Pulm Med 17(1):81

Jacob J, Bartholmai BJ, Rajagopalan S et al (2018) Predicting outcomes in idiopathic pulmonary fibrosis using automated computed tomographic analysis. Am J Respir Crit Care Med 198(6):767–776

Jacob J, Hirani N, van Moorsel CHM et al (2019) Predicting outcomes in rheumatoid arthritis related interstitial lung disease. Eur Respir J 53(1):1800869

Jacob J, Aksman L, Mogulkoc N, Procter AJ, Gholipour B, Cross G, Barnett J, Brereton CJ, Jones MG, van Moorsel CH, van Es W, van Beek F, Veltkamp M, Desai SR, Judge E, Burd T, Kokosi M, Savas R, Bayraktaroglu S, Altmann A, Wells AU (2020) Serial CT analysis in idiopathic pulmonary fibrosis: comparison of visual features that determine patient outcome. Thorax 75(8):648–654

Kim EJ, Elicker BM, Maldonado F, Webb WR, Ryu JH, Van Uden JH, Lee JS, King TE Jr, Collard HR (2010) Usual interstitial pneumonia in rheumatoid arthritis associated interstitial lung disease. Eur Respir J 35:1322

Kim GHJ, Weigt SS, Belperio JA et al (2020) Prediction of idiopathic pulmonary fibrosis progression using early quantitative changes on CT imaging for a short term of clinical 18-24-month follow-ups. Eur Radiol 30(2):726–734

King CS, Shlobin OA (2020) The trouble with group 3 pulmonary hypertension in interstitial lung disease: dilemmas in diagnosis and the conundrum of treatment. Chest 158(4):1651–1664

Lederer DJ, Enright PL, Kawut SM, Hoffman EA, Hunninghake G, van Beek EJ, Austin JH, Jiang R, Lovasi GS, Barr RG (2009) Cigarette smoking is associated with subclinical parenchymal lung disease: the Multi-Ethnic Study of Atherosclerosis (MESA)-lung study. Am J Respir Crit Care Med 180:407–414

Ley B, Elicker BM, Hartman TE et al (2014) Idiopathic pulmonary fibrosis: CT and risk of death. Radiology 273(2):570

Lonzetti L, Zanon M, Pacini GS, Altmayer S, Martins de Oliveira D, Rubin AS, Gazzoni FF, Barros MC, Hochhegger B (2019) Magnetic resonance imaging of interstitial lung diseases: a state-of-the-art review. Respir Med 155:79–85

Lynch DA, Godwin JD, Safrin S, Starko KM, Hormel P, Brown KK, Raghu G, King TE Jr, Bradford WZ, Schwartz DA, Richard Webb W, Idiopathic Pulmonary Fibrosis Study G (2005) High-resolution computed tomography in idiopathic pulmonary fibrosis: diagnosis and prognosis. Am J Respir Crit Care Med 172:488–493

Maher TM, Corte TJ, Fischer A, Kreuter M, Lederer DJ, Molina-Molina M, Axmann J, Kirchgaessler KU, Samara K, Gilberg F, Cottin V (2020) Pirfenidone in patients with unclassifiable progressive fibrosing interstitial lung disease: a double-blind, randomised, placebo-controlled, phase 2 trial. Lancet Respir Med 8(2):147–157

Maldonado F, Moua T, Rajagopalan S et al (2014) Automated quantification of radiological patterns predicts survival in idiopathic pulmonary fibrosis. Eur Respir J 43:204–212

Mogulkoc N, Brutsche MH, Bishop PW, Greaves SM, Horrocks AW, Egan JJ, Greater Manchester Pulmonary Fibrosis C (2001) Pulmonary function in idiopathic pulmonary fibrosis and referral for lung transplantation. Am J Respir Crit Care Med 164:103–108

Perelas A, Silver RM, Arrossi AV, Highland KB (2020) Systemic sclerosis-associated interstitial lung disease. Lancet Respir Med 8(3):304–320

Pitrez EH, Bredemeier M, Xavier RM et al (2006) Oesophageal dysmotility in systemic sclerosis: comparison of HRCT and scintigraphy. Br J Radiol 79(945):719–724

Podolanczuk AJ, Oelsner EC, Barr RG, Hoffman EA, Armstrong HF, Austin JH, Basner RC, Bartels MN, Christie JD, Enright PL et al (2016) High attenuation areas on chest computed tomography in community-dwelling adults: the MESA study. Eur Respir J 48:1442–1452

Podolanczuk AJ, Oelsner EC, Barr RG, Bernstein EJ, Hoffman EA, Easthausen IJ, Hinckley Stukovsky K, RoyChoudhury A, Michos ED, Raghu G et al (2017) High attenuation areas on chest computed tomography and clinical respiratory outcomes in community-dwelling adults. Am J Respir Crit Care Med 196(11):1368–1369

Raghu G, Ghazipura M, Fleming TR et al (2024) Meaningful endpoints for idiopathic pulmonary fibrosis (IPF) clinical trials: emphasis on 'feels, functions, survives'. Report of a collaborative discussion in a symposium with direct engagement from representatives of patients, investigators, the National Institutes of Health, a Patient Advocacy Organization, and a Regulatory Agency. Am J Respir Crit Care Med 209(6):647–669

Raghunath S, Rajagopalan S, Karwoski RA, Bruesewitz MR, McCollough CH, Bartholmai BJ, Robb RA (2013) Landscaping the effect of CT reconstruction parameters: robust interstitial pulmonary fibrosis quantitation. In: Proceedings – international symposium on biomedical imaging, pp 374–377. https://doi.org/10.1109/ISBI.2013.6556490

Remy-Jardin M, Ryerson CJ, Schiebler ML et al (2021) Imaging of pulmonary hypertension in adults: a position paper from the Fleischner Society. Radiology 298(3):531–549

Richardson C, Agrawal R, Lee J et al (2016) Esophageal dilatation and interstitial lung disease in systemic sclerosis: a cross-sectional study. Semin Arthritis Rheum 46(1):109–114

Robbie H, Wells AU, Jacob J, Walsh SLF, Nair A, Srikanthan A, Tazoniero P, Devaraj A (2019) Visual and automated CT measurements of lung volume loss in idiopathic pulmonary fibrosis. AJR Am J Roentgenol 213(2):318–324

Robbie H, Wells AU, Fang C, Jacob J, Walsh SLF, Nair A, Camoras R, Desai SR, Devaraj A (2022) Serial decline in lung volume parameters on computed tomography (CT) predicts outcome in idiopathic pulmonary fbrosis (IPF). Eur Radiol 32(4):2650–2660

Salisbury ML, Lynch DA (2017) Toward early identification of clinically relevant interstitial lung disease. Am J Respir Crit Care Med 196(11):1368–1369

Salisbury ML, Lynch DA, van Beek EJ et al (2017) Idiopathic pulmonary fibrosis: the association between the adaptive multiple features method and fibrosis outcomes. Am J Respir Crit Care Med 195:921–929

Silva CI, Müller NL, Lynch DA et al (2008) Chronic hypersensitivity pneumonitis: differentiation from idiopathic pulmonary fibrosis and nonspecific interstitial pneumonia by using thin-section CT. Radiology 246(1):288–297

Si-Mohamed SA, Nasser M, Colevray M, Nempont O, Lartaud PJ, Vlachomitrou A, Broussaud T, Ahmad K, Traclet J, Cottin V, Boussel L (2022) Automatic quantitative computed tomography measurement of longitudinal lung volume loss in interstitial lung diseases. Eur Radiol 32(6):4292–4303

Sumikawa H, Johkoh T, Colby TV, Ichikado K, Suga M, Taniguchi H, Kondoh Y, Ogura T, Arakawa H, Fujimoto K, Inoue A, Mihara N, Honda O, Tomiyama N, Nakamura H, Muller NL (2008) Computed tomography findings in pathological usual interstitial pneumonia: relationship to survival. Am J Respir Crit Care Med 177:433–439

Sundaram B, Gross BH, Martinez FJ, Oh E, Muller NL, Schipper M, Kazerooni EA (2008) Accuracy of high-resolution CT in the diagnosis of diffuse lung disease: effect of predominance and distribution of findings. AJR Am J Roentgenol 191:1032–1039

Takekoshi D, Arami S, Sheppard TJ et al (2015) Computed tomography of the esophagus in scleroderma and lung disease. Tohoku J Exp Med 237(4):345–352

Thillai M, Oldham JM, Ruggiero A et al (2024) Deep learning-based segmentation of computed tomography scans predicts disease progression and mortality in idiopathic pulmonary fibrosis. Am J Respir Crit Care Med 210(4):465–472

Travis WD, Costabel U, Hansell DM, King TE Jr, Lynch DA, Nicholson AG, Ryerson CJ, Ryu JH, Selman M, Wells AU, Behr J, Bouros D, Brown KK, Colby TV, Collard HR, Cordeiro CR, Cottin V, Crestani B, Drent M, Dudden RF, Egan J, Flaherty K, Hogaboam C, Inoue Y, Johkoh T, Kim DS, Kitaichi M, Loyd J, Martinez FJ, Myers J, Protzko S, Raghu G, Richeldi L, Sverzellati N, Swigris J, Valeyre D, ATS/ERS Committee on Idiopathic Interstitial Pneumonias (2013) An official American Thoracic Society/European Respiratory Society statement: update of the international multidisciplinary classification of the idiopathic interstitial pneumonias. Am J Respir Crit Care Med 188(6):733–748

Tyker A, Ventura IB, Lee CT et al (2021) High-titer rheumatoid factor seropositivity predicts mediastinal lymphadenopathy and mortality in rheumatoid arthritis-related interstitial lung disease. Sci Rep 11(1):22821

Walsh SLF (2019) Mediastinal lymphadenopathy in interstitial lung disease. Time to be counted. Am J Respir Crit Care Med 199(6):685–687

Walsh SLF, Richeldi L (2019) Demystifying fibrotic hypersensitivity pneumonitis diagnosis: it's all about shades of grey. Eur Respir J 54(1):1900906

Walsh SLF, Sverzellati N, Devaraj A et al (2014) Connective tissue disease related fibrotic lung disease: high resolution computed tomographic and pulmonary function indices as prognostic determinants. Thorax 69:216–222. https://doi.org/10.1136/thoraxjnl-2013-203843

Walsh SLF, Humphries SM, Wells AU, Brown KK (2020) Imaging research in fibrotic lung disease; applying deep learning to unsolved problems. Lancet Respir Med 8(11):1144–1153

Walsh SLF, De Backer J, Prosch H et al (2024) Open Source Imaging Consortium (OSIC). Towards the adoption of quantitative computed tomography in the management of interstitial lung disease. Eur Respir Rev 33(171):230055

Watadani T, Sakai F, Johkoh T et al (2013) Interobserver variability in the CT assessment of honeycombing in the lungs. Radiology 266:936–944

Wells AU, Hansell DM, Rubens MB, Cullinan P, Black CM, du Bois RM (1993) The predictive value of appearances on thin section computed tomography in fibrosing alveolitis. Am Rev Respir Dis 148:1076–1082

Winstone TA, Hague CJ, Soon J et al (2018) Oesophageal diameter is associated with severity but not progression of systemic sclerosis-associated interstitial lung disease. Respirology 23(10):921–926

Wu X, Kim GH, Salisbury ML et al (2019) Computed tomographic biomarkers in idiopathic pulmonary fibrosis. The future of quantitative analysis. Am J Respir Crit Care Med 199(1):12–21

Xu Y, van Beek EJ, Hwanjo Y et al (2006) Computer-aided classification of interstitial lung diseases via MDCT: 3D adaptive multiple feature method (3D AMFM). Acad Radiol 13:969–978

Yamaguchi K, Nakajima T, Yamaguchi A et al (2022) Quantitative CT analysis of interstitial pneumonia in anti-melanoma differentiation-associated gene 5 antibody-positive dermatomyositis: a single center, retrospective study. Clin Rheumatol 41(5):1473–1481

Zavaletta VA, Bartholmai BJ, Robb RA (2007) High resolution multidetector CT-aided tissue analysis and quantification of lung fibrosis. Acad Radiol 14:772–787

Thymus

Jeanne B. Ackman

Contents

Abstract

This chapter reviews the use of standard, widely available picture archiving and communication system (PACS) measurement tools to distinguish normal thymus, thymic hyperplasia, and thymic cysts from thymic tumors and lymphoma by computed tomography (CT) and magnetic resonance imaging (MRI), with the aim to reduce the unnecessary or non-therapeutic thymectomy rate and offer further guidance to thoracic surgeons when surgery is indicated. Measurement pitfalls will be discussed, along with the strengths and weaknesses of CT, ^{18}fluorodeoxyglucose positron emission tomography (^{18}FDG PET)/CT, and MRI in this regard. There will also be a brief discussion about the significance of tumor size, as it applies to the staging of thymic epithelial tumors. Caution is urged in ascribing too much significance to specific numbers and cutoff values provided here and in the literature in general, in the absence of other corroborative findings and the use of clinical judgment.

The original version of this chapter has been revised. The missing disclaimer text has been included. A correction to this chapter can be found at https://doi.org/10.1007/174_2025_588

J. B. Ackman (✉)
Harvard Medical School & Massachusetts General Hospital, Boston, MA, USA
e-mail: JACKMAN@mgh.harvard.edu

Med Radiol Diagn Imaging (2026), corrected publication 2025
https://doi.org/10.1007/174_2023_469,

Published Online: 30 December 2023

Abbreviations

^{18}FDG PET/CT	^{18}Fluorodeoxyglucose positron emission tomography/computed tomography
2D	2-Dimensional
3D	3-Dimensional
ADC	Apparent diffusion coefficient
AP	Anteroposterior
CSR	Chemical shift ratio
CT	Computed tomography
DCE	Dynamic contrast enhancement
DIR	Double inversion recovery
DWI	Diffusion-weighted imaging
ECG-gated	Electrocardiogram-gated
GRE	Gradient echo
HU	Hounsfield units
IASLC	International Association for the Study of Lung Cancer
IP	In-phase
ITMIG	International Thymic Malignancy Interest Group
MRI	Magnetic resonance imaging
MTLT	Maximum thymic lobar thickness
OP	Opposed-phase or out-of-phase
PACS	Picture archiving and communication system
ROI	Region-of-interest
SD	Standard deviation
SI	Signal intensity
SII	Signal intensity index
SUV	Standard uptake value
T	Tesla (1.5 T, 3 T …)
T1W	T1-weighted
T2W	T2-weighted
TE	Time-to-echo
TET	Thymic epithelial tumor
TNM	Tumor node metastases
TRV	Transverse
TTP	Time-to-peak

1 Introduction

Since the emergence of computed tomography (CT), there has been a high rate of unnecessary or nontherapeutic thymectomy secondary to the limited ability of CT to distinguish benign from malignant thymic lesions (Ackman et al. 2015; Kent et al. 2014). The thymus has long been considered dispensable in adulthood (Thapa and Farber 2019); however, it may be more important to our immunity in adulthood than we currently recognize (Kooshesh et al. 2023). The spleen had also been considered dispensable until more recently, when its substantive immune functions became more fully appreciated (Bronte and Pittet 2013; Thai et al. 2016; Swirski et al. 2009). The effect of thymectomy on immunity in adult humans has not been rigorously studied. Efforts to retain it, when appropriate and safe to do so, are reasonable. Knowledge of magnetic resonance imaging (MRI) features which distinguish normal thymus, thymic hyperplasia, and thymic cysts from thymic tumors (Inaoka et al. 2007; Priola et al. 2015; Ackman and Wu 2011; Ackman et al. 2013, 2016, 2021; McInnis et al. 2016; Hammer et al. 2019; Ackman 2015; Madan et al. 2018; Heeger and Ackman 2021), in addition to awareness of normal thymic appearance by CT and MRI, more comprehensively informs clinical management and should reduce the occurrence of unnecessary thymectomy. Making these clinically important distinctions often requires measurement. This chapter reviews the rationale behind these measurements, mechanics of acquiring them to avert misdiagnosis (McInnis et al. 2016; Hammer et al. 2019), and proposed measurement threshold values or cutoffs in the literature. Nevertheless, it urges caution in ascribing too much significance to specific numbers and cutoff values provided here and in the literature in general (Lamba et al. 2014), in the absence of other corroborative clinical and imaging findings and the use of clinical judgment.

2 Basic Tenets of Size and Region-of-Interest (ROI) Measurement on CT and MRI

2.1 Size Measurements

- Measurements should always be performed on the series of images that show the borders of the lesion best or most clearly, unobscured by artifacts of whatever kind, including image noise, respiratory motion artifact, pulsatility artifact on both CT and MRI, beam hardening artifact on CT, and susceptibility artifact and chemical shift or India ink artifact on MRI.
  - For example, it is suboptimal to procure size measurements on opposed-phase images, because when a lesion is partially or completely surrounded by chemical shift artifact, it is unclear where the true borders of the lesion are—inside, outside, or in between.
- Size measurements should also not be procured from post-processed, subtracted dynamic contrast-enhanced images because misregistration of the pre- and postcontrast images can confound their accuracy and these images tend to be noisy, so true lesion borders can be difficult to rely upon with confidence.
- As always, care should be taken to place calipers precisely along the margins of the lesion.
- If two perpendicular measurements of a lesion are sought on the same image, the lines drawn must be perpendicular to each other, rather than configured as an "X," because performing the latter yields inclusion of a component of the other dimension in each measurement:
  - For example, inclusion of a transverse dimensional component in an AP measurement and vice versa.

2.2 Region-of-Interest (ROI) Measurements

- When sampling tissue, the ROI should be made as large as possible within the confines of the lesion or a lesion component of interest, including as many pixels as possible and excluding artifacts to the greatest degree possible. The aim is to obtain a representative sample of the tissue of interest. Because an ROI cannot "see through" artifact to measure the intrinsic CT attenuation or MR signal of the lesion itself, it will average the attenuation or signal of the artifact into the reported measurement, yielding misleading information and potentially confounding diagnosis.
  - On CT, this means not trusting or relying on ROI values acquired from parts of lesions partially covered by beam hardening or streak artifact or with significant image noise.
  - On MRI, this means excluding India ink artifact and susceptibility artifact from an ROI's coverage area, for example (Fig. 1).
- ROI morphology should be suited to the lesion of interest, i.e., round for a round lesion and elliptical for an ovoid lesion, in order to maximize the size of the ROI.
- When interpreting ROIs, one must keep in mind that:
  - Hounsfield unit (HU) ROIs on CT are a form of *absolute* measurement, with specific ROI ranges indicative of specific tissue types like water and macroscopic or gross fat.
  - ROIs of signal intensity acquired by MRI are *relative*, rather than absolute, measurements, though still quite useful for tissue characterization.
- One should always attend to the standard deviation (SD) and/or maximum and minimum ROI values, in addition to the mean ROI value, to avoid ascribing too much significance to small changes in ROI measurement.

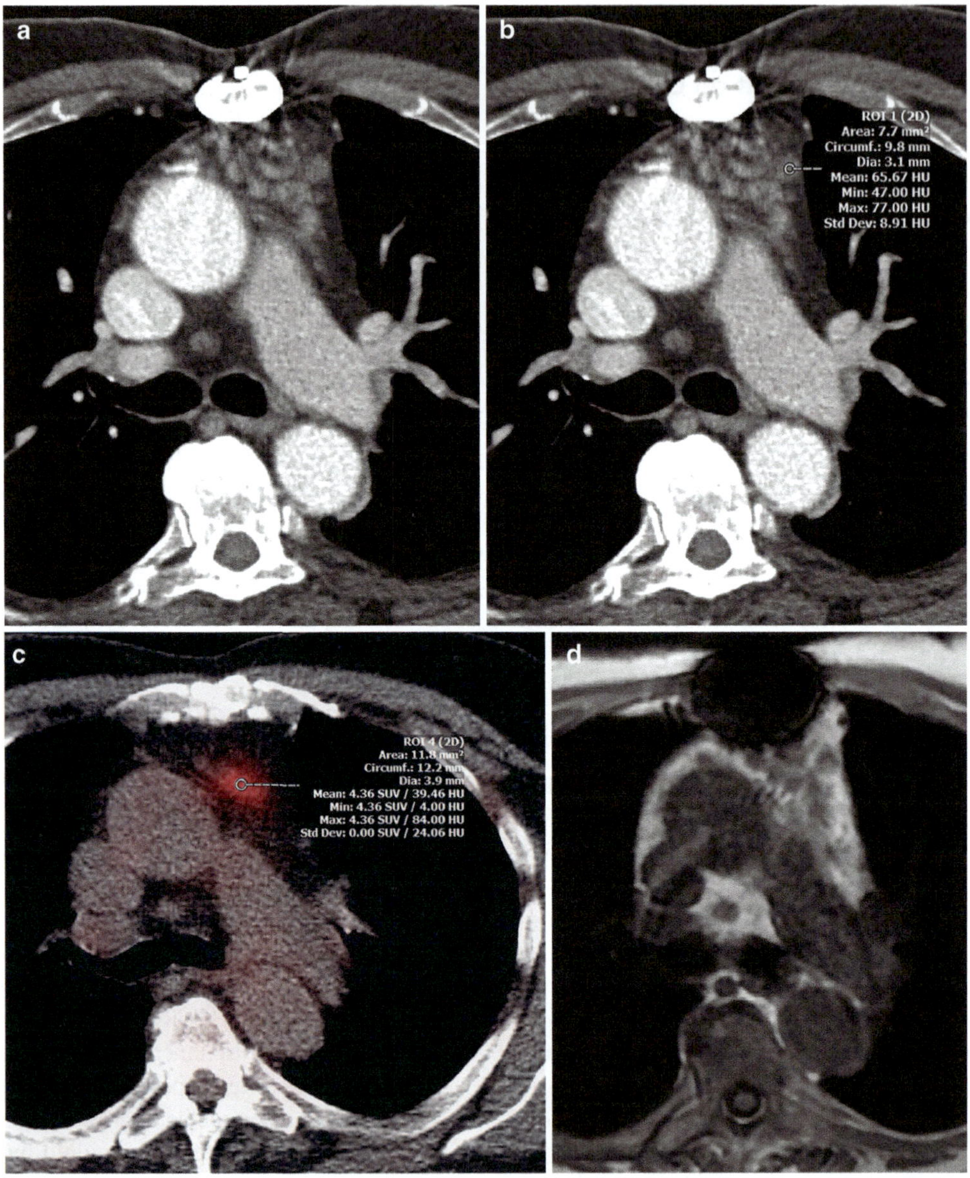

Fig. 1 Seventy-five-year-old man with a history of rheumatoid arthritis and pathology-proven follicular lymphoid hyperplasia. (**a** and **b**) Axial contrast-enhanced CT without and with ROI placed on one of many small clustered thymic nodules in the left prevascular mediastinum, showing an attenuation of 66 HU. (**c**) Axial non-contrast ^{18}FDG PET/CT shows this tissue to be intensely FDG-avid, with a standard uptake value (SUV) of 4.4. (**d** and **e**) In- and opposed-phase T1-weighted (T1W) MR images, respectively, show equivocal qualitative suppression of the central aspect of some of these nodules on opposed-phase imaging. (**f**) ECG-gated double inversion recovery (DIR) T2-weighted (T2-W) image shows the thymic nodules to be T2 hyperintense to muscle. (**g** and **h**) A tiny ROI was placed within one of the thymic nodules, initially on the (**g**) opposed-phase image, avoiding marginal India ink artifact; it was then copied and pasted onto the (**h**) in-phase image, yielding mean ROI values of 211 and 272, respectively, and a signal intensity index (SII) of $[(272 - 211)/272] \times 100 = 22\%$, indicating the presence of microscopic fat. This finding and the morphologic appearance of the thymic tissue (clustered nodularity) favor nodular thymic hyperplasia (excess thymic soft tissue for age) over lymphoma. A thymic epithelial tumor (TET) would not present as multiple small, distinct, clustered nodules. Notably, the majority of these nodules are too small to allow for ROI placement within them, without inclusion of India ink artifact at the margin, which could significantly lower the ROI value and pose a risk of misdiagnosis. The susceptibility artifact in the sternum on the MR images is due to sternotomy wires. Separately, note how the susceptibility artifact blooms on the gradient echo images (**d**, **e**, **g**, **h**) and is minimal on the fast spin echo (DIR) T2-WI (**f**)

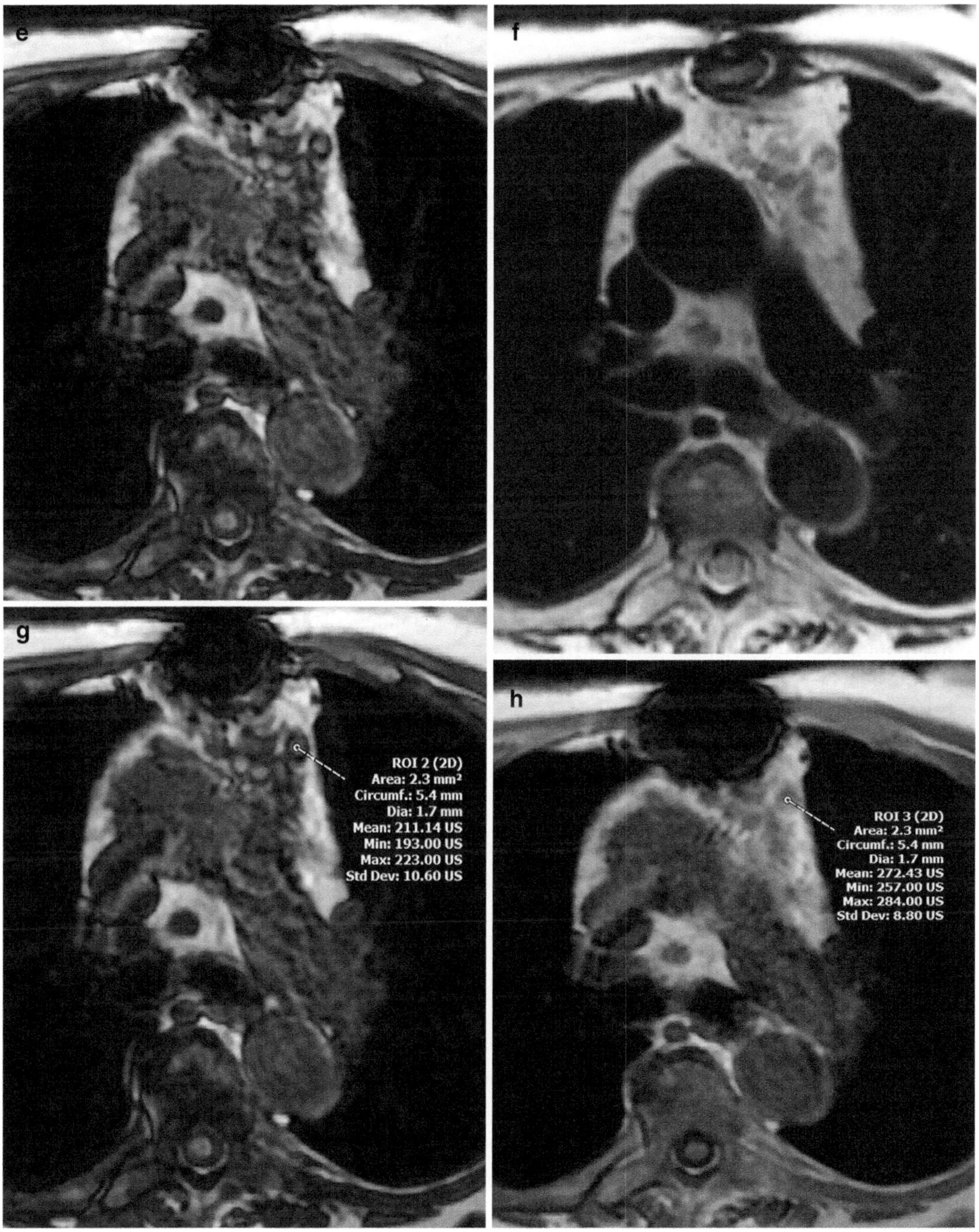

Fig. 1 (continued)

3 Normal Thymus and Thymic Hyperplasia

3.1 Normal Thymus and the Importance of Age for Assessment and Characterization

3.1.1 Location, Morphological and Densitometric/Signal Criteria

- Normal and hyperplastic thymic tissue can be present not only anywhere in the prevascular mediastinum, from thoracic inlet to diaphragm, but also occasionally in the paratracheal space of the visceral mediastinum and in the neck, the latter due to the embryologic path of descent of the thymus from the third pharyngeal pouch in the neck into the prevascular space of the chest.
- Morphology, CT attenuation, and/or MRI signal must all be considered when assessing thymic tissue for benignity.
- Normal thymus exhibits typical morphologic patterns, whether triangular/arrowhead, trapezoidal/quadrilateral, or bipyramidal. The thymus may have straight, concave, or slightly convex margins, depending upon age and individual phenotypes of the gland (Ackman et al. 2013; Francis et al. 1985).
- In humans, the normal thymus reaches maximum weight at puberty and then begins to involute, initially exhibiting microscopic fatty atrophy and, eventually, macroscopic fatty atrophy. By age 40, the thymus is mostly fatty, and by age 60, the thymus is almost completely fatty. Thin, reticulonodular strands of fatty-intercalated thymic tissue may remain, well into the seventh decade, however (Francis et al. 1985; Drabkin et al. 2018). Therefore, the age of the individual must be considered when one is determining whether a given thymus is normal or hyperplastic on imaging (Fig. 2). Of note, rebound thymic hyperplasia and thymic lymphoid hyperplasia can exist without abnormal enlargement or increased mass of the gland, unlike true thymic hyperplasia.
- Fat content:
  - Macroscopic or gross fat, like that found in the subcutaneous fat of the chest wall, is readily discernible by both CT and MRI, with standard fatty attenuation values on CT and with standard T1/T2 hyperintensity and spectral fat suppression on MRI.
  - Microscopic fat, in contradistinction, is not detectable by CT but is discernible by MRI, with the use of in- and opposed-phase T1-weighted chemical shift gradient echo (GRE) imaging. Chemical shift MR imaging identifies the presence of fat and water in the same voxel, the so-called microscopic fat. When microscopic fat is present in tissue, the MRI signal of the lesion suppresses or drops on the opposed-phase image, when compared with the in-phase image. This non-macroscopically fatty component is typically isoattenuating or hypoattenuating to muscle on CT and T1 isointense and T2 hyperintense to muscle on MRI.

    Of note, the signal of macroscopic fat will not suppress on opposed-phase imaging because macroscopic or gross fat is extremely water-poor; hence, sufficient fat and water will not be present in the same voxel of imaged macroscopic fat.
  - Decades earlier, this tissue characterization capability of MRI was demonstrated in the context of adrenal adenomas (Mitchell et al. 1992); more recently, it has been shown to be useful for distinguishing normal and hyperplastic thymus from thymic tumors and lymphoma (Inaoka et al. 2007).
- The CT attenuation and MRI signal of normal thymus and thymic hyperplasia should be homogenous, aside from the presence of any intercalated macroscopic fat amidst thymic tissue. If other forms of signal heterogeneity are found, then the possibility of a concurrent embedded thymic cyst or thymic tumor must be considered and, as always, attention to all

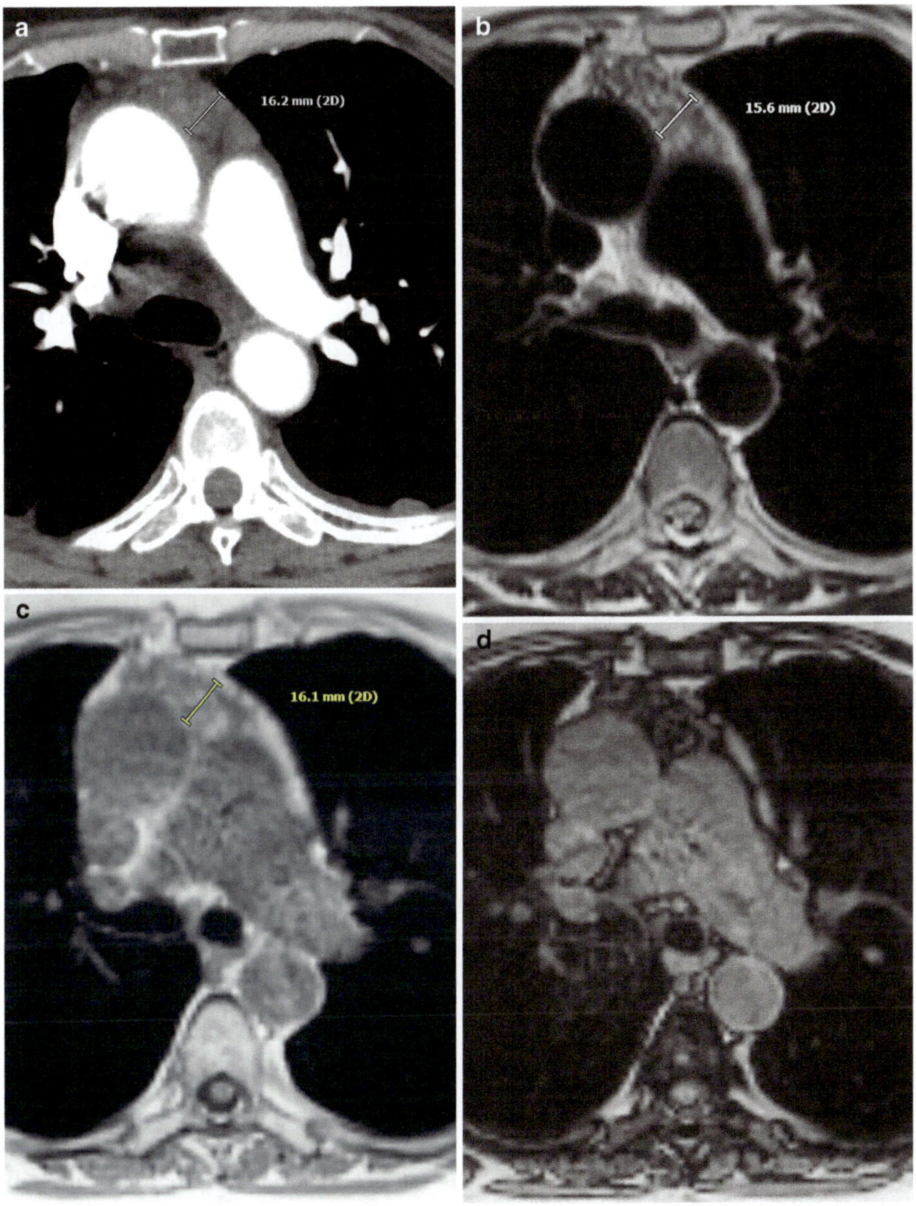

Fig. 2 Seventy-year-old woman with qualitatively suppressing thymic hyperplasia. (**a**) Axial CT with IV contrast showing a maximum thymic lobar thickness (MTLT) measurement of 16 mm, as measured perpendicular to the long axis of the left thymic lobe. (**b**) DIR T2-W image with MTLT measurement of 16 mm. Note that the CT and MRI measurements are the same, as should be expected, provided that the level of inspiratory breath hold is similar between examinations (thymic hyperplasia is soft and pliable). The thymic soft tissue is T2 hyperintense to muscle and is marbled by even more T2-hyperintense tissue, which is isointense to the macroscopic fat in the chest wall. On (**c**) in-phase T1-W imaging, the intercalated macroscopic fat is T1 hyperintense to muscle and T1 isointense to the fat of the chest wall. Note the MTLT measurement of 16 mm on this pulse sequence as well. (**d**) Opposed-phase T1-W image shows a marked, qualitatively appreciable signal suppression of the excess thymic tissue, proving the presence of microscopic fat and that this excess thymic tissue for age represents thymic hyperplasia. (**e**) Postcontrast fat-saturated T1-W imaging shows expected enhancement of this living, cellular tissue, which is not appreciable to the naked eye on the corresponding CT. Had these thymic findings been present in a 20–30-year-old individual, rather than this older woman, they would have indicated normal thymus, rather than thymic hyperplasia

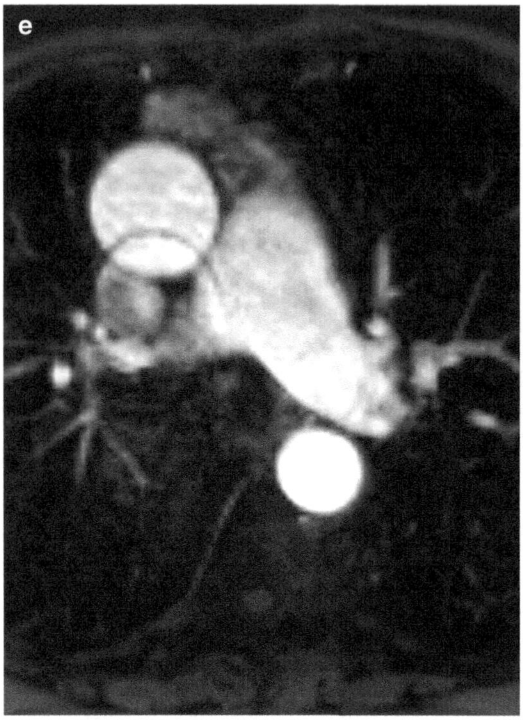

Fig. 2 (continued)

MRI pulse sequences/imaging series is needed to sort this out.

- Enhancement of normal and hyperplastic thymic tissue is readily appreciable by MRI, though not by CT, secondary to the higher soft tissue contrast capabilities of MRI. Table 1 provides the basic components of a thymus MRI protocol.

3.1.2 Maximum Thymic Lobar Thickness (MTLT) and Its Implications

- In 1982, Baron et al. (1982) proposed a standard means of measuring the thymus on 10 mm collimation axial CT, defining thymic width as the long axis of each lobe and maximum thymic lobar thickness (MTLT) as the short axis of each lobe. That is, *the MTLT is measured perpendicular to the long axis of each lobe*. These measurements *differ* from strictly transverse (TRV) and anteroposterior (AP) measurements of the gland, which are often performed in clinical practice, for which no useful cutoff values for normal versus abnormal have been proposed. Araki et al. found intraobserver and interobserver agreement of various thymic measurement parameters on CT to be the poorest for MTLT, with an intraobserver agreement for right and left lobe thickness of 0.61 and 0.65 and with an interobserver agreement for right and left lobe thickness of 0.56 and 0.59, respectively (Araki et al. 2014a). Agreement was better for TRV and AP diameters and what they termed thymic lobe "length," a parameter previously called "width" by Baron et al. in 1982. It is therefore essential to know how to measure the MTLT to use the proposed cutoff values in the literature for distinguishing normal thymus from thymic hyperplasia as a function of age, to avoid the risk of misinterpretation.
- Baron et al. found normal MTLT to be less than or equal to 1.3 cm in all patients over age 20 years. A subsequent study of 20–30-year-old men and women by Ackman et al. 21 years later, employing multidetector CT at 2–2.5 mm slice thickness, found a sex difference in thymic appearance, with the normal thymus of young woman tending to be fuller, more quadrilateral in shape, and of higher CT attenuation than that of men (Ackman et al. 2013), risking misinterpretation as thymic hyperplasia or tumor. This finding infers a slower rate of fatty atrophy in women than men, with potential immunologic implications. The same study also found the MTLT to be greater in the 20–30-year age group than the 1.3 cm cutoff proposed earlier by Baron et al. The new proposed upper limit of normal, allowing for 2 standard deviations (SDs), was found to be $\leq$1.6 cm for triangular thymuses and $\leq$2.2 cm for quadrilateral thymuses in these young adults. An MTLT greater than these values, in the setting of appropriate morphology, CT attenuation, and/or MRI signal, indicates thymic hyperplasia, as opposed to normal thymus.
- When measuring the MTLT, caliper placement must therefore adapt to the shape of the gland. Figure 3 illustrates how to measure

Table 1 Thymus MR imaging protocol

Pulse sequence[a–c]	Acquisition time[d]
BH[e] 3-plane localizer	20 s[f] acquisition
BH axial SSFP[g] water-WI	13 s acquisition
BH axial in- and opposed-phase T1-WI[h]	20 s per acquisition
BH axial ECG-gated[i] double IR[j] T2-WI[k]	20 s *per slice*
BH precontrast axial and sagittal 3D[l] ultrafast GRE[m] fat-sat[n] T1-WI	20 s per acquisition
BH postcontrast[o] 3D ultrafast GRE fat-sat DCE[p] T1-WI at 20 s, 1 min, 3 min, 5 min (all axial, except at 3 min with sagittal plane[q])	20 s per dynamic run
Optional RTr[r], radially acquired T2-WI, instead of double IR T2-WI	≤105 s for coverage of ½ chest
Optional BH or RTr DWI[s] with ADC[t] map with *b* values of 50, 400, 800 s/mm^2	25 s for BH acq, 300–480 s for RTr acq for 10 or 25 slices, respectively
Optional BH or RTr fat-sat T2-WI of desired type	A function of pulse sequence selection

[a] No TR, TE, flip angle, or NEX information has been provided because these vary per examination based on MRI vendor and hardware and software platforms and would therefore be unnecessarily constraining and inaccurate
[b] Default slice thickness for pulse sequences = 4 mm, except for diffusion-weighted imaging (DWI)—5 mm slices
[c] Coils = torso coil, cardiac coil, or interlocking neck and torso coils as needed, depending upon lesion location, to ensure that lesion is in the center of coil (good signal-to-noise ratio or SNR) and absence of phase wrap
[d] Acquisition times are provided for 1.5 Tesla (T) scanners—they can be significantly shorter on 3 T scanners and with software upgrades
[e] *BH* breath hold—all breath holds should be ≤20 s
[f] *s* seconds
[g] *SSFP* Steady-state free precession, a white-blood balanced gradient echo (GRE) sequence (GE/Siemens/Philips acronyms = FIESTA/True FISP/b-FFE)
[h] *T1WI* T1-weighted imaging
[i] *ECG-gated* electrocardiogram-gated
[j] *Double IR* double inversion recovery = black-blood imaging; in general, double-IR T2-weighted imaging should be of lesion only because it takes significantly longer to acquire than the other listed pulse sequences and is labor-intensive from a breath-hold standpoint (20 s per slice, rather than for the whole stack or acquisition). Recommend substituting respiratory-triggered (RTr) radially acquired T2-WI for default DIR T2-WI when more than 10–14 slices are needed to image a given lesion, because RTr imaging is passive and does not require serial breath-hold efforts by the patient
[k] *T2WI* T2-weighted imaging
[l] *3D* 3-dimensional
[m] *GRE* gradient echo
[n] *Fat sat* fat saturated (spectral fat saturation, unless pre/post-DCE imaging is performed with Dixon technique, in which case fat saturation is the result of automated post-processing of initially acquired in- and opposed-phase images)
[o] Intravenous (IV) contrast: 20 cc of ionic, macrocyclic gadolinium such as gadoterate meglumine
[p] *DCE* dynamic contrast-enhanced imaging with GE/Siemens/Philips acronyms LAVA/VIBE/THRIVE or LAVA Flex/Dixon/mDixon—latter Dixon techniques are preferable to avert poor fat saturation around thymic lesions on some scanners
[q] Planes can be altered to optimize evaluation of a particular mass as needed. The proposed planes meet the need of the most prevascular mediastinal/thymic imaging. A third plane can be added precontrast and for postcontrast DCE at 6 min if needed; for example, for surgical planning
[r] *RTr* respiratory-triggered—recommend exchanging RTr radially acquired T2-WI for default DIR T2-WI when more than 10–14 slices are needed to image a given lesion, because RTr imaging is passive and does not require serial breath-hold efforts by the patient. If assessment of pericardial and myocardial invasion is needed, ECG-gated DIR T2-WI can be performed exclusively over the area of interest, to keep breath holds to a minimum and reduce examination acquisition time
[s] *DWI* diffusion-weighted imaging
[t] *ADC* apparent diffusion coefficient

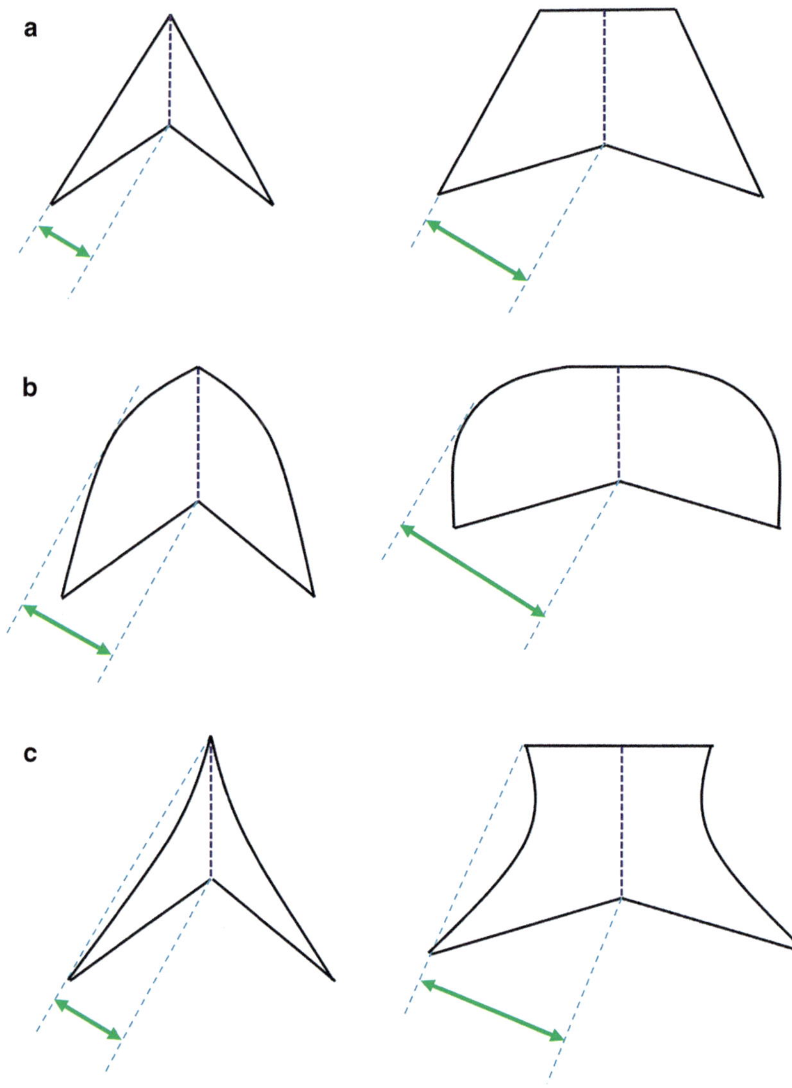

Fig. 3 Measurement of maximum thymic lobar thickness (MTLT) and its adaptation to different thymic shapes, (**a**, straight; **b**, convex; and **c**, concave lateral margins). This measurement is acquired from a line drawn perpendicular to the long axis of the larger of the two thymic lobes (green arrows). When the lobes are inseparable from each other on imaging, then an anteroposteriorly oriented line (dashed purple line) can be drawn to bisect the gland; the MTLT can then be acquired perpendicular to the long axis of the thicker of the two sides. The occasional unilobar thymus must be recognized, in which case, no bisection is needed and the MTLT can be obtained in the axis perpendicular to the long axis of this single lobe. (Diagram modified from Ackman JB et al., Radiology, 2013 (Ackman et al. 2013))

the MTLT, as a function of thymic morphology. Figures 2 and 4 provide in situ examples. It is important to be aware that normal thymus and thymic hyperplasia are malleable soft tissue, so their morphology and thickness can vary to some extent with differences in inspiratory (and expiratory) effort; small differences in measurement between same-day imaging studies can therefore simply be due to the phase of the respiratory cycle in which the images were acquired.

3.2 Thymic Hyperplasia

3.2.1 General Points and Issues

- There are two main histopathological types of thymic hyperplasia—true thymic hyperplasia and thymic lymphoid hyperplasia.
  - True thymic hyperplasia describes greater thymic mass than expected for age and is histopathologically normal.

    Rebound thymic hyperplasia is also histopathologically normal and is therefore

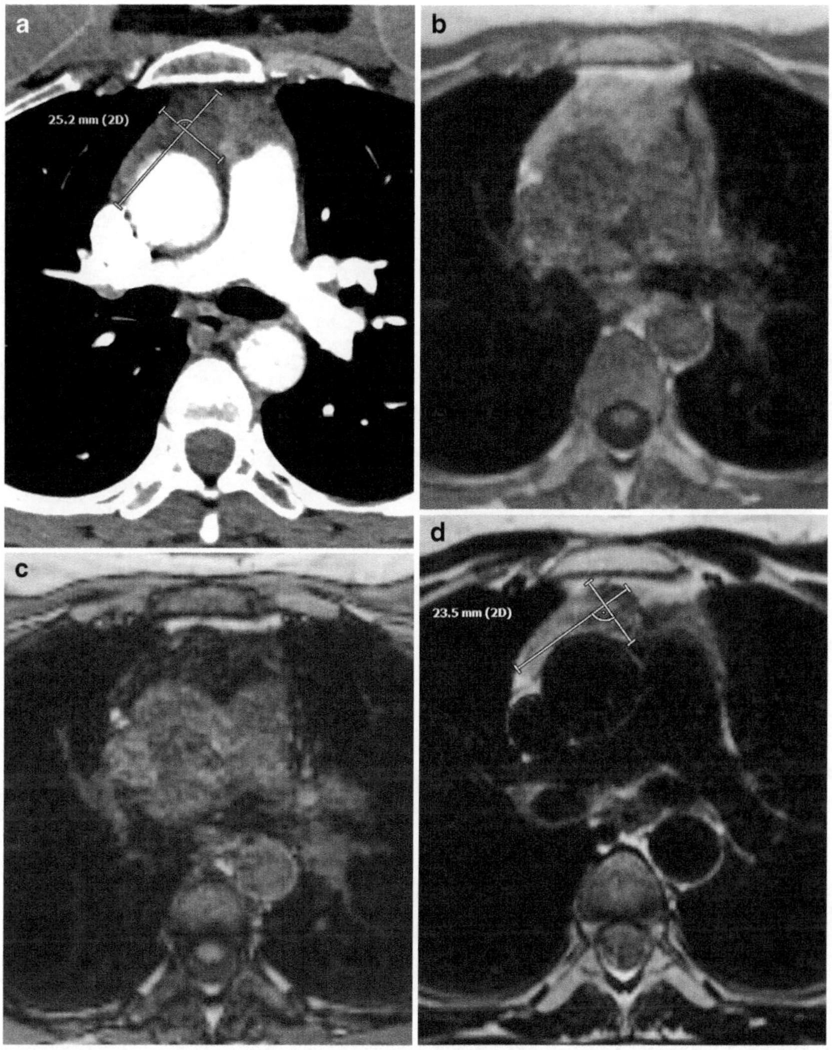

Fig. 4 Thirty-eight-year-old woman with a history of breast cancer—qualitatively suppressing thymic hyperplasia of 25 mm maximum thymic lobar thickness (MTLT). (**a**) Axial CT with IV contrast shows excess thymic tissue for age (by age 38, the thymic tissue should be more macroscopically fatty), with quadrilateral morphology and an MTLT of 25 mm, as measured perpendicular to the long axis of the larger of the two thymic lobes (right lobe). (**b** and **c**) Axial in- and opposed-phase T1-W MR images (performed 5 months later), respectively, show qualitative signal suppression or "signal dropout" throughout the thymic tissue on the opposed-phase image, indicating the presence of microscopic fat and proving this thymic tissue to represent thymic hyperplasia, rather than lymphoma or an advanced thymic epithelial tumor. (**d**) Measurement of the MTLT on the ECG-gated double inversion recovery (DIR) T2-W MR image shows it to be similar (24 mm) to that obtained on the preceding CT. While no calculations are needed to prove the presence of microscopic fat in this case, on account of qualitative signal suppression, appreciable to the naked eye, they have been performed for demonstration purposes. (**e** and **f**) ROI placement on thymic tissue and a nonfatty chest wall muscle on the same image for chemical shift ratio (CSR) calculation on the in-phase (**e**) and opposed-phase images (**f**), respectively—an ROI was placed over an area of relatively higher signal in the thymic tissue on the opposed-phase image (**f**) first. The operator then copied and pasted it onto the in-phase image (**e**), eliciting an ROI of the same size, shape, and location. The same copy-paste method was used to procure ROIs of the same size, shape, and location over nonfatty chest wall musculature on the in- and opposed-phase images. The resultant CSR $= 32/95 \div 124/94 = 0.34/1.32 = 0.3$ proves the presence of microscopic fat in the area sampled. (**g** and **h**) ROI placement on thymic tissue only on the in (**g**)- and opposed (**h**)-phase images for the signal intensity index (SII) calculation. The SII $= [(124 - 32)/124] \times 100 = 74\%$; that is, there is a 74% reduction in signal between the in- and opposed-phase images, again proving the presence of microscopic fat in the area sampled and confirming the excess thymic tissue to represent thymic hyperplasia

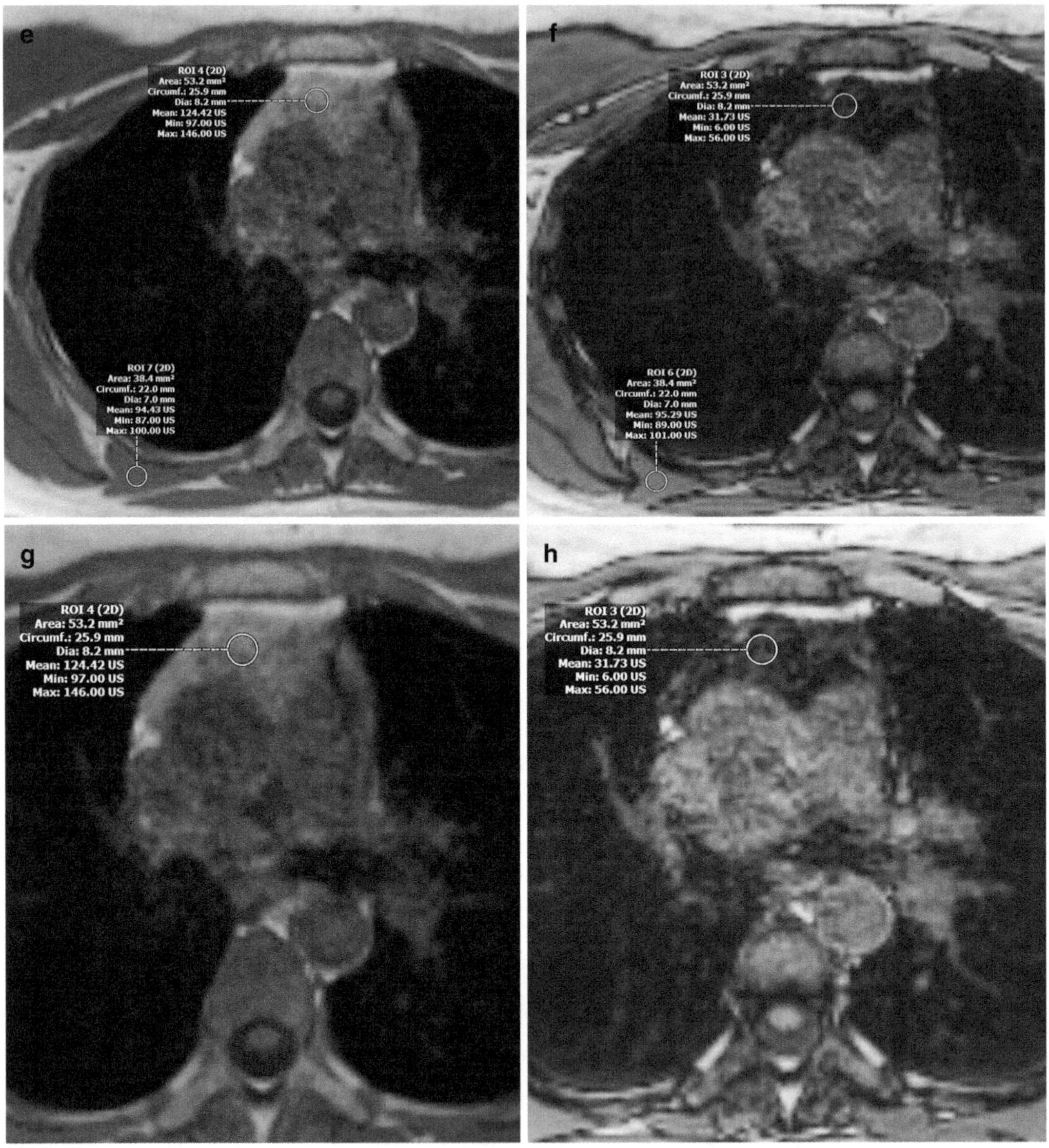

Fig. 4 (continued)

a form of true hyperplasia. It refers to rapid re-emergence of thymic tissue after suppression by various thymic insults, including chemotherapy, radiation therapy, infection, burns, and surgery; it may or may not be of greater mass than expected for age, however.

– By contrast, thymic lymphoid hyperplasia is histopathologically abnormal, exhibiting more germinal centers than expected for age (Goldblum et al. 2018).

- CT attenuation values greater than 41 HU on contrast-enhanced CT have been proposed as indicative of thymic lymphoid hyperplasia, rather than true thymic hyperplasia (Araki et al. 2014b). However, the 41 HU cutoff value was derived from a small sample of 15 patients, and because CT contrast medium bolus timing and enhancement vary and are to some degree dependent on the individual patient's cardiac function, it should only be used, if at all, to favor one form of hyperplasia over the other. It should not be considered diagnostic. Experientially, lymphoid follicular hyperplasia has been histopathologically diagnosed in the setting of predominantly fatty thymus on CT at our quaternary referral institution.

- Chemical shift MRI has been proven to be useful for distinguishing normal and hyperplastic thymus from thymic tumors and lymphoma (Inaoka et al. 2007; Priola et al. 2015) and will be discussed in the next section.

3.2.2 Chemical Shift MR Imaging: The Chemical Shift Ratio (CSR) and the Signal Intensity Index (SII)

- Chemical shift MR imaging refers to in- and opposed-phase gradient echo T1-weighted imaging.
  In the chest, it is performed with breath-hold technique. On a 1.5 Tesla (1.5 T) MRI scanner, two-dimensional (2D) in- and opposed-phase imaging delivers high-quality T1-weighted imaging over a ≤ 20-s breath hold. On a 3 Tesla (3 T) MRI scanner, three-dimensional (3D) in- and opposed-phase MR imaging must be performed to ensure appropriate time-to-echo (TE) selection for the CSR and SII calculations, which depend upon it.
- It is important to be aware that chemical shift MR imaging distinguishes normal and hyperplastic thymus from thymic tumors and lymphoma in most, *but not all*, adults. Non-suppressing thymic hyperplasia has been reported in young adults, especially young women, as the thymic tissue in these instances may not contain sufficient fat to suppress (Inaoka et al. 2007; Priola et al. 2015; Ackman et al. 2012, 2013). Chemical shift MRI should *not* be used to make this distinction in the pediatric population because of insufficient fatty atrophy in this age group. If the thymic tissue does not suppress but exhibits normal MRI signal and is thymiform, even if bulging or abundant, another MRI tool can be used to assist in distinguishing benign thymus from tumor, both in adults and in the pediatric population—specifically, diffusion-weighted imaging (DWI) with apparent diffusion coefficient (ADC) mapping (Priola et al. 2018), which will be discussed further in a subsequent section of this chapter.
- When there is qualitative suppression of the thymiform thymic tissue on opposed-phase imaging, no semiquantitative means of detecting microscopic fat is needed (Figs. 2 and 4). When there is absent *qualitative* suppression of thymic tissue on chemical shift MR imaging, there have been two proposed means of *quantifying* signal loss between in- and opposed-phase imaging in order to detect smaller amounts of microscopic fat than appreciable to the unaided eye. The first proposed method is a calculation of the chemical shift ratio (CSR) (Inaoka et al. 2007), and the second is a calculation of the signal intensity index (SII) (Priola et al. 2015). These calculation methods are described in subsequent Sects. 3.2.3 and 3.2.4 and are briefly summarized here:
  - A CSR calculation can be performed whether the in- and opposed-phase images have been acquired sequentially or simultaneously, the latter, by necessity, in a single breath hold. This ratio of ROI values in thymus and muscle on the same image provides for ROI standardization and averts misregistration issues resulting from sequential breath-hold acquisitions.
  - The SII calculation should only be performed if the in- and opposed-phase MR images were acquired in a single breath hold by dual-echo technique, which averts misregistration issues. When chemical shift MRI is acquired by dual-echo technique, the SII calculation is practically

preferable to the CSR calculation because it requires placement of two, rather than four, ROIs and is therefore less prone to error.

3.2.3 Chemical Shift Ratio (CSR) Calculation

- Given the increased availability and prevalence of *dual-echo* chemical shift MR imaging in current MRI software packages, it is best to reserve the performance of the CSR calculation for the increasingly rare instance in which it is not available and the in- and opposed-phase T1-weighted MR images are acquired with separate breath holds (that is not by dual-echo technique). The ROI placement on musculature in the same image that it requires provides a reference standard and allows for normalization of the thymic ROI value. As mentioned earlier, procurement of the CSR requires proper placement of twice the number of ROIs, increasing the risk of ROI placement error, incorrect divisors and dividends, and thereby an incorrect quotient, with resultant increased risk of diagnostic error. Therefore, care must be taken not only with how and where to place the ROIs on the thymic tissue, but also how and where to place them on the chest wall musculature, when obtaining a CSR.
  - ROIs of the same size and shape should be placed on both the thymic tissue of interest and on the most robust, nonfatty paraspinal muscle or other nonfatty chest wall muscle at the same level of the in- and out-of-phase MRI series (usually the same table position), avoiding chemical shift (India ink) artifact at the interface between macroscopic fat and water-containing soft tissue and any other artifacts (Fig. 4).
  - It is best to position the ROIs on the opposed-phase image first, avoiding the black lines of chemical shift or India ink artifact in the thymus and the chest wall muscle.

    If the low signal of the India ink artifact at the margins is averaged into the ROI value, the ROI value will be markedly reduced and will not accurately reflect the amount of fat within the thymic tissue (Fig. 2).
  - In some PACS, these ROIs can be subsequently copied and pasted onto the in-phase image, better assuring ROIs of the same size, shape, and location. Occasionally, this copy-paste method does not place ROIs precisely, and manual correction is needed.
- If the thymic tissue exhibits variable T1-weighted signal, it is important to assess the tissue of highest T1-weighted signal on the opposed-phase images, in addition to the most suppressing tissue, examining the range of CSRs. While the higher T1 signal tissue on the opposed-phase images is most apt to represent less atrophied thymic tissue, it can alternatively represent a benign thymic cyst or a thymic epithelial tumor (TET) embedded within thymic hyperplasia. Usually, the variability of suppression on opposed-phase images is due to variable or heterogeneous fatty atrophy within the gland, however, rather than coincident diagnoses. Benign thymic cysts, when embedded within normal thymus and thymic hyperplasia, would not be expected to suppress on opposed-phase MR imaging, as they typically do not contain microscopic fat, in contradistinction to dermoid cysts which can suppress. Evaluation of the signal characteristics of the non-suppressing tissue on the other MRI pulse sequences, including pre- and post-contrast dynamic contrast-enhanced imaging, will further assist in differentiation of normal and hyperplastic thymus, benign thymic cysts, and thymic tumors, with or without cystic or necrotic components.
- The CSR is reported as a decimal number. Inaoka et al. (2007) introduced the use of CSR for thymic evaluation and found that a CSR less than or equal to 0.7 indicates the presence of microscopic fat and is diagnostic of normal or hyperplastic thymus, provided that locational, morphologic, and signal criteria are also met. Priola et al. (2015) subsequently found that a CSR less than or equal to 0.8 is

effective for this distinction, with a sensitivity and specificity of 100% and 96.7%, respectively. A CSR greater than or equal to 1.0 signifies tumor in most, but not all, cases in the adult population. CSRs between these numbers are indeterminate.

$$\mathrm{CSR} = \left[\left(\mathrm{OP\,SI\,thymus} \div \mathrm{OP\,SI\,chest\ wall\ muscle}\right)\right] / \left[\left(\mathrm{IP\,SI\,thymus} \div \mathrm{IP\,SI\,chest\ wall\ muscle}\right)\right]$$

IP = in-phase
OP = opposed-phase
SI = signal intensity as measured by ROI
CSR $\leq$ 0.8 indicates normal/hyperplastic thymus
CSR $\geq$ 1.0 indicates tumor, in *most but not all* adults
CSR = 0.9 is indeterminate

3.2.4 Signal Intensity Index (SII) Calculation

- The signal intensity index (SII) is simply a measure of the percentage signal dropout of the thymic tissue of interest between the in- and opposed-phase MR images.
- It does not require a standardization reference within the same image because it is only applicable to chemical shift MRI acquired by *dual-echo* technique.
- It therefore solely requires ROI placement on the thymic tissue of interest, not on a reference skeletal muscle (Fig. 4).
- The method for ROI placement for procurement of the SII is the same as described for the CSR, with the exception that it exclusively requires ROI placement on the thymic tissue, not on chest wall musculature. The SII is reported as a percentage. An SII greater than or equal to 9% indicates the presence of microscopic fat and is diagnostic of normal or hyperplastic thymus, with a sensitivity of 100% and specificity of 100% (Priola et al. 2015), provided that morphologic and other MRI signal criteria are also met:

$$\mathrm{SII} = \left(\left[\left(\mathrm{IP\,SI\,thymus} - \mathrm{OP\,SI\,thymus}\right)\right]\right) / \left(\mathrm{IP\,SI\,thymus}\right) \times 100$$

IP = in-phase
OP = opposed-phase
SI = signal intensity, as measured by ROI
SII $\geq$ 9% = normal thymus or thymic hyperplasia, rather than tumor, in most, *but not all*, adults

3.2.5 Apparent Diffusion Coefficient (ADC) Mapping and Procurement of the ADC Value

- If the thymic tissue of interest exhibits features on CT and/or MRI resembling thymic hyperplasia but does not suppress on opposed-phase MR imaging, diffusion-weighted imaging with ADC mapping can serve as an adjunctive mean of distinguishing normal and hyperplastic thymus from tumor (Fig. 5). While all tissues except water restrict the diffusion of water molecules to some degree, these benign entities restrict water diffusion far less than thymic epithelial tumors and lymphoma. In a study comparing 9–29-year-old subjects with non-suppressing normal thymus on chemical shift MRI to those with prevascular mediastinal lymphoma, Priola et al. found a significant difference in mean ADC value and no overlap in ADC value between the two groups, with mean ADC values of $2.48 \pm 0.38 \times 10^{-3}$ mm²/s and $1.24 \pm 0.23 \times 10^{-3}$ mm²/s, respectively (Priola et al. 2018). Therefore, if non-suppressing thymic tissue resembling thymic hyperplasia on other MRI pulse sequences demonstrates an ADC value in the 2.5 ± 0.4 range, it should represent thymic hyperplasia, rather than lymphoma or a thymic epithelial tumor (Priola et al. 2018; Abdel Razek et al. 2014). The diffusion-weighted images used to create the ADC map should show greater signal *decay* or reduction with increasing *b* values and thereby increased diffusion weighting if the thymic tissue is benign.

- DWI can be performed in a variety of ways. However, in the chest, for a more reliable result, DWI should be performed with breath-hold or respiratory-triggered technique to minimize the compromising effect of movement of the lesion on the accuracy of the ADC map. Construction of the most accurate ADC map would require an infinite number of *b* values; however, this is not clinically practicable. The more numerous the *b* values, the longer the image acquisition time. The minimum practical number of *b* values to ensure a clinically useful ADC map is three, though some believe that two *b* values are sufficient. We use *b* values of 50, 400, and 800 s/mm^2. The *b* values employed for respiratory-triggered DWI in the above-discussed Abdel Razek et al. study were 0, 150, 500, and 800 s/mm^2 (Abdel Razek et al. 2014). A maximum *b* value of 800 s/mm^2 is sufficiently diffusion-weighted and yields reasonable image quality. *B* values greater than 800 s/mm^2, including 1000 s/

Fig. 5 Twenty-nine-year-old man with non-suppressing thymic hyperplasia that regressed and suppressed 2 years later (**a–i** images from 2019, **j–n** images from 2021). (**a**) CT with IV contrast shows excess, mass-like, isoattenuating soft tissue in the thymic bed with a maximum thymic lobar thickness (MTLT), as measured perpendicular to the long axis of the left thymic lobe, of 29 mm. (**b** and **c**) Double inversion recovery (DIR) T2-W and in-phase T1-W MR images show the lesion to be T2 hyperintense and T1 isointense to muscle. (**d**) Opposed-phase T1-W MR imaging shows no qualitative suppression of the tissue. (**e** and **f**) ROIs, initially placed over the area of highest signal within the thymic tissue on the opposed-phase image and then copied and pasted onto the in-phase image, yielded values of 111 and 104, respectively, resulting in a signal intensity index (SII) of $[(104 - 111)/104] \times 100 = -7\%$; the standard deviations of the ROI measurements were 6 and 5, respectively. Thus, there was no discernible microscopic fat in this tissue. Prior to ADC mapping, the differential diagnosis included non-suppressing thymic hyperplasia, a high-risk thymic epithelial tumor (TET), and lymphoma (though no lymphadenopathy was present elsewhere, lowering the likelihood of latter diagnosis). (**g**) A postcontrast 3D ultrafast GRE fat-saturated T1-W image acquired 5 min after IV contrast administration shows this tissue to enhance markedly. Note that the enhancement of this tissue is not appreciable on CT secondary to a combination of the lower soft tissue contrast of CT and the earlier phase of the contrast bolus at which this standard chest CT was acquired. (**h** and **i**) The ADC map, created by breath-hold diffusion-weighted imaging (BH DWI) with *b* values of 50, 400, and 800, showed the lesion to be markedly hyperintense overall, indicating the absence of qualitatively restricted diffusion throughout most of the lesion and strongly favoring non-suppressing thymic hyperplasia over lymphoma and a TET. Nevertheless, there were scattered, multifocal areas of low ADC signal amidst the generalized hyperintensity, such that ROI sampling yielded ADC values of 2.8, 1.1, 1.9, 2.7, and 0.6×10^{-3} mm²/s. This broad range of ADC values, suggesting both nonsignificantly restricted and significantly restricted areas, highlights the hazard of ascribing too much credibility to individual ADC values. In this particular case, the combination of the fairly homogenous signal of this tissue on all other pulse sequences, its morphology, the lack of lymphadenopathy elsewhere, and the overall qualitative lack of restricted diffusion strongly favored non-suppressing thymic hyperplasia over tumor. The patient therefore underwent annual MRI surveillance. Two years later, in 2021, the amount of thymic tissue had significantly decreased, with an MTLT of 15 mm on the (**j**) DIR T2-W image. (**k** and **l**) In- and opposed-phase T1-W MR imaging showed qualitative suppression of tissue signal on the opposed-phase image. (**m** and **n**) ROI placement, initially on the least suppressing tissue on the opposed-phase image (**n**) and then copied and pasted onto the in-phase image (**m**), was expectedly confirmatory, yielding an SII of $[(114 - 80)/114] \times 100 = 30\%$ and proving the presence of microscopic fat within the least suppressing thymic tissue. These findings indicate intervally-regressed thymic hyperplasia. The man's thymus was now within normal limits for age

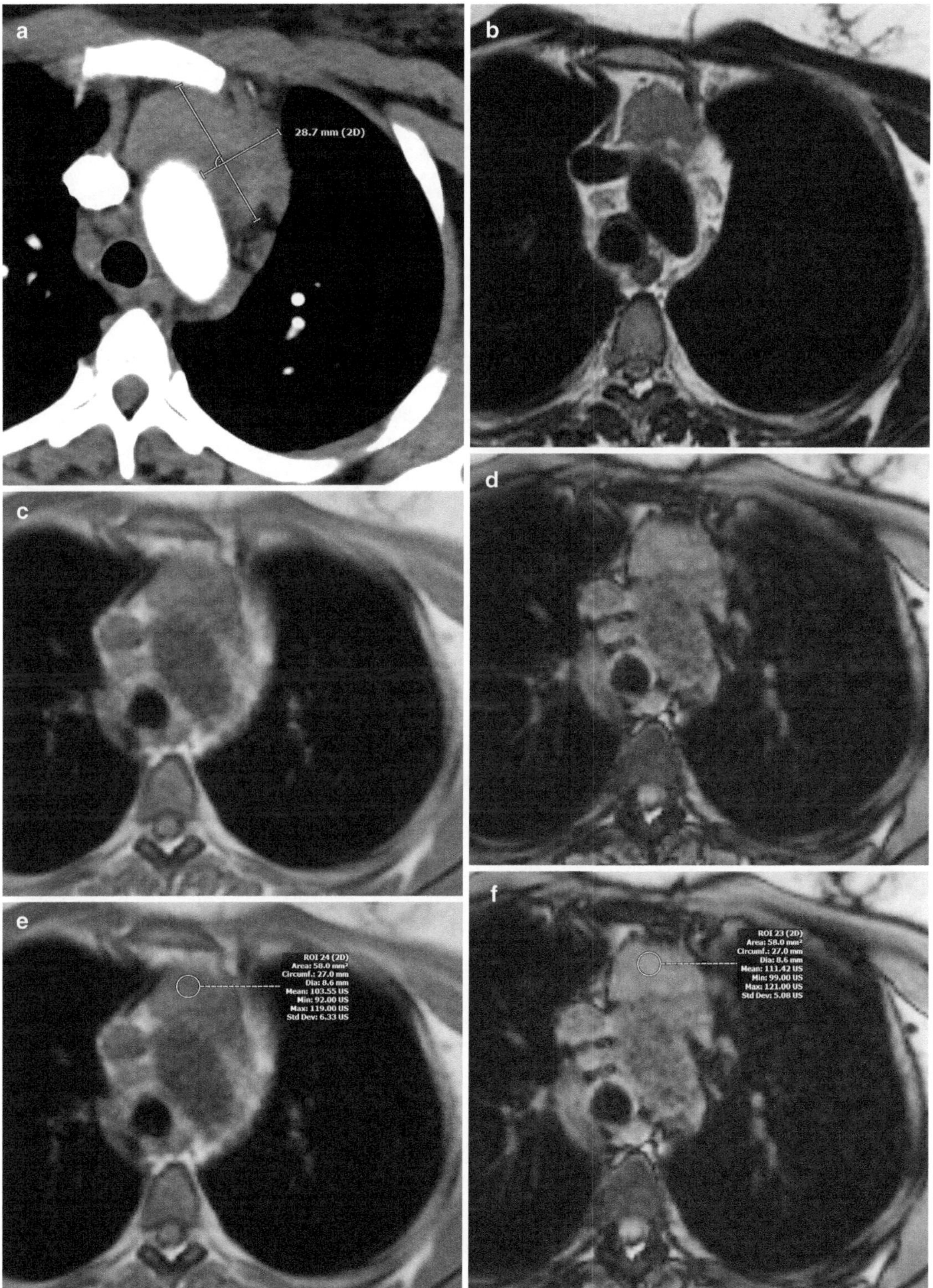
a
28.7 mm (2D)
b
c
d
e
ROI 24 (2D)
Area: 58.0 mm²
Circumf.: 27.0 mm
Dia: 8.6 mm
Mean: 103.55 US
Min: 92.00 US
Max: 119.00 US
Std Dev: 6.33 US
f
ROI 23 (2D)
Area: 58.0 mm²
Circumf.: 27.0 mm
Dia: 8.6 mm
Mean: 111.42 US
Min: 99.00 US
Max: 121.00 US
Std Dev: 5.08 US

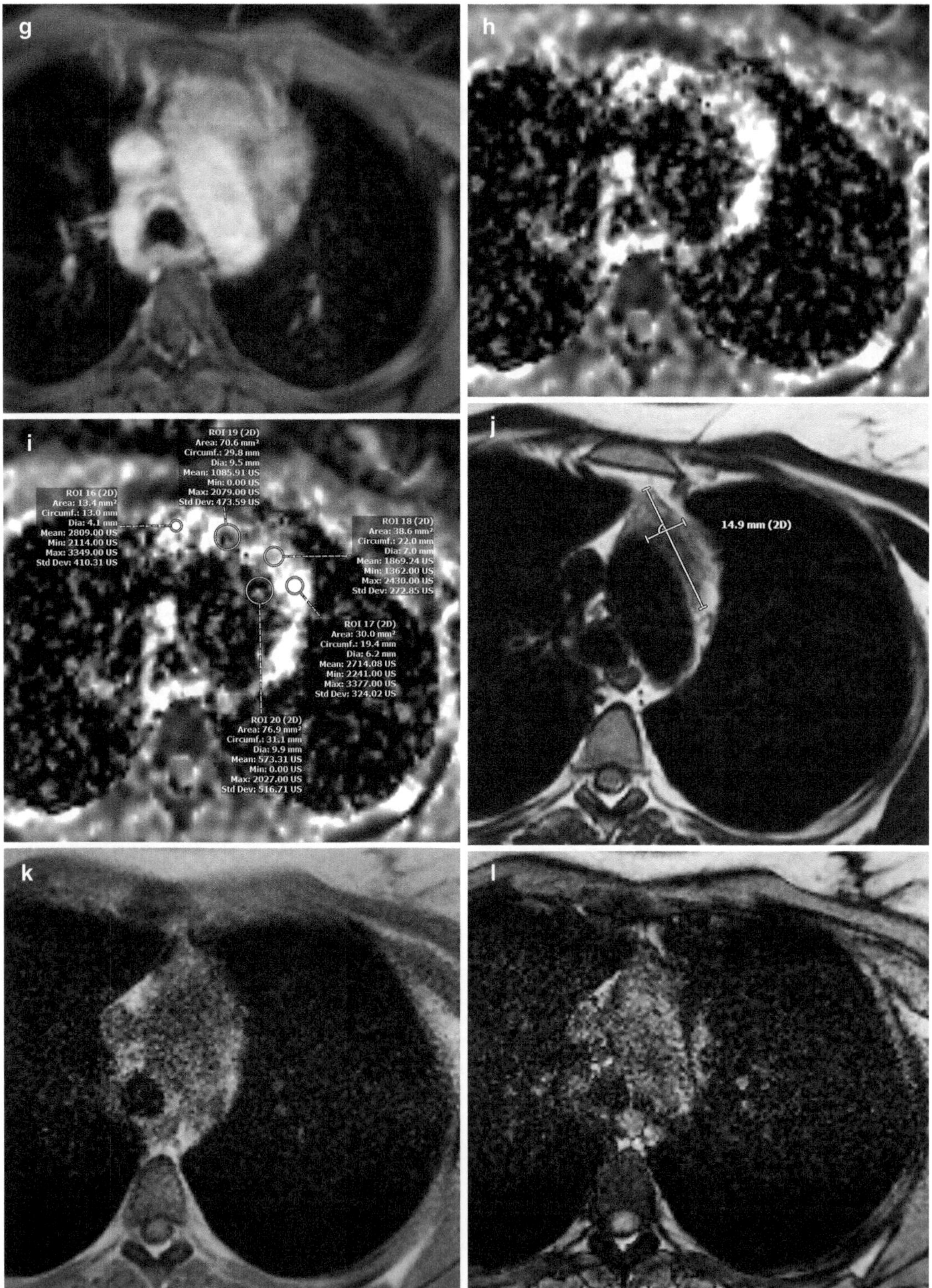

Fig. 5 (continued)

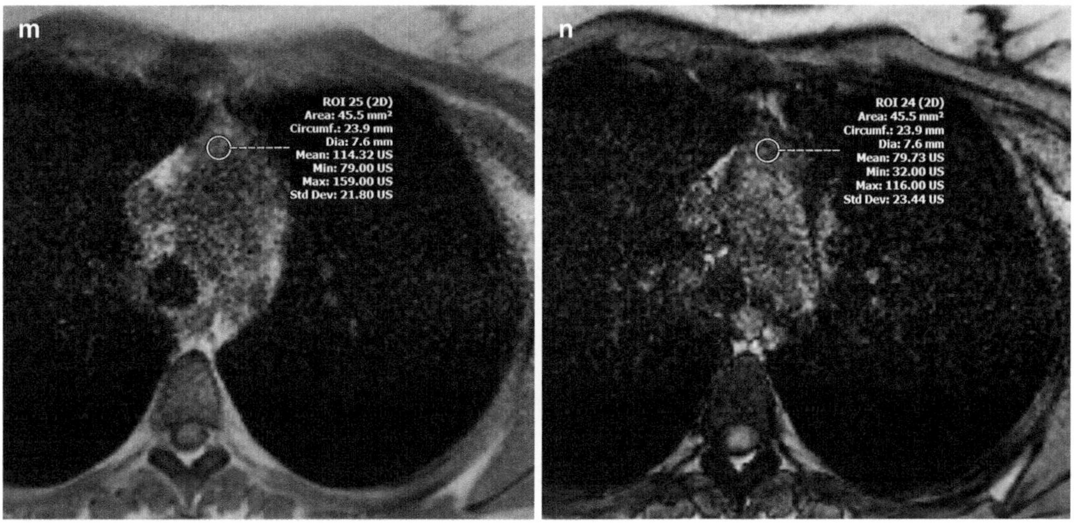

Fig. 5 (continued)

mm^2, often yield poor-quality images, on account of their lower signal-to-noise ratio (SNR) and greater artifact potential. These poorer quality images risk misinterpretation.

- While free breathing yields surprisingly readable diffusion-weighted images in the chest, it can provide inaccurate assessment of the diffusion restriction within tissue and thereby yield an *inaccurate* ADC map. This potential for inaccuracy derives from the fact that on an ADC map, signal loss not only occurs in areas of reduced Brownian motion of water molecules, but can also occur (as can signal gain) in areas of bulk motion. There is resultant risk of misdiagnosis of benign lesions as malignant, and malignant lesions as benign, both of which could adversely impact clinical decision-making. In the abdomen, reliable ADC maps have been achieved during free breathing when multiple DWI acquisitions during free breathing are averaged (deSouza et al. 2018); however, this approach must be validated in the chest before deemed clinically reliable, given greater cardiorespiratory motion-related challenges in the chest than in the abdomen. This averaging approach can also lengthen examination acquisition time.
- For ADC assessment, in order to identify the thymic tissue restricting the diffusion of water the most (which usually correlates with the most hypercellular, malignant, aggressive tissue), the ROI should be placed on the thymic tissue with the most (non-artifact-related) hypointense signal, excluding cystic and necrotic areas which approach water in ADC value (the latter are typically markedly ADC hyperintense). The ROI should be sufficiently large to yield a credible representation or sampling of the tissue and avert disproportionate influence by artifacts including image noise, ghosting, respiratory motion, eddy current artifact, and geometric distortion. The procured mean ROI number must then be multiplied by a vendor-specific factor, which is often 10^{-3}, and reported as an ADC value with the suffix "$\times 10^{-3}$ mm^2/s." Figures 5, 6, and 7 provide examples of ROI placement for ADC value acquisition. If the thymic tissue of interest is still indeterminate, both close MRI surveillance in 3–6 months and diagnostic intervention can be reasonable approaches, depending on the level of clinical suspicion.
- ADC values, like many procured numbers in clinical radiology and medicine in general, should not be interpreted in isolation, but instead, in the context of the other imaging findings and the clinical setting (Fig. 5). Proposed cutoff values in the literature for dis-

tinguishing benign from malignant lesions and less aggressive from more aggressive lesions should only be used as rough guides. When DWI has been standardized across vendors and hardware and software platforms for the purpose of investigation, ADC values have been found to be reproducible. Nevertheless, there has yet to be full standardization of diffusion-weighted imaging across vendors and platforms in clinical practice (Malyarenko et al. 2013; Shukla-Dave et al. 2019).

3.2.6 ^{18}FDG PET/CT

- Because of overlap in maximum standard uptake value (SUV_{max}) between thymic hyperplasia and thymic tumors (Kumar et al. 2009), there is general reluctance to rely on ^{18}FDG PET/CT and SUV values to distinguish between normal thymus, thymic hyperplasia, thymic cysts, and thymic tumors including lymphoma (Fig. 1).
  - For example, a mean SUV_{max} of 2.05 ± 0.6 has been reported for normal thymus (Gawande et al. 2012), and mean SUV_{max} values of 3.73 ± 1.22 (Jerushalmi et al. 2009) and 2.89 ± 0.10 (Gawande et al. 2012) have been reported for thymic hyperplasia.
- A range of SUV_{max} values have been reported for low-risk and high-risk thymomas and thymic carcinoma, with higher SUV_{max} values found in high-risk thymoma and thymic carcinoma than in low-risk thymoma (Hephzibah et al. 2014; Endo et al. 2008).
  - For example, a mean SUV_{max} of 4.8 ± 2.0 has been found for low-risk thymomas, 5.5 ± 2.2 for high-risk thymomas, and 11.8 ± 6.7 for thymic carcinomas (Lee et al. 2021).

Fig. 6 Fifty-eight-year-old woman with atypical carcinoid (neuroendocrine) tumor. (**a**) Axial CT with IV contrast shows a large, well-circumscribed, rounded, T1-isointense mass with its epicenter in the right thymic bed. (**b–e**) Axial in-phase T1-W image without and with ROI and opposed-phase T1-W image without and with ROI, respectively, show the mass to be largely T1 isointense to muscle, albeit with some heterogeneity of T1-W signal. An ROI was first placed over an area of relatively higher T1 signal intensity on the opposed-phase image and then copied and pasted onto the in-phase image—note its same size, shape, and location, yielding ROI values of 99 on the in-phase image and 100 on the opposed-phase image and indicating the lack of suppression or lack of microscopic fat in this area. ROIs placed elsewhere (not shown) also indicated nonsuppression of signal on opposed-phase imaging. (**f**) DIR T2-W image reveals the mass to be heterogeneously T2 hyperintense to muscle. Note the lack of T2 isointensity to fat in the areas of T1 isointensity to fat, proving that these areas of the tumor are not composed of macroscopic fat. (**g–k**) Coronal pre- and coronal and sagittal, post-dynamic contrast-enhanced (DCE) images at 20 s, 1 min, 3 min, and 5 min, respectively, with ROIs placed solely over the solid, cellular, most intensely enhancing part of the tumor (avoiding areas of T1-hypointense necrosis), show mean ROIs of 84 (precontrast) and 129, 162, 170, and 166 postcontrast, respectively. Allowing for the standard deviations provided in concert with the mean ROI value in PACS, a roughly constructed temporal peak enhancement curve (in one's mind) shows that the lesion reached peak enhancement within 1 min and plateaued thereafter, out to 5 min. (**l–n**) Axial postcontrast fat-saturated T1-W imaging at 6 min, post-processed subtracted axial image at 6 min, and post-processed subtracted coronal image: post-processed subtracted imaging confirms multifocal areas of low signal or nonenhancement within the mass that represent areas of necrosis. (**o** and **p**) Axial ADC map, without and with ROI of 738, respectively. A mean ROI of 738 on the ADC map yields an ADC value of $738 \div 1000 = 0.7 \times 10^{-3}$ mm^2/s and indicates marked restricted diffusion within this sampled enhancing, cellular component of the tumor. While the combination of tumor location, morphology, and rapid time-to-peak enhancement would suggest a low-risk thymoma, the very low ADC value or marked water restriction of the tumor is discordant with this diagnosis and favors a more aggressive lesion. Indeed, the mass was a neuroendocrine tumor, rather than a thymoma. Neuroendocrine or carcinoid tumors in the prevascular mediastinum are notoriously more aggressive than their counterparts in the lung (Fukai et al. 1999; Sullivan and Weksler 2017). Black arrows point to the ROIs in the images

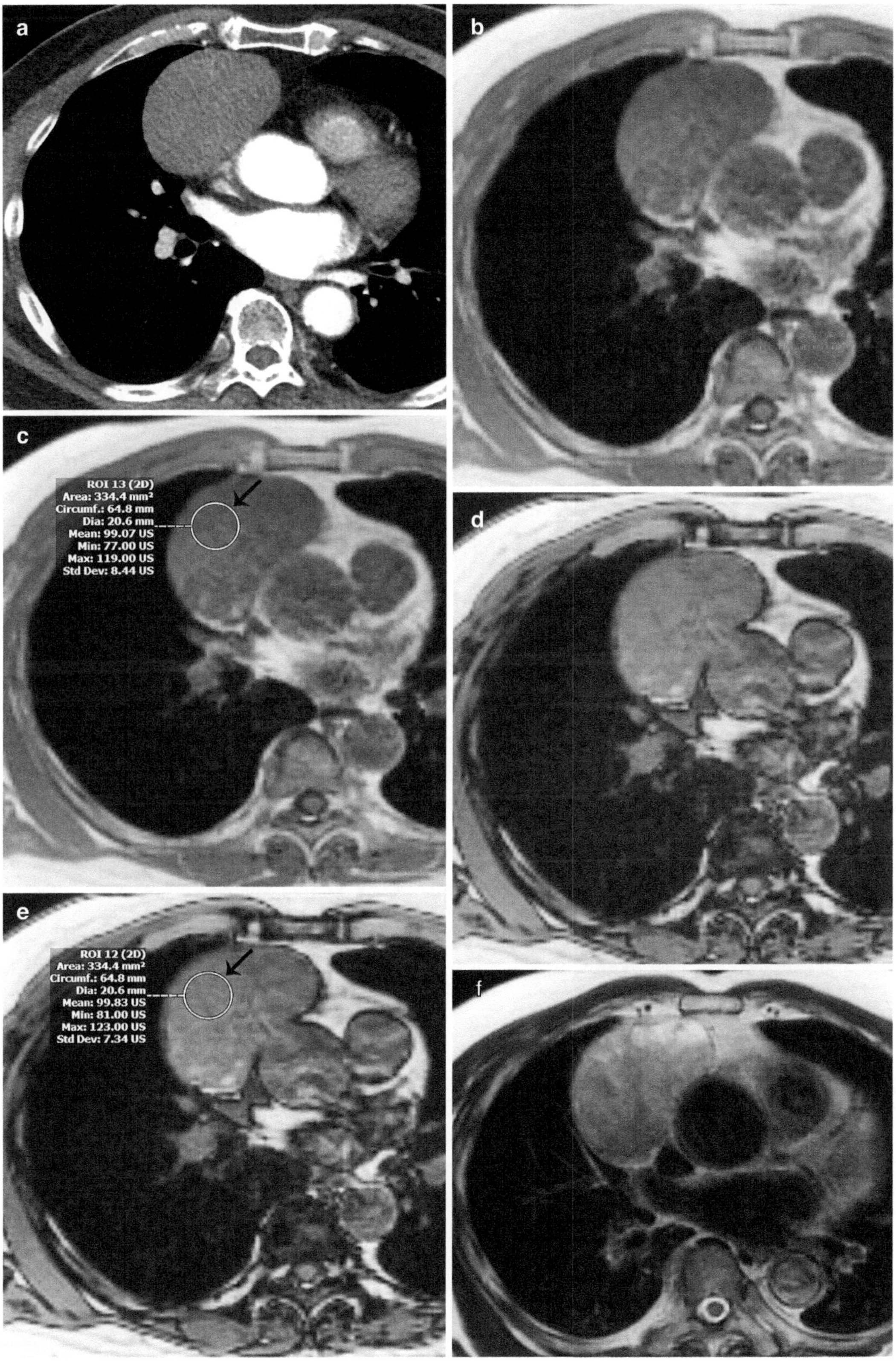
a
b
c
ROI 13 (2D)
Area: 334.4 mm²
Circumf.: 64.8 mm
Dia: 20.6 mm
Mean: 99.07 US
Min: 77.00 US
Max: 119.00 US
Std Dev: 8.44 US
d
e
ROI 12 (2D)
Area: 334.4 mm²
Circumf.: 64.8 mm
Dia: 20.6 mm
Mean: 99.83 US
Min: 81.00 US
Max: 123.00 US
Std Dev: 7.34 US
f

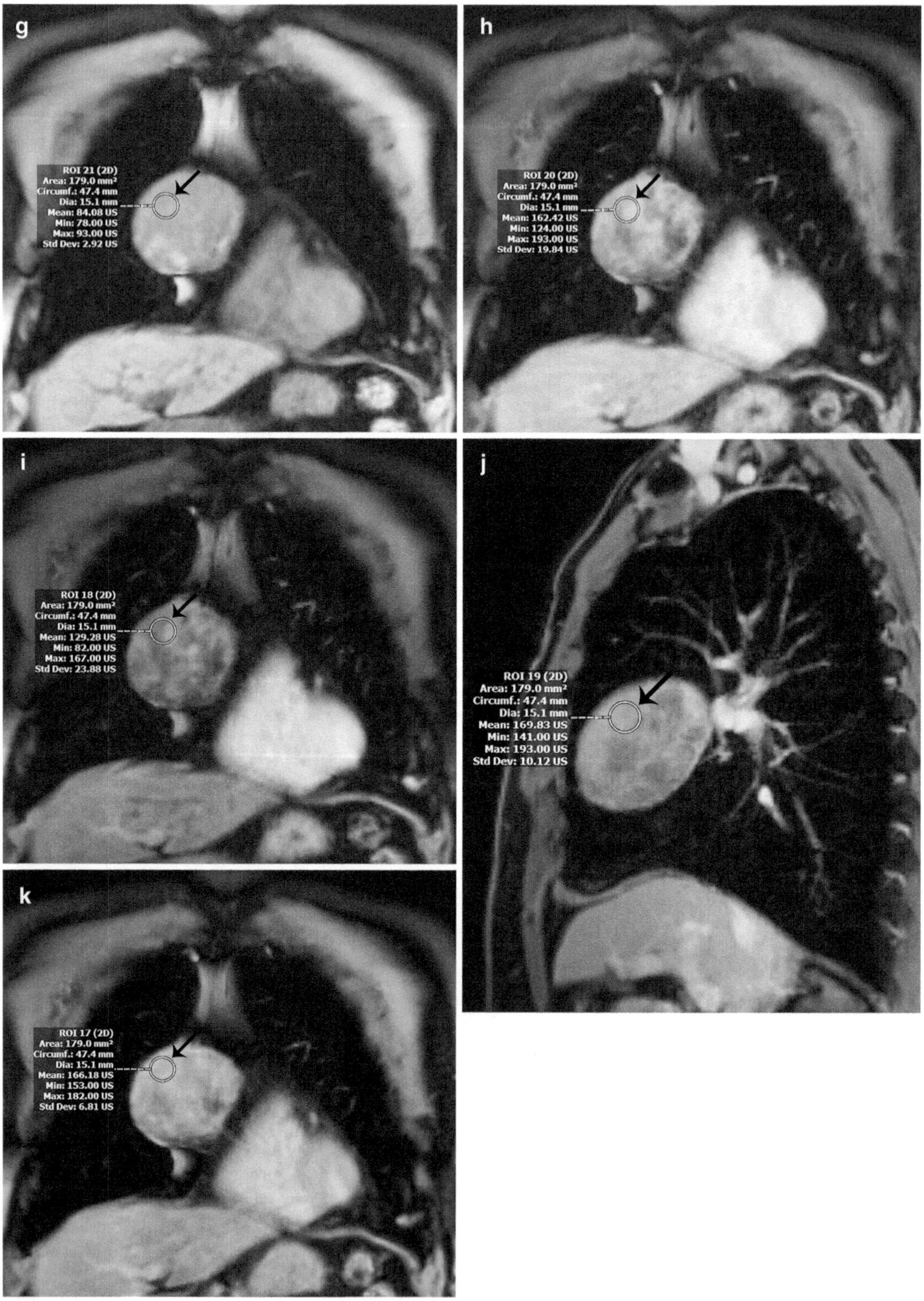

Fig. 6 (continued)

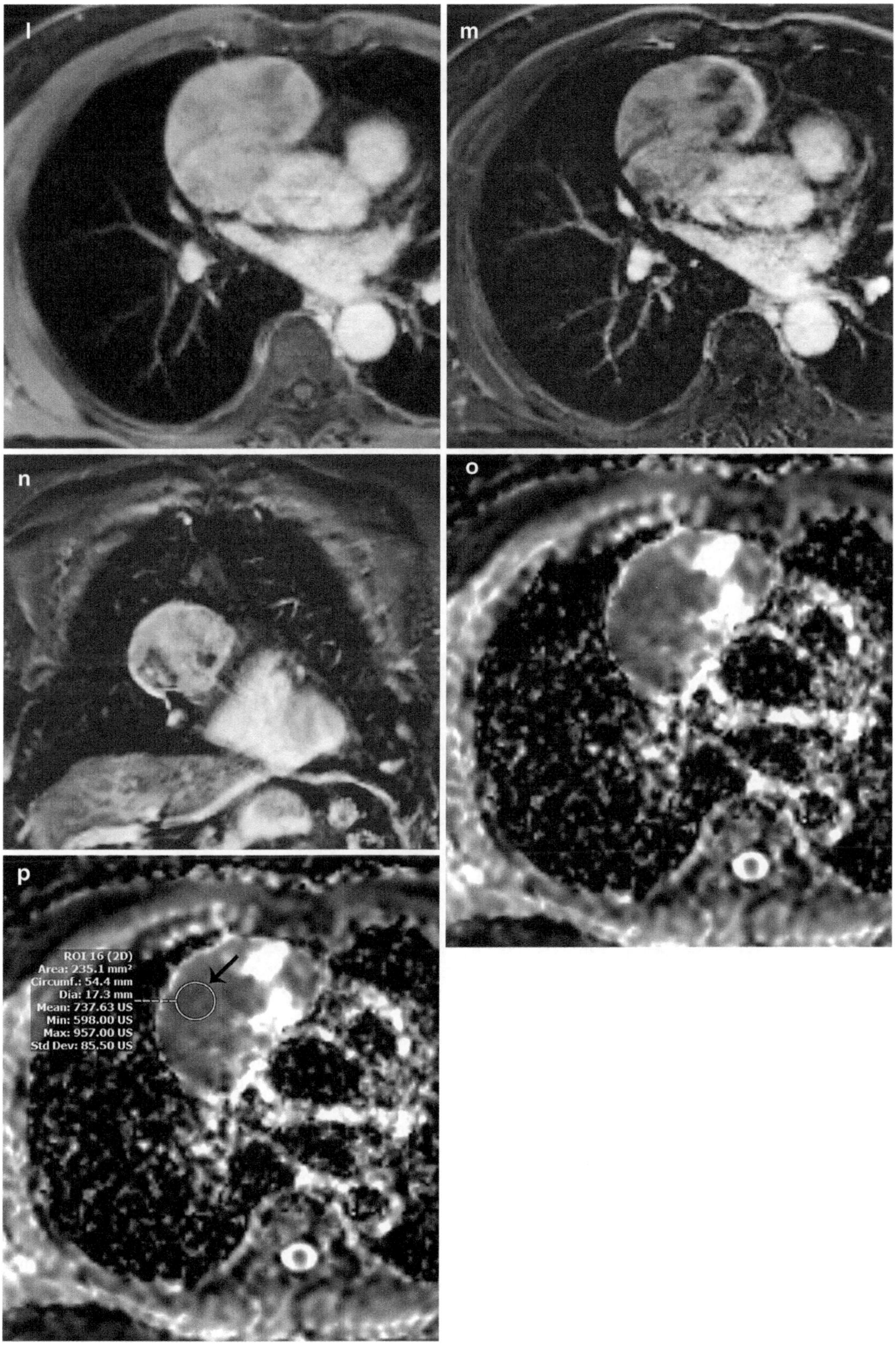

Fig. 6 (continued)

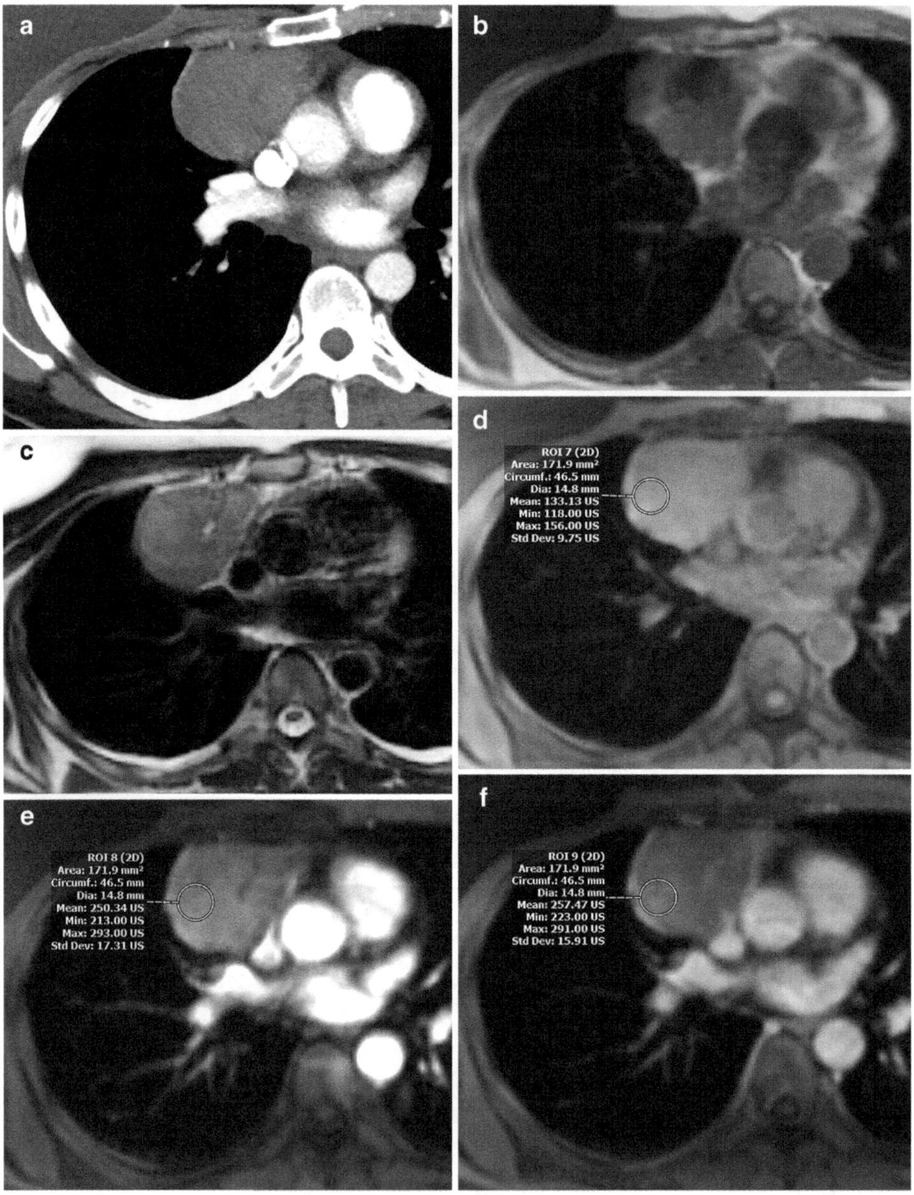

Fig. 7 Forty-five-year-old woman with WHO type B1B2 thymoma. (**a**) Axial CT with IV contrast shows a large, rounded right thymic mass, isoattenuating to muscle. (**b** and **c**) Axial in-phase T1-W (**a**) and respiratory-triggered, radially acquired T2-W (**b**) images, respectively, show the mass to be of heterogeneous T1 and T2 signal, though predominantly T1 isointense and mildly T2 hyperintense to muscle. (**d–h**) Axial precontrast (**d**) and postcontrast fat-saturated T1-W imaging acquired at (**e**) 20 s, (**f**) 1 min, (**g**) 3 min (sagittal), and (**h**) 5 min with ROIs of the same size, shape, and location [triangulated in the picture archiving and communications system (PACS) on the sagittal image]. An ROI was initially placed over the most enhancing part of the tumor and then copied, pasted, and shifted as needed to overlie the same component of the tumor on the other pre- and postcontrast sequences, yielding values of 133 precontrast and 250, 257, 254, and 304 postcontrast. This sequence of ROI values, which are relative, not absolute values on MRI (as opposed to CT Hounsfield units), indicates initially plateaued enhancement from 20 s to 3 min, with maximum enhancement at 5 min. This mixed pattern of enhancement suggests low- and high-risk components to this tumor, the location and morphology of which, especially in the absence of lymphadenopathy, indicate high statistical likelihood of a thymoma. Both low-risk (WHO type B1) and high-risk (WHO type B2) histopathological tissue types were found in the tumor. (**i** and **j**) ADC map without (**i**) and with (**j**) ROI placement over an area of lower signal within the tumor yielded a mean ROI of 738 and therefore an ADC value of 0.7×10^{-3} mm^2/s, a finding compatible with marked restriction of the diffusion of water and a higher risk component to the tumor

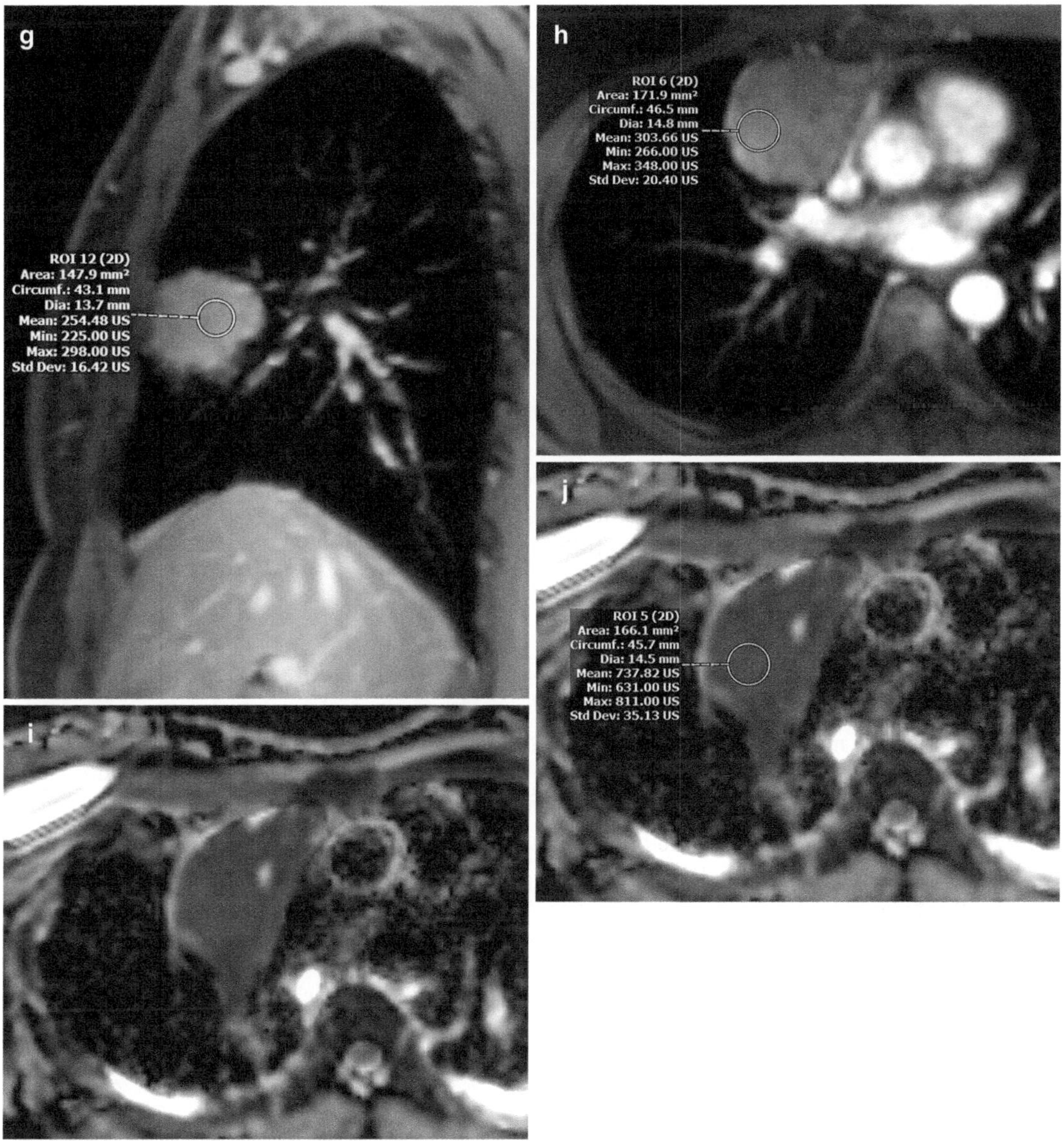

Fig. 7 (continued)

- Another study found that ^{18}FDG PET cannot reliably predict histologic grade of thymoma but can differentiate it from thymic carcinoma (Nakagawa et al. 2017).
- Of note, ^{18}FDG PET avidity has also been reported in benign thymic cysts—e.g., 1.1 ± 0.3 (Lee et al. 2019). For these reasons, reliance on SUV_{max} values for thymic lesion evaluation is problematic.

4 Thymic Cysts

Thymic cysts can be unilocular or multilocular.

4.1 Unilocular Cysts

- Unilocular thymic cysts can fluctuate in size, CT attenuation, and MRI signal over time, occasionally reaching CT attenuation values of 100 HU (Ackman et al. 2021), and have therefore not infrequently been misinterpreted by experienced subspecialist radiologists as thymic tumors (Ackman et al. 2015). Thymic cysts are sacs of fluid, so their size and morphology in a given plane can vary with differences in inspiratory (and expiratory) effort. Therefore, there can be differences in measurement between same-day cross-sectional imaging studies on account of the phase of the respiratory cycle in which the images were acquired.
- While the wall of most benign unilocular thymic cysts is usually imperceptible on CT, an identifiable wall was present in 98% of thymic cysts on MRI. In a retrospective study of unilocular thymic cysts, as initially defined by MRI, the mean wall thickness on MRI was 2 ± 0.5 mm (1 SD). Benign unilocular thymic cyst wall thicknesses of up to 4.2 mm were found (Fig. 8) (Ackman et al. 2021). It is important to be aware that benign unilocular thymic cysts can fluctuate in size, CT attenuation, and MRI signal over time, often on account of chronic, recurrent hemorrhage and resorption. Therefore, it is not the amount of fluid in the lesion or size of the lesion that matters, in terms of weighing a differential diagnosis toward benignity or malignancy, but the amount of solid, enhancing cellular tissue in the wall of the lesion (Ackman et al. 2021; Villalba et al. 2023).
- To be confident of the benign nature of the unilocular thymic cyst, it is important to verify that the cyst wall is smooth and uniform in thickness, without mural nodularity or associated soft tissue mass.

4.2 Multilocular Cysts

- Multilocular thymic cysts are inherently more complex and, to date, remain difficult to distinguish with confidence from cystic thymic neoplasms, even by MRI, because thymic hyperplasia can intercalate between cysts and may thereby mimic irregular wall thickening.

Fig. 8 Seventy-one-year-old man with regressing thymic cyst (arrows) over 3.5 months. (**a** and **b**) Axial CT with IV contrast without and with ROI, respectively, shows a left thymic nodule with an attenuation value of 35 HU. The differential diagnosis by CT includes a hemorrhagic or proteinaceous cyst and a thymic epithelial tumor (TET). (**c**–**f**) Axial DIR T2-W, precontrast fat-saturated T1-W, and postcontrast T1-W images without and with wall thickness measurement, respectively, show a T1-isointense, T2-hyperintense, centrally nonenhancing lesion with a T1/T2-hypointense, smoothly thickened 4.2 mm enhancing wall. (**g**–**j**) 3.5 months later, axial (**g**) in-phase T1-W, (**h**) DIR T2-W, (**i**) precontrast fat-saturated T1-W, and (**j**) postcontrast fat-saturated T1-W images show the lesion to have significantly decreased in size and wall thickness, though with identical signal characteristics. (Images slightly modified from those in Ackman JB et al., Radiology, 2021 (Ackman et al. 2021))

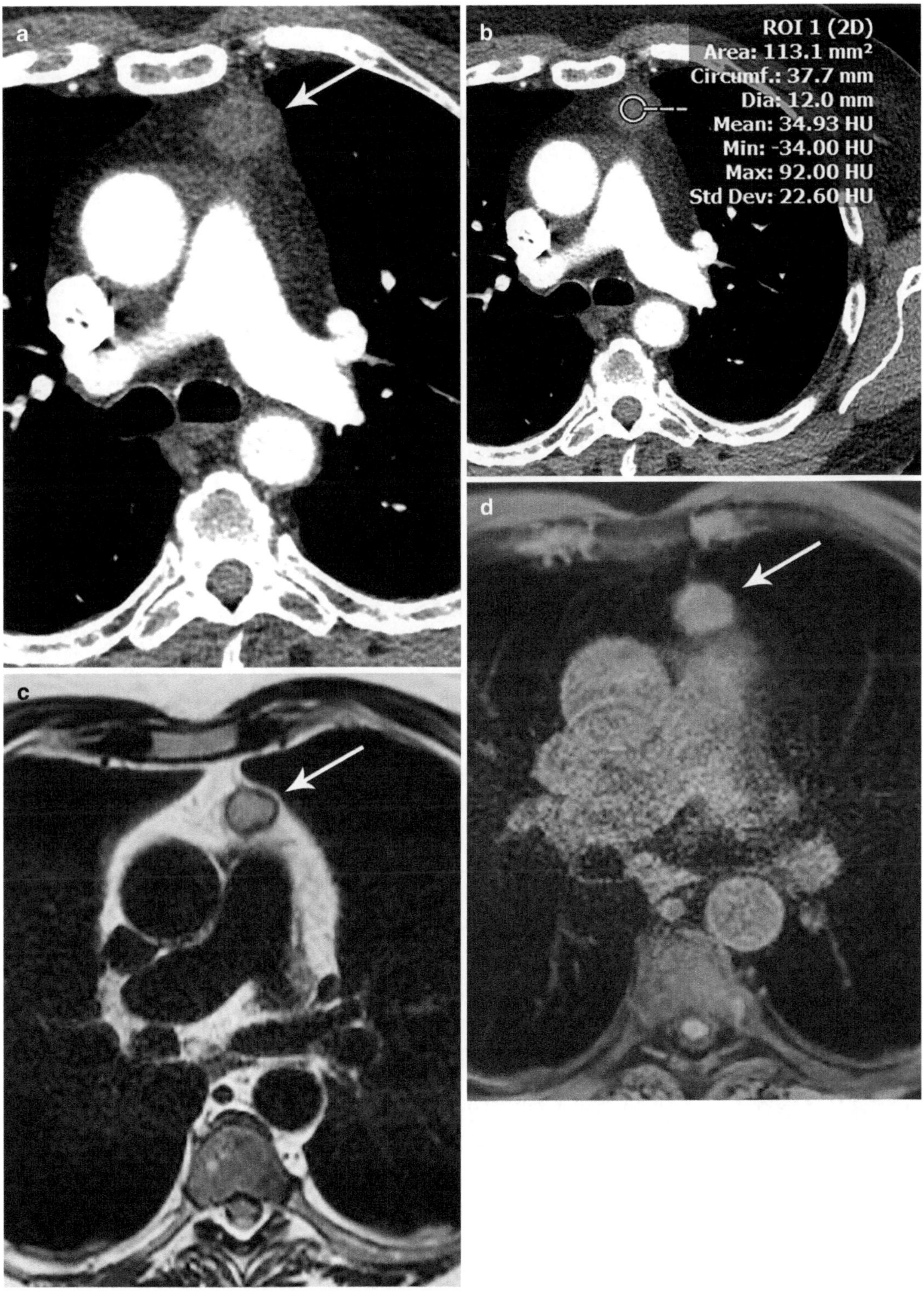
a
b
ROI 1 (2D)
Area: 113.1 mm²
Circumf.: 37.7 mm
Dia: 12.0 mm
Mean: 34.93 HU
Min: -34.00 HU
Max: 92.00 HU
Std Dev: 22.60 HU
c
d

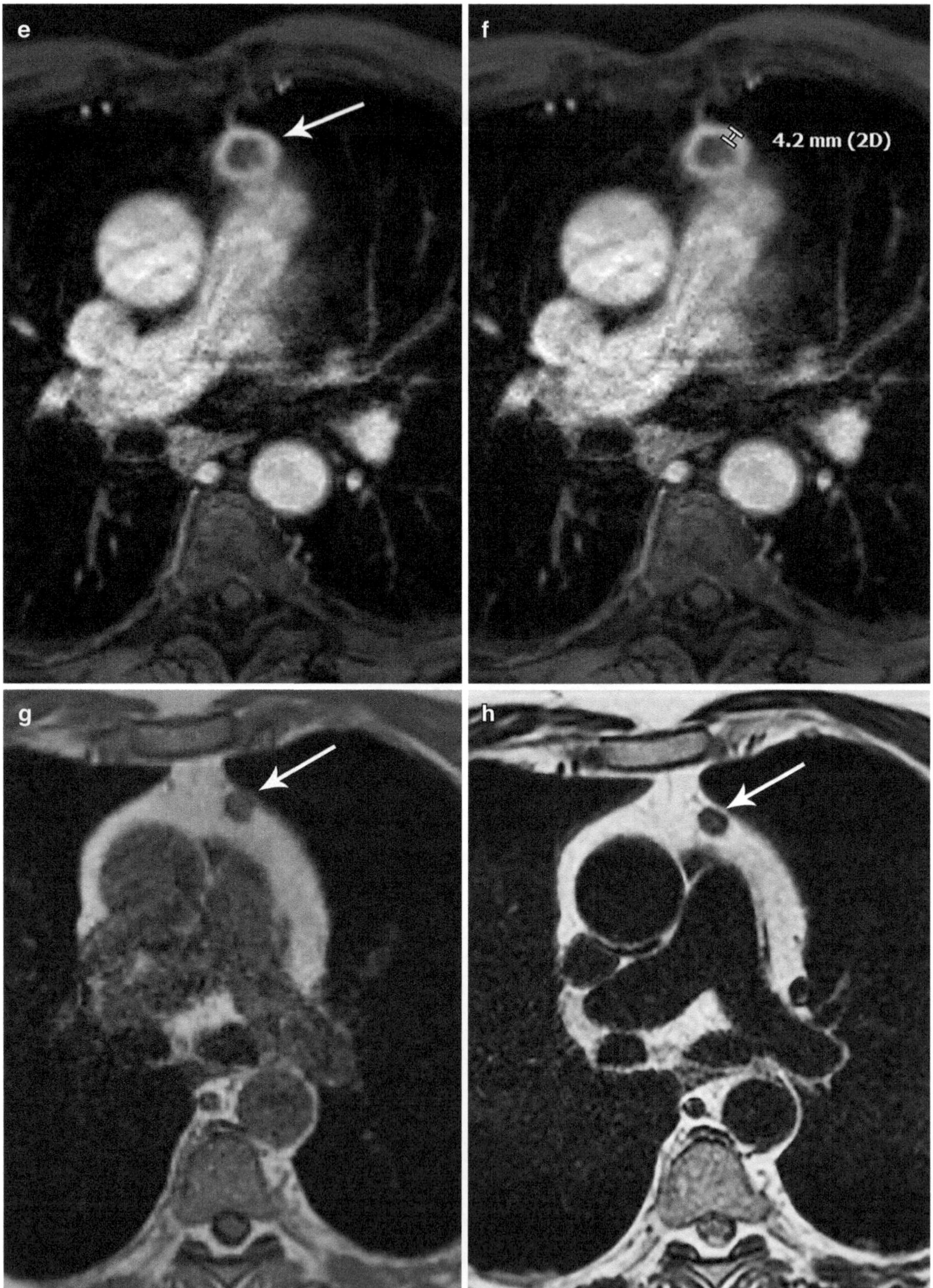

Fig. 8 (continued)

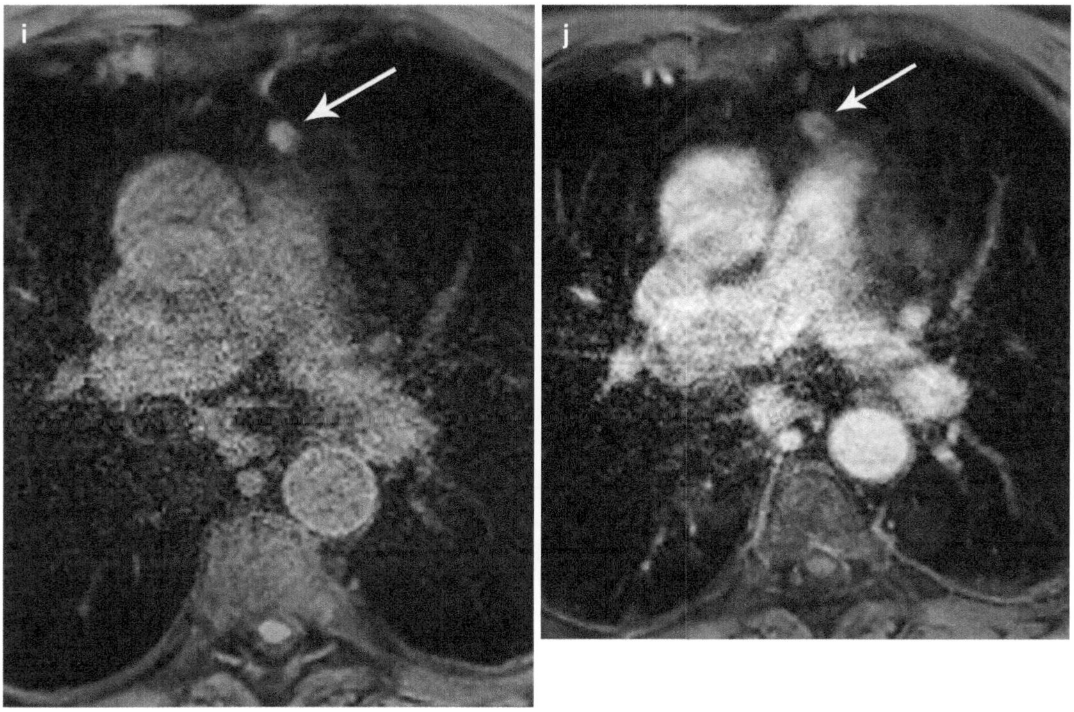

Fig. 8 (continued)

- If the thymic hyperplasia is sufficiently thick that an ROI can be placed within it, in- and opposed-phase imaging may help discern it from irregular or excessive wall thickening of the cyst itself. Nevertheless, because the long-term behavior of multilocular thymic cysts has not, as of yet, been studied with any rigor, it is best to follow these lesions by MRI, with expanded follow-up intervals over time if no concerning changes are detected, or alternatively to resect them, depending upon the level of clinical suspicion for malignancy.
- MRI surveillance offers more benefit than surveillance by CT because it not only will show any change in size and morphology like CT, but also is more apt to detect early changes in wall thickness, mural nodularity, and septations that may be CT occult because of its higher soft tissue contrast and stronger tissue characterization capability.

5 Dermoid Cyst/Mature Teratoma

- Mature teratomas, of which dermoid cysts are a subtype, often contain macroscopic and/or microscopic fat. CT can detect macroscopic fat in a thymic mass and, in the context of other findings compatible with a mature teratoma, including soft tissue attenuation material, a tooth or other calcification, and rounded, rather than draping morphology (latter morphology more typical of a thymolipoma), can make a specific diagnosis of this entity.
- Some mature teratomas or dermoid cysts do not exhibit macroscopic fat however, and, when this is the case on CT, a thymoma should be strongly favored over other tumors, including a teratoma, because thymoma, though rare, is the most common primary prevascular mediastinal neoplasm (Roden et al. 2020). Chemical shift MRI, because of its ability to detect microscopic fat, adds diagnostic specificity in this context (Fig. 9).

Fig. 9 Twenty-seven-year-old woman with mature cystic teratoma. (**a** and **b**) Coronal and axial CT with IV contrast shows a large mixed attenuation cystic mass with irregular wall thickening, internal fluid, a small amount of calcification superiorly, a small amount of macroscopic fatty content, and adjacent pleural thickening. These CT findings are diagnostic of an inflamed cystic teratoma, which has elicited pleural reaction and reactive lymphadenopathy (with or without malignant component). MRI was requested for surgical planning and further tissue characterization. In addition to corroborating the preceding CT findings, (**c** and **d**) the higher soft tissue contrast of the coronal single-shot FSE T2-W images and axial respiratory-triggered radially acquired T2-W MR images highlight the extensive tissue heterogeneity of the mass on account of its various constituents, which are of variable T2 signal; they also better demonstrate the superior septation within the mass, though unable to identify calcification within the septation. The axial MR images additionally show increased left lower lobe atelectasis along the posterior margin of the tumor in the interval between the CT and MRI. (**e** and **f**) In- and opposed-phase T1-W images, respectively, show a greater extent of fatty constitution than the CT would suggest, with areas of T1-hyperintense macroscopic fat that suppress or saturate on (**g** and **h**) postcontrast coronal and axial (latter subtracted) ultrafast GRE fat-saturated T1-W images and with areas of T1-isointense signal on the in-phase image that suppress on the (**f**) opposed-phase T1-W image that represents CT-occult microscopic fat (black arrows). The importance of the latter finding is that dermoid cysts/mature teratomas sometimes lack macroscopic fat and only contain microscopic fat. In such cases, if an MRI is not performed, a specific diagnosis could not be made. White arrows point to macroscopic fat within the mass on all provided CT and MRI images. Black arrows point to microscopic fat (opposed-phase T1-W MR image only) within the mass

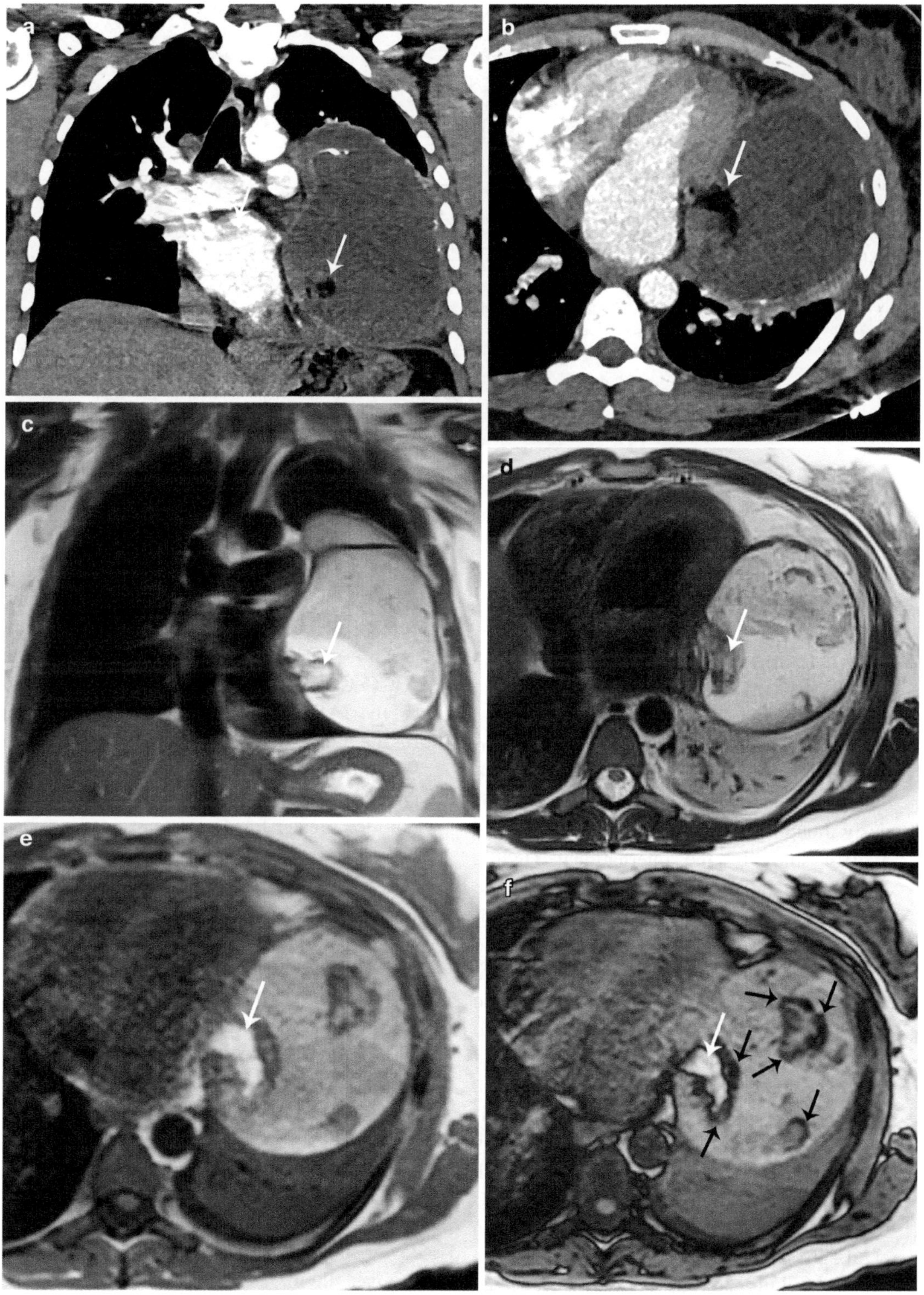
a
b
c
d
e
f

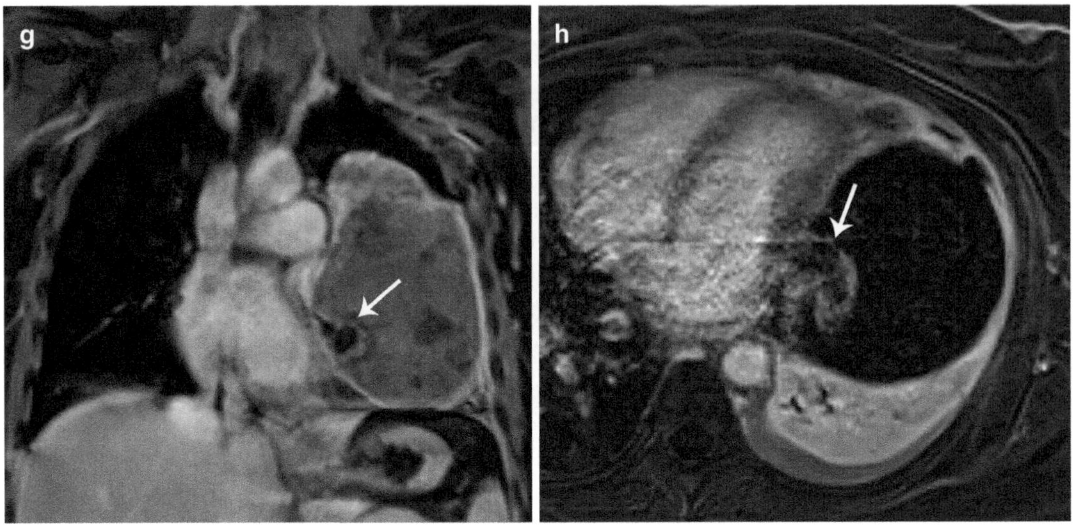

Fig. 9 (continued)

6 Thymic Epithelial Tumors (TETs)

6.1 Is Primary Tumor Size Relevant?

- While tumor measurement remains integral to reporting and treatment planning for thymic epithelial tumors and tumor size was previously thought to have prognostic significance, a 2014 study by the International Thymic Malignancy Interest Group (ITMIG) and the International Association for the Study of Lung Cancer (IASLC) investigators found no significant difference in prognosis or survival of the largest cohort of patients with thymic epithelial tumors yet studied with respect to unidimensional tumor size less than or equal to, versus greater than, 10 cm (Nicholson et al. 2014). Therefore, the inaugural TNM classification system for TETs developed jointly by these two organizations (Detterbeck et al. 2014) and subsequently published in the AJCC Cancer Staging Manual, eighth Edition (Amin et al. 2017), does not take tumor size into account, but instead focuses exclusively on the degree or "level" to which the tumor involves adjacent mediastinal structures (Nicholson et al. 2014). This discounting of tumor size is controversial (Bian et al. 2018; Safieddine et al. 2014), however, and will likely be countered in the imminent ninth edition of the AJCC Cancer Staging Manual, as suggested by the IASLC TET staging project proposal for the tumor (T) component for the upcoming 9th edition of the TNM classification of malignant tumors (Okumura et al. 2023) which reported greater freedom-from-recurrence and overall survival for TETS ≤ 5 cm.

6.2 Use of Temporal (Dynamic) Enhancement Pattern to Distinguish Between Lower and Higher Stage Thymomas, Thymic Carcinoma, Malignant Germ Cell Tumors, and Lymphoma

- Assessment of the temporal enhancement pattern of a thymic tumor by dynamic contrast-enhanced (DCE) MRI can help distinguish lower stage thymomas from higher stage thymomas, thymic carcinoma, lymphoma, and other non-thymomatous tumors (Sakai et al. 2002). Sakai et al. (2002) found statistically significant differences between mean time-to-peak (TTP) enhancement for Masaoka stage I, II, and III thymoma and thymic carcinoma, with TTP values of 1.4 ± 0.6, 1.2 ± 0.9, 2.5 ± 1.0, and 3.5 ± 0.9 min, respectively. The mean TTP for lymphoma was 3.9 ± 0.9 min and for malignant germ cell tumor, 2.1 ± 0.9 min. The method Sakai et al. used was to plot time enhancement curves of the highest ROI value obtained from the solid, enhancing component of the tumor on dynamic contrast-enhanced imaging obtained every 30 s over 5 min.

- Because there is overlap in the TTP enhancement between these tumors, however, such values should only be used as a rough guide for distinguishing between TETs and non-TETs in the prevascular mediastinum, that is, as a means of weighing the differential diagnosis. Combining the TTP results with those of other MRI and/or CT features can further narrow the differential diagnosis (Fig. 6). For example, the presence of lymphadenopathy outside of the prevascular mediastinum would favor lymphoma, high-risk thymoma, and thymic carcinoma over low-risk thymoma. In everyday clinical practice, obtaining a large number of breath-hold DCE acquisitions can be challenging for the patient and MR technologist, and temporal enhancement curves are seldom generated. For this reason, in clinical practice, we perform a more qualitative assessment of these lesions with ROIs placed over the maximum area of enhancement in these lesions on DCE at 20 s and 1, 3, and 5 min (Figs. 6 and 7). We then use this information to help weigh our differential diagnosis.

6.3 Apparent Diffusion Coefficient (ADC) Mapping

- Qualitative assessment of DWI findings and quantitative assessment by procurement of ADC values from the solid, cellular, enhancing component of the thymic tumor can help distinguish low-risk thymomas from high-risk thymoma, thymic carcinoma, and lymphoma (Abdel Razek et al. 2014) (Fig. 7). Abdel Razek et al. (2014) found that cutoff ADC values of 1.25 and 1.22 × 10^{-3} mm^2/s differentiated low-risk thymoma from high-risk thymoma and thymic carcinoma with an area under the curve of 0.804 and 0.851, respectively. Li et al. (2019) used a combination of ADC values and DWI texture analysis to predict TET subtype and stage. The mean ADC values for low-risk, high-risk thymoma and thymic carcinoma were 1.63 ± 0.63, 1.30 ± 0.51, and 0.86 ± 0.20 × 10^{-3} mm^2/s, respectively ($p = 0.002$). Other aggressive prevascular mediastinal tumors, including neuroendocrine tumors (Fukai et al. 1999; Sullivan and Weksler 2017), would be expected to have lower ADC values. In practice, we use these reported TET ADC values and cutoffs as rough guides, recognizing that DWI is not sufficiently standardized across MRI vendors and hardware and software platforms to rely on these ADC values as hard numbers. Please refer to earlier Sect. 3.2.5 regarding the nuts and bolts of ADC value procurement.

7 Conclusion

- Use of widely available measurement tools in PACS can help to distinguish thymic hyperplasia and thymic cysts from thymic tumors on CT and MRI and has the potential to reduce the rate of unnecessary thymectomy and its associated morbidity and health care cost. When a thymic mass is deemed indeterminate on CT or suspected by chest radiography or clinical indicators, MRI, unless contraindicated, should be performed to facilitate a more specific, noninvasive diagnosis (Ackman et al. 2023; Expert Panel on Thoracic Imaging et al. 2021). Making this distinction noninvasively by employing the larger toolset of MRI is worthwhile, given prevalent concern for seeding biopsy tracks with thymoma and thymic carcinoma and increased risk of metastatic pleural dissemination (Fujiwara et al. 2003; Kattach et al. 2005; Nagasaka et al. 1993;

Matsumoto et al. 2007). The aforementioned MRI tools can weigh the differential diagnosis between lower and higher stage thymomas, thymic carcinoma, and lymphoma, further assisting clinical management. It nevertheless remains important not to ascribe too much significance to measured values, in the absence of global assessment of a lesion's imaging features and good clinical judgment.

Acknowledgments The author would like to thank John E. Kirsch, PhD, MRI physicist, at the Athinoula A. Martinos Center for Biomedical Imaging at Massachusetts General Hospital, for his invaluable input regarding high-quality diffusion-weighted MR imaging and ADC mapping in the chest.

Disclaimer All measurements in this book have been obtained from peer-reviewed papers and guidelines from professional organizations, unless explicitly stated otherwise. While the authors, editors, and publisher have gone through a rigorous process to establish their correct reproduction from the original source, each measurement must be interpreted in the correct clinical context, this along with an accurate way of measurement, and taking into account all technical variables, this including follow-up exams with various equipment or software. Neither the authors, the editors, nor the publisher can accept any legal responsibility for any improper application or interpretation of these measurements as well as their potential consequences.

References

Abdel Razek AA, Khairy M, Nada N (2014) Diffusion-weighted MR imaging in thymic epithelial tumors: correlation with World Health Organization classification and clinical staging. Radiology 273:268–275

Ackman JB (2015) MR imaging of mediastinal masses. Magn Reson Imaging Clin N Am 23:141–164

Ackman JB, Wu CC (2011) MRI of the thymus. AJR Am J Roentgenol 197:W15–W20

Ackman JB, Mino-Kenudson M, Morse CR (2012) Nonsuppressing normal thymus on chemical shift magnetic resonance imaging in a young woman. J Thorac Imaging 27:W196–W198

Ackman JB, Kovacina B, Carter BW, Wu CC, Sharma A, Shepard JA, Halpern EF (2013) Sex difference in normal thymic appearance in adults 20–30 years of age. Radiology 268:245–253

Ackman JB, Verzosa S, Kovach AE et al (2015) High rate of unnecessary thymectomy and its cause. Can computed tomography distinguish thymoma, lymphoma, thymic hyperplasia, and thymic cysts? Eur J Radiol 84:524–533

Ackman JB, Gaissert HA, Lanuti M, Digumarthy SR, Shepard JA, Halpern EF, Wright CD (2016) Impact of nonvascular thoracic MR imaging on the clinical decision making of thoracic surgeons: a 2-year prospective study. Radiology 280:464–474

Ackman JB, Chintanapakdee W, Mendoza DP, Price MC, Lanuti M, Shepard JO (2021) Longitudinal CT and MRI characteristics of unilocular thymic cysts. Radiology 301:443–454

Ackman JB, Chung JH, Walker CM et al (2023) ACR Appropriateness Criteria® imaging of mediastinal masses. J Am Coll Radiol 20(5S):S224–S233

Amin MB, American Joint Committee on Cancer, American Cancer Society (2017) AJCC cancer staging manual, 8th edn/editor-in-chief, Amin MB; editors, Edge SB, et al; Gress DM—Technical editor; Meyer LR—Managing editor. ed. American Joint Committee on Cancer, Springer, Chicago IL. xvii, 1024 pages

Araki T, Sholl LM, Gerbaudo VH, Hatabu H, Nishino M (2014a) Thymic measurements in pathologically proven normal thymus and thymic hyperplasia: intraobserver and interobserver variabilities. Acad Radiol 21:733–742

Araki T, Sholl LM, Gerbaudo VH, Hatabu H, Nishino M (2014b) Imaging characteristics of pathologically proven thymic hyperplasia: identifying features that can differentiate true from lymphoid hyperplasia. AJR Am J Roentgenol 202:471–478

Baron RL, Lee JK, Sagel SS, Peterson RR (1982) Computed tomography of the normal thymus. Radiology 142:121–125

Bian D, Zhou F, Yang W et al (2018) Thymoma size significantly affects the survival, metastasis and effectiveness of adjuvant therapies: a population based study. Oncotarget 9:12273–12283

Bronte V, Pittet MJ (2013) The spleen in local and systemic regulation of immunity. Immunity 39:806–818

deSouza NM, Winfield JM, Waterton JC et al (2018) Implementing diffusion-weighted MRI for body imaging in prospective multicentre trials: current considerations and future perspectives. Eur Radiol 28:1118–1131

Detterbeck FC, Stratton K, Giroux D et al (2014) The IASLC/ITMIG Thymic Epithelial Tumors Staging Project: proposal for an evidence-based stage classification system for the forthcoming (8th) edition of the TNM classification of malignant tumors. J Thorac Oncol 9:S65–S72

Drabkin MJ, Meyer JI, Kanth N, Lobel S, Fogel J, Grossman J, Krumenacker JH (2018) Age-stratified patterns of thymic involution on multidetector CT. J Thorac Imaging 33:409–416

Endo M, Nakagawa K, Ohde Y et al (2008) Utility of 18FDG-PET for differentiating the grade of malignancy in thymic epithelial tumors. Lung Cancer 61:350–355

Expert Panel on Thoracic Imaging, Ackman JB, Chung JH et al (2021) ACR Appropriateness Criteria® imaging of mediastinal masses. J Am Coll Radiol 18:S37–S51

Francis IR, Glazer GM, Bookstein FL, Gross BH (1985) The thymus: reexamination of age-related changes in size and shape. AJR Am J Roentgenol 145:249–254
Fujiwara K, Matsumura A, Tanaka H, Ohmori K, Yamamoto S, Iuchi K (2003) [Needle tract implantation of thymoma after transthoracic needle biopsy]. Kyobu Geka 56:448–451
Fukai I, Masaoka A, Fujii Y, Yamakawa Y, Yokoyama T, Murase T, Eimoto T (1999) Thymic neuroendocrine tumor (thymic carcinoid): a clinicopathologic study in 15 patients. Ann Thorac Surg 67:208–211
Gawande RS, Khurana A, Messing S et al (2012) Differentiation of normal thymus from anterior mediastinal lymphoma and lymphoma recurrence at pediatric PET/CT. Radiology 262:613–622
Goldblum JR, Lamps LW, McKenney JK, Myers JL, Ackerman LV, Rosai J (2018) Rosai and Ackerman's surgical pathology, 11th edn. Elsevier, Philadelphia, PA. 2 volumes (xiv, 2142 pages)
Hammer MM, Barile M, Bryson W, Bhalla S, Raptis CA (2019) Errors in interpretation of magnetic resonance imaging for thymic lesions. J Thorac Imaging 34:351–355
Heeger AP, Ackman JB (2021) Added value of magnetic resonance imaging for the evaluation of mediastinal lesions. Radiol Clin North Am 59:251–277
Hephzibah J, Shanthly N, Oommen R (2014) Diagnostic utility of PET CT in thymic tumours with emphasis on 68Ga-DOTATATE PET CT in thymic neuroendocrine tumour—experience at a tertiary level hospital in India. J Clin Diagn Res 8:QC01–QC03
Inaoka T, Takahashi K, Mineta M et al (2007) Thymic hyperplasia and thymus gland tumors: differentiation with chemical shift MR imaging. Radiology 243:869–876
Jerushalmi J, Frenkel A, Bar-Shalom R, Khoury J, Israel O (2009) Physiologic thymic uptake of 18F-FDG in children and young adults: a PET/CT evaluation of incidence, patterns, and relationship to treatment. J Nucl Med 50:849–853
Kattach H, Hasan S, Clelland C, Pillai R (2005) Seeding of stage I thymoma into the chest wall 12 years after needle biopsy. Ann Thorac Surg 79:323–324
Kent MS, Wang T, Gangadharan SP, Whyte RI (2014) What is the prevalence of a "nontherapeutic" thymectomy? Ann Thorac Surg 97:276–282; discussion 282
Kooshesh K, Foy BH, Sykes DB, Gustafsson K, Scadden DT (2023) Health consequences of thymus removal in adults. New Engl J Med 389:406–17.
Kumar A, Regmi SK, Dutta R et al (2009) Characterization of thymic masses using (18)F-FDG PET-CT. Ann Nucl Med 23:569–577
Lamba R, McGahan JP, Corwin MT, Li CS, Tran T, Seibert JA, Boone JM (2014) CT Hounsfield numbers of soft tissues on unenhanced abdominal CT scans: variability between two different manufacturers' MDCT scanners. AJR Am J Roentgenol 203:1013–1020
Lee SH, Yoon SH, Nam JG et al (2019) Distinguishing between thymic epithelial tumors and benign cysts via computed tomography. Korean J Radiol 20:671–682
Lee J, Cho YS, Kim J, Shim YM, Lee KH, Choi JY (2021) Prognostic significance of metabolic parameters by (18)F-FDG PET/CT in thymic epithelial tumors. Cancers (Basel) 13:712
Li B, Xin YK, Xiao G et al (2019) Predicting pathological subtypes and stages of thymic epithelial tumors using DWI: value of combining ADC and texture parameters. Eur Radiol 29:5330–5340
Madan R, Ratanaprasatporn L, Ratanaprasatporn L, Carter BW, Ackman JB (2018) Cystic mediastinal masses and the role of MRI. Clin Imaging 50:68–77
Malyarenko D, Galban CJ, Londy FJ et al (2013) Multi-system repeatability and reproducibility of apparent diffusion coefficient measurement using an ice-water phantom. J Magn Reson Imaging 37:1238–1246
Matsumoto K, Ashizawa K, Tagawa T, Nagayasu T (2007) Chest wall implantation of thymic cancer after computed tomography-guided core needle biopsy. Eur J Cardiothorac Surg 32:171–173
McInnis MC, Flores EJ, Shepard JA, Ackman JB (2016) Pitfalls in the imaging and interpretation of benign thymic lesions: how thymic MRI can help. AJR Am J Roentgenol 206:W1–W8
Mitchell DG, Crovello M, Matteucci T, Petersen RO, Miettinen MM (1992) Benign adrenocortical masses: diagnosis with chemical shift MR imaging. Radiology 185:345–351
Nagasaka T, Nakashima N, Nunome H (1993) Needle tract implantation of thymoma after transthoracic needle biopsy. J Clin Pathol 46:278–279
Nakagawa K, Takahashi S, Endo M, Ohde Y, Kurihara H, Terauchi T (2017) Can (18)F-FDG PET predict the grade of malignancy in thymic epithelial tumors? An evaluation of only resected tumors. Cancer Manag Res 9:761–768
Nicholson AG, Detterbeck FC, Marino M et al (2014) The IASLC/ITMIG Thymic Epithelial Tumors Staging Project: proposals for the T component for the forthcoming (8th) edition of the TNM classification of malignant tumors. J Thorac Oncol 9:S73–S80
Okumura M, Marina M, Cilento V, et al (2023) The international association for the study of lung cancer thymic epithelial tumor staging project: proposal for the T component for the forthcoming (ninth) edition of the TNM classification of malignant tumors. J Thorac Oncol 18:1638–1654
Priola AM, Priola SM, Ciccone G et al (2015) Differentiation of rebound and lymphoid thymic hyperplasia from anterior mediastinal tumors with dual-echo chemical-shift MR imaging in adulthood: reliability of the chemical-shift ratio and signal intensity index. Radiology 274:238–249
Priola AM, Priola SM, Gned D, Giraudo MT, Veltri A (2018) Nonsuppressing normal thymus on chemical-shift MR imaging and anterior mediastinal lymphoma: differentiation with diffusion-weighted MR imaging by using the apparent diffusion coefficient. Eur Radiol 28:1427–1437
Roden AC, Fang W, Yan S et al (2020) The distribution of mediastisnal lesions across multi-institutional,

international, radiology databases. J Thorac Oncol 15:568–579
Safieddine N, Liu G, Cuningham K et al (2014) Prognostic factors for cure, recurrence and long-term survival after surgical resection of thymoma. J Thorac Oncol 9:1018–1022
Sakai S, Murayama S, Soeda H, Matsuo Y, Ono M, Masuda K (2002) Differential diagnosis between thymoma and non-thymoma by dynamic MR imaging. Acta Radiol 43:262–268
Shukla-Dave A, Obuchowski NA, Chenevert TL et al (2019) Quantitative imaging biomarkers alliance (QIBA) recommendations for improved precision of DWI and DCE-MRI derived biomarkers in multicenter oncology trials. J Magn Reson Imaging 49:e101–e121
Sullivan JL, Weksler B (2017) Neuroendocrine tumors of the thymus: analysis of factors affecting survival in 254 patients. Ann Thorac Surg 103:935–939
Swirski FK, Nahrendorf M, Etzrodt M et al (2009) Identification of splenic reservoir monocytes and their deployment to inflammatory sites. Science 325:612–616
Thai LH, Mahevas M, Roudot-Thoraval F et al (2016) Long-term complications of splenectomy in adult immune thrombocytopenia. Medicine (Baltimore) 95:e5098
Thapa P, Farber DL (2019) The role of the thymus in the immune response. Thorac Surg Clin 29:123–131
Villalba JA, Haramati A, Garlin M, Reyes F, Wright CD, Louissaint A Jr, Ackman JB (2023) Intralesional microbleeding in resected thymic cysts indeterminate on imaging. Mediastinum 7:13

Thyroid/Lymph Nodes/Esophagus

Katharina Martini, Lisa Jungblut, and Thomas Frauenfelder

Contents

K. Martini · L. Jungblut · T. Frauenfelder (✉)
Diagnostic and Interventional Radiology, University Hospital Zurich, University Zurich, Zurich, Switzerland
e-mail: katharina.martini@hirslanden.ch; Lisa.Jungblut@usz.ch; Thomas.Frauenfelder@usz.ch

Abstract

In this chapter, measurements relevant in the thyroid gland, lymph nodes, and esophagus will be discussed. First, an overview of the origin and physiological foundation of the anatomic structures as well as the importance and current indications in clinical routine will be discussed. Then, a practical description of how the measurements will be performed and the standard measurement values are given. Finally, the potential pitfalls or possible confounding factors and how to avoid them will be discussed.

1 Thyroid Gland

1.1 Origins and Physiological Foundation

The thyroid gland is located in the anterior aspect of the neck in the visceral space and extends from C5 to T1 vertebra. The organ lies ventrally to the thyroid and cricoid cartilages and the first three tracheal rings (Weissleder et al. 2011). The thyroid gland is a butterfly- or "H"-shaped organ composed by two lobes, each with a superior and inferior pole. Normally, the superior pole is narrower than the inferior pole giving a pear-like shape to each lateral lobe. The two lobes are connected in the midline by a narrow isthmus, which is adherent to the tracheal rings. Each lobe mea-

https://doi.org/10.1007/174_2024_500,
Published Online: 07 August 2024

sures approximately 4–7 cm in length. Average weight is 25 g (Vinh and Zafereo 2021).

The imaging modality of choice for the evaluation of the thyroid gland is ultrasound (US). US is a cheap and straightforward radiation-free imaging modality, which delivers excellent soft tissue contrast. Additionally, US Doppler mode allows to evaluate tissue perfusion and can be used as a tool to guide tissue biopsies or fine needle aspiration of thyroid gland lesions (Grant et al. 2015).

Evaluation of the thyroid gland is normally performed when (1) thyroid hormonal blood values are abnormal or (2) the thyroid gland is abnormal in the clinical evaluation (enlarged gland, nodular impression) (Grant et al. 2015).

1.2 How Is the Measurement Performed?

The first step in the proper US evaluation of the thyroid gland is correct positioning of the patient: (1) the patient should lie in the supine position; (2) the patient should avoid using pillows to sustain the patient's head, since they cause flexion of the head which results in shortening of the neck—this position will make a proper evaluation challenging; and (3) the patient should try to extend the neck as much as possible by flexing the head backwards with his chin pointing to the ceiling. In this way, the anterior part of the neck is extended, and the evaluation of the thyroid gland becomes easier. If necessary, the patient neck can be supported by a small pillow.

US should be performed with a linear high-frequency transducer (~14 MHz). First, an axial B-mode image of the whole thyroid gland should be obtained using the virtual convex option to get a general impression of the gland and its possible lesions. In transverse plane, the thickness of the thyroid gland isthmus can be measured. The isthmus should not be thicker than 5 mm (Fig. 1).

In the second step, each lobe of the thyroid gland should be evaluated separately: axial and sagittal planes should be acquired, and each lobe should be measured in its three dimensions in order to perform volume calculations as follows:

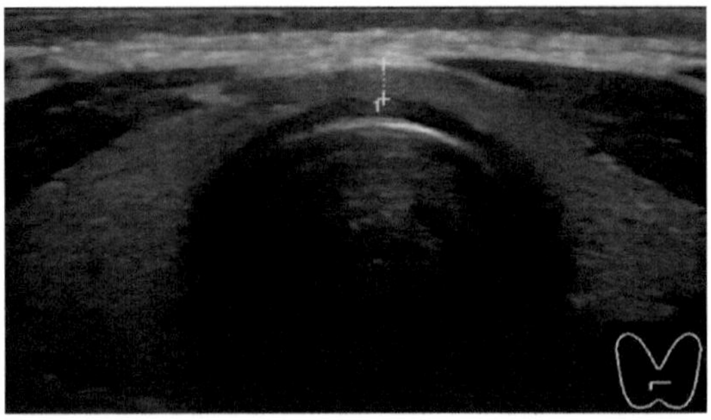

Fig. 1 Measurement of the thyroid gland isthmus in transverse plane (precise plane of view). The isthmus should not be thicker than 5 mm

The width and depth are measured on the transverse section of the lobe: the width is the distance between the most lateral point of the lobe and the acoustic shadowing of the trachea medially, and the depth is the maximum anterior-posterior distance in the middle third of the lobe. The length that is measured on longitudinal section (sagittal view) is the maximum distance from the most cranial to the most caudal part of the lobe. In some cases, an accessory lobe may be found on the upper margin of the isthmus, named Lalouette pyramid, whose volume must be added to that of the lobes (Ghervan 2011).

These measurements are the basis for volume determination of the thyroid. The underlying formula is:

$$V = W \times D \times L \times \text{“correction factor”}$$

V = volume (mL), W = width (cm), D = depth (cm), and L = length (cm).

In the literature, different values were proposed as correction factor. The originally proposed correction factor was 0.479 and has been adopted widely since then, including the WHO (Brunn et al. 1981). Later, a new factor of 0.529 has been proposed based on CT measurements (Shabana et al. 2006). Finally, a last factor "$\pi/6$" was described reflecting the ellipsoid formula (Şeker and Taş 2010). Taking into account the various biological factors influencing the size mentioned above, the simplified use of the correction factor of 0.5 is reasonable in everyday life. The volume of the entire thyroid gland is defined as the sum of the right and left thyroid lobe.

1.3 What Are the Expected Results and Range of Normal Values?

There is a wide range of normal values in thyroid gland measurement. The values depend on age, size, gender, and weight (Heged et al. 1987). The relationship between thyroid volume, body weight, and age in non-goitrous healthy subjects can be described using a formula that allows the calculation of normal thyroid size for a population:

$$\text{Normal thyroid volume}(\text{mL}) = 1.97 + 0.21 \times \text{body weight}(\text{kg}) + 0.06 \times \text{age}(\text{years})$$

Furthermore, there may be seasonal fluctuations with approximately 20% higher values in winter season (Hegedüs et al. 1987). Cyclic alterations of thyroid volume have also been found with 50% higher values in the second half of the menstrual cycle, which may be related to TSH alterations. Therefore, when an examination performed during the second half of the cycle shows a large thyroid volume, a second examination obtained during the first half of the cycle should be performed to confirm the thyroid volume. Lastly, medical conditions like acute hepatic disease or chronic renal disease that may lead to a higher thyroid volume should also be considered when assessing thyroid values (Hegedüs 1990). When evaluating the occurrence rate of goiter, the goitrogenic effects of drugs, and goiter treatment outcomes, these factors should be considered. In children, the upper limits of the thyroid volume correlate with age, as this has been shown by the French ThyroMobile study (Delange et al. 1997). Normal values of the thyroid gland can be found in Table 1. It has to be admitted that there are no minimal volumes defined.

1.4 Confounding Factors

It is important to measure the whole gland. In subjects with short necks, US might be more challenging. As mentioned before, a good retroflection of the neck improves the field of view. In some cases, the thyroid gland or goiter can extend deeply into the upper mediastinum—in these cases, attention should be paid to measure the entire gland. In some cases, this may not be possible with US, and CT or MRI may be necessary to evaluate and measure the entire extension of the gland.

Adjacent lymph nodes or parathyroid glands should not be confounded with thyroid gland and must be excluded from measurements. Measurements should be strictly orthogonal because diagonal measurements result in false higher values.

Last but not least, patient history should always be considered as mentioned earlier, also including previous surgery like thyroidectomy and hemithyroidectomy.

Table 1 Normal values of thyroid gland measurements (adapted from Viduetsky and Herrejon 2019, Dighe et al. 2017, Delange et al. 1997)

Length	40–70 mm
Width	10–30 mm
Depth	10–20 mm
Isthmus	<5 mm
Volume for adult males and females	Male 12–18 mL Female 10–15 mL
Volume at children age	
6	Male <5.4 mL Female <5 mL
7	Male <5.7 mL Female <5.9 mL
8	Male <6.1 mL Female <6.9 mL
9	Male <6.8 mL Female <8 mL
10	Male <7.8 mL Female <9.2 mL
11	Male <9 mL Female <10.4 mL
12	Male <10.4 mL Female <11.7 mL
13	Male <12 mL Female <13.1 mL
14	Male <13.9 mL Female <14.6 mL
15	Male <16 mL Female <16.1 mL

1.5 Clinical Implementation of the Measurement

Size measurements are mostly performed in patients with abnormal thyroid hormonal blood levels: in Graves' disease or Hashimoto thyroiditis, the thyroid gland is often enlarged and can be hyperechogenic.

Thyroid lesions are a common finding in US evaluation of the thyroid gland and range from benign age-related changes to malignant thyroid gland carcinomas. In order to distinguish a benign from a malignant lesion, size criteria are controversial and still continuously evolving. US risk classification systems have been established by several societies: the American Thyroid Association (ATA), the American College of Radiology (ACR), the European Thyroid Association, and the Korean Society of Thyroid Radiology. Several studies have compared the diagnostic performance of those risk stratification systems in which the Korean-TIRADS (K-TIRADS) showed the best specificity, while the ACR-TIRADS presented with the best sensitivity. Meanwhile, another study showed that the ACR-TIRADS outperformed the K-TIRADS in terms of a higher area under the curve (AUC) and lower false-negative rate (Kang et al. 2021). All those risk stratification systems classify thyroid lesions according to composition, echogenicity, shape, and margin as well as echogenic focus. In combination with the size of the lesion, the need of FNA or follow-up is defined (Fig. 2). A taller-than-wide shape (defined as a transverse diameter superior to the anteroposterior diameter) is a useful US feature for predicting thyroid malig-

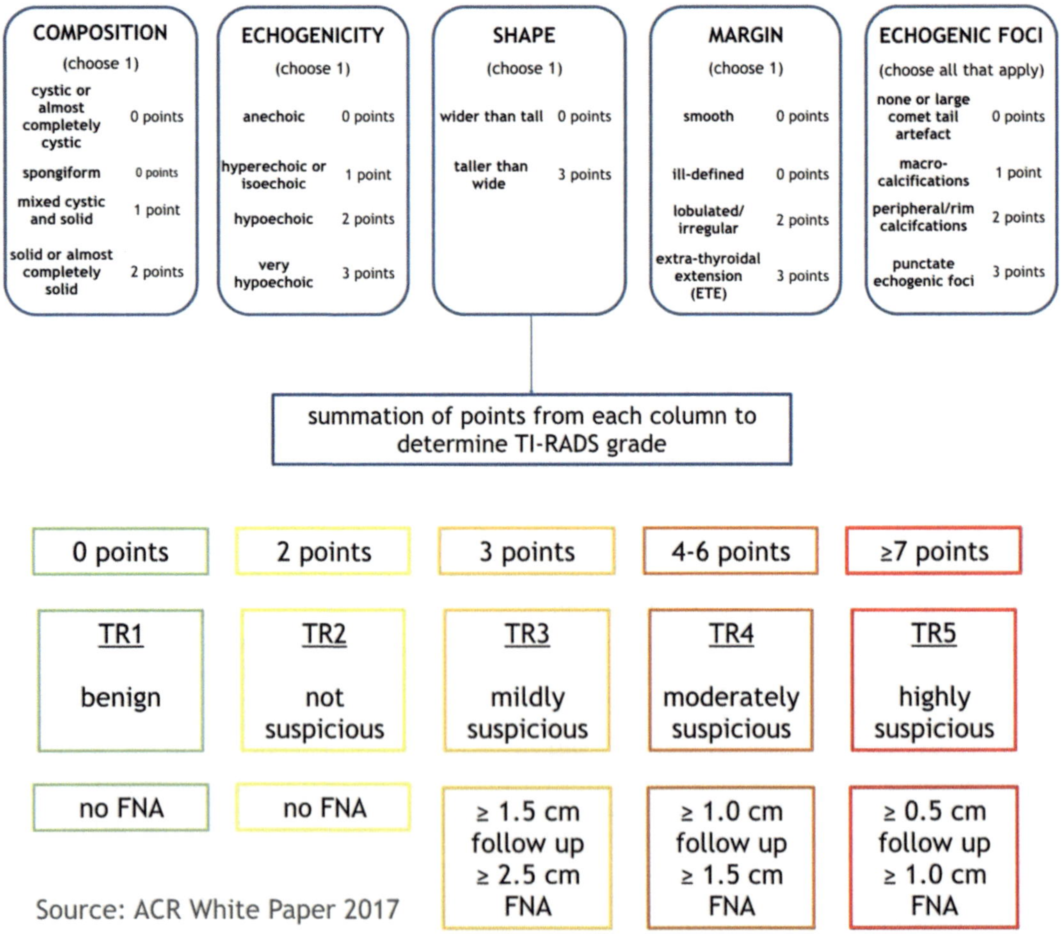

Fig. 2 TI-RADS classification flowchart. Fine needle aspiration (FNA). (Adapted from Tessler et al. 2017)

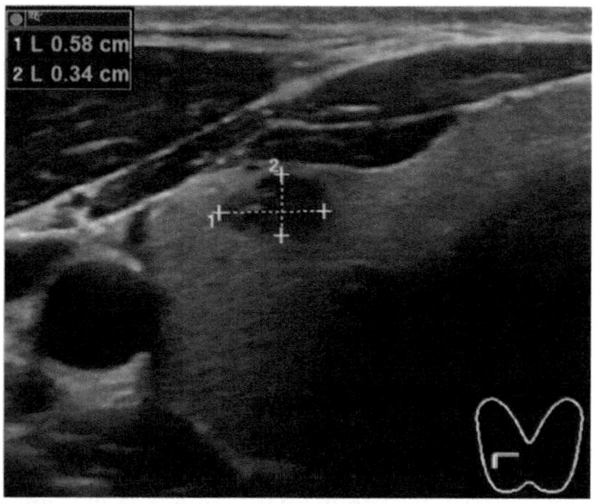

Fig. 3 TI-RADS 2 lesion. Spongiform, hypoechoic, ill-defined, wider-than-tall lesion without echogenic foci in the right thyroid lobe (TI-RADS 2)

nancy in the axial/transverse diameter—similar to breast imaging (Moon et al. 2011). An example is shown in Fig. 3. The higher the TR (TI-RADS) level, the higher the likelihood of malignancy. If the patient presents with multiple nodules, only the four highest-scoring nodules (which are not necessarily the largest) should be scored, reported, and followed up (Tessler et al. 2017).

TI-RADS classification serves as a pivotal guide for the standardized assessment of thyroid nodules, based on their ultrasound features. It facilitates clinical decision-making, particularly concerning the need for fine needle aspiration biopsies. The system aims to reduce unnecessary biopsies of benign nodules, ensuring more efficient allocation of medical resources and decreased patient anxiety. Moreover, it promotes consistent reporting among radiologists, leading to enhanced communication with referring clinicians.

2 Lymph Nodes

2.1 Origins and Physiological Foundation

Lymph nodes are located in almost all parts of the body, including the mediastinum, the axilla, and the neck. Lymph nodes contain immune cells that can help fight infections or react to other pathologies or situations like vaccines (COVID-19) (Suwatanapongched and Gierada 2006; Solomon et al. 2021). An increase in size or a change in lymph node attenuation can be a sign of ongoing infection, chronic diseases, or malignancies and therefore be of interest in many imaging studies (Suwatanapongched and Gierada 2006; Nin et al. 2016).

2.2 How Is the Measurement Performed?

The diagnosis of pathological lymph nodes in the chest relies mainly on morphological criteria and size measurements (Nin et al. 2016). Lymph node abnormalities are depicted on CT as an increase in size and/or number of lymph nodes or changes in lymph node attenuation (Suwatanapongched and Gierada 2006). Commonly used methods for size assessment in lymph nodes include the maximum and minimum axial diameters and the ratio of these two values (Schwartz and Bogaerts 2009). Usually, the short axis of the lymph node is used to define if the node is enlarged or not. There are various thresholds for various lymph node stations in the body (Kiyono et al. 1988; Schwartz and Bogaerts 2009; Ganeshalingam and Koh 2009).

2.3 What Are the Expected Results and Range of Normal Values?

Generally speaking, a normal benign lymph node should be ovoid in shape, the short axis should not exceed 1 cm, and the node should contain a centrally located fatty hilum. If the lymph node shows one of the following criteria, it might be considered suspicious: round, larger than 1 cm in the short axis and a loss of fatty hilus (Ganeshalingam and Koh 2009).

For the chest, the generally accepted size threshold for pathological enlargement in cancer patients is of >10 mm along the short axis of the node (Suwatanapongched and Gierada 2006). Other authors propose different standard maximum normal short-axial diameters for nodal stations: station 7, 12 mm; stations 4 and 10R, 10 mm; and other stations, 8 mm (Nin et al. 2016). Regarding the internal mammary lymph node, there is no clear cutoff, but breast MR-related studies show 4 mm for short axis length and 10 mm for long axis length to predict metastasis (Lee and Kim 2016). There is very little data in the literature on what constitutes a normal sized cardiophrenic lymph node. Dorfman et al. (1991) evaluated this type of lymph node and concluded that lymph nodes that exceeded a short axis diameter of 8 mm in the paracardiac region were abnormal and should be considered suspicious, especially if more than one node was present. A study by Farmakis et al. (2013) found that FDG PET/CT is more accurate in the detection of pathologic cardiophrenic lymph nodes than CT, especially when they are subcentimeter in size. Normal values of thoracic lymph nodes are shown in Table 2.

Of note, lymph nodes may be enlarged due to a variety of conditions, including inflammatory, infectious, or malignant diseases. Therefore, it is important to distinguish benign from malignant entities (Kumar et al. 2011). Although CT and MRI provide good structural details, their diagnostic criteria might overlook microscopic metastases or partial tumoral infiltration of the node. In addition, in a malignant clinical condition, enlarged lymph nodes may correspond to malignant as well as inflammatory/infectious causes. For these reasons, CT has only low sensitivity and specificity (64% and 62%, respectively) in detecting malignant lymph nodes (McLoud et al. 1992). ^{18}F-fluorodeoxy glucose positron emission tomography (^{18}F-FDG PET) can be used as a problem solver, with a sensitivity of 84% and a specificity of 89% in detecting malignant mediastinal lymph nodes in lung cancer patients (Toloza et al. 2003). Most of the studies conducted in developed countries have shown high sensitivity and specificity if maximum standardized uptake value (SUVmax) of 2.5 was used as the cutoff value to differentiate benign from malignant nodes. However, these high diagnostic values of PET and PET/CT cannot be extrapolated to countries where mediastinal lymph node involvement due to granulomatous diseases is common, and in these countries, higher SUVmax value thresholds might be recommended (Kumar et al. 2011). In addition, some disorders like sarcoidosis or silicosis may also display high uptake values, as well as postoperative changes. Fungal disease may also give rise to high values of SUVmax. Overlapping of SUV between malignant and benign lymph nodes explains why histopathological proof may be required in any case of high SUVmax.

Table 2 Normal values of thoracic lymph nodes (Glazer et al. 1985)

Generally short axis	≤10 mm
Region 7	≤12 mm
Regions 4 and 10R	≤10 mm
Other thoracic stations	≤8 mm, but recommend FDG PET/CT in a context of known malignancy

2.4 Confounding Factors

Not only the localization of the lymph node but also patients' age has to be considered in lymph node measurements: In children under the age of 10 years, most lymph nodes are ≤7 mm. In older pediatric patients, lymph node sizes are comparable to values in adult individuals (De Jong and Nievelstein 2012).

2.5 Clinical Implementation of the Measurement

US is the first-line imaging modality to assess palpable superficial lymph nodes in the axilla and the clavicular region (Suwatanapongched and Gierada 2006). Additionally, US Doppler mode poses the possibility to evaluate tissue perfusion and can be used as a tool to guide tissue biopsies or fine needle aspiration in unclear or suspicious lesions. When it is up to evaluate mediastinal or hilar lymph nodes, normally CT or MR is used (Suwatanapongched and Gierada 2006). PET in combination with CT or MRI is used to detect lymph node disease in cancer patients (Toloza et al. 2003). Measuring a newly appearing lymph node in patients with cancer holds significant clinical importance. First and foremost, it can indicate the spread or progression of the disease, helping clinicians determine the stage and aggressiveness of the cancer with regard to RECIST. Accurate measurement also aids in monitoring the node over time to evaluate treatment efficacy. Consequently, measuring of lymph nodes is important for guiding treatment decisions and forecasting patient prognosis. It also reduces the number of interventional procedures.

3 Esophagus

3.1 Origins and Physiological Foundation

The esophagus is a muscular tube that extends from the oropharynx to the cardia of the stomach. The esophagus begins at the hypopharynx and descends mostly to the left of the midline. In its course to the abdominal cavity, the esophagus can be divided into three parts (Weissleder et al. 2011):

- The cervical part: beginning at the upper esophageal sphincter, the esophagus is located in the anterior aspect of the neck in the so-called visceral space.
- The thoracic part: from the thoracic inlet to the esophageal hiatus of the diaphragm and is located in the middle or posterior mediastinum, pending of the mediastinal compartments' classification considered.
- The abdominal part: from the esophageal hiatus to the junction with the cardia of the stomach.

Depending on the patient size, the length of the esophagus varies from 23 to 37 cm with a diameter of 1–2 cm (Pearson et al. 2019).

Different imaging modalities can be used to evaluate the esophagus: with CT as well as MRI, the esophagus can be evaluated in its entire course. Observing the normal appearance and wall thickness of the esophagus in CT scans aids in diagnosing esophageal diseases and precisely identifying the tumor target in esophageal carcinomas for modern radiotherapy (Xia et al. 2009). MRI might have a higher soft tissue contrast to better evaluate the extent of possible lesions. Barium esophagography plays an important role in the time-resolved evaluation of the motility. In addition, it allows to examine the patient in the "normal" upright position.

3.2 How Is the Measurement Performed?

Because the esophagus may be collapsed in supine position, measurements of the dimension of the esophagus lumen are usually not performed routinely in CT or MRI. Measurements of the esophageal wall are possible, but standard normal values for esophageal wall thickness have not been established. However, some studies report that the wall thickness is approximately 5 mm during contraction and 2 mm during dilation of the esophagus (Xia et al. 2009). For esophagitis, a threshold of 5 mm and a target sign of the esophageal wall were proposed (Berkovich et al. 2000). Normal values for esophageal measurements are shown in Table 3.

However, measurements are more frequently obtained in barium swallows, especially in the setting of diverticula evaluation, evaluation of hiatal hernia, or evaluation of the presence and severity of achalasia.

3.2.1 Barium Swallow

Before starting, assessment of a risk of aspiration (i.e., wet voice, recurrent pneumonia, or aspiration) should be performed, and if unsure, let the patient swallow some water and observe. If there are signs of aspiration or the patient has had any kind of intervention/surgery which could have harmed the integrity of the esophagus or the gastrointestinal tract, use a nonionic water-soluble contrast agent instead of barium (Dodds et al. 1990).

Table 3 Esophageal measurements (Butler et al. 2012)

Length	23–37 cm
Width	1–2 cm
Length of phrenic ampulla	2–4 cm
Three anatomic constrictions	
Cervical	C 5/6 (due to cricoid cartilage)
Thoracic	T 4/5 (due to aortic arch)
Abdominal	T 10/11 (due to esophageal hiatus)

3.2.1.1 Achalasia

Achalasia is a motility disorder of the esophagus characterized by the inability of the lower esophageal sphincter to relax properly and a loss of esophageal peristalsis. This results from degeneration of the myenteric plexus neurons in the esophageal wall, leading to food and liquid retention in the esophagus and difficulty of swallowing. Currently, three different manometric subtypes of achalasia are defined: classic achalasia, achalasia with esophageal compression, and spastic achalasia (Oude Nijhuis et al. 2020).

The examination procedure of the barium esophagography is as follows. First, a scout film without contrast agent of the entire esophagus in the anteroposterior plane is performed (in tall patients where the cranio-caudal extension of the esophagus exceeds the detector size, perform one image for the cranial and a second one for the caudal portion of the esophagus). Then image series/fluoroscopy videos while swallowing the contrast agent is performed. Four stages of achalasia have been described based on the maximum diameter and shape of the esophagus above the functional stenosis on barium swallow: stage 1 > 4 cm; stage 2 = 4–6 cm; stage 3 > 6 cm, with a straight esophagus; and stage 4 > 6 cm, with a sigmoid-shaped esophagus (Riccio et al. 2022). Another technique is the "timed" barium swallow. In a person with normal esophageal function, the esophagus should be emptied of 250 mL of barium within 10–20 s and have no residual barium at 1 min. If there is a delay in the passage of contrast agent, a contrast column will build in the esophagus. Images at 1, 3, and 5 min should be performed in order to document and measure the contrast column in height and width at these time points (Riccio et al. 2022). The size and persistence of the contrast column correspond to the severity of the achalasia, but to date, there is no classification system for those measurements (Fig. 4).

3.2.1.2 Diverticula

First, a scout film without contrast agent of the entire esophagus in the anteroposterior and lateral plane is performed which includes the digestive tract from the hard palate to the gastric fundus (in tall patients, two images should be obtained to capture the entire cranio-caudal extension). Then, image series/fluoroscopy videos while swallowing the contrast agent are performed, first in the lateral and then in the anteroposterior plane. In this way, if the patient aspirates and the examination should be interrupted, the diagnostically more important lateral planes are registered. Size and location of the diverticula, if any, should be registered (Fig. 5).

3.2.1.3 Hiatal Hernias

Although nowadays predominantly diagnosed and measured with CT or MRI, there still are hiatal hernias which are first diagnosed on barium swallow.

First, a scout film without contrast agent of the esophagus including the upper abdomen in the anteroposterior and lateral plane is performed. Then, image series/fluoroscopy videos while swallowing the contrast agent are performed, first in the lateral and then in the anteroposterior plane. Additional imaging should be performed while the patient performs the Valsalva maneuver. If a hiatal hernia is encountered, measure the size of the hiatal hernia in two planes (Fig. 6). In primary intervention, recurrence of hiatal hernia is more likely the larger the hiatal surface area is on the so-called hiatal surface area. The size of this area is the major contributing factor regarding the possibility of reherniation with indication

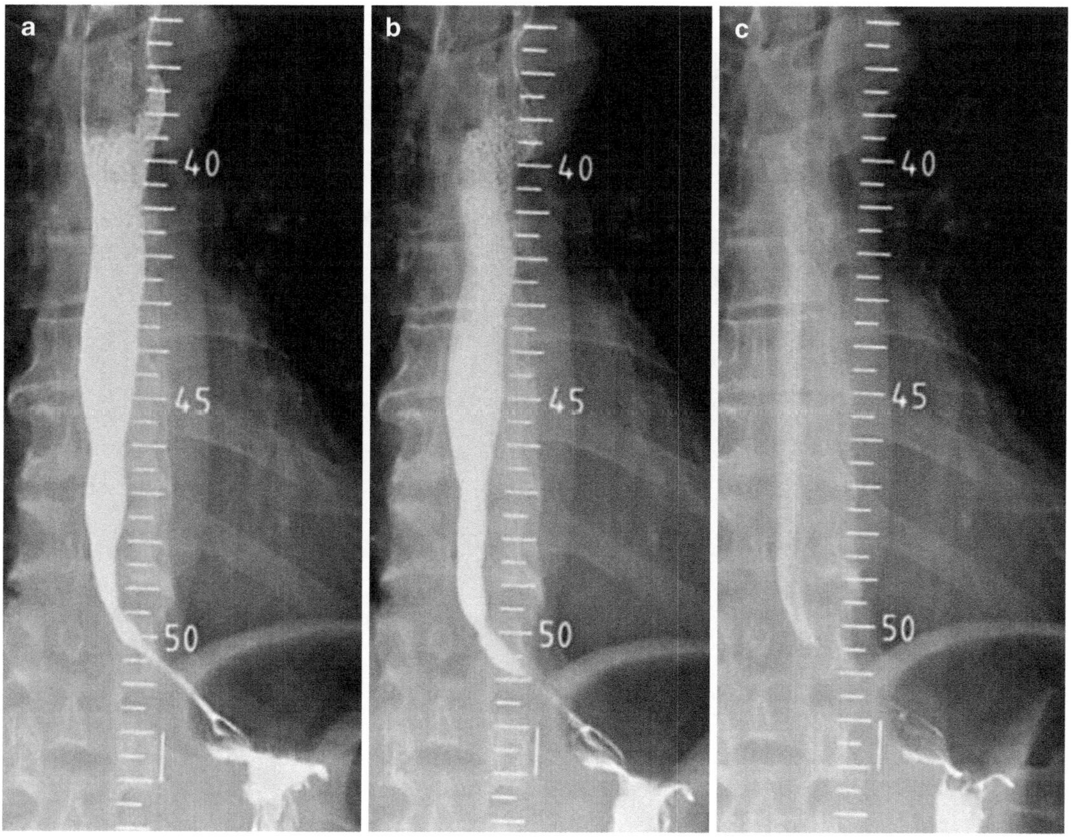

Fig. 4 Achalasia. After barium swallow, a contrast agent column formed and persisted at (**a**) 1 and (**b**) 3 min. (**c**) At 5 min, the column diminished

for mesh hiatoplasty with a cutoff of at least 5.6 cm^2 (Koch et al. 2011). This area is measured intra-abdominally with a ruler.

3.3 What Are the Expected Results and Range of Normal Values?

3.4 Confounding Factors

Since the esophagus is normally collapsed, it can be challenging to evaluate the esophageal wall for lesions on CT or MRI. Based on personal experience rather than literature, it can be helpful to let the patient drink diluted contrast medium directly before the CT or MRI examination in order to have some contrast in the tubular organ, which makes wall lesions more conspicuous.

3.5 Clinical Implementation of the Measurement

While an enlarged esophagus (>3 cm) is mostly due to failed or prolonged transition of food or fluids to the stomach, a too narrow esophagus (small-caliber esophagus) is a characteristic finding in eosinophilic esophagitis and lichen planus, a chronic inflammatory condition involving the skin, mucus membranes, and esophagus.

A small-caliber esophagus is defined as an esophagus with a caliber <1 cm. Similarly, short-

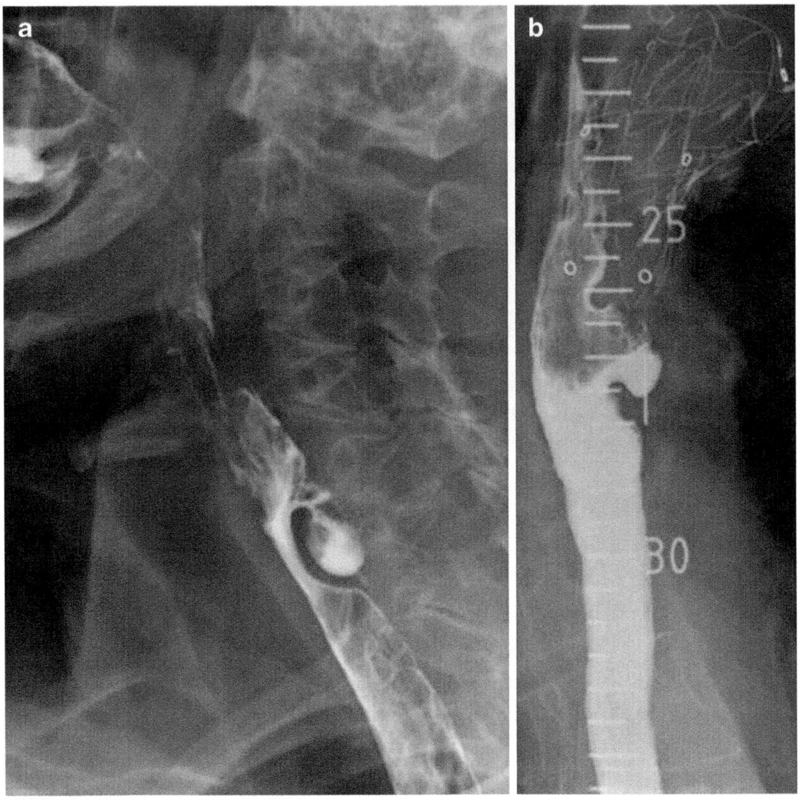

Fig. 5 Diverticula. (**a**) Posteriorly located diverticulum protruding through the horizontal and oblique components of the cricopharyngeus muscle (Zenker diverticulum). In this image, the measurement scale was not placed in the field of view, which makes diverticulum measurement difficult. (**b**) Laterally located diverticulum in the middle third of the esophagus. In this patient, the measurement scale was superimposed to the pathology. This should normally be avoided. Note an aortic endoprosthesis in (**b**)

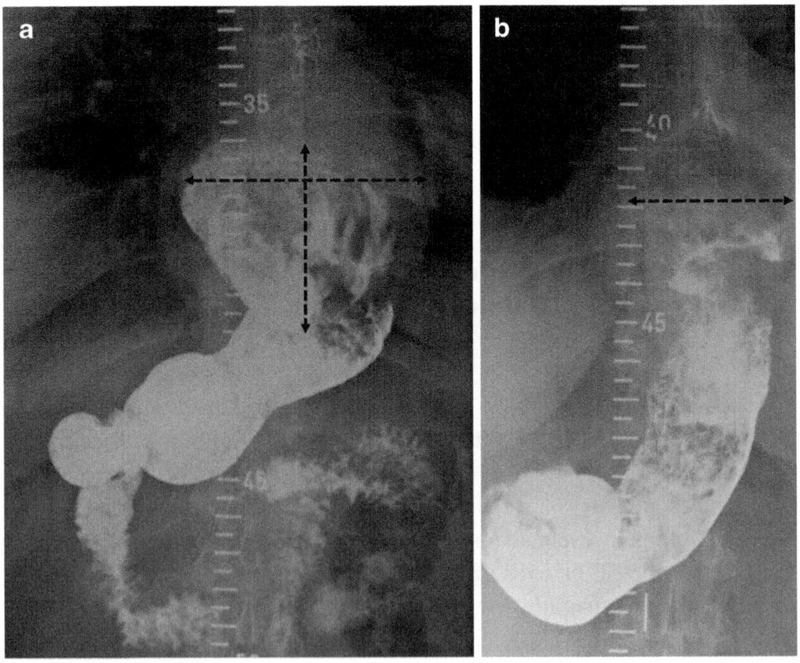

Fig. 6 Hiatal hernia. (**a**) Anteroposterior and (**b**) lateral-oblique view of an axial hiatal hernia with protrusion of portions of the stomach into the thoracic cavity. Measurement in two planes is indicated with dotted lines and arrows

segment strictures are a known finding that may be physiological due to anatomic compression. In pathological conditions, it is more important to focus on the irregularity in caliber with a transition point rather than absolute measurements to define strictures, as this better indicates the underlying pathology. Recognizing esophageal dilation on a CT scan is important because its presence may suggest an underlying disease process that requires further investigation, treatment, or both. Although measuring of the esophagus diameter and wall thickness might be of importance for various clinical scenarios, there is no general agreed-upon "cutoff" for abnormal esophageal diameter.

Disclaimer All measurements in this book have been obtained from peer-reviewed papers and guidelines from professional organizations, unless explicitly stated otherwise. While the authors, editors, and publisher have gone through a rigorous process to establish their correct reproduction from the original source, each measurement must be interpreted in the correct clinical context, this along with an accurate way of measurement, and taking into account all technical variables, this including follow-up exams with various equipment or software. Neither the authors, the editors, nor the publisher can accept any legal responsibility for any improper application or interpretation of these measurements as well as their potential consequences.

References

Berkovich GY, Levine MS, Miller WT (2000) CT findings in patients with esophagitis. AJR Am J Roentgenol 175(5):1431–1434. https://doi.org/10.2214/ajr.175.5.1751431

Brunn J, Block U, Ruf G, Bos I, Kunze WP, Scriba PC (1981) Volumetrie der Schilddrüsenlappen mittels real-time-sonographie [Volumetric analysis of thyroid lobes by real-time ultrasound (author's transl)]. Dtsch Med Wochenschr 106(41):1338–1340. https://doi.org/10.1055/s-2008-1070506

Butler P, Mitchell A, Healy JC (2012) Applied radiological anatomy. Cambridge University Press. ISBN: 0521766664

De Jong PA, Nievelstein R-JA (2012) Normal mediastinal and hilar lymph nodes in children on multi-detector row chest computed tomography. Eur Radiol 22:318–321. https://doi.org/10.1007/s00330-011-2253-9

Delange F, Benker G, Caron P et al (1997) Thyroid volume and urinary iodine in European schoolchildren: standardization of values for assessment of iodine deficiency. Eur J Endocrinol 136:180–187. https://doi.org/10.1530/eje.0.1360180

Dighe M, Barr R, Bojunga J et al (2017) Thyroid US: state of the art. Part 1—thyroid US reporting and diffuse thyroid diseases. Med Ultrason 19(1):79–93. https://doi.org/10.11152/mu-980

Dodds WJ, Logemann JA, Stewart ET (1990) Radiologic assessment of abnormal oral and pharyngeal phases of swallowing. AJR Am J Roentgenol 154:965–974. https://doi.org/10.2214/ajr.154.5.2108570

Dorfman RE, Alpern MB, Gross BH, Sandler MA (1991) Upper abdominal lymph nodes: criteria for normal size determined with CT. Radiology. 180(2):319–22. https://doi.org/10.1148/radiology.180.2.2068292. PMID: 2068292.

Farmakis S, Vejdani K, Muzaffar R, Parkar N, Osman MM (2013) Detection of metastatic disease in cardiophrenic lymph nodes: FDG PET/CT versus contrast-enhanced CT and implications for staging and treatment of disease. Front Oncol 3:260. Published 2013 Oct 1. https://doi.org/10.3389/fonc.2013.00260

Ganeshalingam S, Koh D-M (2009) Nodal staging. Cancer Imaging 9:104–111. https://doi.org/10.1102/1470-7330.2009.0017

Ghervan C (2011) Thyroid and parathyroid US. Med Ultrason 2011(13):80–84

Glazer GM, Gross BH, Quint LE, Francis IR, Bookstein FL, Orringer MB (1985) Normal mediastinal lymph nodes: number and size according to American Thoracic Society mapping. AJR Am J Roentgenol 144(2):261–265. https://doi.org/10.2214/ajr.144.2.261

Grant EG, Tessler FN, Hoang JK et al (2015) Thyroid US reporting lexicon: white paper of the ACR Thyroid Imaging, Reporting and Data System (TIRADS) Committee. J Am Coll Radiol 12:1272–1279. https://doi.org/10.1016/j.jacr.2015.07.011

Heged L, Rasmussen N, Knudsen N (1987) Seasonal variation in thyroid size in healthy males. Horm Metab Res 19:391–392. https://doi.org/10.1055/s-2007-1011833

Hegedüs L (1990) Thyroid size determined by US. Influence of physiological factors and non-thyroidal disease. Dan Med Bull 37(3):249

Hegedüs L, Rasmussen N, Knudsen N (1987) Seasonal variation in thyroid size in healthy males. Horm Metab Res 19(8):391–392. https://doi.org/10.1055/s-2007-1011833

Kang S, Ki Kwon S, Choi HS, Kim MJ, Park YJ, Park DJ, Cho SW (2021) Comparison of Korean vs. American thyroid imaging reporting and data system in malignancy risk assessment of indeterminate thyroid nodules. Endocrinol Metab (Seoul) 36(5):1111–1120. https://doi.org/10.3803/EnM.2021.1208

Kiyono K, Sone S, Sakai F et al (1988) The number and size of normal mediastinal lymph nodes: a postmortem study. AJR Am J Roentgenol 150:771–776. https://doi.org/10.2214/ajr.150.4.771

Koch O, Asche KU, Berger J, Weber E, Franderath FA, Pointner R (2011) Influence of the size of the hiatus on the rate of reherniation after laparoscopic fundoplication and refundoplication with mesh hiatoplasty. Surg Endosc 5(4):1024–1030. https://doi.org/10.1007/s00464-010-1308-3

Kumar A, Dutta R, Kannan U et al (2011) Evaluation of mediastinal lymph nodes using 18F-FDG PET-CT scan and its histopathologic correlation. Ann Thorac Med 6:11–16. https://doi.org/10.4103/1817-1737.74270

Lee HW, Kim SH (2016) Breast magnetic resonance imaging for assessment of internal mammary lymph node status in breast cancer. J Breast Cancer 19(2):191–8. https://doi.org/10.4048/jbc.2016.19.2.191. Epub 2016 Jun 24. PMID: 27382396; PMCID: PMC4929261.

McLoud TC, Bourgouin PM, Greenberg RW et al (1992) Bronchogenic carcinoma: analysis of staging in the mediastinum with CT by correlative lymph node mapping and sampling. Radiology 182:319–323. https://doi.org/10.1148/radiology.182.2.1732943

Moon HJ, Kwak JY, Kim E-K, Kim MJ (2011) A taller-than-wide shape in thyroid nodules in transverse and longitudinal ultrasonographic planes and the prediction of malignancy. Thyroid 21:1249–1253. https://doi.org/10.1089/thy.2010.0372

Nin CS, de Souza VVS, do Amaral RH et al (2016) Thoracic lymphadenopathy in benign diseases: a state of the art review. Respir Med 112:10–17. https://doi.org/10.1016/j.rmed.2016.01.021

Oude Nijhuis RAB, Zaninotto G, Roman S, Boeckxstaens GE, Fockens P, Langendam MW, Plumb AA, Smout A, Targarona EM, Trukhmanov AS, Weusten B, Bredenoord AJ (2020) European guidelines on achalasia: United European Gastroenterology and European Society of Neurogastroenterology and Motility recommendations. United European Gastroenterol J 8(1):13–33. https://doi.org/10.1177/2050640620903213

Pearson WG, Griffeth JV, Ennis AM (2019) Functional anatomy underlying pharyngeal swallowing mechanics and swallowing performance goals. Perspect ASHA Special Interest Groups 4:648–655. https://doi.org/10.1044/2019_PERS-SIG13-2018-0014

Riccio F, Costantini M, Salvador R (2022) Esophageal achalasia: diagnostic evaluation. World J Surg 46:1516–1521. https://doi.org/10.1007/s00268-022-06483-3

Schwartz LH, Bogaerts J, Ford R et al (2009) Evaluation of lymph nodes with RECIST 1.1. Eur J Cancer 45:261–267. https://doi.org/10.1016/j.ejca.2008.10.028

Şeker S, Taş İ (2010) Determination of thyroid volume and its relation with isthmus thickness. Eur J Gen Med 7(2):125–129. https://doi.org/10.29333/ejgm/82838

Shabana W, Peeters E, De Maeseneer M (2006) Measuring thyroid gland volume: should we change the correction factor? AJR Am J Roentgenol 186(1):234–236. https://doi.org/10.2214/AJR.04.0816

Solomon JJ, Heyman B, Ko JP, Condos R, Lynch DA (2021) CT of post-acute lung complications of COVID-19. Radiology 301(2):E383–E395. https://doi.org/10.1148/radiol.2021211396

Suwatanapongched T, Gierada DS (2006) CT of thoracic lymph nodes. Part I: anatomy and drainage. BJR 79:922–928. https://doi.org/10.1259/bjr/26411607

Tessler FN, Middleton WD, Grant EG et al (2017) ACR Thyroid Imaging, Reporting and Data System (TI-RADS): white paper of the ACR TI-RADS Committee. J Am Coll Radiol 14:587–595. https://doi.org/10.1016/j.jacr.2017.01.046

Toloza EM, Harpole L, McCrory DC (2003) Noninvasive staging of non-small cell lung cancer: a review of the current evidence. Chest 123:137S–146S. https://doi.org/10.1378/chest.123.1_suppl.137s

Viduetsky A, Herrejon CL (2019) Sonographic evaluation of thyroid size: a review of important measurement parameters. J Diagn Med Sonogr 35(3):206–210. https://doi.org/10.1177/8756479318824290

Vinh D, Zafereo M (2021) Surgical considerations in thyroid cancer: what the radiologist needs to know. Neuroimaging Clin N Am 31:327–335. https://doi.org/10.1016/j.nic.2021.04.010

Weissleder R, Wittenberg J et al (2011) Primer of diagnostic imaging. Expert consult-online and print. Mosby

Xia F, Mao J, Ding J, Yang H (2009) Observation of normal appearance and wall thickness of esophagus on CT images. Eur J Radiol 72(3):406–411. https://doi.org/10.1016/j.ejrad.2008.09.002

The Pleura

Anand Sundaralingam, Najib Rahman,
and Fergus Gleeson

Contents

A. Sundaralingam (✉)
Oxford Respiratory Trials Unit, Churchill Hospital, Headington, UK

Oxford Pleural Unit, Oxford Centre for Respiratory Medicine, Oxford University Hospitals NHS Trust, Oxford, UK

Imperial College Healthcare NHS Trust, London, UK
e-mail: anand.sundaralingam@ndm.ox.ac.uk

N. Rahman
Oxford Respiratory Trials Unit, Churchill Hospital, Headington, UK

Oxford Pleural Unit, Oxford Centre for Respiratory Medicine, Oxford University Hospitals NHS Trust, Oxford, UK

Chinese Academy of Medical Health Sciences, University of Oxford, Oxford, UK

NIHR Oxford Biomedical Research Centre, University of Oxford, Oxford, UK
e-mail: najib.rahman@ndm.ox.ac.uk

F. Gleeson
Department of Radiology, Oxford University Hospitals, Oxford, UK
e-mail: Fergus.gleeson@oncology.ox.ac.uk; Fergus.gleeson@ouh.nhs.uk

Med Radiol Diagn Imaging (2026)
https://doi.org/10.1007/174_2025_590,
Published Online: 24 August 2025

1 Introduction

The pleural lining is a crucial component of the thoracic cavity and a common site for pathology. Imaging of this vital structure is therefore of great importance, as both a diagnostic and therapeutic aid. This chapter discusses the imaging of the pleura, with a particular focus on measurements and other tools to evaluate this important structure.

2 Anatomy and Normal Appearance

The pleural lining consists of two thin membranes, the visceral pleura and the parietal pleura. The visceral pleura covers the entire surface of the lung whilst the parietal pleura covers the inner surface of the thoracic cage (Hallifax and Rahman 2016).

The parietal pleura can be subdivided into different anatomical divisions (Fig. 1):

- The costal pleura (lining the inner surface of the ribs and intercostal muscles)
- The diaphragmatic pleura (covering the convex surface of the diaphragm)
- The cervical pleura (extending above the first rib and rising into the neck)
- The mediastinal pleura (adherent to the mediastinal structures)

Superiorly, the parietal pleura extends for 2–3 cm above the first rib, along the medial third of the clavicle, deep to the sternocleidomastoid, forming the cervical pleura.

Inferiorly, the pleura reflects at the lower boundary of the thoracic cage. On the right-hand side, anteriorly it will often extend beyond the costal margin in the infrasternal region, whilst on both sides, posteriorly it will reflect at the costovertebral angles, forming the diaphragmatic pleura.

There are two recesses within the pleural cavity, where the space is not entirely filled by lung parenchyma. These are the costomediastinal recess, which is found between the mediastinal pleura and the costal pleura, located posterior to the sternum and the costodiaphragmatic recess which is the space between the costal pleura and the diaphragmatic pleura.

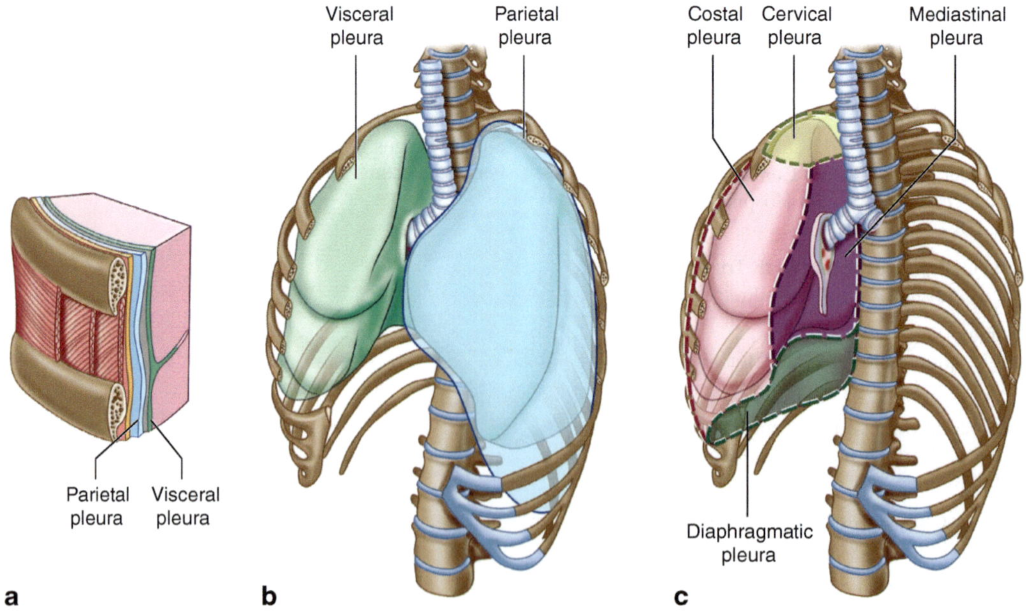

Fig. 1 Anatomical divisions of the pleura

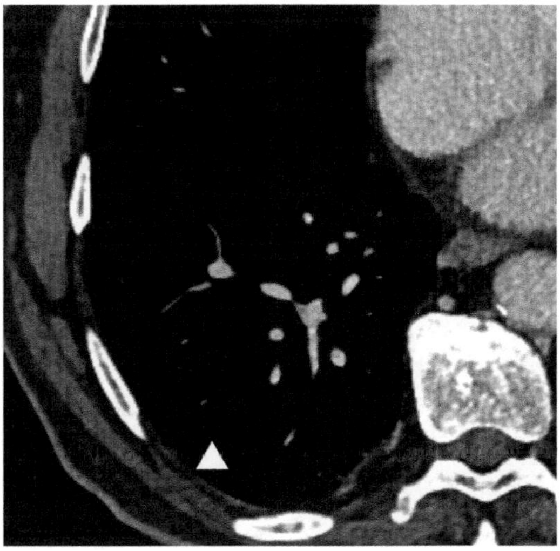

Fig. 2 The extra-pleural space indicated by the 'intercostal stripe' (white arrowhead) on CT. This space consists of the extra-pleural fat, endothoracic facia and innermost intercostal muscle

The pleural cavity represents the space between the visceral pleura and the parietal pleura. It is an entirely sealed cavity, with no connection between the right or left hemithorax (in humans) and usually measures 10–20 μm in diameter. In healthy subjects, the pleural cavity is estimated to contain 0.26 mL/kg of fluid per hemithorax (Noppen 2016).

Whilst the pleura can be visualised through a variety of imaging modalities, for an overview of the whole pleura, computed tomography (CT) is the mainstay imaging tool of choice. In healthy subjects, most of the pleura is not visible on CT; however, the 'intercostal stripe' may be visible in the intercostal spaces, and it represents the extra-pleural space (EPS) and acts as a surrogate marker for the pleura. It is not usually seen internal to the ribs on CT. The EPS or 'intercostal stripe' is a 1–2 mm line made up of extra-pleural fat, endothoracic fascia and the innermost intercostal muscle (Fig. 2) (Duerden et al. 2020; Santamarina et al. 2017). The parietal pleura is not usually visible on CT; therefore, any visible soft tissue seen internal to the ribs or causing thickening of the intercostal stripe usually represents abnormal pleural thickening. Exceptions to this rule are where intrathoracic muscles (e.g. transversus thoracis, subcostal muscles) may be seen internal to the ribs, and in some instances, the intercostal vessels may extend from the intercostal space, where they may be visible, internal to the rib, and mimic intercostal stripe thickening, particularly in examinations obtained without contrast medium administration. Intrathoracic muscles may be identified by a smooth and regular lung-chest wall interface on lung window (Fig. 3) (Alfudhili et al. 2016). The other structure that may be seen internal to the ribs is fat in extra-pleural lipomatosis that is usually located posterolaterally between the 4th and 8th ribs.

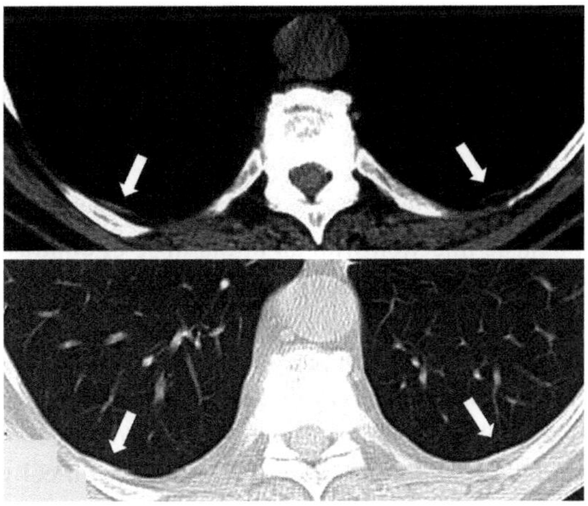

Fig. 3 The smooth and regular lung-chest wall interface on lung windows indicating intrathoracic muscles (white arrowhead)

3 Imaging Technique

3.1 Plain Chest Radiograph

The most frequently performed imaging test, the chest X-ray provides limited information about the normal pleura. However, it remains very useful in the detection of air and to some extent fluid within the pleural space. It is best to acquire images in the posteroanterior (PA) projection, although supine anteroposterior (AP) images are often taken in the acutely unwell patient but have a poorer sensitivity for detecting pleural disease.

3.2 Computed Tomography

The pleura, particularly in the presence of pleural fluid, is better visualised on CT with the use of iodinated intravenous contrast. It is recommended that either: an acquisition at 90 s using a biphasic injection with an initial dose of contrast followed by an arterial bolus which enables pleural (portal tissue phase enhancement) enhancement plus arterial enhancement if the pulmonary arteries also require review to exclude for instance a pulmonary embolus as the cause of an effusion; or a delayed phase (90 s) scan which specifically targets and optimises pleural enhancement. Indeed, arterial phase (CT Pulmonary Angiogram) scans, may even reduce the sensitivity for detection of pleural-based malignancy (Tsim et al. 2017; Arenas-Jiménez et al. 2018; Raj et al. 2011). CTs should be performed as volumetric scans, using thin sections (sub 1 mm) to enable multiplanar reconstruction. For optimal viewing of the pleura, images should be reviewed using a mediastinal window setting (40/400) on a soft tissue algorithm. The fissures are better viewed on a lung window (−500/1500 or −600/1600) (Hallifax et al. 2017).

Scanning in the supine position is the usual convention; however, this may overestimate pleural thickening in the posterobasal regions due to adjacent atelectasis or subpleural lymphatic fluid accumulation or small pleural effusions may be mistaken for thickening. Occasionally, additional prone imaging may help differentiate between these differing conditions (Alfudhili et al. 2016; Claude-Desroches et al. 2012; Goo et al. 2003).

Often debated is whether to drain pleural effusions prior to performing a CT scan, due to concerns surrounding the sensitivity for detecting parenchymal pathology in the presence of an effusion. In fact, scanning in the presence of a pleural effusion may even aid in the identification of pleural thickening (Fig. 4) (Corcoran et al. 2016).

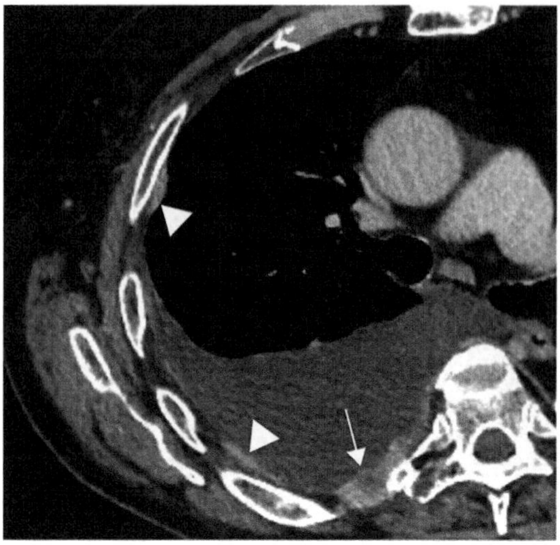

Fig. 4 Pleural thickening accentuated in the presence of effusion with difference in Hounsfield units differentiating pleural abnormality from effusion (white arrowheads) and grossly abnormal nodular pleural thickening likely extending into chest wall metastases (white arrow)

3.3 Thoracic Ultrasound

Ultrasound (US) has rapidly become one of the most useful imaging tools in the management of pleural disease. Its portability and real-time image acquisition lends itself not just to procedural guidance, but it also has great utility for diagnostic purposes. A curvilinear probe (3.5–5 MHz) is the optimal transducer for the initial assessment of the pleura, as most pleural pathology requires reasonable depth to visualise in full, and the resolution this transducer provides is more than adequate to guide most pleural interventions (Hallifax et al. 2017). In certain circumstances, a linear probe (8–12 MHz) may be useful in providing additional information. Its higher resolution and shallow depth of field is optimally placed to visualise chest wall structures (e.g. intercostal vascular and nerve bundles), and may facilitate advanced procedures, such as regional anaesthesia. Most of the scanning with US will be in ‘B-mode’ (‘Brightness-mode’). This will scan a plane through the body and the echoes are converted into a 2-D image. Pathology such as a pleural effusion can be readily visualised in this mode (Fig. 5). M-mode (‘Movement-mode’) can also be of use in pleural disease. By taking a cross-sectional plane across a region of interest, movement over time can be assessed. This can be particularly useful in assessing diaphragmatic excursion, but other use cases have also been discovered (e.g. identification of pneumothorax). Both colour flow and pulse wave Doppler modes

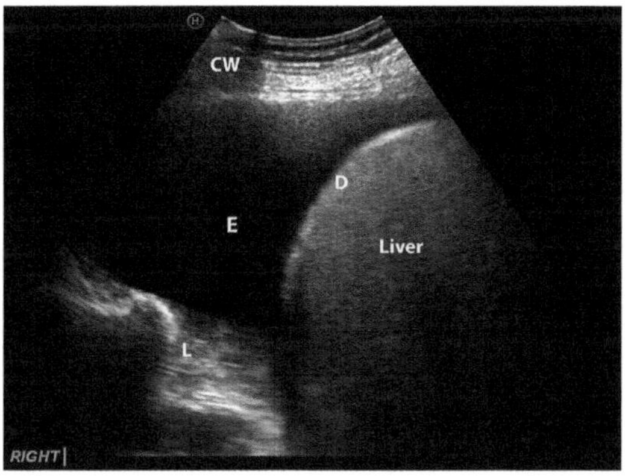

Fig. 5 Pleural effusion on thoracic US. CW = chest wall, E = effusion, D = diaphragm, L = lung

can be useful adjuncts in the assessment of vascular structures prior to intervention. Increasingly more novel US techniques are entering the clinical domain in pleural medicine (Banka et al. 2020).

This includes contrast-enhanced US which relies on differential tissue enhancement with contrast, between malignant and non-malignant lesions (delayed 'arrival time' or AT of contrast >8 s in malignant tissue or a lesion compared to lung AT of >2.5 s). The lesion-lung AT has been shown to have greater overall diagnostic accuracy (97%) compared to an absolute AT value (86%) (Bai et al. 2016; Hong-Xia et al. 2016).

US elastography is another technique, which differentiates malignant and benign lesions through a difference in 'tissue-stiffness', which can be quantitatively calculated with 'shear-wave elastography' or SWE (using a SWE_{mean} of >47.25 kPa to diagnose a malignant pleural lesion). Using this SWE_{mean} threshold has been shown to have a sensitivity of 84% and specificity of 91% (Jiang et al. 2019).

3.4 Magnetic Resonance Imaging

The role of MRI in pleural disease is an emerging field; T1-weighted, contrast-enhanced images on MRI allow for better visualisation of the tissue planes involved in the thoracic cavity and chest wall. It is therefore particularly of value in assessing the degree of tumour invasion in malignancies such as MPM (Heelan et al. 1999; Tsim et al. 2020). To date it remains an area of academic interest and reserved for more troublesome cases rather than routine care. In addition to contrast-enhanced MRI, diffusion-weighted MRI, which measures an 'apparent diffusion coefficient' (ADC), a measure of tissue cellularity, has been shown to be of use in differentiating between benign and malignant pleural lesions. Using an ADC threshold of $<1.5 \times 10^{-3}$ mm^2 s^{-1} to identify malignant pleural lesions has been shown to have a sensitivity of 100%, specificity of 92% and an overall diagnostic accuracy of 98% (Revelli et al. 2016).

3.5 PET-CT

PET-CT provides functional information on the metabolic activity of pleural abnormalities, with the use of 18F-fluorodeoxyglucose (FDG), reported as of value in differentiating benign from malignant lesions. Whilst PET-CT can be quite sensitive at detecting malignant pleural disease (sensitivity 81–95%), false-positives due to infection, inflammation or post-talc pleurodesis and false-negatives due to low-grade tumours (such as epithelioid mesothelioma) remain an issue (Treglia et al. 2014; Porcel et al. 2015). Recently published data does not support its use in directing targeted biopsies over contrast CT, and current guidelines do not recommend its routine use for staging in malignant pleural mesothelioma (MPM), but it may be reserved for those being considered for multimodality treatment (de Fonseka et al. 2024; Woolhouse et al. 2018; Popat et al. 2022; Tschopp et al. 2015).

4 Radiological Measurements

Precise measurements based on radiological appearance are often sought by clinicians, and this is no different in pleural disease. Whilst it remains debatable as to whether this should affect treatment decisions or indeed if it does affect clinical outcomes; nonetheless, there have been some efforts made to provide precise radiological measurements for clinicians and these will be outlined below.

4.1 Pneumothorax

CT remains the gold standard in both diagnosing the presence and the size of a pneumothorax (Tschopp et al. 2015). However, it is neither practical nor recommended to subject all patients with possible pneumothoraces to CT and most patients will be diagnosed from a chest X-ray. Consequently, much of the literature has focused on using the chest X-ray to estimate the size of a pneumothorax. All methods to quantitatively measure the size of a three-dimensional structure based on two-dimensional imaging are subject to a degree of error; nonetheless, the most often used are described below.

4.1.1 Collin's Method

Collin's method is perhaps one of the best recognised and calculates the 'percentage pneumothorax size' (% of the hemithorax) based on taking measurements of distance from the lung edge to the chest wall (Fig. 6). The method was derived from comparing calculations based on chest X-ray to CT, using the following formula (Collins et al. 1995).

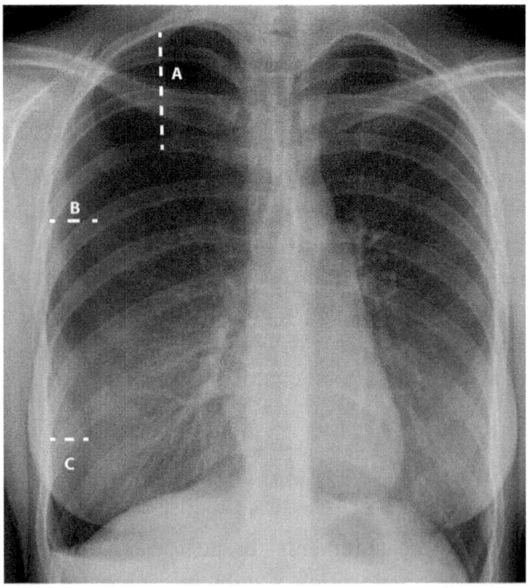

Fig. 6 Collin's method
% Collins = 4.2 + 4.7(*A* + *B* + *C*)
A = maximum intrapleural distance at the apex
B = intrapleural distance at the midpoint of the upper half of the lung
C = intrapleural distance at the midpoint of the lower half of the lung
*Also used in Rhea's method: [(*A* + *B* + *C*)/3]

$$\% \text{ Collins} = 4.2 + 4.7(A + B + C)$$

A = maximum intrapleural distance at the apex
B = intrapleural distance at the midpoint of the upper half of the lung
C = intrapleural distance at the midpoint of the lower half of the lung

This method is considered more accurate at estimating size in large pneumothoraces (e.g. if $A + B + C > 4$ cm) (Jouneau et al. 2023).

4.1.2 Rhea's Method

Rhea's method uses a similar technique and measurements as the Collins' method (Fig. 6).

$$\text{Rhea's method for calculating intrapleural distance} = (A + B + C)/3$$

However, Rhea's method uses a normogram to convert the average intrapleural distance into a percentage of hemithorax pneumothorax size. This method was derived from comparing calculations based on chest X-ray to hemithorax and collapsed lung volumes based on lateral and PA chest radiographs (Rhea et al. 1982). The normogram shows that an intrapleural distance of 1, 2, 3, 4 and 5 cm corresponds roughly to pneumothoraces of 14%, 23%, 32%, 40% and 50%, respectively. Rhea's method is considered more accurate at estimating smaller pneumothoraces and may underestimate the size of larger pneumothorax (Jouneau et al. 2023; Salazar et al. 2014; Kelly et al. 2006).

4.1.3 Light's Index

Light's index uses a ratio of the average diameter of the lung compared to the hemithorax using the following formula (Fig. 7) (Light 1988)

$$\% \text{ Light} = \left[1 - \left(b^3 / a^3\right)\right] \times 100$$

b = average diameter of the collapsed lung
a = average diameter of the hemithorax

There appears to be poor agreement between all three of these methods for estimation of size of pneumothorax (Salazar et al. 2014; Hoi et al. 2007).

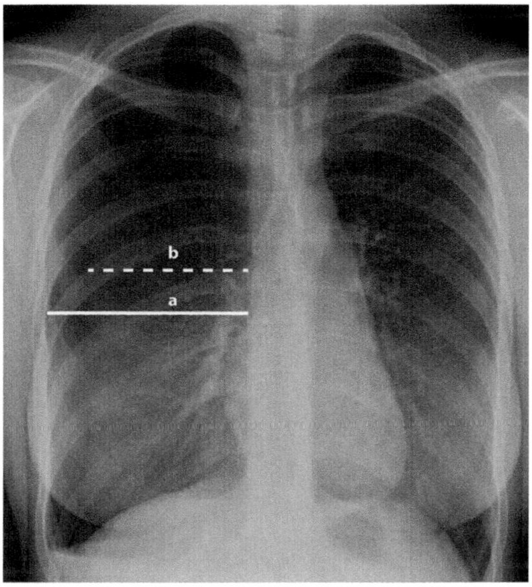

Fig. 7 Light's method: Ratio of the average diameter of the collapsed lung (*b*) to the hemithorax (*a*)
% Light = $[1 - (b^3/a^3)] \times 100$

For simplicity, most society guidelines have tended to use single variable thresholds to determine if a pneumothorax is significant (such as 'large') and requires intervention. The 2010 British Thoracic Society (BTS) guidelines used a cut-off of 2 cm between the lung edge and chest wall at the level of the hilum (MacDuff et al. 2010), whilst the American College of Chest Physicians (ACCP) used a cut-off of 3 cm between the lung edge and apex of the thorax (also referred to as cupola) (Fig. 8) (Baumann et al. 2001). Both the Belgian Society of Pulmonology and the Spanish Society of Pulmonology and Thoracic Surgery suggest a displacement of the pleural line along the entire lateral chest wall would constitute a 'large' pneumothorax (Aguinagalde et al. 2018; De Leyn et al. 2005).

Recent landmark studies into the management of pneumothorax have questioned the practice of management according to the size of the pneumothorax (Hallifax et al. 2020; Brown et al. 2020). Of greater importance in decision-making around the need for intervening in a pneumothorax is the overall clinical picture and how well patients are tolerating the pneumothorax in terms of physiological parameters and symptom burden. Certainly, underlying medical comorbidities (e.g. COPD or other chronic lung disease) will also affect the clinical picture.

The most recent society guidelines no longer recommend this approach of measuring pneumothorax size. Size of pneumothorax only becomes a relevant consideration if it is in fact felt to be too small to be safely intervened in based on CXR, at which point image guidance (i.e. CT guided) should be sought for safe insertion of a chest drain (Roberts et al. 2023).

4.2 Pleural Effusion

4.2.1 Volume

Similar to pneumothorax, the initial imaging of choice in pleural effusion is likely to be the chest X-ray. However, unlike in pneumothorax, the appearances on chest X-ray are neither specific nor sensitive (Zaki et al. 2024). A PA chest X-ray is thought to only reveal a visible meniscus once 200 mL of pleural fluid have accumulated in the pleural space, whilst a lateral decubitus chest X-ray, is a little more sensitive, and can detect as little as 50 mL (Blackmore et al. 1996). Differentiating between dense consolidation, or lung collapse from effusion may not always be possible and because of this, thoracic US as a point-of-care test has become commonly used to help this differentiation. US is both more sensitive and specific at detecting pleural effusion compared to chest X-ray (95% vs. 68% and 98% vs. 85%, for sensitivity and specificity, respectively) (Zaki et al. 2024).

4.2.1.1 Ultrasound

Quantifying the volume of effusion based on ultrasound appearances has been the subject of interest, with various different methodologies described.

Balik Formula

In this prospective study of an intensive care population, patients were scanned supine, with a mild trunk elevation of 15°, using a curvilinear

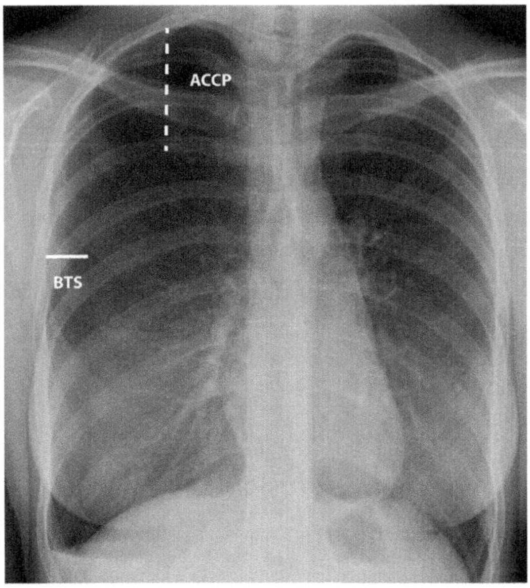

Fig. 8 BTS (solid line) uses the intrapleural distance at the hilum whilst ACCP (dashed line) uses the lung edge to apex of chest wall (or 'cupola') distance

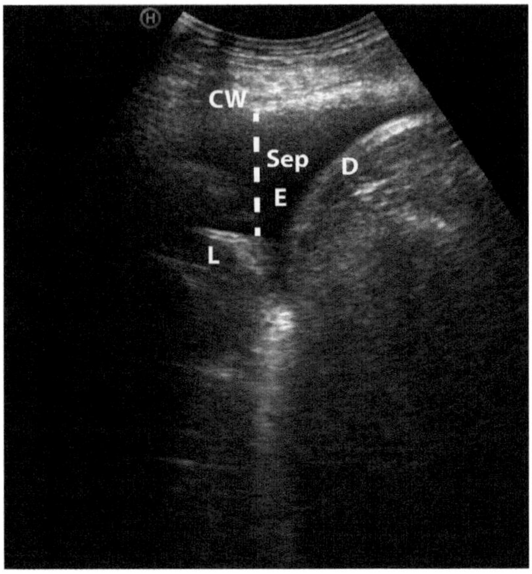

Fig. 9 Balik formula, the distance between the visceral pleura (at lung base) and parietal pleura (at chest wall) is the 'Sep' (or 'maximum separation')
Volume of effusion (mL) = 20 × Sep (mm)
CW = chest wall, D = diaphragm, E = effusion, L = lung

probe. The probe was held in the posterior axillary line, at an oblique angle, running parallel to the rib space. The distance between the visceral pleura (at lung base) and the parietal pleura (at chest wall) was measured at end-expiration ('maximum separation', Fig. 9) (Balik et al. 2006). The relationship between this value ('Sep') and the volume of effusion is expressed as follows:

$$\text{Volume of effusion}\left(\text{mL}\right) = 20 \times \text{Sep}\left(\text{mm}\right)$$

Sep = maximal separation

Eibenberger Formula

In this study, patients were scanned whilst supine during maximum inspiration in the posterolateral part of the chest wall, using a curvilinear probe. The maximum perpendicular distance between the posterior surface of the lung and the posterior chest wall was measured (Eibenberger et al. 1994). The relationship between the maximum perpendicular distance and volume of effusion drained was almost linear, and this is expressed as follows:

$$\text{Volume of effusion}\left(\text{mL}\right) = 47.6\left(\text{maximum perpendicular distance, mm}\right) - 837\,\text{mL}$$

At lower volumes, this formula becomes less accurate, and in fact produces non-plausible (negative) values.

Goecke Formula

Two variants of this formula in which patients are scanned in the erect position with a curvilinear probe placed against the posterolateral chest wall exist (Goecke and Schwerk 1990). The probe is held in a longitudinal orientation, with the index marker directed cephalad. Measurements are taken at end-expiration. With the first variant (Goecke 1), the cranio-caudal height of the effusion in cm is measured (from costophrenic angle

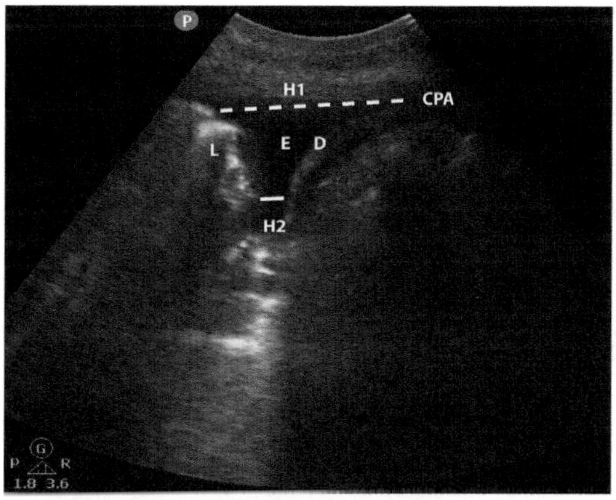

Fig. 10 The Goecke formulae, can either take just the measurement cranio-caudally from the costophrenic angle to lung base, $H1$ or take an additional measurement from the mid-diaphragm point to lung base, $H2$
Goecke 1: Volume (mL) = 90($H1$)
Goecke 2: Volume (mL) = 70($H1$ + $H2$)
CPA = costophrenic angle, L = lung, E = effusion, D = diaphragm

to lung base, '$H1$', Fig. 10). The Goecke 1 calculation is as follows:

$$\text{Volume}(\text{mL}) = 90(H1)$$

$H1$ = distance from costophrenic angle to lung base

In the second variant (Goecke 2), an additional measurement is also taken from the mid-diaphragm (subpulmonary region) to lung base, in cm ('$H2$', Fig. 10). Here the equation is as follows:

$$\text{Volume}(\text{mL}) = 70(H1 + H2)$$

$H1$ = distance from costophrenic angle to lung base
$H2$ = distance from the mid-diaphragm to lung base

Usta Formula

In this study of post-cardiac surgical patients, patients were scanned in an erect position with a linear probe (Usta et al. 2010). The probe was placed in the mid-scapular line and orientated longitudinally. The distance between the mid-diaphragm and the lung base is measured in mm ('D'). The equation is as follows:

$$\text{Volume}(\text{mL}) = 16(D)$$

D = distance from the mid-diaphragm to lung base

Whilst there is not much to separate these different methods, scanning in the erect position with the Goecke 2 formula appears to yield slightly more accurate estimates of effusion volume than Balik and Eibenberger formulas (Ibitoye et al. 2018; Hassan et al. 2017).

4.2.1.2 Computed Tomography

CT has often been viewed as the gold standard for estimating the volume of a pleural effusion. However, most reporting refers to subjective grading systems of volume. Techniques have been developed that use volumetric analysis or quantitative characteristics (such as cranio-caudal length, AP depth) that can categorise effusions into small, medium or large categories (Fig. 11) (Moy et al. 2013; Chiao et al. 2015). More complex calculations have also been developed. We will summarise them below.

Hazlinger Formula

In the Hazlinger formula, b represents the greatest effusion depth in cm, perpendicular to the parietal pleura on transversal scan (Fig. 12) (Hazlinger et al. 2014).

$$\text{Volume}(\text{mL}) = 0.365(b^3) - 4.529(b^2) + 159.723(b) - 88.377$$

b = greatest effusion depth in cm, perpendicular to the parietal pleura on transversal scan (i.e. axial)

Given the complexity of this equation, the authors also provide a useful conversion table (Table 1).

Of note, the precise definition of 'greatest effusion depth' is debatable, given the location

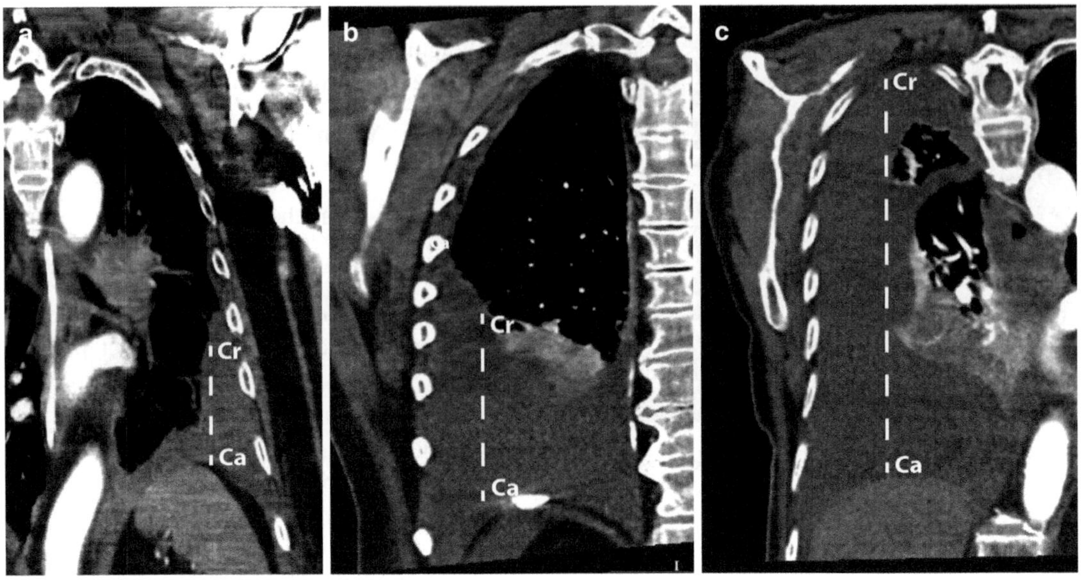

Fig. 11 Coronal CTs demonstrating different cranio-caudal (Cr-Ca) length of pleural effusions (**a** small, **b** moderate, **c** large)

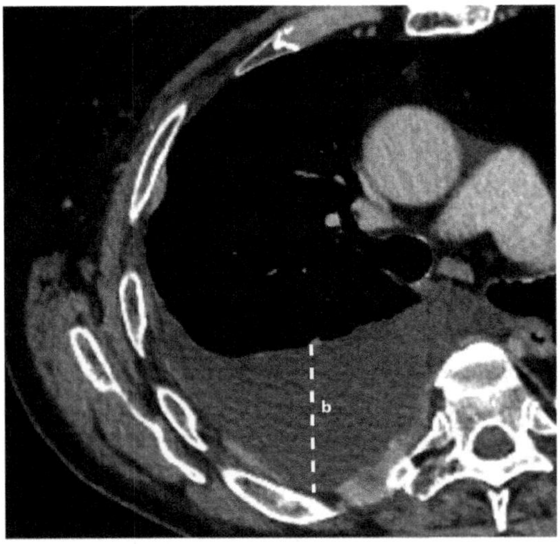

Fig. 12 The Hazlinger formula is a calculation based on CT, where *b* represents the greatest depth of effusion, perpendicular to the parietal pleura on axial view

you choose to measure the effusion depth from can lead to varying results. It is the authors' practice to, therefore, measure the depth of effusion (on axial view) at the midpoint of the effusion, based on its appearance in cranio-caudal view.

Table 1 Hazlinger conversion table

Dimension '*b*' (cm)	Pleural effusion volume (mL)
1	67
2	216
3	360
4	501
5	643
6	786
7	933
8	1086
9	1248
10	1421

Mergo Formula

In the Mergo formula, both the depth of effusion of transverse scan and length, on cranio-caudal measurement are required (Fig. 13) (Mergo et al. 1999).

$$\text{Volume}(\text{mL}) = d^2 \times l$$

d = greatest effusion depth in cm, perpendicular to the parietal pleura on axial orientation

l = greatest effusion length in cm, when measured cranio-caudally on coronal orientation

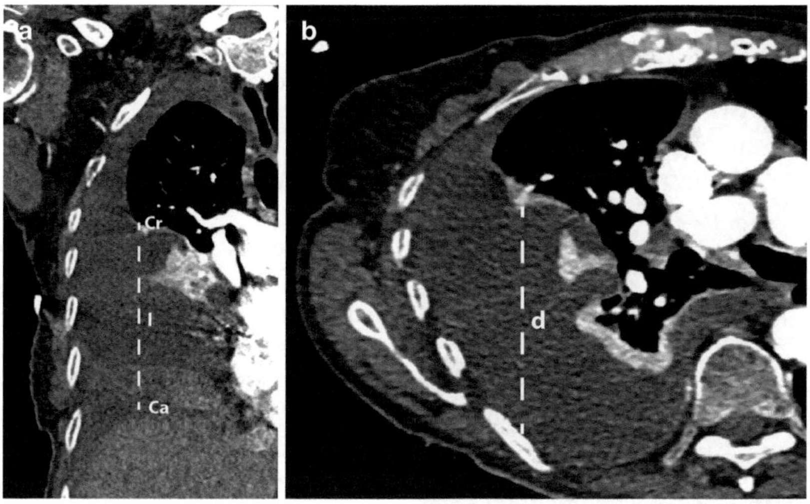

Fig. 13 The Mergo formula is a calculation based on CT, where 'l' represents the greatest length of effusion measured cranio-caudally (Cr-Ca) on coronal orientation (**a**) and 'd' represents the greatest depth of effusion measured perpendicular from the parietal pleura on axial orientation (**b**). This figure illustrates some of the limits of volume assessment of pleural fluid when using imaging. The 'd' and 'l' measurements may be difficult to position on the CT images, particularly in multiloculated effusions, potentially resulting in under- or overestimation of the pleural fluid volume and in substantial interobserver variability

Guo Formula

In the Guo formula (Guo et al. 2013), the authors used a CT volume-rendering technology to calculate volume of pleural effusion. They initially used the technology on a self-designed pleural cavity model with a known quantity of 'effusion', then on patients pre- and post-thoracocentesis to ensure the difference in effusion volume calculated by the technique correlated to actual volume removed and finally on a validation cohort of patients to produce a regression equation to calculate effusion volume based on greatest depth of effusion, using an identical measurement as the Hazlinger technique (Fig. 12) (Hazlinger et al. 2014).

The formula is as follows:

$$\text{Volume}(\text{mL}) = (158.16 \times d) - 116.01$$

d = greatest depth of effusion in cm, perpendicular to the parietal pleura on axial orientation

More recently, machine learning techniques have helped automate this process and pleural effusion detected on CT can be segmented to produce accurate estimates of volume, though this is not widely used in clinical practice (Sexauer et al. 2022).

4.2.2 Echogenicity

There are other properties of pleural effusion that are clinically relevant beyond volume. Whilst CT and chest X-ray have their uses, thoracic US is the key imaging modality used to characterise pleural fluid. Pleural effusions are traditionally classified according to whether they are transudates or exudates, based on their biochemical properties. Exudates are protein and LDH rich, indicating parietal pleural inflammation or obstruction of pleural fluid outflow, whilst transudates indicate changes in the hydrostatic and oncotic pressure balance between the systemic circulation and the pleural space. This can be a useful classification system as it can also aid in identifying the cause of the effusion (Mercer et al. 2019). Therefore, imaging that can help differentiate between these categories is valuable.

Pleural effusion on US can be described as echogenic or anechoic (Fig. 14). The precise mechanism for echogenicity is unknown, but it has been theorised that echogenicity is indicative of fluid that contains protein, cellular content

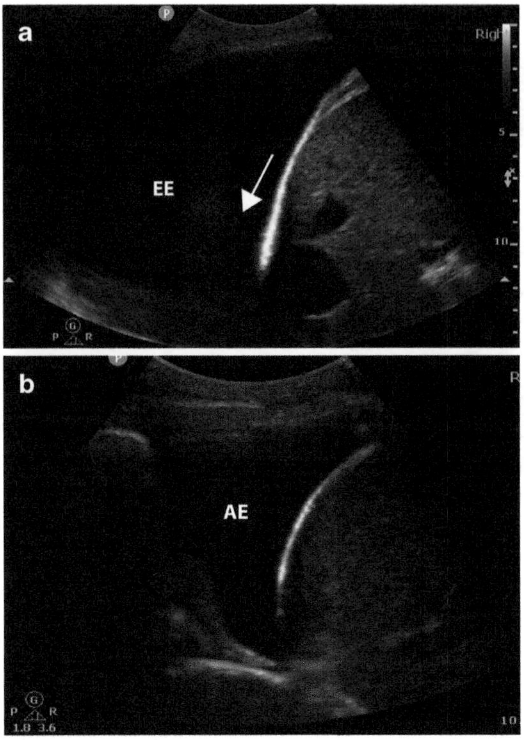

Fig. 14 Patterns of echogenicity. (**a**) Echogenic effusion (EE), with typical echogenic swirling pattern (arrow). (**b**) Anechoic effusion (AE)

(including blood) and other solid debris (e.g. exudates) that reflect the ultrasound back to the probe, generating 'echos', compared to fluid that is more dilute (such as transudates). A number of studies have attempted to draw associations between this feature of pleural effusion on ultrasound and eventual diagnoses; however, the results have been mixed and at sometimes contradictory (Yang et al. 1992; Chen et al. 2008; Asciak et al. 2019; Shkolnik et al. 2020).

One problem with the approaches adopted by these earlier studies was the use of subjective grading systems, another was the use of binary categories (such as echogenic or not). More recent studies have attempted to quantify the degree of 'echogenicity', through the use of post-processing pixel density analysis, with a suggestion that this more objective marker of echogenicity and analysis as a continuous variable may be more discerning at differentiating exudates from transudates, though this methodology is still in its infancy (Soni et al. 2022; Kalkanis et al. 2017).

4.3 Malignant Pleural Disease

Malignancy is the leading cause of exudative effusions, but some of the imaging features of malignant pleural disease can overlap with benign disease, making it difficult at times to differentiate between the two (Roberts et al. 2023).

In its recent comprehensive guideline, the BTS performed a meta-analysis of the diagnostic accuracy of various imaging modalities in diagnosing malignant pleural disease and concluded that the pooled sensitivity of thoracic US vs. CT vs. PET-CT was 79.8% vs. 89.5% vs. 81.3% whilst the specificity was 89.5% vs. 81.3% vs. 92.2%, respectively (Tsim et al. 2017; Porcel et al. 2015; Bugalho et al. 2014; Qureshi et al. 2009; Hallifax et al. 2015; Luo et al. 2001; Tsim et al. 2018; Sun et al. 2016; Yang et al. 2019).

Features that indicate malignant pleural disease on thoracic US include the following: parietal pleural thickening >1 cm, nodular pleural thickening, visceral pleural thickening, diaphragmatic thickening >7 mm, loss of resolution of five layers of the diaphragm and diaphragmatic nodules (Fig. 15) (Qureshi et al. 2009).

CT features of malignant pleural disease include the following: nodular pleural thickening, pleural thickening extending along mediastinal surfaces, thickening of the parietal pleura >1 cm and circumferential pleural thickening encasing the lung (Fig. 16) (Arenas-Jiménez et al. 2018; Kim et al. 2014; Leung et al. 1990; Hierholzer et al. 2000; Metintas et al. 2002; Traill et al. 2001). To note, any thickening of the mediastinal pleura is considered pathologic irrespective of the thickness.

4.3.1 Interventions in Malignant Pleural Disease

Pleural effusion secondary to malignancy represents metastatic disease for most primary cancers (with the exception of malignant pleural meso-

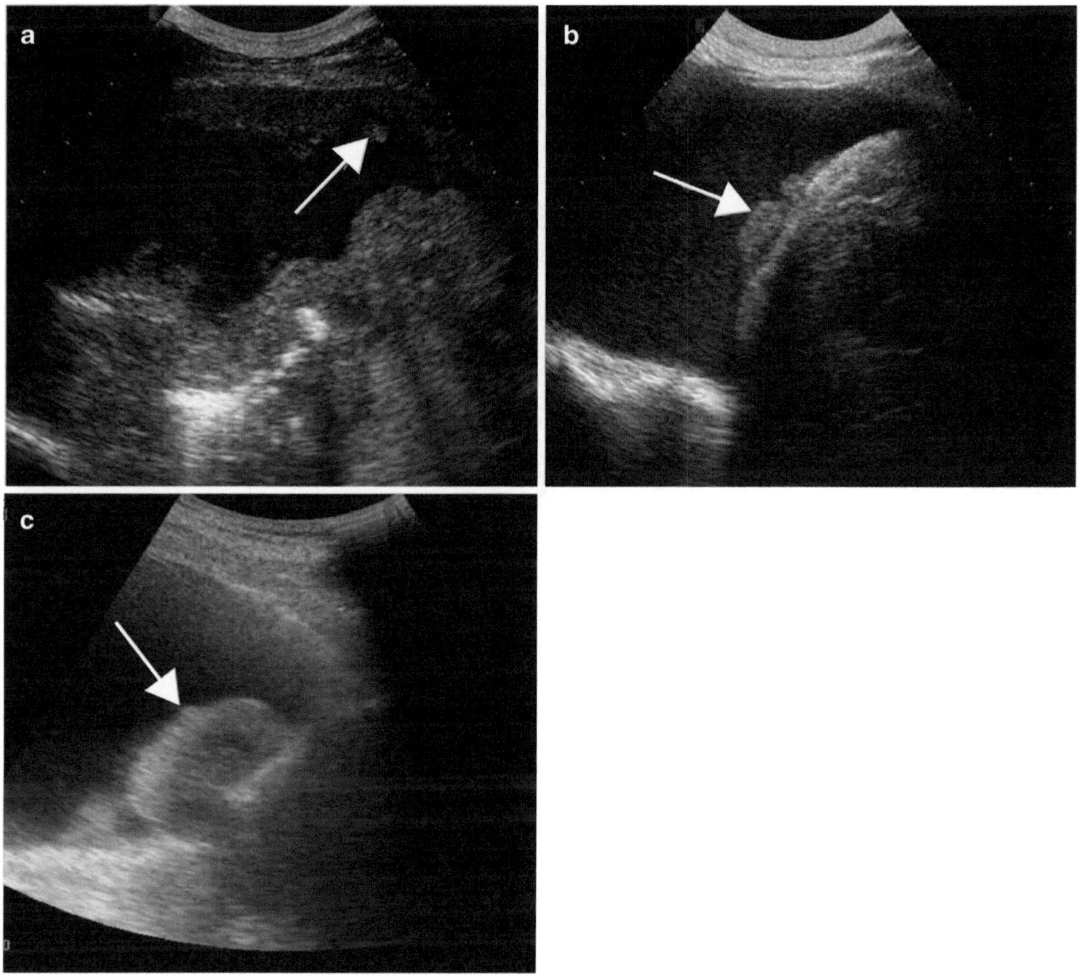

Fig. 15 Some features of malignancy on thoracic ultrasound. (**a**) Parietal pleural thickening and nodularity (white arrow). (**b**) Diaphragmatic nodularity (white arrow). (**c**) Large diaphragmatic nodule (white arrow)

thelioma (MPM) or pleural sarcoma, where pleural effusion is a feature of locally advanced disease) (Goldstraw et al. 2016; Berzenji et al. 2018). Therefore, much of the treatment paradigm in managing these patients is with effective palliation in mind. Patients with pleural effusion due to malignancy may often be symptomatic with profound dyspnoea and therefore require both diagnostic and therapeutic interventions. Although pleural fluid cytology can be diagnostic for malignancy, studies have shown that the overall sensitivity from cytology can be poor, particularly for certain primary cancers (e.g. MPM or squamous cell lung cancer) (Arnold et al. 2018; Mercer et al. 2020). Furthermore, whilst therapeutic thoracocentesis may offer short-term relief of dyspnoea, it does not represent definitive management of a malignant pleural effusion (MPE), which is likely to recur. As a result, guidelines now recommend a more expedited pathway for patients with consideration of pleural biopsy upfront, either via an US-guided approach or through medical thoracoscopy (MT) (Roberts et al. 2023). Patients benefit not just from improved diagnostic yields from histology, and importantly from greater 'actionable' pathological information, in the era of precision therapies (Sundaralingam et al. 2022), but with the latter intervention, patients have the opportunity to also receive definitive effusion control in the same sit-

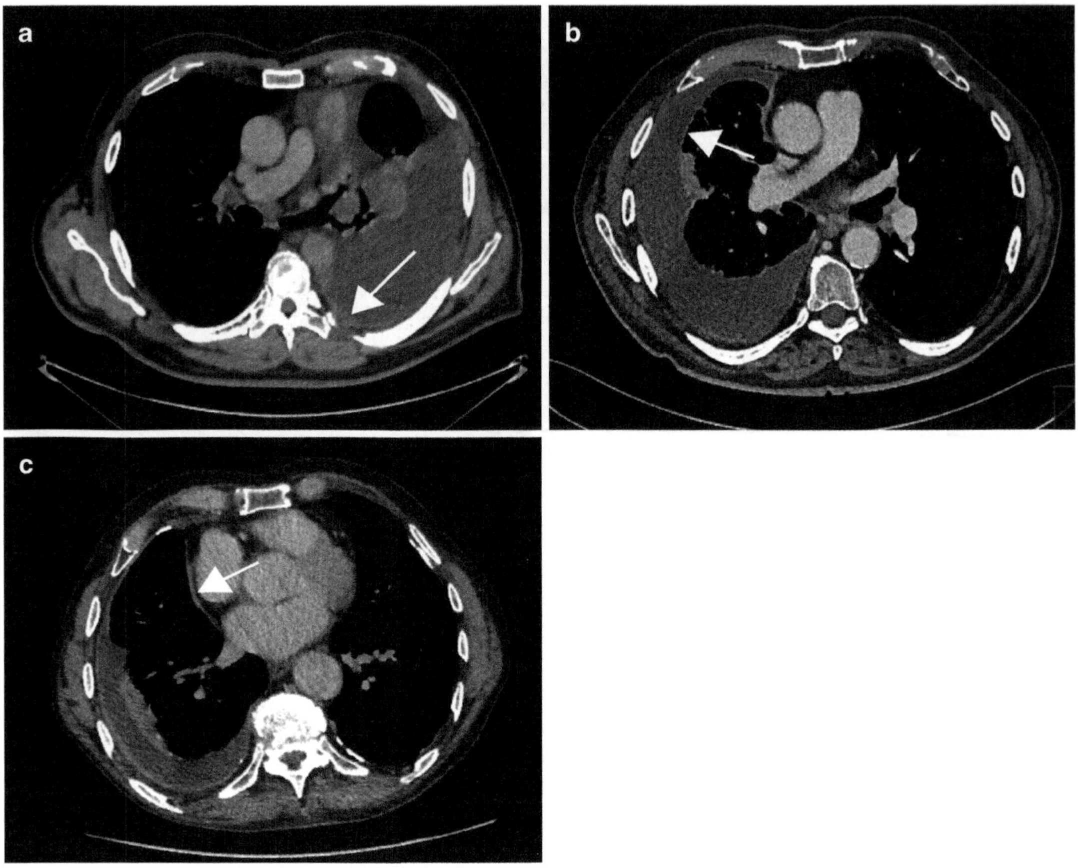

Fig. 16 CT features of malignancy. (**a**) Parietal pleural nodularity >1 cm (white arrow). (**b**) Circumferential pleural thickening encasing the lung (white arrow). (**c**) Mediastinal pleural thickening (white arrow)

ting, via thoracoscopic poudrage. Whilst many different agents have been shown to be effective in achieving pleurodesis, sterile graded talc has been shown to be one of the most effective (Dipper et al. 2020). Talc may be delivered via thoracoscopic poudrage or as a talc slurry via chest drain, and the two approaches have been shown to have similar pleurodesis success rates (78% vs. 76%, respectively) and therefore one is not favoured over another (Bhatnagar et al. 2020). For talc slurry, usually 4–5 g of graded, sterile talc mixed with 50 mL 0.9% saline and 20 mL 1% Lidocaine is instilled into the pleural space via chest drain (Asciak et al. 2023). An alternative to pleurodesis for definitive effusion control is an indwelling pleural catheter (IPC). Patients can be discharged with these devices in situ for further drainage at home. In studies to date, both dyspnoea and quality of life appear to be similar for patients with MPE managed with pleurodesis or an IPC (Davies et al. 2012; Sivakumar et al. 2024). Pleurodesis may not be an option for certain groups of patients, particularly those who have 'trapped lung' or 'non-expansile lung'. This term describes a situation whereby the lung fails to re-expand despite evacuation of the pleural effusion; instead, a hydropneumothorax often replaces the evacuated fluid. It is thought to be secondary to visceral pleural thickening, fibrosis and contraction because of malignant infiltration. Due to poor visceral and parietal pleural apposition, attempts at pleurodesis are futile (Roberts et al. 2023). Some patients managed with an IPC may develop an 'auto-pleurodesis' whereby visceral and parietal pleura achieve symphysis without any artificial pleurodesis agents, and this is thought to occur in approximately 20% of patients (not including those with trapped lung). This baseline rate of auto-pleurodesis can be improved upon further, either by adopting a more aggressive home drainage regime (daily) or by instilling talc slurry via the IPC (Wahidi et al. 2017; Bhatnagar et al. 2018).

4.4 Pleural Infection

Both US and CT can be useful tools in the assessment of this condition, whilst chest X-ray is less helpful. US can more accurately identify septations and loculations within pleural fluid (Fig. 17), compared to CT and therefore indicate pleural infection at a more mature stage and potentially at greater risk of treatment failure at time of initial intervention (Sundaralingam et al. 2020; McLoud and Flower 1991; Svigals et al. 2017). CT is often reserved for more advanced cases, or following treatment failure. It can identify tube thoracostomy positioning, aid in surgical planning if treatment escalation is required or identify complications such as bronchopleural fistula or lung abscess (Duerden et al. 2020). The classical CT features of empyema include the 'split-pleura' sign and >30 mm separation between the parietal pleura and the visceral pleura (Fig. 18), other features include pleural enhancement, thickening of the parietal pleura, extra-pleural fat hypertrophy and infiltration, intrapleural air bubble collection (in the absence of recent pleural intervention) and loculation of pleural fluid (Sundaralingam et al. 2020; Tsujimoto et al. 2015; Porcel et al. 2017).

4.4.1 Interventions in Pleural Infection

The key pillars in the management of pleural infection are prompt antimicrobial therapy and effective drainage of the infected collection (Roberts et al. 2023). Whilst there has been much debate on the optimum size of chest tube in managing empyema, to date there is little evidence to support using a large bore tube over a smaller one (Mei et al. 2023). Of greater importance is the careful siting of the tube into the infected collection, which can often be loculated and difficult to access. In such cases, direct US guidance or CT guidance may be necessary to correctly place the drainage catheter. Once correctly inserted, a further problem that may be encountered is poor drainage. This is because the pleural effusion in empyema has a tendency to septate and eventually loculate, largely due to activation of the coagulation cascade, excessive fibrin deposition and impaired breakdown of fibrin. In addition, the fluid itself is viscous and frankly purulent due to bacterial cellular content (Sundaralingam et al. 2021). Intrapleural enzyme therapies (IETs) have been shown to aid drainage in such situations. It is theorised that intrapleural fibrinolytic may disrupt the fibrin-rich adhesions via activation of

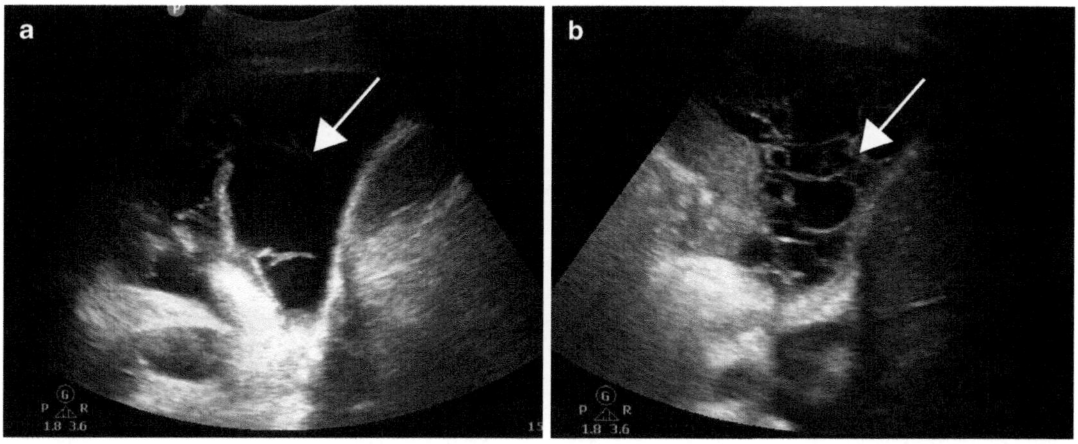

Fig. 17 Thoracic US features in pleural infection. (**a**) Septations (white arrow). (**b**) Dense loculations (white arrow)

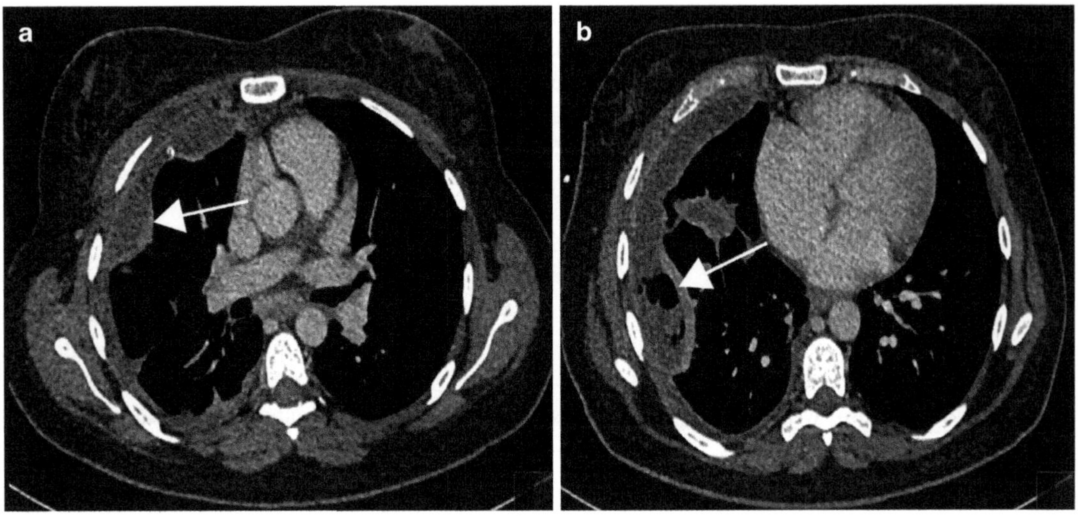

Fig. 18 Some CT features of pleural infection. (**a**) Split-pleura sign (white arrow). (**b**) Intrapleural air within the pleural effusion (white arrow), in the absence of recent pleural intervention this would indicate gas forming organisms within the pleural space

plasminogen and exerting a lavage effect by stimulating pleural fluid formation, whilst DNase reduces pleural fluid viscosity through the breakdown of extracellular DNA and biofilm formation (Simpson et al. 2000). The MIST-2 trial, a randomised controlled trial (RCT) comparing the effects of a single agent recombinant tissue plasminogen activator (t-PA) to single agent DNase, as well as dual therapies to placebo, demonstrated that it was the dual action of the t-PA and DNase that resulted in improved drainage and radiological clearance, length of stay and surgical referral rates in patients with confirmed empyema (Rahman et al. 2011). As a result of this landmark trial, intrapleural enzyme therapies have become the standard of care in managing non-draining empyema. In the study an empirical dosing regimen of 10 mg t-PA and 5 mg DNase administered intrapleurally twice daily for 3 days was used (Asciak et al. 2023; Rahman et al. 2011). There has been understandable concern around the risk of bleeding from such a regime; however, this concern appears to be exaggerated. In a recent retrospective cohort study, the risk of intrapleural haemorrhage following IET was found to be 4.1% (Akulian et al. 2022). Nonetheless, many dose de-escalation regimes have been proposed both for safety and cost concerns, and appear to retain efficacy, albeit in non-RCT study settings (Piccolo et al. 2014; Popowicz et al. 2017; Mehta et al. 2016; McClune et al. 2016; Majid et al. 2016). Whilst surgery remains a cornerstone in the management of pleural infection, its precise role with regard to when and in whom it should be considered remains unclear, and there is much variation in practice. Reserving it for only the most advanced and late-stage empyema in which other therapies have failed seems intuitive; however, this may place patients at greater risk of surgical complications or the need for more invasive surgical approaches (Sundaralingam et al. 2021). Therefore, head-to-head trials of early surgery vs. IET are needed. Following promising results of a feasibility study, which demonstrated acceptability of early surgery in pleural infection to both patients and surgeons, definitive trials are planned (Bedawi et al. 2023).

5 Conclusion

There are a range of radiological tools available when managing pleural pathology, each with its own advantages and shortcomings, depending on the task at hand. Whilst measurement tools have been developed to provide more precise information, such data is not commonly useful of itself in clinical practice and must be used in combination with the overall clinical picture. Potentially, the increasing development and future use of Artificial Intelligence tools in medicine may change their value by enabling more consistent quantification than is currently possible, and make them more reliable as predictors of disease severity, the need for interventions and as prognostic markers.

With widespread adoption of point-of-care US in many healthcare settings, increasing use cases for advanced modes of US such as CEUS and SWE to both direct biopsies as well as assess for treatment response in MPE and MPM, the incoming wave of CTs from lung cancer screening that is sure to also identify pleural pathologies and the burgeoning role of MRI in accurate staging of MPM as well as other pleural-based lesions, it is suffice to say the future of imaging in pleural disease is fast moving and looks bright.

Disclaimer All measurements in this book have been obtained from peer-reviewed papers and guidelines from professional organizations, unless explicitly stated otherwise. While the authors, editors, and publisher have gone through a rigorous process to establish their correct reproduction from the original source, each measurement must be interpreted in the correct clinical context, this along with an accurate way of measurement, and taking into account all technical variables, this including follow-up exams with various equipment or software. Neither the authors, the editors, nor the publisher can accept any legal responsibility for any improper application or interpretation of these measurements as well as their potential consequences.

References

Aguinagalde B, Aranda JL, Busca P et al (2018) SECT Clinical practice guideline on the management of patients with spontaneous pneumothorax. Cir Esp 96(1):3–11

Akulian J, Bedawi EO, Abbas H et al (2022) Bleeding risk with combination intrapleural fibrinolytic and enzyme therapy in pleural infection – an international, multicenter, retrospective cohort study. Chest 162(6):1384–1392

Alfudhili KM, Lynch DA, Laurent F, Ferretti GR, Dunet V, Beigelman-Aubry C (2016) Focal pleural thickening mimicking pleural plaques on chest computed tomography: tips and tricks. Br J Radiol 89(1057):20150792

Arenas-Jiménez JJ, García-Garrigós E, Escudero-Fresneda C et al (2018) Early and delayed phases of contrast-enhanced CT for evaluating patients with malignant pleural effusion. Results of pairwise comparison by multiple observers. Br J Radiol 91(1089):20180254

Arnold DT, De Fonseka D, Perry S et al (2018) Investigating unilateral pleural effusions: the role of cytology. Eur Respir J 52(5):1801254

Asciak R, Hassan M, Mercer RM et al (2019) Prospective analysis of the predictive value of sonographic pleural fluid echogenicity for the diagnosis of exudative effusion. Respiration 97(5):451–456

Asciak R, Bedawi EO, Bhatnagar R et al (2023) British Thoracic Society Clinical Statement on pleural procedures. Thorax 78(Suppl 3):s43–s68

Bai J, Yang W, Wang S et al (2016) Role of arrival time difference between lesions and lung tissue on contrast-enhanced sonography in the differential diagnosis of subpleural pulmonary lesions. J Ultrasound Med 35(7):1523–1532

Balik M, Plasil P, Waldauf P et al (2006) Ultrasound estimation of volume of pleural fluid in mechanically ventilated patients. Intensive Care Med 32(2):318

Banka R, Skaarup S, Mercer R, Laursen C (2020) Thoracic ultrasound: a key tool beyond procedure guidance [Internet]. In: Maskell NA, Laursen CB, Lee YCG, Rahman NM (eds) Pleural disease (ERS monograph). European Respiratory Society, Sheffield, pp 73–89. Available from: https://doi.org/10.1183/2312508X.10023819

Baumann MH, Strange C, Heffner JE et al (2001) Management of spontaneous pneumothorax: an American College of Chest Physicians Delphi consensus statement. Chest 119(2):590–602

Bedawi EO, Stavroulias D, Hedley E et al (2023) Early video-assisted thoracoscopic surgery or intrapleural enzyme therapy in pleural infection: a feasibility randomized controlled trial. The Third Multicenter Intrapleural Sepsis Trial—MIST-3. Am J Respir Crit Care Med 208(12):1305–1315

Berzenji L, Van Schil PE, Carp L (2018) The eighth TNM classification for malignant pleural mesothelioma. Transl Lung Cancer Res 7(5):543–549

Bhatnagar R, Keenan EK, Morley AJ et al (2018) Outpatient talc administration by indwelling pleural catheter for malignant effusion. N Engl J Med 378(14):1313–1322

Bhatnagar R, Piotrowska HEG, Laskawiec-Szkonter M et al (2020) Effect of thoracoscopic talc poudrage vs talc slurry via chest tube on pleurodesis failure rate among patients with malignant pleural effusions: a randomized clinical trial. JAMA 323(1):60–69

Blackmore CC, Black WC, Dallas RV, Crow HC (1996) Pleural fluid volume estimation: a chest radiograph prediction rule. Acad Radiol 3(2):103–109

Brown SGA, Ball EL, Perrin K et al (2020) Conservative versus interventional treatment for spontaneous pneumothorax. N Engl J Med 382(5):405–415

Bugalho A, Ferreira D, Dias SS et al (2014) The diagnostic value of transthoracic ultrasonographic features in predicting malignancy in undiagnosed pleural effusions: a prospective observational study. Respiration 87(4):270–278

Chen H-J, Tu C-Y, Ling S-J et al (2008) Sonographic appearances in transudative pleural effusions: not always an anechoic pattern. Ultrasound Med Biol 34(3):362–369

Chiao D, Hanley M, Olazagasti JM (2015) CT volumetric analysis of pleural effusions: a comparison with thoracentesis volumes. Acad Radiol 22(9):1122–1127

Claude-Desroches M, Bierry G, Touitou-Gottenberg D, Golmard J-L, Grenier PA, Beigelman-Aubry C (2012) Focal dependent pleural thickening at MDCT: pleural lesion or functional abnormality. Diagn Interv Imaging 93(5):360–364

Collins CD, Lopez A, Mathie A, Wood V, Jackson JE, Roddie ME (1995) Quantification of pneumothorax size on chest radiographs using interpleural distances: regression analysis based on volume measurements from helical CT. AJR Am J Roentgenol 165(5):1127–1130

Corcoran JP, Acton L, Ahmed A et al (2016) Diagnostic value of radiological imaging pre- and post-drainage of pleural effusions. Respirology 21(2):392–395

Davies HE, Mishra EK, Kahan BC et al (2012) Effect of an indwelling pleural catheter vs chest tube and talc pleurodesis for relieving dyspnea in patients with malignant pleural effusion: the TIME2 randomized controlled trial. JAMA 307(22):2383–2389

Fonseka D de, Arnold DT, Smartt HJM et al (2024) PET-CT-guided versus CT-guided biopsy in suspected malignant pleural thickening: a randomised trial. Eur Respir J [Internet]. [cited 2024 Feb 7];63(2). Available from: https://erj.ersjournals.com/content/63/2/2301295

De Leyn P, Lismonde M, Ninane V et al (2005) Guidelines Belgian Society of Pneumology. Guidelines on the management of spontaneous pneumothorax. Acta Chir Belg 105(3):265–267

Dipper A, Jones HE, Bhatnagar R, Preston NJ, Maskell N, Clive AO (2020) Interventions for the management of malignant pleural effusions: a network meta-analysis. Cochrane Database Syst Rev [Internet]. [cited 2021 Apr 1]. Available from: http://doi.wiley.com/10.1002/14651858.CD010529.pub3

Duerden L, Benamore R, Edey A (2020) Radiology: what is the role of chest radiographs, CT and PET in modern management? [Internet]. In: Maskell NA, Laursen CB, Lee YCG, Rahman NM (eds) Pleural disease (ERS monograph). European Respiratory Society, Sheffield, pp 48–72. Available from: https://doi.org/10.1183/2312508X.10023819

Eibenberger KL, Dock WI, Ammann ME, Dorffner R, Hörmann MF, Grabenwöger F (1994) Quantification of pleural effusions: sonography versus radiography. Radiology 191(3):681–684

Goecke W, Schwerk WB (1990) Ultraschall-diagnostik '89 [Internet]. In: Die Real-Time Sonographie in der Diagnostik von Pleuraergüssen. Springer Link. [cited 2024 Feb 19], pp 385–387. Available from: https://link.springer.com/chapter/10.1007/978-3-642-93467-4_98

Goldstraw P, Chansky K, Crowley J et al (2016) The IASLC lung cancer staging project: proposals for revision of the TNM stage groupings in the forthcoming (eighth) edition of the TNM classification for lung cancer. J Thorac Oncol 11(1):39–51

Goo JM, Chung MJ, Lee HJ, Im J-G (2003) Posterior subpleural nodules in patients with underlying malignancies: value of prone computed tomography. J Comput Assist Tomogr 27(2):274–278

Guo Z-J, Lin Q, Liu H-T et al (2013) The preliminary exploration of 64-slice volume computed tomography in the accurate measurement of pleural effusion. Acta Radiol 54(7):765–769

Hallifax R, Rahman N (2016) Pleural embryology and gross structure, circulation, lymphatics, and nerves. In: Light RW, Lee YCG (eds) Textbook of pleural diseases. CRC Press, Boca Raton, pp 13–24

Hallifax RJ, Haris M, Corcoran JP et al (2015) Role of CT in assessing pleural malignancy prior to thoracoscopy. Thorax 70(2):192–193

Hallifax RJ, Talwar A, Wrightson JM, Edey A, Gleeson FV (2017) State-of-the-art: radiological investigation of pleural disease. Respir Med 124:88–99

Hallifax RJ, McKeown E, Sivakumar P et al (2020) Ambulatory management of primary spontaneous pneumothorax: an open-label, randomised controlled trial. Lancet 396(10243):39–49

Hassan M, Rizk R, Essam H, Abouelnour A (2017) Validation of equations for pleural effusion volume estimation by ultrasonography. J Ultrasound 20(4):267–271

Hazlinger M, Ctvrtlik F, Langova K, Herman M (2014) Quantification of pleural effusion on CT by simple measurement. Biomed Pap Med Fac Univ Palacky Olomouc Czech Repub 158(1):107–111

Heelan RT, Rusch VW, Begg CB, Panicek DM, Caravelli JF, Eisen C (1999) Staging of malignant pleural mesothelioma: comparison of CT and MR imaging. AJR Am J Roentgenol 172(4):1039–1047

Hierholzer J, Luo L, Bittner RC et al (2000) MRI and CT in the differential diagnosis of pleural disease. Chest 118(3):604–609

Hoi K, Turchin B, Kelly A-M (2007) How accurate is the Light index for estimating pneumothorax size? Australas Radiol 51(2):196–198

Hong-Xia Z, Wen H, Ling-Gang C et al (2016) A new method for discriminating between bronchial and pulmonary arterial phases using contrast-enhanced ultrasound. Ultrasound Med Biol 42(7):1441–1449

Ibitoye BO, Idowu BM, Ogunrombi AB, Afolabi BI (2018) Ultrasonographic quantification of pleural effusion: comparison of four formulae. Ultrasonography 37(3):254–260

Jiang B, Li X, Yin Y et al (2019) Ultrasound elastography: a novel tool for the differential diagnosis of pleural effusion. Eur Respir J 54(2):1802018
Jouneau S, Ricard J-D, Seguin-Givelet A et al (2023) SPLF/SMFU/SRLF/SFAR/SFCTCV Guidelines for the management of patients with primary spontaneous pneumothorax. Ann Intensive Care 13(1):88
Kalkanis A, Varsamas C, Gourgoulianis K (2017) Correlation of pleural effusions' grayscale sonographic parameters with fluid's analysis results. J Thorac Dis 9(3):543–546
Kelly A-M, Weldon D, Tsang AYL, Graham CA (2006) Comparison between two methods for estimating pneumothorax size from chest X-rays. Respir Med 100(8):1356–1359
Kim JS, Shim SS, Kim Y, Ryu YJ, Lee JH (2014) Chest CT findings of pleural tuberculosis: differential diagnosis of pleural tuberculosis and malignant pleural dissemination. Acta Radiol 55(9):1063–1068
Leung AN, Müller NL, Miller RR (1990) CT in differential diagnosis of diffuse pleural disease. AJR Am J Roentgenol 154(3):487–492
Light R (1988) Pneumothorax. In: Textbook of respiratory medicine. WB Saunders, Philadelphia, p 1754
Luo L, Hierholzer J, Bittner RC, Chen J, Huang L (2001) Magnetic resonance imaging in distinguishing malignant from benign pleural disease. Chin Med J 114(6):645–649
MacDuff A, Arnold A, Harvey J, BTS Pleural Disease Guideline Group (2010) Management of spontaneous pneumothorax: British Thoracic Society Pleural Disease Guideline 2010. Thorax 65 Suppl 2:ii18–ii31
Majid A, Kheir F, Folch A et al (2016) Concurrent intrapleural instillation of tissue plasminogen activator and DNase for pleural infection. A single-center experience. Ann Am Thorac Soc 13(9):1512–1518
McClune JR, Wilshire CL, Gorden JA et al (2016) Safety and efficacy of intrapleural tissue plasminogen activator and DNase during extended use in complicated pleural space infections. Can Respir J 2016:1–6
McLoud TC, Flower CD (1991) Imaging the pleura: sonography, CT, and MR imaging. AJR Am J Roentgenol 156(6):1145–1153
Mehta HJ, Biswas A, Penley AM, Cope J, Barnes M, Jantz MA. Management of Intrapleural Sepsis with Once Daily Use of Tissue Plasminogen Activator and Deoxyribonuclease. Respiration. 2016;91(2):101–6. https://doi.org/10.1159/000443334. Epub 2016 Jan 14. PMID: 26761711.
Mei F, Rota M, Bonifazi M et al (2023) Efficacy of small versus large-bore chest drain in pleural infection: a systematic review and meta-analysis. Respiration 102(3):247–256
Mercer RM, Corcoran JP, Porcel JM, Rahman NM, Psallidas I (2019) Interpreting pleural fluid results. Clin Med 19(3):213–217
Mercer RM, Varatharajah R, Shepherd G et al (2020) Critical analysis of the utility of initial pleural aspiration in the diagnosis and management of suspected malignant pleural effusion. BMJ Open Respir Res 7(1):e000701
Mergo PJ, Helmberger T, Didovic J, Cernigliaro J, Ros PR, Staab EV (1999) New formula for quantification of pleural effusions from computed tomography. J Thorac Imaging 14(2):122–125
Metintas M, Ucgun I, Elbek O et al (2002) Computed tomography features in malignant pleural mesothelioma and other commonly seen pleural diseases. Eur J Radiol 41(1):1–9
Moy MP, Levsky JM, Berko NS, Godelman A, Jain VR, Haramati LB (2013) A new, simple method for estimating pleural effusion size on CT scans. Chest 143(4):1054–1059
Noppen M (2016) Normal physiological fluid and cellular contents. In: Light RW, Lee YCG (eds) Textbook of pleural diseases. CRC Press, Boca Raton, pp 45–48
Piccolo F, Pitman N, Bhatnagar R et al (2014) Intrapleural tissue plasminogen activator and deoxyribonuclease for pleural infection. An effective and safe alternative to surgery. Ann Am Thorac Soc 11(9):1419–1425
Popat S, Baas P, Faivre-Finn C et al (2022) Malignant pleural mesothelioma: ESMO Clinical Practice Guidelines for diagnosis, treatment and follow-up☆. Ann Oncol 33(2):129–142
Popowicz N, Bintcliffe O, De Fonseka D et al (2017) Dose de-escalation of intrapleural tissue plasminogen activator therapy for pleural infection. The alteplase dose assessment for pleural infection therapy project. Ann Am Thorac Soc 14(6):929–936
Porcel JM, Hernández P, Martínez-Alonso M, Bielsa S, Salud A (2015) Accuracy of fluorodeoxyglucose-PET imaging for differentiating benign from malignant pleural effusions: a meta-analysis. Chest 147(2):502–512
Porcel JM, Pardina M, Alemán C, Pallisa E, Light RW, Bielsa S (2017) Computed tomography scoring system for discriminating between parapneumonic effusions eventually drained and those cured only with antibiotics: CT for parapneumonic effusions. Respirology 22(6):1199–1204
Qureshi NR, Rahman NM, Gleeson FV (2009) Thoracic ultrasound in the diagnosis of malignant pleural effusion. Thorax 64(2):139–143
Rahman NM, Phil D, Maskell NA et al (2011) Intrapleural use of tissue plasminogen activator and DNase in pleural infection. N Engl J Med 365(6):518–526
Raj V, Kirke R, Bankart MJ, Entwisle JJ (2011) Multidetector CT imaging of pleura: comparison of two contrast infusion protocols. Br J Radiol 84(1005):796–799
Revelli M, Chiesa F, Del Prato A et al (2016) Role of respiratory-triggered diffusion-weighted MRI in the assessment of pleural disease. Br J Radiol 89(1064):20160289
Rhea JT, DeLuca SA, Greene RE (1982) Determining the size of pneumothorax in the upright patient. Radiology 144(4):733–736
Roberts ME, Rahman NM, Maskell NA et al (2023) British Thoracic Society Guideline for pleural disease. Thorax 78(Suppl 3):s1–s42

Salazar AJ, Aguirre DA, Ocampo J, Camacho JC, Díaz XA (2014) Evaluation of three pneumothorax size quantification methods on digitized chest X-ray films using medical-grade grayscale and consumer-grade color displays. J Digit Imaging 27(2):280–286

Santamarina MG, Beddings I, Lermanda Holmgren GV, Opazo Sanchez H, Volpacchio MM (2017) Multidetector CT for evaluation of the extrapleural space. Radiographics 37(5):1352–1370

Sexauer R, Yang S, Weikert T et al (2022) Automated detection, segmentation, and classification of pleural effusion from computed tomography scans using machine learning. Investig Radiol 57(8):552–559

Shkolnik B, Judson MA, Austin A et al (2020) Diagnostic accuracy of thoracic ultrasonography to differentiate transudative from exudative pleural effusion. Chest 158(2):692–697

Simpson G, Roomes D, Heron M (2000) Effects of streptokinase and deoxyribonuclease on viscosity of human surgical and empyema pus. Chest 117(6):1728–1733

Sivakumar P, Fitzgerald DB, Ip H et al (2024) The impact of outpatient *versus* inpatient management on health-related quality of life outcomes for patients with malignant pleural effusion: the OPTIMUM randomised clinical trial. Eur Respir J 63(2):2201215

Soni NJ, Dreyfuss ZS, Ali S et al (2022) Pleural fluid echogenicity measured by ultrasound image pixel density to differentiate transudative versus exudative pleural effusions. Ann Am Thorac Soc 19(5):857–860

Sun Y, Yu H, Ma J, Lu P (2016) The role of 18F-FDG PET/CT integrated imaging in distinguishing malignant from benign pleural effusion. PLoS One 11(8):e0161764

Sundaralingam A, Bedawi EO, Rahman NM (2020) Diagnostics in Pleural Disease. Diagnostics (Basel) 10(12):1046

Sundaralingam A, Banka R, Rahman NM (2021) Management of pleural infection. Pulm Ther 7(1):59–74

Sundaralingam A, Aujayeb A, Akca B et al (2022) Achieving molecular profiling in pleural biopsies. Chest S0012369222041691

Svigals PZ, Chopra A, Ravenel JG, Nietert PJ, Huggins JT (2017) The accuracy of pleural ultrasonography in diagnosing complicated parapneumonic pleural effusions. Thorax 72(1):94–95

Traill ZC, Davies RJ, Gleeson FV (2001) Thoracic computed tomography in patients with suspected malignant pleural effusions. Clin Radiol 56(3):193–196

Treglia G, Sadeghi R, Annunziata S et al (2014) Diagnostic accuracy of 18F-FDG-PET and PET/CT in the differential diagnosis between malignant and benign pleural lesions: a systematic review and meta-analysis. Acad Radiol 21(1):11–20

Tschopp JM, Bintcliffe O, Astoul P et al (2015) ERS task force statement: diagnosis and treatment of primary spontaneous pneumothorax. Eur Respir J 46(2):321–335

Tsim S, Stobo DB, Alexander L, Kelly C, Blyth KG (2017) The diagnostic performance of routinely acquired and reported computed tomography imaging in patients presenting with suspected pleural malignancy. Lung Cancer 103:38–43

Tsim S, Humphreys CA, Cowell GW et al (2018) Early contrast enhancement: a novel magnetic resonance imaging biomarker of pleural malignancy. Lung Cancer 118:48–56

Tsim S, Cowell GW, Kidd A et al (2020) A comparison between MRI and CT in the assessment of primary tumour volume in mesothelioma. Lung Cancer 150:12–20

Tsujimoto N, Saraya T, Light RW et al (2015) A simple method for differentiating complicated parapneumonic effusion/empyema from parapneumonic effusion using the split pleura sign and the amount of pleural effusion on thoracic CT. PLoS One 10(6):e0130141

Usta E, Mustafi M, Ziemer G (2010) Ultrasound estimation of volume of postoperative pleural effusion in cardiac surgery patients. Interact Cardiovasc Thorac Surg 10(2):204–207

Wahidi MM, Reddy C, Yarmus L et al (2017) Randomized trial of pleural fluid drainage frequency in patients with malignant pleural effusions. The ASAP Trial. Am J Respir Crit Care Med 195(8):1050–1057

Woolhouse I, Bishop L, Darlison L et al (2018) BTS guideline for the investigation and management of malignant pleural mesothelioma. BMJ Open Respir Res 5(1):e000266

Yang PC, Luh KT, Chang DB, Wu HD, Yu CJ, Kuo SH (1992) Value of sonography in determining the nature of pleural effusion: analysis of 320 cases. AJR Am J Roentgenol 159(1):29–33

Yang M-F, Tong Z-H, Wang Z et al (2019) Development and validation of the PET-CT score for diagnosis of malignant pleural effusion. Eur J Nucl Med Mol Imaging 46(7):1457–1467

Zaki HA, Albaroudi B, Shaban EE et al (2024) Advancement in pleura effusion diagnosis: a systematic review and meta-analysis of point-of-care ultrasound versus radiographic thoracic imaging. Ultrasound J 16(1):3

Diaphragm

Samia Boussouar, Martin Dres,
and Alban Redheuil

Contents

Supplementary Information The online version contains supplementary material available at https://doi.org/10.1007/174_2024_517.

S. Boussouar (✉) · A. Redheuil
Cardiovascular and Thoracic Imaging Unit, Hôpital Pitié Salpêtrière, Assistance Publique-Hôpitaux de Paris (APHP), Paris, France

Laboratoire d'Imagerie Biomédicale, Sorbonne Université, INSERM, CNRS, Institute of Cardiometabolism and Nutrition, Paris, France
e-mail: samia.boussouar@aphp.fr

M. Dres
Sorbonne Université, INSERM, UMRS1158 Neurophysiologie Respiratoire Expérimentale et Clinique, Paris, France

Service de Médecine Intensive et Réanimation, Département R3S, AP-HP, Groupe Hospitalier Pitié-Salpêtrière Charles Foix, Paris, France

The diaphragm is the chief muscle of inspiration and the most powerful of the respiratory muscles. The diaphragm also serves as a mechanical barrier separating the thorax from the abdomen and maintains the pressure gradient between both compartments (Nason et al. 2012). Under normal conditions, this thin dome-shaped muscular structure acts like a piston within a syringe, generating airflow within airways as its dome descends and enabling tidal breathing. The pressure generated across the dome between the thoracic and abdominal cavities is called the transdiaphragmatic pressure and is proportional to the tension developed within the muscle fibers. Therefore, in terms of physiological meaning, the diaphragm function can be estimated by its capacity to generate this transdiaphragmatic pressure. Diaphragm dysfunction can be associated with the presence of respiratory symptoms, in particular dyspnea, exercise intolerance, and sleep disturbances, and, in the more severe cases, may have a negative impact on survival. Uni- and bilateral diaphragm dysfunction diagnosis and management may be problematic for the clinician because of its relative rarity, its sometimes-subtle clinical manifestations, and difficulties in obtaining a physiologically confirmed diagnosis. As such, diaphragm dysfunction is probably underdiagnosed, but should not be neglected, as it may negatively impact the quality of life, can be a marker of disease severity, and, in some instances such as in the intensive care unit, can be a prognostic marker.

Med Radiol Diagn Imaging (2026)
https://doi.org/10.1007/174_2024_517,
Published Online: 01 December 2024

Despite their importance, diaphragm dysfunction etiologies are often underestimated by clinicians and radiologists (Celli 2002). Therefore, in clinical practice, a routine evaluation of its mobility should be emphasized.

1 When?

Diaphragm dysfunction can be suspected in various clinical scenarios: after surgery in case of an abnormally elevated hemidiaphragm on a chest X-ray, in a dyspneic patient without obvious respiratory or cardiac cause, and during the weaning from mechanical ventilation in critically ill patients. It can also be secondary to a trauma or to a phrenic nerve paralysis of any cause. Diaphragmatic eventration is characterized by the thinning of a segment or the entire diaphragm, where muscle tissue is replaced predominantly by fibroelastic tissue, typically due to muscle atrophy.

Diaphragm dysfunction can be unilateral or, more rarely, bilateral. Symptoms are more likely to occur in patients with comorbidities or underlying acute or chronic cardiopulmonary disease. Symptoms may worsen in the supine position due to higher pressure from the abdominal content on the diaphragm. Traumatic lesions are one of the most common causes of "true" unilateral diaphragm paralysis (McDonald et al. 2018). In particular, coronary artery bypass grafting surgery is frequently associated with lesions of the phrenic nerves resulting in postoperative diaphragmatic paralysis.

Unilateral involvement is often asymptomatic and discovered incidentally, while bilateral diaphragmatic dysfunction can lead to respiratory failure. Pulmonary function tests show a pattern of restriction (Dubé and Dres 2016). The etiological research of diaphragmatic disorders is mainly based on anamnesis and electromyographic study. However, functional imaging with fluoroscopy, ultrasonography, or magnetic resonance imaging is a simple and effective method to diagnose diaphragmatic dysfunction.

2 How? Why?

2.1 Chest X-Ray

Chest X-ray is a noninvasive and easily accessible method. It allows a static evaluation of the two hemidiaphragms (Saltiel et al. 2013). Hemidiaphragms are dome-shaped structures visible up to the midline on a frontal view. The upper contours of the hemidiaphragms do not delimit the bottom of the lungs that is seen through the hemidiaphragms.

In normal conditions, the dome of the right hemidiaphragm projects anteriorly over the fifth or sixth rib and posteriorly over the tenth rib. The right hemidiaphragm is usually a little higher than the left up to one-half intercostal space or 0–25 mm (Chetta et al. 2005) because of the liver. The anterior and medial portions of the diaphragm are normally higher than the posterior and lateral portions (Toledo et al. 2003). On a lateral (left side) view, the two domes intersect, and the left dome can be notably distinguished from the right dome by its anterior obliteration by the cardiac opacity due to silhouette sign (Fig. 1). Hemidiaphragm position is often considered pathological on chest X-ray if the difference in the z-axis between the two domes exceeds 2 cm or if the left hemidiaphragm is higher as the right one (Chetta et al. 2005) (Fig. 2). Furthermore, the top of the normal diaphragm should be located at the junction between its medial third and middle third. Any lateral displacement of this point should suggest a subpulmonic pleural effusion, usually associated with an increased opacity at the level of the diaphragmatic dome (Chest X-Ray).

Diaphragmatic mobility can be investigated on chest X-rays using two X-ray images: the first at maximum inspiration and the second at maximum expiration. The images are then superimposed. The diaphragm motion is either the distance between the highest points of a hemidiaphragm between expiration and maximum inspiration or less relevantly the surface area between inspiration and expiration (Toledo et al. 2003; Fernandes et al. 2007). Diaphragmatic mobility is variable

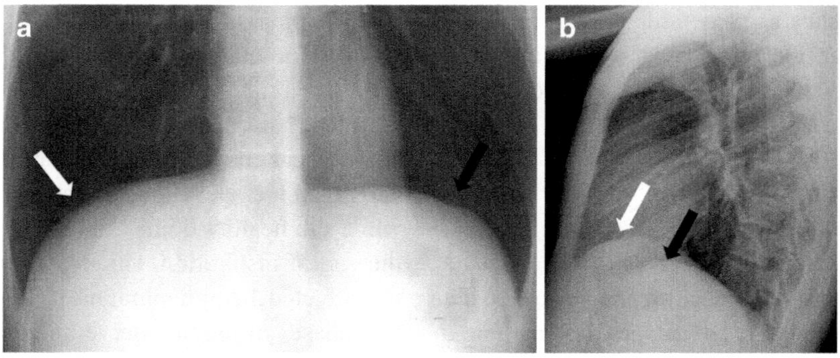

Fig. 1 Frontal (**a**) and left side (**b**) chest radiographs centered on the diaphragm. The right hemidiaphragm is slightly higher compared to the left one (less than 2 cm). On lateral view, note that the right diaphragmatic dome (white arrow) is visible in full continuity whereas the left diaphragmatic dome (black arrow) is masked due to contact with the cardiac structure (silhouette sign)

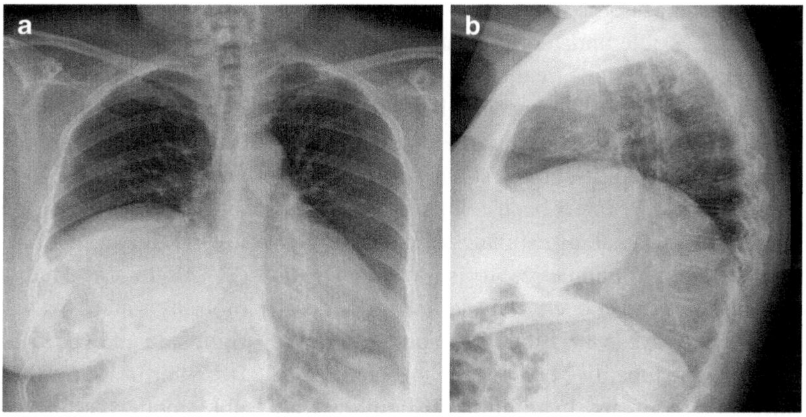

Fig. 2 Frontal (**a**) and left side (**b**) chest radiographs show a pathological elevation of the right hemidiaphragm of more than one intercostal space or more than 2 cm compared to the left one

ranging from 0 to 97 mm or from 40 to 120 cm^2. The measurement method is reproducible, and the reasons for different measurement results are mainly related to the individual, especially age and obesity which can alter the respiratory mechanics (Gierada et al. 1998; Zerah et al. 1993). Yamada et al. (2017) demonstrated that the average diaphragmatic excursions during tidal breathing in standing position using dynamic chest radiography with a flat-panel detector system are 11.0 mm (right) and 14.9 mm (left). The left diaphragm displays notably greater and quicker motion in contrast to the right. Higher BMI and tidal volume are linked with increased excursions of both diaphragms (Yamada et al. 2017). Unilateral diaphragmatic disease usually manifests as elevation at chest X-ray. The dome of the affected diaphragm is elevated, and the costophrenic and costovertebral sulci are deeper on the affected side. It should be differentiated from eventration that most commonly involves the anteromedial portion of the right hemidiaphragm. When the eventration is complete, the left hemidiaphragm is more commonly affected than the right hemidiaphragm (Nason et al. 2012). In the clinical context, chest X-ray is mainly used to screen for diaphragmatic abnormalities, and its relevance for precise measurements is not expected. The radiological assessment of unilateral paralysis presents a potential pitfall due to the considerable variability in the normal height of the hemidiaphragm. In adults with normal pulmonary function, significant variability in the position and shape of the diaphragm is also observed, partly attributable to factors such as weight, age, and thoracic dimensions (Suwatanapongched et al. 2003). Therefore, the elevation of the hemidiaphragm on a chest radiograph is not a reliable diagnostic indicator of hemidiaphragm dysfunction. However, the presence of a normally positioned hemidiaphragm substantially reduces the likelihood of such dysfunction.

2.2 Fluoroscopy

Fluoroscopy provides dynamic images of the diaphragm and offers the advantage of being able to visualize the motion of the domes in real time (Gierada et al. 1998). Although it is not used anymore nowadays (replaced by US or MRI), this test was simple to perform, and the results were easy to interpret. Dynamic evaluation of diaphragmatic motion using fluoroscopy has long been used to evaluate possible unilateral diaphragmatic weakness. During a sniff maneuver, a paradoxical upward motion of the abnormal hemidiaphragm may be observed, which confirms the diagnosis. Despite its ease of use, the test has several drawbacks: it has only rarely been compared to a reference technique, making estimates of its sensitivity and specificity imprecise; it is dependent on patient effort and cooperation and only provides a semiquantitative evaluation of diaphragm function, making repetitive prospective measurements difficult to compare. In addition, it should not be used in the setting of bilateral diaphragm weakness, as the abnormal breathing pattern observed in this setting may obscure radiological findings and lead to false-negative results.

Sniff test: To sniff, the patient first takes a deep breath in, then exhales completely, and inhales as hard, quickly, and deeply as possible with the mouth closed. The maneuver is repeated quickly a few times. Images are taken from the front and in profile with sequences of calm breaths, deep breaths, and sniffles with video recordings. This may be nowadays applied by MRI.

The normal excursion of the diaphragm during a deep inspiration is at least one intercostal space in adults. The excursion can be something a little asymmetrical. In lateral projection, the excursion of the posterior part of the hemidiaphragm is usually greater than that of the anterior part, especially on the right side. When sniffling, both hemidiaphragms move downward simultaneously.

In diaphragmatic dysfunction, the excursion is reduced or canceled during a calm and deep inspiration in the affected portion of the diaphragm (Nason et al. 2012; Qureshi 2009). A paradoxical movement is defined by an abrupt and anarchic elevation of the diseased dome, while the healthy dome continues to lower with the end of inspiration. Paradoxical movement of the affected hemidiaphragm can be seen in the late phases of phrenic nerve unilateral paralysis. Although fluoroscopy is generally considered the preferred modality for real-time evaluation of diaphragmatic motion, its complexity and interpretation challenges can be problematic for its use in clinical routine. In order to address this issue, Leal et al. developed a simplified approach based on digital radiography fluoroscopy (Leal et al. 2017). The objective was to assess the validity and reliability of this method for measuring diaphragmatic mobility. This method involves measuring the distance between the diaphragmatic domes at expiration and inspiration, following the protocol as described by Saltiel et al. (2013). In this study, the mean diaphragmatic mobility values were 64.90 ± 12.9 mm for the right side and 63.95 ± 11.7 mm for the left side. It is worth noting that reference values for diaphragmatic mobility are not yet defined in the literature. However, it is observed that most healthy adults have global diaphragmatic mobility values above 30 mm (Gierada et al. 1998; Unal et al. 2000; Simon et al. 1969).

Fluoroscopy is rarely used in clinical practice for that purpose. The decrease in diaphragmatic mobility is subjective, suffering from a strong dependence on the cooperation of the patient, the experience of the radiologist, and a limited reproducibility. The drawback of the unavoidable radiation makes this method much less relevant nowadays, due to the strength of the following methods.

2.3 Ultrasound

Direct examination of the morphology and mobility of the diaphragm has been nearly impossible for a long time at patient bedside. The ideal tool candidate would have to be noninvasive, free of radiation exposure, easily available at the bedside, portable, easy to use, and low cost. Ultrasound (US) fits almost all the above features (Gierada et al. 1998). When a muscle contracts, it shortens, displaces, and thickens. Diaphragmatic US allows a dynamic approach of the contraction of each hemidiaphragm separately thanks to its direct visualization. US can also be used in the supine position; the latter can exaggerate the inability of the diaphragm to move during inspiration, thereby enhancing the ability to detect paralysis or weakness.

US can measure the thickness, thickening, and excursion of the diaphragm. The diaphragm is located between the peritoneal and pleural layers, which appears as a thick echogenic line (Fig. 3).

Normal hemidiaphragms move downward during inspiration, which lowers the intrathoracic pressure and increases the abdominal pressure. The excursion of the hemidiaphragms is globally similar on both sides. For reasons of feasibility, the right approach is often preferred using subcostal and intercostal approach since the left window is less convenient to image the diaphragm. The intercostal approach analyzes the diaphragm at the level where it adheres to the rib cage, known as the zone of apposition, and provides information on the thickness and thickening of the muscle, while the subcostal approach, more practical and feasible, analyzes its excursion (or displacement). The subcostal approach visualizes the caudal displacement of the hemidiaphragm that is called diaphragmatic excursion (Fig. 4). Measurement of the excursion of the right hemidiaphragm is associated with high intra- and interobserver reliability (Kim et al. 2011; Boussuges et al. 2009). The normal diaphragmatic excursion should be greater than 36 mm in women and 47 mm in men during maximal inspiratory effort. The optimal threshold of diaphragmatic excursion defining diaphragmatic dysfunction varies between studies. In the ICU context, it has been reported that diaphragmatic motion of less than 10 mm is in favor of diaphragmatic dysfunction in the subcostal approach, and diaphragmatic motion of more than 25 mm excludes diaphragmatic dysfunction (Dres et al. 2017; Dres and Demoule 2020; Grosu et al. 2012). A paralyzed hemidiaphragm will demonstrate no orthograde motion during calm breathing and may show a paradoxical movement.

Diaphragm US can detect a decrease in diaphragm thickness over time, suggesting muscle atrophy. This has been shown in critically ill patients exposed to mechanical ventilation (Goligher et al. 2018). Changes in thickness between expiration and inspiration can also be used to determine fractional diaphragm thickening expressed as a percentage. A thickening fraction <20%, in spontaneous inspiration, is frequently used as a surrogate of diaphragmatic dysfunction and is considered normal if >30% (Jorens and Schepens 2016; Dubé et al. 2017). Poudlard et al. showed however a poor correlation between fractional diaphragm thickening and transdiaphrag-

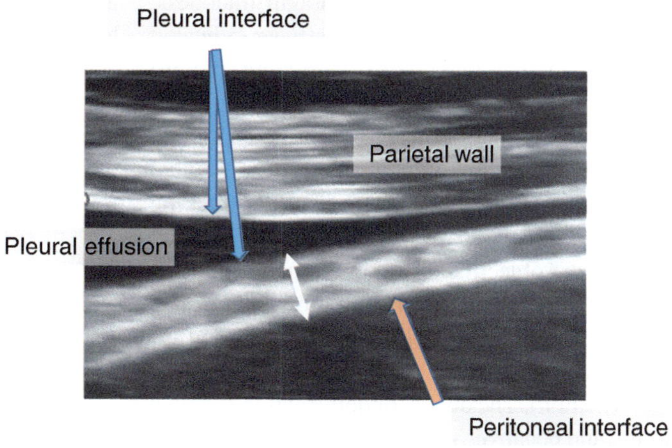

Fig. 3 The B-mode (2D) ultrasound identifies the diaphragm as a hyperechoic (white arrow) structure composed of three superimposed layers when using a high-frequency linear probe (8–13 MHz). The diaphragm is positioned between the peritoneal and parietal pleural layers

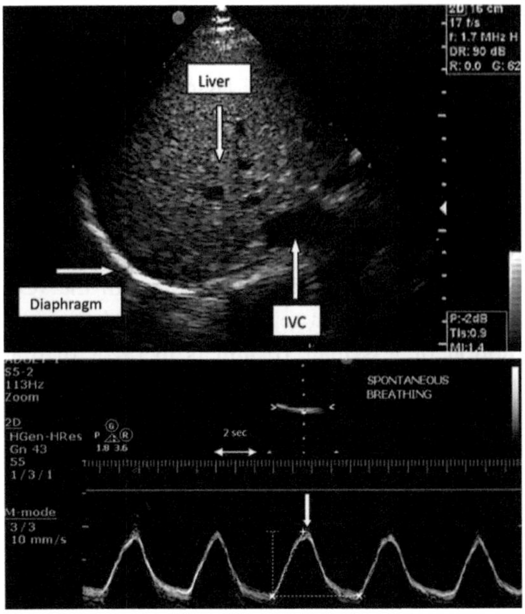

Fig. 4 The subcostal approach uses a low-frequency probe (<5 MHz), typically an abdominal probe. The probe is positioned under the right costal margin, perpendicular to the midclavicular line, and directed toward the liver. In B mode, the diaphragm appears as a hyperechoic line diametrically opposite to the probe, surrounding the liver. After adjusting the depth and contrast, the marking line is placed perpendicularly to the apex of the diaphragmatic dome. In TM mode: the elevation of the base line reflects the diaphragmatic excursion that can be measured. In intensive care unit, a motion less than 1 cm is in favor of diaphragmatic dysfunction

matic pressure because thickening is a one-dimensional parameter, while diaphragm contraction results from an active three-dimensional motion (Kim et al. 2011; Poulard et al. 2022).

In addition to assessing diaphragm thickness, thickening, and excursion, studies have indicated that longitudinal diaphragm shortening (strain) can be analyzed using speckle tracking, and diaphragm stiffness can be quantified through shear wave elastography (shear modulus) (Bachasson et al. 2019). The speckle tracking technique is derived from the echocardiography and has the objective to follow unique groups of pixels ("kernels") between expiration and inspiration to measure their displacement and how different kernels move in relation to one another (deformation). The degree of deformation is called strain, and negative value indicates kernels coming closer together. The more negative the strain, the greater the degree of deformation and the greater the contraction. The correlation between diaphragm thickening fraction and diaphragm strain is moderate (coefficient of determination, $r^2 = 0.44$, $p < 0.001$), whereas the correlation between diaphragm strain and diaphragm excursion is weak ($r^2 = 0.14$, $p < 0.001$) (Bachasson et al. 2019). By contrast, the correlation between strain and transdiaphragmatic pressure is higher ($r^2 = 0.72$, $p < 0.0001$) (Orde et al. 2016).

Shear wave elastography is an ultrasound-based imaging technique that can noninvasively measure shear wave velocity propagating in a target tissue, and the shear wave velocity can be directly linked to shear modulus. Because of the strong linear relationship between muscle shear modulus and active muscle force, ultrasound shear wave elastography provides an index of change in individual muscle force. The correlation between submaximal inspiratory mouth pressure and diaphragmatic shear modulus is high ($r^2 > 0.95$) (Oppersma et al. 2017) in healthy subjects as well is the correlation between transdiaphragmatic pressure and shear modulus ($r^2 = 0.82$) during isovolumetric inspiratory effort against closed airways and the correlation between transdiaphragmatic pressure and shear modulus during ventilation ($r^2 = 0.70$) against inspiratory loading (Chino et al. 2018).

Despite a good interobserver reproducibility reported by research studies, main limitations of diaphragmatic US are the partial nature of the exploration of the diaphragm, particularly on the left (digestive interpositions) with medial zones less well explored than the peripheral zones, the dependence on the US conditions related to the patient with low echogenicity and the operator expertise, and lastly, the impossibility to evaluate the motion of the two domes simultaneously (Dubé and Dres 2016; Fossé et al. 2020).

2.4 CT

Chest CT is an essential examination for the exploration of a proven or suspected diaphragmatic pathology with three main objectives:

1. Look for a lesion on the cervical and thoracic pathway of the phrenic nerve, i.e., anterior scalene muscle, vertical on the right side, oblique on the left side along the mediastinum (tumor of the pulmonary apex, thymoma, lymph nodes …) (Fig. 5).
2. Excluding other etiologies associated with an elevated hemidiaphragm (subpleural or subphrenic effusion, collection/abscess, or mass) and conditions that mimic respiratory muscle weakness (restriction due to interstitial lung disease) or alter the diaphragm itself like in shrinking lung in lupus or Sjögren disease or in myositis.
3. Precise the anatomy of the diaphragm. The development of imaging techniques and the possibilities of MPR reconstruction make it possible to distinguish between a diaphragmatic hernia, a diaphragmatic rupture, and eventration despite absence of quantitative values. The signs of rupture are of two types: direct by the demonstration of a defect in the dome thanks to multiplanar reformat and indirect signs including the ascent of the abdominal organs toward the thorax and the presence of "dependent viscera" sign (Hassankhani et al. 2023; Bergin et al. 2001; Desir and Ghaye 2012). In case of an elevated hemidiaphragm, demonstration of its completeness allows a diagnosis of eventration.

Chest CT also allows assessment of diaphragm thickness, which is most reliably measured at the level of the diaphragmatic crura often measured at the L1 vertebral level on CT. Values below 1.5 mm and an obvious disparity in thickness between one side and the other suggest diaphragm atrophy (Sukkasem et al. 2017) (Figs. 6 and 7). However, thinning of the diaphragmatic crura on the affected side may not be reliably seen in early paralysis, and exact parameters of normal diaphragm thickness are poorly defined (Sukkasem et al. 2017; Lallement et al. 2024). Lallement et al. report that for left diaphragmatic weakness, a threshold of less than 5.0 mm at the L1 level has excellent diagnostic performance (100% specificity and 100% PPV) (Lallement et al. 2024). It is also possible to obtain CT scan evaluation of the diaphragm volume, which is potentially of interest to detect changes over time (Jung et al. 2014).

Nevertheless, despite its good spatial resolution allowing an exhaustive analysis of the diaphragmatic silhouette, the analysis of the diaphragm remains imperfect with CT as it suf-

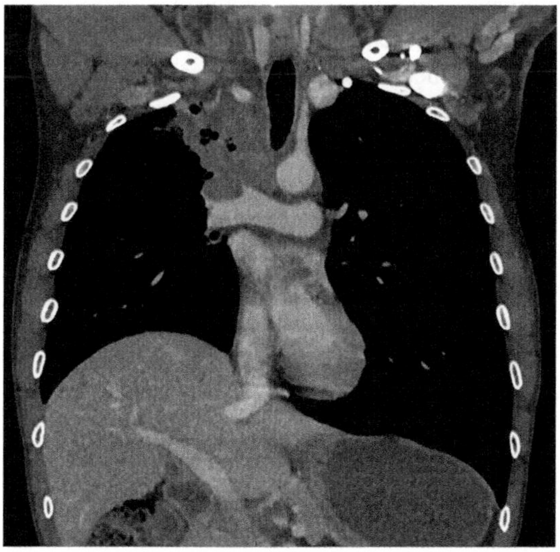

Fig. 5 Elevation of more than 2 cm of the right hemidiaphragm secondary to an apical tumor mass of the right upper lobe invading the right phrenic nerve along the superior vena cava

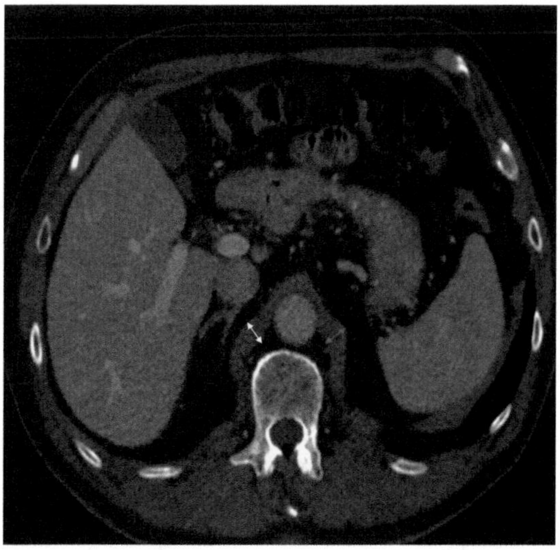

Fig. 6 Normal thickness of both diaphragmatic crura, 8 mm for the right crura (white arrow) and 9 mm for the left (blue arrow)

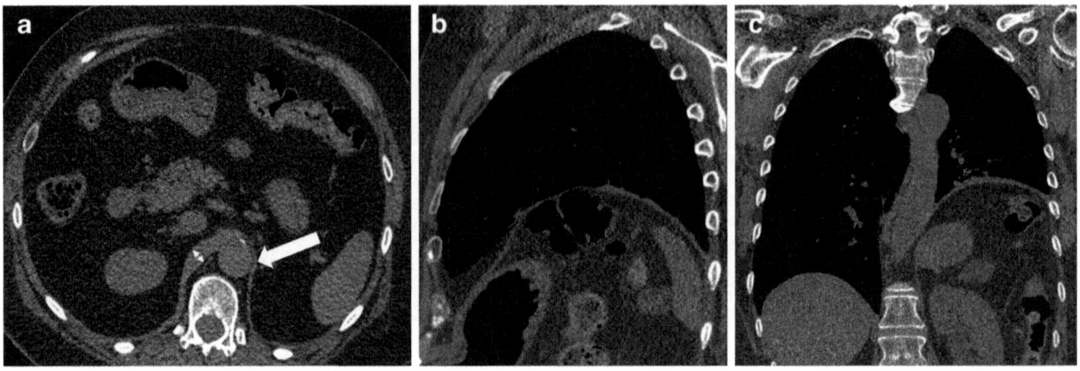

Fig. 7 Elevation of the left hemidiaphragm secondary to diaphragmatic muscle atrophy, resulting in complete eventration. The left crus is significantly thinned (arrow, <2 mm) compared to the right crus (measuring 7 mm). Note the presence of a small passive atelectasis in contact with the elevated dome of the left hemidiaphragm

fers from its lack of contrast resolution between the soft tissues and its radiating character, which limits the possibilities of performing a dynamic study. In a study of 226 patients, a quantitative measurement of diaphragmatic excursion was conducted to assess the adequacy of expiratory phase CT images. Azour et al. demonstrated that the average diaphragmatic excursion was 2.5 cm between inspiratory and expiratory scans (2.7 cm in men, 2.3 cm in women) (Azour et al. 2021).

2.5 MRI

Compared to computed tomography (CT) and fluoroscopy, dynamic magnetic resonance imaging (MRI) offers several advantages, such as better soft tissue contrast, absence of ionizing radiation, and greater flexibility in selecting scanning planes. Dynamic MRI is an emerging technique that allows quantitative assessment of excursion, synchronicity, and velocity of diaphragmatic motion, but its use is constrained by the limited availability of the technique and its high cost (Kondo et al. 2000; Nason et al. 2012; Gaeta et al. 2013; Le Pimpec-Barthes et al. 2019).

MRI provides morphological (diaphragmatic ruptures, hernias …) (Fig. 8) and dynamic information (Supplementary Videos 1 and 2). The protocol for diaphragmatic MRI typically includes T2-weighted sequences for static imaging during inspiration and expiration, assessing diaphragm morphology and position. Dynamic cine MRI is used to capture real-time diaphragm movement during free or forced respiration, with coronal or sagittal planning and optimized parameters to minimize motion artifacts. Optional T1-weighted sequences and mapping can be added to detect additional structural anomalies. MRI motion analysis can identify localized diaphragmatic dysfunctions, which are then a strong argument for a distal involvement of the dividing branches of the phrenic nerve. This particular case of damage to the distal dividing branches of the phrenic nerve is one of the limitations of electromyographic exploration.

The measurement of diaphragmatic motion can be performed according to two main methods: cranio-caudal height variations between the pulmonary apex and the diaphragmatic dome or distance traveled by the top of the diaphragmatic dome between inspiration and expiration (Suga et al. 1999; Plathow et al. 2009; Dinkel et al. 2009; Kiryu et al. 2006; Gierada et al. 1995; Iwasawa et al. 2002). Other studies focused on the antero-posterior diameter of the rib cage as well as the area of the diaphragm to assess the pathophysiology of the inspiratory mechanics as a whole with a good correlation between spirometry and measured chest areas (Suga et al. 1999; Iwasawa et al. 2002; Freeman et al. 2006; Cluzel et al. 2000).

MRI measurements of diaphragm thickness are poorly reproducible due to its very small thickness, and it is not used in daily practice (Fig. 9).

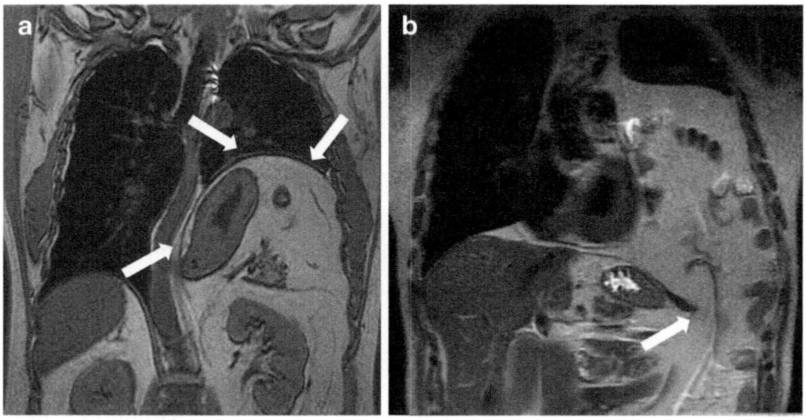

Fig. 8 Continuous diaphragmatic muscle in relation to a complete left-sided eventration (**a**) (white arrows). On the opposite, discontinuous diaphragmatic muscle in relation to a phrenic rupture in another patent (**b**) (white arrow)

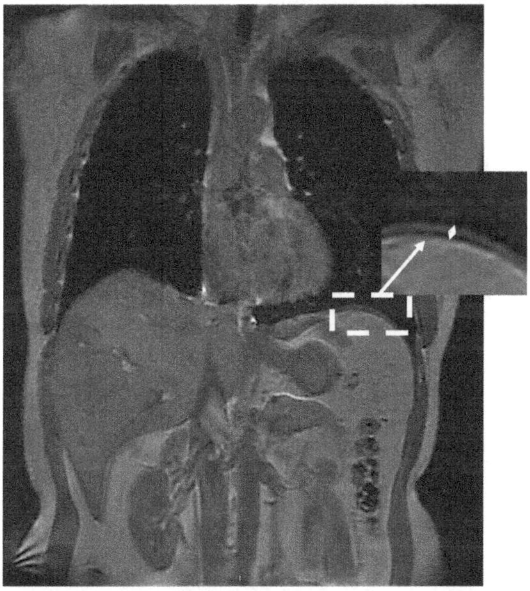

Fig. 9 In the coronal plane on T1 SE MRI, the thickness of the left hemidiaphragm dome is noted to be thin (double arrow). Measurement accuracy is limited by the low spatial resolution of the MRI. The delineation of the right hemidiaphragm is more complex due to the iso-signal interface with the liver, making the diaphragm contours harder to define

The absolute value of diaphragmatic excursion is difficult to interpret because of the many factors that may be responsible for variation (patient cooperation, physiological state, age of the patient, etc.). For example, an absolute quantification of diaphragmatic function in the supine position may range from 44 mm on the right to 42 mm on the left (mean values) (Gierada et al. 1995), from 30 to 90 mm in a study using an open MRI system (Unal et al. 2000), and in another study 55 mm in young healthy controls, 44 mm in 60–80-year-old controls, and 12 mm in emphysematous patients ($p < 0.0001$) (Iwasawa et al. 2002). Open MRI systems enhance patient comfort and accommodate individuals with larger body sizes while reducing claustrophobia more effectively than traditional closed MRI machines. They also facilitate reduced abdominal pressure on the diaphragm while offering imaging capabilities that closely replicate natural breathing.

The evaluation of the respiratory function in supine position is not strictly directly comparable to that in a standing upright position. Diaphragmatic course is indeed significantly greater in the sitting position than in supine position (mean difference of 20 mm on the right and 8 mm on the left according to Takazakura et al. 2004) with a mean right motion of 93 mm in sitting and 89 mm in supine position and a mean left motion of 81 mm in sitting and 75 mm in supine position (i.e., a significant difference between positions $p < 0.05$) according to Kiryu et al. (2006).

The diaphragmatic motion increases from front to back (anteroposterior gradient). As an example, Le Pimpec-Barthes et al. reported median normal values on the right between 36 and 55/66 and 75/69 and 95 mm (anterior/middle/posterior) and on the left between 24 and 50/58 and 70/57 and 90 mm (anterior/middle/posterior). Thus, the cranio-caudal displacement of the diaphragm is more pronounced posteriorly than anteriorly, with an excursion of the anterior portion of the diaphragm averaging 56% of that of the posterior portion (Gierada et al. 1995) (Fig. 10). In addition, the cranio-caudal displacement of the diaphragm is greater laterally than medially.

Dynamic MRI correlates well with US measurements of diaphragmatic excursion with normal deep breathing values of 70 mm in men and 57 mm in women in a study by Boussuges et al. (2009).

Hao et al. proposed a new method for comprehensive analysis of diaphragmatic motion using free-breathing dynamic MRI. After constructing 4D MRI images, manually delineated at end inspiration and end expiration, they observed that the regional velocities of the right hemidiaphragm, which ranged from 4.28 to 9.83 mm/s, were almost always significantly higher than those of the left hemidiaphragm, which ranged from 3.73 to 8.18 mm/s, at corresponding locations (Hao et al. 2022, 2024). Hao et al. demonstrated in their latest study on a population of 177 healthy children that the velocity ranges were between −2 and −13 mm/s (caudo-cranial displacement), without difference in velocity between genders (Hao et al. 2024). The same authors reported that excursion and maximum velocity of the right diaphragm are significantly greater than those of the left diaphragm in Hao's study evaluated with supine MRI (Hao et al. 2022). In contrast, Yamada's study of 103 adult patients showed faster motion on the left during upright radiographic imaging (Yamada et al. 2017). Anatomical asymmetry of the diaphragm may influence respiratory dynamics, as well as the positioning of internal organs such as the liver in adults and the spleen in children. Although a precise scientific explanation for this observed diaphragmatic asymmetry is currently lacking, it is plausible that the presence of these organs limits respective diaphragmatic excursion.

Hao et al. observed a significant difference in sagittal curvatures between the two hemidiaphragms, but no notable difference in coronal curvatures, using the method for comprehensive diaphragmatic motion analysis with free-breathing dynamic MRI (Hao et al. 2022). Using the diaphragm segmentation model, the same group demonstrated in their latest study that sag-

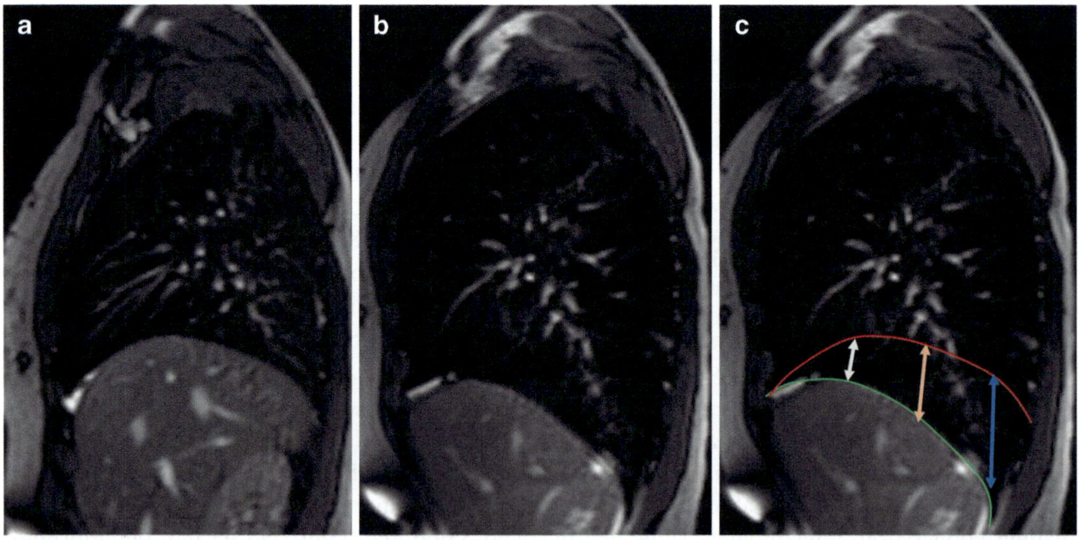

Fig. 10 Normal diaphragmatic magnetic resonance imaging findings in sagittal cine SSFP sequence with images at full expiration (**a**) and full inspiration (**b**) demonstrating the physiologic diaphragmatic excursion. (**c**) Normal dynamic MR diaphragmatic course measured between full expiration (red) and full inspiration (green). Anterior-posterior gradient of the diaphragm showing heights of 24 mm at the anterior (white arrow), 44 mm in the midsection (orange arrow), and 65 mm at the posterior (blue arrow), highlighting the maximum difference in the posterior portion

ittal curvature ranges were between −3 and −27 m^{-1}, and coronal curvature ranges were between −6 and −20 m^{-1}. This unit (m^{-1}) indicates the amount of curvature per unit length along the curve, enabling assessment of the configuration and angle of curvature in the specific region analyzed (Hao et al. 2024).

The variability of diaphragmatic course values, between the various publications and between different populations of patients, must thus be considered when interpreting the results for each patient. It is possible to consider each subject as his or her own control, allowing matching on data such as age and sex, but above all to be free of variations in terms of examination conditions, in particular the patient's understanding of the breathing instructions.

3 Perspectives/Future

A simple and fast MRI protocol should be performed as the first imaging method to assess the diaphragm owing to its noninvasive property, its performance for any pathological uni- or bilateral hemidiaphragm, and its better reproducibility than US. A primary focus on dynamic assessment of the diaphragm should be performed first before morphological assessment, especially in fragile patients, with the latter being commonly firstly assessed with CT. PET/CT imaging with 18F-FDG could also be a promising technique for detecting increased uptake in respiratory muscles during acute respiratory distress (Bondeelle et al. 2023).

4 Key Points

- **Chest X-ray**: There is no scientifically established consensus on a specific recommended measurement.
- **Fluoroscopy**: Not recommended and currently not used in clinical practice.
- **Ultrasound**: Often used in intensive care units. Hemidiaphragm is pathological if diaphragmatic motion of less than 10 mm (normal >25 mm) and thickening fraction <20% (normal >30%).
- **Chest computed tomography**: Used to analyze morphological diaphragmatic anatomy and surrounding structures.
- **MRI**: The most commonly reported values in the literature are those indicating normal diaphragmatic motion exceeding 25 mm with an anteroposterior gradient.

Disclaimer All measurements in this book have been obtained from peer-reviewed papers and guidelines from professional organizations, unless explicitly stated otherwise. While the authors, editors, and publisher have gone through a rigorous process to establish their correct reproduction from the original source, each measurement must be interpreted in the correct clinical context, this along with an accurate way of measurement, and taking into account all technical variables, this including follow-up exams with various equipment or software. Neither the authors, the editors, nor the publisher can accept any legal responsibility for any improper application or interpretation of these measurements as well as their potential consequences.

References

Azour L, Mendelson DS, Rogers L, Salvatore MM (2021) Diaphragmatic excursion: quantitative measure to assess adequacy of expiratory phase CT chest images. Eur J Radiol 136:109527. https://doi.org/10.1016/j.ejrad.2021.109527. Epub 2021 Jan 8

Bachasson D, Dres M, Niérat MC, Gennisson JL, Hogrel JY, Doorduin J, Similowski T (2019) Diaphragm shear modulus reflects transdiaphragmatic pressure during isovolumetric inspiratory efforts and ventilation against inspiratory loading. J Appl Physiol (1985) 126(3):699–707. https://doi.org/10.1152/japplphysiol.01060.2018. Epub 2019 Feb 7

Bergin D, Ennis R, Keogh C, Fenlon HM, Murray JG (2001) The "dependent viscera" sign in CT diagnosis of blunt traumatic diaphragmatic rupture. AJR. Am J Roentgenol 177(5):1137–1140. https://doi.org/10.2214/ajr.177.5.1771137

Bondeelle L, Vercellino L, Dres M, Bachasson D, Demoule A, Morélot-Panzini C, Similowski T, Bergeron A (2023) 18F-FDG uptake by respiratory muscles in acute respiratory insufficiency in a patient with graft versus host disease. Respir Med Res 84:101023. https://doi.org/10.1016/j.resmer.2023.101023. Epub 2023 May 19

Boussuges A, Gole Y, Blanc P (2009) Diaphragmatic motion studied by m-mode ultrasonography: methods, reproducibility, and normal values. Chest

135(2):391–400. https://doi.org/10.1378/chest.08-1541. Epub 2008 Nov 18

Celli BR (2002) Respiratory management of diaphragmatic paralysis. Semin Respir Crit Care Med 23(3):275–281

Chetta A, Rehman AK, Moxham J, Carr DH, Polkey MI (2005) Chest radiography cannot predict diaphragm function. Respir Med 99(1):39–44. https://doi.org/10.1016/j.rmed.2004.04.016

Chino K, Ohya T, Katayama K, Suzuki Y (2018) Diaphragmatic shear modulus at various submaximal inspiratory mouth pressure levels. Respir Physiol Neurobiol 252–253:52–57. https://doi.org/10.1016/j.resp.2018.03.009. Epub 2018 Mar 19

Cluzel P, Similowski T, Chartrand-Lefebvre C, Zelter M, Derenne J-P, Grenier PA (2000) Diaphragm and chest wall: assessment of the inspiratory pump with MR imaging—preliminary observations 1. Radiology 215(2):574–583

Desir A, Ghaye B (2012) CT of blunt diaphragmatic rupture. Radiographics 32(2):477–498

Dinkel J, Hintze C, Tetzlaff R, Huber PE, Herfarth K, Debus J et al (2009) 4D-MRI analysis of lung tumor motion in patients with hemidiaphragmatic paralysis. Radiother Oncol 91(3):449–454

Dres M, Demoule A (2020) Monitoring diaphragm function in the ICU. Curr Opin Crit Care 26(1):18–25. https://doi.org/10.1097/MCC.0000000000000682

Dres M et al (2017) Critical illness-associated diaphragm weakness. Intensive Care Med 43:1441–1452

Dubé B-P, Dres M (2016) Diaphragm dysfunction: diagnostic approaches and management strategies. J Clin Med 5(12):113 [cited 2019 Sep 16]

Dubé BP, Dres M, Mayaux J, Demiri S, Similowski T, Demoule A (2017) Ultrasound evaluation of diaphragm function in mechanically ventilated patients: comparison to phrenic stimulation and prognostic implications. Thorax 72(9):811–818. https://doi.org/10.1136/thoraxjnl-2016-209459. Epub 2017 Mar 30

Fernandes M, Cukier A, Ambrosino N, Leite JJ, Feltrim MI (2007) Respiratory pattern, thoracoabdominal motion and ventilation in chronic airway obstruction. Monaldi Arch Chest Dis 67(4):209–216

Fossé Q, Poulard T, Niérat MC, Virolle S, Morawiec E, Hogrel JY, Similowski T, Demoule A, Gennisson JL, Bachasson D, Dres M (2020) Ultrasound shear wave elastography for assessing diaphragm function in mechanically ventilated patients: a breath-by-breath analysis. Crit Care 24(1):669. https://doi.org/10.1186/s13054-020-03338-y

Freeman RK, Wozniak TC, Fitzgerald EB (2006) Functional and physiologic results of video-assisted thoracoscopic diaphragm plication in adult patients with unilateral diaphragm paralysis. Ann Thorac Surg 81(5):1853–1857

Gaeta M, Barca E, Ruggeri P, Minutoli F, Rodolico C, Mazziotti S et al (2013) Late-onset Pompe disease (LOPD): correlations between respiratory muscles CT and MRI features and pulmonary function. Mol Genet Metab 110(3):290–296

Gierada DS, Curtin JJ, Erickson SJ, Prost RW, Strandt JA, Goodman LR (1995) Diaphragmatic motion: fast gradient-recalled-echo MR imaging in healthy subjects. Radiology 194(3):879–884

Gierada DS, Slone RM, Fleishman MJ (1998) Imaging evaluation of the diaphragm. Chest Surg Clin N Am 8(2):237–280

Goligher EC, Dres M, Fan E, Rubenfeld GD, Scales DC, Herridge MS et al (2018) Mechanical ventilation-induced diaphragm atrophy strongly impacts clinical outcomes. Am J Respir Crit Care Med 197(2):204–213

Grosu HB, Lee YI, Lee J, Eden E, Eikermann M, Rose KM (2012) Diaphragm muscle thinning in patients who are mechanically ventilated. Chest 142(6):1455–1460. https://doi.org/10.1378/chest.11-1638

Hao Y, Udupa JK, Tong Y, Wu C, McDonough JM, Lott C, Clark A, Anari JB, Cahill PJ, Torigian DA (2022) Regional diaphragm motion analysis via dynamic MRI. Proc SPIE Int Soc Opt Eng 12031:120313F. https://doi.org/10.1117/12.2611951. Epub 2022 Apr 4

Hao Y, Udupa JK, Tong Y, Wu C, McDonough JM, Gogel S, Mayer OH, Alnoury M, Cahill PJ, Anari JB, Torigian DA (2024) Quantifying normal diaphragmatic motion and shape and their developmental changes via dynamic MRI. medRxiv [Preprint]. https://doi.org/10.1101/2024.05.12.24306850

Hassankhani A, Amoukhteh M, Valizadeh P, Jannatdoust P, Eibschutz LS, Myers LA, Gholamrezanezhad A (2023) Diagnostic utility of multidetector CT scan in penetrating diaphragmatic injuries: a systematic review and meta-analysis. Emerg Radiol 30(6):765–776. https://doi.org/10.1007/s10140-023-02174-1. Epub 2023 Oct 4

Iwasawa T, Kagei S, Gotoh T, Yoshiike Y, Matsushita K, Kurihara H et al (2002) Magnetic resonance analysis of abnormal diaphragmatic motion in patients with emphysema. Eur Respir J 19(2):225–231

Jorens PG, Schepens T (2016) Ultrasound: a novel translational tool to study diaphragmatic dysfunction in critical illness. Ann Transl Med 4(24):515. https://doi.org/10.21037/atm.2016.12.49

Jung B, Nougaret S, Conseil M, Coisel Y, Futier E, Chanques G, Molinari N, Lacampagne A, Matecki S, Jaber S (2014) Sepsis is associated with a preferential diaphragmatic atrophy: a critically ill patient study using tridimensional computed tomography. Anesthesiology 120(5):1182–1191. https://doi.org/10.1097/ALN.0000000000000201

Kim WY, Suh HJ, Hong S-B et al (2011) Diaphragm dysfunction assessed by ultrasonography: influence on weaning from mechanical ventilation. Crit Care Med 39:2627–2630. https://doi.org/10.1097/CCM.0b013e3182266408

Kiryu S, Loring SH, Mori Y, Rofsky NM, Hatabu H, Takahashi M (2006) Quantitative analysis of the velocity and synchronicity of diaphragmatic motion:

dynamic MRI in different postures. Magn Reson Imaging 24(10):1325–1332
Kondo T, Kobayashi I, Taguchi Y, Ohta Y, Yanagimachi N (2000) A dynamic analysis of chest wall motions with MRI in healthy young subjects. Respirology (Carlton, Vic) 5(1):19–25
Lallement P, Boussuges A, Habert P, Bermudez J, Reynaud-Gaubert M, Delliaux S, Bregeon F, Coiffard B (2024) Evaluation of computed tomography in the diagnosis of ultrasound-proven diaphragm dysfunction. Respir Res 25(1):135. https://doi.org/10.1186/s12931-024-02770-w
Le Pimpec-Barthes F, Hernigou A, Mazzella A et al (2019) Dynamic magnetic resonance imaging in unilateral diaphragm eventration: knowledge improvement before and after plication. J Thorac Dis 11:3467
Leal BE, Gonçalves MA, Lisboa LG, Linné LMS, Tavares MGS, Yamaguti WP, Paulin E (2017) Validity and reliability of fluoroscopy for digital radiography: a new way to evaluate diaphragmatic mobility. BMC Pulm Med 17(1):62. https://doi.org/10.1186/s12890-017-0402-x
McDonald AA, Robinson BRH, Alarcon L, Bosarge PL, Dorion H, Haut ER, Juern J, Madbak F, Reddy S, Weiss P, Como JJ (2018) Evaluation and management of traumatic diaphragmatic injuries: a practice management guideline from the Eastern Association for the Surgery of Trauma. J Trauma Acute Care Surg 85(1):198–207. https://doi.org/10.1097/TA.0000000000001924
Nason LK, Walker CM, McNeeley MF, Burivong W, Fligner CL, Godwin JD (2012) Imaging of the diaphragm: anatomy and function. Radiographics 32(2):E51–E70
Oppersma E, Hatam N, Doorduin J, van der Hoeven JG, Marx G, Goetzenich A, Fritsch S, Heunks LMA, Bruells CS (2017) Functional assessment of the diaphragm by speckle tracking ultrasound during inspiratory loading. J Appl Physiol (1985) 123(5):1063–1070. https://doi.org/10.1152/japplphysiol.00095.2017. Epub 2017 May 18
Orde SR, Boon AJ, Firth DG, Villarraga HR, Sekiguchi H (2016) Diaphragm assessment by two dimensional speckle tracking imaging in normal subjects. BMC Anesthesiol 16(1):43. https://doi.org/10.1186/s12871-016-0201-6
Plathow C, Schoebinger M, Herth F, Tuengerthal S, Meinzer H-P, Kauczor H-U (2009) Estimation of pulmonary motion in healthy subjects and patients with intrathoracic tumors using 3D-dynamic MRI: initial results. Korean J Radiol 10(6):559–567
Poulard T, Bachasson D, Fossé Q, Niérat MC, Hogrel JY, Demoule A, Gennisson JL, Dres M (2022) Poor correlation between diaphragm thickening fraction and transdiaphragmatic pressure in mechanically ventilated patients and healthy subjects. Anesthesiology 136(1):162–175. https://doi.org/10.1097/ALN.0000000000004042
Qureshi A (2009) Diaphragm paralysis. Semin Respir Crit Care Med 30(3):315
Saltiel RV, Grams ST, Pedrini A, Paulin E (2013) High reliability of measure of diaphragmatic mobility by radiographic method in healthy individuals. Braz J Phys Ther 17(2):128–136. https://doi.org/10.1590/S1413-35552012005000076
Simon G, Bonnell J, Kazantzis G, Waller RE (1969) Some radiological observations on the range of movement of the diaphragm. Clin Radiol 20(2):231–233. https://doi.org/10.1016/S0009-9260(69)80181
Suga K, Tsukuda T, Awaya H, Takano K, Koike S, Matsunaga N et al (1999) Impaired respiratory mechanics in pulmonary emphysema: evaluation with dynamic breathing MRI. J Magn Reson Imaging 10(4):510–520
Sukkasem W, Moftah SG, Kicska G, Godwin JD, Pipavath S, Stern E (2017) Crus atrophy: accuracy of computed tomography in diagnosis of diaphragmatic paralysis. J Thorac Imaging 32:383–390. https://doi.org/10.1097/RTI.0000000000000276
Suwatanapongched T, Gierada DS, Slone RM et al (2003) Variation in diaphragm position and shape in adults with normal pulmonary function. Chest 123:2019–2027
Takazakura R, Takahashi M, Nitta N, Murata K (2004) Diaphragmatic motion in the sitting and supine positions: healthy subject study using a vertically open magnetic resonance system. J Magn Reson Imaging 19(5):605–609
Toledo NS, Kodaira SK, Massarollo PC, Pereira OI, Mies S (2003) Right hemidiaphragmatic mobility assessment with US measurement of craniocaudal displacement of left branches of portal vein. Radiology 228(2):389–394. https://doi.org/10.1148/radiol.2282011554
Unal O, Arslan H, Uzum K, Osbay B, Sakaria ME (2000) Evaluation of diaphragmatic movement with MR fluoroscopy in chronic obstructive pulmonary disease. J Clin Imaging 24:347–350
Yamada Y, Ueyama M, Abe T, Araki T, Abe T, Nishino M, Jinzaki M, Hatabu H, Kudoh S (2017) Time-resolved quantitative analysis of the diaphragms during tidal breathing in a standing position using dynamic chest radiography with a flat panel detector system ("Dynamic X-ray phrenicography"). Acad Radiol 24:393–400
Zerah F, Harf A, Perlemuter L, Lorino H, Lorino AM, Atlan G (1993) Effects the obesity on respiratory resistance. Chest 103(5):1470–1476. https://doi.org/10.1378/chest.103.5.1470

The Chest Wall

Chiara Pozzessere and Patrick Omoumi

Contents

1 Introduction

The chest wall, the boundary of the thoracic cavity, is a complex structure composed of bones, joints, muscles and subcutaneous tissues with a crucial role in respiratory mechanics and protection of intrathoracic organs. The bone thoracic wall comprises the sternum anteriorly, 12 pairs of ribs laterally for each side and 12 thoracic vertebras posteriorly. The sternum is jointed to the clavicula by the sternoclavicular joint and to the first seventh ribs by the sterno-chondro-costal joints. Each vertebra is connected to the other by the intervertebral disc and to the ribs by the costovertebral and costo-transverse joints.

Chest wall metrics serve two main purposes. Clinically, they are useful for diagnosing and assessing the severity of some congenital and acquired conditions, including evaluation of congenital deformities, trauma, tumour, inflammation and infection, as well as for treatment planning. Moreover, the chest wall metrics are often used for forensic analysis, both anthropologic and crime-related ones. Imaging plays a major role in these settings. In clinical practice, the imaging modalities to study the chest wall include conventional radiology (CR), computed tomography (CT), ultrasound (US) and magnetic resonance imaging (MRI), the choice of which depends on the setting, the structure to evaluate, their availability and cost/effectiveness considerations. CR, US and CT are widely available in most countries, but CT and MRI more expensive

C. Pozzessere (✉) · P. Omoumi
Department of Diagnostic and Interventional Radiology, Lausanne University Hospital and University of Lausanne, Lausanne, Switzerland
e-mail: Chiara.Pozzessere@chuv.ch; Patrick.Omoumi@chuv.ch

Med Radiol Diagn Imaging (2026)
https://doi.org/10.1007/174_2025_615,
Published Online: 30 December 2025

than CR and US. By using the appropriate projections, CR allows a good evaluation of chest bones and joints, quickly, at low cost and with minimal radiation exposure, but it does not provide information on soft tissues. US is a low-cost and non-ionizing modality useful in the assessment of joints and soft-tissue structures. However, its effectiveness is limited by bone interference, which restricts the penetration window of US waves, and by operator dependency which can affect the consistency and accuracy of the results. CT offers a detailed assessment of chest wall structures yielding higher spatial resolution and cross-sectional view compared to CR and allows for 2D and 3D reformats and density measurements. MRI allows excellent soft-tissue contrast and tissue component quantification with no radiation exposure, making it ideal for chest wall assessment; however, due to its high costs, long examination time and lower availability relative to other modalities, it represents a third-level examination reserved to specific cases. For the above-mentioned reasons, to date CT is the modality of choice in most cases, while the use of the other modalities for chest wall measurements is reserved to few limited conditions. The recent introduction of CT photon-counting detectors is portending a revolutionary change in medical imaging, as they allow for notable radiation dose reduction while increasing image quality as well as for spectral imaging (Mourad et al. 2024). As far as costs will be reduced, photon-counting CT will probably replace the other modalities in more clinical conditions.

Historically, the first application of radiological imaging in forensic sciences dates back to the early 1900s when the paleoanthropologist Gorjanovic-Kramberger used this technique to investigate the bone structures of the Kapina Neanderthals (Gorjanovic-Kramberger 1902). Nowadays, forensic investigations often rely on imaging and specifically use chest imaging metrics for age estimation in the living (e.g. migrants and asylum seekers) through CR or CT and employ post-mortem computed tomography (PMCT) for virtual autopsy, skeletal identification and anthropological studies (Filograna et al. 2019; Franklin et al. 2016). Indeed, for the post-mortem studies, imaging acquisition is quicker than anatomic preparation and allows for noninvasive assessment of a large number of specimens and analysis of internal structures without dissection, also in case of fossilized, decomposed, partially destroyed or macerated skeletal remains (Filograna et al. 2019). Moreover, compared to the dry bones which eventually undergo post-mortem process such as desiccation and shrinkage, images of radiologic "fresh bones" reflect morpho-volumetric parameters of "in vivo" ones (Kieffer 2010). Finally, images can be digitally available in archiving systems, which allows rapid image storage of human remains and reproducible measurements.

This chapter will discuss the *when, how and why* of chest wall measurements with emphasize on the clinical and forensic relevance for each different structure.

2 The Sternum

The sternum is a long and flat bone located in the middle line of the anterior thoracic wall that consists of three parts: manubrium, sternal body and xyphoid process. The manubrium is located at the level of the T3–T4 vertebral bodies and is jointed to the clavicula by the sternoclavicular joint (SCJ) and to the costal cartilages of the first ribs and the upper part of the second ribs. Inferiorly, the manubrium articulates with the sternal body by a synarthrosis at the manubriosternal junction (MSJ), also called sternal angle or angle of Louis. During deep breathing, the MSJ angle increases up to 4.4°, allowing energy storage to facilitate thoracic cage deflation in the following passive exhalation. A manubriosternal fusion occurs in around 20% of population. The sternal body is located at the level of the T5–T9 vertebral bodies and is articulated with the inferior part of the second ribs and down up to the seventh ribs. The xyphosternal junction joins the sternal body to the xyphoid process. The xyphoid process ranges from 2 to 5 cm in length and modifies its structure during development, transitioning from cartilaginous in childhood to ossified in adulthood.

2.1 Measurements in Clinical Practice

Variations in the MSJ angle or angle of Louis (normal values: 145°–175°; 163° in males and 165° in female) may be associated with chest wall deformities, such as *pectus excavatum* and *pectus carinatum* (Mak et al. 2016; Restrepo et al. 2009).

2.1.1 Pectus Abnormalities

Pectus excavatum (also called funnel chest) is the most common congenital anomaly of the sternum and occurs in 1/300–1000 subjects. Due to a rapid and misdirect growth of lower costal cartilages, the chest presents with a concave deformity characterized by the anterior protrusion of the ribs and the posterior displacement of the lower part of the sternum. This deformity may lead to an abnormal redistribution of the position of structures of the chest such as leftward displacement and axial rotation of the heart (that may be responsible for a silhouette sign with the right lower border of the mediastinum) and reduction of the left lung space and prevertebral space. This condition may be isolated or associated with other syndromes such as Marfan, Ehlers-Danlos or Poland syndromes, congenital heart diseases and scoliosis.

In *pectus carinatum* (also called pigeon breast), a deformity occurring in up to 5% of subjects, a part of the sternum is bulging anteriorly. Also, it may be isolated or associated with congenital heart diseases and scoliosis. As for *pectus excavatum*, it may cause cardiorespiratory symptoms in addition to esthetical deformity. Rarely, both abnormalities can be present together in the so-called *pectus arcuatum*, for a premature sternal ossification that involves the MSJ and the first ribs.

These conditions can be corrected surgically, and CT is the standard of reference for preoperative measurements. Since this population undergoing surgical treatment is usually young, we strongly encourage to perform low dose or ultra-low dose CT, delivering an effective dose <0.5 mSv. For reference, the effective dose delivered with a CXR in the PA projection is about 0.02 mSv and 0.1 mSv when a lateral view is also acquired (“Table” n.d.).

2.1.1.1 Haller Index

Haller index (HI), also known as *pectus index*, provides an objective assessment of deformity severity on CT. The HI is obtained on CT images acquired during full inspiration by dividing the largest transverse thoracic diameter by the smallest anteroposterior diameter in *pectus excavatum* or by the largest antero-posterior diameter for *pectus carinatum*:

$$\begin{aligned}\text{HI} = {} & \text{largest transverse thoracic diameter} / \\ & \text{smallest}\left(\text{for pectus excavatum}\right) \\ & \text{or largest}\left(\text{for pectus carinatum}\right) \\ & \text{antero} \quad \text{posterior diameter}\end{aligned}$$

The measurements are performed at the inner aspect of the ribs, the most posterior border of the sternum and the anterior aspect of the thoracic vertebra (Haller et al. 1987). Normal sternal index ranges from 2.5 to 2.7; higher values are consistent with *pectus excavatum* of mild (<3.2), moderate (3.2–3.5) and severe (>3.5) grades. Surgery is indicated for HI greater than 3.25 in *pectus excavatum* and lower than 1.8 in *pectus carinatum* (Haller et al. 1987; Mak et al. 2016) (Figs. 1 and 2). Differently, in *pectus arcuatum*, surgical intervention may be indicated in patients with MSJ angles <130° (normal values: 145°–175°) (Mak et al. 2016).

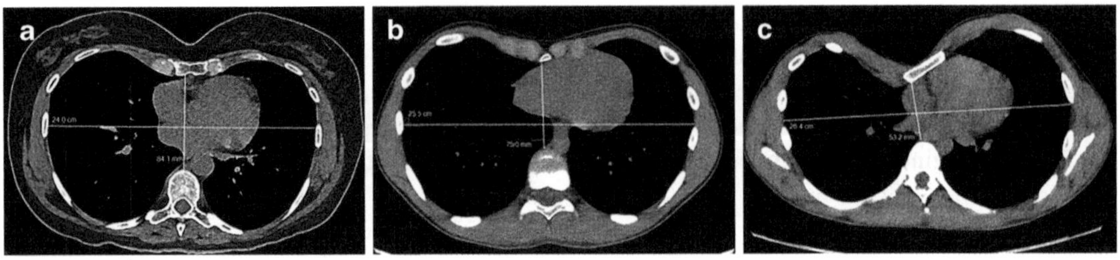

Fig. 1 Haller index (HI) measurements in patients with *pectus excavatum*. The HI is measured by the ratio of the maximal inner transverse chest diameter (internal edge of the ribs at the largest point) to the minimal anterior-posterior diameter (from the posterior wall of the sternum to the anterior wall of the vertebra) on the axial CT images, as following: HI = maximal transverse thoracic diameter/minimal anteroposterior diameter. (**a**) Mild *pectus excavatum*, HI 2.8, (**b**) moderate *pectus excavatum*, HI 3.3, and (**c**) severe *pectus excavatum*, HI 5. In case of tilted sternum or other deformities causing chest obliquity, the measurements are oblique maintaining an angle close to 90° between the two lines

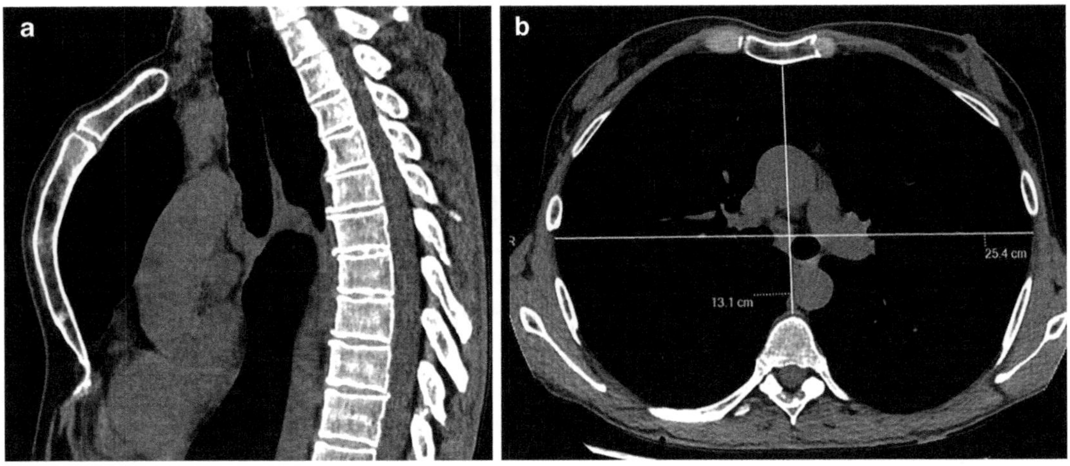

Fig. 2 Haller index (HI) measurement in *pectus carinatum*. (**a**) The sagittal view of a patient shows the typical appearance of a *pectus carinatum*. (**b**) The HI is measured by the ratio of the maximal inner transverse chest diameter (internal edge of the ribs at the largest point) to the maximal anterior-posterior diameter (from the posterior wall of the sternum to the anterior wall of the vertebra) on the axial CT images, as following: HI = maximal transverse thoracic diameter/maximal anteroposterior diameter. In this patient, the HI is 1.9 (normal values 2.5–2.7)

2.1.1.2 Correction Index

Since the HI may not accurately reflect the severity of bone deformity in patients with disproportionate chest dimensions including overly broad, narrow, or tilted sternum, several modified indices have been proposed, including the correction index (CI) (St. Peter et al. 2011; Poston et al. 2014). The CI measures the percentage of required sternal correction to normalize the chest wall. A virtual normal antero-posterior chest diameter (in other words, the virtual anteroposterior chest diameter if the pectus excavatum was corrected) is assumed as the distance between the most anterior aspect of the vertebral body and a line crossing the level of the most anterior rib at the site of deepest depression of the sternum. The formula to calculate the CI is the following (Fig. 3):

$$\mathrm{CI} = \left[\left(A - B \right) / A \times 100 \right].$$

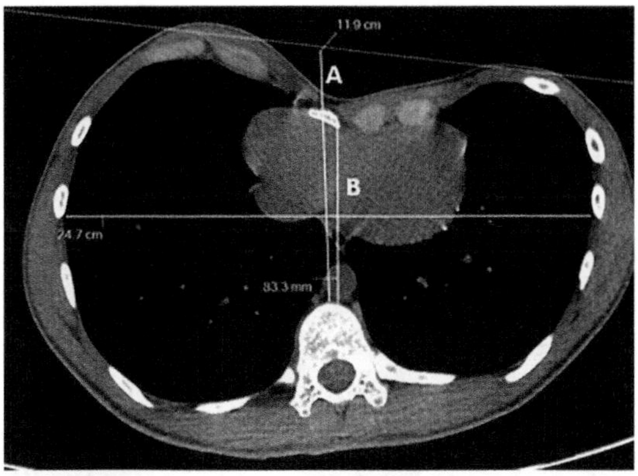

Fig. 3 The correction index (CI) may be more reliable than Haller index (HI) in non-standard chest morphology. To calculate it, a virtual line (dashed line) is drawn between the anterior margins of the anterior ribs at the level where the deformation is maximal. The distance between the most anterior aspect of the vertebral body and this line, passing through the mid-point of the sternum, is called *A* and represents the virtual normal antero-posterior chest diameter. This distance *A* is then subtracted by the measurement of the minimal antero-posterior distance used for the HI *in pectus excavatum* (*B*). This value is then divided by the virtual antero-posterior diameter (*A*) and the results multiplied by 100, to obtain chest depression percentage. CI = [(*A* – *B*) / *A* x 100]. In this case, despite a visually significant pectus excavatum with titled sternum, HI is 2.9, consistent with a mild deformity, and would not require surgery. Conversely, the CI result of 30% may indicate surgery (normal value <28%)

A = virtual normal anteroposterior chest diameter

B = distance between the most posterior aspect of the sternum at the site of the deepest depression and anterior vertebra

A HI of 3.25 corresponds to a CI of 28%, suggesting that a CI ≥28% is a reliable threshold for surgical indication. Nevertheless, CI is a more complicated and time-consuming measurement method, typically reserved for non-standard chest morphologies, such as patients with an overly broad, narrow, or tilted sternum.

2.1.1.3 Depression Index

In the depression index (DI), the vertebral body diameter is used as main metric rather than the thoracic diameter (Fagelman et al. 2015). To obtain the DI, a line across the most anterior rib is drawn at the level of the maximal depression of the sternum and the distance from this line, and the middle point of the sternum is then divided by the transverse diameter of the vertebral body at that level. The formula to calculate the CI is the following:

DI = distance between the level of the most anterior rib at the site of deepest depression of the sternum and the mid sternum / transverse diameter of the vertebral body at that level.

Other measurements include the asymmetry index, the chest shape index and the sternal torsion angle (Cartoski et al. 2006).

2.1.2 Sternal Foramen

The *sternal foramen* is a developmental round or oval bone defect of the sternal body or the xyphoid process detected in up to 10% of patients undergoing chest imaging that should not be confused as bone lesion or gunshot lesions in both clinical practice and forensic examinations (Babinski et al. 2015) (Fig. 4). Complications such as pneumothorax, intrathoracic haemorrhage and pericardial tamponade may occur in case of trauma, bone marrow biopsy or acupuncture. For this reason, its presence and size as well as the distance between the skin and the pericardium should be mentioned whenever detected. It usually measures about 6 mm (3–16 mm) of diameter, and the average distance from the skin and the anterior part of the pericardium is about 4 cm (4.2 ± 0.5 cm vs. 3.4 ± 0.8 cm for females and males, respectively) (Babinski et al. 2015).

2.2 Measurements in Forensic Studies

The sternum is a reference bone especially for sex determination in unidentified human remains relying on the *Hyrtl's Law*, which defines that the manubrium length exceeds half the length of the sternal body in female, while in males the sternal body length exceeds twice the length of the manubrium (Hyrtl 1871). In the past, CR frontal projections were often used for sternum measurements (Table 1).

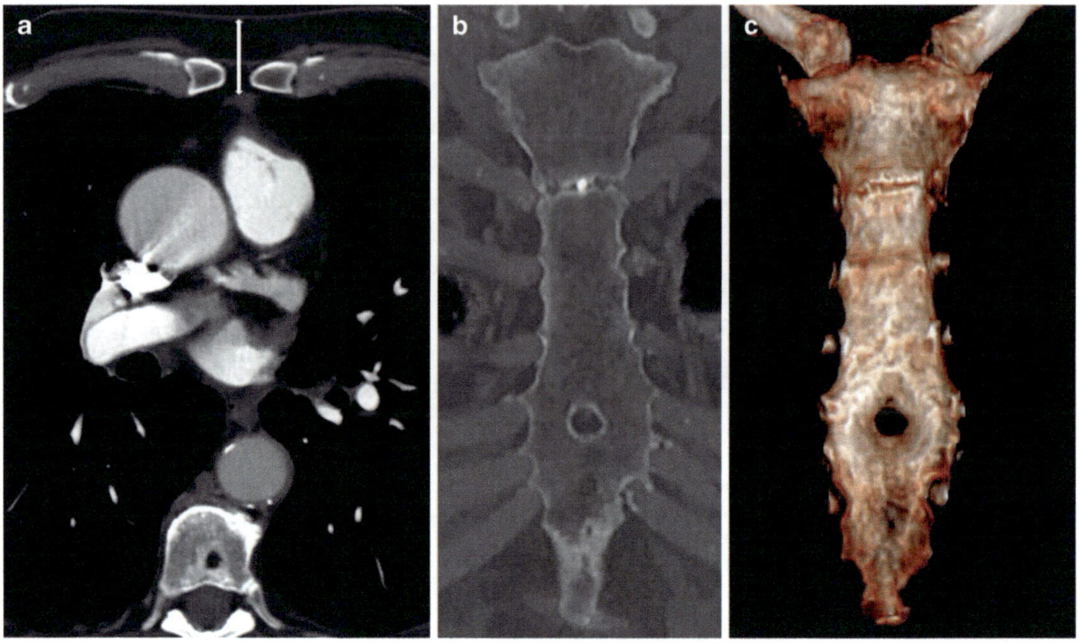

Fig. 4 Sternal foramen on CT. (**a**) On axial plane, a 10 mm large bony defect in the midline of the sternal body is depicted. The arrow shows the distance between the skin and the anterior part of the pericardium; (**b**) multiplanar reformat reconstruction (MPR) shows the typical round appearance of the sternal foramen; (**c**) sternal foramen on 3D-reconstruction

Table 1 CR anthropologic reference values for sex assessment in >25-year-old males and >21-year-old females

Measurement	All	Male	Female
Sternal length (mm)	143–168	157–183	133–148
Manubrial length (mm)	50 ± 5	55 ± 5	50 ± 5
Sternal area (mm^2)	5754 ± 1156	6380 ± 926	4752 ± 689

Today, however, CT is more commonly used, as it offers 3D-reconstructions and reproducible sternal measurements such as (a) manubrium width, measured at the level of the first incisura costalis; (b) manubrium length, obtained from the highest midpoint of the manubrium to the manubriosternal junction; (c) upper sternal body width, measured at the level of the midpoint of the 2–3 *incisurae costales*; (d) lower sternal body width, obtained at the level of the midpoint of the 4–5 *incisurae costales*; (e) sternal body length, measured from the manubriosternal junction and mesoxiphoid junction; (f) fourth rib width, measured from the superior to the inferior edge of the fourth rib, lateral to the *fossa costalis* (Fig. 5). The sternal area can also be calculated as following: (manubrium length + sternal body length) × (manubrium width + upper sternal body width + lower sternal body width)/3. Anthropological CT values for both sexes are reported in Table 2 (Uysal Ramadan et al. 2010).

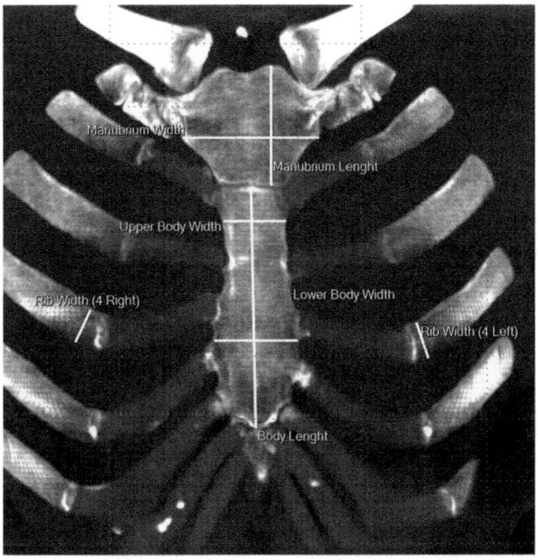

Fig. 5 CT multiplanar reconstruction (MPR) with maximum intensity projection (MIP) image showing the different sternal measurements used in forensic studies to establish age and sex

Table 2 CT mean and average values of sternal metrics

Measurement	Female (± SD)	Male (± SD)
Sternal length (mm)	135.4 ± 9.5	154.6 ± 12.3
Manubrium length (mm)	50.3 ± 4.9	53.9 ± 5.5
Body length (mm)	85.1 ± 8.7	100.7 ± 10.7
Manubrium width (mm)	54.0 ± 5.2	61.4 ± 6.0
Upper Body width (mm)	25.2 ± 3.3	28.7 ± 3.8
Lower Body width (mm)	30.7 ± 5.0	34.9 ± 5.9
Sternal area (mm^2)	4971.7 ± 661	6454.5 ± 905.3

Adapted from Uysal Ramadan et al. (2010)

3 The Clavicle

The clavicles are a pair of long, slightly curved bones articulating the sternum through the sternoclavicular joint and the scapula through the acromioclavicular joint, thus connecting the thorax to the shoulder and participating in the protection of the chest organs.

The assessment of medial clavicle ossification, the part connecting to the sternum, assumes an important role in age estimation since the clavicle is the latest bone to reach a complete ossification. The Group on Forensic Age Diagnostics (Arbeitsgemeinschaft für Forensische Altersdiagnostik; AGFAD) recommends staging its ossification when wrist and/or dental development assessment is not reliable, such as in case of alleged unaccompanied minors as the hand bones ossification is completed at 18 years of age, thus limiting the determination of legal adulthood (Lossois et al. 2022; Schmeling et al. 2016).

CT has recently replaced CR as the modality of choice thanks to the more detailed information provided. Thin slice thickness (<1 mm) and bone kernel reconstruction allows an optimal evaluation (Mühler et al. 2006). Today, MRI is not routinely used due to the lower spatial resolution compared to CT, but the recent implementation of low-field MR strength may open the door for the use of this modality in the future (Widek et al. 2023).

Historically, ossification stages were scored on a 5-point scale; subcategories have been introduced in the last few years in the attempt of differentiating the subtle development changes detected at CT (Fig. 6) (Kellinghaus et al. 2010; Schmeling et al. 2016). Although bone maturation is affected by several factors including sex, ethnicity, socio-economic and nutritional status, complete ossification of the epiphyseal cartilage correlates with a high probability of adulthood (Fig. 6) (Madentzoglou et al. 2025; Reder et al. 2024). Nevertheless, discrepancies due to the reader experience might be overcome in the future through the artificial intelligence systems (Wesp et al. 2024).

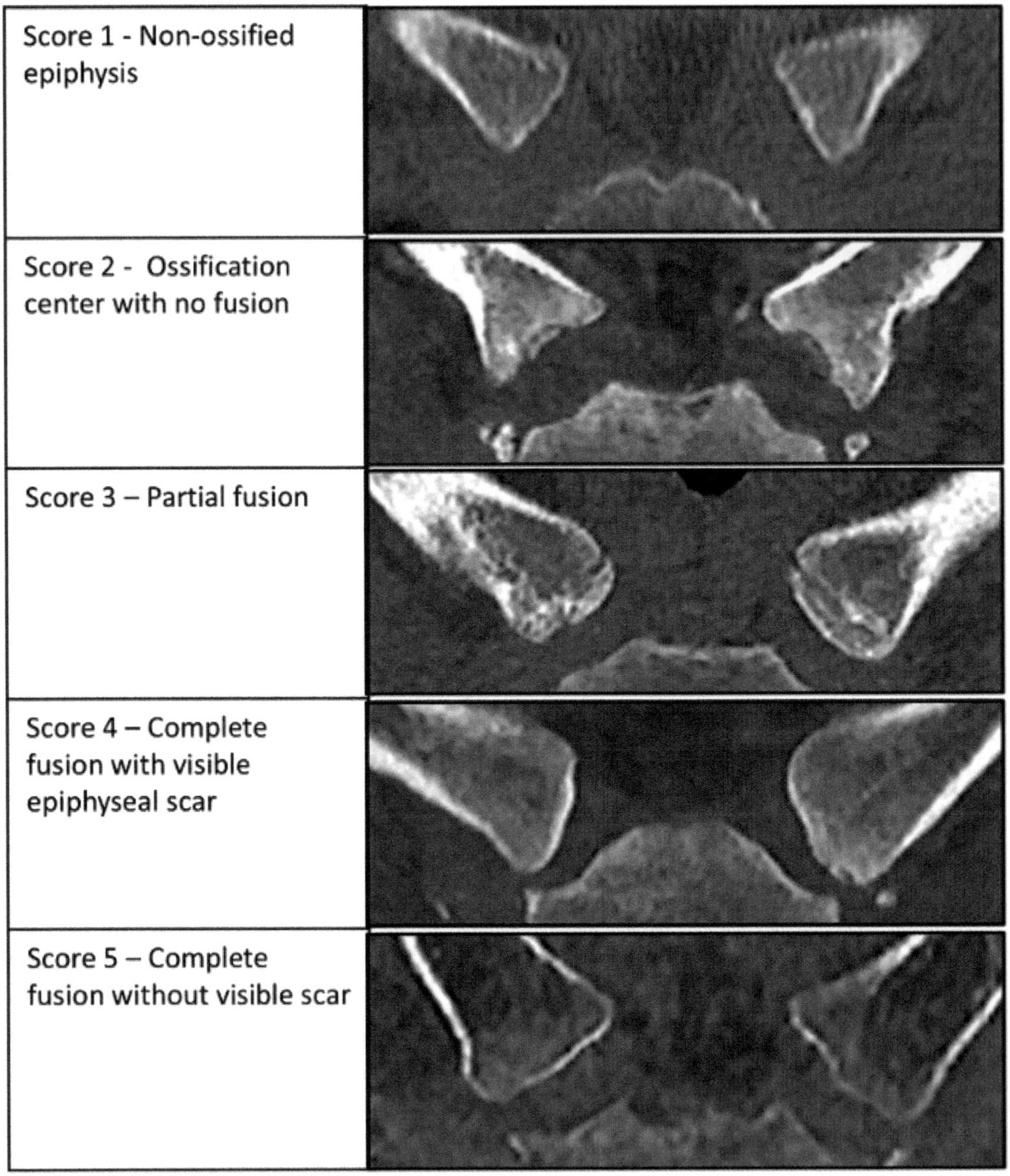

Fig. 6 CT images of the five stages of the medial clavicle ossification

4 The Ribs

The rib cage consists of 12 pairs of ribs that encircle and protect the thorax. Posteriorly, the ribs articulate with the corresponding vertebral bodies through the costovertebral joints and with the transverse processes of the vertebrae through the costotransverse joints. Anteriorly, the first seven ribs articulate with the sternum, while the eighth to tenth ribs (also known as false ribs) articulate with the seventh costal cartilage, and the last two pairs of ribs remain "floating". The neurovascular bundle (containing the intercostal vein, artery and nerve) usually runs in the inter-

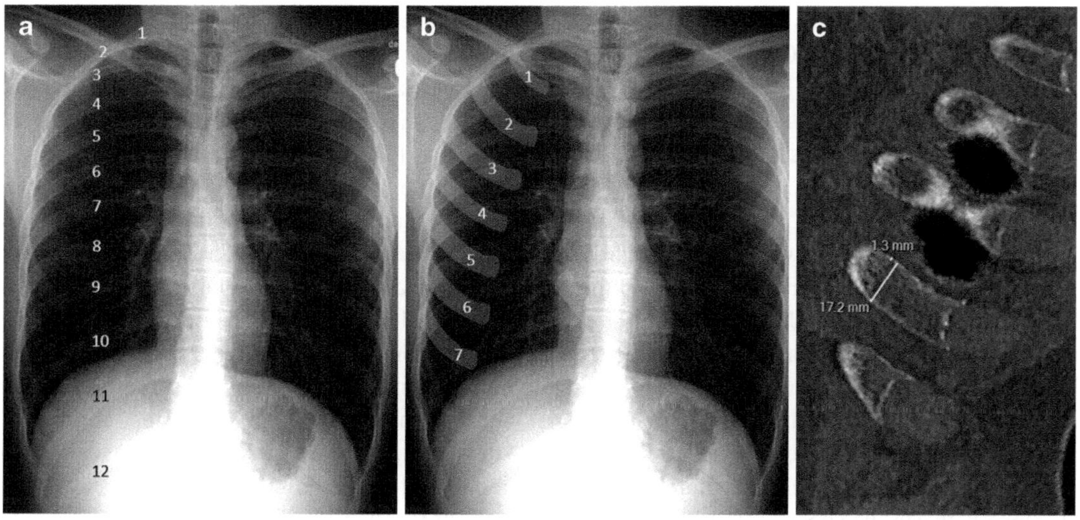

Fig. 7 (**a**, **b**) Posterior-anterior (PA) projection chest X-ray in erect position with labelled rib count. Chest radiography inspirium quality criteria are fulfilled. (**a**) Twelve posterior arcades are counted, ten of which (labelled in white) are above the diaphragm. (**b**) Seven anterior arcades are labelled at the midline over the diaphragm. (**c**) Multiplanar reconstruction (MPR) CT image of the anterior arch of the 4th right rib showing regular cortical (1.3 mm) and cranio-caudal rib thickness values (17.2 mm)

costal space below the lower edge of the ribs; thus, access in invasive procedures should ideally be made a few millimetres above the upper edge of a rib. However, with ageing, the neurovascular bundle may present with a meandering course particularly in the posterior intercostal area.

4.1 Measurements in Clinical Practice

Anatomic variants include variations in number, length and thickness. The presence of supernumerary ribs or a reduced number of rib pairs (generally 11 instead of 12) can be sporadic or associated with some trisomies, such as trisomy 21, and has no significant clinical impact (Kurihara et al. 1999). CR, performed with dedicated views (typically including an AP view and occasionally right and left anterior oblique views for specific purposes), is sufficient for visualization of the entire rib cage and ribs count (Fig. 7a). A cervical rib, either unilateral or bilateral arising from the 7th cervical vertebra, is an incidental finding reported in up to 8% of humans (Glass et al. 2002). Usually asymptomatic, it can be responsible for compression of the brachial plexus or the subclavian vessels causing a thoracic outlet syndrome. In such a condition, MRI is the modality of choice allowing for a radiation-free evaluation of the cause of the neurovascular bundle compression at different arms positions (Gilcrease-Garcia et al. 2020). Short ribs may be detected in up to 16% of adults and has no clinical significance. Newborns with known rib-polydactyly syndrome may have significant variations in rib length, which can lead to severe respiratory mechanics alterations (Glass et al. 2002). As note, ribs count is routinely used as a technical quality criterion at chest X-ray to establish adequate maximum inspirium: as shown in Fig. 7a, in posterior-anterior (PA) projection, at least 5–6 anterior arches or 10 posterior arches should be visible above the midline of the dome of the right diaphragm (Kelly 2012).

Regular ribs cranio-caudal thickness in adults is approximately 15–20 mm, and the cortical bone thickness ranges from approximately 1–2 mm (Fig. 7b) (Weaver et al. 2014). Diffuse alterations in rib thickness may be rarely observed in adults, such as thinning in trisomy 18 and thickening in severe forms of major thalassemia, respectively (Glass et al. 2002).

4.2 Measurements in Forensic Studies

The rib cage is affected by age, sex, height and weight. Although this is no relevant in clinical practice, it may be used to establish human remains characteristics in anthropomorphic studies. As previously mentioned, rib cranio-caudal thickness ranges between 15 and 20 mm (Weaver et al. 2014). The 4th rib is often used as reference and its caudo-cranial thickness, defined as the distance between the superior and inferior edges of the rib laterally to the costo-chondral articulation, varies by sex, averaging about 18 mm in men and 15 mm in women (Figs. 5 and 7b) (Uysal Ramadan et al. 2010). The rib cage significantly increases in all three dimensions during the development, reaching its maximal volume at the age of 30, and remaining almost stable afterwards (Weaver et al. 2014). At the same time, the thoracic index, representing the ratio between the average antero-posterior and lateral measurements, decreases during the first 20 years of life, and then it remains stable until the age of 70. The rib orientation changes with age, following kyphotic changes overtime. Generally, in women, the rib cage is 10% smaller than in men (Bellemare et al. 2006).

5 The Vertebrae

The thoracic spine lies in the posterior midline of the thoracic wall and is composed of 12 vertebrae. It plays a crucial role in maintaining thoracic posture, supporting the upper body and protecting the posterior aspect of the thoracic organs, particularly the spinal cord. The thoracic vertebrae share a common anatomical structure (Waxenbaum et al. 2024). Each vertebra consists of an anterior portion, called the body, and a posterior portion, known as the neural arch, which is formed by two pedicles, two laminae and one spinous process. The vertebrae are connected to each other by fibrocartilaginous intervertebral discs and facet joints through their superior and inferior articular processes. Each thoracic vertebra has six facets: two on the transverse processes and four demifacets. These facets articulate with the corresponding rib through the costovertebral and costotransverse joints. The inferior demifacet of a thoracic vertebra articulates with the rib located below, which also articulates with the superior demifacet of the adjacent inferior vertebra. The size of the vertebrae varies with age, with an increase in height during childhood. After the age of 40, age-related changes due to the mineral bone and muscle tone reduction lead to slight to severe vertebral body height loss (de Reuver et al. 2022).

5.1 Measurements in Clinical Practice

Vertebral and discal morphometry can be influenced by various conditions, including post-traumatic changes, osteoporosis, degenerative changes, congenital malformations, metabolic disorders and oncologic diseases. There are no standard reference values for measuring vertebrae nor intervertebral discs; their assessments rely on comparing different parts of the same vertebra, adjacent vertebrae and discs. Typically, the height of the anterior wall of the vertebra is slightly less than that of the posterior wall, except in the distal thoracic part where they are of equal size. This characteristic contributes to the physiological kyphotic curve. Imaging plays a crucial role in diagnosing, assessing the severity and planning the treatment of various dorsal spine conditions.

5.1.1 Spine Angulation

CR is the first-line examination for evaluating kyphosis and scoliosis, performed in PA and lateral views in standing position or AP in supine position when standing is not possible. The Cobb angle is the standard method for quantifying the anterior and lateral curvature of the thoracic spine, defining severity of kyphotic and scoliotic deformities (Katzman et al. 2010; Kim et al. 2010). Cobb method has some intrinsic pitfalls (Kim et al. 2010). First, it relies only on two-dimensional measurements, while different spine deformities may often coexist in the same patient (e.g. scoliosis + hyperkyphosis). Moreover, these abnormal spine conditions rotations may cause difficulties in correct patient positioning that may lead to up to 20% calculation differences. Differences up to 10° in Cobb angle values measurements may occur due to technical or physiological conditions as well as interobserver variability. To overcome angle calculation difficulties, digital measurements through dedicated software are suggested.

5.1.1.1 Kyphosis: Straight Back Syndrome

Physiologically, thoracic spine has a slight, physiological, kyphotic curve, meaning an anterior curvature ranging between 20° and 29°. This angle depends on age and gender, and from the fourth decade, due to the mineral bone and muscular tone changes as well as intervertebral disc degeneration and thinning, the curvature increases of about 3% per decades, leading to an age-related *hyperkyphosis* up to 50° in 20–40% of elderly (Fon et al. 1980). *Hyperkyphosis*, defined as an angle over 40°, may be (i) age-related, mainly caused by posture, osteoporosis and fractures; (ii) caused by Scheuermann's disease, also known as juvenile kyphosis, a curvature deformity due to an abnormal vertebral development causing anterior wedging greater than 5° and endplate irregularities of at least 3 consecutive vertebral bodies (Fig. 8b); (iii) congenital, secondary to developmental failure (type 1) or segmentation failure (type 2) of vertebral bodies, a rare but severe condition leading to a deformity with neurological compression; and (iv) secondary to vertebral body deformity after fracture or infection (Katzman et al. 2010; Urrutia et al. 2019). Lateral CR projection of the thoracic spine is routinely used to measure the Cobb angle. The Cobb angle is obtained by measuring the angle between lines perpendicular to the superior endplate of the upper vertebra (usually T2, or T4 when T2 is not visible) and the inferior endplate of the lower vertebra (usually T12) forming the beginning and the end of the curve, respectively (Fig. 8a, b).

Inversely, *Straight Back Syndrome (SBS)* refers to a loss of the physiological thoracic kyphosis and is often associated with cardiovascular manifestations (Kong et al. 2023). Similarly, SBS is evaluated on lateral CR view, by calculating the distance from the midpoint of the anterior edge of T8 to a line connecting the anterior endplates of T4 and T12 (Fig. 8c); a distance less than 1.2 cm is consistent with SBS (Kong et al. 2023).

5.1.1.2 Scoliosis

Scoliotic curvature is usually evaluated for the entire spine on the AP dorsal projection in erect position (Dickson 2004). The entire spine is usually involved; hence, measurements usually include both the dorsal and lumbar tracts. Severity scoliosis assessment relies on Cobb angle measurement, which is defined between lines perpendicular to the superior endplate of the uppermost tilted vertebra and the inferior endplate of the lowermost tilted vertebra (Fig. 9). Table 3 provides a grading scale for Cobb angle measurements of scoliotic curves. Another method, less used, for measuring spinal curvature is the Ferguson angle, which assesses the angle between two lines passing through the midpoint of the apical vertebra (the most deviated vertebra) and the midpoints of the end vertebrae (Waldt et al. 2014). Other methods, including the Lenke Classification, a reliable system for adolescent idiopathic scoliosis assessment, as well as Nash-Moe method introduced to grading vertebral rotations, are not limited to the thoracic spine assessment ("Manuals and Presentations | Scoliosis Research Society" n.d.). EOS imaging enables the measurement of spinal static parameters and is ideal for monitoring children and young adults due to its low radiation dose (De Leucio et al. 2023). In recent years, the application of 3D-US for scoliosis assessment has been investigated; however, its use is not yet widespread (Kumar et al. 2024).

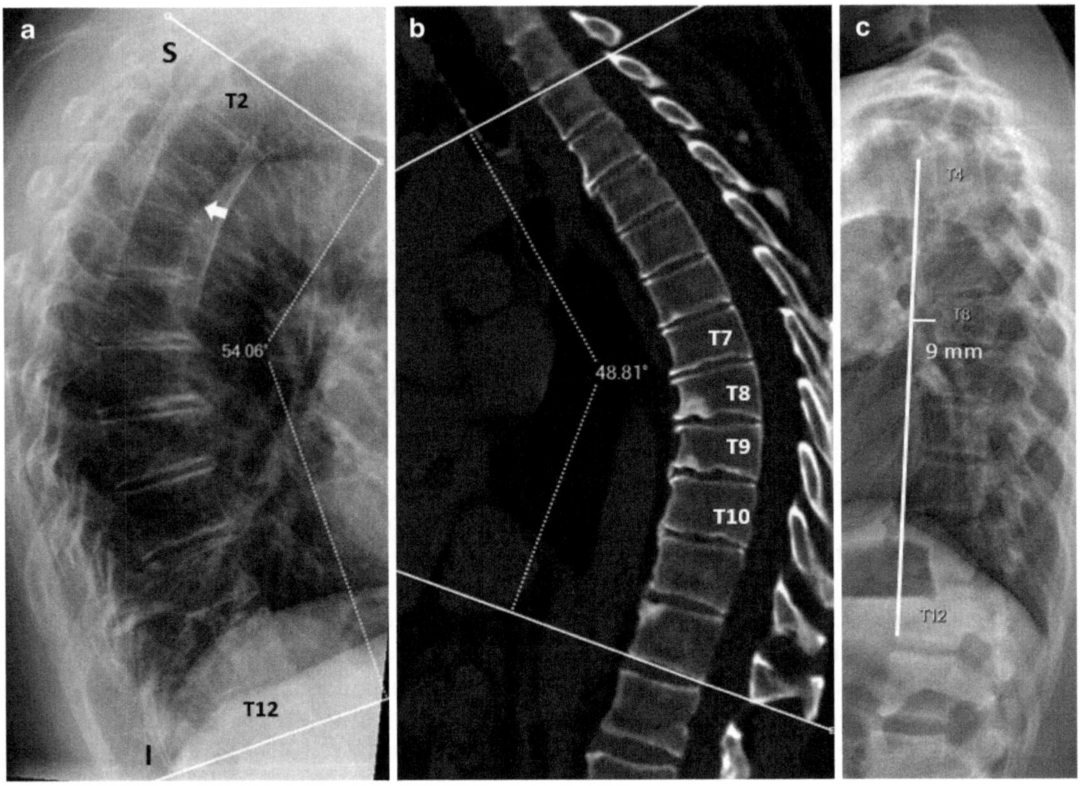

Fig. 8 Kyphosis and straight back syndrome. (**a**) Hyperkyphosis of the thoracic spine caused by a T4 fracture (arrow). Radiography on lateral projection shows the Cobb method for kyphosis deformity assessment, which consists in calculating the angle between the beginning and the end of the kyphotic curve. In this patient, a line at the superior endplate of T2 and the inferior endplate of T12 are drawn, and the angle is obtained by drawing two perpendicular dotted lines from lines S and I. (**b**) Hyperkyphosis secondary to Scheuermann's disease. CT image in sagittal plane showing anterior wedging greater than 5° of the vertebral bodies from T7 to T10, vertebral endplate irregularity and signs of disc degeneration, causing thoracic spine kyphosis of about 49°. (**c**) Radiography on lateral view of the thoracic spine showing Straight Back Syndrome. A line connecting the anterior edges of the superior endplate of T4 and of the inferior endplate of T12 is drawn and the distance between this line and the midpoint of the anterior edge of T8 midpoint is obtained, being 9 mm

5.1.2 Vertebral Body

Fractures are generally secondary to trauma, osteoporosis, malignancy and more rarely infection. Vertebral deformity following fractures can lead to changes in mechanical support, potentially resulting in hyperkyphosis depending on the number and severity of the vertebral fractures. Imaging is the standard reference for fracture detection, assessment and planning management (Miao et al. 2024). CR, including the antero-posterior (AP) and the lateral projections, is usually performed in low-energy or osteoporotic fractures. It is important to note that CR has several limitations. Particularly in patients with scoliosis, minimal fractures may be misdiagnosed due to the obliquity of the spine; moreover, the superimposition of bony structures in the cervicothoracic region can lead to CR underdiagnosis of T1 and T2 fractures. CT is the modality of choice especially for high-energy fracture assessment, as it allows for an accurate fracture detection, classification, vertebral body height loss quantification, evaluation of retropulsed fragments and assessment of spinal canal, including epidural hematoma and spinal cord involvement. MRI is, however, more sensitive than CT, especially in the evaluation of trauma complications and establish the nature of the fracture. MRI allows for the quantification of bone marrow fat replacement by malignancy through T2-weighted Dixon sequence. In malignant fractures, both the signal intensity

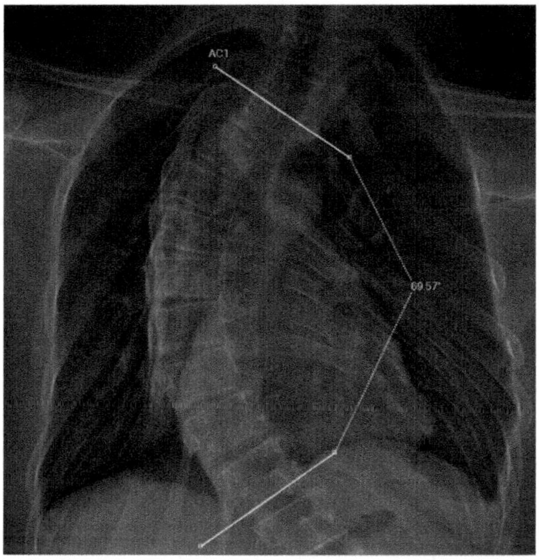

Fig. 9 Severe scoliosis of the thoracic spine. A line parallel to the superior endplate of T4 and the inferior endplate of T12, representing the uppermost and lowermost tilted vertebrae, respectively, are drawn. Two perpendicular lines (dotted lines) between the aforementioned lines are then added to calculate the Cobb angle, resulting in 70°, which is consistent with severe scoliosis

Table 3 Scoliotic curve grading according to Cobb angle measurement

Angle	Grading
0°–10°	Normal curve
10°–20°	Mild scoliosis
20°–40°	Moderate scoliosis
>40°	Severe scoliosis

drop between in-phase and out-of-phase images as well as the fat fraction obtained from water-only and fat-only images are lower compared to benign fractures (Bacher et al. 2021). The loss of height (LOH) assessment is a widely used method to quantify the reduction in vertebral body height (Miao et al. 2024). This semi-quantitative assessment is obtained by measuring the anterior, middle, and posterior heights of the vertebral body. According to Genant et al. system, fractures are graded as follows based on LOH: mild (20–25%; grade 1), moderate (25–40%; grade 2), and severe (>40%; grade 3) (Genant et al. 1993) (Fig. 10). The location of the height reduction, along with bone density, is useful in identifying the cause of the

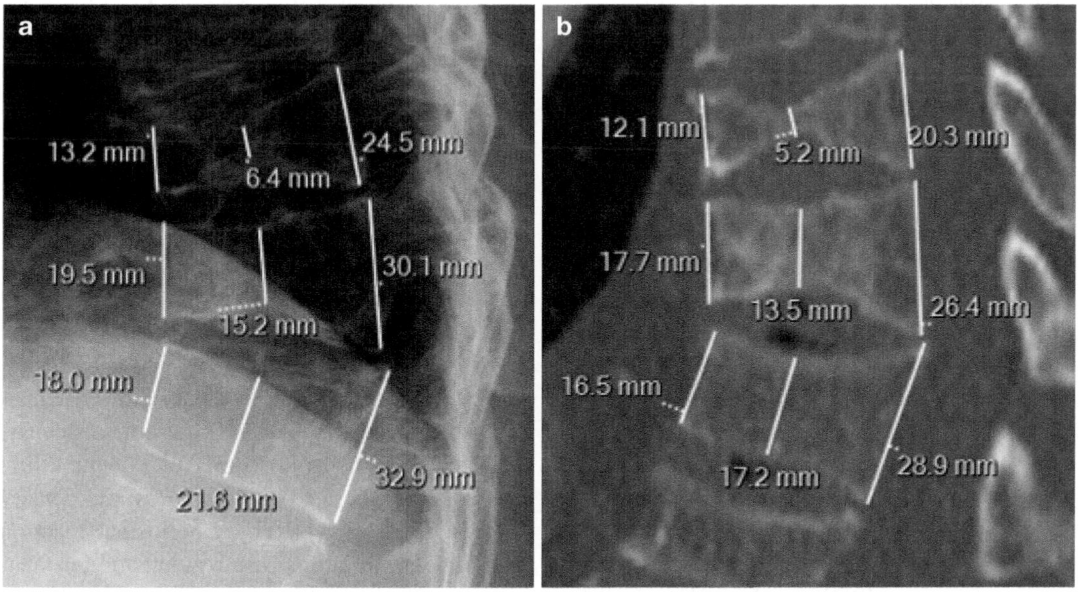

Fig. 10 (**a**) Dorsal spine CR depicting a grade 3 biconcave fracture of T10 (loss of height 46%), grade 2 wedge fracture of T11 (loss of height 35%) and grade 3 wedge fracture of T12 (loss of height 45%), according to Genant et al. semi-quantitative assessment. (**b**) Same patient, loss of height severity assessment at CT, confirming a grade 3 fracture of T10 (loss of height 40%), a grade 2 fracture of T11 (loss of height 33%) and a grade 3 fracture of T10 (loss of height 43%). See the slight measurement difference due to the intrinsic CR limitations

fracture. Minimal body deformities (LOH <20%) may be anatomical variants or indicative of degenerative spondylosis.

6 Bone Density

Osteoporosis is the fourth leading cause of chronic disease morbidity in Europe, affecting up to 21% of women and 6% of men over 50 years old. It consists in the loss of bone density and mass, which results in a higher bone fragility and fracture risk. Dual-Energy X-ray Absorptiometry (DXA or DEXA) is a widely used method to assess osteopenia and osteoporosis in individuals at risk by measuring bone mineral density (BMD) primarily at the lumbar spine and hip (Krugh and Langaker 2025). Bone density can be also evaluated on CT images and, in particular, Quantitative Computed Tomography (QCT) and Dual-Energy Computed Tomography (DECT) provide a detailed 3D evaluation of trabecular and cortical bone and correlate with fracture risk; however, its higher costs, the need of phantom calibration and the high radiation exposure compared to DEXA limit its use as primary tool in osteoporosis screening (Gruenewald et al. 2022). MRI offers a radiation-free alternative, and the few data available so far show a lower accuracy compared to CT. Despite the easy access to DEXA, its use depends on local practice and the importance of osteoporosis screening is sometimes underestimated. With the aim to increase osteoporosis early detection and fracture prevention, the opportunistic assessment of direct bone attenuation or through software assistance on CT performed for other indications, including chest CT for lung cancer screening, has more recently raised high interest among the radiology community (Cheng et al. 2021; Zhu et al. 2021). A direct measurement of bone attenuation values can be easily obtained by drawing a region of interest (ROI) on the trabecular bone of the first lumbar vertebral body (L1) on non-contrast enhanced CT. Hounsfield units (HU) do not significantly change on the various reconstruction planes neither with various reconstruction kernels; however, bone-sharpening kernel is preferred as it allows better visualization of vessels or lesions that should be not included in the ROI. Conversely, attenuation may be influenced by several factors including scanner vendor, kV, slice thickness, contrast-medium agent, patient size, vertebra level and vertebral abnormality (fracture, lesions, external material for osteosynthesis, etc.) (Boutin and Lenchik 2020; Eggermont et al. 2018; Zou et al. 2019). Generally, at 120 kV images, values of less than 100 HU are likely consistent with osteoporosis, while a 160 HU cut-off generally excludes osteopenia (Fig. 11) (Boutin and Lenchik 2020). Importantly, HU values correlate with fracture risk and post-operative failure, such as pedicle screw loosening, cage subsidence, lack of vertebral fusion and iatrogenic fracture of an adjacent vertebra (Boutin and Lenchik 2020). On contrast-enhanced CT, a physiological attenuation increase of about 20–30 HU should be considered due to the bone vascularization. When L1 attenuation is not measurable or the vertebra is not included in the acquisition, comparable measurements can be done at different levels, such as T7, T12 or L2 (Boutin and Lenchik 2020). The ongoing implementation of artificial intelligence (AI) and machine learning models opens the door to an automated opportunistic screening in the near future (Ong et al. 2023).

Imaging plays a pivotal role in bone lesions identification, characterization and treatment response assessment. Whereas CT is superior to CR and US for lesion detection, size measurement and characterization, MRI surpasses the performance of CT for the detection and characterization of bone marrow lesions. Nevertheless, CT is often sufficient in various clinical scenarios such as cancer follow-up. At CT, bone lesion evaluation is based on tumour matrix, density and margins, as well as on periosteal reaction and bone destruction. Lesion attenuation is measured in Hounsfield unit (HU). The sclerotic lesions are defined as those with higher attenuation than the surrounding normal trabecular bone, the lucent/lytic ones as those with lower attenuation than normal trabecular bone, while

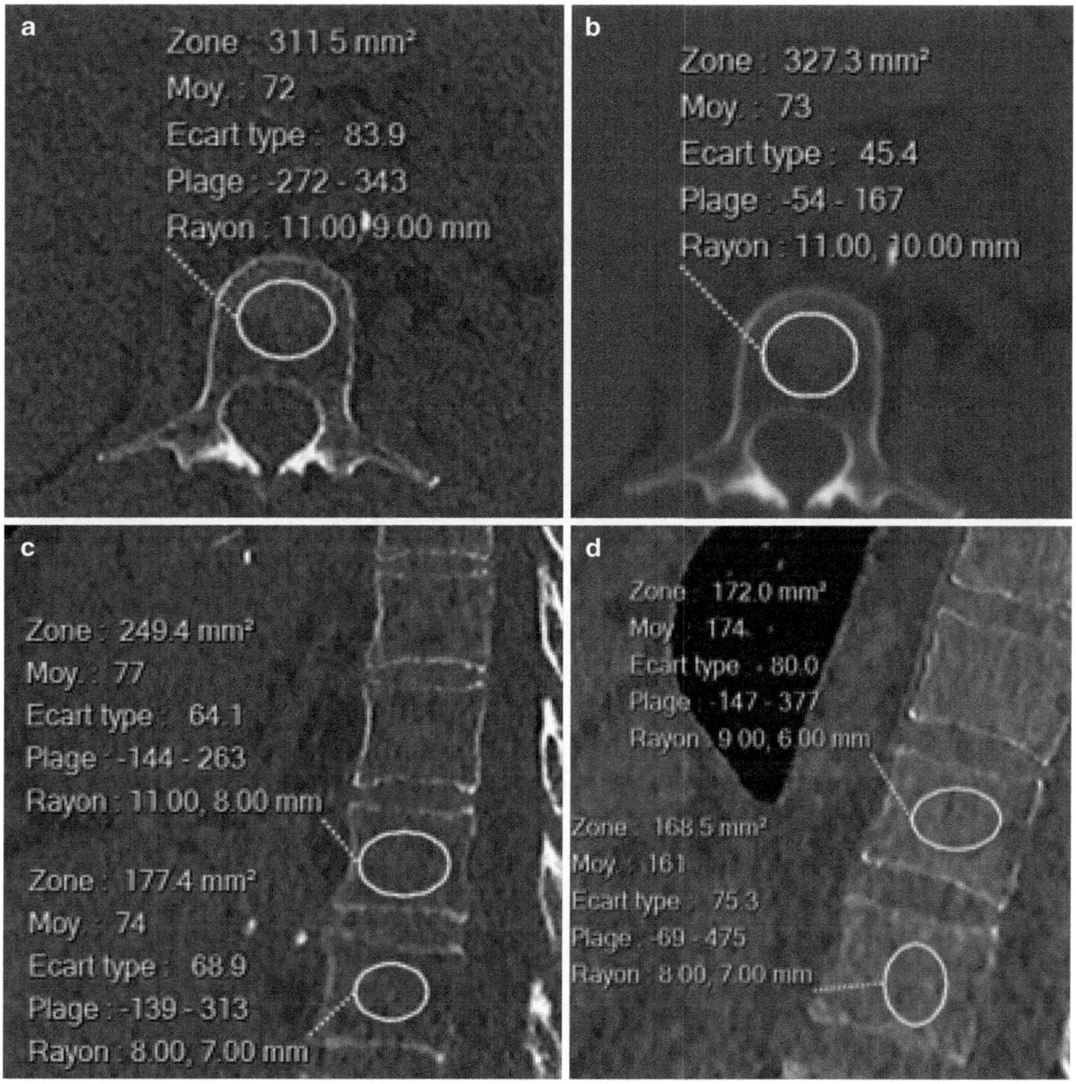

Fig. 11 Vertebral bone density measurements on chest CT at 120 kV. (**a**) L1 attenuation value measured by a region of interest (ROI) on bone kernel reconstruction on axial plane is 72 HU, consistent with osteoporosis; (**b**) same patient, L1 attenuation value measured on soft-tissue kernel on axial plane is 73 HU; (**c**) same patient, attenuation value on L1 and T12 is 74 HU and 77 HU, respectively, on bone-kernel reconstruction on sagittal plane. Bone density can be assessed on different planes and different kernels reconstructions, with no significant differences. HU may slightly vary on different vertebral bodies: if L1 attenuation cannot be measured, T12 is a reliable alternative. Please note the low density of the vertebra bodies in this patient, due to the loss of bone mass and density. (**d**) Different patient, L1 and T12 attenuation values on bone-kernel reconstruction on sagittal plane are 161 HU and 174 HU, respectively, compatible with normal bone density. Please note the visually higher density of the body vertebrae in this patient

mixed ones combine features of both types (Chang et al. 2022). Fatty lesion attenuation ranges between −30 and −120 HU, and lesions containing fat may be characterized as benign. Benign sclerotic lesions, such as bone islands or enostoses, typically exhibit attenuation levels averaging above 885 HU, with maximum levels often exceeding 1060 HU (Chang et al. 2022). Below these thresholds, sclerotic lesions should be considered as metastatic. It should be men-

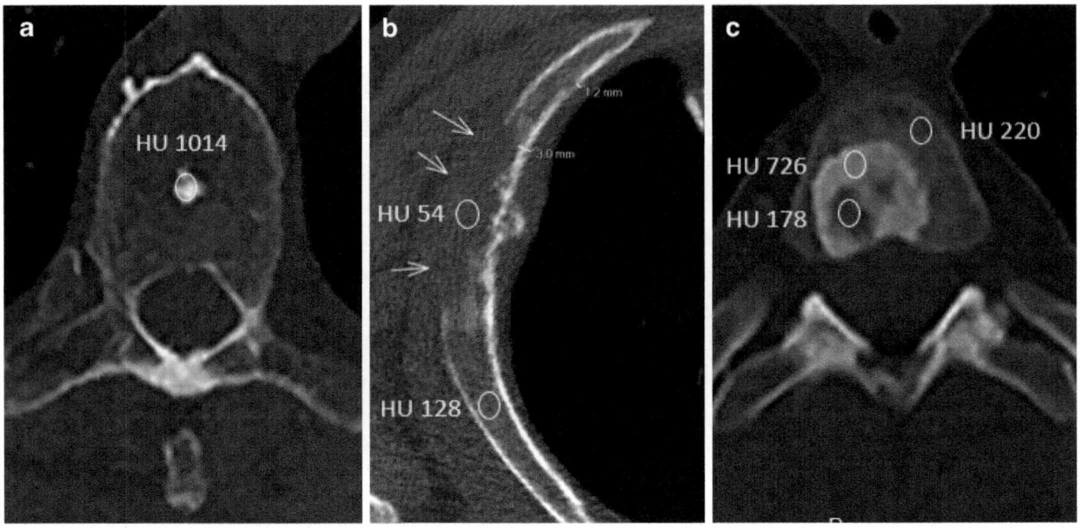

Fig. 12 (**a**) Sclerotic bone lesion of the 7th thoracic vertebral body with high attenuation values (HU 1014), consistent with enostosis/bone island. (**b**) Metastatic lytic lesion of the 2nd rib causing irregular cortical thickening and thinning along with extensive bone destruction. The attenuation values (HU 54) within the lesion are lower than the surrounding non-pathological rib values (HU 128), which is consistent with soft tissue metastatic replacement. (**c**) Mixed, well defined metastasis of the 3rd vertebral body, characterized by sclerotic (HU 726) and lytic (HU 178) densities compared to the adjacent normal bone (HU 220)

tioned that these thresholds have to be used with care (Fig. 12). It is to note that enostosis may evolve with time, basically 1 mm per year, varying in density or increasing in size.

7 The Anterior Chest Wall Joints

The sterno-costo-clavicular junction is formed by the manubriosternal joint (MSJ), the sternoclavicular joint (SCJ) and the two first costosternal joints (see above). The SCJ is a synovial joint with two non-congruent articular surfaces. It is composed of a joint capsule, a fibrocartilage disc, and is reinforced by the anterior and posterior sternoclavicular ligaments, the interclavicular ligament and the costoclavicular ligament to ensure stability. The subclavius, sternocleidomastoid, sternohyoid and pectoralis major muscles participate in joint stabilization.

7.1 Measurements in Clinical Practice

Although some conditions including traumatic injuries, inflammation, infection, degenerative disorders may affect the SCJ space, the interest of the SCJs measurements is limited in clinical practice due to its great interreader variability as well as its intrareader variability depending on the joint position (Tuscano et al. 2009). Asymmetrical maturation and size of SCJ may be observed in up to 10–15% of healthy subjects and should be not confused as pathological condition (Tuscano et al. 2009). While US and MRI are preferred for congenital and inflammatory or infectious conditions, CT is the modality of choice in post-traumatic and instability assessment. MRI protocol requires T2w and fat-suppressed images for tissue characterization and assessment of the articular surface and the periarticular tissues, while T1w are required for bones and anatomic evaluation. Post-contrast

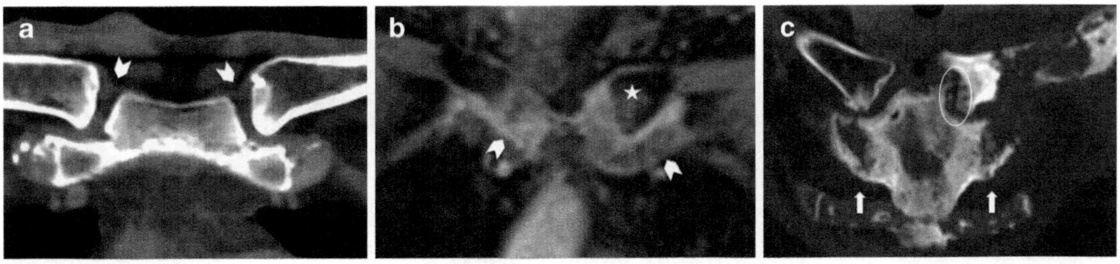

Fig. 13 Normal and pathologic sternoclavicular joints (SCJ). (**a**) CT on coronal view showing physiological SCJ space. (**b**) Contrast-enhanced MRI T1 Fat Sat Vibe sequence on coronal plane of septic arthritis depicting notable enhancement of the synovia (arrowheads) and symmetrical distention of the SCJ (not shown), as well as inflammatory enhancement of the clavicular epiphysis (star). (**c**) Coronal CT reconstruction of chronic SAPHO with secondary SCJ osteoarthrosis, characterized by subchondral cyst and hyperostosis of the left SCJ (circle) and costosternal joint of the first pair of ribs (arrows)

acquisitions are performed for assess synovial enhancement due to inflammatory/infectious hyperaemia. For CT images analysis, reconstructed images with thin sections and both bone and soft-tissue kernels are needed for a comprehensive evaluation of the SCJ. In case of trauma, contrast agent provides important information on the status of the mediastinal structures and some life-threatening complications such as bleeding. SCJ distention may occur in degenerative disease and arthritis (Fig. 13). Diagnosis differential relies on associated signs rather than measurements, such as the presence of subchondral sclerosis, subchondral cysts and osteophytes (signs of arthrosis) or marginal erosions (sign of arthritis). In arthrosis, joint distention is generally mild (3–8 mm) (Johnson et al. 2010). In septic arthritis, a rare but severe complication that may occur in intravenous drug abusers, diabetes, inflammatory arthritis or after thoracic surgery, SCJ involvement is often asymmetric and severe, with important inflammatory capsular distension (10–20 mm) extending over the sternum and clavicles, associated with bone marrow oedema and bone destruction (Fig. 13b) (Johnson et al. 2010; Restrepo et al. 2009).

Tietze syndrome and rheumatoid arthritis are the inflammatory arthritis most frequently affecting the SCJ. The articular involvement is usually symmetric and characterized by joint inflammation with moderate capsular distension compared to septic arthritis (Volterrani et al. 2008). SAPHO syndrome (acronym for Synovitis, Acne, Pustulosis, Hyperostosis and Osteitis) is a rare polyostotic and cutaneous inflammatory condition mainly involving the SCJ, the costochondral and manubriosternal joints as well as the thoracic spine. Although in early phase, SAPHO shares inflammatory changes similar to the other inflammatory/infection conditions such as joint effusion, oedema and bone erosions, the asymmetric involvement and the presence of costoclavicular enthesopathy and hyperostotic foci of more than 5 mm at the costosternal part of the first pair of ribs are highly suggestive of the diagnosis. In the advanced phase, the chronic inflammation leads to hyperostosis, enthesopathies, bone destruction along with secondary arthrosis and ankylosis (Fig. 13c) (Depasquale et al. 2012).

SCJ instability is a rare condition that can result from high-energy trauma, congenital clavicle malformations, Ehlers-Danlos syndrome, infections and arthritis. Management, whether conservative or surgical, depends on the cause, severity and direction of the instability. Severity ranges from sprain with no ligamentous laxity (grade 1) to subluxation (grade 2) and dislocation (grade 3) (Fig. 14). The posterior dislocation, where the medial clavicle is displaced posteriorly to the manubrium, is less frequent than the anterior one. However, it is more severe due to the potential injuries on the mediastinal structures behind, such as vessels, phrenic nerve and trachea, and often requires surgical intervention. Conversely, anterior instability is generally not critical and managed conservatively. In trauma,

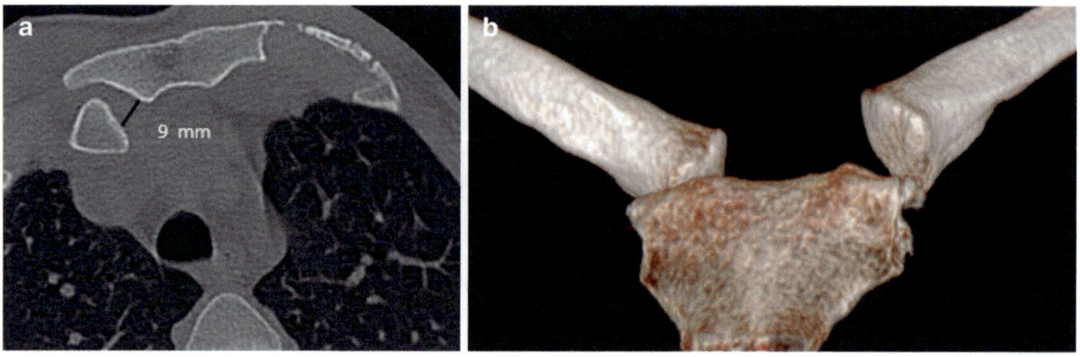

Fig. 14 Post-traumatic grade 2 instability of the right sternoclavicular joint (SCJ). (**a**) Axial CT shows a subluxation in the posteroinferior direction of the right clavicle associated with a widening of the right SCJ (9 mm). (**b**) 3D reconstruction CT. In clinical practice, the measurement is not straightforward due to the orientation of the joint, and the diagnosis relies on the position of the articular surface

SCJ instability should be suspected in case of widening >2 mm of the SCJ compared to the contralateral joint when in association with rib fractures or pneumothorax or haemothorax (Çakmak et al. 2020).

8 Sarcopenia

Sarcopenia, defined as the muscle mass reduction with fatty replacement, is observed in several conditions such as malnutrition, physical inactivity, some chronic diseases such as chronic obstructive pulmonary disease (COPD) and malignancy. Since it is associated with poor outcome and decreased overall survival, its quantification has been receiving increasing interest in the last few years to better evaluate pre-treatment risk in order to reduce morbidity and mortality in fragile patients (Cruz-Jentoft et al. 2019; Hasenauer et al. 2023). Currently, it is not routinely assessed in clinical practice due to the lack of standardization and validated tools, but it may be reported in radiological reports in the future thanks to the increasing implementation of automated segmentation through dedicated AI software. Muscle quantity can be measured on non-contrast images with semi-automated or automated software, after segmentation of the all skeletal muscles at the level of L3, including the psoas, the paraspinal and the abdominal wall muscles on axial CT (Tagliafico et al. 2022). The following threshold ranges are defined for the skeletal muscle and the subcutaneous and intramuscular adipose tissues: 29 to 150 HU and −30 to −190 HU, respectively. The presence of intramuscular adipose tissue content (IMAC) can be calculated dividing the mean muscular attenuation value by the mean subcutaneous fat attenuation value. The cross-sectional muscle area, defined as the muscle area on the CT slice, is adjusted to the patient's height to obtain the SMI. Cross-sectional muscle area (CSMA) and skeletal muscle index (SMI) are the most used CT-derived measurements to determine the presence and the absence of sarcopenia (Hasenauer et al. 2023). In the absence of abdominal acquisition, sarcopenia may be calculated at the level of T10 on axial chest CT, as SMI values at this level are comparable with those obtained at the L3 level, defining sarcopenia as SMI <28.8 cm^2/m^2 for men and <20.4 cm^2/m^2 for women (Kaltenhauser et al. 2023).

9 The Breast

Gynecomastia is a common condition in males, characterized by an increase in mammary gland tissue beneath the nipple-areolar complex. It results from an elevated oestrogens-to-androgens ratio and can be either physiological, occurring due to natural hormonal fluctuations, or pathological, associated with conditions such as liver cir-

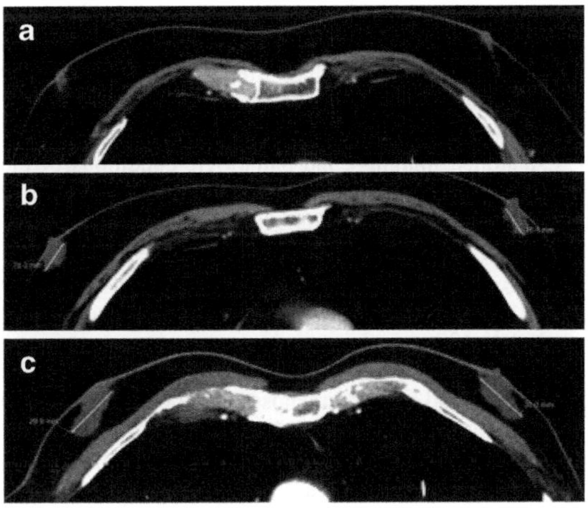

Fig. 15 (**a**, **b**) Normal breast tissue measuring <2 cm on axial CT. (**c**) Gynecomastia on axial CT

rhosis, obesity, hormone-secreting tumours, endocrine disorders and medications. It is important not to confuse with pseudogynecomastia, commonly seen in obese individuals, which involves an increase in fat deposition without glandular increase. At imaging, glandular breast tissue exceeding 2 cm in maximum diameter is considered indicative of gynecomastia (Fig. 15) (Iuanow et al. 2011). This condition is often bilateral, though when unilateral, distinguishing it from breast cancer can be challenging. Mammography is generally sufficient to confirm gynecomastia. US serves as additional imaging when mammography is not conclusive or malignancy is suspected (Mannix et al. 2024). Measurements in female breast have no clinical interest.

10 Conclusion

In conclusion, imaging metrics of the chest wall components have clinical, forensic and anthropomorphic undeniable interests. In clinical practice, CT represents the modality of choice in the majority of cases. Measurements may be useful for diagnosis, severity assessment and pre- and post-treatment planning. In forensic studies, imaging metrics, mainly through CT, are used for age and sex determination in alleged unaccompanied minors, virtual autopsy and human remains identification.

References

Babinski MA, de Lemos L, Babinski MSD, Gonçalves MVT, De Paula RC, Fernandes RMP (2015) Frequency of sternal foramen evaluated by MDCT: a minor variation of great relevance. Surg Radiol Anat 37:287–291. https://doi.org/10.1007/s00276-014-1339-x

Bacher S, Hajdu SD, Maeder Y, Dunet V, Hilbert T, Omoumi P (2021) Differentiation between benign and malignant vertebral compression fractures using qualitative and quantitative analysis of a single fast spin echo T2-weighted Dixon sequence. Eur Radiol 31:9418–9427. https://doi.org/10.1007/s00330-021-07947-1

Bellemare F, Fuamba T, Bourgeault A (2006) Sexual dimorphism of human ribs. Respir Physiol Neurobiol 150:233–239. https://doi.org/10.1016/j.resp.2005.04.002

Boutin RD, Lenchik L (2020) Value-added opportunistic CT: insights into osteoporosis and sarcopenia. Am J Roentgenol 215:582–594. https://doi.org/10.2214/AJR.20.22874

Çakmak V, Türkoğlu S, Özen M, Çakmak P (2020) Widening of sternoclavicular joint distances in blunt chest trauma. Cukurova Med J 45:1713–1719. https://doi.org/10.17826/cumj.779481

Cartoski MJ, Nuss D, Goretsky MJ, Proud VK, Croitoru DP, Gustin T, Mitchell K, Vasser E, Kelly RE (2006) Classification of the dysmorphology of pectus excavatum. J Pediatr Surg 41:1573–1581. https://doi.org/10.1016/j.jpedsurg.2006.05.055

Chang CY, Garner HW, Ahlawat S, Amini B, Bucknor MD, Flug JA, Khodarahmi I, Mulligan ME, Peterson JJ, Riley GM, Samim M, Lozano-Calderon SA, Wu JS (2022) Society of Skeletal Radiology– white paper. Guidelines for the diagnostic management of incidental solitary bone lesions on CT and MRI in adults: bone reporting and data system (Bone-RADS). Skeletal Radiol 51:1743–1764. https://doi.org/10.1007/s00256-022-04022-8

Cheng X, Zhao K, Zha X, Du X, Li Y, Chen S, Wu Y, Li S, Lu Y, Zhang Y, Xiao X, Li YH, Ma X, Gong X, Chen W, Yang Y, Jiao J, Chen B, Lv Y, Gao J, Hong G, Pan

Y, Yan Y, Qi H, Ran L, Zhai J, Wang L, Li K, Fu H, Wu J, Liu S, Blake GM, Pickhardt PJ, Ma Y, Fu X, Dong S, Zeng Q, Guo Z, Hind K, Engelke K, Tian W, For the China Health Big Data (China Biobank) project investigators (2021) Opportunistic screening using low-dose CT and the prevalence of osteoporosis in China: a nationwide, multicenter study. J Bone Miner Res 36:427–435. https://doi.org/10.1002/jbmr.4187

Cruz-Jentoft AJ, Bahat G, Bauer J, Boirie Y, Bruyère O, Cederholm T, Cooper C, Landi F, Rolland Y, Sayer AA, Schneider SM, Sieber CC, Topinkova E, Vandewoude M, Visser M, Zamboni M, Writing Group for the European Working Group on Sarcopenia in Older People 2 (EWGSOP2), and the E.G. for E (2019) Sarcopenia: revised European consensus on definition and diagnosis. Age Ageing 48:16–31. https://doi.org/10.1093/ageing/afy169

De Leucio A, Tenisch E, Zambelli PY, Omoumi P (2023) EOS imaging. In: Simoni P, Aparisi Gómez MP (eds) Essential measurements in pediatric musculoskeletal imaging. Springer International Publishing, Cham, pp 263–298. https://doi.org/10.1007/978-3-031-17735-4_12

de Reuver S, Costa L, van Rheenen H, Tabeling CS, Lemans JVC, Schlösser TPC, Kruyt MC, van Stralen M, Castelein RM (2022) Disc and vertebral body morphology from birth to adulthood. Spine 47:E312. https://doi.org/10.1097/BRS.0000000000004278

Depasquale R, Kumar N, Lalam RK, Tins BJ, Tyrrell PNM, Singh J, Cassar-Pullicino VN (2012) SAPHO: what radiologists should know. Clin Radiol 67:195–206. https://doi.org/10.1016/j.crad.2011.08.014

Dickson RA (2004) (i) Spinal deformity—basic principles. Curr Orthop 18:411–425. https://doi.org/10.1016/j.cuor.2004.12.001

Eggermont F, Derikx LC, Free J, van Leeuwen R, van der Linden YM, Verdonschot N, Tanck E (2018) Effect of different CT scanners and settings on femoral failure loads calculated by finite element models. J Orthop Res 36:2288–2295. https://doi.org/10.1002/jor.23890

Fagelman KM, Methratta S, Cilley RE, Wilson MZ, Hollenbeak CS (2015) The Depression Index: an objective measure of the severity of pectus excavatum based on vertebral diameter, a morphometric correlate to patient size. J Pediatr Surg 50:1130–1133. https://doi.org/10.1016/j.jpedsurg.2014.11.043

Filograna L, Pugliese L, Muto M, Tatulli D, Guglielmi G, Thali MJ, Floris R (2019) A practical guide to virtual autopsy: why, when and how. Semin Ultrasound CT MRI, Forensic Radiology 40:56–66. https://doi.org/10.1053/j.sult.2018.10.011

Fon GT, Pitt MJ, Thies AC (1980) Thoracic kyphosis: range in normal subjects. AJR Am J Roentgenol 134:979–983. https://doi.org/10.2214/ajr.134.5.979

Franklin D, Swift L, Flavel A (2016) 'Virtual anthropology' and radiographic imaging in the Forensic Medical Sciences. Egypt J Forensic Sci, Advances in Forensic Anthropology 6:31–43. https://doi.org/10.1016/j.ejfs.2016.05.011

Genant HK, Wu CY, van Kuijk C, Nevitt MC (1993) Vertebral fracture assessment using a semiquantitative technique. J Bone Miner Res 8:1137–1148. https://doi.org/10.1002/jbmr.5650080915

Gilcrease-Garcia BM, Deshmukh SD, Parsons MS (2020) Anatomy, imaging, and pathologic conditions of the brachial plexus. Radiographics 40:1686–1714. https://doi.org/10.1148/rg.2020200012

Glass RBJ, Norton KI, Mitre SA, Kang E (2002) Pediatric ribs: a spectrum of abnormalities. Radiographics 22:87–104. https://doi.org/10.1148/radiographics.22.1.g02ja1287

Gorjanovic-Kramberger D (1902) Del Pal∗ olithische Mensch und seine Zeitgenossen aus dem Dilivium von Krapina in Kroatien, II. MAGW 31:189–216

Gruenewald LD, Koch V, Martin SS, Yel I, Eichler K, Gruber-Rouh T, Lenga L, Wichmann JL, Alizadeh LS, Albrecht MH, Mader C, Huizinga NA, D'Angelo T, Mazziotti S, Wesarg S, Vogl TJ, Booz C (2022) Diagnostic accuracy of quantitative dual-energy CT-based volumetric bone mineral density assessment for the prediction of osteoporosis-associated fractures. Eur Radiol 32:3076–3084. https://doi.org/10.1007/s00330-021-08323-9

Haller JA, Kramer SS, Lietman SA (1987) Use of CT scans in selection of patients for pectusexcavatum surgery: a preliminary report. J Pediatr Surg 22:904–906. https://doi.org/10.1016/S0022-3468(87)80585-7

Hasenauer A, Forster C, Hungerbühler J, Perentes JY, Abdelnour-Berchtold E, Koerfer J, Krueger T, Becce F, Gonzalez M (2023) CT-derived sarcopenia and outcomes after thoracoscopic pulmonary resection for non-small cell lung cancer. Cancer 15:790. https://doi.org/10.3390/cancers15030790

Hyrtl J (1871) Handbuch der topographischen Anatomie,: Enthält die topographische anatomie des Koppes, des Halses, der Brust, und des Unterleibes. W. Braumüller

Iuanow E, Kettler M, Slanetz PJ (2011) Spectrum of disease in the male breast. Am J Roentgenol 196:W247–W259. https://doi.org/10.2214/AJR.09.3994

Johnson MC, Jacobson JA, Fessell DP, Kim SM, Brandon C, Caoili E (2010) The sternoclavicular joint: can imaging differentiate infection from degenerative change? Skeletal Radiol 39:551–558. https://doi.org/10.1007/s00256-009-0802-y

Kaltenhauser S, Niessen C, Zeman F, Stroszczynski C, Zorger N, Grosse J, Großer C, Hofmann H-S, Robold T (2023) Diagnosis of sarcopenia on thoracic computed tomography and its association with postoperative survival after anatomic lung cancer resection. Sci Rep 13:18450. https://doi.org/10.1038/s41598-023-45583-5

Katzman WB, Wanek L, Shepherd JA, Sellmeyer DE (2010) Age-related hyperkyphosis: its causes, consequences, and management. J Orthop Sports Phys Ther 40:352–360. https://doi.org/10.2519/jospt.2010.3099

Kellinghaus M, Schulz R, Vieth V, Schmidt S, Pfeiffer H, Schmeling A (2010) Enhanced possibilities to make statements on the ossification status of the medial clavicular epiphysis using an amplified stag-

ing scheme in evaluating thin-slice CT scans. Int J Legal Med 124:321–325. https://doi.org/10.1007/s00414-010-0448-2
Kelly B (2012) The chest radiograph. Ulster Med J 81:143–148
Kieffer CL (2010) Tibia and fibula stature formulae for modern female populations based on digital radiographic measurements. J Forensic Sci 55:695–700. https://doi.org/10.1111/j.1556-4029.2010.01362.x
Kim H, Kim HS, Moon ES, Yoon C-S, Chung T-S, Song H-T, Suh J-S, Lee YH, Kim S (2010) Scoliosis imaging: what radiologists should know. Radiographics 30:1823–1842. https://doi.org/10.1148/rg.307105061
Kong M-W, Pei Z-Y, Zhang X, Du Q-J, Tang Q, Li J, He G-X (2023) Related mechanisms and research progress in straight back syndrome. World J Cardiol 15:479–486. https://doi.org/10.4330/wjc.v15.i10.479
Krugh M, Langaker MD (2025) Dual-energy X-ray absorptiometry. In: StatPearls. StatPearls Publishing, Treasure Island (FL)
Kumar S, Awadhiya B, Ratnakumar R, Thalengala A, Areeckal AS, Nanjappa Y (2024) A review of 3D modalities used for the diagnosis of scoliosis. Tomography 10:1192–1204. https://doi.org/10.3390/tomography10080090
Kurihara Y, Yakushiji YK, Matsumoto J, Ishikawa T, Hirata K (1999) The ribs: anatomic and radiologic considerations. Radiographics 19:105–119. https://doi.org/10.1148/radiographics.19.1.g99ja02105
Lossois M, Cyteval C, Baccino E, Peyron P-A (2022) Forensic age assessments of alleged unaccompanied minors at the Medicolegal Institute of Montpellier: a 4-year retrospective study. Int J Legal Med 136:853–859. https://doi.org/10.1007/s00414-022-02813-1
Madentzoglou MS, Nathena D, Sinatkas V, Karantanas A, Kontakis G, Papadomanolakis A, Kranioti EF (2025) CT-assisted age estimation from the medial clavicular epiphysis in the Greek population according to Schmeling and Kellinghaus classification. Legal Med 73:102589. https://doi.org/10.1016/j.legalmed.2025.102589
Mak SM, Bhaludin BN, Naaseri S, Di Chiara F, Jordan S, Padley S (2016) Imaging of congenital chest wall deformities. Br J Radiol 89:20150595. https://doi.org/10.1259/bjr.20150595
Mannix J, Duke H, Almajnooni A, Ongkeko M (2024) Imaging the male breast: gynecomastia, male breast cancer, and beyond. Radiographics 44:e230181. https://doi.org/10.1148/rg.230181
Manuals and Presentations | Scoliosis Research Society [WWW Document] (n.d.). URL https://www.srs.org/Education/Manuals-and-Presentations. Accessed 4 Oct 25
Miao KH, Miao JH, Belani P, Dayan E, Carlon TA, Cengiz TB, Finkelstein M (2024) Radiological diagnosis and advances in imaging of vertebral compression fractures. J Imaging 10:244. https://doi.org/10.3390/jimaging10100244
Mourad C, Gallego Manzano L, Viry A, Booij R, Oei EHG, Becce F, Omoumi P (2024) Chances and challenges of photon-counting CT in musculoskeletal imaging. Skeletal Radiol 53:1889–1902. https://doi.org/10.1007/s00256-024-04622-6
Mühler M, Schulz R, Schmidt S, Schmeling A, Reisinger W (2006) The influence of slice thickness on assessment of clavicle ossification in forensic age diagnostics. Int J Legal Med 120:15–17. https://doi.org/10.1007/s00414-005-0010-9
Ong W, Liu RW, Makmur A, Low XZ, Sng WJ, Tan JH, Kumar N, Hallinan JTPD (2023) Artificial intelligence applications for osteoporosis classification using computed tomography. Bioengineering 10:1364. https://doi.org/10.3390/bioengineering10121364
Poston PM, Patel SS, Rajput M, Rossi NO, Ghanamah MS, Davis JE, Turek JW (2014) The correction index: setting the standard for recommending operative repair of pectus excavatum. Ann Thorac Surg 97:1176–1180. https://doi.org/10.1016/j.athoracsur.2013.12.050
Reder SR, Fritzen I, Brockmann MA, Hardt J, Elsner K, Petrowski K, Bjelopavlovic M (2024) Comparing a common clavicle maturation-based age estimation method to ordinary regression analyses with quadratic and sex-specific interaction terms in adolescents. Sci Rep 14:2754. https://doi.org/10.1038/s41598-024-52980-x
Restrepo CS, Martinez S, Lemos DF, Washington L, McAdams HP, Vargas D, Lemos JA, Carrillo JA, Diethelm L (2009) Imaging appearances of the sternum and sternoclavicular joints. Radiographics 29:839–859. https://doi.org/10.1148/rg.293055136
Schmeling A, Dettmeyer R, Rudolf E, Vieth V, Geserick G (2016) Forensic age estimation. Dtsch Ärztebl Int 113:44–50. https://doi.org/10.3238/arztebl.2016.0044
St. Peter SD, Juang D, Garey CL, Laituri CA, Ostlie DJ, Sharp RJ, Snyder CL (2011) A novel measure for pectus excavatum: the correction index. J Pediatr Surg 46:2270–2273. https://doi.org/10.1016/j.jpedsurg.2011.09.009
Table: Typical Radiation Doses* [WWW Document] (n.d.) MSD Man. Prof. Ed. URL https://www.msdmanuals.com/professional/multimedia/table/typical-radiation-doses. Accessed 9 Nov 25
Tagliafico AS, Bignotti B, Torri L, Rossi F (2022) Sarcopenia: how to measure, when and why. Radiol Med (Torino) 127:228–237. https://doi.org/10.1007/s11547-022-01450-3
Tuscano D, Banerjee S, Terk MR (2009) Variations in normal sternoclavicular joints; a retrospective study to quantify SCJ asymmetry. Skeletal Radiol 38:997–1001. https://doi.org/10.1007/s00256-009-0689-7
Urrutia J, Narvaez F, Besa P, Meissner-Haecker A, Rios C, Piza C (2019) Scheuermann's disease in patients 15–40 years old: a study to determine its prevalence and its relationship with age and sex using chest radiographs as screening tool. J Orthop Sci 24:776–779. https://doi.org/10.1016/j.jos.2018.12.024
Uysal Ramadan S, Türkmen N, Dolgun NA, Gökharman D, Menezes RG, Kacar M, Koşar U (2010) Sex deter-

mination from measurements of the sternum and fourth rib using multislice computed tomography of the chest. Forensic Sci Int 197:120.e1–120.e5. https://doi.org/10.1016/j.forsciint.2009.12.049

Volterrani L, Mazzei MA, Giordano N, Nuti R, Galeazzi M, Fioravanti A (2008) Magnetic resonance imaging in Tietze's syndrome. Clin Exp Rheumatol 26:848–853

Waldt S, Gersing A, Brügel M (2014) Measurements and classifications in spine imaging. Semin Musculoskelet Radiol 18:219–227. https://doi.org/10.1055/s-0034-1375565

Waxenbaum JA, Reddy V, Futterman B (2024) Anatomy, back, thoracic vertebrae. In: StatPearls. StatPearls Publishing, Treasure Island (FL)

Weaver AA, Schoell SL, Stitzel JD (2014) Morphometric analysis of variation in the ribs with age and sex. J Anat 225:246–261. https://doi.org/10.1111/joa.12203

Wesp P, Schachtner BM, Jeblick K, Topalis J, Weber M, Fischer F, Penning R, Ricke J, Ingrisch M, Sabel BO (2024) Radiological age assessment based on clavicle ossification in CT: enhanced accuracy through deep learning. Int J Legal Med 138:1497–1507. https://doi.org/10.1007/s00414-024-03167-6

Widek T, De Tobel J, Ehammer T, Genet P (2023) Forensic age estimation in males by MRI based on the medial epiphysis of the clavicle. Int J Legal Med 137:679–689. https://doi.org/10.1007/s00414-022-02924-9

Zhu Y, Triphuridet N, Yip R, Becker BJ, Wang Y, Yankelevitz DF, Henschke CI (2021) Opportunistic CT screening of osteoporosis on thoracic and lumbar spine: a meta-analysis. Clin Imaging 80:382–390. https://doi.org/10.1016/j.clinimag.2021.08.005

Zou D, Li W, Deng C, Du G, Xu N (2019) The use of CT Hounsfield unit values to identify the undiagnosed spinal osteoporosis in patients with lumbar degenerative diseases. Eur Spine J 28:1758–1766. https://doi.org/10.1007/s00586-018-5776-9

Part III
Clinical Part - Vessels

CT and MR Measurements in Pulmonary Hypertension

Gabriel Galea and Nick Screaton

Contents

G. Galea
Mater Dei Hospital, Msida, Malta

N. Screaton (✉)
Royal Papworth Hospital, Cambridge, UK
e-mail: n.screaton@nhs.net

1 Introduction

1.1 History and Definition

Pulmonary hypertension (PH) is diagnosed by finding a mean pulmonary arterial pressure (mPAP) of more than 20 mmHg at rest when measured invasively at right heart catheterisation (RHC) (Humbert et al. 2022). The haemodynamics of mPAP at RHC are a function of both diastolic and systolic pulmonary artery pressure (dPAP and sPAP, respectively) and are calculated as mPAP = (2/3 × dPAP) + (1/3 × sPAP).

Pulmonary vascular resistance (PVR) describes the resistance against blood flow from the pulmonary artery through the pulmonary circulation to the left atrium. PVR is measured in Woods' units (WU) invasively at cardiac catheterisation. The normal PVR is usually less than 2 WU (sometimes reported as <160 dynes/s/cm^{-5}); an elevated PVR is defined as ≥3 WU (<240 dynes/s/cm^{-5}). Patients with pathological remodelling of the small pulmonary arteries (i.e. pre-capillary PH) have an elevated PVR. Conversely, post-capillary PH defines PH due to an increase in pulmonary venous pressure in left-sided heart disease; PVR in these patients is initially normal (PVR can be elevated in end-stage disease in this cohort).

Pulmonary arterial wedge pressure (PAWP) is used a surrogate marker of left ventricular/left atrial end-diastolic pressure and therefore, pul-

https://doi.org/10.1007/174_2025_602,
Published Online: 03 September 2025

Table 1 Haemodynamic definitions of pulmonary hypertension

Definition	Haemodynamic characteristics
Pulmonary hypertension (PH)	mPAP >20 mmHg
Pre-capillary pulmonary hypertension	mPAP >20 mmHg PAWP ≤15 mmHg PVR ≥3 WU
Isolated post-capillary pulmonary hypertension	mPAP >20 mmHg PAWP >15 mmHg PVR ≤2 WU
Combined post- and pre-capillary pulmonary hypertension pulmonary hypertension	mPAP >20 mmHg PAWP >15 mmHg PVR >2 WU
Exercise-induced pulmonary hypertension	mPAP/CO slope between rest and exercise >3 mmHg/L/min

CO cardiac output, *mPAP* mean pulmonary arterial pressure, *PAWP* pulmonary arterial wedge pressure, *PVR* pulmonary vascular resistance, *WU* Wood units

monary venous pressure. A normal PAWP implies normal left ventricular diastolic function and normal pulmonary *venous* pressure and effectively excludes left heart disease as the cause for PH; an elevated PAWP suggests significant left heart disease.

Pre-capillary PH, found in patients in groups 1, 3 and 4 and some from group 5 (Table 1), is formally defined as the presence of mPAP >20 mmHg with a pulmonary artery wedge pressure (PAWP) ≤15 mmHg and PVR ≥3 WU (Naeije and Chin 2019; Simonneau et al. 2019). Isolated post-capillary PH, predominantly in patients in group 2 and some in group 5, is defined as a PAWP >15 mm Hg alongside an mPAP >20 mm Hg. There may be some overlap between the two groups, particularly in patients with chronic congenital heart disease (Humbert et al. 2022; Naeije and Chin 2019; Simonneau et al. 2019; Currie et al. 2018).

The definition of PH has changed multiple times over the years. In 1961, a World Health Organisation (WHO) expert committee stated that the mPAP in a healthy, supine subject at rest is usually 15 mmHg and never more than 20 mmHg (Qaiser et al. 2023). Following this, at the first World Symposium on Pulmonary Hypertension (WSPH) organised by the WHO in 1973, PH was formally defined as an mPAP ≥25 mmHg measured by RHC in the supine patient at rest (Simonneau et al. 2019). This definition remained unchanged over subsequent WSPH meetings from 1998 to 2013 (Hoeper et al. 2016; Engelfriet et al. 2007; Coghlan and Handler 2006).

More recently, this was challenged by data based on a retrospective review of over 1100 patients from 47 studies which suggested that mPAP at rest in normal subjects is 14.0 ± 3.3 mmHg, independent of sex and ethnicity and with little variability with posture and age (Lettieri et al. 2006). An mPAP of 20 mmHg is two standard deviations (SD) above 14.0 mmHg, which further suggests that the upper limit of normal is truly 20 mmHg. This was additionally supported by increasing the amounts of data showing that certain patient groups with a mPAP 21–24 mmHg (i.e. previously considered as 'borderline' PH) had worse outcomes than matched patients with a mPAP of <20 mmHg (Simonneau et al. 2019; Nunes et al. 2006; Peacock et al. 2007). To this extent, in two recent major updates on PH and for the foreseeable future, the current commonly accepted definition of PH remains a resting mPAP of ≥20 mmHg at RHC (Humbert et al. 2022; Simonneau et al. 2019; Humbert et al. 2012).

This common definition of PH is usually associated with a normal or decreased cardiac output (CO). Less commonly and less well understood, PH can occur in the context of a hyperdynamic circulation which is characterised by an increased circulatory volume and decreased systemic vascular resistance. There are various causes of a hyperdynamic state including high output heart failure, cirrhosis, obesity, hyperthyroidism and chronic anaemia. Regardless of aetiology, PH in the context of a hyperdynamic state is characterised by finding an mPAP of >20 mmHg, a high CO (>8 L/min) and/or cardiac index ≥4 L/min/m^2 and variable PAWP and PVR depending on the specific aetiology. It is beyond the scope of this chapter to discuss each of the aetiologies in detail; however, it is thought that PH in a hyperdynamic circulation, regardless of underlying aetiology, is driven by a dynamic process that is caused by increased blood flow, leading to continuous sheer stress on the pulmonary circulation (Qaiser et al. 2023).

1.2 Classification of Pulmonary Hypertension

PH has been classified into groups based on each group's similar pathophysiology, clinical features, haemodynamics and therapeutic profiles (Table 2) (Humbert et al. 2022).

1.3 Clinical Relevance of PH

PH is a significant global health issue with an estimated prevalence of 1% (Humbert et al. 2022); the incidence of PH depends on the subtype and the patient population in question. Globally, the commonest cause of PH is left heart disease (Hoeper et al. 2016). The second commonest cause worldwide for PH is lung disease, particularly severe COPD (Humbert et al. 2022). PH is also common in patients with congenital heart disease with up to 30% of these patients eventually developing PH (Engelfriet et al. 2007). It is a frequent complication in patients with connective tissue disease—up to 10% of patients with a connective tissue disease will develop PH and of this cohort, approximately half will die within a year of diagnosis (Coghlan and Handler 2006). PH is also found in as many as 30% of patients with idiopathic pulmonary fibrosis (IPF), and the presence of PH in this patient population confers a two- to three-fold increased risk of death (Lettieri et al. 2006). PH in advanced sarcoidosis can lead to near doubling in the mortality rate compared to similar stage sarcoidosis without PH (Nunes et al. 2006). PAH, previously

Table 2 Updated clinical classification of PH (Humbert et al. 2022)

1. PAH (Pulmonary arterial hypertension)
1.1 Idiopathic PAH
1.1.1 Non-responders at vasoreactivity testing
1.1.2 Acute responders at vasoreactivity testing
1.2 Heritable PAH
1.3 Drug- and toxin-induced PAH
1.4 PAH associated with
1.4.1 Connective tissue disease
1.4.2 Human Immunodeficiency Virus (HIV)
1.4.3 Portal hypertension
1.4.4 Congenital heart disease
1.4.5 Schistosomiasis
1.5 PAH with features of venous/capillary (PVOD/PCH) involvement
1.6 Persistent PH of the newborn syndrome
2. PH due to left heart disease
2.1 Heart failure
2.1.1 With preserved ejection fraction
2.1.2 With reduced or mildly reduced ejection fraction (reduced ejection fraction ≤40%; mildly reduced ejection fraction 41–49%)
2.2 Valvular heart disease
2.3 Congenital/acquired cardiovascular conditions leading to post-capillary PH
3. PH due to lung diseases and/or hypoxia
3.1 Obstructive lung disease or emphysema
3.2 Restrictive lung disease
3.3 Other lung disease with mixed restrictive/obstructive pattern
3.4 Hypoventilation syndromes
3.5 Hypoxia without lung disease (e.g. high altitude)
3.6 Developmental lung disorders
4. PH due to pulmonary artery obstruction
4.1 Chronic thromboembolic PH (CTEPH)
4.2 Other pulmonary artery obstruction
5. PH with unclear and/or multifactorial mechanisms
5.1 Haematological disorders
5.2 Systemic disorders
5.3 Metabolic disorders
5.4 Chronic renal failure with or without haemodialysis
5.5 Pulmonary tumour thrombotic microangiopathy
5.6 Fibrosing mediastinitis

known as primary PH, is a rare disorder with an estimated incidence of 2–7 cases per million depending on the population studied (Peacock et al. 2007).

Despite the clear clinical importance and the impact on quality of life and life expectancy, PH is clinically silent and therefore frequently undiagnosed or diagnosed at a late stage in the disease (Humbert et al. 2012). The increasing availability of disease modifying therapies can improve the prognosis for patients with PH and emphasises the importance of timely diagnosis (Coghlan and Handler 2006). While RHC with direct measurement of mPAP and PVR remains the gold standard for PH diagnosis, it is an expensive procedure, slows the diagnostic pathway due to the need for referral to tertiary centres and carries a 1% risk of serious complication. Consequently, cross-sectional imaging, namely, computed tomography (CT) and magnetic resonance imaging (MRI), plays an increasingly important role in the early detection and non-invasive monitoring of patients.

The aim of this chapter is to outline important measurements in different modalities in cardiovascular imaging that might suggest or confirm a diagnosis of PH as well as to describe important limitations of these modalities. A brief discussion of novel/research measurements will also be included.

2 Chest Radiograph Measurements in PH

The chest radiograph (CXR) is recommended in the early stages of work-up of patients with suspected PH (McGoon et al. 2004) giving information on heart size, pulmonary vasculature, lung parenchyma and chest wall abnormalities. CXRs are ubiquitous in the assessment of PH and are abnormal in 90% of patients at the time of diagnosis of PH.

The severity of PH does not, however, necessarily correlate with the severity of findings at CXR (Galiè et al. 2015). Additionally, the measurements on CXR that can contribute to a diagnosis of PH on CXR have moderate to good sensitivity but are non-specific. Moreover, cardiac measurements on CXR that suggest PH, namely, the finding of dilated right heart chambers, occur late in the disease process—by the time RV dilatation is evident on CXR, PH is often advanced with significant clinical decompensation, less treatment options and worse prognosis.

2.1 Pulmonary Vascular Measurements

The main pulmonary artery (MPA) diameter is frequently increased on PH patients at cross-sectional imaging and correlates with invasively measured mPAP (Mahammedi et al. 2013). The MPA is not visible on CXR; however, the right and left pulmonary artery diameters and hilar dimensions on CXR can be used as surrogate markers of MPA diameter and can help predict PH.

Pulmonary vasculature measurements on posteroanterior (PA) CXR suggestive of PH are:

- Right descending/interlobar pulmonary artery diameter >16 mm or left descending pulmonary artery diameter >18 mm (Matthay et al. 1981). Finding *both* in combination raises the positive predictive value (PPV) of underlying PH to 93% (Altschul et al. 2019). Figure 1 shows the measurement of the right descending/interlobar and left descending pulmonary arteries in blue and red, respectively.
- A hilar width, measured as the distance between the lateral points of the left and right hilum, of >112 mm can diagnose PH with a sensitivity of 82%, specificity of 31%, PPV of 78% and negative predictive value (NPV) of 38% (Mirsadraee et al. 2013). Measurement of hilar width is demonstrated on Fig. 2.
- Hilum-thoracic ratio >0.44, where 'hilum' is the distance between the lateral points of the left and right hilum and 'thoracic' is the largest internal thoracic diameter, has a sensitivity of 86%, specificity of 44%, PPV of 85% and

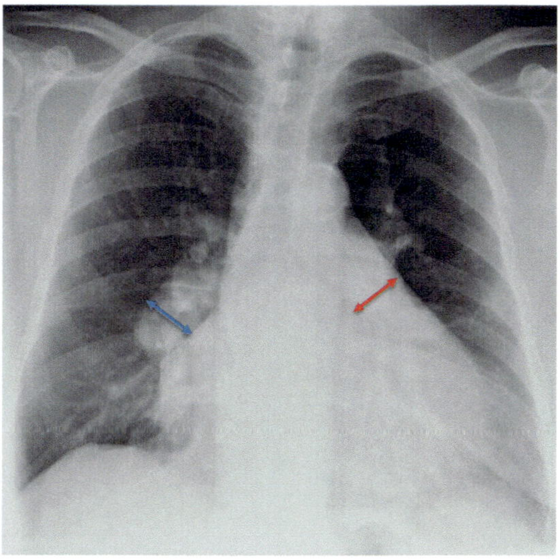

Fig. 1 Frontal CXR showing dilated right (blue) and left (red) descending pulmonary arteries. Right descending/interlobar pulmonary artery diameter >16 mm or left descending pulmonary artery diameter >18 mm are abnormal

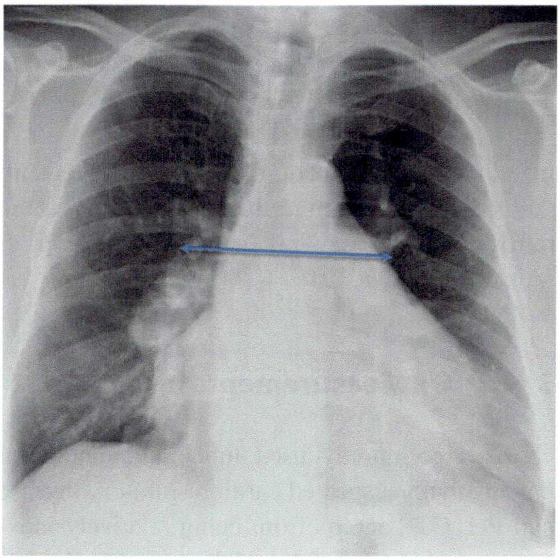

Fig. 2 Frontal CXR showing the measurement of the hilar width. A hilar width of >112 mm is abnormal, suggesting PH

NPV of 33% for the diagnosis of PH (Mirsadraee et al. 2013). Measurement of the hilum-thoracic ratio is outlined in Fig. 3.

There are some significant limitations to the above measurements. First, accurately outlining

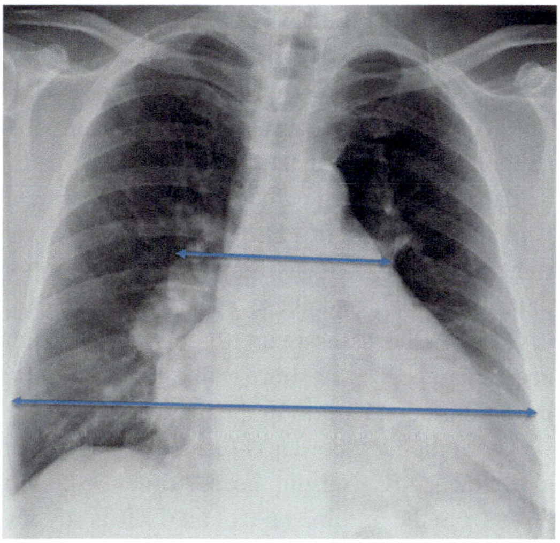

Fig. 3 Frontal CXR showing the measurement of the hilum-thoracic ratio. A hilum-thoracic ratio >0.44 suggests PH

and measuring the right and left descending pulmonary arteries may not always be possible on CXR, particularly on rotated radiographs. Additionally, the data regarding the cut-off values for branch pulmonary artery diameters is limited and variable with different authors, suggesting 17 mm or 20 mm to be more sensitive cut-off values for the right descending pulmonary artery diameter (Bush et al. 1988; Chang 1962; Chetty et al. 1982). This uncertainty is also supported by data showing that the diameters of the branch pulmonary arteries on CXR can vary with sex, age and BSA (Teichmann et al. 1970).

Assessing hilar width and hilum-thoracic ratio is therefore easier to do and more reproducible (Altschul et al. 2019; Mirsadraee et al. 2013) than measuring the diameters of the descending pulmonary arteries although limitations also exist in the measurement of hilar width and hilum-thoracic ratio. Hilar margins may not always be well-defined or clearly delineable on CXR, particularly if there is underlying interstitial lung disease, introducing inter- and intra-observer variability. Moreover, while an elevated hilar width or hilum-thoracic ratio may suggest a diagnosis of PH, they offer little information regarding the aetiology and severity and further imaging is almost always indicated.

2.2 Right Heart Chamber Measurements

The cardiothoracic ratio is the conventional method of assessing heart size, but this gives little data about specific chamber enlargement and is of limited value in PH. Right atrial (RA) and right ventricular (RV) dilatation are common findings in PH, and these can be evaluated on CXR. Specific assessment for dilation of right heart chambers is of more value than assessing the cardiothoracic ratio in the diagnosis of PH.

The right heart border is formed by the RA on a frontal CXR. A right heart border ≥45 mm away from the midline on frontal CXR is suggestive of RA dilatation, and this can diagnose PH with a sensitivity of 75%, specificity of 42%, PPV of 40% and NPV of 75% (Altschul et al. 2019; Mirsadraee et al. 2013). Figure 4 shows the measurement of the projection of the right heart border. A boot-shaped heart with upward tilt of the cardiac apex on a frontal CXR suggests RV dilatation. The RV is in an immediate retrosternal position and is therefore better assessed on a lateral view. On a normal lateral CXR, the craniocaudal extent of the RV occupies less than 1/3 the length from the inferior border of the heart to the manubriosternal junction. In RV enlargement, the heart takes up more than 1/3 and fills in the retrosternal space. This is shown on Fig. 5 (Altschul et al. 2019).

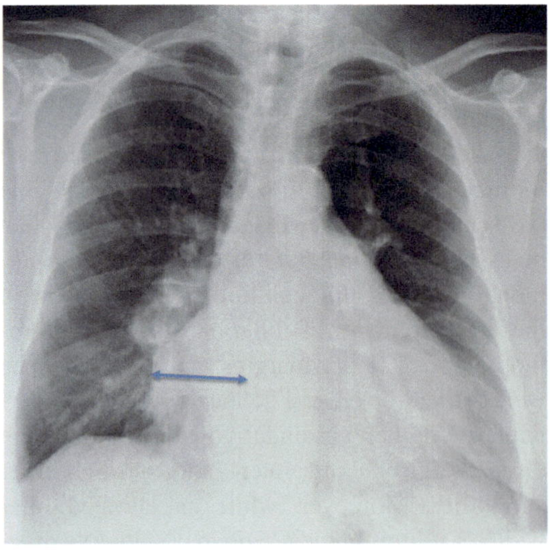

Fig. 4 Frontal CXR showing the measurement of projection of right heart border. A right heart border ≥45 mm away from the midline on frontal CXR is suggestive of RA dilatation

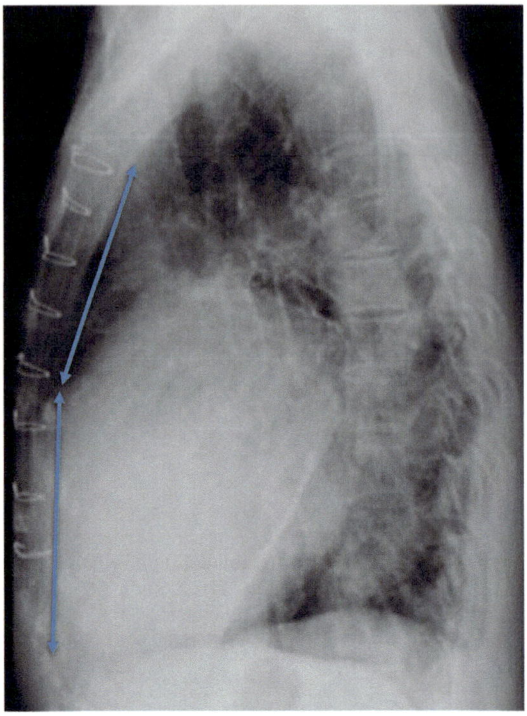

Fig. 5 In RV enlargement, the heart occupies more than 1/3 of the length from the inferior border of the heart to the sternomanubrial junction

3 CT Measurements in PH

CT is a commonly used imaging modality in patients with suspected cardiorespiratory disease and PH. CT benefits from being relatively inexpensive, well-tolerated, widely available, having high spatial resolution and multi-planar reconstruction capabilities. Additionally, CT images cardiac and pulmonary vascular anatomy as well as lung parenchyma in exquisite detail in a single examination and therefore is of great value in classifying the underlying cause of PH. CT may be performed either in patients with non-specific symptoms, as part of the work-up of patients at risk of PH (such as COPD and interstitial lung disease (ILD)), or specifically for the evaluation of PH. There are numerous robust, quantitative measurements that can be performed on CT to aid in the non-invasive diagnosis of PH.

Various CT imaging techniques exist for the work-up of suspected PH which can be tailored to the clinical scenario. In suspected chronic lung disease, an unenhanced, high-resolution CT is best to quantify lung parenchymal changes. Single or dual-energy contrast-enhanced CT for more accurate assessment of cardiac and vascular structures as well as chronic thromboembolism is also of value. Acquisitions may be done in systemic arterial or pulmonary arterial phases. It is also possible to opacify both right and left sides of the heart, including the pulmonary arterial tree, simultaneously using higher contrast doses and longer injections. A suggested protocol is 0.8–1 mL/kg of contrast, 0.8–1 mL/kg of 1:1 contrast:saline and 1 mL/kg saline. Bolus-tracking technique is used to trigger the start of image acquisition, with region of interest (ROI) placement either in the left atrium (LA) or in the ascending aorta (Ao) and an ROI threshold of 120 HU. The scan should be performed in gentle inspiration.

3.1 Pulmonary Vasculature Measurements on CT

3.1.1 Main Pulmonary Artery Diameter

The association between MPA dilatation and PH is well-established and has been shown to hold true across the various subtypes of PH (Tan et al. 1998; Ackman Haimovici et al. 1997; Lange et al. 2013; Boerrigter et al. 2010; Heinrich et al. 2005; Walsh et al. 2014; Zyłkowska et al. 2012; Colin et al. 2018). Increased pulmonary artery pressures lead to remodelling of the MPA with mural thickening mediated by elastin and collagen deposition and dilatation of the vessel as a response to increased mural shear stress (Botney 1999). The diameter of the MPA is not solely affected by pulmonary artery pressure (PAP) but also depends on age, gender, BSA, genetic factors and the presence of lung fibrosis (Raymond et al. 2014).

There have been numerous studies investigating the diameter of the normal MPA. However, the most robust data comes from the Framingham Heart Study and from Severance Hospital in Seoul, South Korea, where pulmonary artery diameters were measured in 706 healthy volunteers and 813 healthy individuals, respectively. The Framingham Heart study showed a mean (SD) pulmonary artery diameter of 25.1 (2.8) mm with an upper limit of normal (defined as the 90th percentile) of 28.9 mm in men and 26.9 mm in women (Truong et al. 2012). The study from South Korea showed a mean MPA diameter of 25.9 mm and an upper limit of normal of 31.3 mm in males and 29.6 mm in females (Lee et al. 2015).

The diameter of the pulmonary artery on CT imaging should be measured on axial images at the widest portion of the MPA within 3 cm of the bifurcation (Fig. 6). Measurements do not differ significantly between inspiratory and expiratory CT (Ratanawatkul et al. 2020). The vascular lumen alone should be measured on contrast-enhanced studies, whereas the vessel wall should be included on non-contrast studies (Raymond et al. 2014).

The diameter of the MPA correlates strongly with mPAP ($R = 0.67$, $p < 0.0001$). It also correlates with indexed PVR (PVRi) ($R = 0.78$, $p < 0.0001$) (Devaraj et al. 2008) which is a marker relating the absolute value of PVR to the

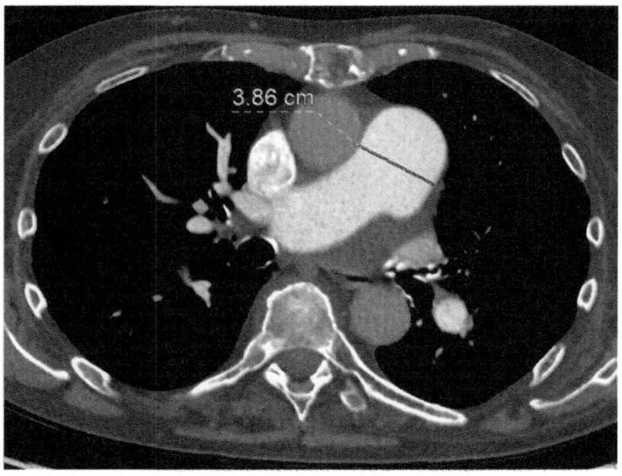

Fig. 6 Axial image from a CT pulmonary angiogram showing the measurement of the diameter of the main pulmonary artery, measured at the widest portion of the MPA within 3 cm of the bifurcation

patient's body surface area to account for differences in body size on blood flow. An MPA diameter of ≥29 mm has an 87% sensitivity, 89% specificity and 97% PPV for PH (Tan et al. 1998; Liu et al. 2023). Due to a low NPV, MPA diameters smaller than 29 mm do not necessarily exclude PH. Increasing the MPA threshold to 32 mm increases the specificity to 93% with a NPV of 90%, but sensitivity decreases to 47%, missing milder cases of PH (Alhamad et al. 2011). Due to difficulties in establishing a definite single threshold for MPA diameter, the Fleischner society issued a position paper on PH in 2021 which proposed different thresholds of PA diameter for suggesting underlying PH in different risk populations (low risk >34 mm, intermediate risk >32 mm and high risk >30 mm). These thresholds require further validation (Remy-Jardin et al. 2021).

The clinical importance of a dilated MPA goes beyond its correlation with mPAP. Severe MPA dilatation itself carries its own risks and complications. An MPA diameter of >48 mm is an independent risk factor for sudden death in patients with CTEPH and PAH. The contribution of MPA dilatation towards an increased risk of death is not entirely understood. Compression of the left main coronary artery is a recognised complication of severe MPA dilatation (Zyłkowska et al. 2012; Kawut et al. 1999; Mesquita et al. 2004), and in patients presenting with cardiac symptoms including angina, palpitations or syncope, and an MPA of >40 mm, the possibility of left main coronary artery compression by an enlarged MPA should be raised. However, death also occurs due to pulmonary artery dissection, pulmonary artery rupture and possibly due to an increased risk of malignant arrhythmia caused by severe MPA dilatation (Zyłkowska et al. 2012).

Measurement of MPA diameter is a quick and easy measurement to perform, and finding an elevated MPA diameter on CT should prompt a more concerted and formal work-up for PH. Nevertheless, it has its limitations. In patients with ILD and established lung fibrosis, MPA diameter does not correlate with mPAP or indexed PVR (PVRi) ($R = 0.23$, $p = 0.22$ for mPAP and $R = 0.23$, $p = 0.28$ for PVRi) and is therefore an unreliable marker for PH. This is thought likely due to lung fibrosis causing tractional dilation of the MPA giving false positive measurements. Other measurements (see below) should be used to assess for PH in the context of lung fibrosis. Dilatation of the MPA in the *absence* of PH may also be idiopathic or also seen in the context of other conditions including pulmonary valve stenosis (with post-stenotic dilatation), scenarios where there is increased pulmonary blood flow such as in large arteriovenous malformations, in connective tissue diseases such as Marfan's and Ehlers-Danlos syndromes and in inflammatory vasculitides such as Takayasu and Behcet's disease.

3.1.2 Pulmonary Artery: Ascending Aortic Size

Multiple studies have also demonstrated a strong correlation between an increased main pulmonary artery:ascending aorta (MPA:Ao) diameter and mPAP (Mahammedi et al. 2013; Ng et al. 1999; Kuriyama et al. 1984; Bouchard et al. 1985; Murray et al. 1994). In essence, it could be argued that assessing MPA diameter relative to ascending aortic diameter is a form of 'internal normalisation' as it corrects for gender, age, BSA, phase of the cardiac cycle and other technical factors (Raymond et al. 2014; Truong et al. 2012; Ng et al. 1999).

In assessing MPA:Ao ratio, MPA diameter is measured as previously described. The aortic diameter is measured as the largest diameter of the ascending aorta on axial images (not necessarily at the same level as the MPA), with the vascular lumen alone measured on a contrast-enhanced study and the vessel wall included in the measurement on a non-contrast study. Figure 7 demonstrates the measurement of the MPA:Ao ratio.

Data from the Framingham Heart study shows that in healthy individuals, the mean (SD) MPA:Ao diameter ratio is 0.77, while data from the Korean study shows a slightly higher mean MPA:Ao diameter ratio of 0.87 (Lee et al. 2015; Remy-Jardin et al. 2021). When an MPA:Ao ratio of >1 is found, PH can be diagnosed with a sensitivity of 70%, specificity of 92%, PPV of 96%

and NPV of 52% (Ng et al. 1999; Devaraj and Hansell 2009; Devaraj et al. 2010).

MPA:Ao diameter ratio correlates strongly with mPAP and PVRi in PH patients ($R = 0.72$, $p < 0.0001$ for mPAP and $R = 0.71$, $p < 0.0001$ for PVRi) and is a better predictor of PH than the absolute diameter of the MPA (Devaraj et al. 2008; Murray et al. 1994). Importantly, MPA:Ao ratio also correlates well with pulmonary haemodynamic parameters ($R = 0.54$, $p < 0.005$ for mPAP and $R = 0.48$, $p = 0.04$ for PVRi) in patients with lung fibrosis, and therefore, an increased MPA:Ao ratio remains a reliable marker for PH across all PH subtypes (Devaraj et al. 2008; Ng et al. 1999). In the context of interstitial lung disease, MPA:Ao ratio should be quoted alone and not in conjunction with absolute MPA diameter.

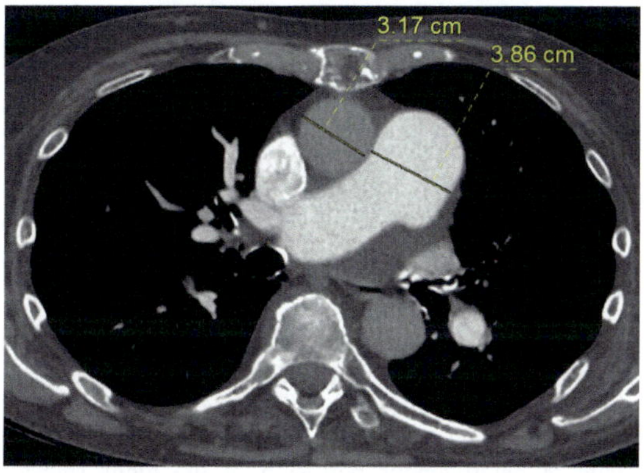

Fig. 7 Axial image from a CT pulmonary angiogram showing an elevated mean pulmonary artery to aortic ratio

The ratio of the cross-sectional area (CSA) of the MPA to the diameter of the ascending aorta can also be assessed on CT. The ascending aortic diameter is measured as previously described. The MPA CSA is measured on a double oblique reconstruction through the MPA just proximal to its bifurcation. Figure 8 outlines the measurement of the MPA CSA on double oblique reconstruction through the MPA. The MPA CSA to aortic diameter ratio correlates as strongly with mPAP as the MPA:Ao diameter ratio ($R^2 = 0.45$, $p < 0.001$) (Devaraj et al. 2010). This same study also showed a link between mPAP and the diameter of a thoracic vertebral body at the same level although the correlation was weaker than the MPA CSA:Ao diameter or MPA:Ao diameter ratios.

When using an abnormal MPA:Ao ratio to suggest a diagnosis of PH, a degree of caution should be exercised. Disease unrelated to PH such as bicuspid aortic valve, pulmonary stenosis and connective tissue diseases can cause dilatation of the ascending aorta or MPA resulting in false positive or negative results. Also, aorta fre-

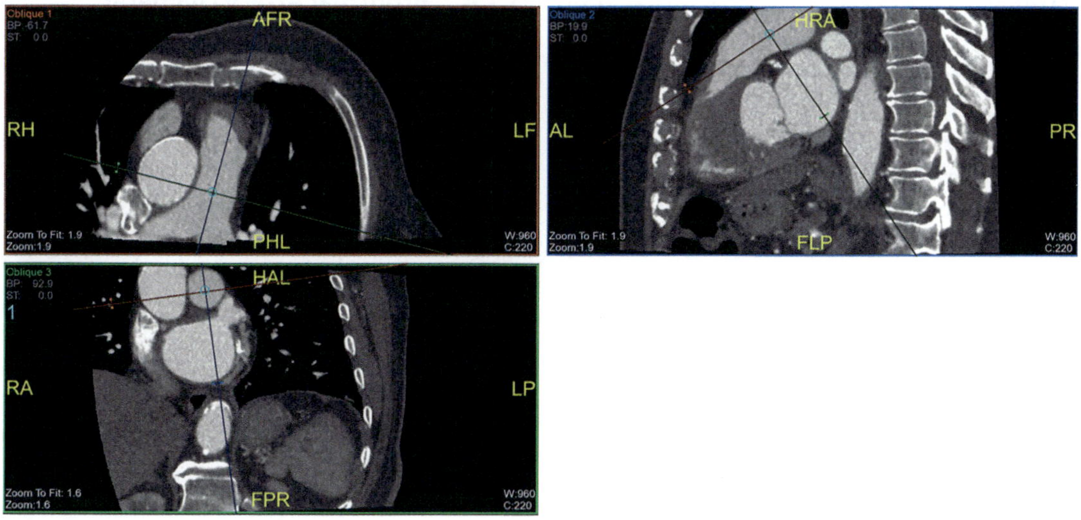

Fig. 8 Double oblique reconstruction through the MPA just proximal to its bifurcation demonstrating measurement of MPA CSA (blue outline on bottom left image)

quently dilates with age, and MPA:Ao ratio should be used cautiously in patient above 50 years.

3.1.3 Segmental Pulmonary Artery Diameter

Like the MPA, the segmental pulmonary arteries are also remodelled in PH. Numerous studies have shown a correlation between the absolute diameter of more peripheral pulmonary arteries and mPAP, although this is weaker than the correlation between mPAP and MPA diameter (Ackman Haimovici et al. 1997; Kuriyama et al. 1984; Schmidt et al. 1996). There is, however, a strong correlation between the diameter of the segmental pulmonary artery relative to the adjacent bronchus when measured in vertically oriented bronchovascular bundles of the apical upper lobe segments and the superior and posterior lower lobe segments. In healthy subjects on an inspiratory CT, the segmental pulmonary arteries are equal to or smaller in diameter than the adjacent bronchi when bronchial diameter is measured from outer wall to outer wall. However, the segmental pulmonary arteries frequently dilate in PH and in the presence of an MPA ≥29 mm; a segmental pulmonary artery:bronchial diameter ratio of ≥1:1 in 3 or more lobes suggests PH (Tan et al. 1998) with a specificity of 87% and a sensitivity of 68% (Devaraj et al. 2010); this can be applied across all groups of PH including patients with established interstitial fibrosis (Tan et al. 1998). Figure 9 shows the appropriate measurement of this ratio.

There are certain drawbacks to this parameter. In particular, the ratio is affected by the phase of the respiratory cycle with the diameter of the bronchi being significantly smaller in expiration. Other limitations to measuring this ratio include the presence of bronchiectasis, lung infiltrative conditions, chronic thrombosis of segmental pulmonary arteries in CTEPH and diseases with hypoxaemic vasoconstriction. The value of this parameter therefore remains controversial and warrants further evaluation in the future.

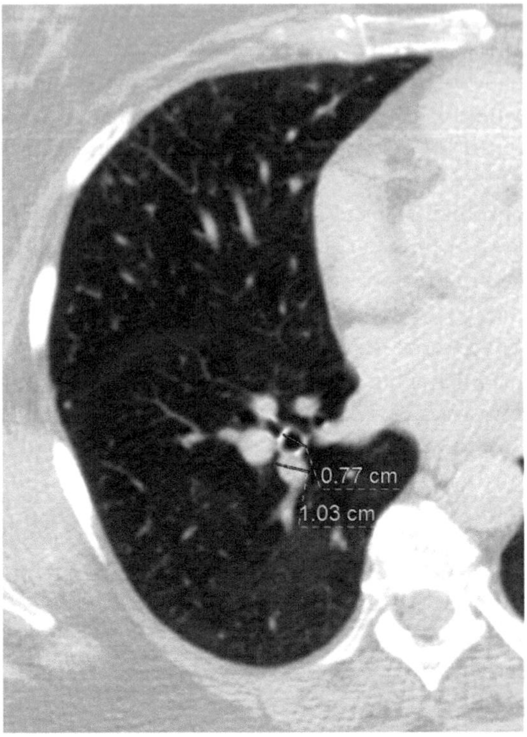

Fig. 9 An axial image from a CT pulmonary angiogram demonstrating the measurement of dilated, vertically oriented posterior segment right lower lobe pulmonary artery relative to the accompanying segmental bronchus. Note is made of heterogenous perfusion of the lungs (mosaic attenuation)

3.1.4 Bronchial Artery Diameter

Normal bronchial arteries are not usually identifiable in healthy patients. Hypertrophied bronchial arteries may be found in PH (Devaraj and Hansell 2009). This is particularly true in patients with CTEPH where there is a higher frequency of bronchial artery hypertrophy than in other forms of PH; however, bronchial artery dilatation occurs sufficiently frequently in other forms of PH to render this as an unreliable sign of CTEPH specifically. What constitutes an abnormally dilated bronchial artery is subjective although data from small study populations suggests that the upper limit of normal is 1.5 mm (Remy-Jardin et al. 2005).

3.1.5 Other Signs

There are various other quantitative and qualitative signs described in the literature that suggests the presence of PH on CT.

The MPA volume is calculated on CT as follows: a centre line is drawn from the centre of the pulmonary valve to the MPA bifurcation. The length of the centre line is considered the MPA length. CSA is measured at each 10 mm segment of the centre line and a mean CSA calculated. The MPA volume is defined as the product of the mean CSA and the MPA length. Measurement of MPA volume is cumbersome and shows modest correlation with mPAP (r = 0.30, p < 0.001). There is early experimental data suggesting that MPA volume based on automated 3D volumetry correlates strongly with mPAP and can even be used to non-invasively and accurately calculate mPAP found at RHC using regression models based on MPA volume and echo-derived sPAP. These models are promising but require further investigation and validation (Melzig et al. 2019; Colin et al. 2020a).

The egg-and-banana sign describes the appearances of the MPA on the same axial slice as the lower level of the aortic arch. It has a sensitivity of 39% and specificity of 85% for the detection of PH according to some data; other studies have shown no difference in the detection of PH using this sign, and in isolation, it is of slightly limited value. It may be used in conjunction with other traditional signs to add strength to suspicions of the presence of PH in appropriate patients (Colin et al. 2018; Scelsi et al. 2018).

3.2 Cardiac Measurements on CT

Advances in CT technology mean that full retrospective cardiac imaging can be performed with significantly lower doses than the prohibitive doses seen in the early days of cardiac imaging. While not routine, retrospective CT can accurately assess cardiac volumes and function in PH. More frequently, however, the heart is imaged on ungated studies. Despite motion artefact, important observations on the heart can also be made on ungated imaging which are of value in the assessment of patients with PH.

3.2.1 Right Atrial Dimensions

Elevated RA pressures and RA dilatation reflect RV overload in PH and are markers of adverse outcomes (Querejeta Roca et al. 2015). RA diameter can be assessed on ungated, axial CT imaging by measuring the transverse or longitudinal diameter; both measurements compare well with RA size at MRI although the transverse diameter matches MRI data more closely and has better interobserver agreement (Eifer et al. 2018). RA transverse diameter is measured as the largest diameter perpendicular to the interatrial septum and parallel to the tricuspid annular plane (Fig. 10). The RA appendage and coronary sinus should be excluded from the measurement (Eifer et al. 2018; Gopalan 2011). For men, a RA transverse diameter ≥67 mm has 91.5% specificity, 58.6% sensitivity and 82.8% accuracy for diagnosing RA enlargement, when compared to MRI as the gold standard. For women, a RA transverse diameter threshold ≥64 mm has a 92.9% specificity, 75.0% sensitivity and 90.1% accuracy for diagnosing RA enlargement (Eifer et al. 2018). Both measurements show no significant

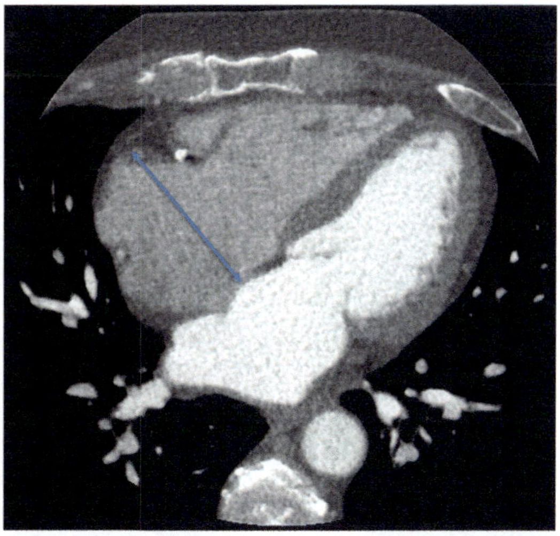

Fig. 10 Axial CT image showing the measurement of the transverse diameter of the right atrium, measured as the largest diameter perpendicular to the interatrial septum and parallel to the tricuspid annular plane

variation with changes in BSA (Eifer et al. 2018). It is important to note that on ungated CT imaging, a 'small' RA diameter can still be seen in the presence of significant PH if the heart is imaged at a point in the cardiac cycle where the atria are yet to fill.

RA area is a commonly measured metric on echocardiography with an established correlation with mPAP, sPAP, dPAP, PVR and N-terminal prohormone of brain natriuretic peptide (NT-proBNP) levels (Fischer et al. 2018) as well as a recognised link between increasing RA area and increased mortality in PH (Liu et al. 2020). Measurement of RA area on ungated CT is also possible with good correlation with echocardiographic values. A CT equivalent of the echocardiographic 4-chamber view is created on CT using multiplanar reformatting of axial images as outlined in Fig. 11. The long axis reference line is initially aligned through the left ventricular (LV) apex and mid mitral valve with the short axis reference line parallel and aligned with the mitral annular plane. Imaging slice height is adjusted to remove the LV outflow tract (which would create the echocardiographic equivalent of a 5-chamber view). The RA area is then measured by drawing a freehand ROI around the RA with exclusion of the RA appendage (Fig. 11). The normal RA area on CT is 17.0 ± 4.1 cm^2 (Gopalan et al. 2022). While measuring RA area on CT is a theoretically attractive tool to help diagnose and risk-stratify patients, there are some important limitations to this measurement. Firstly, the recommended reference values are based on a well-designed study but with limited sample size. Secondly, accurately measuring RA area can be challenging due to significant streak artefact from intravenous contrast medium entering the RA. Additionally, RA size may be spuriously altered by the high flow rates of IV contrast media used in CT and by alterations in venous return by the inspiratory breath hold of CT. Finally, RA size can be underestimated on ungated CT imaging if the imaged phase of the cardiac cycle is not at or close to ventricular end-systole.

Measuring atrial volumes volume on CT pulmonary angiogram (CTPA) is possible using newer-generation automated software. It has been done in smaller studies with success for left atrial (LA) volume, but no large dataset exists for RA volume. Measuring RA volume on retrospective, ECG-gated cardiac CT is also possible using automated and semi-automated software, the latter being time consuming with relatively high inter-observer variability, possibly due to complex RA geometry (Rheinheimer et al. 2016). Additionally, no normal reference range exists

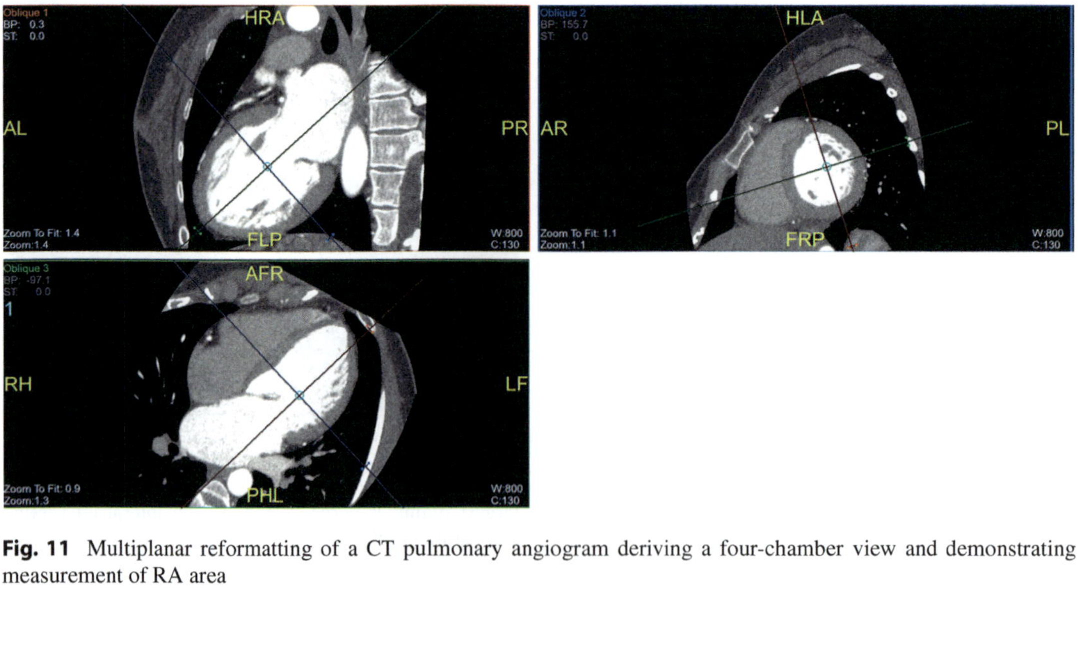

Fig. 11 Multiplanar reformatting of a CT pulmonary angiogram deriving a four-chamber view and demonstrating measurement of RA area

for measuring RA volume on retrospective cardiac CT. Applying MRI reference ranges to CT should be done with caution. While there is a correlation between the two modalities, there is also considerable intermodality variability with data from a small population showing significantly higher RA volumes on CT than MR (Rheinheimer et al. 2016), potentially due to the higher venous return in inspiration during CT acquisition and high flow and volumes of intravascular contrast agents, both found in CT. Routine measurement of RA volumes is therefore not yet recommended pending larger trials.

3.2.2 Left Atrial Size

Pulmonary hypertension due to left heart disease (PH-LHD) is the most common cause of PH (Galiè et al. 2015). As previously described, PH-LHD is diagnosed at RHC on finding a PAWP >15 mm Hg alongside an mPAP >20 mm Hg (Naeije and Chin 2019; Simonneau et al. 2019; Currie et al. 2018).

LA area measured on thoracic CT is the most accurate CT measurement for predicting an elevated PAWP and can contribute towards the non-invasive diagnosis of PH-LHD. LA area is measured on axial images on the slice where the chamber appears the largest. The atrial endocardial borders are traced, excluding the LA appendage and pulmonary veins (Fig. 12). This method is quick and has excellent interobserver reproducibility (intra-class correlation = 0.972, $p < 0.001$). LA areas $\geq$26.8 cm^2 and $\geq$30 cm^2 can diagnose PAWP of >15 mmHg and >18 mmHg with specificities of 89% and 94% and sensitivities of 60% and 53%, respectively (Currie et al. 2018).

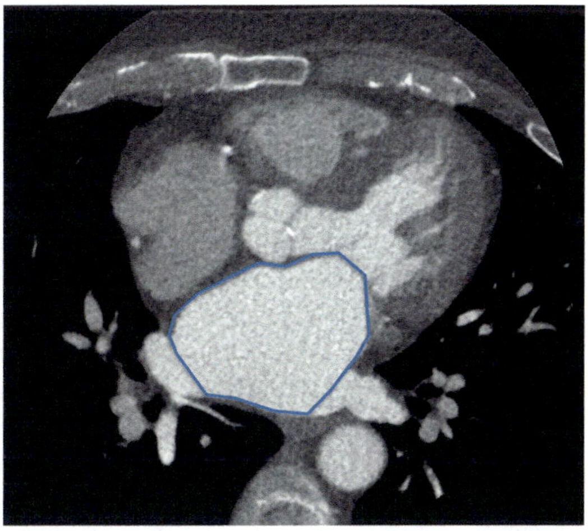

Fig. 12 Axial image from narrow field of view reconstruction of a cardiac CT demonstrating the measurement of left atrial area excluding pulmonary veins and left atrial appendage

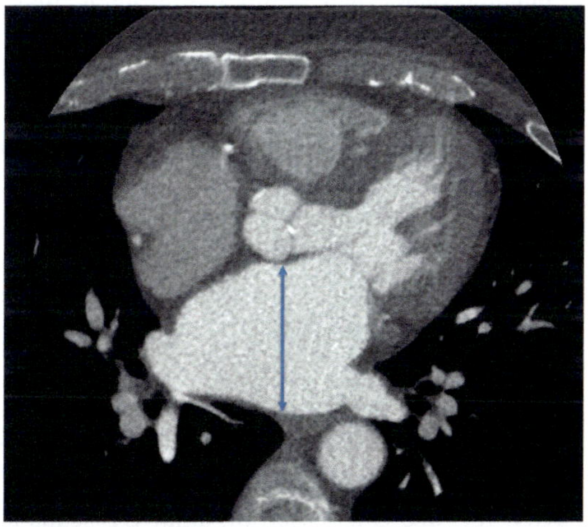

Fig. 13 Axial image from narrow field of view reconstruction of a cardiac CT demonstrating the measurement of left atrial AP diameter

LA enlargement can also be assessed by measuring anteroposterior (AP) LA diameter on axial, ungated CT images. On the slice where the chamber is largest, the AP diameter is measured in the anteroposterior plane, excluding the pulmonary veins and the LA appendage (Fig. 13). For men, an LA AP diameter threshold $\geq$50 mm diagnoses LA enlargement (compared to MRI as gold standard) with 92% specificity and 47% sensitivity. For women, an LA AP diameter threshold $\geq$45 mm diagnoses LA enlargement with 96% specificity and 54% sensitivity (Eifer et al. 2018).

LA volume is routinely measured on MRI and echocardiography and can reliably distinguish PH-LHD from others forms of PH (Crawley et al. 2013). LA volumes and function can also be measured on retrospective cardiac CT using automated and semi-automated software. Semi-automated packages require the endocardial borders of the LA to be outlined on successive slices through the chamber at the point in the cardiac cycle of smallest and largest atrial size; however, it is a time-consuming process, taking approximately 15–20 min per scan, and is not routinely performed in clinical practice (Stojanovska et al. 2011). More recently developed, automated software has allowed rapid, automated 3D segmentation of atrial (and ventricular) sizes on CT. The importance of finding an enlarged LA is that this is commonly found in group 2 PH patients (PH-LHD), whereas it is an uncommon finding in other groups. A LA volume of ≥110 mL can differentiate group 2 PH patients from other groups with a sensitivity of 79% and a specificity of 90%. This is significantly more accurate than previous recommendations to use LA diameter ($p = 0.009$) (Melzig et al. 2022).

The above data is promising, although fairly recent, and needs further validation; this is likely to become easier once automated atrial segmentation and volume calculation becomes more widespread. Unlike on echocardiography and MRI, there is no data correlating LA volume measured on CT with PAWP. Nevertheless, when echocardiography and MRI are inconclusive (e.g. normal LV ejection fraction but severe diastolic dysfunction) or contraindicated, in the appropriate context, increased LA volume can contribute to a diagnosis of PH-LHD.

3.2.3 Right Ventricular Diameter

One of the earliest pathological responses of the right ventricle (RV) to PH is dilatation of the RV cavity. RV size is assessed on axial CT scans at the mid ventricular level where the chamber is the largest, on the slice with least motion artefact (Fig. 14). The maximum transverse RV diameter is measured from the interventricular septum to the RV free wall, perpendicular to the interventricular septum and parallel to the plane of the tricuspid annulus (Eifer et al. 2018). Transverse diameters ≥60 mm in men and ≥57 mm in women diagnose RV dilatation with specificities of 93% and 91% and sensitivities of 67% and 53%, respectively, when compared to MRI as gold standard (Eifer et al. 2018).

RV size on axial CT can also be assessed by measuring the RV:LV diameter ratio. The normal axial diameter of the RV is smaller than the left ventricle (LV); an RV:LV ratio of >1 implies RV dilatation. Transverse RV diameter is assessed at the widest point in the mid-ventricle, as above. LV diameter is measured at the widest point in the cavity (not necessarily on the same slice as the widest RV diameter), perpendicular to the interventricular septum and parallel to the mitral annulus. An RV:LV diameter >1.0 identifies PH with a sensitivity of 90% and a specificity of 35% (Bax et al. 2020). It is also a predictor of increased mortality at 5 years in patients with ILD-related PH (HR, 3.26; $p = 0.003$) (Bax et al. 2020), while an RV:LV diameter >1.2 is a marker of adverse outcomes in inoperable CTEPH (Ema et al. 2017).

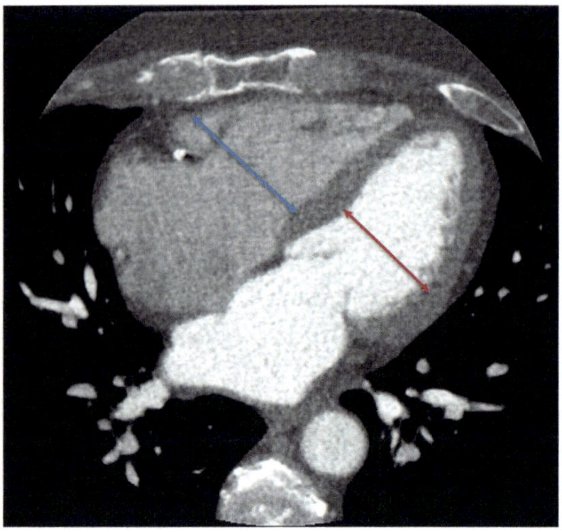

Fig. 14 Axial image from narrow field of view reconstruction of a cardiac CT demonstrating the measurement of right ventricular transverse diameter (blue arrow); the red arrow shows the measurement of left ventricular transverse diameter for the purpose of calculating RV:LV diameter ratio (note the LV measurement does not necessarily need to be on the same slice as the RV transverse diameter measurement)

3.2.4 RV Volume and Function

Cardiac MRI is the gold standard for assessing cardiac volumes and function (Bellenger et al. 2000). However, there is very good correlation between retrospective cardiac CT and cardiac MRI for the assessment of ventricular size and function (Maffei et al. 2012; Wai et al. 2013; Raman et al. 2006; Guo et al. 2010). Retrospective cardiac CT is a useful tool in assessing RV volume and function with only a moderate dose penalty on more modern scanners, and it is helpful when echocardiography is non-diagnostic and MRI is contraindicated or not tolerated.

Conventional cardiac CT contrast injection protocols are designed to optimise contrast in the left side of the heart. If retrospective imaging is being performed to specifically assess right chamber volume and function, the contrast bolus should be timed to maximise contrast resolution between the ventricular myocardium and RV cavity (Taylor et al. 2010). A triphasic contrast injection protocol of 50–70 mL of contrast media, 30–50 mL of a 70:30 contrast:saline mix and a 30–40 mL of saline flush results in good quality and prolonged RV opacification without beam-hardening artefact (Kerl et al. 2008; Lu et al. 2010). The administration of β-blockers prior to CT for ventricular function analysis is not recommended—data comparing ventricular volumes and function in the same patients assessed on the same day on both CT and MRI showed significantly, and spuriously, higher ventricular volumes and lower ejection fractions on CT. The reason for this may be the negative inotropic effects of the β-blocker given prior to the CT (Schlosser et al. 2007).

Retrospective cardiac CT images the entire cardiac cycle. Evaluation of the reconstructed data set as a cine loop allows visual analysis of ventricular function and regional wall motion. RV contraction involves both radial contraction and longitudinal shortening, with the longitudinal component contributing proportionately more to systolic function. Semi-quantitative analysis of RV function can be performed by assessing the tricuspid annular plane systolic excursion (TAPSE) as a surrogate marker of longitudinal RV contractility. TAPSE is a well-established and accurate semi-quantitative measurement of RV function in echocardiography and cardiac MRI and can easily be assessed on CT (Dupont et al. 2011). The CT equivalents of the 4-chamber echocardiographic view are reconstructed as described above using multiplanar reformat. TAPSE is then measured as the difference between the lengths of a line drawn from the tricuspid annular plane to the RV apex in end-diastole and a similar line drawn in end-systole (Fig. 15a, b).

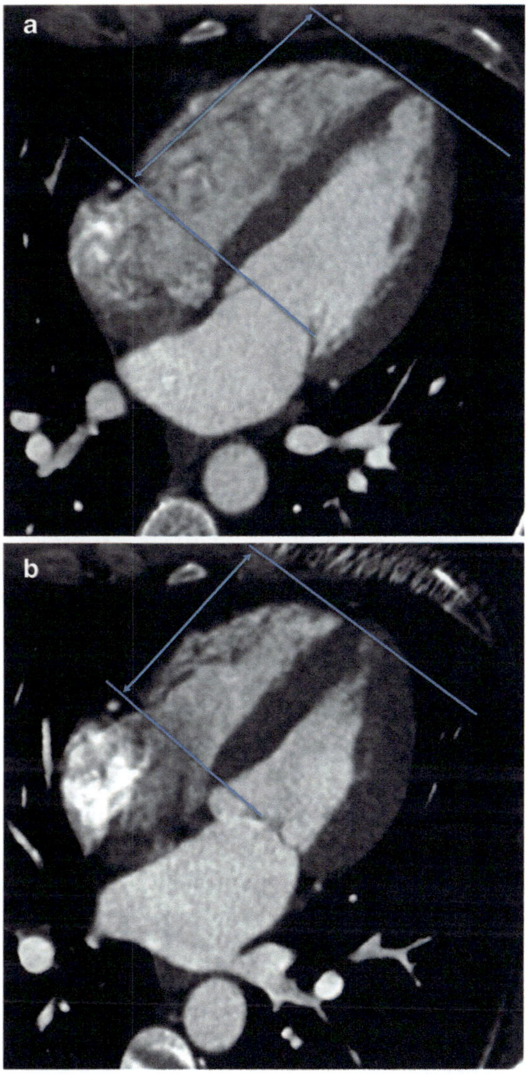

Fig. 15 (**a**, **b**) Images from a retrospectively ECG-gated cardiac CT in end-diastole (above) and end-systole (below). TAPSE is measured as the difference between the lengths of the two arrowed lines

The normal TAPSE when measured on M-mode echocardiography is ≥20 mm. A TAPSE of <18 mm is a strong indicator of RV systolic dysfunction and in patients with PAH, is an adverse marker of survival. The unadjusted risk of death (hazard ratio) for patients with a TAPSE of <18 mm compared to those with a TAPSE of ≥18 mm is 5.7 and for every 1 mm decrease in

TAPSE below this, the unadjusted risk of death increases by 17% (Forfia et al. 2006). However, an established measurement tool, particularly at echocardiography, TAPSE assessment has several limitations. It measures motion of only a small portion of RV myocardium and cannot be considered a comprehensive representation of the entire RV function. Basal RV longitudinal motion is also increased in the presence of significant tricuspid regurgitation, which may falsely elevate TAPSE. Finally, due to ventricular interdependence, LV systolic function may also affect TAPSE (Kind et al. 2010; López-Candales et al. 2006).

The same data set can also be used for volumetric analysis; this can be done in the short-axis orientation or in the true axial plane. While the analysis can be performed, in a similar fashion to cardiac MRI, on contiguous slices of up to 8 mm thickness, using thinner slices allows increased accuracy of RV endocardial and epicardial contouring, particularly around the tricuspid valve and right ventricular outflow tract (RVOT). The downside of using thinner slices for volumetric analysis is the longer post-processing time needed if contouring is done manually (Gopalan 2011) although, given the inherent high contrast between RV myocardium and contrast-enhanced blood pool, most advanced cardiac CT processing packages can automatically segment RV contours with little input needed by the user. Figures 16 and 17b show typical, automated LV and RV segmentation including accurate segmentation at the geometrically complex RVOT.

RV volumes are calculated by outlining endocardial contours on short axis/axial stack images (using horizontal and vertical long axis planes to correlate anatomy) at end-diastole and end-systole. This allows calculation of RV stroke volume, ejection fraction and cardiac output. Trabeculations and the RVOT are, by convention, included as part of the ventricular volume (Stojanovska et al. 2014).

Ventricular volumes and function on CT correlate closely with those on MRI although due to minor differences in temporal and spatial resolution and signal to noise levels, these cannot be directly extrapolated (Lin and Min 2008; Van Der Vleuten et al. 2006). Due to the dose implications

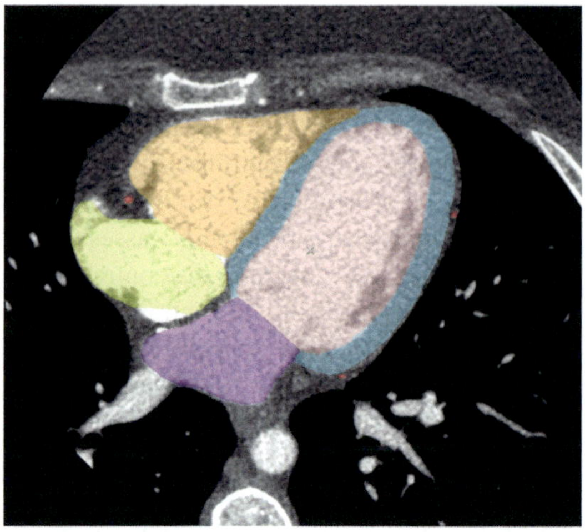

Fig. 16 Snapshot of a 4-chamber reconstruction slice from a single phase of the cardiac cycle of a retrospective cardiac CT showing accurate, automated segmentation of cardiac chambers

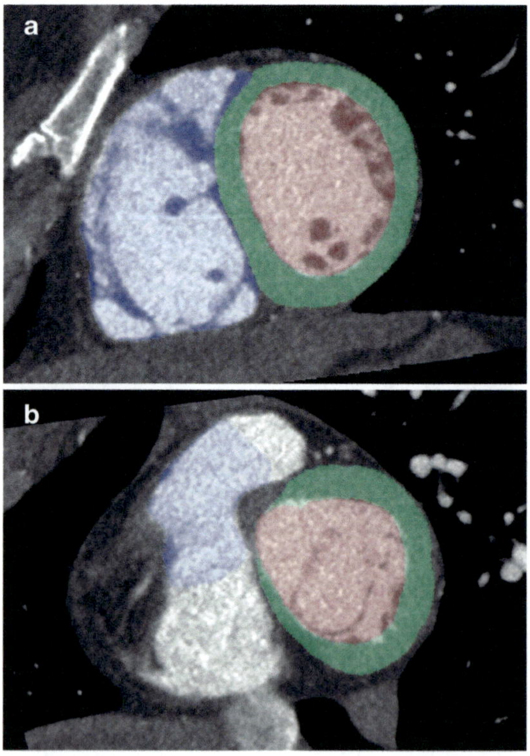

Fig. 17 (**a**, **b**) Images from short axis view reconstructions through the ventricles at the mid ventricular level (above) and basal ventricular level (below) showing automated segmentation of ventricular volumes. Modern, commercially available software is capable of quick and accurate segmentation of the complex geometry at the RVOT (below)

of assessing ventricular function by CT, scant data is available for normative values for RV volume and function. The largest study population to date using conventional methods of functional analysis consists of 74 patients (Stojanovska et al. 2014). Normal RV parameters, calculated from this study population, are given in Tables 3 and 4.

3.2.5 RV Wall Thickness

RV myocardial thickness is measured on ECG-gated imaging at the free wall of the RV in end-diastole. Measurements performed on non-ECG gated chest imaging should be used with caution as they may overestimate myocardial thickness if the scan was acquired at any point other than end-diastole. The normal RV wall thickness is <4 mm (Lin et al. 2008) measured as shown in Fig. 18. An RV free-wall myocardial thickness of >4 mm is abnormal, and a free wall thickness of ≥6 mm is a strong predictor of PH with an odds ratio (OR) of 30.5, sensitivity of 81% and specificity of 92% (Chan et al. 2011; Mortani Barbosa et al. 2012).

3.2.6 Septal Deviation

The normal position of the interventricular septum (IVS) is convex to the right. In the development of cor pulmonale, the RV pressure rises, equalling and eventually exceeding systemic pressures. Mirroring this, the IVS initially becomes straight and eventually, convex to the left, bowing into the left ventricle. Leftward deviation of the IVS during systole can diagnose an mPAP ≥30 mmHg with 86% sensitivity and 91% specificity (Alunni et al. 2010).

Table 3 Right ventricular volumes and function in females by age

Age (years)	30–39	40–49	50–59	60–70
Absolute				
EDV (mL)	173 (146–200)	157 (138–176)	169 (150–187)	155 (133–177)
ESV (mL)	74 (56–92)	56 (32–80)	79 (57–99)	57 (36–78)
SV (mL)	99 (83–115)	101 (87–115)	91 (80–102)	97 (82–112)
EF (%)	58 (51–65)	66 (53–79)	54 (46–62)	64 (52–76)
Indexed				
EDV/BSA (mL/m^2)	88 (75–100)	85 (78–92)	92 (85–99)	88 (78–97)
ESV/BSA (mL/m^2)	38 (28–48)	30 (18–42)	42 (33–51)	32 (20–44)
SV/BSA (mL/m^2)	50 (45–55)	55 (47–63)	50 (44–56)	56 (47–64)

All values given as mean (95% confidence interval)
BSA body surface area, *EDV* end-diastolic volume, *EF* ejection fraction, *ESV* end-systolic volume, *SV* stroke volume (Stojanovska et al. 2014)

Table 4 Right ventricular volumes and function in males by age

Age (years)	30–39	40–49	50–59	60–70
Absolute				
EDV (mL)	214 (197–230)	197 (169–225)	182 (160–204)	203 (74–131)
ESV (mL)	100 (71–128)	84 (52–115)	71 (47–95)	91 (58–124)
SV (mL)	113 (96–130)	113 (91–135)	111 (98–124)	112 (97–126)
EF (%)	54 (42–66)	59 (45–72)	62 (51–73)	57 (45–67)
Indexed				
EDV/BSA (mL/m^2)	101 (94–107)	96 (84–107)	86 (77–95)	99 (84–114)
ESV/BSA (mL/m^2)	47 (34–60)	41 (26–56)	34 (22–45)	45 (27–63)
SV/BSA (mL/m^2)	54 (43–65)	56 (44–67)	52 (45–58)	54 (47–61)

All values given as mean (95% confidence interval)
BSA body surface area, *EDV* end-diastolic volume, *EF* ejection fraction, *ESV* end-systolic volume, *SV* stroke volume (Stojanovska et al. 2014)

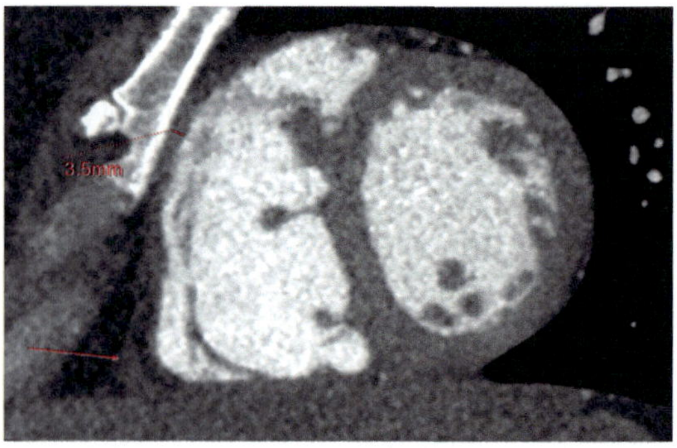

Fig. 18 Short axis reconstructed image at the mid ventricular level showing the measurement of the RV free wall. A small amount of pericardial fluid is also shown (red arrow). Caution should be taken to not include pericardial fluid in measuring the RV wall thickness. Altering window width and level to make pericardial fat insinuated between RV myocardium and fluid more prominent can help

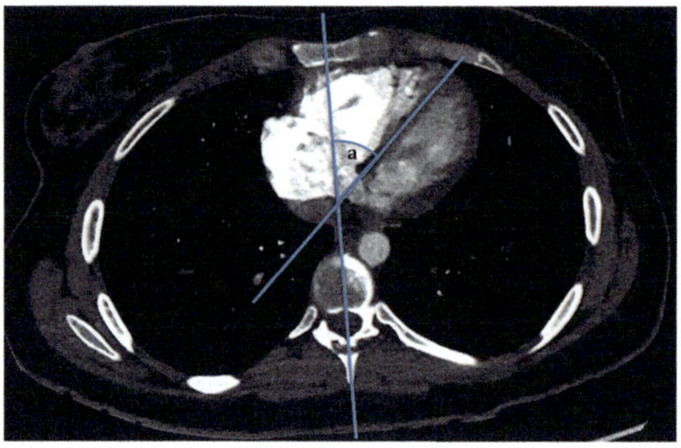

Fig. 19 Axial image from a CTPA demonstrating the measurement of the septal angle, an angle drawn between the interventricular septum and a line drawn from the midpoint of the sternum to the thoracic spinous process on the same axial image

The degree of leftward deviation of the IVS can be quantified by measuring the septal angle. The septal angle refers to the angle between the interventricular septum and a line drawn from the midpoint of the sternum to the thoracic spinous process on the same axial image (Fig. 19). This angle increases with RV overload and dilatation. A septal angle of >68° is a strong predictor of diagnosing PH at RHC, and the angle also correlates strongly with PVR and NT-proBNP levels (Tang et al. 2013). This suggests that an elevated septal angle is a sign of adverse cardiac remodelling and may be linked to worse outcomes

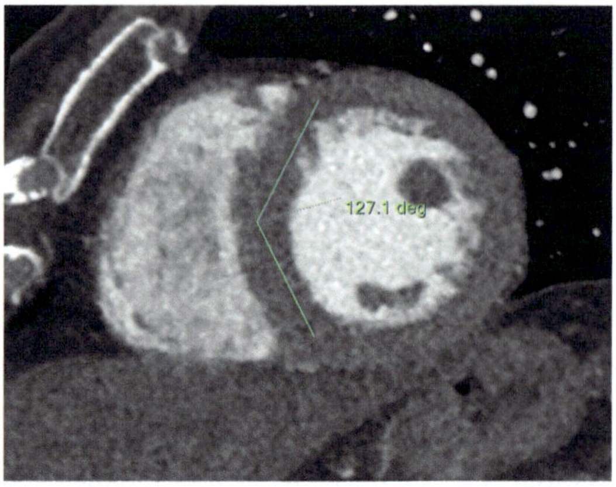

Fig. 20 Short axis reconstructed image at the mid ventricular level showing the measurement of the interventricular septal angle, defined as the angle from the RV insertion points to the mid-interventricular septum

although larger studies with longer follow-up are needed.

The interventricular septal angle can also be measured on a short-axis reconstruction of the heart. Using multiplanar reformat software to generate a mid-chamber short-axis image, the interventricular septal angle which is defined as the angle from the RV insertion points to the mid-interventricular septum can be measured, as outlined in Fig. 20. An interventricular septal angle of ≥ 130° diagnoses PH with a sensitivity of 93%, specificity of 35% and a positive predictive value of 91%. Finding an angle of ≥140° diagnoses PH with a sensitivity of 78%, specificity of 97% and a positive predictive value of 99% (Swift et al. 2020).

3.3 Advanced CT Imaging Techniques

CT approaches to the evaluation of PH are rapidly evolving. The following section includes several techniques that are still in development and that will likely not be available and ready for widespread clinical use for some time. However, these novel imaging approaches can provide unique insight into the pathophysiology of PH and should be examined in prospective research studies (including clinical trials) to determine their utility relative to conventional imaging approaches.

3.3.1 Pulmonary Artery Distensibility

The PA changes CSA in healthy subjects during the cardiac cycle, predictably increasing in area in systole and decreasing in diastole. This distensibility is reduced in patients with PH when measured at the right pulmonary artery (RPA) due to remodelling and decreased compliance of the pulmonary artery vasculature (Revel et al. 2009).

Measurement of RPA distensibility requires retrospective ECG-gated CT imaging. The CSA of the RPA is obtained by using double-oblique multiplanar reconstructions at the midway point between the origin of the RPA and its first anterior branch with the plane of reconstruction perpendicular to the long axis on both axial and coronal views. This is demonstrated in Fig. 21.

The largest area (CSA_{max}) and the smallest area (CSA_{min}) are found and RPA distensibility is defined as:

$$\frac{CSA_{max} - CSA_{min}}{CSA_{max}}$$

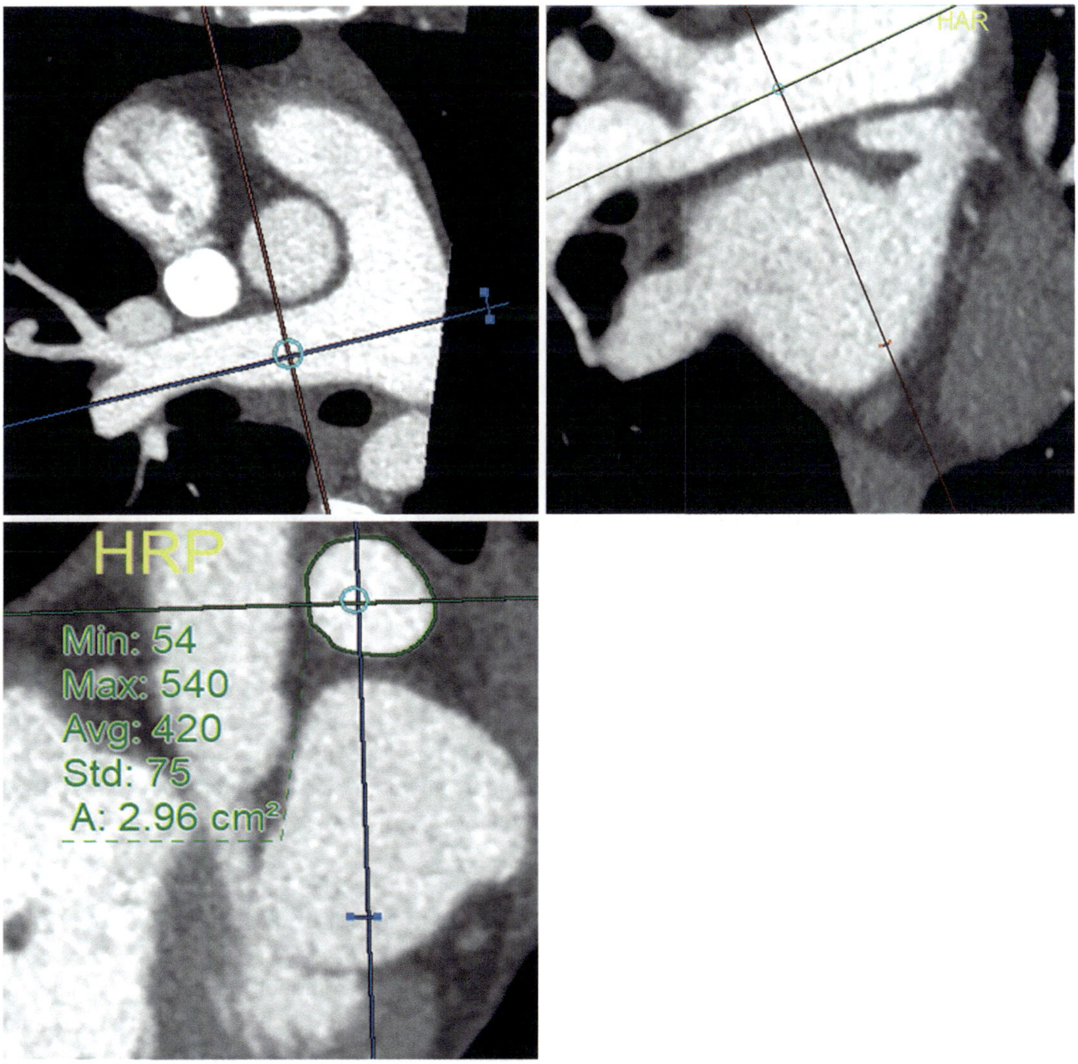

Fig. 21 Double oblique multiplanar reconstructions to obtain a true short axis through the RPA (third image) on which RPA is measured

RPA distensibility as assessed by this method correlates with mPAP, and using a cut-off of 17% or lower for RPA distensibility is a good predictor of pulmonary hypertension (Colin et al. 2020a; Revel et al. 2009). The importance of this is further highlighted by data showing that pulmonary artery distensibility of <16% is a predictor of increased mortality in patients with PAH (Gan et al. 2007). While retrospective CT gating permits assessment of vascular distensibility, the radiation dose means that MRI is likely the optimal modality to gain this data.

Pulmonary artery pulsatility index (PAPi) is a novel haemodynamic measurement that reflects right ventricular and pulmonary arterial coupling; it is indirectly linked to PA distensibility. In PH, the increased RV afterload impairs contractility leading to RV failure and death. PAPi is marker of the RV adaptive response to afterload—the lower the PAPi, the lower the RV contractile reserve (i.e. lower PAPi is a marker of RV dysfunction). PAPi is measured at RHC and defined as [(pulmonary artery systolic pressure − diastolic pulmonary artery pressure)/mean right atrial pressure].

In one group of PAH patients, a PAPi of <3.7 was linked with a one-year survival of 51% compared with 75% for a PAPi of >3.7. Three-year survival is 33% with a PAPi of <3.7 compared to 59% in patients with a PAPi of >3.7. Data from a smaller group of patients confirmed the importance of PAPi as a prognostic marker and showed that this remains significant even over long follow-up periods—a PAPi of <5.3 is associated with survival of 77.2% (1 year), 58.6% (3 years), 50.4% (5 years), 39.6% (7 years), and 31.7% (10 years) compared with survival rates of 95.7%, 86.2%, 80.4%, 71.2%, and 53.4%, respectively, for a PAPi of >5.3.

3.3.2 Pulmonary Artery Volumes

Measuring pulmonary artery diameters on CT is an established practice, but at borderline measurements, the sensitivity and specificity drops. With advanced, semi-automated image processing techniques, 3D measurements of the main and branch pulmonary arteries can be extracted and their respective volumes calculated. Several small studies have indicated the potential of these techniques to offer higher sensitivity and specificity for the diagnosis of PH as well as a close correlation with mPAP (Rengier et al. 2019) although larger studies with more robust data as well as software packages offering quick and easy automated volume measurements are required before this enters mainstream clinical practice.

3.3.3 Pulmonary Transit Time on Cardiac CT

In patients with advanced heart failure with reduced ejection fraction (HFrEF), PH is common and results from increased LV end-diastolic pressure transmitted to the left atrium and eventually to the pulmonary circulation. The elevated left heart filling pressures are associated with a worse outcome but cannot easily be measured at transthoracic echocardiography. Assessing pulmonary transit time can be a surrogate for assessing LV filling pressure (and by correlation, elevated pulmonary capillary bed pressure).

Pulmonary transit time (PTT) defines the time interval necessary for a contrast bolus to pass from the right side to the left side of the heart. It can easily be measured on cardiac CT using commercially available software. Circular ROIs are placed in the RV and LV, and time-attenuation curves are generated for each of the ROIs. PTT is calculated by subtracting the time to peak (maximal attenuation) of the first (RV) curve from time to peak of the second (LV) curve. A PTT of 14 s detects an elevated PAWP with a sensitivity, specificity, positive predictive value and negative predictive value of 83%, 90%, 94% and 76%, respectively. A PTT of 14 s also detects PH with a sensitivity, specificity, positive predictive value and negative predictive value of 91%, 88%, 91% and 88%, respectively (Colin et al. 2020b).

3.3.4 Contrast Haemodynamics in the Main Pulmonary Artery on CTPA

In PH, vascular remodelling leads to changes in haemodynamics through the pulmonary vascular bed. As mPAP and PVR rise, the increased backpressure at the prearteriolar level leads to delayed transit and pooling of blood in the MPA. This can be assessed on imaging by finding a greater relative peak of contrast in the MPA in PH patients when compared to healthy subjects (Altschul et al. 2019).

When using bolus tracking techniques to trigger the start of the scan on a CTPA, the peak density of contrast in the MPA and the aorta can be quantified using regions of interest placed in both vessels. A peak contrast density ratio between the MPA and aorta of 1.5 or more is a strong predictor of PH with a sensitivity of 88.5% and specificity of 79.2% (Siegel and Mirpuri 2014). This measurement is of particular value as, assuming bolus tracking is routinely performed, it is easily calculated on already available data without the need for additional radiation, contrast and only minimal user input.

The slow transit of contrast through the pulmonary vascular bed in PH also leads to delayed scan initiation (increased time to threshold) when using bolus tracking techniques in patients with PH. Time to threshold is defined as the time from the beginning of contrast injection to the contrast density in the MPA reaching a specific point. A time to threshold of ≥7.75 s for a contrast density of 100 HU has 80% sensitivity and 82% specificity for diagnosing PH (Davarpanah et al. 2011). Using time to threshold of ≥7.75 s and finding an MPA diameter of >27.6 mm in tandem increase the specificity for PH to 94% with a positive predictive value of 96%, although sensitivity declines to 75%. A time to threshold of ≥8.75 s has a sensitivity of 85% and specificity of 78% for diagnosing pulmonary hypertension *with* RV dilatation (Davarpanah et al. 2011). The latter measurement is of particular value as it can allow the radiologist to be more confident of reporting RV dilatation even if the scan is degraded by motion.

3.3.5 Vessel Tortuosity and Distance Metric

Tortuosity is a measure of twistedness of vessels and is a well-documented sequela of hypertension and vasculopathy in any arterial circulation (Han 2012). *Subjectively* increased tortuosity of the peripheral pulmonary arterial tree on CTPA is a recognised but soft radiological sign of pulmonary hypertension; this can also be quantified. Of note, this is best measured on inspiratory CT as scans obtained in expiration may show normal, increased tortuosity of vessel, particularly in the lower lobes. The most common method of quantifying vascular tortuosity is the "distance metric", which provides a ratio of the actual vessel path length to the linear distance between its endpoints (Smedby et al. 1993). In essence, the higher the distance metric, the more bending in a vessel as it courses between two points.

Advanced software, currently in use in the pre-clinical setting, allows rapid, automated segmentation and calculation of the tortuosity of the pulmonary vascular tree (Helmberger et al. 2014). A significant correlation exists between increased tortuosity of the pulmonary vascular tree and PH with a distance metric of >1.213 having a sensitivity and specificity of 83% for diagnosing PH on CT. Moreover, there is also a good correlation between distance metric and mPAP, PVR and WHO functional status (Helmberger et al. 2014).

Initial studies on the assessment of distance metric show promise although the current data pool remains small, the software has not reached widespread clinical use nor has it been externally validated. Nevertheless, it is an automated measurement that requires no user intervention and can therefore be run on thoracic CTs/CTPAs without additional data acquisition and no additional workload for the radiologist opening up a promising avenue for assessment of the presence of PH and potentially, assessing prognosis and response to treatment.

3.3.6 Dual-Energy CTPA

In recent years, CT systems capable of dual energy CT (DECT) imaging have become increasingly common although widespread clinical implementation remains limited due to cost. Using dual-source systems or highly responsive detector materials that allow rapid switching between different kilovoltages (kV) from a single source, near simultaneous acquisition of volumetric datasets of varying kV is now possible (Johnson et al. 2007). Dual energy scanning exploits the difference in photoelectric absorption of iodinated contrast media at different energy levels to derive the iodine content in each voxel imaged. This data can then be used to provide a map of pulmonary blood volume (PBV), which is a surrogate indicator of pulmonary perfusion (Johnson et al. 2007; Ameli-Renani et al. 2014). The main interest of DECT in PH is in CTEPH, where derived perfusion maps help quantify regional blood flow and assess perfusion defects due to both proximal and distal disease, giving information regarding the proximal and distal extents of disease burden, guiding potential surgical intervention and following up post-operative patients.

In PH, PBV can be formally quantified using commercially available software. The software quantifies PBV by measuring the enhancement of lung parenchyma relative to a reference point in a central vessel, usually the pulmonary trunk on axial images. PBV is then calculated as:

$$\text{PBV} = \left(\text{mean enhancement of lung parenchyma in HU} / \text{mean enhancement of reference point in HU}\right) \times \text{calibration factor } 0.15$$

Lung isolation and partitioning into right/left and upper/middle/lower is automatically performed and PBV is displayed for each region.

Global PBV is reduced in patients with CTEPH-PH, and PBV inversely correlates with both sPAP ($R = -0.64$, $p = 0.001$) and mPAP ($r = -0.57$, $p = 0.004$) (Meinel et al. 2013). Larger studies giving more robust data are needed to truly assess the importance of assessing PBV on DECT and to define precise PBV values below, which PH can be diagnosed with confidence and the implications on prognosis. Nevertheless, automated quantification of PBV requires little user input while offering quick results, and there is tremendous scope for further research in this area.

The iodine maps derived from DECT can also be used to assess, qualitatively and semi-quantitatively, iodine content and, therefore, collateral blood flow via bronchial arteries to lung segments with occluded pulmonary arteries. CTEPH patients with enlarged bronchial arteries bypassing occluded bronchial arteries and providing collateral flow to the lung have reduced mortality post-pulmonary thromboendarterectomy than patients without collateral flow (Kauczor et al. 1994). No established thresholds exist for what constitutes good collateral flow on DECT to guide surgeons re the utility of intervention, and future work in DECT should also focus on assessing such thresholds as well as predicting haemodynamic response post-surgery.

4 Magnetic Resonance Imaging in Pulmonary Hypertension

Cardiac MRI and contrast-enhanced MR pulmonary angiography are powerful tools with several advantages over CT and echocardiography in the work-up of patients with suspected PH. MRI allows reproducible and accurate dynamic assessment of flow parameters in the pulmonary vascular tree that are challenging to obtain on echocardiography, primarily due to the frequently poor echo-windows to the pulmonary vasculature. Cardiac MRI is considered the gold standard for the evaluation of RV volumes, function and mass due to high definition of the blood pool-myocardium interface, reproducibility and the fact that, unlike echocardiography, no geometric assumptions are required (Pennell et al. 2004; Peña et al. 2012). Moreover, MRI is largely unaffected by body habitus, lung disease and chest wall deformity. The lack of ionising radiation in MRI is of value as it allows repeated examinations without accumulating radiation exposure.

4.1 Pulmonary Vascular Measurements on MRI

4.1.1 Pulmonary Artery Diameter

Main and branch pulmonary artery diameters can be assessed on MRI using axial black blood imaging, white blood steady-state free precession (SSFP) imaging or MR angiography. Diameters are measured from outer wall to outer wall in the axial plane or if 3-d data is obtained, through double oblique reconstructions at the MPA and branch pulmonary arteries. Although no studies have been performed specifically correlating pulmonary arterial diameters on MRI with mPAP and PVR, the values quoted for CT are likely to hold true for MRI. Therefore, in the appropriate clinical and radiological context, an MPA diameter of >29 mm and an MPA:ascending aortic diameter of >1 are both suggestive of PH.

4.1.2 Pulmonary Artery Area

In PH, the progressive distention of the pulmonary arterial tree leads to an increase in the minimal cross-sectional area of the MPA, reduction in the compliance of the pulmonary vascular bed and increased wall stiffening. Pulmonary artery stiffness, which is inversely proportional to vessel distensibility (Reiter et al. 2016), is associated with RV dysfunction and increased mortality in PH (Gan et al. 2007; Swift et al. 2012a; Stevens et al. 2012; Sanz et al. 2009); therefore, assessing vessel distensibility or relative area change is an important MR parameter in the evaluation of PH.

Minimal and maximal CSA of the MPA can be assessed on MRI by segmenting the vessel area throughout the cardiac cycle. A cross section through the MPA is acquired as outlined in Fig. 22. Commercially available software allows the semi-automated contouring of ROIs defining the area of a cross section of the MPA. The minimum area (A_{min}) occurs in diastole and the maximal area occurs in systole (A_{max}). MPA distensibility is defined by area change (AC), i.e. $A_{max} - A_{min}$, and by relative area change (RAC), i.e. $(A_{max} - A_{min})/A_{min}$ (Reiter et al. 2016).

Regardless of the underlying cause for PH, there is robust data correlating both an increased A_{min} as well as reduced RAC (and therefore distensibility) with PH. An A_{min} ≥6.0 cm² can identify an mPAP ≥25 mmHg with a sensitivity of 88% and specificity of 66% and a PVR >3 WU with a sensitivity of 96% and specificity of 85%. Increasing the threshold to A_{min} ≥6.6 cm² diagnoses PH with a sensitivity of 93% and specificity of 88% (Sanz et al. 2009; Swift et al. 2012b). An RAC <15% shows good sensitivity (84%) and

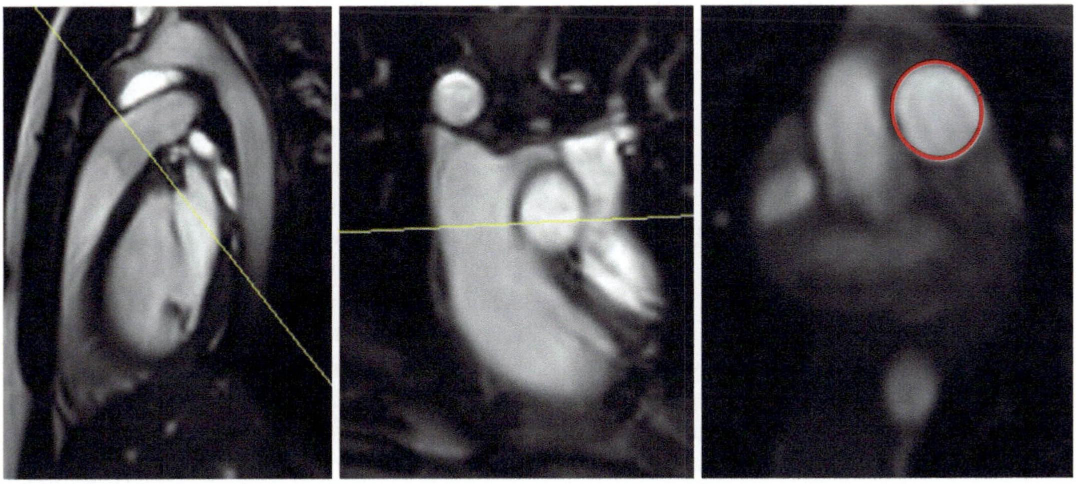

Fig. 22 The first two pictures show still images from cines acquired in the longitudinal plane through the RVOT and MPA. The yellow lines indicate the planning planes for acquisition of a cine of a true cross-section through the MPA, shown in the third picture in red

specificity (74%) for a diagnosis of PH with a positive predictive value of 94% (Swift et al. 2012b). Finally, RAC is also an important prognostic marker in PH with an RAC <15% an important predictor of mortality with a hazard ratio of 0.85, $p = 0.03$ (Swift et al. 2012b).

4.1.3 Pulmonary Artery Flow

ECG-gated black blood imaging is a technique that nulls the signal from flowing blood using a dual-inversion recovery, fast spin echo sequence. Axial, ECG- and respiratory-gated black blood imaging through the chest is routinely performed in cardiac MRI to plan further sequences as well as to assess thoracic and cardiac anatomy. Good signal suppression is achieved in fast-flowing blood, for instance, in the aorta. Signal suppression is less effective in areas of slower or more turbulent blood flow with intraluminal high signal at these areas such as at the bifurcation of vessels and in the pulmonary arteries of patients with PH (von Schulthess 1985). In PH, the slow-flowing blood in the proximal pulmonary vasculature and resultant artefact is thought to occur as a result of the decreased cardiac output secondary to elevated PVR and RV dysfunction.

The severity of pulmonary blood flow artefact (PFA) on axial black-blood MR images can be assessed using a visual, semi-quantitative scoring system (Swift et al. 2012c). The presence of PFA in the pulmonary arterial tree is scored as below and as shown in Fig. 23:

Segmental vessels = 1
Lobar vessels = 2
Distal right/left main vessels = 3
Proximal right/left main vessels = 4
Pulmonary trunk = 5

No PFA is assigned a score of 0. The total PFA score is the average of the PFA scores of the right and left pulmonary vessels.

A total PFA score of >1 can diagnose PH with a sensitivity of 86% and specificity of 85%. Additionally, a PFA score >2.5 is a predictor of mortality in PH patients. Higher PFA scores also correlate directly with mPAP ($r = 0.65$, $p < 0.0001$) and PVR ($r = 0.70$, $p < 0.0001$) and negatively with cardiac index ($r = -0.53$, $p < 0.0001$) (Swift et al. 2012c).

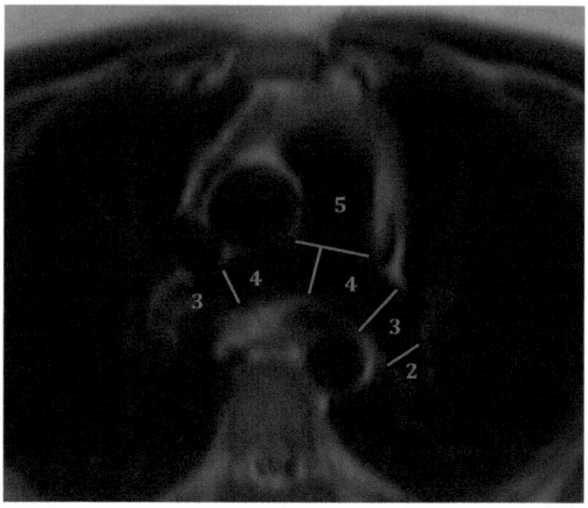

Fig. 23 Image from an axial black blood sequence through the chest at the level of the MPA. There is flow artefact in the distal right main pulmonary artery giving a score of 3. Schematic representation of scores 2–5 is also shown (a score of 1 is not shown—this corresponds to segmental pulmonary artery flow artefact)

4.1.4 Flow Velocity Assessment

Phase contrast MRI (PC-MRI) is used to measure blood flow and intravascular velocities and can therefore be used as a surrogate marker for cardiac output and stroke volume. The standard 2-D phase contrast technique, with single-direction velocity encoding along the through-plane direction, is a valuable tool in the assessment of PH.

As a vessel dilates, a decrease in flow velocities in the vessel is typically seen—decreased blood flow velocities in the MPA in PH patients have consequently been widely described (Reiter et al. 2016). While reduced peak MPA velocities correlate only moderately with mPAP and PVR, mean MPA velocity correlates strongly with mPAP ($r = -0.73$) and PVR ($r = -0.86$) and is a promising marker for the non-invasive diagnosis of PH (Sanz et al. 2007). A mean MPA flow velocity of <11.7 cm/s identifies an mPAP of ≥25 mmHg with a sensitivity and specificity of 93% and 82%, respectively, and a PVR of >3 WU with a sensitivity and specificity of 91% and 93%, respectively (Sanz et al. 2007).

The flow velocity waveform on phase-contrast imaging is also of value in the diagnosis of PH. A prominent characteristic of the MPA flow velocity waveform in PH patients is an abnormal mid-systolic velocity deceleration or notch, with the notch occurring slightly earlier in systole in CTEPH than in PAH (Castelain et al. 2001). Interestingly, in the majority of CTEPH patients post-pulmonary endarterectomy, the notch disappears as flow velocities in the MPA normalise, although this has not yet been shown to correlate with long-term outcomes (Rolf et al. 2015). A rapid upstroke indicating a shorter time interval from the beginning of anterograde flow to peak systolic flow correlates with mPAP >40 mmHg, while a ratio of maximal change in flow rate during ejection to acceleration volume is strongly correlated with a PVR of ≥6 mm WU (Tardivon et al. 1994; Mousseaux et al. 1999) although neither of these parameters are routinely quantified in clinical practice.

4.1.5 Flow Volume Assessment

The blood volume flow through the MPA in the cardiac cycle (Qp) reflects the RVSV minus, if present, any tricuspid regurgitant flow and therefore, the flow through the pulmonary circulation per heartbeat. Multiplying by heart rate allows calculation of RV cardiac output and RV cardiac index. These measures directly correspond with those measured at RHC, and studies with simultaneous PC-MRI and RHC in PH patients have shown good agreement between both modalities (Reiter et al. 2016; Kreitner et al. 2013).

Assessing flow volume also plays an important role in the evaluation of cardiac shunts which are an important cause of PH. Systemic and coronary flow (Qs) can be assessed in a similar method to pulmonary flow by placing an ROI over the ascending aorta with minimal time delay to the pulmonary flow measurement (Nayak et al. 2015). In the absence of significant shunting and employing velocity-offset corrections for both values, pulmonary and systemic flow should be roughly equal with a Qp:Qs ratio of approximately 1 for both adults and children (0.98–1.05) (Rigsby et al. 2014; Chernobelsky et al. 2007; Holland et al. 2010). Current guidelines recommend assessing Qp:Qs in the workup of all PH patients to ensure no atrial septal defect or anomalous pulmonary venous drainage is present as causes for PH.

4.2 Cardiac Measurements on MRI

4.2.1 RA Size

Elevated RA pressure reflects the increased RV afterload in PH. Elevated RA pressure and increased RA size on echocardiography are important predictors of mortality in PH (Querejeta Roca et al. 2015; Raymond et al. 2002). No similar data is available linking RA size on MRI to outcomes, but the routine measurement of RA size on MRI at baseline and on follow-up studies in PH patients is nevertheless of clinical importance.

Atrial remodelling is most accurately measured by assessing atrial volumes; however, in practice, this is rarely done. 2-D atrial measurements are reliable, easier and quicker to obtain in the clinical setting and are therefore more commonly used in cardiac MRI. Atrial parameters on MRI are measured on the 4-chamber (horizontal long axis) view in the phase of the cardiac cycle where atrial size is largest. Atrial area is measured by drawing a region of interest outlining the endocardium of the right atrium, excluding the inferior vena cava (Fig. 24). Atrial diameter is measured in two planes—longitudinal diameter is obtained from the posterior wall of the right atrium to the centre of the tricuspid plane, and transverse diameter is obtained perpendicular to the longitudinal diameter, at the mid level of the right atrium. Measurement of atrial diameters is shown in Fig. 25. Normal RA size ranges are given in Table 5.

4.2.2 Interventricular Septum Position

The physiological position of the IVS is convex to the right. As previously discussed, with increasing mPAP and RV pressures, the IVS initially flattens and eventually, bows towards the LV.

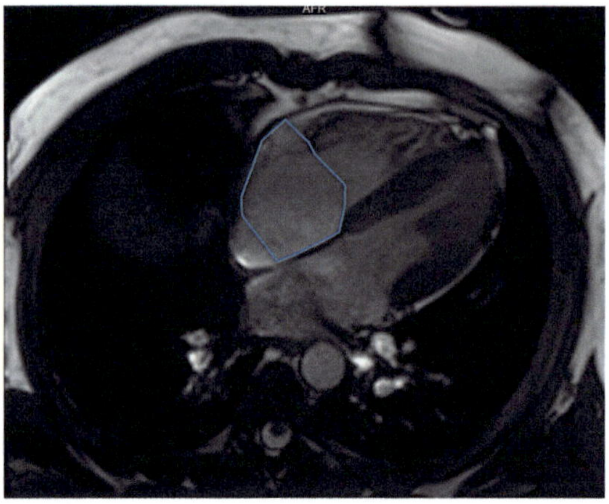

Fig. 24 Four-chamber view showing the measurement of RA area. Atrial area is measured by drawing a free-hand or polygonal region of interest outlining the endocardium of the right atrium, excluding the inferior vena cava

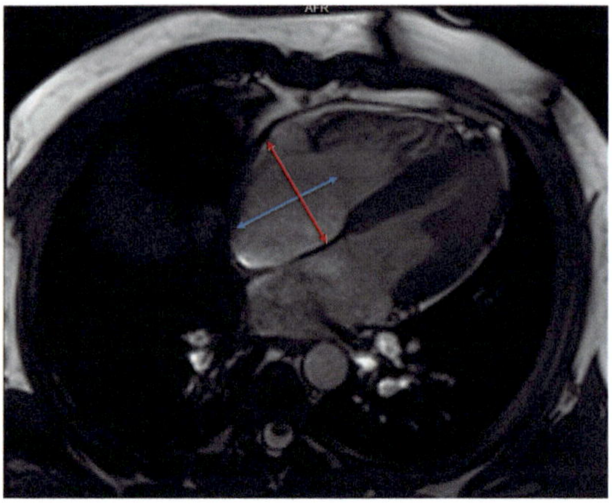

Fig. 25 Four-chamber view showing the measurement of RA longitudinal (blue line) and transverse (red line) diameters. Longitudinal diameter is obtained from the posterior wall of the right atrium to the centre of the tricuspid plane, and transverse diameter is obtained perpendicular to the longitudinal diameter, at the mid level of the right atrium

Table 5 Normal right atrial size (mean, lower/upper limits) (Maceira et al. 2013)

	All	Male	Female
Area (cm^2)	22 (15, 30)	24 (15, 33)	20 (15, 26)
Area/BSA (cm^2/m^2)	12 (8, 15)	12 (8, 16)	12 (9, 15)
Longitudinal diameter (cm)	5.5 (4.3, 6.6)	5.6 (4.6, 6.7)	5.3 (4.3, 6.4)
Longitudinal diameter/ BSA (cm/m^2)	3.0 (2.4, 3.6)	2.9 (2.5, 3.3)	3.1 (2.6, 3.6)
Transverse diameter (cm)	4.7 (3.7, 5.8)	5.0 (3.7, 6.4)	4.5 (3.6, 5.4)
Transverse diameter/BSA (cm/m^2)	2.6 (2.0, 3.2)	2.6 (1.9, 3.3)	2.6 (2.2, 3.1)

The position of the IVS is best assessed on short-axis images at the mid ventricular level (at the level of the papillary muscles of the LV). Flattening of the IVS in diastole is an early marker of PH and leads to impaired diastolic LV filling and reduced LV cardiac output. The degree of flattening and eventual IVS bowing to the left correlates well with severity of PH ($r = 0.77$, $p < 0.001$): above an sPAP of 67 mmHg, IVS bowing to the left is expected (Roeleveld et al. 2005; Dellegrottaglie et al. 2007). The point in the cardiac cycle at which the bowing occurs also correlates with the severity of PH. In a study performed in 43 patients with RHC-proven PH, an abnormal IVS position in *diastole only* was found in patients with a median (interquartile range [IQR]) mPAP of 37 (21–43) mmHg and PVR of 4.5 (2.3–6.5) WU, while an abnormal IVS position in *both systole and diastole* was found in patients with a median (IQR) mPAP of 43 (40–49) mmHg and PVR of 8.0 (5.7–10.6) WU (Alunni et al. 2010).

The degree of flattening of the IVS can be measured quantitatively as the IVS angle. This is measured on short-axis cine images as the angle formed between the insertion points of the ventricles and the midpoint of the septum at the point of maximal septal displacement (Fig. 26). When measured in systole, an IVS angle of >160° can diagnose PH with a sensitivity of 67% and speci-

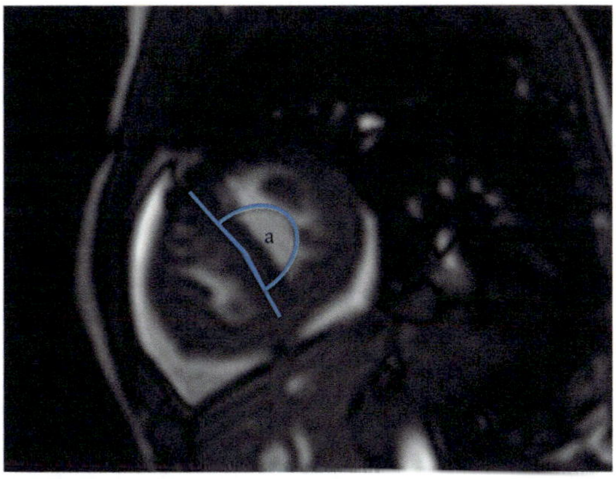

Fig. 26 Still from a short axis cine through the left ventricle at mid ventricular level. The interventricular septal angle is measured as the angle formed between the insertion points of the ventricles to the midpoint of the septum at the point of maximal septal displacement

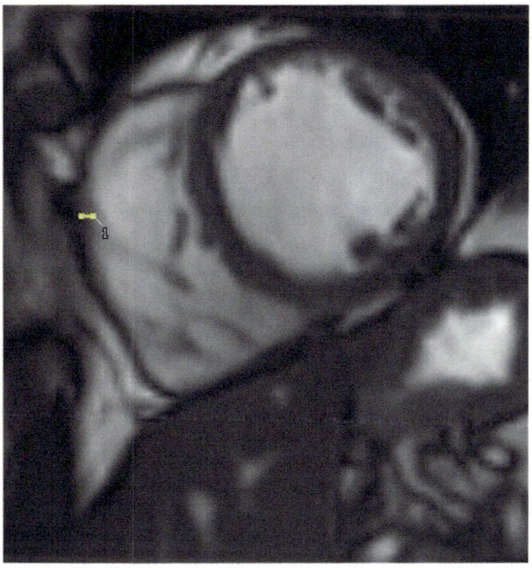

Fig. 27 Short-axis image at the mid ventricular level showing measurement of RV wall measured in end-diastole as the shortest distance between endocardium and epicardium

ficity of 93%. Additionally, an IVS angle of >160° is a marker of adverse outcomes predicting an increased risk of death within 2 years (Johns et al. 2018).

4.2.3 Right Ventricular Wall Thickness

As previously discussed, the initial RV remodelling response to PH is RV hypertrophy due to the increased afterload. RV thickness is measured in end-diastole as the shortest distance between endocardium and epicardium of the RV free wall on axial or short-axis images, where the RV appears thickest (Fig. 27). Trabeculae should not be included in the measurement. RV hypertrophy is diagnosed on MRI when myocardial thickness is >4 mm although more severe RV hypertrophy is diagnosed above a free wall thickness of >7 mm (Goerne et al. 2018; van Wolferen et al. 2007a). The severity of RV hypertrophy correlates with mPAP although RV thickness is not a predictor of mortality.

4.2.4 RV Mass and Ventricular Mass Index

In chronic PH, increased RV mass, representing underlying RV hypertrophy, is a frequent finding. An elevated ventricular mass index (VMI) is also a frequent finding in PH where VMI defines the ratio of RV mass:LV mass. In essence, VMI is a form of internal normalisation of RV mass against LV mass (which does not hypertrophy in PH) with all other variables such as age, gender, BMI, conditioning being equal.

Assessing RV mass (and LV mass for the calculation of VMI) can be performed on short-axis or axial stack images. The respective masses are calculated by outlining RV and LV endo- and epicardial contours using commercially available semi-automated software. RV mass is significantly affected by the inclusion or exclusion of trabeculae and papillary muscles as part of the myocardium (Kawel-Boehm et al. 2015). Excluding the trabeculae and papillary muscles from RV mass results in higher reproducibility; however, it is less accurate at measuring the true mass. Regardless of which method is used for the RV, the same method should then be used for the LV.

RV mass is elevated in PH patients but correlates only weakly with mPAP ($r = 0.56$). The normal values for RV mass are given in Table 6. There is a far stronger correlation between mPAP and VMI ($r = 0.81$) and a VMI of >0.6 diagnoses PH with a sensitivity of 84% and specificity of 71% (Saba et al. 2002; Katz et al. 1993).

RV mass and VMI are particularly promising indices in the work up of PH as they do not reflect

Table 6 Right ventricular mass and indexed mass by age and gender [mean ± SD (lower/upper limits)] (Kawel-Boehm et al. 2015)

	Men		Women	
Age	<60	>60	<60	>60
RVM (g)	68 ± 14 (40, 96)	63 ± 14 (35, 91)	50 ± 11 (28, 72)	44 ± 11 (22, 66)
RVM/BSA (g/m^2)	35 ± 7 (29, 49)	32 ± 7 (18, 46)	30 ± 5 (20, 40)	25 ± 5 (15, 35)

RVM right ventricular mass, *BSA* body surface area

a one-off measurement of a parameter that varies significantly in the short term but rather, are measures of long-term remodelling. They are also of value in assessing response to treatment. The main drawback of these measurements is that outlining RV epi- and endocardial contours is time-consuming and technically challenging, particularly where RV myocardium is thin. More advanced software packages have made this a more efficient process in recent years although there is still scope for improvement.

4.2.5 Semi Quantitative Assessment of RV Function

Semi-quantitative assessment of RV function may be useful in cardiac MRI (CMRI) if formal quantification on short-axis or axial imaging is not possible due to poor image quality, technical issues or aborted scans due to claustrophobia. The main driver of RV function is longitudinal shortening. Assessing the degree of excursion of the lateral tricuspid annular plane between end-diastole and end-systole, i.e. TAPSE, is useful.

Measurement of TAPSE has been described above (see Sect. 3.2.4). On MRI, a TAPSE above 23 mm is normal (Bulluck et al. 2014), while values between 18 and 23 mm suggest mild RV systolic impairment. A TAPSE of <18 mm is a strong indicator of RV dysfunction with TAPSE of <10 mm suggestive of severe dysfunction and adverse outcomes (Forfia et al. 2006; Goerne et al. 2018).

4.2.6 Ventricular Volumes and Function

CMRI is the gold standard in measuring biventricular volumes and function, and these measurements provide valuable information in the work-up of suspected and follow-up of confirmed PH patients.

Ventricular volumes and function are measured on retrospective steady-state free precession (SSFP) cine imaging. In patients with arrhythmia, prospective imaging can be beneficial; this mildly underestimates the true end-diastolic volumes but usually not to a clinically significant degree. Images can be acquired in the short-axis or axial planes. The short axis plane is more commonly used as it allows accurate quantification of biventricular function using a single series of images. The caveat to this is that identification of the tricuspid plane in RV analysis can be challenging on short-axis views and requires some experience. Identification of the tricuspid plane and the RVOT/pulmonary valve interface is easier on axial images although this requires the acquisition of an additional set of SSFP images lengthening scanning time by at least 8–10 min.

Quantification of ventricular volumes and function is based on the semi-automated outlining of endocardial contours in end-diastole and end-systole and has been extensively described in the literature (Schulz-Menger et al. 2013). End-diastole is the image with the largest blood volume; end-systole is the image with the smallest blood volume. For end-diastolic and end-systolic image identification, the full image stack should be evaluated and the same phase chosen for all end-diastolic images and separately, end-systolic images. The pulmonary and aortic valves may be visualised, and endocardial volumes are included just up to but not above this level. Trabeculations are ignored and considered part of endocardial volume, and a smooth contour is drawn to improve reader reproducibility (Schulz-Menger et al. 2013). Total volumes are taken as the sum of volumes from individual 2D slices, accounting for any interslice gap and slice thickness.

Various reference ranges exist for normal ventricular volumes and function. The two largest patient cohorts are those evaluated by Foppa et al. in the Framingham Heart Study and those evaluated by Petersen et al. in the United Kingdom Biobank study. There is no worldwide consensus as to which reference range should be the standard with all references ranges having their drawbacks. The results published by Foppa et al. (2016) were based on a larger patient cohort ($n = 1336$); however, the participants in this study included patients with hypertension, diabetes, hypercholesterolaemia and those who were current smokers. The cohort analysed by Petersen et al. (2017) comprised less patients ($n = 804$) although all were free of cardiovascular disease but also of classic cardiovascular risk factors such as hypertension, smoking, diabetes and hypercholesterolaemia. In the authors' opinion, the ranges described by Petersen et al. are currently the most comprehensive and are listed in Tables 7, 8, 9 and 10.

Despite being the most comprehensive ranges currently available, the data does have certain limitations. First, RV volumes were calculated on short axis imaging. There is conflicting evidence that RV values derived on axial imaging may be more accurate with less inter-observer variability than those derived on short-axis imaging. On balance however, acquiring both axial and short-axis images is time-consuming particularly if patients are short of breath and unable to lie flat for long periods and in experienced hands, assessing RV function on short-axis imaging is sufficiently accurate, particularly in patients without complex congenital heart disease (Kawel-Boehm et al. 2015; Schulz-Menger et al. 2013; Alfakih et al. 2003a; James et al. 2013). Another limitation to the above dataset is that the study cohort comprised a Caucasian-only population aged 45–74. To our knowledge, no large-scale study using SSFP-imaging in multi-ethnic populations has been performed thus far so, in the absence of such data, using the above ranges would be acceptable. Studies have been performed for patients younger than 45 and older than 74 (Alfakih et al. 2003b; Hudsmith et al. 2005; Maceira et al. 2006; van der Ven et al. 2020); however, even the largest study by *Van der Ven* et al. included only 141 patients across all ages and more data is needed for these age groups.

RV size and function are critical barometers of cardiovascular health in PH. The degree of RV dysfunction is related to the severity of PH as

Table 7 Right ventricular reference ranges for males detailing mean, lower reference limit and upper reference limit by age group

	Age range								
	45–54			55–64			65–74		
	Lower	Mean	Upper	Lower	Mean	Upper	Lower	Mean	Upper
RVEDV (mL)	124	192	260	109	181	252	99	173	248
RVESV (mL)	47	91	135	42	82	123	34	81	129
RVSV (mL)	62	101	140	60	98	136	54	92	131
RVEDVi (mL/m^2)	68	97	126	56	92	128	55	90	125
RVESVi (mL/m^2)	25	46	67	21	42	63	19	42	66
RVSVi (mL/m^2)	34	51	68	31	50	69	30	48	67
RVEF (%)	40	53	65	45	55	65	40	54	68

Reference limits are derived by the upper and lower bounds of the 95% prediction interval for each parameter at each age group

RVEDV right ventricular end-diastolic volume, *RVESV* right ventricular end-systolic volume, *RVSV* right ventricular stroke volume, *RVEDVi* right ventricular end-diastolic volume indexed to BSA, *RVESVi* right ventricular end-systolic volume indexed to BSA, *RVSVi* right ventricular stroke volume indexed to BSA, *RVEF* right ventricular ejection fraction

Table 8 Right ventricular reference ranges for females detailing mean, lower reference limit and upper reference limit by age group

	Age range								
	45–54			55–64			65–74		
	Lower	Mean	Upper	Lower	Mean	Upper	Lower	Mean	Upper
RVEDV (mL)	85	138	192	83	125	168	84	128	171
RVESV (mL)	27	61	95	27	52	77	26	54	82
RVSV (mL)	48	78	107	47	73	100	48	74	99
RVEDVi (mL/m^2)	53	81	110	51	75	99	53	77	101
RVESVi (mL/m^2)	17	36	55	16	31	46	17	32	48
RVSVi (mL/m^2)	30	46	61	29	44	59	30	44	59
RVEF (%)	45	56	68	47	59	70	46	58	70

Reference limits are derived by the upper and lower bounds of the 95% prediction interval for each parameter at each age group

RVEDV right ventricular end-diastolic volume, *RVESV* right ventricular end-systolic volume, *RVSV* right ventricular stroke volume, *RVEDVi* right ventricular end-diastolic volume indexed to BSA, *RVESVi* right ventricular end-systolic volume indexed to BSA, *RVSVi* right ventricular stroke volume indexed to BSA, *RVEF* right ventricular ejection fraction

Table 9 Left ventricular reference ranges for males detailing mean, lower reference limit and upper reference limit by age group

	Age range								
	45–54			55–64			65–74		
	Lower	Mean	Upper	Lower	Mean	Upper	Lower	Mean	Upper
LVEDV (mL)	109	170	232	108	169	230	93	156	218
LVESV (mL)	39	71	103	39	71	102	34	66	97
LVSV (mL)	58	99	140	59	98	137	49	90	132
LVEDVi (mL/m^2)	60	86	112	55	86	117	52	81	110
LVESVi (mL/m^2)	21	36	51	20	36	52	19	34	49
LVSVi (mL/m^2)	32	50	68	30	50	70	28	47	67
LVEF (%)	47	58	70	48	58	69	47	58	69

Reference limits are derived by the upper and lower bounds of the 95% prediction interval for each parameter at each age group

LVEDV left ventricular end-diastolic volume, *LVESV* left ventricular end-systolic volume, *LVSV* left ventricular stroke volume, *LVEDVi* left ventricular end-diastolic volume indexed to BSA, *LVESVi* left ventricular end-systolic volume indexed to BSA, *LVSVi* left ventricular stroke volume indexed to BSA, *LVEF* left ventricular ejection fraction

well as the symptomatic class. An increased RV volume is a predictor of poor survival. *Progressive* RV dilatation is an even stronger predictor of poor survival, and this is potentially of greater clinical importance—increasing RV dilatation despite treatment is a direct predictor of treatment failure and offers an important opportunity to change treatment or list patients for transplantation (van Wolferen et al. 2007a). Reduced stroke volume (i.e. <30–34 mL/m^2 for males and <29–30 mL/m^2 for females, depending on age range) on MRI at baseline, as well as at one year following the initiation of treatment, is also predictive of poor survival in PH, whilst a stroke vol-

Table 10 Left ventricular reference ranges for females detailing mean, lower reference limit and upper reference limit by age group

	Age range								
	45–54			55–64			65–74		
	Lower	Mean	Upper	Lower	Mean	Upper	Lower	Mean	Upper
LVEDV (mL)	88	131	175	80	121	161	81	122	163
LVESV (mL)	31	52	73	26	47	68	25	48	70
LVSV (mL)	49	79	110	47	74	100	47	74	100
LVEDVi (mL/m^2)	54	78	101	50	72	94	50	73	96
LVESVi (mL/m^2)	19	31	43	16	28	40	16	29	42
LVSVi (mL/m^2)	30	47	63	29	44	59	29	45	60
LVEF (%)	50	60	70	51	61	72	50	61	72

Reference limits are derived by the upper and lower bounds of the 95% prediction interval for each parameter at each age group

LVEDV left ventricular end-diastolic volume, *LVESV* left ventricular end-systolic volume, *LVSV* left ventricular stroke volume, *LVEDVi* left ventricular end-diastolic volume indexed to BSA, *LVESVi* left ventricular end-systolic volume indexed to BSA, *LVSVi* left ventricular stroke volume indexed to BSA, *LVEF* left ventricular ejection fraction

ume of <25 mL/m^2 for both males and females is strongly suggestive of a poor prognosis (van Wolferen et al. 2007a).

A decreased LVEDV is a marker of impaired LV diastolic filling and is also a strong predictor of poor survival in PH patients. Impaired LV filling may be a result of a reduced RVSV or due to compression of the LV by a dilated RV. Since both reduced RVSV and increased RVEDV are strong predictors of adverse outcome and mortality in PH patients, it is understandable that a low LVEDV at baseline or a decrease in LVEDV despite treatment is also poor prognostic marker in PH (van Wolferen et al. 2007a).

4.3 Advanced MRI Imaging Techniques

In addition to the conventional measurements described above, more advanced MR imaging techniques allow assessment of multiple parameters related to blood flow topology, pulse wave propagation and contrast kinetics. Most of these measurements were defined in specific patient groups in single-centre studies, and therefore, their applicability to routine clinical practice requires further investigation; however, the data shows significant promise, even beyond RHC.

4.3.1 Vortical and Retrograde Flow in the MPA

Early studies, both on echocardiography and PC-MRI, showed a heterogeneous flow profile in the MPA when mPAP exceeded 16 mmHg with retrograde flow in mid-to-end systole (Kondo et al. 1992). The origin of this retrograde flow was later clarified using 3-d time-resolved PC-MRI, which showed the presence of a vortex of blood flow in the MPA, with forward flow in the ventral side and reverse flow in the dorsal side of the vessel (Reiter et al. 2008; Helderman et al. 2011). The duration of the vortical flow in the MPA relative to the duration of the cardiac cycle (t_{vortex}) has been found to be related to mPAP.

A recently proposed model assessing vortical flow is based on the acquisition of retrospectively gated, segmented, 2-d, spoiled-gradient-echo–based cine PC sequence with 3-d velocity encoding by a four-point velocity encoding scheme acquired in free-breathing in the RVOT plane and a multi-directional velocity encoding set to 90 cm/s (adjusted in case of aliasing). Dedicated software is used to extract the data acquired to derive and view time-resolved, 3-d velocity fields allowing analysis of vortical flow direction, velocity and duration. The model defines a linear correlation between the duration of vortical flow in the MPA and mPAP, where $t_{vortex} = 0\%$ of the cardiac cycle correlates with an mPAP of 16 mmHg. Linear, segmented increases in t_{vortex} are seen with increasing mPAP with a gradient of 1.59% per mmHg (Reiter et al. 2015). Using this model, vortical blood flow in the MPA lasting for >14.3% of the cardiac cycle can diagnose PH with sensitivity of 97% and specificity of 96%.

Data also shows that retrograde flow in the MPA (which, if of sufficient volume and velocity, contributes to the formation of a vortex) is seen at earlier points in the cardiac cycle in PH compared to healthy subjects. Similar data sets to those acquired above can be used to assess the time of onset of retrograde flow (rROT) in the MPA relative to the cardiac cycle. An rROT of ≤25% can distinguish patients with an mPAP of 25 mmHg from those with lower pulmonary artery pressures with a sensitivity and specificity of 100% (Helderman et al. 2011).

4.3.2 Pulse Wave Velocity

RV contraction ejects blood into the MPA creating a pressure wave which propagates through the pulmonary vasculature with pulse-wave velocity (PWV) (Reiter et al. 2016). An increase in PWV occurs when there is decreased compliance and distensibility of the pulmonary vasculature (Nayak et al. 2015), both of which are early markers of PH.

The PWV can be estimated using various techniques on MRI; the transit time (TT) method is one of these methods and is reliable and reproducible. In this approach, free-breathing, non-respiratory gated PC-imaging is used to assess the TT of the flow wave between two levels in the pulmonary vascular tree, usually the pulmonary trunk and proximal left/right pulmonary arteries. The distance between these two points is measured from anatomical MR data. The PWV is then defined by

$$\mathrm{PWV} = \Delta x / \Delta T$$

where Δx defines the distance between the two points and ΔT defines the time difference between onset of flow velocity at the respective points (Bradlow et al. 2007). The PWV in PH patients (5.2 ± 0.5 m s^{-1}) is more than double the PWV in healthy subjects (2.1 ± 0.6 and 2.3 ± 0.4 m s^{-1} between the mPA and the proximal left or right pulmonary artery, respectively) (Bradlow et al. 2007; Ibrahim et al. 2011). PWV is a promising parameter in PH; it can be assessed fairly rapidly and is a reproducible measurement; however, more data is needed before it can be applied to routine clinical practice.

4.3.3 First-Pass Bolus Kinetic Parameters

In patients with PH, the altered PVR and mPAP and the resultant deleterious effect on RV function slow pulmonary transit time of a contrast material bolus (Jones et al. 1972). Contrast-enhanced MRI can be used to assess kinetic parameters of a bolus of contrast as it travels from the right to the left ventricle via the pulmonary circulation.

On motion-corrected saturation-recovery gradient-echo images, ROIs are placed in the RV and LV cavities excluding myocardium, papillary muscle and trabeculations. Using dedicated software packages, time vs average signal intensity curves are generated for passage of the contrast material bolus through the RV and LV which are then used to calculate first-pass kinetic parameters.

Right-to-left ventricle PTT is calculated by subtracting the time of peak enhancement in the RV from that in the LV. LV full width at half maximum (FWHM) is defined as the width of the time-intensity curve at half its maximum signal intensity. LV time-to-peak (TTP) calculated as the time interval between the first appearance of the contrast material bolus (where *first appearance* is defined as the time of 20% peak signal intensity) and peak signal intensity can also be defined (Skrok et al. 2012).

The above parameters have only been measured in small study populations thus far. In healthy subjects in the largest population, median (IQR) PTT 6.4 s (5.7–7.1), FWHM 5.7 s (5.3–7.9) and TTP 3.2 s were significantly shorter than in patients with established PH (8.2 s (6.9–9.9),

9.0 s (6.6–12.3), 4.8 s (3.9–6.5)), for each parameter, respectively. The importance of this data in PH is that PTT, FWHM and TTP correlate with biventricular volumes and function, PVR, indexed PVR and mPAP as measured on RHC and established survival predictors including VMI and RV cardiac index (Skrok et al. 2012; Swift et al. 2014).

While highly promising, measurement parameters have several limitations. First, the calculation of these indices requires dedicated software which is not widely commercially available. Secondly, the analysis is fairly time-consuming requiring approximately 2–4 min of user-input per parameter. Thirdly, first pass kinetics have only been examined in small patient cohorts (Skrok et al. 2012; Sergiacomi et al. 2010; Lakoma et al. 2010), and studies confirming their validity in the follow-up of PH patients (which is where their true value probably lies) have not been performed. Finally, assessing these parameters requires the use of intravenous gadolinium-based contrast agents, with its inherent risks and contraindications, although this is likely to be a standard part of most MR examinations performed in routine clinical practice.

4.3.4 Non-invasive Quantitative Assessment of Pulmonary Vasculature Haemodynamics

The non-invasive estimation of mPAP and PVR is highly desirable for several reasons. RHC is an invasive and expensive investigation, not without its complications. Additionally, in severe PH, severe RV systolic dysfunction may give spuriously low measurements for mPAP and PVR giving the impression of an improving clinical course and false reassurance.

Using multivariate linear regression analysis, Swift et al. (2013) derived a formula based exclusively on MR-derived parameters to estimate mPAP non-invasively:

$$\text{CMR predicted MPAP} = -4.6 + (\text{IVS angle} \times 0.23) + (\text{VMI} \times 16.3)$$

IVS angle is measured as described above, i.e. the angle between the mid-point of the IVS and the two ventricular hinge points at the phase of maximal septal displacement on mid-chamber short-axis cine images. VMI is the ratio of RV mass:LV mass; measurement of VMI has also been described above.

Using the above, mPAP can be estimated with good correlation ($R = 0.7$, $p < 0.0001$) with invasively derived mPAP. The formula predicts an mPAP of ≥32 mmHg with 87% specificity and 90% sensitivity and has an area under the receiver operating characteristic (ROC) curve of 0.96 ($p < 0.0001$) for the detection of the presence of PH (Swift et al. 2013).

4.3.5 Right Ventricular Perfusion

An important component of progressive RV failure in PH is a decline in RV coronary perfusion (Freed et al. 2016; van Wolferen et al. 2007b). Right coronary artery (RCA) perfusion can be assessed using an established method (Marcus et al. 1999) which, summarily, involves obtaining axial localisers at the level of the ascending aorta to identify the origins of the left anterior descending (LAD) and RCA followed by an oblique localiser cutting a longitudinal section through the RCA. Phase contrast imaging with velocity encoding set at 40 cm/s is used for flow quantification with an image plane adjusted orthogonally to the longitudinal section of the RCA at ~20 mm from its origin.

Using this method, peak and mean systolic RCA flow can be assessed, and these are usually significantly decreased in PH patients with changes correlating inversely with RV mass and RV pressure (van Wolferen et al. 2007b). Semi-automated software packages can also be used to analyse ventricular perfusion under both stress and rest, with calculation of RV and LV myocardial perfusion maps and perfusion reverse indices. Reduced biventricular perfusion reverses are significantly correlated with increasing mPAP, decreasing RVEF and VMI (Vogel-Claussen et al. 2011). Additionally, PH patients have significantly lower RV at-rest myocardial blood flow per gram of myocardial tissue compared with the LV.

The implication of decreased RV perfusion on guiding treatment and on patient outcomes is unknown. However, decreased perfusion indices suggest microvascular dysfunction which is likely to be an important predictor of eventual RV failure. More data is needed to explore the importance of myocardial perfusion and create ranges to guide intervention and prognostication.

4.3.6 Dynamic Perfusion MRI

Pulmonary perfusion abnormalities, commonly found in patients with PH due to heterogeneity in the pulmonary vascular bed, were classically demonstrated using scintigraphy. More recently, due to advances in gradient systems and 3D gradient-recalled echo MR sequences with very short TR and TE (<3.0 ms and 1.0 ms, respectively), it has also become possible to assess global and regional pulmonary perfusion using MRI. The technique is based on rapid, sequential scans through the whole chest following the injection of a contrast bolus. The contrast kinetics through the lungs can then be assessed using dedicated software based on indicator dilution theory and fuzzy cluster analysis to derive quantitative pulmonary perfusion parameters, namely, pulmonary blood flow (PBF), mean transit time (MTT) and PBV.

In small studies performed on patients with PAH and connective tissue-related PH (Ohno et al. 2007, 2012), dynamic perfusion MRI demonstrated reduced PBF and increased MTT in patients with PH with a significant negative correlation between PBF and both mPAP and PVR and significant positive correlation between MTT and PVR. Dynamic perfusion MRI looks to be a promising technique with robust and reproducible scan parameters and reasonable scanning times and may play an increasingly prominent role in the work-up and follow-up of PH in the future but is currently limited by small pool of data and the experimental nature of software needed for analysis.

4.3.7 Native T1 Mapping

Native myocardial T1 mapping is a promising MRI technique where the *T1* relaxation times within a tissue are assessed on a pixel-by-pixel basis. Normal native *T1* times are elevated in the presence of oedema or collagen (scar tissue) in the extracellular space. An elevated *T1* value is therefore a marker for myocarditis, myocardial infarction, non-ischaemic cardiomyopathy and diastolic heart failure (Alabed et al. 2021).

Normal *T1* relaxation times are unique to individual scanner models and acquisition parameters; however, numerous studies have shown that patients with pulmonary hypertension have elevated native *T1* values relative to healthy controls on the same machines and using identical protocols. This is particularly true when measured at the RV insertion points into the interventricular septum with precapillary PH patients having a mean difference of 108 ms at these locations, significantly higher than patients with hypertrophic or dilated cardiomyopathies. Elevated *T1* values also correlate with increasing RV volumes and decreasing ventricular function. Additionally, one study performed on a small number of PH patients scanned on a 3.0-T MRI machine using a modified Look-Locker inversion-recovery pulse sequence showed that patients with very elevated native *T1* values, ≥1385 ms in this study, had significantly increased hospitalisation rates and lower survival compared with PH patients with less markedly elevated *T1* values (Alabed et al. 2021; Asano et al. 2021). This will require validation on future, larger datasets.

Inter- and intraobserver variability in the manual quantification of native *T1* values is good. Additionally, most current MRI analysis software packages have robust tools for the automatic quantification of native *T1* values with good reproducibility. The true value of native *T1* mapping may lie in the long-term follow-up of PH patients as the assessment of developing fibrosis, even before it manifests as visually appreciable late gadolinium enhancement may help alter management at an earlier stage. Unfortunately, reproducibility of native *T1* values between different scanners varies considerably even when using the same sequences and field strengths. This is particularly troublesome when a patient's care is transferred to another centre or if new machines are acquired. MRI harmonisation techniques have been proposed to reduce variability between scanners although these have not been widely implemented thus far. Despite these limitations, there is hope that *T1* mapping will become a mainstream technique in cardiac MRI in the near future and serve as an important diagnostic, therapeutic and prognostic decision-making tool.

5 Conclusion

Despite advances in treatment options and improved survival in recent years, pulmonary hypertension remains a common disease with considerable morbidity and mortality. Importantly, it is a challenging diagnosis to make requiring invasive and expensive right heart catheterisation. This chapter has described important measurements on both CT and MRI, which may help make an earlier diagnosis of PH, guide response to treatment and contribute towards overall improved patient outcomes.

Disclaimer All measurements in this book have been obtained from peer-reviewed papers and guidelines from professional organizations, unless explicitly stated otherwise. While the authors, editors, and publisher have gone through a rigorous process to establish their correct reproduction from the original source, each measurement must be interpreted in the correct clinical context, this along with an accurate way of measurement, and taking into account all technical variables, this including follow-up exams with various equipment or software. Neither the authors, the editors, nor the publisher can accept any legal responsibility for any improper application or interpretation of these measurements as well as their potential consequences.

References

Ackman Haimovici JB, Trotman-Dickenson B, Halpern EF, Dec GW, Ginns LC, Shepard JAO et al (1997) Relationship between pulmonary artery diameter at computed tomography and pulmonary artery pressures at right-sided heart catheterization. Acad Radiol 4(5):327–334

Alabed S, Saunders L, Garg P, Shahin Y, Alandejani F, Rolf A et al (2021) Myocardial T1-mapping and extracellular volume in pulmonary arterial hypertension: a systematic review and meta-analysis. Magn Reson Imaging 79:66–75

Alfakih K, Plein S, Bloomer T, Jones T, Ridgway J, Sivananthan M (2003a) Comparison of right ventricular volume measurements between axial and short axis orientation using steady-state free precession magnetic resonance imaging. J Magn Reson Imaging 18(1):25–32

Alfakih K, Plein S, Thiele H, Jones T, Ridgway JP, Sivananthan MU (2003b) Normal human left and right ventricular dimensions for MRI as assessed by turbo gradient echo and steady-state free precession imaging sequences. J Magn Reson Imaging 17(3):323–329

Alhamad EH, Al-Boukai AA, Al-Kassimi FA, Alfaleh HF, Alshamiri MQ, Alzeer AH et al (2011) Prediction of pulmonary hypertension in patients with or without interstitial lung disease: reliability of CT findings. Radiology 260(3):875–883

Altschul E, Remy-Jardin M, Machnicki S, Sulica R, Moore JA, Singh A et al (2019) Imaging of pulmonary hypertension: pictorial essay. Chest 156(2):211–227

Alunni JP, Degano B, Arnaud C, Tétu L, Blot-Soulétie N, Didier A et al (2010) Cardiac MRI in pulmonary artery hypertension: correlations between morphological and functional parameters and invasive measurements. Eur Radiol 20(5):1149–1159

Ameli-Renani S, Rahman F, Nair A, Ramsay L, Bacon JL, Weller A et al (2014) Dual-energy CT for imaging of pulmonary hypertension: challenges and opportunities. Radiographics 34(7):1769–1790

Asano R, Ogo T, Morita Y, Kotoku A, Aoki T, Hirakawa K et al (2021) Prognostic value of right ventricular native T1 mapping in pulmonary arterial hypertension. PLoS One 16(11):e0260456

Bax S, Jacob J, Ahmed R, Bredy C, Dimopoulos K, Kempny A et al (2020) Right ventricular to left ventricular ratio at CT pulmonary angiogram predicts mortality in interstitial lung disease. Chest 157(1):89–98

Bellenger NG, Burgess MI, Ray SG, Lahiri A, Coats AJS, Cleland JGF et al (2000) Comparison of left ventricular ejection fraction and volumes in heart failure by echocardiography, radionuclide ventriculography and cardiovascular magnetic resonance. Are they interchangeable? Eur Heart J 21(16):1387–1396

Boerrigter B, Mauritz GJ, Marcus JT, Helderman F, Postmus PE, Westerhof N et al (2010) Progressive dilatation of the main pulmonary artery is a characteristic of pulmonary arterial hypertension and is not related to changes in pressure. Chest 138(6):1395–1401

Botney MD (1999) Role of hemodynamics in pulmonary vascular remodeling: implications for primary pulmonary hypertension. Am J Respir Crit Care Med 159:361–364

Bouchard A, Higgins CB, Byrd BF, Amparo EG, Osaki L, Axelrod R (1985) Magnetic resonance imaging in pulmonary arterial hypertension. Am J Cardiol 56(15):938–942

Bradlow WM, Gatehouse PD, Hughes RL, O'Brien AB, Gibbs JSR, Firmin DN et al (2007) Assessing normal pulse wave velocity in the proximal pulmonary arteries using transit time: a feasibility, repeatability, and observer reproducibility study by cardiovascular magnetic resonance. J Magn Reson Imaging 25(5):974–981

Bulluck H, Ngamkasem H, Sado D, Treibel TA, Fontana M, Maestrini V et al (2014) A simple technique to

measure TAPSE and MAPSE on CMR and normal values. J Cardiovasc Magn Reson 16(S1):1–2
Bush A, Gray H, Denison DM (1988) Diagnosis of pulmonary hypertension from radiographic estimates of pulmonary arterial size. Thorax 43(2):127–131
Castelain V, Hervé P, Lecarpentier Y, Duroux P, Simonneau G, Chemla D (2001) Pulmonary artery pulse pressure and wave reflection in chronic pulmonary thromboembolism and primary pulmonary hypertension. J Am Coll Cardiol 37(4):1085–1092
Chan AL, Juarez MM, Shelton DK, MacDonald T, Li CS, Lin TC et al (2011) Novel computed tomographic chest metrics to detect pulmonary hypertension. BMC Med Imaging 11:7
Chang CH (1962) The normal roentgenographic measurement of the right descending pulmonary artery in 1,085 cases and its clinical application. II. Clinical application of the measurement of the right descending pulmonary artery in the radiological diagnosis of pulmonary h. Am J Roentgenol Radium Therapy, Nucl Med 87:929–935
Chernobelsky A, Shubayev O, Comeau CR, Wolff SD (2007) Baseline correction of phase contrast images improves quantification of blood flow in the great vessels. J Cardiovasc Magn Reson 9(4):681–685
Chetty KG, Brown SE, Light RW (1982) Identification of pulmonary hypertension in chronic obstructive pulmonary disease from routine chest radiographs. Am Rev Respir Dis 126(2):338–341
Coghlan JG, Handler C (2006) Connective tissue associated pulmonary arterial hypertension. Lupus 15:138–142
Colin GC, Gerber BL, de Meester de Ravenstein C, Byl D, Dietz A, Kamga M et al (2018) Pulmonary hypertension due to left heart disease: diagnostic and prognostic value of CT in chronic systolic heart failure. Eur Radiol 28(11):4643–4653
Colin GC, Verlynde G, Pouleur AC, Gerber BL, Beauloye C, Kefer J et al (2020a) Pulmonary hypertension due to left heart disease: diagnostic value of pulmonary artery distensibility. Eur Radiol 30(11):6204–6212
Colin GC, Pouleur AC, Gerber BL, Poncelet PA, de Meester C, D'Hondt AM et al (2020b) Pulmonary hypertension detection by computed tomography pulmonary transit time in heart failure with reduced ejection fraction. Eur Heart J Cardiovasc Imaging 21(11):1291–1298
Crawley SF, Johnson MK, Dargie HJ, Peacock AJ (2013) LA volume by CMR distinguishes idiopathic from pulmonary hypertension due to HFpEF. JACC Cardiovasc Imaging 6(10):1120–1121
Currie BJ, Johns C, Chin M, Charalampopolous T, Elliot CA, Garg P et al (2018) CT derived left atrial size identifies left heart disease in suspected pulmonary hypertension: derivation and validation of predictive thresholds. Int J Cardiol [Internet] 260:172–177. Available from: https://linkinghub.elsevier.com/retrieve/pii/S0167527317369085
Davarpanah AH, Hodnett PA, Farrelly CT, Shah SJ, Cuttica M, Ragin AB et al (2011) MDCT bolus tracking data as an adjunct for predicting the diagnosis of pulmonary hypertension and concomitant right-heart failure. Am J Roentgenol 197(5):1064–1072
Dellegrottaglie S, Sanz J, Poon M, Viles-Gonzalez JF, Sulica R, Goyenechea M et al (2007) Pulmonary hypertension: accuracy of detection with left ventricular septal-to-free wall curvature ratio measured at cardiac MR. Radiology 243(1):63–69
Devaraj A, Hansell DM (2009) Computed tomography signs of pulmonary hypertension: old and new observations. Clin Radiol 64:751–760
Devaraj A, Wells AU, Meister MG, Corte TJ, Hansell DM (2008) The effect of diffuse pulmonary fibrosis on the reliability of CT signs of pulmonary hypertension. Radiology 249(3):1042–1049
Devaraj A, Wells AU, Meister MG, Corte TJ, Wort SJ, Hansell DM (2010) Detection of pulmonary hypertension with multidetector CT and echocardiography alone and in combination. Radiology 254(2):609–616
Dupont MVM, Drăgean CA, Coche EE (2011) Right ventricle function assessment by MDCT. Am J Roentgenol 196:77–86
Eifer DA, Nguyen ET, Thavendiranathan P, Hanneman K (2018) Diagnostic accuracy of sex-specific chest CT measurements compared with cardiac MRI findings in the assessment of cardiac chamber enlargement. Am J Roentgenol [Internet] 211(5):993–999. Available from: https://www.ajronline.org/doi/10.2214/AJR.18.19805
Ema R, Sugiura T, Kawata N, Tanabe N, Kasai H, Nishimura R et al (2017) The dilatation of main pulmonary artery and right ventricle observed by enhanced chest computed tomography predict poor outcome in inoperable chronic thromboembolic pulmonary hypertension. Eur J Radiol 94:70–77
Engelfriet PM, Duffels MGJ, Möller T, Boersma E, Tijssen JGP, Thaulow E et al (2007) Pulmonary arterial hypertension in adults born with a heart septal defect: the Euro Heart Survey on adult congenital heart disease. Heart 93(6):682–687
Fischer L, Benjamin N, Blank N, Egenlauf B, Fischer C, Harutyunova S et al (2018) Right heart size and function significantly correlate in patients with pulmonary arterial hypertension – a cross-sectional study. Respir Res 19(1):216
Foppa M, Arora G, Gona P, Ashrafi A, Salton CJ, Yeon SB et al (2016) Right ventricular volumes and systolic function by cardiac magnetic resonance and the impact of sex, age, and obesity in a longitudinally followed cohort free of pulmonary and cardiovascular disease: the Framingham Heart Study. Circ Cardiovasc Imaging 9(3):e003810
Forfia PR, Fisher MR, Mathai SC, Housten-Harris T, Hemnes AR, Borlaug BA et al (2006) Tricuspid annular displacement predicts survival in pulmonary hypertension. Am J Respir Crit Care Med 174(9):1034–1041
Freed BH, Collins JD, François CJ, Barker AJ, Cuttica MJ, Chesler NC et al (2016) MR and CT imaging for the evaluation of pulmonary hypertension. JACC Cardiovasc Imaging 9(6):715–732

Galiè N, Humbert M, Vachiery JL, Gibbs S, Lang I, Torbicki A et al (2015) ESC/ERS Guidelines for the diagnosis and treatment of pulmonary hypertension. Eur Respir J 2015:903–975

Gan CTJ, Lankhaar JW, Westerhof N, Marcus JT, Becker A, Twisk JWR et al (2007) Noninvasively assessed pulmonary artery stiffness predicts mortality in pulmonary arterial hypertension. Chest 132(6):1906–1912

Goerne H, Batra K, Rajiah P (2018) Imaging of pulmonary hypertension: an update. Cardiovasc Diagn Ther 8:279–296

Gopalan D (2011) Right heart on multidetector CT. Br J Radiol 84(SPEC. ISSUE 3):S306–S323

Gopalan D, Riley J, Leong K, Alsanjari S, Ariff B, Auger W et al (2022) Biatrial volumetric assessment by non-ECG-gated CT pulmonary angiography correlated with transthoracic echocardiography in patients with normal diastology. Tomography 8(6):2761–2771

Guo YK, Gao HL, Zhang XC, Wang QL, Yang ZG, Sen ME (2010) Accuracy and reproducibility of assessing right ventricular function with 64-section multi-detector row CT: comparison with magnetic resonance imaging. Int J Cardiol 139(3):254–262

Han HC (2012) Twisted blood vessels: symptoms, etiology and biomechanical mechanisms. J Vasc Res 49:185–197

Heinrich M, Uder M, Tscholl D, Grgic A, Kramann B, Schäfers HJ (2005) CT scan findings in chronic thromboembolic pulmonary hypertension: predictors of hemodynamic improvement after pulmonary thromboendarterectomy. Chest 127(5):1606–1613

Helderman F, Mauritz GJ, Andringa KE, Vonk-Noordegraaf A, Marcus JT (2011) Early onset of retrograde flow in the main pulmonary artery is a characteristic of pulmonary arterial hypertension. J Magn Reson Imaging 33(6):1362–1368

Helmberger M, Pienn M, Urschler M, Kullnig P, Stollberger R, Kovacs G et al (2014) Quantification of tortuosity and fractal dimension of the lung vessels in pulmonary hypertension patients. PLoS One 9(1):e87515

Hoeper MM, Humbert M, Souza R, Idrees M, Kawut SM, Sliwa-Hahnle K et al (2016) A global view of pulmonary hypertension. Lancet Respir Med 4(4):306–322

Holland B, Printz B, Lai W (2010) Baseline correction of phase-contrast images in congenital cardiovascular magnetic resonance. J Cardiovasc Magn Reson 12(1):11

Hudsmith LE, Petersen SE, Francis JM, Robson MD, Neubauer S (2005) Normal human left and right ventricular and left atrial dimensions using steady state free precession magnetic resonance imaging. J Cardiovasc Magn Reson 7(5):775–782

Humbert M, Coghlan JG, Khanna D (2012) Early detection and management of pulmonary arterial hypertension. Eur Respir Rev 21:306–312

Humbert M, Kovacs G, Hoeper MM, Badagliacca R, Berger RMF, Brida M et al (2022) 2022 ESC/ERS Guidelines for the diagnosis and treatment of pulmonary hypertension. Eur Heart J 43(38):3618–3731

Ibrahim ESH, Shaffer JM, White RD (2011) Assessment of pulmonary artery stiffness using velocity-encoding magnetic resonance imaging: evaluation of techniques. Magn Reson Imaging 29(7):966–974

James SH, Wald R, Wintersperger BJ, Jimenez-Juan L, Deva D, Crean AM et al (2013) Accuracy of right and left ventricular functional assessment by short-axis vs axial cine steady-state free-precession magnetic resonance imaging: Intrapatient correlation with main pulmonary artery and ascending aorta phase-contrast flow measurements. Can Assoc Radiol J 64(3):213–219

Johns CS, Wild JM, Rajaram S, Tubman E, Capener D, Elliot C et al (2018) Identifying at-risk patients with combined pre- and postcapillary pulmonary hypertension using interventricular septal angle at cardiac MRI. Radiology 289(1):61–68

Johnson TRC, Krauß B, Sedlmair M, Grasruck M, Bruder H, Morhard D et al (2007) Material differentiation by dual energy CT: initial experience. Eur Radiol 17(6):1510–1517

Jones RH, Sabiston DC, Bates BB, Morris JJ, Anderson PAW, Goodrich JK (1972) Quantitative radionuclide angiocardiography for determination of chamber to chamber cardiac transit times. Am J Cardiol 30(8):855–864

Katz J, Whang J, Boxt LM, Barst RJ (1993) Estimation of right ventricular mass in normal subjects and in patients with primary pulmonary hypertension by nuclear magnetic resonance imaging. J Am Coll Cardiol 21(6):1475–1481

Kauczor HU, Schwickert HC, Mayer E, Schweden F, Schild HH, Thelen M (1994) Spiral CT of bronchial arteries in chronic thromboembolism. J Comput Assist Tomogr 18(6):855–861

Kawel-Boehm N, Maceira A, Valsangiacomo-Buechel ER, Vogel-Claussen J, Turkbey EB, Williams R et al (2015) Normal values for cardiovascular magnetic resonance in adults and children. J Cardiovasc Magn Reson 17:29

Kawut SM, Silvestry FE, Ferrari VA, Denofrio D, Axel L, Loh E et al (1999) Extrinsic compression of the left main coronary artery by the pulmonary artery in patients with long-standing pulmonary hypertension. Am J Cardiol 83(6):984–986

Kerl JM, Ravenel JG, Nguyen SA, Suranyi P, Thilo C, Costello P et al (2008) Right heart: Split-bolus injection of diluted contrast medium for visualization at coronary CT angiography. Radiology 247(2):356–364

Kind T, Mauritz GJ, Marcus JT, van de Veerdonk M, Westerhof N, Vonk-Noordegraaf A (2010) Right ventricular ejection fraction is better reflected by transverse rather than longitudinal wall motion in pulmonary hypertension. J Cardiovasc Magn Reson 12(1):35

Kondo C, Caputo GR, Masui T, Foster E, O'Sullivan M, Stulbarg MS et al (1992) Pulmonary hypertension: pulmonary flow guantification and flow profile analysis with velocity-encoded cine MR imaging. Radiology 183(3):751–758

Kreitner KF, Wirth GM, Krummenauer F, Weber S, Pitton MB, Schneider J et al (2013) Noninvasive assessment of pulmonary hemodynamics in patients with chronic thromboembolic pulmonary hypertension by high temporal resolution phase-contrast MRI: correlation with simultaneous invasive pressure recordings. Circ Cardiovasc Imaging 6(5):722–729

Kuriyama K, Gamsu G, Stern RG, Cann CE, Herfkens RJ, Brundage BH (1984) CT-determined pulmonary artery diameters in predicting pulmonary hypertension. Investig Radiol 19(1):16–22

Lakoma A, Tuite D, Sheehan J, Weale P, Carr JC (2010) Measurement of pulmonary circulation parameters using time-resolved MR angiography in patients after Ross procedure. Am J Roentgenol 194(4):912–919

Lange TJ, Dornia C, Stiefel J, Stroszczynski C, Arzt M, Pfeifer M et al (2013) Increased pulmonary artery diameter on chest computed tomography can predict borderline pulmonary hypertension. Pulm Circ 3(2):363–368

Lee SH, Kim YJ, Lee HJ, Kim HY, Kang YA, Park MS et al (2015) Comparison of CT-determined pulmonary artery diameter, aortic diameter, and their ratio in healthy and diverse clinical conditions. PLoS One 10(5):e0126646

Lettieri CJ, Nathan SD, Barnett SD, Ahmad S, Shorr AF (2006) Prevalence and outcomes of pulmonary arterial hypertension in advanced idiopathic pulmonary fibrosis. Chest 129(3):746–752

Lin FY, Min JK (2008) Assessment of cardiac volumes by multidetector computed tomography. J Cardiovasc Comput Tomogr 2(4):256–262

Lin FY, Devereux RB, Roman MJ, Meng J, Jow VM, Jacobs A et al (2008) Cardiac chamber volumes, function, and mass as determined by 64-multidetector row computed tomography. Mean values among healthy adults free of hypertension and obesity. JACC Cardiovasc Imaging 1(6):782–786

Liu K, Zhang C, Chen B, Li M, Zhang P (2020) Association between right atrial area measured by echocardiography and prognosis among pulmonary arterial hypertension: a systematic review and meta-analysis. BMJ Open 10(9):e031316

Liu A, Xu W, Xi L, Deng M, Yang H, Huang Q et al (2023) Cardiovascular metrics on CT pulmonary angiography in patients with pulmonary hypertension — re-evaluation under the updated guidelines of pulmonary hypertension. Insights Imaging 14(1):179

López-Candales A, Rajagopalan N, Saxena N, Gulyasy B, Edelman K, Bazaz R (2006) Right ventricular systolic function is not the sole determinant of tricuspid annular motion. Am J Cardiol 98(7):973–977

Lu JG, Lv B, Chen XB, Tang X, Jiang SL, Dai RP (2010) What is the best contrast injection protocol for 64-row multi-detector cardiac computed tomography? Eur J Radiol 75:159–165

Maceira AM, Prasad SK, Khan M, Pennell DJ (2006) Reference right ventricular systolic and diastolic function normalized to age, gender and body surface area from steady-state free precession cardiovascular magnetic resonance. Eur Heart J 27(23):2879–2888

Maceira AM, Cosín-Sales J, Roughton M, Prasad SK, Pennell DJ (2013) Reference right atrial dimensions and volume estimation by steady state free precession cardiovascular magnetic resonance. J Cardiovasc Magn Reson 15(1):29

Maffei E, Messalli G, Martini C, Nieman K, Catalano O, Rossi A et al (2012) Left and right ventricle assessment with Cardiac CT: Validation study vs. Cardiac MR. Eur Radiol 22(5):1041–1049

Mahammedi A, Oshmyansky A, Hassoun PM, Thiemann DR, Siegelman SS (2013) Pulmonary artery measurements in pulmonary hypertension: the role of computed tomography. J Thorac Imaging 28(2):96–103

Marcus JT, Smeenk HG, Kuijer JPA, Van der Geest RJ, Heethaar RM, Van Rossum AC (1999) Flow profiles in the left anterior descending and the right coronary artery assessed by MR velocity quantification: effects of through-plane and in-plane motion of the heart. J Comput Assist Tomogr 23(4):567–576

Matthay RA, Schwarz MI, Ellis JH, Steele PP, Siebert PE, Durrance JR et al (1981) Pulmonary artery hypertension in chronic obstructive pulmonary disease: determination by chest radiography. Investig Radiol 16(2):95–100

McGoon M, Gutterman D, Steen V, Barst R, McCrory DC, Fortin TA et al (2004) Screening, early detection, and diagnosis of pulmonary arterial hypertension: ACCP evidence-based clinical practice guidelines. Chest 126(1 SUPPL):14S–34S

Meinel F, Graef A, Thierfelder K, Armbruster M, Schild C, Neurohr C et al (2013) Automated quantification of pulmonary perfused blood volume by dual-energy CTPA in chronic thromboembolic pulmonary hypertension. Röfo 186(02):151–156

Melzig C, Wörz S, Egenlauf B, Partovi S, Rohr K, Grünig E et al (2019) Combined automated 3D volumetry by pulmonary CT angiography and echocardiography for detection of pulmonary hypertension. Eur Radiol 29(11):6059–6068

Melzig C, Do TD, Egenlauf B, Partovi S, Grünig E, Kauczor HU et al (2022) Diagnostic accuracy of automated 3D volumetry of cardiac chambers by CT pulmonary angiography for identification of pulmonary hypertension due to left heart disease. Eur Radiol 32(8):5222–5232

Mesquita SMF, Castro CRP, Ikari NM, Oliveira SA, Lopes AA (2004) Likelihood of left main coronary artery compression based on pulmonary trunk diameter in patients with pulmonary hypertension. Am J Med 116(6):369–374

Mirsadraee M, Nazemi S, Hamedanchi A, Naghibi S (2013) Simple screening of pulmonary artery hypertension using standard chest X ray: an old technique, new landmark. Tanaffos 12(3):17–22

Mortani Barbosa EJ, Gupta NK, Torigian DA, Gefter WB (2012) Current role of imaging in the diagnosis and management of pulmonary hypertension. Am J Roentgenol 198:1320–1331

Mousseaux E, Tasu JP, Jolivet O, Simonneau G, Bittoun J, Gaux JC (1999) Pulmonary arterial resistance: noninvasive measurement with indexes of pulmonary flow estimated at velocity-encoded MR imaging preliminary experience. Radiology 212(3):896–902

Murray TI, Boxt LM, Katz J, Reagan K, Barst RJ (1994) Estimation of pulmonary artery pressure in patients with primary pulmonary hypertension by quantitative analysis of magnetic resonance images. J Thorac Imaging 9(3):198–204

Naeije R, Chin K (2019) Differentiating precapillary from postcapillary pulmonary hypertension. Circulation 140(9):712–714

Nayak KS, Nielsen JF, Bernstein MA, Markl M, Gatehouse PD, Botnar RM et al (2015) Cardiovascular magnetic resonance phase contrast imaging. J Cardiovasc Magn Reson 17(1):71

Ng CS, Wells AU, Padley SPG (1999) A CT sign of chronic pulmonary arterial hypertension: the ratio of main pulmonary artery to aortic diameter. J Thorac Imaging 14(4):270–278

Nunes H, Humbert M, Capron F, Brauner M, Sitbon O, Battesti JP et al (2006) Pulmonary hypertension associated with sarcoidosis: mechanisms, haemodynamics and prognosis. Thorax 61(1):68–74

Ohno Y, Hatabu H, Murase K, Higashino T, Nogami M, Yoshikawa T et al (2007) Primary pulmonary hypertension: 3D dynamic perfusion MRI for quantitative analysis of regional pulmonary perfusion. Am J Roentgenol 188(1):48–56

Ohno Y, Koyama H, Yoshikawa T, Nishio M, Matsumoto S, Matsumoto K et al (2012) Contrast-enhanced multidetector-row computed tomography vs. time-resolved magnetic resonance angiography vs. contrast-enhanced perfusion MRI: assessment of treatment response by patients with inoperable chronic thromboembolic pulmonary hypertension. J Magn Reson Imaging 36(3):612–623

Peacock AJ, Murphy NF, McMurrey JJV, Caballero L, Stewart S (2007) An epidemiological study of pulmonary arterial hypertension. Eur Respir J 30(1):104–109

Peña E, Dennie C, Veinot J, Muñiz SH (2012) Pulmonary hypertension: how the radiologist can help. Radiographics 32(1):9–32

Pennell DJ, Sechtem UP, Higgins CB, Manning WJ, Pohost GM, Rademakers FE et al (2004) Clinical indications for cardiovascular magnetic resonance (CMR): consensus panel report. Eur Heart J 25:1940–1965

Petersen SE, Aung N, Sanghvi MM, Zemrak F, Fung K, Paiva JM et al (2017) Reference ranges for cardiac structure and function using cardiovascular magnetic resonance (CMR) in Caucasians from the UK Biobank population cohort. J Cardiovasc Magn Reson 19(1):18

Qaiser KN, Sahay S, Tonelli AR (2023) Pulmonary hypertension due to high cardiac output. Respir Med 206:107034

Querejeta Roca G, Campbell P, Claggett B, Solomon SD, Shah AM (2015) Right atrial function in pulmonary arterial hypertension. Circ Cardiovasc Imaging 8(11):e003521

Raman SV, Shah M, McCarthy B, Garcia A, Ferketich AK (2006) Multi-detector row cardiac computed tomography accurately quantifies right and left ventricular size and function compared with cardiac magnetic resonance. Am Heart J 151(3):736–744

Ratanawatkul P, Oh A, Richards JC, Swigris JJ (2020) Performance of pulmonary artery dimensions measured on high-resolution computed tomography scan for identifying pulmonary hypertension. ERJ Open Res 6(1):00232–02019

Raymond RJ, Hinderliter AL, Willis PW, Ralph D, Caldwell EJ, Williams W et al (2002) Echocardiographic predictors of adverse outcomes in primary pulmonary hypertension. J Am Coll Cardiol 39(7):1214–1219

Raymond TE, Khabbaza JE, Yadav R, Tonelli AR (2014) Significance of main pulmonary artery dilation on imaging studies. Ann Am Thorac Soc 11:1623–1632

Reiter G, Reiter U, Kovacs G, Kainz B, Schmidt K, Maier R et al (2008) Magnetic resonance-derived 3-dimensional blood flow patterns in the main pulmonary artery as a marker of pulmonary hypertension and a measure of elevated mean pulmonary arterial pressure. Circ Cardiovasc Imaging 1(1):23–30

Reiter G, Reiter U, Kovacs G, Olschewski H, Fuchsjäger M (2015) Blood flow vortices along the main pulmonary artery measured with MR imaging for diagnosis of pulmonary hypertension. Radiology 275(1):71–79

Reiter U, Reiter G, Fuchsjäger M (2016) MR phase-contrast imaging in pulmonary hypertension. Br J Radiol 89:20150995

Remy-Jardin M, Duhamel A, Deken V, Bouaziz N, Dumont P, Remy J (2005) Systemic collateral supply in patients with chronic thromboembolic and primary pulmonary hypertension: Assessment with multi-detector row helical CT angiography. Radiology. 235:274–281

Remy-Jardin M, Ryerson CJ, Schiebler ML, Leung ANC, Wild JM, Hoeper MM et al (2021) Imaging of pulmonary hypertension in adults: a position paper from the Fleischner Society. Eur Respir J 57(1):2004455

Rengier F, Melzig C, Derlin T, Marra AM, Vogel-Claussen J (2019) Advanced imaging in pulmonary hypertension: emerging techniques and applications. Int J Cardiovasc Imaging 35:1407–1420

Revel MP, Faivre JB, Remy-Jardin M, Delannoy-Deken V, Duhamel A, Remy J (2009) Pulmonary hypertension: ECG-gated 64-section CT angiographic evaluation of new functional parameters as diagnostic criteria. Radiology 250(2):558–566

Rheinheimer S, Reh C, Figiel J, Mahnken AH (2016) Assessment of right atrium volume by conventional CT or MR techniques: which modality resembles in vivo reality? Eur J Radiol 85(5):1040–1044

Rigsby CK, Hilpipre N, McNeal GR, Zhang G, Boylan EE, Popescu AR et al (2014) Analysis of an automated background correction method for cardiovascular MR phase contrast imaging in children and young adults. Pediatr Radiol 44(3):265–273

Roeleveld RJ, Marcus TJ, Faes TJC, Gan TJ, Boonstra A, Postmus PE et al (2005) Interventricular septal configuration at MR imaging and pulmonary arterial pressure in pulmonary hypertension. Radiology 234(3):710–717

Rolf A, Rixe J, Kim WK, Guth S, Körlings N, Möllmann H et al (2015) Pulmonary vascular remodeling before and after pulmonary endarterectomy in patients with chronic thromboembolic pulmonary hypertension: a cardiac magnetic resonance study. Int J Cardiovasc Imaging 31(3):613–619

Saba TS, Foster J, Cockburn M, Cowan M, Peacock AJ (2002) Ventricular mass index using magnetic resonance imaging accurately estimates pulmonary artery pressure. Eur Respir J 20(6):1519–1524

Sanz J, Kuschnir P, Rius T, Salguero R, Sulica R, Einstein AJ et al (2007) Pulmonary arterial hypertension: noninvasive detection with phase-contrast MR imaging. Radiology 243(1):70–79

Sanz J, Kariisa M, Dellegrottaglie S, Prat-González S, Garcia MJ, Fuster V et al (2009) Evaluation of pulmonary artery stiffness in pulmonary hypertension with cardiac magnetic resonance. JACC Cardiovasc Imaging 2(3):286–295

Scelsi CL, Bates WB, Melenevsky YV, Sharma GK, Thomson NB, Keshavamurthy JH (2018) Egg-and-Banana Sign: a novel diagnostic CT marker for pulmonary hypertension. Am J Roentgenol 210(6):1235–1239

Schlosser T, Mohrs OK, Magedanz A, Voigtländer T, Schmermund A, Barkhausen J (2007) Assessment of left ventricular function and mass in patients undergoing Computed Tomography (CT) coronary angiography using 64-detector-row CT: comparison to magnetic resonance imaging. Acta Radiol 48(1):30–35

Schmidt HC, Kauczor HU, Schild HH, Renner C, Kirchhoff E, Lang P et al (1996) Pulmonary hypertension in patients with chronic pulmonary thromboembolism: chest radiograph and CT evaluation before and after surgery. Eur Radiol 6(6):817–825

Schulz-Menger J, Bluemke DA, Bremerich J, Flamm SD, Fogel MA, Friedrich MG et al (2013) Standardized image interpretation and post processing in cardiovascular magnetic resonance: Society for Cardiovascular Magnetic Resonance (SCMR) Board of Trustees Task Force on Standardized Post Processing. J Cardiovasc Magn Reson 15(1):35

Sergiacomi G, Bolacchi F, Cadioli M, Angeli ML, Fucci F, Crusco S et al (2010) Combined pulmonary fibrosis and emphysema: 3D time-resolved MR angiographic evaluation of pulmonary arterial mean transit time and time to peak enhancement. Radiology 254(2):601–608

Siegel Y, Mirpuri T (2014) Pulmonary hypertension detection using dynamic and static measurable parameters on CT angiography. J Comput Assist Tomogr 38(4):586–590

Simonneau G, Montani D, Celermajer DS, Denton CP, Gatzoulis MA, Krowka M et al (2019) Haemodynamic definitions and updated clinical classification of pulmonary hypertension. Eur Respir J 53(1):1801913

Skrok J, Shehata ML, Mathai S, Girgis RE, Zaiman A, Mudd JO et al (2012) Pulmonary arterial hypertension: MR imaging-derived first-pass bolus kinetic parameters are biomarkers for pulmonary hemodynamics, cardiac function, and ventricular remodeling. Radiology 263(3):678–687

Smedby O, Hogman N, Nilsson S, Erikson U, Olsson AG, Walldius G (1993) Two-dimensional tortuosity of the superficial femoral artery in early atherosclerosis. J Vasc Res 30(4):181–191

Stevens GR, Garcia-Alvarez A, Sahni S, Garcia MJ, Fuster V, Sanz J (2012) RV dysfunction in pulmonary hypertension is independently related to pulmonary artery stiffness. JACC Cardiovasc Imaging 5(4):378–387

Stojanovska J, Cronin P, Patel S, Gross BH, Oral H, Chughtai K et al (2011) Reference normal absolute and indexed values from ECG-gated MDCT: left atrial volume, function, and diameter. Am J Roentgenol 197(3):631–637

Stojanovska J, Prasitdumrong H, Patel S, Sundaram B, Gross BH, Yilmaz ZN et al (2014) Reference absolute and indexed values for left and right ventricular volume, function and mass from cardiac computed tomography. J Med Imaging Radiat Oncol 58(5):547–558

Swift AJ, Rajaram S, Condliffe R, Capener D, Hurdman J, Elliot C et al (2012a) Pulmonary artery relative area change detects mild elevations in pulmonary vascular resistance and predicts adverse outcome in pulmonary hypertension. Investig Radiol 47(10):571–577

Swift AJ, Rajaram S, Condliffe R, Capener D, Hurdman J, Elliot CA et al (2012b) Diagnostic accuracy of cardiovascular magnetic resonance imaging of right ventricular morphology and function in the assessment of suspected pulmonary hypertension results from the ASPIRE registry. J Cardiovasc Magn Reson 14(1):40

Swift AJ, Rajaram S, Marshall H, Condliffe R, Capener D, Hill C et al (2012c) Black blood MRI has diagnostic and prognostic value in the assessment of patients with pulmonary hypertension. Eur Radiol [Internet] 22(3):695–702. Available from: http://link.springer.com/10.1007/s00330-011-2306-0

Swift AJ, Rajaram S, Hurdman J, Hill C, Davies C, Sproson TW et al (2013) Noninvasive estimation of PA pressure, flow, and resistance with CMR imaging. JACC Cardiovasc Imaging 6(10):1036–1047

Swift AJ, Telfer A, Rajaram S, Condliffe R, Marshall H, Capener D et al (2014) Dynamic contrast–enhanced magnetic resonance imaging in patients with pulmonary arterial hypertension. Pulm Circ 4(1):61–70

Swift AJ, Dwivedi K, Johns C, Garg P, Chin M, Currie BJ et al (2020) Diagnostic accuracy of CT pulmonary angiography in suspected pulmonary hypertension. Eur Radiol 30(9):4918–4929

Tan RT, Kuzo R, Goodman LR, Siegel R, Haasler GB, Presberg KW (1998) Utility of CT scan evaluation for predicting pulmonary hypertension in patients with parenchymal lung disease. Chest 113(5):1250–1256

Tang Q, Liu M, Ma Z, Guo X, Kuang T, Yang Y (2013) Non-invasive evaluation of hemodynamics in pulmonary hypertension by a Septal angle measured by computed tomography pulmonary angiography: comparison with right-heart catheterization and association with N-terminal pro-B-type natriuretic peptide. Exp Ther Med 6:1350–1358

Tardivon AA, Mousseaux E, Brenot F, Bittoun J, Jolivet O, Bourroul E et al (1994) Quantification of hemodynamics in primary pulmonary hypertension with magnetic resonance imaging. Am J Respir Crit Care Med 150(4):1075–1080

Taylor AJ, Cerqueira M, Hodgson JMB, Mark D, Min J, O'Gara P et al (2010) ACCF/SCCT/ACR/AHA/ASE/ASNC/NASCI/SCAI/SCMR 2010 appropriate use criteria for cardiac computed tomography. J Am Coll Cardiol 56:1864–1894

Teichmann V, Jezek V, Herles F (1970) Relevance of width of right descending branch of pulmonary artery as a radiological sign of pulmonary hypertension. Thorax 25(1):91–96

Truong QA, Massaro JM, Rogers IS, Mahabadi AA, Kriegel MF, Fox CS et al (2012) Reference values for normal pulmonary artery dimensions by noncontrast cardiac computed tomography the Framingham heart study. Circ Cardiovasc Imaging 5(1):147–154

van der Ven JPG, Sadighy Z, Valsangiacomo Buechel ER, Sarikouch S, Robbers-Visser D, Kellenberger CJ et al (2020) Multicentre reference values for cardiac magnetic resonance imaging derived ventricular size and function for children aged 0–18 years. Eur Heart J Cardiovasc Imaging 21(1):102–113

Van Der Vleuten PA, Willems TP, Götte MJW, Tio RA, Greuter MJW, Zijlstra F et al (2006) Quantification of global left ventricular function: comparison of multidetector computed tomography and magnetic resonance imaging. A meta-analysis and review of the current literature. Acta Radiol 47(10):1049–1057

van Wolferen SA, Marcus JT, Boonstra A, Marques KMJ, Bronzwaer JGF, Spreeuwenberg MD et al (2007a) Prognostic value of right ventricular mass, volume, and function in idiopathic pulmonary arterial hypertension. Eur Heart J 28(10):1250–1257

van Wolferen SA, Marcus JT, Westerhof N, Spreeuwenberg MD, Marques KMJ, Bronzwaer JGF et al (2007b) Right coronary artery flow impairment in patients with pulmonary hypertension. Eur Heart J 29(1):120–127

Vogel-Claussen J, Skrok J, Shehata ML, Singh S, Sibley CT, Boyce DM et al (2011) Right and left ventricular myocardial perfusion reserves correlate with right ventricular function and pulmonary hemodynamics in patients with pulmonary arterial hypertension. Radiology 258(1):119–127

von Schulthess GK (1985) Pathologic blood flow in pulmonary vascular disease as shown by gated magnetic resonance imaging. Ann Intern Med 103(3):317

Wai B, Thai WE, Brown H, Truong QA (2013) Novel phase-based noise reduction strategy for quantification of left ventricular function and mass assessment by cardiac CT: comparison with cardiac magnetic resonance. Eur J Radiol 82(8):e337–e341

Walsh SLF, Wells AU, Sverzellati N, Keir GJ, Calandriello L, Antoniou KM et al (2014) An integrated clinicoradiological staging system for pulmonary sarcoidosis: a case-cohort study. Lancet Respir Med 2(2):123–130

Zyłkowska J, Kurzyna M, Florczyk M, Burakowska B, Grzegorczyk F, Burakowski J et al (2012) Pulmonary artery dilatation correlates with the risk of unexpected death in chronic arterial or thromboembolic pulmonary hypertension. Chest 142(6):1406–1416

Pulmonary Embolism

Naama R. Bogot and Galit Aviram

Contents

Abbreviations

CM	Contrast medium
CTOI	CT obstruction index
CTPA	Computed tomographic pulmonary angiogram
DVT	Deep vein thrombosis
IVC	Inferior vena cava
LA	Left atrium
LV	Left ventricle
NPV	Negative predictive value
PA	Pulmonary artery
PBV	Pulmonary blood volume
PD	Perfusion-like defects
PE	Pulmonary embolism
PPV	Positive predictive value
RA	Right atrium
RV	Right ventricle
RV/LV	Right-to-left ventricular ratio
RVD	Right ventricular dysfunction
SVC	Superior vena cava
TAPSE	Tricuspid annular plane systolic excursion
VTE	Venous thromboembolism

Pulmonary embolism (PE) is a potentially life-threatening disease (Barco et al. 2020a). Clinical presentation of acute PE has a wide spectrum, varying from acute hemodynamic shock or cardiac arrest in a minority of patients (about 5–10%) to a stable condition in most of the cases, or it may even be asymptomatic.

N. R. Bogot
Department of Radiology, Shaare Zedek Medical Center, Jerusalem, Israel

G. Aviram (✉)
Department of Diagnostic Radiology, Tel Aviv Sourasky Medical Center, Tel Aviv University, Faculty of Medicine, Tel Aviv, Israel

Med Radiol Diagn Imaging (2026)
https://doi.org/10.1007/174_2025_677,
Published Online: 23 January 2026

1 Assessment of Clinical (Pre-test) Probability

Because symptoms associated with PE are nonspecific, the clinical identification of patients presenting with PE can be challenging. Standard diagnostic strategies for PE consist three successive steps: evaluating PE clinical probability, D-dimer testing when indicated, and chest imaging if indicated. The first step of the diagnostic strategy is thus to estimate the clinical probability of PE as low, moderate, or high. PE prevalence is <15% among persons with low clinical probability, 15–40% among persons with moderate clinical probability, and >40% among persons with high clinical probability (Van Belle et al. 2006).

Two structured scores have been validated for identifying the clinical probability of PE: the Wells score and the revised Geneva score (Wolf et al. 2004; Le Gal et al. 2006) (Tables 1 and 2). These scores include consideration of predisposing factors (recent immobilization, malignancy, and history of venous thromboembolism (VTE)) and clinical characteristics at presentation (age, heart rate, signs of deep vein thrombosis (DVT), hemoptysis). The revised Geneva score includes only objective components, whereas the Wells score also includes one subjective item—PE is the most likely diagnosis. In addition to these two structured scores, the clinical probability can also be estimated by unstructured clinical impression entitled as the "gestalt."

D-dimers are fibrin degradation products showing high sensitivity and low specificity for the diagnosis of PE. In patients with low or intermediate clinical probability, PE can be excluded without imaging studies if the D-dimer levels are negative. Below the age of 50 years, the usual threshold is 500 ng/mL. Above 50 years of age, a threshold of age × 10 ng/mL has been shown to safely reduce the number of patients undergoing CTPA (Righini et al. 2014). In patients with high probability or positive D-dimer levels, further evaluation by imaging is required.

Table 1 Wells Score (Wolf et al. 2004)

Variables	Score
Clinically suspected DVT (leg swelling, pain with palpation)	3.0
Alternative diagnosis is less likely than PE	3.0
Immobilization/surgery in previous 4 weeks	1.5
Previous history of DVT or PE	1.5
Tachycardia (heart rate more than 100 bpm)	1.5
Malignancy (treatment for within 6 months, palliative)	1.0
Hemoptysis	1.0

Interpretation of Wells Score:
The pretest probability of PE according to Wells criteria:
Score <2.0: Low probability (Rate of PE: ~3.6%)
Score 2.0–6.0: Moderate probability (Rate of PE: ~20.5%)
Score >6.0: High probability (Rate of PE: ~66.7%)

Table 2 Revised Geneva score (Le Gal et al. 2006)

Variables	Score
Age more than 65 years	1.0
Prior history of DVT or PE	3.0
Surgery under general anesthesia or fracture of the lower limbs within the last month	2.0
Active malignant condition (currently active or cured less than 1 year ago)	2.0
Unilateral lower limb pain	3.0
Hemoptysis	2.0
Heart rate 75–94 beats per minute	3.0
Heart rate 95 or more beats per minute	5.0
Pain on deep palpation of lower limb and unilateral edema	4.0

Interpretation of the Revised Geneva Score:
Score 0–3 points: Low probability (Rate of PE: 8%)
Score 4–10 points: Intermediate probability (Rate of PE: 28%)
Score ≥11 points: High probability (Rate of PE: 74%)

Computed tomographic pulmonary angiogram (CTPA) is the imaging study of choice for the diagnosis of PE in stable patients because it has a high diagnostic performance and has the advantage of identifying alternative diagnoses such as pneumonia or pleural effusions or other disorders. Nowadays CTPA is readily available around the clock in most centers and has a low inconclusive rate (Konstantinides et al. 2020).

2 Assessment of PE Severity and Risk Stratification

Following the positive diagnosis of acute PE, risk stratification is an important step to determine the appropriate therapeutic approach and management of patients with PE.

2.1 How to Obtain Risk Stratification in Patients with Acute PE?

Risk stratification in acute PE is based on the estimated PE-related early mortality risk, which is defined by in-hospital or 30-day mortality (Konstantinides et al. 2020).

2.1.1 Patients with High Risk

Patients with high risk present with hemodynamic instability and constitute around 5–10% of all PE patients. They are in shock or present with persistent arterial hypotension <90 mmHg for at least 15 min or systolic pressure drop >40 mmHg, not caused by arrythmia, hypovolemia, or sepsis. As an immediately life-threatening situation, high-risk PE requires an emergency diagnostic (upon suspicion) and therapeutic (upon confirmation, or if the level of clinical suspicion is sufficiently high) strategies. The most useful initial test in this condition is bedside transthoracic echocardiography, which will yield evidence of acute right ventricular dysfunction (RVD) and rarely right heart thrombi when acute PE is the cause of the patient's hemodynamic instability, while also excluding other etiologies for hemodynamic instability such as aortic dissection or pericardial tamponade. No further risk stratification is required. Immediate reperfusion therapy should be issued if not contraindicated.

2.1.2 Patients with Intermediate and Low Risk

In the large remaining group of patients with PE who are hemodynamically stable, management is based on risk stratification, which requires the assessment of two sets of prognostic criteria: (i) clinical evaluation mostly based on the simplified pulmonary embolism severity index (sPESI) (Table 3) (Jimenez et al. 2010), and the presence of comorbidity and any other worsening conditions that may adversely affect early prognosis, and (ii) imaging and laboratory indicators of PE severity, mostly related to the presence of RVD (Fig. 1).

Table 3 Simplified Pulmonary Embolism Severity Index (sPESI) (Jimenez et al. 2010)

Age >80 years old (1 point)
History of cancer (1 point)
Chronic cardiopulmonary disease (1 point)
Cardiac pulse ≥110 beats/min (1 point)
Systolic blood pressure <100 mmHg (1 point)
Oxygen saturation <90% at diagnosis of PE (1 point)
Interpretation: 0 point: Low risk of 30-day mortality 1–6 points: Patient is not in low risk of 30-day mortality

Current guidelines from the European Society of Cardiology (Konstantinides et al. 2020) further subclassify patients of the *intermediate risk* group into intermediate-high risk, which need admission to intensive care unit to promptly begin thrombolysis in case of hemodynamic deterioration, and intermediate–low risk, which are simply monitored in regular hospitalization wards.

Patients with sPESI > 0 with both RVD on imaging *and* elevated cardiac biomarkers are classified as Intermediate-high risk.

Patients with sPESI > 0 with either RVD on imaging *or* elevated cardiac biomarkers, but not both, are classified as Intermediate-low risk.

Patients with low risk based on sPESI = 0, but RVD on imaging are re-classified to Intermediate-low risk.

Low risk patients are those with sPESI = 0 without evidence of RVD on imaging nor elevated cardiac biomarkers (if checked, not obligatory to check). They might benefit from home care in the era of PE treatment with direct oral anticoagulants (Fig. 1) (Becattini et al. 2021; Barco et al. 2020b).

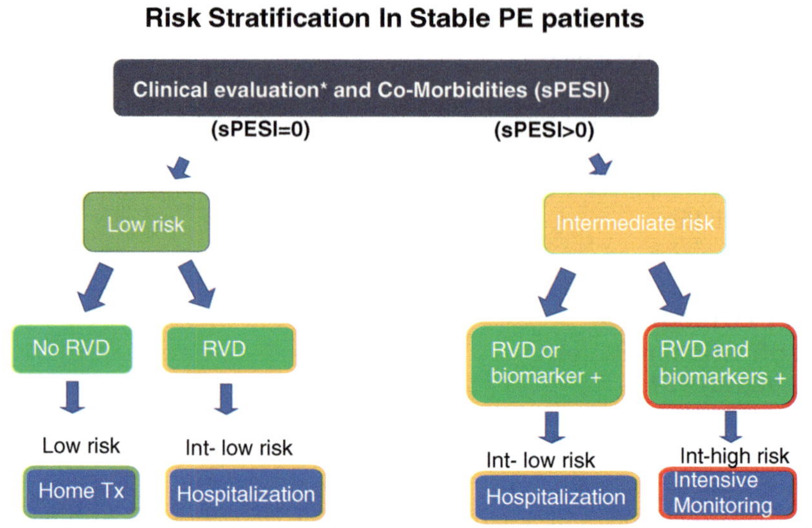

Fig. 1 Risk-adjusted management strategy for acute pulmonary embolism in hemodynamically stable patients. *Clinical evaluation should be done using clinical gestalt or models like pulmonary embolism severity index (PESI/simplified PESI (age >80 years, with cancer, CHF pulmonary disease, HR >110, BP <100, Sat <90%)) scores or Hestia criteria. Right ventricle dysfunction (RVD) is evaluated by transthoracic echocardiography or CTPA. Cardiac biomarkers refer to cardiac troponin level, BNP or NT pro BNP. Int = Intermediate, PESI = Pulmonary Embolism Severity Index, RVD = right ventricle dysfunction, Tx = treatment

2.2 RVD and PE Severity Assessment

RVD can be assessed either at imaging (echocardiography or CT/MR) or by elevated laboratory biomarkers of RV dysfunction or cardiac injury including BNP (B-type natriuretic peptide), NT-pro BNP (N-terminal pro B-type natriuretic peptide), or troponin.

2.2.1 Echocardiographic Assessment of RVD

Echocardiographic assessment of the morphology and function of the RV is widely recognized as a valuable tool for the prognostic assessment in clinical practice with a variety of parameters, including right-to-left ventricular (RV/LV) diameter ratio ≥1.0 and a tricuspid annular plane systolic excursion (TAPSE) <16 mm (Pruszczyk et al. 2014).

2.2.2 CT Assessment of RVD

CTPA is not only the modality of choice for the diagnosis of PE due to its ability to show directly and accurately the presence and extent of thrombi within the pulmonary arteries, and it can also show the cardiac structures and thus can contribute to risk stratification by the assessment of RVD (Table 3).

2.2.2.1 RV/LV Diameter Ratio

The current guidelines recommend the value of RV/LV diameter ratio ≥1 on CTPA as the imaging marker for determination of RVD (Konstantinides et al. 2020). In 2004, a RV/LV diameter ratio >0.9 on reconstructed 4-chamber (4-ch) CT view was reported to predict early death (Schoepf et al. 2004). Later, easier and faster measurement on the original axial slices was shown to have equally valuable prognostic information when compared with 4-ch diameter measurements (Kumamaru et al. 2012). In a prospective multicentric trial using axial RV/LV diameter, a ratio ≥0.9 was reported as an independent predictor for in-hospital death or clinical deterioration with a hazard ratio of 3.5 in the overall acute PE population and with a hazard ratio of 3.8 in hemodynamically stable patients (Becattini et al. 2011). Since then, large series with rather conflicting data have been published

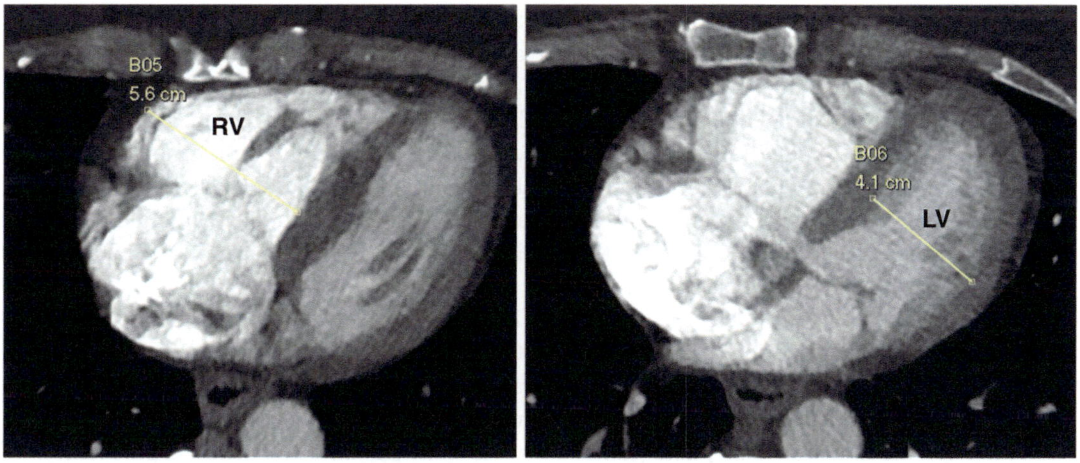

Fig. 2 Right ventricle (RV) and left ventricle (LV) diameter measurements on axial slices. The largest diameter of each ventricle from endocardium to endocardium, most of the time located 1 cm distal to the tricuspid/mitral valves plane and perpendicular to the interventricular septum, or at the chamber's widest diameter. In this example, the RV/LV ratio is 56/41 = 1.4, suggesting a right ventricle dysfunction

regarding the prognostic value of an increased RV/LV ratio as measured on CTPA to predict the overall mortality among patients diagnosed with acute PE, due to many variations across studies, i.e., variable studied populations, measurement techniques, and outcomes. Yet, most meta-analysis found supporting results for this parameter (Bova et al. 2014; Meinel et al. 2015; Trujillo-Santos et al. 2013; Barco et al. 2019); the largest meta-analysis reported that patients with a diameter ratio ≥1.0 should be considered to have an approximately 2.5-fold risk for all-cause mortality and adverse outcome and a five-fold risk for PE-related mortality (Meinel et al. 2015). Other large studies (Jiménez et al. 2014; Aviram et al. 2012a; Cozzi et al. 2021) and an older meta-analysis, however, reported conflicting results regarding the use of RV/LV as a prognostic factor (Coutance et al. 2011). Though RV/LV diameter ratio ≥1 on CTPA is the most widely used marker for mortality, studies show so much conflicting results due to the overall low rate of mortality among stable PE patients, and the variety of confounding factors that may influence any adverse outcome, including terminal oncological disease or sepsis that often coexist among acute PE patients and may be the leading cause of mortality. Therefore, the positive predictive value (PPV) of RV/LV diameter ratio ≥1 is only 8% for short-term mortality after acute PE, which is similar to that of echocardiography. On the other hand, patients with RV/LV diameter ratio <1.0 have excellent short-term outcomes with a negative predictive value (NPV) of 93–100% (Konstantinides et al. 2020; Becattini et al. 2011).

How to Measure the RV/LV Diameter Ratio?

Manual diameter measurements of the ventricles are obtained on axial views, using the maximal diameter of each ventricle from endocardium to endocardium (not necessarily on the same axial slice for both ventricles), most of the time located 1 cm distal to the tricuspid/mitral valves plane and perpendicular to the interventricular septum, or at the chamber's widest diameter (Fig. 2).

Advantage of CT RV/LV Diameter Ratio

It is easily obtained on the original axial slices using manual electronic caliper. Reproducibility in the same center is good (Ende-Verhaar et al. 2017).

Limitations of CT RV/LV Diameter Ratio

- Studies report a high prevalence (48–70%) of increased RV/LV diameter ratio when measured at CT (either ≥0.9 or 1.0) in patients with acute PE: thus, these parameters have both low specificity and positive predictive value for patient outcome. Moreover, in a consecutive series of 862 patients undergoing CTPA for suspected acute PE, where 142/862 patients eventually had PE, the overall prevalence of a RV/LV diameter ratio ≥1 was high (64%) in the whole population; thus, an RV/LV diameter ratio ≥1 is frequent also in patients without acute PE (Hadad et al. 2021). However, in cases where there is a previous CT (negative for PE) available for comparison, the interval increase in RV/LV diameter ratio is more accurate for predicting 30-day mortality (Lu et al. 2008).

- Variation in the measurements plane (same or different axial slices for the RV and LV) or differences in the point of diameter measurements with respect to the atrio-ventricular valve plan may also exist. We recommend measuring 1 cm distal to the tricuspid/mitral valves plane.
- The inspiratory state during the acquisition of CT, which is related to the breath-hold instructions, may also have some influence on the angle of the heart and possibly on the RV/LV diameter ratio when measured on axial images.
- Routine CTPA is acquired without ECG-gating, which may result in some blurring of the endocardial borders due to motion artefacts. The use of ECG-gating may eliminate these artifacts, nevertheless at the expense of an increased radiation dose. The benefit from ECG-gated CT scan for the evaluation of RV ventricular diameter, area, and volume measurements was reported as minimal and does not justify its routine clinical use (Lu et al. 2009). Moreover, both ventricles are found approximately on the same position in the z-axis on the CTPA scan and thus will be scanned while they are in the same phase of the cardiac cycle without gating; thus, the RV/LV diameter ratio is assumed to be similar to that evaluated by an ECG-gated scan.

Abnormal Features Without Definite Proof of Quantitative Criteria

Interventricular straightening or septal bowing toward the left ventricle has also been suggested as a qualitative imaging finding reflecting RVD and thus associated with increased mortality in acute PE (Meinel et al. 2015; Becattini et al. 2014; Lyhne et al. 2019). Some other authors however did not find such an association with outcome (Ghaye et al. 2006; Araoz et al. 2003). Interventricular septal straightening or bowing, indeed, was found to have a high degree of interobserver variability (Araoz et al. 2007).

2.2.2.2 Cardiac Chambers Volumetry

Compared to unidimensional measurements, volumetric analysis is more accurate for size assessment. A dedicated software is necessary for three-dimensional (3D) heart segmentation of cardiac structures and calculations of their respective volumes.

How to Assess Cardiac Chamber Volumes?

Semi-automated or fully automated volumetric measurements of the RV, right atrium (RA), LV, and left atrium (LA) can be obtained by commercially available software. Using a semiautomatic tool for ventricular volume analysis, the endocardial contours are segmented from the valvular plane to the apex of both ventricles. The volumes of each cavity are subsequently calculated (Kang et al. 2011). In the case of fully automated algorithm, the software adapts an anatomical model of the heart chambers to the CT image volume (Aviram et al. 2016). The output consists of a 3D graphic display of the heart segmented into its main structures. The volume of each cardiac chamber is automatically calculated as the sum of all voxels included inside the volume (Fig. 3). Visual confirmation of the segmentation correctness can be easily obtained in every reformation as the segmentation is superimposed over the CT images. In case of inaccurate segmentation, 3D tools are available for manual corrections.

Right/Left Ventricle Volume Ratio

A few retrospective studies reported that increased RV/LV volume ratio is more accurate for the identification of RVD using echocardiography as the reference standard (Henzler et al. 2012) and for prediction of adverse outcome of PE (Kang et al. 2011; Meyer et al. 2012) (Table 4). As a high degree of concordance have been reported between

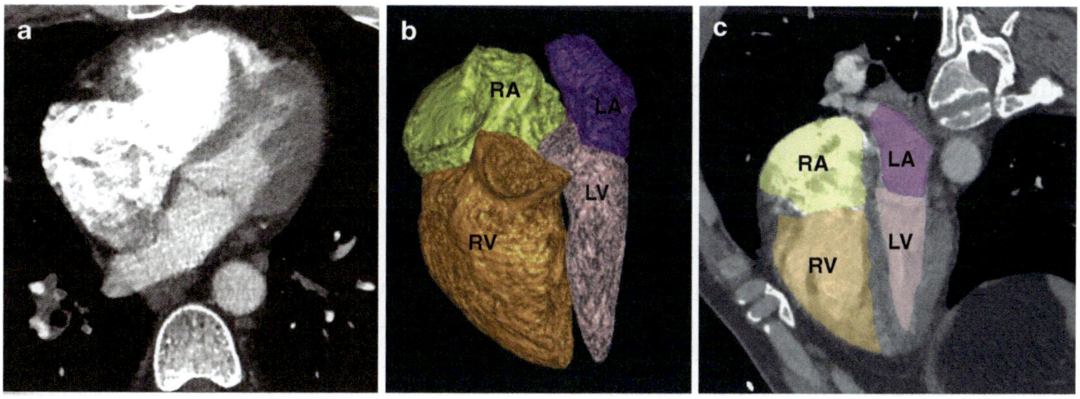

Fig. 3 Volumetric segmentation of the heart. Representative case showing CT volumetric segmentation of the 4 cardiac chambers of a 50-year-old male with intermediate-high risk PE, who eventually underwent reduced dose thrombolysis. (**a**) Axial image showing the dilated RA and RV compressing the LA and LV. (**b**) Volumetric model of the 4 cardiac chambers. (**c**) Horizontal long axis reformation (4-chamber view). LA—purple; LV—pink; RA—yellow; RV—orange. Volumes of the left atrium (LA): 45 mL; left ventricle (LV): 63 mL; right atrium (RA): 156 mL; right ventricle (RV): 227 mL. RV/LV volume ratio = 3.6, RA/LA volume ratio = 3.5

Table 4 Cardiovascular parameters associated with increased 30 days mortality in acute pulmonary embolism

Parameter	All-cause mortality risk	Source
RV/LV diameter ≥1 (Meinel et al. 2015)	2.5 (1.8–3.5)	Meta-analysis
RV/LV volume ≥1.2 (Kang et al. 2011)	6.5 (1.8–23.8)	Retrospective
RA/LA volume ≥1.2 (Aviram et al. 2016)	2.1 (1.3–3.4)	Retrospective
RA/LA volume ≥1.8 (Lerchbaumer et al. 2021)	3.1 (1.9–5.2)[a]	Prospective
LA volume ≤62 mL (Aviram et al. 2016)	2.4 (1.5–3.9)	Retrospective
IVC CM reflux (substantial[b]) (Meinel et al. 2015)	2.2 (1.5–3.2)	Meta-analysis

[a]Adverse events including mortality
[b]Substantial IVC CM reflux is defined as CM reflux into the IVC and the hepatic veins

ECG-gated and non-gated cardiac volume ratio measurements, the routine use of ECG-gating is not justified in clinical use for this purpose (Lu et al. 2009). A threshold value of RV/LV volume ratio >1.2 was suggested as predictive of 30-day death (Kang et al. 2011). In the largest retrospective series which investigated the association between the cardiac chamber volume and mortality, RV/LV volume ratio was however not found to be a significant predictor (Aviram et al. 2016).

Right/Left Atrial Ratio

When RVD is present, the decrease in stroke volume of the RV can lead to a decrease in pulmonary venous return with sudden underfilling of the LA, contributing to the decrease of LV preload, cardiac output, systemic blood pressure, and coronary perfusion, which may eventually cause circulatory collapse. In addition, RVD may be associated with RA enlargement. The RA walls are thin membranous structures, altered by minor pressure changes of up to 5 mmHg, while higher pressures are needed to induce RV dilation (the RV wall is more muscular and stiffer than that of the RA). Thus, any increase in RA volume and decrease in LA volume resulting from the increased hemodynamic load related to the sudden increased pulmonary vascular resistance secondary to acute PE may be more pronounced or even precede any change at the ventricular level.

Patients with a RA/LA volume ratio >1.2 had a higher 30-day mortality rate (17% vs. 9.4%; HR, 2.1; $p = 0.002$) in a study on 636 acute PE patients (Aviram et al. 2016). LA volume ≤62 mL was associated with around twice the mortality rate when compared to patients with LA volume

>62 mL (19.6% vs. 8.9%; HR adj 2.44, 95% CI 1.5–3.9, $p < 0.001$) (Aviram et al. 2016). On a different cohort of 609 prospectively registered PE patients, using the same volumetric software, a calculated cut-off value of 1.8 (AUC 0.64, 95% CI 0.56–0.71) predicted an adverse outcome, both in unselected (OR 3.1, 95% CI 1.9–5.2) and normotensive patients (OR 2.7, 95% CI 1.3–5.6) (Lerchbaumer et al. 2021). LA volume was also the only atrial measurement associated with PE-related mortality in another cohort of patients with more severe PE (Kirkbride et al. 2022).

Advantages of Cardiac Chamber Volumes

- 3D, objective, and reproducible when using the automatic tools without manual corrections, the automatic volumetric software always provided the same measurement (less than a 1 mL difference) (Aviram et al. 2016).

Limitations

- Software is required.

2.2.3 Reflux of Contrast Medium in the IVC

Substantial reflux of contrast medium (CM) into the inferior vena cava (IVC) when detected on CTPA may serve as a pathophysiological marker of RVD (Aviram et al. 2012b). IVC CM reflux is a radio-dynamic sign, which can be easily identified on the original axial slices, requiring no special reformation. Groves et al. suggested 6 grades of IVC reflux as a semi-quantitative method to assess by CT evidence of tricuspid regurgitation (Groves et al. 2004).

2.2.3.1 How to Assess Reflux?

IVC CM reflux is considered moderate or severe, when the supra-hepatic IVC is completely opacified by CM (grade 3), or when there is opacification of the central, mid, or peripheral hepatic veins (grades 4–6), according to Groves et al. (2004).

In the context of acute PE risk assessment, Aviram et al. reported that substantial reflux (moderate or severe grades according to Grove's descriptions) is related to an increased 30-day mortality by a factor of 2.2 (Aviram et al. 2008) (Fig. 4) (Table 4). Other studies reported the association between the presence of reflux and adverse outcome with or without quantifying the reflux grade (Meinel et al. 2015; Ghaye et al. 2006; Bach et al. 2015).

2.2.3.2 Advantage of IVC CM Reflux

- Immediate visual assessment on the axial images.

2.2.3.3 Limitations of IVC Reflux

- IVC CM reflux grade is highly dependent on technical factors including the injection rate of CM (Yeh et al. 2004) and CM volume relative to the patient's BMI. Thus, high CM injection rate in small persons may result a substantial IVC reflux in patients without RVD.
- Reflux may also appear in case of tricuspid regurgitation and atrial fibrillation (Aviram et al. 2012b).
- Reflux cannot be determined when CM is injected through femoral veins or central lines.

2.2.3.4 Vessels Measurements

Pulmonary Artery Diameter

PA diameter is measured as the widest diameter of the pulmonary artery (PA) trunk perpendicular to its long axis approximately halfway between the pulmonary valve and the bifurcation of the pulmonary trunk. PA diameter is not considered as a reliable tool for risk stratification in the acute PE setting. The value of 29.0 mm has been established as the maximal normal value of main PA diameter and suggested as cutoff to detect pulmonary hypertension (PHT) (Truong et al. 2012; Mahammedi et al. 2013). However, in normal population, older age, male sex, and higher body surface area are each correlated with larger PA diameter. There are many threshold measurements for PA diameter in PHT found in the literature, with various sensitivity and specificities; thus, it is also a questionable marker for PHT. The

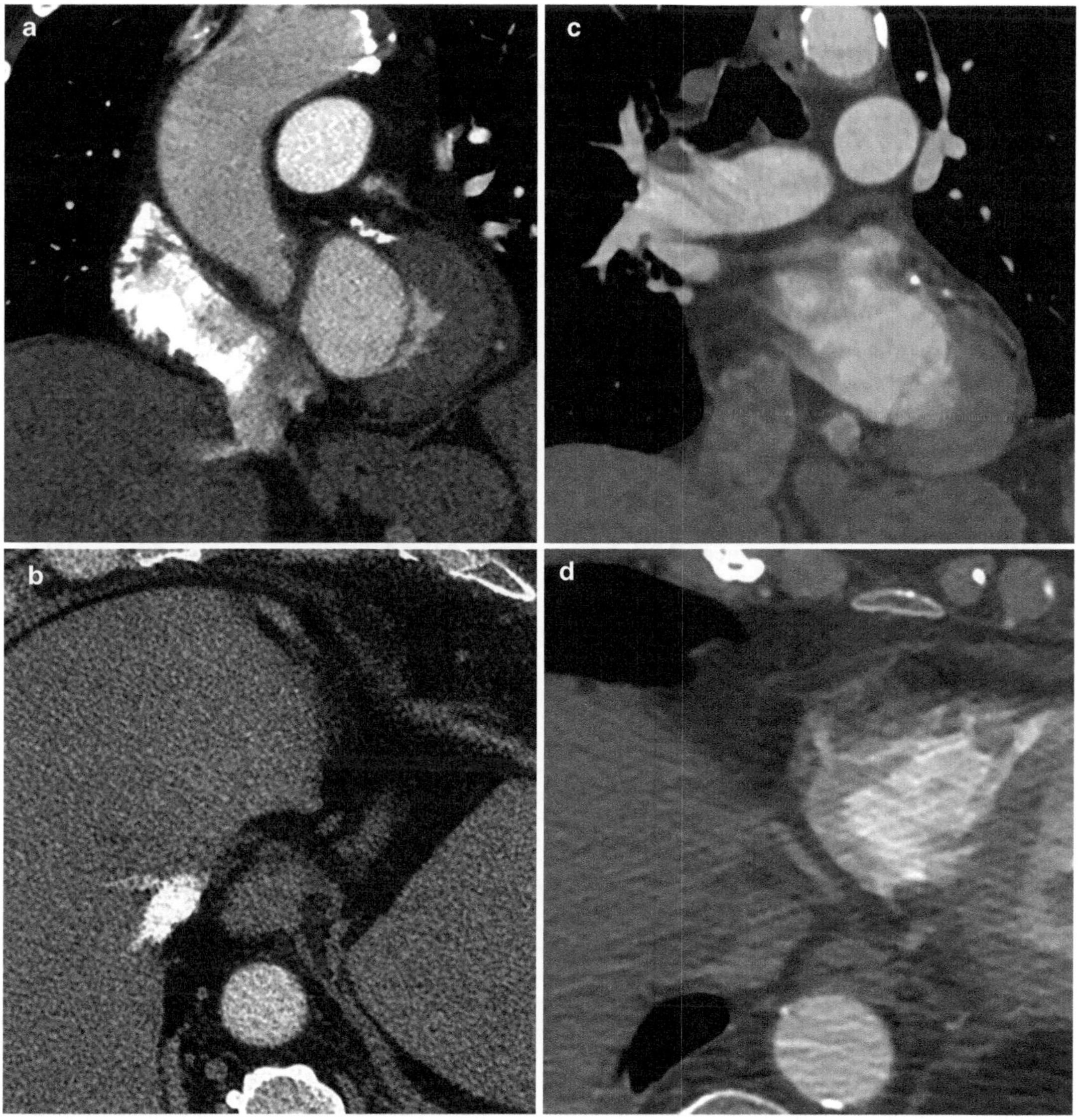

Fig. 4 Reflux of contrast medium into IVC. (**a**, **b**) Substantial reflux into the IVC and the central hepatic veins. (**c**, **d**) no significant reflux

position paper from the Fleischner Society proposed various thresholds of PA diameter for suggesting underlying PHT according to the clinical context (Remy-Jardin et al. 2021). In the acute setting, the PA dilates minimally (around 1 mm) and thus does not correlate to prognosis. In a single retrospective study, a median PA diameter of 29.9 mm correlated with adverse outcome, but this was with a broad range, and thus, authors admit that the PA diameter is not a useful measurement clinically (Lyhne et al. 2019).

Advantages:

- PA diameter is easy to measure.

Limitations:

- Not a reliable measurement. May represent background of underlying PHT.

Other Vascular Measurements

Other vascular measurements have been investigated. Similar to PA diameter, conflicting results have been reported concerning their value for risk stratification of patients with PE.

Increased diameter of SVC, azygos vein, coronary sinus, and IVC may result from right heart dysfunction. For each of those parameters, almost an equivalent number of studies showed them as significantly correlated or not with adverse outcomes, and very rarely as independent predictors (Cozzi et al. 2021; Ghaye et al. 2006; Araoz et al. 2003). Therefore, those contrasted results should considered them as of low interest in predicting patient outcome in clinical routine.

2.2.4 Thrombus Load-CT Obstruction Index (CTOI)

It was shown that the thrombus obstruction burden in the pulmonary arteries calculated on conventional angiography correlates with PE severity and may be used to guide treatment (Miller et al. 1971; Walsh et al. 1973). Bankier et al. adapted one of these angiographic indexes (Miller index) to CTPA by evaluating the embolic burden in the main, lobar, and segmental pulmonary arteries. Their PE severity CT obstruction index (CTOI) showed excellent interobserver agreement (≥ 0.85; $p = 0.001$) and good correlation with the angiographic indexes (Bankier et al. 1997).

Mastora et al. suggested a new CTOI system taking into account the level and number of involved pulmonary arteries with the severity of vascular obstruction (on a 5-point scale) to represent the percentage of obstructed vascular bed (Mastora et al. 2003). They divided the pulmonary arteries into 31 subdivisions. Percentage of obstructed pulmonary circulation may be calculated for the entire pulmonary arterial (PA) bed, central PA bed, and peripheral PA bed. The score was compared to PA pressure measured using echocardiography. The PA pressure was found to be significantly higher in patients with CTOI higher than 50% ($p < 0.001$).

Qanadli et al. proposed a CTOI using a simplified approach (Qanadli et al. 2001). They divided the lungs in 20 segments and refined the index to assess the degree of obstruction (partial vs. complete) to evaluate lung perfusion beyond the clot as a marker of RV load. They found that CTOI >40% predicts RV dilatation ($p = 0.01$).

Multiple other cohorts using the Qanadli CTOI reported conflicting results. Wu et al. and Van der Meer et al. found that CTOI index ≥60% or ≥40%, respectively, was associated with short-term mortality, while Pech et al. and Ghaye et al. did not find such correlation to patient survival (Ghaye et al. 2006; Wu et al. 2004; Pech et al. 2007; van der Meer et al. 2005). In a different cohort, CTOI was found to predict survival in patient subgroup without cardiopulmonary disease (Rotzinger et al. 2020).

Finally, a meta-analysis showed no correlation between the Qanadli CTOI and 30 days mortality (Vedovati et al. 2013).

2.2.4.1 How to Calculate Mastora and Qanadli CTOI

In the Mastora CTOI, the PA are considered to have 31 subdivisions: 5 mediastinal (pulmonary trunk, right and left main PA, and right and left interlobar PA), 6 lobar PA, and 20 segmental PA. A central PE is defined if there is one or more clot(s) at mediastinal or lobar level. The percentage of vascular obstruction for each artery is determined using a 5-point scale (1 < 25%; 2 = 25–49%; 3 = 50–74%; 4 = 75–99%; 5 = 100%), yielding a maximal score of 155. The percentage of pulmonary circulation obstructed is calculated by dividing the observed score for each level by the maximal possible score for this level. The score may be calculated for the entire PA bed, central PA bed (mediastinal and lobar arteries), and peripheral PA bed (Mastora et al. 2003).

In the Qanadli CTOI, each lung is considered to have 10 segments (3 upper lobes, 2 right middle lobe/lingual, and 5 in the lower lobes), resulting in a total of 20 segments. A score is assigned to every segment, 1 for partial and 2 for complete occlusion, resulting in a maximal score of 40. As an example, partially occluding clot in the main right PA will be calculated as 10, but if there is also complete occlusion of a right lower lobar segmental PA, the score for the right lung will be 11 (10 for the partial occlusion of the main PA + 1 for complete occlusion of a segmental branch). A clot in a subsegmental PA, without a proximal clot, will be assigned a score of 1. In order to calculate the CTOI as percent, the total cal-

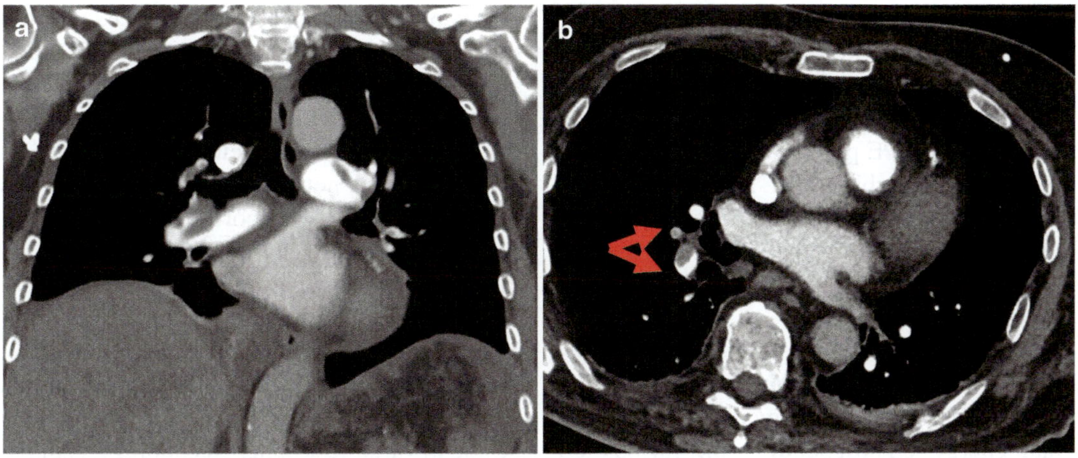

Fig. 5 Example of Qanadli CTOI score in two different patients. (**a**) Coronal CT pulmonary angiography shows non obstructive bilateral central pulmonary emboli. CTOI is 20, CTOI percentage is 50%. (**b**) Axial CT pulmonary angiography demonstrates partially occluding clot in the descending right lower lobe artery leading to the 4 basal segments and total occlusion of right middle lobe lateral segment artery (red arrows). Yielded CTOI is 6, and CTOI percentage is 15%

culated score is then divided by 40 and multiplied by 100 (Fig. 5) (Qanadli et al. 2001).

2.2.4.2 Advantages of CTOI

- Both scores are reproducible (Mahammedi et al. 2013; Meyer et al. 2021).
- No software required.

2.2.4.3 Limitations of CTOI

- Both scores are cumbersome to calculate. However, the Qanadli score involves less pulmonary subdivisions (20 vs. 31), and the occlusion degree is simplified (2-point vs. 5-point scale), is more intuitive to understand and calculate, and is faster to obtain than the Mastora score (Meyer et al. 2021). A more practical approach may be to mention specifically the size and number of involved arteries and, when the clot burden is heavy, to state it in the conclusion.
- In addition, the CT resolution nowadays is significantly better than at the times that the index was created. Therefore, even for emboli previously considered as fully obstructive, some contrast can be seen surrounding them due to improved image resolution, which can change obstructing grade, particularly when thinner slice thickness is used.
- Studies regarding the correlation of CTOI and prognosis are mainly retrospective and reported conflicting results (Wu et al. 2004; van der Meer et al. 2005; Vedovati et al. 2013; Norton et al. 2021; Apfaltrer et al. 2012; Chaosuwannakit et al. 2021).

2.2.5 Localization of Clots

2.2.5.1 Localization of the Most Proximal Clot

Easier than CTOI calculation, the simple localization of the most proximal clot has shown to be predictor of outcome in a few studies. A multicentric study showed that central PE (clots located in main PA) on one side and segmental or subsegmental PE on the other side were associated with HR of 8.3 and 0.12 for adverse outcome in stable patients, respectively (Vedovati et al. 2012). The localization of the most proximal clot is recommended in structured reporting for PE.

2.2.5.2 Saddle Embolus

Saddle PE, namely, clot straddling the bifurcation of the pulmonary trunk, has been reported in 3–5% of PE patients at CTPA. No worse prognosis in patients showing central saddle embolus was reported in the vast majority of studies (Gandara et al. 2011).

2.2.5.3 Intracardiac Clots

Also called as clots in transit (in the right heart), intracardiac clots occur in 4–18% of patients with PE. They have been reported to be associated with worse PE prognosis and higher risk of PE recurrence (Torbicki et al. 2003; Barrios et al. 2016). No accurate quantification has been reported. It is recommended that intracardiac clots depicted on CTPA should be confirmed by echocardiography.

2.2.6 Iodine Maps in Multi-energy CT

Multi-energy CT, also termed spectral CT or Dual energy CT (depending on various CT technologies: Dual source CT, kVp switching, detector-based single source detector CT, dual scans, or photon-counting CT), allows better identification of iodine, as different materials exhibit different X-ray absorption on various X-ray energies (Rajiah et al. 2019; Rassouli et al. 2017; Rajiah 2020). Increased absorption by iodine on low X-ray energy (e.g., low tube voltage) can be used to create iodine-map overlay which are superimposed on the standard CT images and to create pulmonary blood volume (PBV) images that represent iodine distribution within the lung as an indicator of regional blood flow (Fig. 6). Iodine maps may be considered as surrogates of lung perfusion and identify blood-flow "perfusion-like" defects (PD), similar to lung perfusion scintigraphy (Thieme et al. 2008).

2.2.6.1 Clinical Value of Iodine Maps

PBV iodine maps provide functional information, demonstrating whether a thrombus is responsible for any local blood flow decrease or stop (Pontana et al. 2008). Direct assessment of parenchymal blood flow, showing obstruction at the parenchymal level beyond the clot, may be a more direct marker of PE pathophysiological effect on RV overload compared to thrombus load in the pulmonary arteries (Fig. 7) (Chae et al. 2010). It also considers perfusion defects due to other causes as underlying cardio-pleuro-pulmonary disease (i.e., emphysema, bronchiolar disease, previous PE scars) and functional vascular tone modifications due to reflex vasoconstriction or release of vasoactive agents as a consequence of PE or due to peripheral clots not detected by CTPA. Studies evaluating various PD scores for PE risk stratification demonstrated variable correlation of PD score severity with RV/LV ratio, CTOI, D-dimer values, and adverse outcome (Apfaltrer et al. 2012; Chae et al. 2010; Bauer et al. 2011; Im et al. 2017; Meinel et al. 2013; Jawad et al. 2021) (Table 5). Inconsistency in results may be due to variable scanners technology, acquisition technique, particularly related to contrast medium injection, and PBV defects assessment method. Yet, it has been shown that PD scores can distinguish from low- to intermediate-risk groups (Bauer et al. 2011; Im et al. 2017; Kong et al. 2017).

2.2.6.2 How to Assess Perfusion Defects on PBV Iodine Maps?

PBV iodine maps may be generated automatically on CT workstations, using predefined thresholds (standard for each vendor). PDs appear as wedge-shaped peripheral areas with reduced iodine content (Figs. 6 and 7). Common methods to calculate PD: PD score can be calculated based on qualitative assessment of PD for each segment. Alternatively, PD volume can be derived (semi-automatically or automatically). The lung is segmented, and its total volume calculated. Areas showing PDs are either manually traced or automatically calculated (based on pre-set HU threshold), summed, and divided by total lung volume to calculate the relative PD volume (Fig. 8).

2.2.6.3 Advantages of PBV Iodine Maps

- Increases sensitivity for PE detection.
- Areas of decreased blood-flow are demonstrated.
- Subjective PBV assessment do not vary significantly across various CM injections protocols (Kosmala et al. 2020).

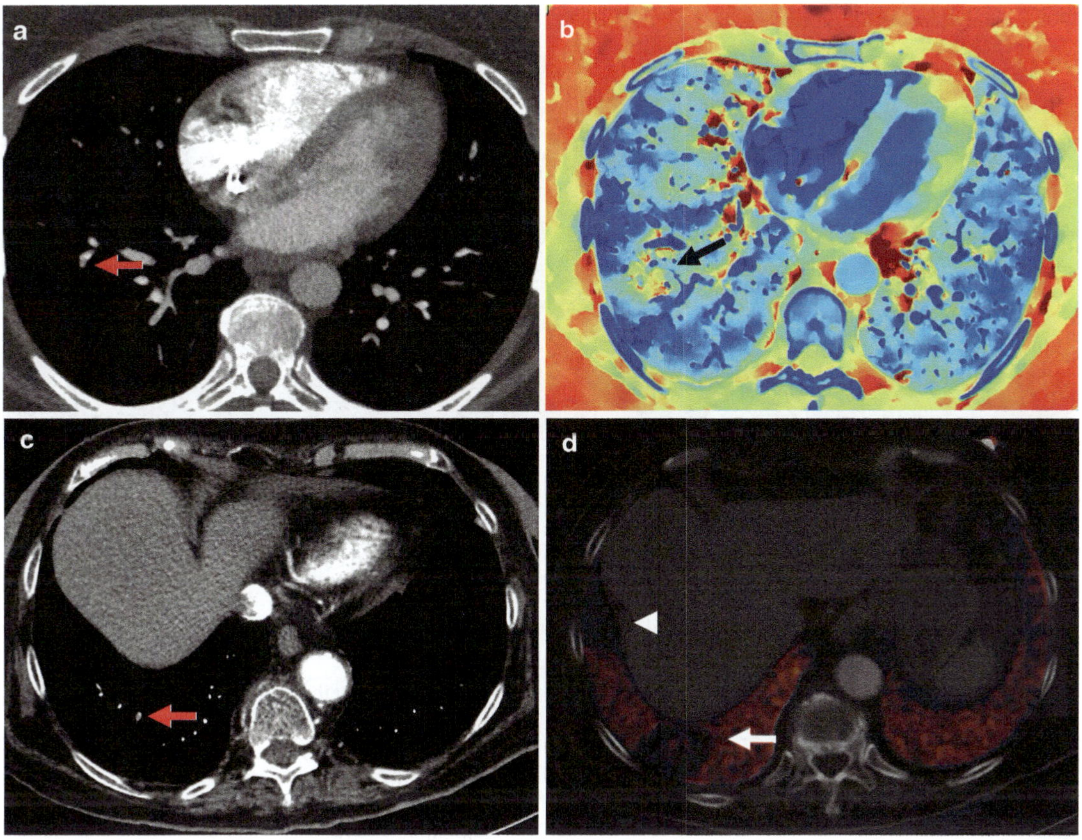

Fig. 6 Pulmonary blood volume (PBV) images and perfusion defects using two different spectral modalities. (**a**, **b**) Detector-based dual energy spectral detector CT (IQon, Philips Healthcare, Best, The Netherlands). (**a**) Axial CT pulmonary angiography showing filling defect in a small subsegmental branch of the right lower lobe (red arrow). (**b**) Z-effective atomic number map image, showing a perfusion defect in the corresponding area in the right lower lobe (black arrow). (**c**, **d**) Dual-source dual energy CT (Somatom Flash, Siemens Healthcare, Forchheim, Germany). (**c**) Axial CT pulmonary angiography showing filling defect in a small subsegmental branch of the right lower lobe (red arrow). (**d**) Iodine color-coded map overlay in red. Perfusion defect in the corresponding area (white arrow) and additional perfusion defect located more anteriorly (white arrowhead). The image with corresponding occluded vessel is not shown

2.2.6.4 Limitations of PBV Iodine Maps

- Wedge-shaped PD can result from hypoxemic arterial vasoconstriction due to airway disease, sometimes without obvious signs of bronchial or bronchiolar disease (Fig. 9).
- In cases of airspace disease, lung consolidation, which shows a higher attenuation than normal aerated lung, may be not processed in the PBV iodine maps and can be mistaken for a PD. In such cases, the PBV maps settings may be manually changed.
- Inhomogeneity of PBV maps can be seen in emphysema or due to artifacts. Breathing or motion artifacts, areas next to the heart or diaphragm or close to dense CM in superior vena cava or heart, may render PBV maps less specific for PE-related PD (Fig. 9).
- There is no standardized PD scoring method.
- Studies regarding the correlation of iodine maps and outcome are limited, retrospective, and small.

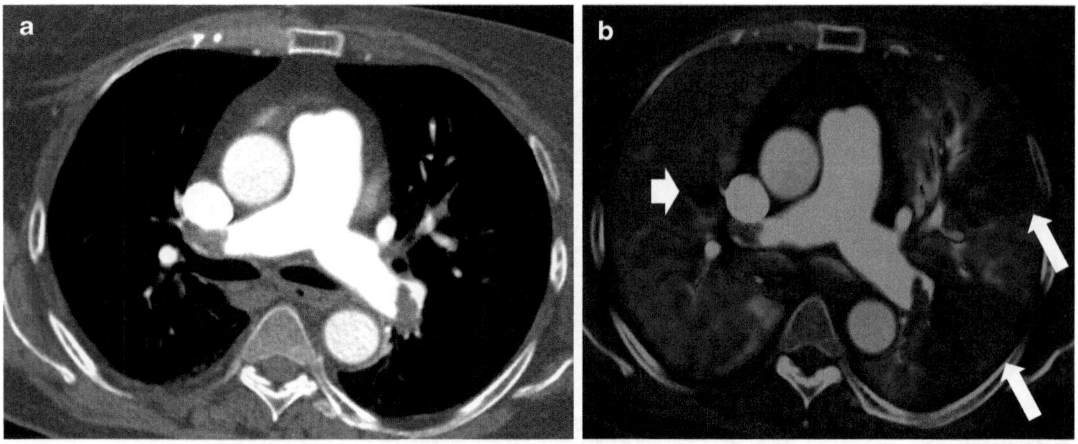

Fig. 7 Perfusion defects resulting from central pulmonary embolism. (**a**) Axial CT pulmonary angiography shows bilateral central pulmonary emboli. (**b**) On the PBV iodine map, there are two segmental perfusion defects in the left upper and left lower lobes (white arrows), and there is no perfusion defects in the right lung. The dark line in the right lung (white arrowhead) is a streak artifact from concentrated contrast material in SVC

Table 5 Correlation between pulmonary blood volume perfusion defects (PD) and various parameters associated with increased PE risk

Parameter	Correlation[a]	PD assessment method	Scanning technique
RV/LV ratio (Chae et al. 2010)	$r = 0.66, 0.69$	Qualitative segmental score	DS
RV/LV ratio (Meinel et al. 2013)	$r = -0.52$	Quantitative PD volume (automated)	DS
RV/LV ratio (Apfaltrer et al. 2012)	$r = 0.2166$	Quantitative PD volume (semi-automated)	DS
RV/LV ratio (Jawad et al. 2021)	$r = 0.45$	Quantitative PD volume (automated)	SS switching kVp
	$r = 0.56$	Quantitative PD volume (semi-automated)	SS switching kVp
Obstruction index (Chae et al. 2010)	$r = 0.85, 0.87$	Qualitative segmental score	DS
Obstruction index (Meinel et al. 2013)[b]	$r = -0.46$	Quantitative PD volume (automated)	DS
Obstruction index (Apfaltrer et al. 2012)	$r = 0.5$	Quantitative PD volume (semi-automated)	DS
Obstruction index (Jawad et al. 2021)	$r = 0.51$	Quantitative PD volume (automated)	SS switching kVp
	$r = 0.85$	Quantitative PD volume (semi-automated)	SS switching kVp
D-Dimer value (Bauer et al. 2011)	$r = 0.43–0.47$	Quantitative PD volume (manual)	DS
Thirty days all-cause mortality risk (Im et al. 2017)	HR 1.044	Quantitative PD volume (semi-automated)	DS
ICU admission (Meinel et al. 2013)[b]	$r = -0.39$	Quantitative PD volume (automated)	DS
Adverse outcome (ICU admission or death) (Apfaltrer et al. 2012)	Auc = 0.838	Quantitative PD volume (semi-automated)	DS

Studies were retrospective
[a]All correlations are statistically significant and mainly weak
[b]Inverse correlation was calculated

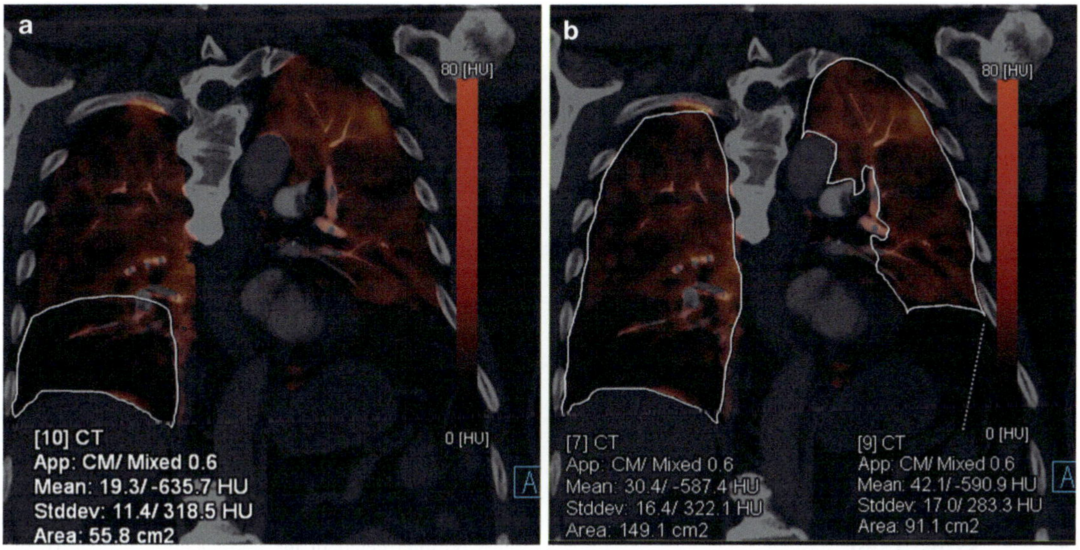

Fig. 8 Assessment of relative perfusion defect volume on pulmonary blood volume iodine maps. (**a**) Area of perfusion defect is manually traced on consecutive PBV images. (**b**) Semi-automated or manual tracing of both lungs on the coronal image. Total lung volume is calculated by propagating the trace through the whole lungs. The relative perfusion defect volume is calculated by dividing the sum of perfusion defects by total lung volume

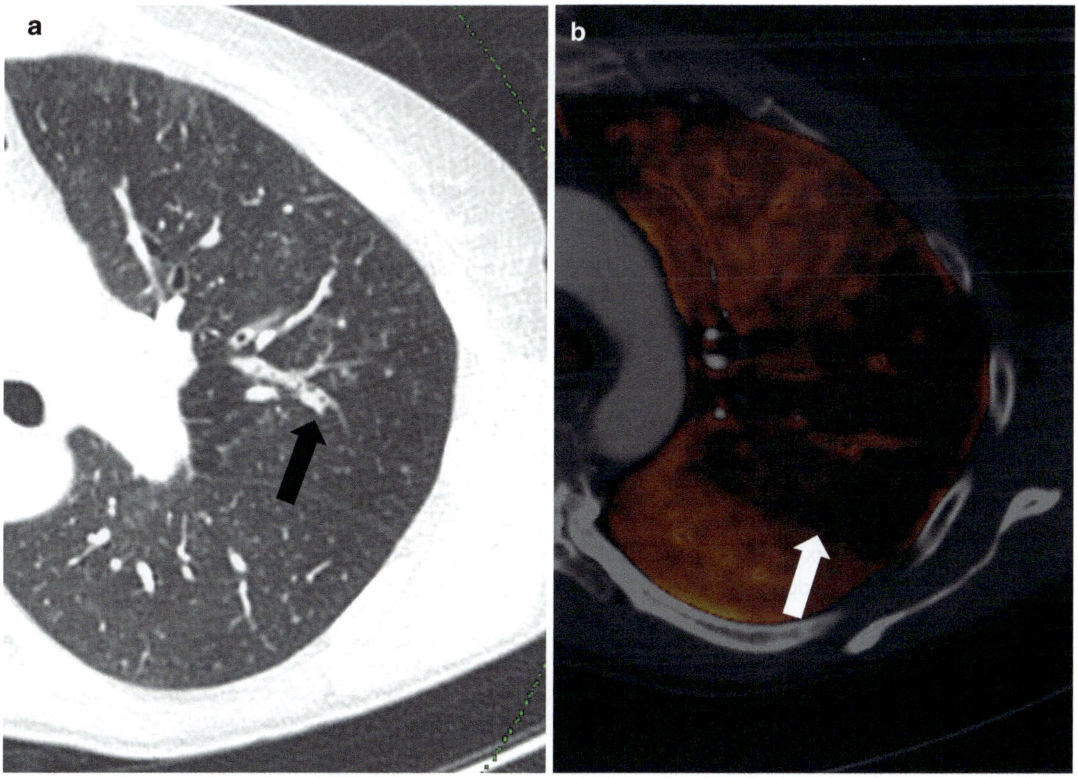

Fig. 9 Perfusion defect due to airway disease. (**a**) Axial image on lung window settings shows dilation and mucous plugging in left upper lobe bronchi (black arrow). (**b**) Pulmonary blood volume iodine map shows a large associated perfusion defect due to associated hypoxemic vasoconstriction (white arrow)

3 Future Perspectives

Artificial intelligence with deep learning models is currently developed and increasingly used in imaging. Machine-based learning and tasks can be used for risk stratification in patients with acute PE. Zhang et al. recently used deep learning models for pulmonary embolism detection and for clot burden calculation using the Qanadli and Mastora scores and correlated them with RV/LA ratio (Zhang et al. 2022). Use of AI for automatic segmentation and measurements and deep learning models for risk stratification are promising fields yet to be explored.

4 Summary

PE is a potentially life-threatening condition requiring fast and accurate diagnosis and risk stratification to establish the appropriate monitoring and treatment. Correct implementation of clinical decision rules in diagnostic workup for PE, such as the Wells score and revised Geneva score, improves adequate use of CTPA for the more highly suspected patients.

In addition to clinical assessment and cardiac biomarkers, CTPA can contribute to risk stratification by imaging findings that are associated with RVD and early mortality. However, all suggested CTPA parameters have limited prognostic power by themselves and need to be used in combination with clinical parameters and cardiac biomarkers.

RV/LV diameter ratio ≥1.0 is the most widely used fast and simple parameter to assess RVD. It predicts risk for increased risk of adverse outcome, which mandates hospitalization, whereas ratios <1.0 can safely exclude adverse outcome and, consequently, help identify patients who are potential candidates for treatment at home.

Other parameters, which are supported by the literature, include substantial reflux of CM to the IVC and the hepatic veins, increased RV/LV volume ratio ≥1.2 and RA/LA volume ratio ≥1.2, as well as reduced LA volume to ≤62 mL.

High CTOI score is a marker of adverse outcome but is cumbersome to calculate.

PBV maps can be easily incorporated into CTPA interpretation. After looking at the pulmonary vessel, looking at the PBV maps for PDs as a sign of functionally occluding clot burden and in order to suspect smaller clots, which may be overlooked at initial inspection.

Use of AI for automatic segmentation and measurements and deep learning models for risk stratification are promising fields yet to be explored.

Disclaimer All measurements in this book have been obtained from peer-reviewed papers and guidelines from professional organizations, unless explicitly stated otherwise. While the authors, editors, and publisher have gone through a rigorous process to establish their correct reproduction from the original source, each measurement must be interpreted in the correct clinical context, this along with an accurate way of measurement, and taking into account all technical variables, this including follow-up exams with various equipment or software. Neither the authors, the editors, nor the publisher can accept any legal responsibility for any improper application or interpretation of these measurements as well as their potential consequences.

References

Apfaltrer P, Bachmann V, Meyer M et al (2012) Prognostic value of perfusion defect volume at dual energy CTA in patients with pulmonary embolism: correlation with CTA obstruction scores, CT parameters of right ventricular dysfunction and adverse clinical outcome. Eur J Radiol 81(11):3592–3597

Araoz PA, Gotway MB, Trowbridge RL et al (2003) Helical CT pulmonary angiography predictors of in-hospital morbidity and mortality in patients with acute pulmonary embolism. J Thorac Imaging 18(4):207–216

Araoz PA, Gotway MB, Harrington JR et al (2007) Pulmonary embolism: prognostic CT findings. Radiology 242(3):889–897

Aviram G, Rogowski O, Gotler Y et al (2008) Real-time risk stratification of patients with acute pulmonary embolism by grading the reflux of contrast into the inferior vena cava on computerized tomographic pulmonary angiography. J Thromb Haemost 6(9):1488–1493

Aviram G, Sirota-Cohen C, Steinvil A et al (2012a) Automated volumetric analysis of four cardiac chambers in pulmonary embolism: a novel technology for fast risk stratification. Thromb Haemost 108(2):384–393

Aviram G, Cohen D, Steinvil A et al (2012b) Significance of reflux of contrast medium into the inferior vena cava on computerized tomographic pulmonary angiogram. Am J Cardiol 109(3):432–437

Aviram G, Soikher E, Bendet A et al (2016) Prediction of mortality in pulmonary embolism based on left atrial volume measured on CT pulmonary angiography. Chest 149(3):667–675

Bach AG, Nansalmaa B, Kranz J et al (2015) CT pulmonary angiography findings that predict 30-day mortality in patients with acute pulmonary embolism. Eur J Radiol 84(2):332–337. https://doi.org/10.1016/j.ejrad.2014.11.023. Epub 2014 Nov 27. PMID: 25487818

Bankier AA, Janata K, Fleischmann D et al (1997) Severity assessment of acute pulmonary embolism with spiral CT: evaluation of two modified angiographic scores and comparison with clinical data. J Thorac Imaging 12(2):150–158

Barco S, Mahmoudpour SH, Planquette B et al (2019) Prognostic value of right ventricular dysfunction or elevated cardiac biomarkers in patients with low-risk pulmonary embolism: a systematic review and meta-analysis. Eur Heart J 40(11):902–910

Barco S, Mahmoudpour SH, Valerio L et al (2020a) Trends in mortality related to pulmonary embolism in the European Region, 2000–15: analysis of vital registration data from the WHO Mortality Database. Lancet Respir Med 8(3):277–287. https://doi.org/10.1016/S2213-2600(19)30354-6. PMID: 31615719

Barco S, Schmidtmann I, Ageno W et al (2020b) Early discharge and home treatment of patients with low-risk pulmonary embolism with the oral factor Xa inhibitor rivaroxaban: an international multicentre single-arm clinical trial. Eur Heart J 41(4):509–518. https://doi.org/10.1093/eurheartj/ehz367. PMID: 31120118

Barrios D, Rosa-Salazar V, Jiménez D et al (2016) Right heart thrombi in pulmonary embolism. Eur Respir J 48(5):1377–1385. https://doi.org/10.1183/13993003.01044-2016. Epub 2016 Oct 6. PMID: 27799388

Bauer RW, Frellesen C, Renker M et al (2011) Dual energy CT pulmonary blood volume assessment in acute pulmonary embolism – correlation with D-dimer level, right heart strain and clinical outcome. Eur Radiol 21(9):1914–1921

Becattini C, Agnelli G, Vedovati MC et al (2011) Multidetector computed tomography for acute pulmonary embolism: diagnosis and risk stratification in a single test. Eur Heart J 32(13):1657–1663. https://doi.org/10.1093/eurheartj/ehr108. PMID: 21504936

Becattini C, Agnelli G, Germini F, Vedovati MC (2014) Computed tomography to assess risk of death in acute pulmonary embolism: a meta-analysis. Eur Respir J 43(6):1678–1690

Becattini C, Maraziti G, Vinson DR, Ng ACC et al (2021) Right Ventricular assessment in patients with pulmonary embolism at low risk for death based on clinical models: an individual patient data meta-analysis. Eur Heart J 42(33):3190–3199. https://doi.org/10.1093/eurheartj/ehab329. PMID: 34179965

Bova C, Sanchez O, Prandoni P et al (2014) Identification of intermediate-risk patients with acute symptomatic pulmonary embolism. Eur Respir J 44(3):694–703. https://doi.org/10.1183/09031936.00006114. PMID: 24696111

Chae EJ, Seo JB, Jang YM et al (2010) Dual-energy CT for assessment of the severity of acute pulmonary embolism: pulmonary perfusion defect score compared with CT angiographic obstruction score and right ventricular/left ventricular diameter ratio. AJR Am J Roentgenol 194(3):604–610

Chaosuwannakit N, Soontrapa W, Makarawate P, Sawanyawisuth K (2021) Importance of computed tomography pulmonary angiography for predict 30-day mortality in acute pulmonary embolism patients. Eur J Radiol Open 25(8):100340. https://doi.org/10.1016/j.ejro.2021.100340. PMID: 33855129; PMCID: PMC8027691

Coutance G, Cauderlier E, Ehtisham J et al (2011) The prognostic value of markers of right ventricular dysfunction in pulmonary embolism: a meta-analysis. Crit Care 15(2):R103

Cozzi D, Moroni C, Cavigli E et al (2021) Prognostic value of CT pulmonary angiography parameters in acute pulmonary embolism. Radiol Med 126(8):1030–1036. https://doi.org/10.1007/s11547-021-01364-6. Epub 2021 May 7. PMID: 33961187

Ende-Verhaar YM, Kroft LJM, Mos ICM et al (2017) Accuracy and reproducibility of CT right-to-left ventricular diameter measurement in patients with acute pulmonary embolism. PLoS One 12(11):e0188862

Gandara E, Bose G, Erkens P, Rodgers M, Carrier M, Wells P (2011) Outcomes of saddle pulmonary embolism: a nested case-control study. J Thromb Haemost 9(4):867–869. https://doi.org/10.1111/j.1538--7836.2011.04189.x. PMID: 21232009

Ghaye B, Ghuysen A, Willems V et al (2006) Severe pulmonary embolism: pulmonary artery clot load scores and cardiovascular parameters as predictors of mortality. Radiology 239(3):883–891

Groves AM, Win T, Charman SC et al (2004) Semi-quantitative assessment of tricuspid regurgitation on contrast-enhanced multidetector CT. Clin Radiol 59(8):715–719

Hadad Y, Iluz M, Ziv-Baran T et al (2021) High prevalence of right ventricular/left ventricular ratio ≥ 1 among patients undergoing computed tomography pulmonary angiography. J Thorac Imaging 36(4):231–235

Henzler T, Roeger S, Meyer M et al (2012) Pulmonary embolism: CT signs and cardiac biomarkers for predicting right ventricular dysfunction. Eur Respir J 39(4):919–926

Im DJ, Hur J, Han KH et al (2017) Acute pulmonary embolism: retrospective cohort study of the predictive value of perfusion defect volume measured with dual-energy CT. AJR Am J Roentgenol 209(5):1015–1022

Jawad S, Ulriksen PS, Kalhauge A, Hansen KL (2021) Acute pulmonary embolism severity assessment evaluated with dual energy CT perfusion compared to conventional CT angiographic measurements. Diagnostics (Basel) 11(3):495

Jimenez D, Aujesky D, Moores L, RIETE Investigators et al (2010) Simplification of the pulmonary embolism severity index for prognostication in patients with acute symptomatic pulmonary embolism. Arch Intern Med 170(15):1383–1389. https://doi.org/10.1001/archinternmed.2010.199. PMID: 20696966

Jiménez D, Lobo JL, Monreal M et al (2014) Prognostic significance of multidetector CT in normotensive patients with pulmonary embolism: results of the protect study. Thorax 69(2):109–115

Kang DK, Thilo C, Schoepf UJ et al (2011) CT Signs of right ventricular dysfunction: prognostic role in acute pulmonary embolism. JACC Cardiovasc Imaging 4(8):841–849

Kirkbride RR, Heidinger BH, Monteiro Filho AC et al (2022) Evidence for left atrial volume being an indicator of adverse events in patients with acute pulmonary embolism: retrospective case-control pilot study. J Thorac Imaging 37(3):173–180

Kong WF, Wang YT, Yin LL, Pu H, Tao KY (2017) Clinical risk stratification of acute pulmonary embolism: comparing the usefulness of CTA obstruction score and pulmonary perfusion defect score with dual-energy CT. Int J Cardiovasc Imaging 33(12): 2039–2047

Konstantinides SV, Meyer G, Becattini C, ESC Scientific Document Group et al (2020) 2019 ESC Guidelines for the diagnosis and management of acute pulmonary embolism developed in collaboration with the European Respiratory Society (ERS). Eur Heart J 41(4):543–603. https://doi.org/10.1093/eurheartj/ehz405. PMID: 31504429

Kosmala A, Gruschwitz P, Veldhoen S, Weng AM, Krauss B, Bley TA, Petritsch B (2020) Dual-energy CT angiography in suspected pulmonary embolism: influence of injection protocols on image quality and perfused blood volume. Int J Cardiovasc Imaging 36(10):2051–2059. https://doi.org/10.1007/s10554-020-01911-8

Kumamaru KK, Hunsaker AR, Wake N et al (2012) The variability in prognostic values of right ventricular-to-left ventricular diameter ratios derived from different measurement methods on computed tomography pulmonary angiography: a patient outcome study. J Thorac Imaging 27(5):331–336. https://doi.org/10.1097/RTI.0b013e3182350a35. PMID: 22139353

Le Gal G, Righini M, Roy PM et al (2006) Prediction of pulmonary embolism in the emergency department: the revised Geneva score. Ann Intern Med 144(3):165–171. https://doi.org/10.7326/0003-4819-144-3-200602070-00004. PMID: 16461960

Lerchbaumer MH, Ebner M, Ritter CO et al (2021) Prognostic value of right atrial dilation in patients with pulmonary embolism. ERJ Open Res 7(2):00414–02020

Lu MT, Cai T, Ersoy H et al (2008) Interval increase in right-left ventricular diameter ratios at CT as a predictor of 30-day mortality after acute pulmonary embolism: initial experience. Radiology 246(1):281–287

Lu MT, Cai T, Ersoy H et al (2009) Comparison of ECG-gated versus non-gated CT ventricular measurements in thirty patients with acute pulmonary embolism. Int J Cardiovasc Imaging 25(1):101–107

Lyhne MD, Schultz JG, MacMahon PJ et al (2019) Septal bowing and pulmonary artery diameter on computed tomography pulmonary angiography are associated with short-term outcomes in patients with acute pulmonary embolism. Emerg Radiol 26(6):623–630

Mahammedi A, Oshmyansky A, Hassoun PM et al (2013) Pulmonary artery measurements in pulmonary hypertension: the role of computed tomography. J Thorac Imaging 28(2):96–103

Mastora I, Remy-Jardin M, Masson P, Galland E, Delannoy V, Bauchart JJ, Remy J (2003) Severity of acute pulmonary embolism: evaluation of a new spiral CT angiographic score in correlation with echocardiographic data. Eur Radiol 13(1):29–35

Meinel FG, Graef A, Bamberg F et al (2013) Effectiveness of automated quantification of pulmonary perfused blood volume using dual-energy CTPA for the severity assessment of acute pulmonary embolism. Investig Radiol 48(8):563–569

Meinel FG, Nance JW Jr, Schoepf UJ et al (2015) Predictive value of computed tomography in acute pulmonary embolism: systematic review and meta-analysis. Am J Med 128(7):747–759

Meyer M, Fink C, Roeger S et al (2012) Benefit of combining quantitative cardiac CT parameters with troponin I for predicting right ventricular dysfunction and adverse clinical events in patients with acute pulmonary embolism. Eur J Radiol 81(11):3294–3299

Meyer HJ, Bailis N, Surov A (2021) Time efficiency and reliability of established computed tomographic obstruction scores in patients with acute pulmonary embolism. PLoS One 16(12):e0260802. https://doi.org/10.1371/journal.pone.0260802

Miller GA, Sutton GC, Kerr IH, Gibson RV, Honey M (1971) Comparison of streptokinase and heparin in treatment of isolated acute massive pulmonary embolism. Br Med J 2(5763):681–684

Norton L, Cooper G, Sheerins O et al (2021) Clinical and radiological characteristics of acute pulmonary embolus in relation to 28-day and 6-month mortality. PLoS One 16(12):e0258843. https://doi.org/10.1371/journal.pone.0258843. PMID: 34962922; PMCID: PMC8714121

Pech M, Wieners G, Dul P et al (2007) Computed tomography pulmonary embolism index for the assessment of survival in patients with pulmonary embolism. Eur Radiol 17(8):1954–1959

Pontana F, Faivre JB, Remy-Jardin M et al (2008) Lung perfusion with dual-energy multidetector-row CT (MDCT): feasibility for the evaluation of acute pulmonary embolism in 117 consecutive patients. Acad Radiol 15(12):1494–1504

Pruszczyk P, Goliszek S, Lichodziejewska B et al (2014) Prognostic value of echocardiography in normotensive patients with acute pulmonary embolism. JACC Cardiovasc Imaging 7(6):553–560. https://doi.org/10.1016/j.jcmg.2013.11.004. PMID: 24412192

Qanadli SD, El Hajjam M, Vieillard-Baron A et al (2001) New CT index to quantify arterial obstruction in pulmonary embolism: comparison with angiographic index and echocardiography. AJR Am J Roentgenol 176(6):1415–1420

Rajiah P (2020) Dual-energy computed tomography in thoracic imaging-current practices and utility: survey of the Society of Thoracic Radiology. J Thorac Imaging 35(2):W43–W50

Rajiah P, Tanabe Y, Partovi S, Moore A (2019) State of the art: utility of multi-energy CT in the evaluation of pulmonary vasculature. Int J Cardiovasc Imaging 35(8):1509–1524

Rassouli N, Etesami M, Dhanantwari A, Rajiah P (2017) Detector-based spectral CT with a novel dual-layer technology: principles and applications. Insights Imaging 8(6):589–598

Remy-Jardin M, Ryerson CJ, Schiebler ML et al (2021) Imaging of pulmonary hypertension in adults: a position paper from the Fleischner Society. Eur Respir J 57(1):2004455

Righini M, van Es J, den Exter PL et al (2014) Age-adjusted D-dimer cutoff levels to rule out pulmonary embolism: the ADJUST-PE study. JAMA 311:1117–1124

Rotzinger DC, Knebel JF, Jouannic AM, Adler G, Qanadli SD (2020) CT pulmonary angiography for risk stratification of patients with nonmassive acute pulmonary embolism. Radiol Cardiothorac Imaging 2(4):e190188

Schoepf UJ, Kucher N, Kipfmueller F et al (2004) Right ventricular enlargement on chest computed tomography: a predictor of early death in acute pulmonary embolism. Circulation 110(20):3276–3280. https://doi.org/10.1161/01.CIR.0000147612.59751.4C. PMID: 15533868

Thieme SF, Becker CR, Hacker M, Nikolaou K, Reiser MF, Johnson TRC (2008) Dual energy CT for the assessment of lung perfusion—correlation to scintigraphy. Eur J Radiol 68(3):369–374

Torbicki A, Galié N, Covezzoli A, Rossi E, De Rosa M, Goldhaber SZ, ICOPER Study Group (2003) Right heart thrombi in pulmonary embolism: results from the International Cooperative Pulmonary Embolism Registry. J Am Coll Cardiol 41(12):2245–2251. https://doi.org/10.1016/s0735-1097(03)00479-0. PMID: 12821255

Trujillo-Santos J, den Exter PL, Gómez V et al (2013) Computed tomography-assessed right ventricular dysfunction and risk stratification of patients with acute non-massive pulmonary embolism: systematic review and meta-analysis. J Thromb Haemost 11(10):1823–1832

Truong QA, Massaro JM, Rogers IS et al (2012) Reference values for normal pulmonary artery dimensions by noncontrast cardiac computed tomography: the Framingham Heart Study. Circ Cardiovasc Imaging 5(1):147–154

Van Belle A, Büller HR, Huisman MV, Huisman PM, Kaasjager K, Kamphuisen PW et al (2006) Effectiveness of managing suspected pulmonary embolism using an algorithm combining clinical probability, D-dimer testing, and computed tomograph. JAMA 295(2):172–179. https://doi.org/10.1001/jama.295.2.172. PMID 16403929

van der Meer RW, Pattynama PM et al (2005) Right ventricular dysfunction and pulmonary obstruction index at helical CT: prediction of clinical outcome during 3-month follow-up in patients with acute pulmonary embolism. Radiology 235(3):798–803. https://doi.org/10.1148/radiol.2353040593. Epub 2005 Apr 21. PMID: 15845793

Vedovati MC, Becattini C, Agnelli G et al (2012) Multidetector CT scan for acute pulmonary embolism: embolic burden and clinical outcome. Chest 142(6):1417–1424. https://doi.org/10.1378/chest.11-2739. PMID: 22628491

Vedovati MC, Germini F, Agnelli G, Becattini C (2013) Prognostic role of embolic burden assessed at computed tomography angiography in patients with acute pulmonary embolism: systematic review and meta-analysis. J Thromb Haemost 11(12):2092–2102

Walsh PN, Greenspan RH, Simon M et al (1973) An angiographic severity index for pulmonary embolism. Circulation 47–48(Suppl):101–108

Wolf SJ, McCubbin TR, Feldhaus KM, Faragher JP, Adcock DM (2004) Prospective validation of Wells Criteria in the evaluation of patients with suspected pulmonary embolism. Ann Emerg Med 44(5):503–510. https://doi.org/10.1016/j.annemergmed.2004.04.002. PMID: 15520710

Wu AS, Pezzullo JA, Cronan JJ, Hou DD, Mayo-Smith WW (2004) CT pulmonary angiography: quantification of pulmonary embolus as a predictor of patient outcome—initial experience. Radiology 230(3):831–835

Yeh BM, Kurzman P, Foster E, Qayyum A, Joe B, Coakley F (2004) Clinical relevance of retrograde inferior vena cava or hepatic vein opacification during contrast-enhanced CT. AJR Am J Roentgenol 183(5):1227–1232

Zhang H, Cheng Y, Chen Z, Cong X, Kang H, Zhang R, Guo X, Liu M (2022) Clot burden of acute pulmonary thromboembolism: comparison of two deep learning algorithms, Qanadli score, and Mastora score. Quant Imaging Med Surg 12(1):66–79. https://doi.org/10.21037/qims-21-140

The Thoracic Aorta

Sara Boccallini

Contents

S. Boccallini (✉)
Department of Cardiovascular and Thoracic Radiology of the Hôpital Louis Pradel, Hospices Civils de Lyon, Lyon, France

Université Claude Bernard Lyon 1, Lyon, France
e-mail: sara.boccalini@yahoo.com

1 Origins and Physiological Foundation

The thoracic aorta originates from the left ventricle, from which pulsation waves are propagated, presents an elaborate 3D structure at the level of the sinus of Valsalva, curves defining an arch that gives origin to the arteries vascularizing the head and upper limbs and then descends toward the diaphragm (Fig. 1). Its function and specific anatomy make of it a complex organ and deeply influence imaging methods trying to depict it, in regard of both acquisition and analysis.

Among the different quantifiable characteristics of the thoracic aorta, its diameters are by far the most important in all the phases of aortic pathology management. Non-invasive imaging modalities are the most commonly employed method to assess this parameter. With an incidence of 10.4 per 100,000 persons/year and a global death rate per 100,000 raising from 2.49 in 1990 to 2.78 in 2010, aneurysms are the second most common aortic disease (after atherosclerosis), a burden for public health and their diagnosis relies solely on the measurement of diameters (Sampson et al. 2014; Clouse et al. 1998). Furthermore, therapeutic management is based almost exclusively on aortic diameters both at diagnosis and during follow-up. These recommendations rely on the knowledge that larger aortic diameters yield a higher risk of potentially

Med Radiol Diagn Imaging (2026)
https://doi.org/10.1007/174_2023_438,
Published Online: 06 September 2024

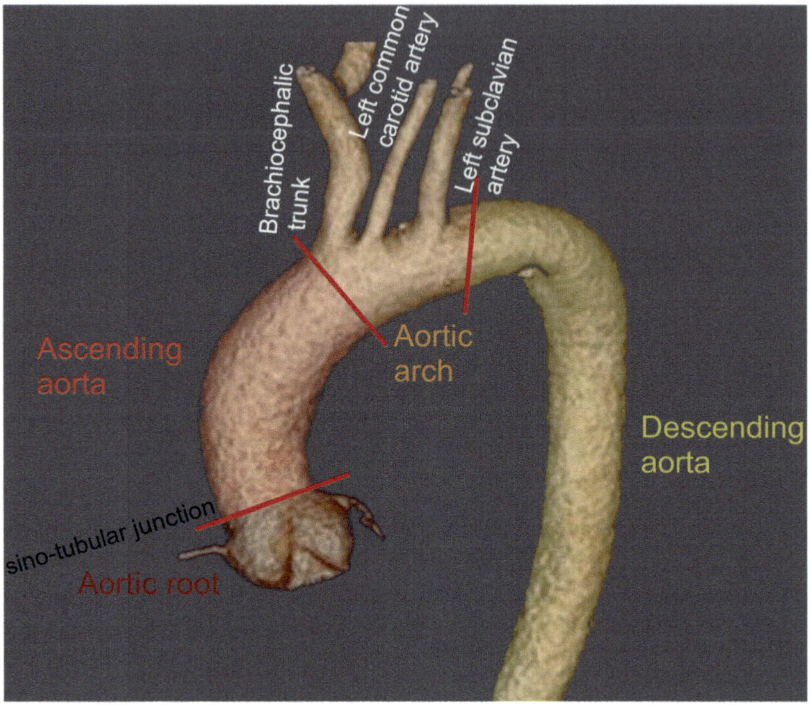

Fig. 1 Volume rendering of a thoracic aorta with the different parts shown in different colors and with anatomic notes

lethal complications such as rupture and dissection. For other pathologies, such as dissection and intramural hematoma, the diagnosis relies on morphological characteristics of the aorta. However, aortic size and its evolution over time are an important prognostic factor and guide successive therapeutic decisions also for these pathologies.

Increasingly more performed, transcutaneous aortic valve implantation/replacement (TAVI/R) requires precise assessment of several structures' dimensions before the procedure, to avoid potentially lethal complications. The most important parameters to be derived are the dimensions of the so-called aortic annulus which corresponds to the plane of deployment of the valve, and the distance from this plane to the ostia of the coronary arteries (Blanke et al. 2019).

The thickness of the aortic wall is an important parameter in the follow-up of IMH as well as aortitis, its increase representing an active phase of the disease.

Other measurements of the thoracic aorta, including volume, length, angulation, and tortuosity are possible with non-invasive imaging techniques but are not routinely employed in clinical practice and their use is mainly limited to research settings.

Due to technical advancement in image acquisitions and subsequent post-processing, aortic hemodynamic parameters are more and more easily obtained and their role in clinical and research settings is in constant development. Velocity, peak velocity, and flow measurements in the aortic root and ascending aorta have been routinely employed in clinical practice for years to estimate the function of the aortic valve as detailed in specific chapters of this book. Other aortic hemodynamic factors have been shown to be important predictors of aortic pathology development and progression and to yield prognostic implications. For instance, abnormal aortic flow patterns due to valvular anomalies (congenital, as in patients with bicuspid aortic valves, or acquired) are associated with subsequent aortic dilation. In fact an eccentric flow in the aorta determines an increased wall shear stress that is believed to be the trigger factor for extracellular matrix rearrangement, aortic wall remodeling, and dilatation (Della Corte et al. 2008; Markl et al. 2012). Of the measurements proposed to quantify abnormal aortic flow wall, shear stress and flow displacement are among the most commonly employed and most accurate, respectively. Considering their potential to influence treatment paradigms, these parameters are likely to have a growing role also in clinical practice in the near future.

2 How to Perform Different Measurements

2.1 Aortic Diameters

Non-invasive imaging modalities are generally employed to assess aortic diameters. The most indicated ones are echocardiography, CT, and MRI. In Table 1, a comparison among different techniques is provided. While echography is a great instrument for a first approach, it has important limitations as it does not allow visualization of the entire length of the aorta and it is mainly a 2D modality. MRI can overcome these limitations but is expensive and its availability is limited due to long examinations. CT allows imaging the entire aorta in a few seconds, 3D evaluation, and assessment of the aortic wall at the expense of radiation exposure and iodine contrast administration. Therefore, in routine clinical practice, CT is considered the modality of reference. MRI should be privileged for all those patients that are young, due to the absence of ionizing radiation, and for whom the injection of iodine contrast material is contraindicated.

In Tables 2 and 3, specifics of CT and MRI acquisitions and reconstructions are provided, respectively. Although several MRI sequences can be employed to measure aortic diameters, 3D acquisitions with isotropic or nearly isotropic voxel should be preferred as they allow multiplanar reconstructions and assessment at multiple levels of the aorta. Therefore, we have limited our attention to these sequences. Figure 2 provides examples of different MRI acquisitions with the respective advantages and pitfalls.

It has to be stressed that for imaging of the ascending aorta cardiac synchronization is always required. Motion artifacts at this level can be so important as to prevent correct visual-

Table 1 Summary of the characteristics of echocardiography, CT, and MRI for thoracic aorta evaluation

	Availability	Rapidity	Imaging of the entire thoracic aorta	Aortic wall	X-rays	Contrast	Patient tolerance
Echo	+ + +	+ +	− − −	− −			+ + +
			Only the aortic root and proximal ascending aorta are generally visible in adults				
CT	+ +	+ + +	+ + +	+ +	+ +	− −	+ +
				Characterization of aortic wall thickening usually requires additional acquisitions, namely before contrast administration and during a portal phase			
MRI	−	− −	+ +	+ +		−	−
			Generally possible in a single acquisition. However, at the limit of the FOV image quality can be deteriorated	Characterization of aortic wall thickening is possible but with additional sequences			

Table 2 Recommended characteristics of CT protocols for aortic diameters assessment

CT	Feature	Specifics
Acquisition	Unenhanced:	• Allows measuring external aortic diameters where the aorta is surrounded by adipose tissue. At the level of the sinuses of Valsalva, the contiguity of the aorta to other cardiac structures can hamper correct measurements
		• Visualization of the aortic wall is limited to cases of IMH and otherwise not possible
	After contrast injection:	• Contrast material should be injected on the right arm to avoid streak artifacts at the level of the aortic arch
		• Contrast injection protocols should be tailored in accordance to the speed of acquisition, as faster scanners require higher injection rates
		• If the patient is known to have a large (e.g., 6–7 cm) and/or long aneurysm, a bigger dose of contrast should be administered to fill the entire aorta
		• Bolus tracking is advised. Standard threshold to trigger the acquisition is of 130–150 HU in the descending aorta
		• Cardiac synchronization is necessary for the ascending aorta
Reconstruction	Phase of the cardiac cycle:	Although larger diameters have been reported in systolic phase at the level of the ascending aorta, diastolic images are preferable as they are often of better quality
	Slice thickness:	≤1 mm
	Kernel:	Soft tissue
Additional reconstructions	Mono-energetic reconstructions:	On dual energy CT scanners, images at low energy can highlight the iodine contained in the voxels since its highest attenuation value is of 33.2 keV. These images can be useful in case of impaired image quality on conventional images due to the poor opacification of the aorta

Table 3 Characteristics of the three most commonly employed sequences for aortic imaging

MRI	Sequence	Details sequence	Details	Acquisition time	Advantages	Limitations
Without contrast	3D bSSFP	Standard balanced gradient echo steady state precession pulse sequence with a T2-preparation pre-pulse and a spectral pre-saturation pulse	• Respiratory navigation • Cardiac gating • Isotropic voxel 1–2 mm	3–6 min		• Sensitivity to flow and susceptibility artifacts • These artifacts are increased at 3T
	Dixon-based methods	Unbalanced fast gradient echo sequence that achieves fat suppression through chemical shift-based water-fat separation with the modified Dixon technique	• Respiratory navigation • Cardiac gating • Isotropic voxel 1–2 mm	3–4 min	Less susceptible to field inhomogeneity	
With gadolinium chelates contrast	CE-CMRA	Fast gradient echo sensible to T1 variation	• Inspiratory breath hold • Usually without cardiac gating • Isotropic voxel 1–2 mm • Bolus detection systems • 0.1–0.2 mmol/kg of contrast at 2–3 mL/s	~10 s Possibility to perform time-resolved acquisitions with a single acquisition in the order of a few seconds	Very resistant to dephasing artifacts	• Lack of cardiac gating can result in artifacts at the level of the sinuses of Valsalva • Timing dependent

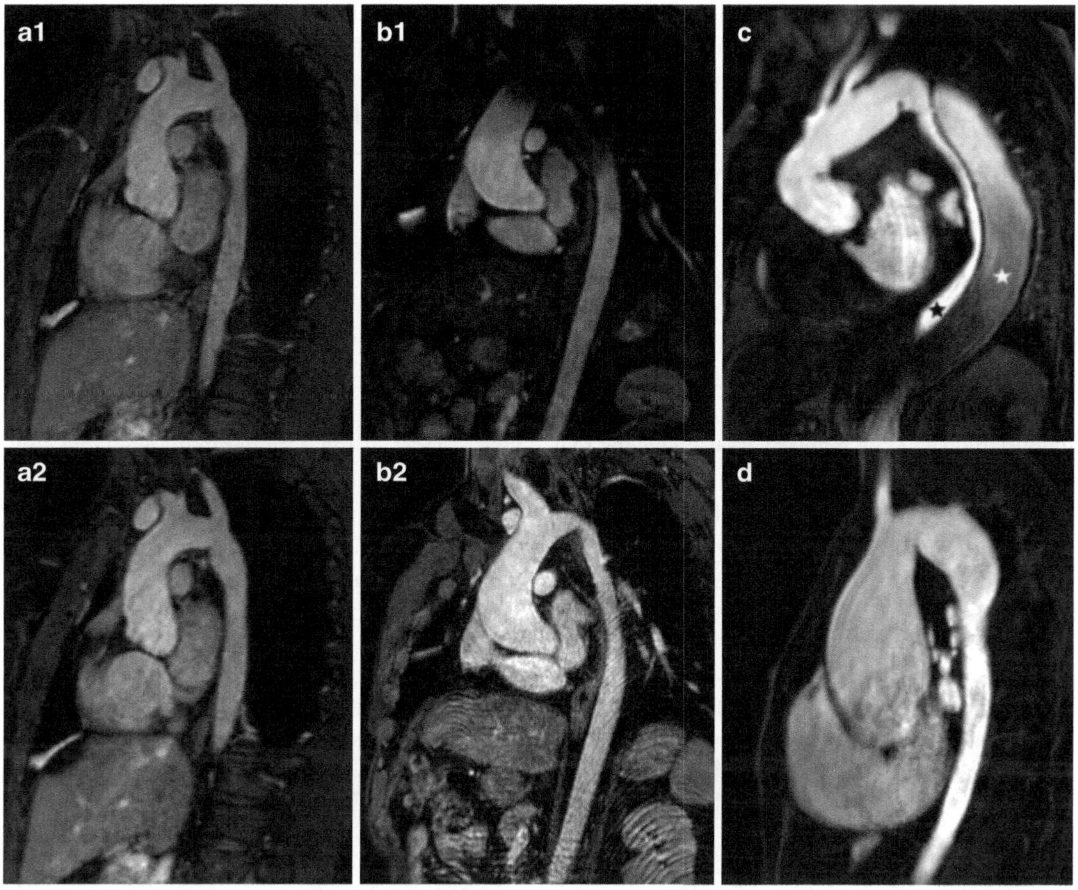

Fig. 2 Different MRI techniques to assess thoracic aorta diameters. **a** and **b** show two examples of two patients for whom two types of acquisitions each were performed (BTFE in **a1** and **b1** and Dixon in **a2** and **b2**). In the first case, both acquisitions were of good quality (**a1** and **a2**), while in the second case, the BTFE (**b1**) showed a typical black band artifact at the limit of the field of view, whereas the Dixon (**b2**) was of good quality. **c** and **d** illustrate two different cases of CE-MRA performed after the injection of Gadolinium-based contrast media. In the case of type A dissection treated with ascending aorta replacement and residual dissection of the descending aorta presented in **c**, it is evident how well the injection can help highlight the different timing of true (black star) and false (white star) channels perfusion. However, this sequence is also prone to artifacts due to the absence of respiratory navigation and cardiac gating affecting the image quality of the abdominal aorta in this case and, very typically, the sinus of Valsalva, as shown in another example in panel **d**. *BTFE* balanced turbo field echo

ization of the aortic wall and therefore a correct evaluation of diameters. The addition of synchronization to CT scan protocols adds concerns about radiation dose that should be lowered as much as possible in these patients who will undergo lifelong surveillance, often starting at a young age. Nowadays, all vendors offer some kind of dose modulation option that, if not automatic, should be implemented for all aortic protocols. Furthermore, available synchronization options, partially different for each vendor, should be reviewed and compared at each center. Although prospective gating is available on most scanners, other more recently introduced techniques, such as prospective dose reduction of retrospective acquisitions or very high pitch prospective acquisitions in a single heartbeat with dual source CT scanners, offer attractive alternatives. For the evaluation of the thoracic descending aorta cardiac synchronization is not essential as movements in this part of the aorta are generally very limited.

Once the reconstructions are available, diameters can be measured.

For both imaging modalities, different planes and techniques can be employed to measure aortic diameters.

The quickest and most simple way is to scroll through axial images and measure the aortic diameter on the selected level. This method has been regarded as inaccurate. It is evident that as the angle between the aorta and the *z*-axis of the patient increases, the maximum aortic diameter identified on an axial plane overestimates the real dimensions of the aorta.

Therefore, most guidelines indicate that measurements should be performed on a plane perpendicular to the long axis of the vessel also named "cross-axial plane." The first prerequisite is to have reconstructions with isotropic (or nearly isotropic) voxels. Thereafter, the desired plane can be identified manually or with the aid of a dedicated software. In both cases, a workstation allowing for multiplanar reconstructions is needed.

The manual technique to identify the correct cross-axial plane is illustrated in Fig. 3. This method has been referred to in many ways, the most common of which is "double oblique." It has to be kept in mind that it is a rather time-consuming method and, even more importantly, it requires some training and experience.

Software can be semi-automatic or fully automatic. Most of the commercially available solutions are based on the integration of different algorithms that permit the identification of the set of points located in the center of the vessel, thereby determining the "centerline" of the aorta (Fig. 4). Multiple views of the aorta are usually

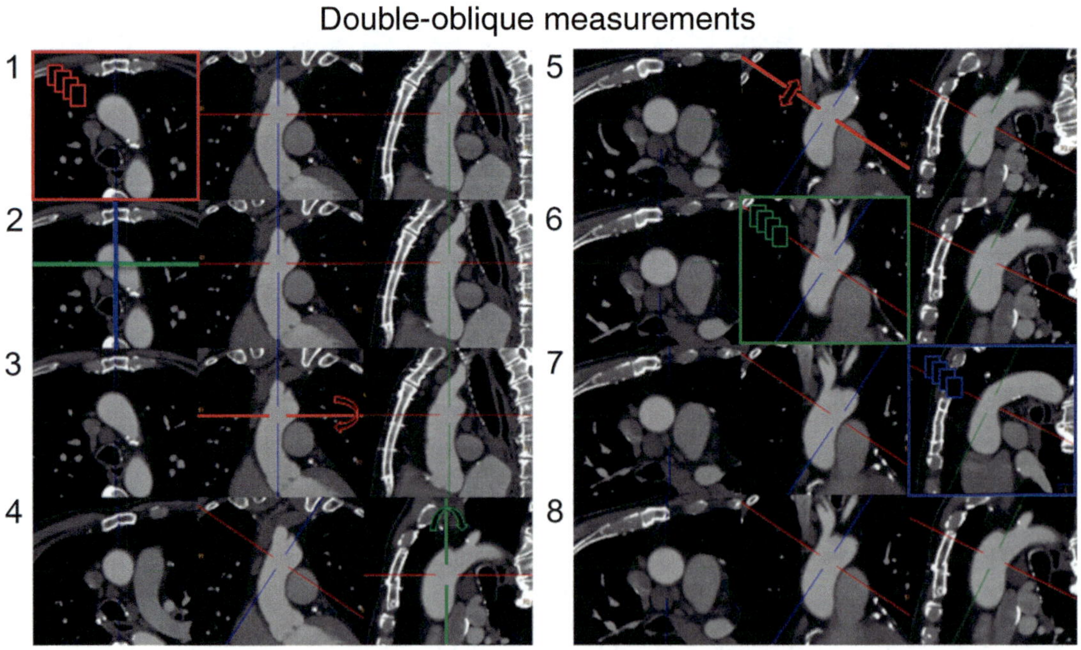

Fig. 3 Description of the steps to perform double oblique measurements. To start the procedure the images should be manipulated with a multiplanar workstation with visualization of the axial, sagittal, and coronal plane. By following the instructions as illustrated, the axial plane (panels of step "1," image on the left) will be transformed in a cross-sectional (or cross-axial) plane of the aorta (panels of step "8," image on the left). Step 1: scroll through axial images until the desired level is reached. In this example, the measure of the proximal aortic arch was the aim. Step 2: move the crosshairs formed by the two axis at the center of the aorta on the axial plane. Step 3: rotate the axis corresponding to the axial plane on one of the other two planes to reach the inclination of the desired final cross-axial plane. Step 4: repeat the same action as in the previous step on the other plane. Step 5: adjust the height of the so-obtained cross-axial plane by adjusting the corresponding axis on one of the other plane. Step 6: scroll through images of this plane to confirm the correct inclination and height of the desired cross-axial plane. Step 7: repeat the previous step on the other plane. Step 8: the correct cross-axial plane has been identified

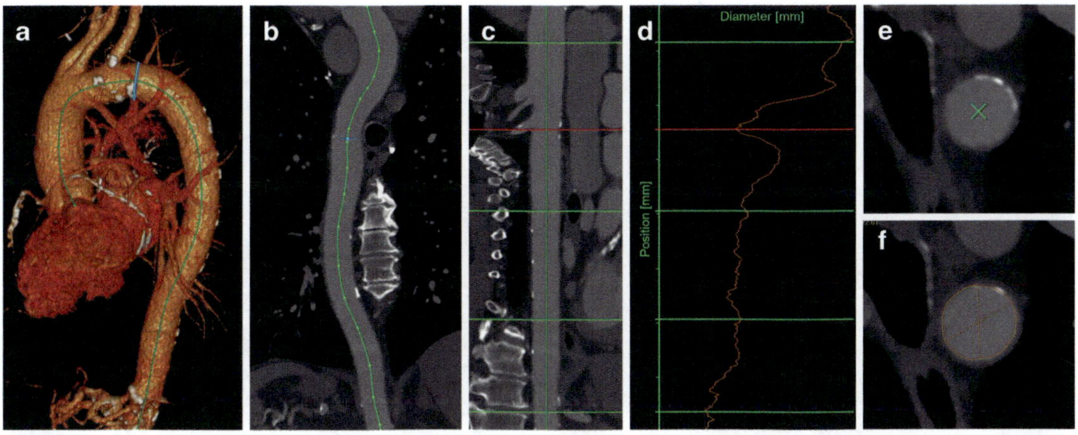

Fig. 4 Automatic or semi-automatic aortic measurements. (**a**) Volume rendering of the aorta with the centerline superposed in green. (**b**) CPR (curved plane reconstruction) showing all the points of the centerline (in green) of the thoracic aorta on a single plane. The aorta, and the rest of the image, can be turned around the centerline. The dots along the centerline are the proposed control points that can be employed to manually adjust the centerline. (**c**) Straightened multiplanar reconstruction displaying all the points of the centerline (in green) of the aorta in a single plane and on a line. The horizontal red and green lines represent levels of interest along the aorta. (**d**) The orange line represents the diameter (in mm, on the *x*-axis) at different locations along the long axis of the aorta (*y*-axis). The user can scroll back and forth along the aorta and find the diameter at that level. (**e**) A cross-sectional image of the aorta as defined by the software, where the green crosshair represents the centerline. By repositioning these centerpoints, which are supposed to be in the center of all cross-axial planes of the aorta by definition, the user can eventually correct the centerline. (**f**) Cross-sectional plane of the aorta with automatically detected contours and showing how minimum and maximum diameter have been calculated by the software

provided by the software and are detailed in Fig. 4. With semi-automatic software, the operator is expressly required to perform some actions to obtain the desired measures. Human tasks vary in number and content depending on the employed product. They usually involve one or more of the following steps: identification of the aortic lumen, modification of the centerline, identification of the exact location for measurements, and adjustment of luminal external contours. With fully automatic solutions, the operator is supposed to obtain all the desired results without active participation in the process. However, we strongly recommend always checking the centerline. Since the aorta has a complex shape and a lot of variability between subjects, errors in segmentation are known to occur and should be rectified (Fig. 5). The stretched MPR is particularly useful for this purpose. In this type of reconstruction, the centerline is a straight line placed in the middle of the image and it is easy to see if the two borders of the aorta have an equal distance from it. Most software allows modifying the centerline either with control points that can be moved as desired or manually tracing the correct centerline. To settle doubts, cross-axial images, where each point of the centerline can be checked and moved, are particularly handy.

Importantly, software have been shown to reduce variability especially for inexperienced operators (Quint et al. 2013). On the other hand, although one often cited advantage of software is time consumption reduction, this has not been consistently proven in real-life scenarios.

Since the aorta can present the maximum dilation at any level, the location and the diameter at this level should be clearly indicated in the report. Additional measurements need to be performed at specific, reproducible, and multiple landmarks along the aorta at each control. In Fig. 6, we report the landmarks described in the most recent guidelines from the ESC and AHA (Hiratzka et al. 2010; Erbel et al. 2014). It is important the aorta to be regarded as an organ since aneurysms

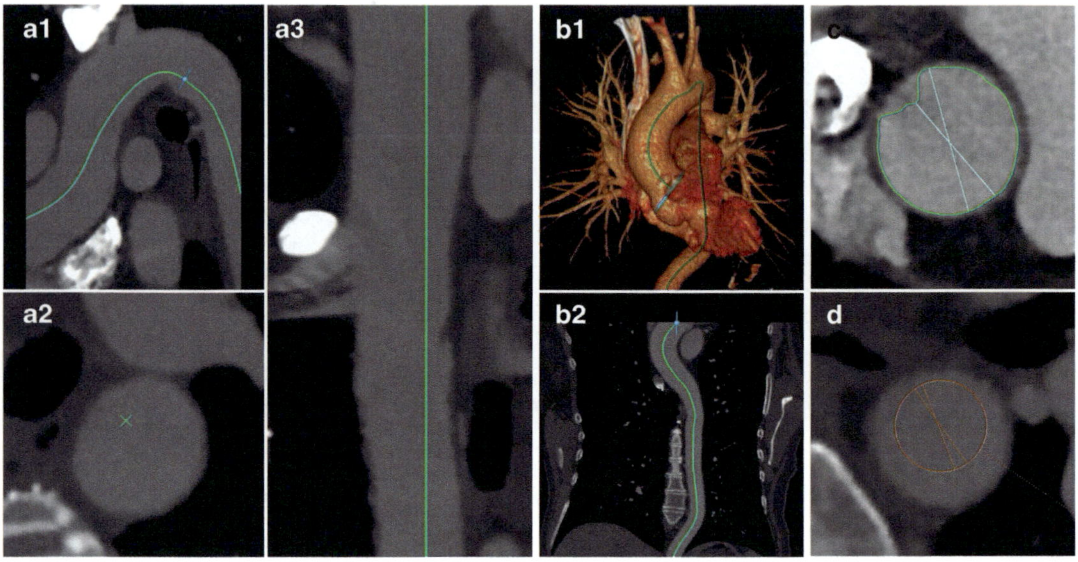

Fig. 5 Most common errors of automatic or semi-automatic software for the assessment of aortic diameters assessment. (**a1**–**a3**) Miscalculation of the centerline. This type of mistake is more likely to occur where the aorta describes steep curves as in the illustrated example at the level of the aortic arch. The centerline is closer to the inner than to the outer curve of the aorta as well visible on the CPR (**a1**) and on the cross-sectional image (**a2**) at the level indicated by the blue pointer on the CPR. Straightened MPR (**a3**) allows a quick overview of possible wrong centerline detection since the centerline is represented as the central line and, therefore, the two aortic walls shown on the plane have to be equally distant from the centerline. (**b1**–**b2**) Too short centerline. This is a rather common error that result in an incomplete centerline with part or the entirety of the sinus of Valsalva not taken into account. The centerline can be prolonged manually or the measurements at the missing levels can be manually calculated with the double oblique technique. (**c** and **d**) Two different examples of erroneous automatic border detection. Since this step is usually based on the difference in attenuation between the inside and the outside of the aorta, aorta with insufficient opacification are more prone to result in this error

are often multiple and are associated with other aortic pathologies. This is why the aorta has to be imaged in its entirety at least once after the patient has been diagnosed with aortic pathology and why the aorta has to be measured at multiple locations at every imaging follow-up.

Once the correct plane has been identified, the diameter can be measured. The maximum aortic diameter should always be reported since size thresholds for patient management are based on this parameter. One exception is at the level of the sinuses of Valsalva where the complex anatomical structure, due to the presence of the three cusps, requires a different technique. Different ways to perform these measurements are illustrated in Fig. 7. It has been shown that cusp-to-commissure method is the most reproducible one and has shown the best correlation with regard to echocardiography (Bons et al. 2019). Therefore, we recommend employing this method of measurement. Dilation at the level of the sinuses of Valsalva can be predominant on a single cusp. In this case, we recommend indicating the affected cusp as this could be useful for echocardiographic follow-up.

Many software programs can not only identify the centerline, but can also identify the borders of its lumen and thus provide diameter measurements. However, as for the centerline, errors can occur, especially in poorly enhanced scans since the identification of the lumen is mainly based on the identification of pixels with high attenuation (Fig. 5). Therefore, also external contours should be checked at least at the level of the desired landmarks.

Diameters are commonly reported in "mm." Reporting decimal values does not seem necessary and values can be approximated to the unit.

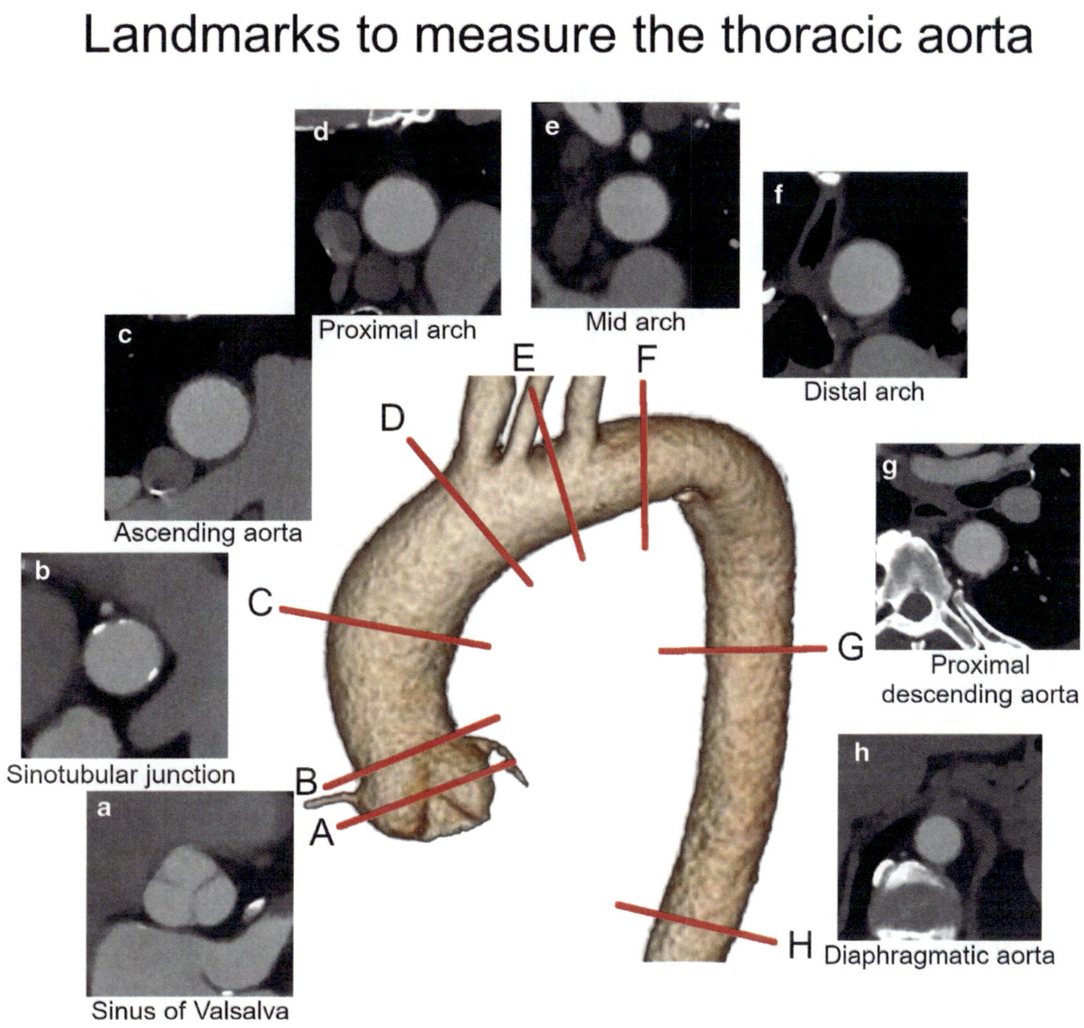

Fig. 6 Landmarks where to measure aortic diameters according to the ESC and AHA (Hiratzka et al. 2010; Erbel et al. 2014; Trimarchi et al. 2014). (**a**) Sinus of Valsalva. Measurements should be performed on the plane where all three leaflets are depicted and form the so-called Mercedes sign. (**b**) Sinotubular junction. (**c**) Ascending aorta. Midway between the sinotubular junction and the proximal aortic arch, normally corresponding at the level of the pulmonary trunk. (**d**) Proximal aortic arch. Just before the origin of the brachiocephalic trunk. (**e**) Mid aortic arch. Between the origin of the left common carotid artery and the left subclavian artery. (**f**) Proximal descending thoracic aorta. Corresponding to the isthmus, about 2 cm after the origin of the left subclavian artery. (**g**) Mid descending aorta. Corresponding to the level of the pulmonary arteries that can be used as an easy landmark according to the ESC guidelines. AHA guidelines suggest to identify this level as the one halfway between the proximal descending aorta and the diaphragmatic aorta. (**h**) Diaphragmatic aorta. Differences between the two societies are mainly found for the abdominal aorta where both recommend measuring the aorta at the origin of the celiac trunk while the ESC includes one more measurements just before the bifurcation

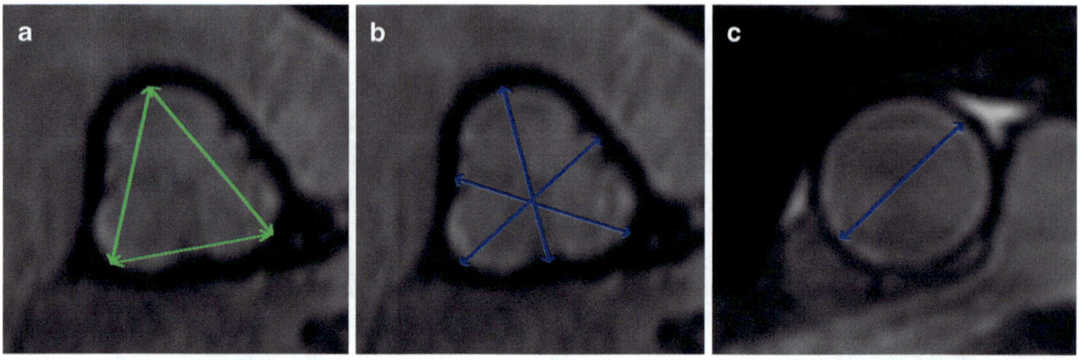

Fig. 7 How to perform aortic measurements at the level of the sinus of Valsalva (**a** and **b**) and at the other landmarks (**c**). In **a**, the three green lines with arrows show cusp-to-cusp measurements of the sinus of Valsalva. In **b**, the three blues lines with arrows show commissure-to-cusp measurements of the sinus of Valsalva (recommended methodology). In **c**, the blue line shows an inner-edge to inner-edge maximum diameter measurement as it can be performed at all other aortic landmarks

2.2 Aortic Annulus Sizing and Distance Between the Coronary Ostia and the Aortic Annulus

The "aortic annulus," also called "virtual basal ring," is the desired plane of deployment of percutaneous aortic valves and corresponds to the part of the left ventricular outflow tract (LVOT) with the smallest surface. As in this location there is no annular anatomical structure, the current spatial definition of the aortic annulus relies on the identification of the plane passing through the three lowest points, the hinge points, of the three aortic cusps (Achenbach et al. 2012; Francone et al. 2020), as illustrated in Fig. 8.

As for aortic diameters, this plane can be identified in different ways, manually or with dedicated software.

Manually, the aortic annulus can be identified by following the same steps illustrated in Fig. 3 with some additional tricks and steps. First, the central cross of the axis in one of the cusps (the one of the non-coronary cusp is the easiest to identify and, therefore, we suggest to start from this one). In addition, the two axes should be rotated so that the cross-axial plane passes through the other two hinge points as well. This can be checked by scrolling through the images. If the plane does not pass through all three hinge points, the step of axis rotation/scrolling must be reiterated. As a final or intermediary step, the resulting cross-sectional plane should be checked. In most aortic valves, the three cusps are almost equally sized and thus while scrolling through images on the selected cross-sectional plane all cusps should appear at the same time and look approximately of the same size.

Software can be based on three principles: identification of a plane perpendicular to the LVOT just before the aortic valve, identification of the plane with the smallest area along the centerline of the LVOT and aortic root, or the identification of the three hinge points. The latter is the most anatomically precise one as it corresponds to the geometric definition of the annulus plane. All automatic steps of all kinds of software should be carefully checked as they are prone to errors considering the anatomical complexity of the aortic root.

One particular case is the definition of the annulus in patients with bicuspid aortic valves (BAV). For these patients, three possible scenarios can be encountered.

The first one is in case of bicuspid valves of type 0 according to the classification of Sievers (Sievers and Schmidtke 2007), meaning valves that are anatomically made of two cusps. In this case, the identification of the three hinge points is clearly impossible, as there are only two

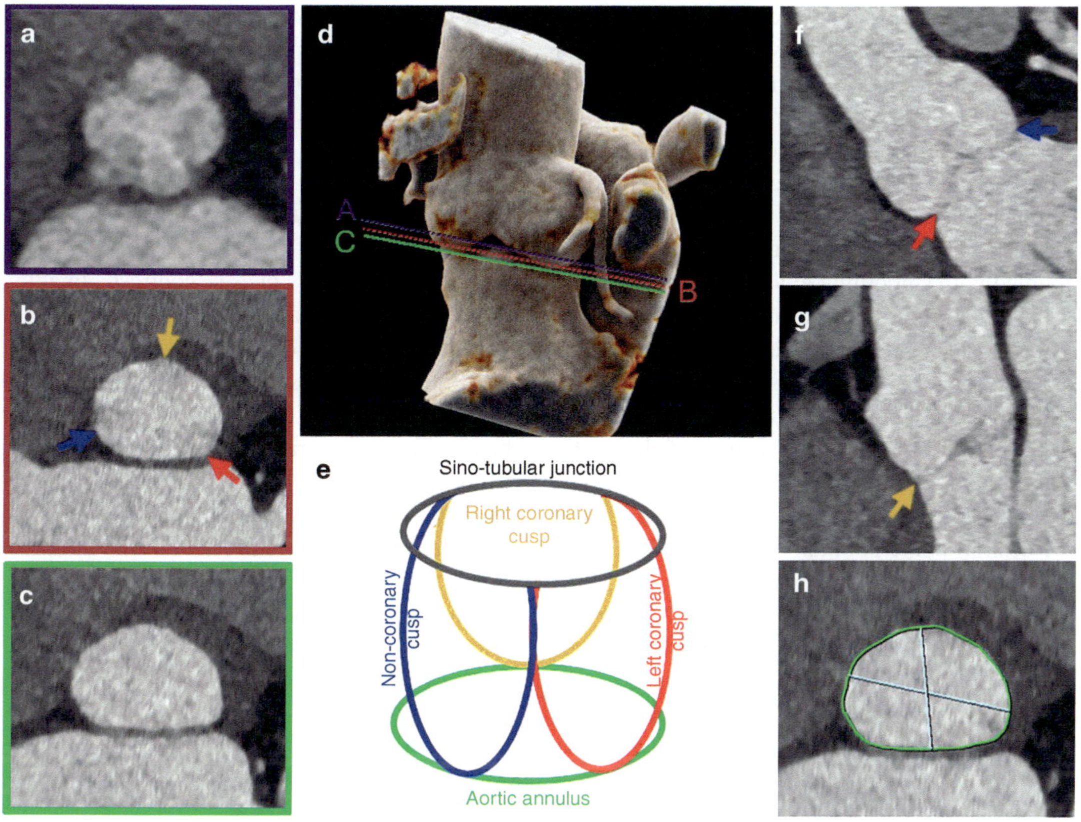

Fig. 8 The aortic annulus. **a**, **b**, and **c** represent three cross sections of the lower part of the sinus of Valsalva, where the lower part of the three cusps is still well visible (**a**), at the level of the three hinge points of the three cusps (three arrows in **b**; yellow arrow = hinge point of the right coronary cusp, blue arrow = hinge point of the non-coronary cusp, red arrow = hinge point of the left coronary cusp) and the plane just below (**c**) that corresponds to the aortic annulus. These three planes are also represented on the 3D rendering in **d**. The green line, corresponding to the aortic annulus is also shown on the diagram in **e** that has a schematic representation of the sinotubular joint (gray), the three cusps (yellow, blue, red) and, as mentioned, the aortic annulus in green. **f** and **g** show the three hinge points the cusps (blue and red arrows in **f**; yellow arrow in **g**) on long-axis views of the aorta. In panel **h**, an example of automatic segmentation of the annulus with automatic calculation of the maximum and minimum diameter of the annulus. Based on this automatic segmentation of the border, also the area-derived diameter can be calculated

(Frangieh et al. 2019). The other two possibilities regard the other two types of bicuspid valves, namely type 1 and type 2, where three cusps are present that are fused along one or two commissures. If the three cusps are symmetric, BAVs type 1 and 2 look like tricuspid valves. However, the cusps are sometimes asymmetric so that the plane passing through the three hinge points is skewed and not representative of the desired plane of deployment of the valve. To take into account these variations, a more tailored approach is needed. This can be based on the identification of the plane passing through the two hinge points in type 0 BAV or the hinge points of the two larger cusps in asymmetric type 1 and 2 that is then tilted until a plane perpendicular to the LVOT and with the lowest possible surface is obtained (Boccalini et al. 2021a).

Once the correct plane has been identified, several dimensions can be calculated manually, semi-automatically, or automatically. Manually, it is possible to trace calipers to calculate maximum and minimum diameters although this is not recommended, as manual measurements are less reproducible than semi-automatic ones (Blanke et al. 2019). It is also possible to draw a line along the wall of the annulus diameter and to derive the effective diameter based on the perimeter or the area. Also these measurements are more reproducible if they are calculated based on automatic detection of the contours of the annulus, especially if automatic measurements are coupled with smoothing algorithms.

Another important measure for TAVI planning is the distance between the annulus and the ostia of the coronary arteries. This distance can be calculated manually by putting the center of the axes in the middle of the cross section of the aortic annulus and then rotating one of the axes to reach the plane of one of the coronary arteries. Once the desired plane is obtained in one of the long axes, a line from, and perpendicular to, the annulus plane (taking the axes passing through the annulus plane as a guide) to the ostium of a coronary artery can be traced and the distance measured. Software can identify the same plane and perform the measurement automatically.

2.3 Aortic Wall Thickness

CT and MRI are the modality of choice for the assessment aortic wall thickness, echocardiography being of limited value in this regard. Acquisition and reconstruction parameters previously described for the measurement of aortic diameters are valid also for the measurement of aortic wall thickness. In addition, other acquisitions can be informative in the context of aortitis but are not strictly necessary to measure the thickness of the aortic wall. Among these, we enumerate a venous CT acquisition, T2w black blood and T1w Gd sequence to confirm the presence of edema and contrast enhancement indicating an active phase of the disease.

At present, there are no recommendations on how to perform these measurements. Aortic wall thickness has been measured on axial as well as on cross-axial planes in different studies. Since in these patients aortic diameters have to be measured nonetheless, we suggest to measure them on cross-axial planes together with aortic diameters and to indicate both parameters on the report for each landmark.

2.4 Hemodynamic Parameters

MRI time-resolved phase contrast imaging allows measuring many dynamic parameters of the aorta including velocity, peak velocity, flow, and compliance. 3D sequences, the so-called 4D flow sequences, not only allow to calculate the above-mentioned parameters in any desired plane but also wall shear stress (WSS) and visualization of flow trajectory (Fig. 9).

Velocity, peak velocity, and flow measurements in the aortic root and ascending aorta are commonly performed in clinical practice to estimate the function of the aortic valve as well as for the detection of shunts as detailed in specific chapters.

Other parameters have been used mainly in research setting.

2.4.1 Wall Shear Stress (WSS)

Stress is a physical entity defined as the internal distribution of forces within a body that balance and react to the external loads applied to it. The walls of arteries are subject to (a) circumferential stress due to pulse pressure variation inside the vessel; (b) shear stress due to blood flow. The direction of the shear stress vector is determined by the direction of the blood flow velocity vector very close to the vessel wall (Papaioannou and Stefanadis 2005). To calculate WSS several formulae have been proposed, depending on the assumptions considered. One assumption of fluid mechanics, also implemented in the formulas employed in aortic imaging, is that the velocity of fluid upon the surface is zero, implying that a gradient of velocities moving away from the surface can be identified. There are several other assumptions that can be taken into consideration, or not, depending on the formula: the fluid is Newtonian (constant viscosity), the vessel is straight, cylin-

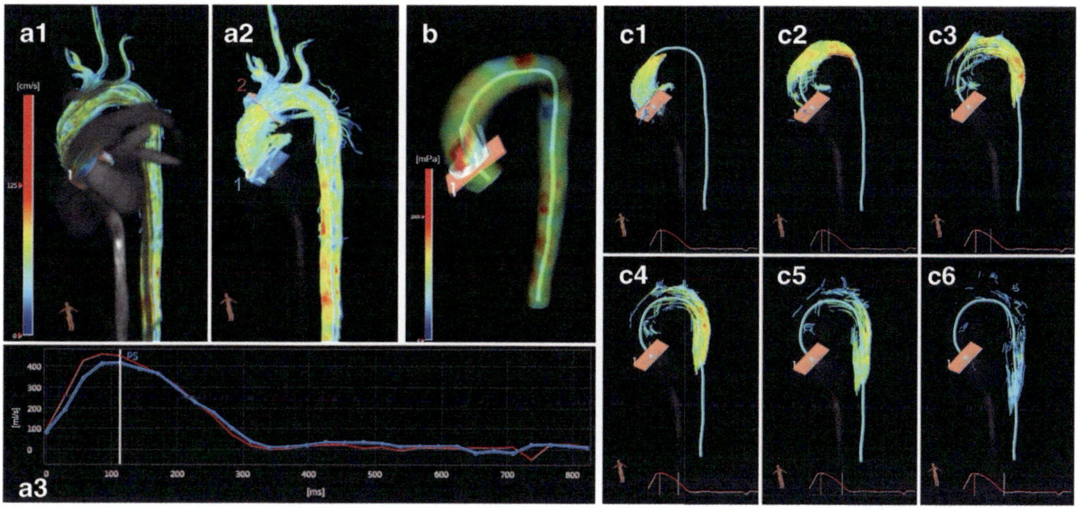

Fig. 9 An example of 4D flow measurements on the thoracic aorta. (**a1–a3**) Streamlines representing velocity color coded tangents to the trajectory lines of the flow are one of the most common visualization tool on which specific levels (e.g., the planes labeled as 1 and 2 in **a2**) can be analyzed in detail (**a3**, blue line for plane 1 and red line for plane 2) regarding the parameter of interest during the entire cardiac cycle. (**b**) shear stress represented with colors along the aorta can be analyzed in detail on the plane of interest. (**c1–c6**) Path lines, indicating the direction of particles at different time points. (Image courtesy of Monica Sigovan, PhD, Creatis)

drical, and inelastic, the flow is laminar and constant (Papaioannou and Stefanadis 2005). The precise description of these parameters and of the formulae goes beyond the scope of this chapter and we invite interested readers to refer to specific publications.

WSS is a force and thus the measurement unit is Pascal (Pa).

2.4.2 Flow Trajectory and Flow Displacement

The trajectory of aortic flow can be highlighted and assessed throughout the cardiac cycle in a subjective way based on vector graph, streamline encoding, and other visualization tools. One of the most reliable ways to quantify flow eccentricity is by means of the so-called flow displacement. Flow displacement was defined as the distance between the center of the lumen and the "center of velocity" of the forward flow (Sigovan et al. 2011).

2.4.3 Compliance and Pulse Wave Velocity

Compliance of a vessel wall is an inverse function of pulse wave velocity. Pulse wave velocity is the difference of onset of flow in two different locations divided by the distance along the centerline of the vessel. Therefore, compliance can be calculated from a 2D phase contrast sequence that passes through the ascending and descending aorta, from an in-plane 2D phase contrast sequence of the thoracic aorta as well as from 3D flow sequences (Nayak et al. 2015).

3 Expected Results and Range of Normal Values

3.1 Aortic Diameters

The aorta can be regarded as a tube gradually tapering downstream from the sinus of Valsalva. As a general (and easy to remember) rule, any value exceeding 40 mm at any location for women of any age and for men <60 years old should prompt further verification.

More precise values are reported in Table 4 for the aortic root, the ascending and descending aorta. To approach this table, some clarifications are needed. We reported only some of the many available studies having decided to focus on the

Table 4 Papers reporting aortic diameters expressed in [mm] at the level of the sinus of Valsalva and/or ascending aorta (AA) and/or descending thoracic aorta (DA) with characteristics of the study

	Population	Method	Measurement details	Sinus of Valsalva			AA			DA		
				Overall	Women	Men	Overall	Women	Men	Overall	Women	Men
Wolak et al. (2008)	Low risk *N* = 2952 for AA *N* = 1931 for DA	CT	• Non-enhanced • Axial plane • Lower level of pulmonary bifurcation				33 ± 4	31.4 ± 3.2	33.5 ± 3.6	24 ± 3	22.6 ± 2.2	25.1 ± 2.5
Rogers et al. (2013)	Low risk *N* = 2343	CT	• Non-enhanced • Axial • Lower level of pulmonary bifurcation					31.9 ± 3.5	34.1 ± 3.9		23.1 ± 2.6	25.8 ± 3.0
Mao et al. (2008)	Healthy *N* = 1612	CT	• Axial plane • Right pulmonary artery mid-slice height									
			• CTA • Inner edge-inner edge				32.8 ± 3.8					
			• CTA • Outer edge-outer edge				35.2 ± 3.8					
			• Non-enhanced CT				35.1 ± 3.8					
Lin et al. (2008)	Healthy *N* = 103	CT	• CTA • Inner edge-inner edge • Sinus of Valsalva • PA bifurcation	31 ± 0.3	29 ± 5	32 ± 6	28 ± 4	28 ± 4	28 ± 4	21 ± 2	20 ± 2	22 ± 2
Devereux et al. (2012)	Healthy *N* = 1207	Echo	• Leading-edge • Parasternal or occasionally apical long-axis	31.8 ± 3.9	3.34 ± 0.34	29.8						
Turkbey et al. (2014)		MRI	• Phase-contrast ECG gated • Right pulmonary level • Inner-edge to inner-edge				31.4					

ones with the largest cohorts of healthy patients. As detailed in the table, different studies have employed different imaging techniques and measurement methods, which might have contributed to the slightly different values.

Furthermore, many variables influence aortic calibers. The aorta is known to dilate over time and, therefore, diameters increase with age. Aortic dimensions are also related to body surface area (BSA). Males have been shown to have larger aortas when absolute values are normalized for BSA.

In Table 5, we report values for the ascending aorta for different age-groups and either normalized for BSA or for different BSA values. In Fig. 10, a graph summarizes results from two studies that adopted a similar methodology (Wolak et al. 2008; Rogers et al. 2013). In addition, whenever possible, we have reported normal aortic diameter values as well as normal upper limits. Because of its statistical implications, the so-defined lower and upper values of a normally distributed population can be calculated as the average ± 2SD and comprise 95.4% of values. Therefore, the upper normal limit can be easily employed as a cutoff in clinical practice.

Based on their observations, several authors have proposed formulas to calculate the expected diameter value of a specific patient based on its gender, age, and BSA. These formulas are reported in Table 6. At present, we do not dispose of sufficient validation data to recommend one over the other, besides the suggestion to use one from a study where authors employed a measurement method similarly to the intended one.

For children, a linear correlation between height and aortic diameter has been demonstrated. On the contrary, the correlation to BSA yielded different results in different studies (Sheil et al. 1995; Gautier et al. 2010). This difference could be linked to the different age range or measurement method between the two studies. Besides using nomograms based on sex and BSA, the *Z*-score has been proposed to ease comparison of values during subsequent follow-up exams in children. The *Z*-score expresses the number of standard deviations of normalized values below or above the expected normal mean.

The relationship between sex and aortic size is not as straightforward as one might expect and as we resumed above. Indeed, although some studies found larger absolute values of aortic diameters in males, also when normalized for BSA (Rogers et al. 2013; Mao et al. 2008), others have reported similar results in the two sexes when normalized for BSA (Lin et al. 2008) except for older people where larger diameters for males have been confirmed (Wolak et al. 2008).

3.2 Aortic Annulus

Several papers have shown that the aortic annulus is mostly elliptical and undergoes morphological and dimensional changes during the cardiac cycle, with bigger dimensions and more circular shape in systole. The variation in morphology has been explained by the simultaneous changes in conformation of the mitral valve apparatus, responsible for the change in shape and even convexity of the posterior part of the aortic annulus. Due to these specific and twofold changes, sizing parameters are not affected by dynamic changes in the same way. The maximum diameter is not as affected by dynamic changes as the minimum diameter, which has been shown to vary between 7.8% and 12.3% in controls. Similarly, in patients with aortic stenosis, differences of <1–9.8% between diastole and systole have been reported for the minimum diameter. Also, the area is greatly affected by the phase of the cardiac cycle with differences of 11.2–28% for healthy annuli and 6.2–21% for stenotic valves. On the contrary, the perimeter is less effected by dynamic changes in both controls (2.2%) and stenotic valves (0.56–7.3%). Absolute values are reported in Table 7, summarized based on data reported in the review by Suchá et al. (2015).

In patients with BAV and no clinically relevant valve dysfunction, the annulus appears to be larger than in patients with TAV with maximum diameter values of 30.42 ± 3.83 mm for valves type 0; 30.04 ± 4.61 mm for valves type 1; 32.34 ± 2.93 mm for valves type 2. Conformational and sizing changes in BAV are also similar to those described for TAV (Boccalini et al. 2021a).

Table 5 Diameter values expressed in [mm] of the ascending aorta in relation to BSA, sex, and age

		All			Women										Men									
	BSA	<40	40–64	65–84	<45		45–54		55–64		65–74		75–84		<45		45–54		55–64		65–74		75–84	
Lin et al. (2008)	mm	26 ± 3	28 ± 3	31 ± 4																				
	mm/m²	13 ± 3	15 ± 2	18 ± 3																				
Rogers et al. (2013)	<1.7				28.8	32.1	29.7	33.5	32.1	36.4	33.6	37.7			30.1	33.8	32.1	35.6	34.0	38.1	36.5	42.4		
	1.7–1.89				30.0	33.7	31.1	34.9	33.3	37.1	33.4	37.3			31.0	34.0	33.3	37.1	34.1	37.5	36.5	40.7		
	≥1.9				31.2	35.1	32.7	36.4	33.3	37.6	35.1	38.5			33.0	36.9	34.3	38.6	36.2	40.2	38.3	43.1		
Wolak et al. (2008)	<1.7				28.4 ± 2.7		29.6 ± 2.8		31.1 ± 2.9		32.5 ± 2.5				28.6 ± 2.2		31 ± 3.8		31.5 ± 2.4		33.9 ± 2.3			
	1.7–1.89				30.0 ± 2.2		31.4 ± 2.9		31.8 ± 2.6		33.4 ± 2.9				30.1 ± 3.1		31.7 ± 3.2		33.5 ± 3.1		35 ± 3			
	1.9–2.09				29.8 ± 2.6		32.5 ± 3.2		33 ± 3		34.3 ± 4.2				30.9 ± 2.7		33.1 ± 3.3		34.6 ± 3.3		35.8 ± 3.2			
	≥2.1				31.3		34.4 ± 3.1		35.4 ± 3.3		32.8				32.3 ± 3		34.4 ± 3.1		36.1 ± 3.5		36.8 ± 2.8			
Turkbey et al. (2014)	mm						28.8	34.4	30.1	36.4	30.6	36.3	31.1	37.1			31.6	37.3	32.8	40.7	34.2	41.0	34.7	40.8
	mm/m²						16.7	20.7	17.6	22.1	18.1	22.1	19.7	28.2			15.9	19.5	16.8	21.1	17.8	21.8	18.6	22.6

Values are reported as provided by the authors of the publications: Lin and Wolak: average and standard deviation; Rogers: mean and 90th centile; Turkbey: median and 95th centile

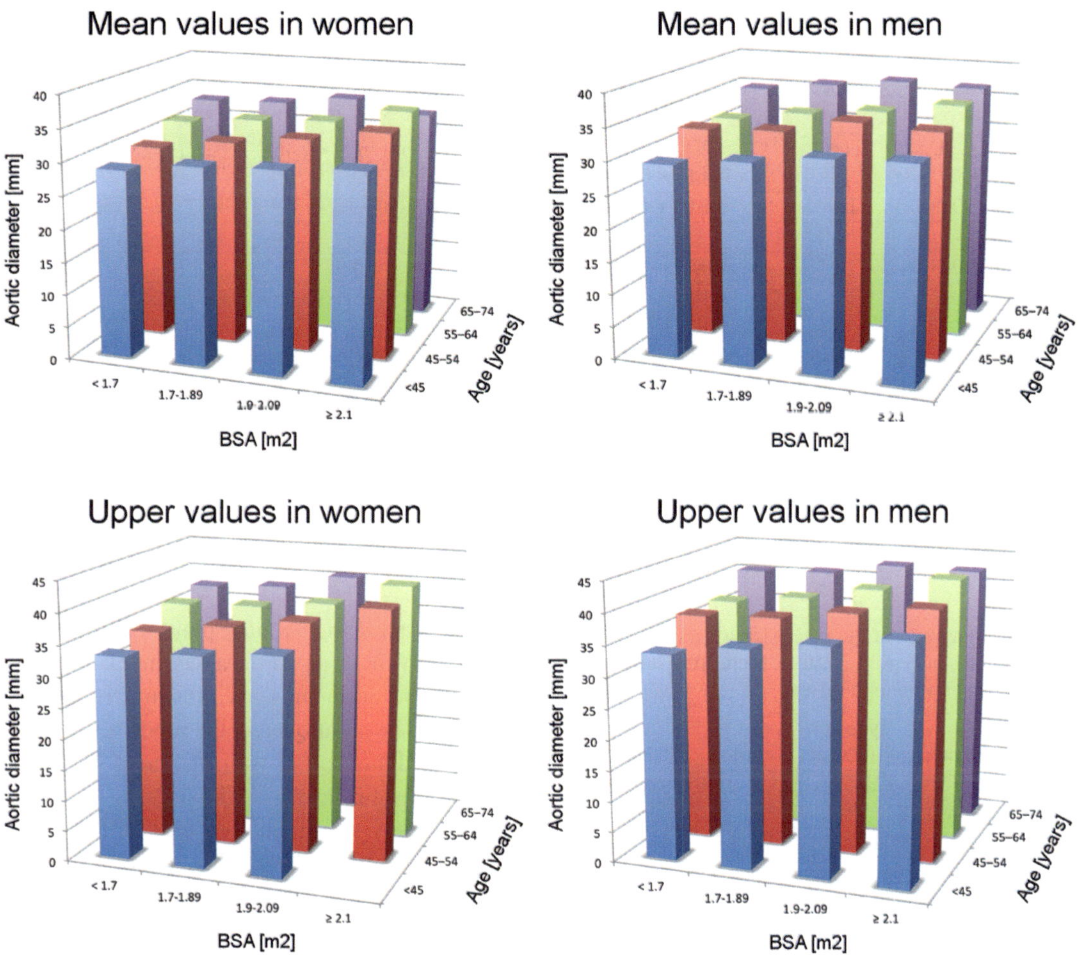

Fig. 10 Graphs summarizing data from the literature regarding mean (top row) and upper (bottom row) values of the ascending aorta in women (on the left) and in men (on the right) per classes of age and BSA

The distance between the annulus and the ostia of the coronary arteries appears to be very variable. Examples of reported distance values from the annulus to the ostia of the coronary arteries in studies performed on CTA scans are of 12.1 ± 3.7 and 16.9 ± 3.3 (Lu et al. 2009; Elattar et al. 2016) and, when reported separately for the right and left ostium, 14.4 ± 2.9 mm, with a range of 7.1–22.7 mm for the left main and 17.2 ± 3.3 mm, with a range of 9.2–26.3 mm for the right coronary (Achenbach et al. 2012).

3.3 Aortic Wall Thickness

The thickness of normal aortic wall is around 3 mm.

For IMH, an aortic wall thickness of 5 mm has been considered as one of the criteria for diagnosis by some authors (Erbel et al. 2014; Haensig 2019; Goldstein et al. 2015). An aortic wall thickness of the intramural hematoma >10 mm is considered a risk factor for disease progression.

3.4 Wall Shear Stress

The average peak systolic WSS magnitude value in the arch of normal subjects was found to be 1.79 Pa, increasing to 2.23 Pa in the descending aorta. The anterior wall of the arch presents higher values that extend all the way to the descending thoracic aorta. Velocity was the strongest predictor of WSS magnitude and axial WSS

Table 6 Formulas to calculate patient's specific normal aortic diameters

Aortic segment	Imaging method	Formula
Aortic root		
Devereux et al. (2012)	Echo	= 2.423 + (age [years] × 0.009) + (bsa [m^2] × 0.461) − (sex [1 = M, 2 = F] × 0.267)
Lin et al. (2008)	CTA	= 1.02 + (0.99 × BSA) + (0.004 × age) ± 0.50
Ascending aorta		
Lin et al. (2008)	CTA	= 0.59 + (0.72 × BSA) + (0.02 × age) ± 0.62
Wolak et al. (2008)	CT	= 14.10 + 0.13 × age (years) − 1.09 (if male) + 0.04 × age (if male) + 5.80 × BSA
Rogers et al. (2013)		= 14.8 + 0.16 (age) ± 1.04 (sex) + 5.34 (BSA)
Descending aorta		
Lin et al. (2008)	CTA	= 0.59 + (0.44 × BSA) + (0.01 × age) + (0.02 + SV) ± 0.38
Wolak et al. (2008)	CT	= 7.73 + 0.11 × age (years) + 0.41 (if male) + 0.02 × age (if male) + 4.91 × BSA
Rogers et al. (2013)	CT	= 8.86 + 0.16 (age) ± 1.79 (sex) + 4.25 (BSA)

Table 7 Summary of the main sizing parameters of the aortic annulus in systole, diastole, for healthy subjects and for patients with stenotic valves

Sizing parameters	Type of patients	Systole	Diastole
Minimum diameter (mm)	Controls	18.8–25.1	19.1–24
	Stenotic valve	18.7–24.8	19.1–23
Maximum diameter (mm)	Controls	20.1–29.7	20.1–30.1
	Stenotic valve	24.7–28.7	24.8–28.7
Area (mm^2)	Controls	370–540	390–460
	Stenotic valve	397–510	396–450
Perimeter (mm)	Controls	69.5–86.6	74.1–88.1
	Stenotic valve	78.5–86.7	74.2–87.5

Based on values reported in Suchá et al. (2015)

in both the arch and descending aorta while values decreased with age (Callaghan and Grieve 2018).

4 Confounding Factors

4.1 Aortic Diameters and Aortic Wall Thickness

Multiple confounding factors can be enumerated regarding aortic diameter assessment.

First of all, *image quality* plays a fundamental role in non-invasive aortic assessment. If a segment of the aorta presents movement artifacts, this should be mentioned in the report and no values about diameters or wall thickness should be provided, as they are not reliable.

As already mentioned, *cardiac synchronization* is recommended for CT acquisitions targeting the ascending aorta. It is known that aortic diameters are significantly different between systole and diastole and more so the closest to the valve (Lin et al. 2008). Although higher values have been reported in systole, diastole is usually employed due to its generally better image quality.

Slice thickness > 1 mm is deemed reducing the quality of multiplanar reconstructions and could potentially influence the accuracy of diameter assessment. Multiples parameters such as MR sequence, kV and keV, Kernel, FOV, zoom, window levels are also likely to have an impact on measurements. However, the influence of all these parameters has not been throughout evaluated and their impact on clinical practice is still unknown.

The *importance of the plane* (axial vs. cross-axial) where to perform the measurement has already been discussed in the previous sections. In addition, it has to be noted that using axial planes results in inaccurate and hardly reproducible choice of exact measurement location. In fact, recommended landmark is easily identifiable on cross-sectional images but correspond to multiple slices on axial images.

Although the aorta has mainly a circular cross-sectional shape, it can often present an elliptic shape. In this case reporting the maximum and minimum diameter can be a more accurate depiction of the actual shape of the vessel. However, as mentioned above, all guidelines' recommendations are based on maximum aortic diameters.

While the aortic maximum diameter measured on axial planes is clearly an overestimation of aortic size, the same cannot be affirmed for the axial minimum diameter. On the contrary, two studies did not find significant differences between minimum axial diameter and corresponding cross-sectional maximum diameter (Rengier et al. 2011; Müller-Eschner et al. 2013). Nonetheless, at present, there is not enough evidence to support the routine use of this faster and easier measurement technique.

While, as seen before, the *thickness of the aortic wall* is an independent parameter of disease for IMH and aortitis and as such it should be reported separately, it is still unclear if and how normal or atherosclerotic wall thickness should be assessed. We have previously indicated that CT and MRI measurements should be performed inner-edge to inner-edge thereby excluding the thickness of the aortic wall. This recommendation is based on different reasons. First of all, most normal values employed for clinical recommendations are based on diameters obtained on non-enhanced CT images, and thus with outer-edge to outer-edge method. However, most of these patients were without known aortic pathology and, therefore, with a thin aortic wall the thickness of which can be disregarded. Secondly, these measurements have been demonstrated having the best correlation to echocardiographic diameters (Bons et al. 2019). Furthermore, on MRI images the aortic wall is depicted in different ways depending on the sequence employed and is particularly prone to chemical shift artifacts due to its position at the interface of different tissues. Probably due to this behavior of the aortic wall as well as to its 2D nature, T2w black blood sequences have been reported as the ones for which operators had the highest degree of confidence for the measurement of aortic diameters (Potthast et al. 2010). Finally, on CE-CEMRA only the aortic lumen is depicted.

Nevertheless, the paradigm of healthy aortic wall not influencing overall aortic measurements due to its very small thickness might be overturned in the next few years due to the introduction of spectral photon counting CT scanners (Fig. 11). These systems provide an increased spatial resolution of about 0.25 mm allowing better visualization not only of the aortic wall but also of the wall of coronary arteries (Boccalini et al. 2021b; Si-Mohamed et al. 2022).

Overall inter-modality, inter-method, interobserver, and intraobserver variability for aortic diameter assessment is high as reported by several authors. For instance, average differences of 2 ± 1.2 mm (LAO: −4.8 to 0.5 mm) (Quint et al. 2013) have been reported between measurements performed with the double oblique technique and an automatic software on the same CT images. Single differences have shown even higher values. Inter-modality variations are even higher with average difference of up to 5.4 mm at the level of the sinus of Valsalva (Bons et al. 2019). Such high values have very important clinical repercussions that will be discussed in the next chapter. In order to reduce this variability, standardization of each step of aortic diameters measurements is of the utmost importance. Since in clinical practice, it is not unusual patients being followed in different centers and/or by different clinicians, it is strongly recommended to always evaluate not only the scan of one's competence but also the previous one and possibly reporting both measures. Moreover, if aortic diameters have been described as stable over a long period of time without reported values, it is wise to check the first exam to confirm the stability and to report absolute diameter values.

4.2 TAVI Planning

Most of the above-mentioned cofounding factors can also be applied to pre-TAVI annulus sizing.

Two particular aspects that deserve separate discussion are: what is the most appropriate phase of the cardiac cycle to perform measurements;

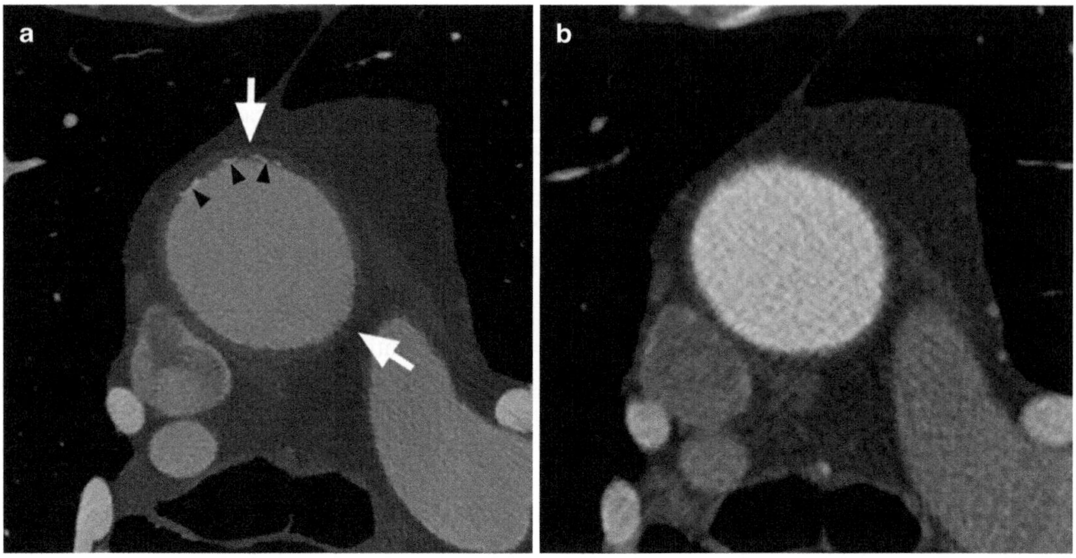

Fig. 11 Potential influence of aortic wall thickness on diameter measurements with the use of Spectral Photon Counting CT (SPCCT). In **a**, an axial image of an ECG gated CTA scan of the ascending aorta performed with a SPCCT scanner. In **b**, an image of the ascending aorta of the same patient obtained with an ECG gated CTA scan with a dual energy dual-layer CT (DEDLCT) scanner equipped with energy-integrating detectors. The wall of the aorta is clearly visible all around its circumference with SPCCT (arrows in **a**) but not with DEDLCT. Furthermore, some tiny calcifications of the anterior aortic wall are very clearly depicted with SPCCT but not even visible with DEDLCT

what to do about the thickness of the wall and how to derive measurements in the presence of annular calcifications. While, as for the rest of the aorta, the image quality of the aortic annulus is normally better in diastole, according to several papers systole yields significantly bigger dimensions that might affect prosthesis sizing (Suchá et al. 2015; Hamdan et al. 2012; De Heer et al. 2012). Therefore, as discussed also in the previous paragraph, measurements should be derived in systole if image quality of this phase allows for it. As a general consideration, the prosthesis has to be chosen based on the inner-edge to inner-edge diameter leaving out the wall thickness. An exception can be made in the presence of calcifications. In this case, authors have suggested different possibilities, the easiest of which is to draw the annulus contour over the calcifications as if they were not there (Blanke et al. 2019).

4.3 Hemodynamic Parameters

4D-flow sequences are known to have a series of technical limitations affecting their applicability and reliability on clinical practice. Some of these limitations are the same encountered with other phase contrast sequences, such as eddy current effects, Max-well terms, and gradient field distortions, that should be corrected according to published criteria, as is normally done for the 3D flow acquisitions (Markl et al. 2012).

In addition, owing to the limited spatial and temporal resolution of 4D-flow, WSS is known to be underestimated. In addition, limited spatial and temporal resolution have been advocated to explain inferior velocity values as compared to echocardiography (Frydrychowicz et al. 2011). Moreover, noise can be so important as to oblige authors to average several phases for calculations

(Rodríguez-Palomares et al. 2018). Importantly, clinical employment of these sequences is greatly limited by all the assumptions on which the calculations are founded, including importantly that of the linearity of the flow (Garcia et al. 2019).

5 Clinical Implementation of the Measurement

5.1 Aortic Diameters

5.1.1 Aneurysm

5.1.1.1 Absolute Diameter

Decisions on therapeutic management of aortic aneurysms rely almost solely on aortic diameters. Thresholds for intervention based on absolute maximum diameter are reported in Table 8 and are based on the recommendation from the ESC regarding aortic and valve pathology of 2014 and 2017, respectively (Erbel et al. 2014; Baumgartner et al. 2017).

It has to be noticed that for patients with Loeys-Dietz syndrome as well as aneurysms-osteoarthritis syndrome, a cutoff value of 42 mm has been proposed by some authors but is not yet implemented in guidelines.

If intervention thresholds are not met, imaging follow-up is recommended. While ultrasound can be employed for aneurysms of the aortic root, with the above-mentioned limitations, CT or MRI is required for assessment of the ascending aorta and aortic arch. However, there are no current indications regarding the best timing. Suggestions of appropriate timing range from every year to

Table 8 Cutoff values prompting interventions on the thoracic aorta

Aortic segment	Cutoff	Target population		
Ascending aorta	55 mm	• General population		
	55 mm	• Bicuspid valve without other risk factors		
	50 mm	• Bicuspid valve with one or more other risk factors[a] or coarctation		
		• Marfan syndrome without risk factors	• Patients with Marfanoid manifestations and other connective tissue disease without risk factors	• TGFBR1 or TGFBR2 mutation (including Loeys Dietz syndrome) without risk factors
	45 mm	• Marfan patients with risk factors[b]	• Patients with Marfanoid manifestations and other connective tissue disease with risk factors	• TGFBR1 or TGFBR2 mutation (including Loeys Dietz syndrome) with risk factors
		• Patients with aortic valve dysfunction requiring surgery and dilation of the aortic root or tubular aorta		
	27.5 mm/m2	• Turner syndrome		
Aortic arch	55 mm			
Descending aorta	55 mm	• If TEVAR is feasible		
	60 mm	• If surgery is the only possible treatment		

[a] Additional risk factors, such as family history, systemic hypertension, coarctation of the aorta, or increase in aortic diameter 0.3 mm/year, and also according to age, body size, comorbidities

[b] Including family history of dissection, size increase 0.3 mm/year (in repeated examinations using the same technique and confirmed by another technique), severe aortic regurgitation, or desire for pregnancy

2–3 years depending on the last measured diameter, family history, and other comorbidities (Goldstein et al. 2015). For BAV patients, the time-schedule is more defined: echocardiographic reports of diameters >45 mm and/or growth of 3 mm/year have to be confirmed by either CT or MRI and patients with >45 mm diameter should be re-controlled annually (Borger et al. 2018).

Growth Rate

The use of growth thresholds to guide aortic aneurysms treatment is one of the most debated topics in the field. The AHA 2010 guidelines on aortic pathology stated that a growth rate of more than 2.5 mm/year should be considered as pathologic and prompt intervention (Hiratzka et al. 2010). However, the authors of the ESC 2014 guidelines acknowledged the high variability in aortic diameters measurements and challenged this concept prompting for more caution (Erbel et al. 2014). Their conclusion was that only a difference of 5 mm or more should be considered clinically significant. However, there are exceptions such as for Marfan patients for whom a growth >3 mm/year is considered a risk factor and indicate surgery for lower absolute aortic diameters.

5.1.2 Dissection

While at diagnosis the treatment for aortic dissection is decided based on its location, diameters play an important role in chronic type B dissection. In this context, a growth of >10 mm/year as well as a total aortic diameter of >60 mm requires interventional or surgical treatment (Trimarchi et al. 2014).

It is well known that the ratio between the diameter of the true lumen/false lumen yields important prognostic implications. Indeed, one of the main causes of death in patients with dissection is visceral complications that can be a consequence of the phenomenon of dynamic hypoperfusion (Evangelista et al. 2018; Rampoldi et al. 2007). Although a small size of the true lumen as well as an intimal flap concave toward the false lumen has been described as signs of the higher pressure exerted by the false lumen, more recent studies have shown that the relationship between the two lumen as well as the appearance of the intimal flap change during the cycle (Fig. 12) relativizing the prognostic value of these signs (Williams et al. 1997; Yang et al. 2014).

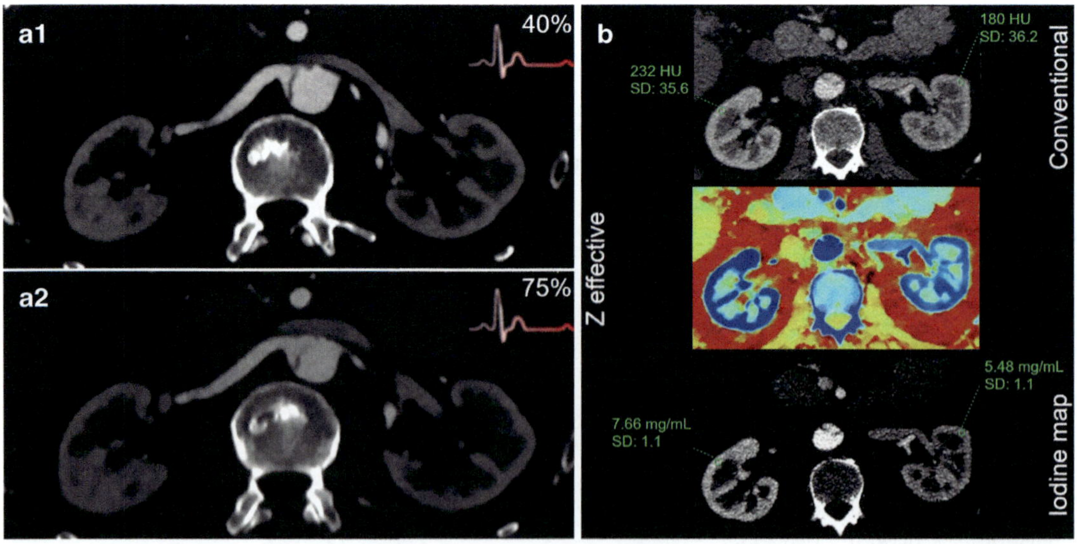

Fig. 12 **a1** and **a2** show an example of variation of true and false lumen diameters at the level of the renal arteries depending on the cardiac phase (systole in **a1** and diastole in **a2**). In **b**, one conventional image and two spectral reconstructions, Z-effective and iodine map, of the two kidneys of a patient with an aortic dissection extending in the left renal artery. Already visible on the conventional image, the different perfusion of the two kidneys is better detectable on Z-effective and can be quantified in terms of mg/mL of iodine on iodine maps

5.1.3 IMH

Regarding maximum aortic size, a diameter of >50 mm is considered a mortality risk factor for type A IMH in the first 3 months of the disease (Evangelista et al. 2004). On the other hand, for type B IMH a diameter >45 mm has been defined as the cutoff value to identify the high-risk population (Evangelista et al. 2014). In the chronic phase of IMH type B absolute diameters >55 mm should prompt surgery (Evangelista et al. 2014).

5.1.4 TAVI Planning

Measurements of the aortic annulus and the distance between the annulus and the ostia are analyzed to establish the best type and size of the TAVI valve. The possible complications after the placement of the valve are the rarely occurring rupture of the LVOT, in case of oversizing, and the more common paravalvular leakages, in case of under-sizing. Indeed leakages occur every time the valve is too small, whereas the small flexibility of the LVOT allows for accommodation of slightly too big valves without further complications. Therefore, in clinical practice, among the few available options of size of each type of TAVI valve, the choice goes for one that is slightly oversized (around 31% oversizing based on the area and 15% based on perimeter) (Abdel-Wahab et al. 2014).

Although in most centers, the annulus represents the most important sizing parameter also in patients with bicuspid valves, it should be mentioned that according to some authors other structures should be assessed instead for BAV patients (Kim et al. 2019). According to these works, the measure of the annulus is not relevant in this specific group due to their more complex and variegated anatomy and, thus, other parameters are more relevant. However, at the moment there is no general consensus on any of the proposed alternatives and the annulus size is still considered the most appropriate (Tchetche et al. 2019).

Another potentially lethal complication is coronary artery ostium obstruction by the valve itself or by the native cusps that are crushed against the wall of the aorta and, if the ostia are low or the annulus is small, can reach the ostia and block blood flow. Self-expandable valves are associated with lower frequencies of coronary occlusion while being more prone to paravalvular leakage especially in the presence of calcifications, although this risk seems reduced with newer generation valves (Thiele et al. 2020; Mahtta et al. 2017).

The access route is also particularly important, as the sheath of TAVI valves is particularly voluminous ranging between 5 mm, for newer models, and 8 mm. If femoral arteries are not accessible, subclavian arteries or carotid arteries can be employed.

5.1.5 Aortic Wall Thickness

5.1.5.1 IMH

Although it is generally recognized that a thicker aortic wall at the moment of diagnosis of IMH is a risk factor for pathology progression and complications, a cutoff has proven difficult to identify and different values have been proposed (Evangelista et al. 2003, 2014; Sueyoshi et al. 2002). A value of 10 mm has shown a PPV of 78.6% and a NPV of 81% (Sueyoshi et al. 2002).

5.1.5.2 Aortitis

For great vessels disease that can affect the aorta, namely giant cell arteritis and Takayasu arteritis, thickening of the aortic wall is one of the main diagnostic criteria at non-invasive imaging (Matsunaga et al. 1997; Dejaco et al. 2018). Restoration of normal aortic thickness has been shown as a sign of inactive disease and wall thickness reduction has been considered as a marker of effective therapy (Choe et al. 1999; Aluquin et al. 2002). However, at the present time, 18FDG PET/CT is the preferred imaging modality to establish whether the disease is active or not (Puppo et al. 2014), as illustrated in the example of Fig. 13.

5.2 Hemodynamics Parameters

Hemodynamic parameters derived from through-plane contrast phase acquisitions placed in the

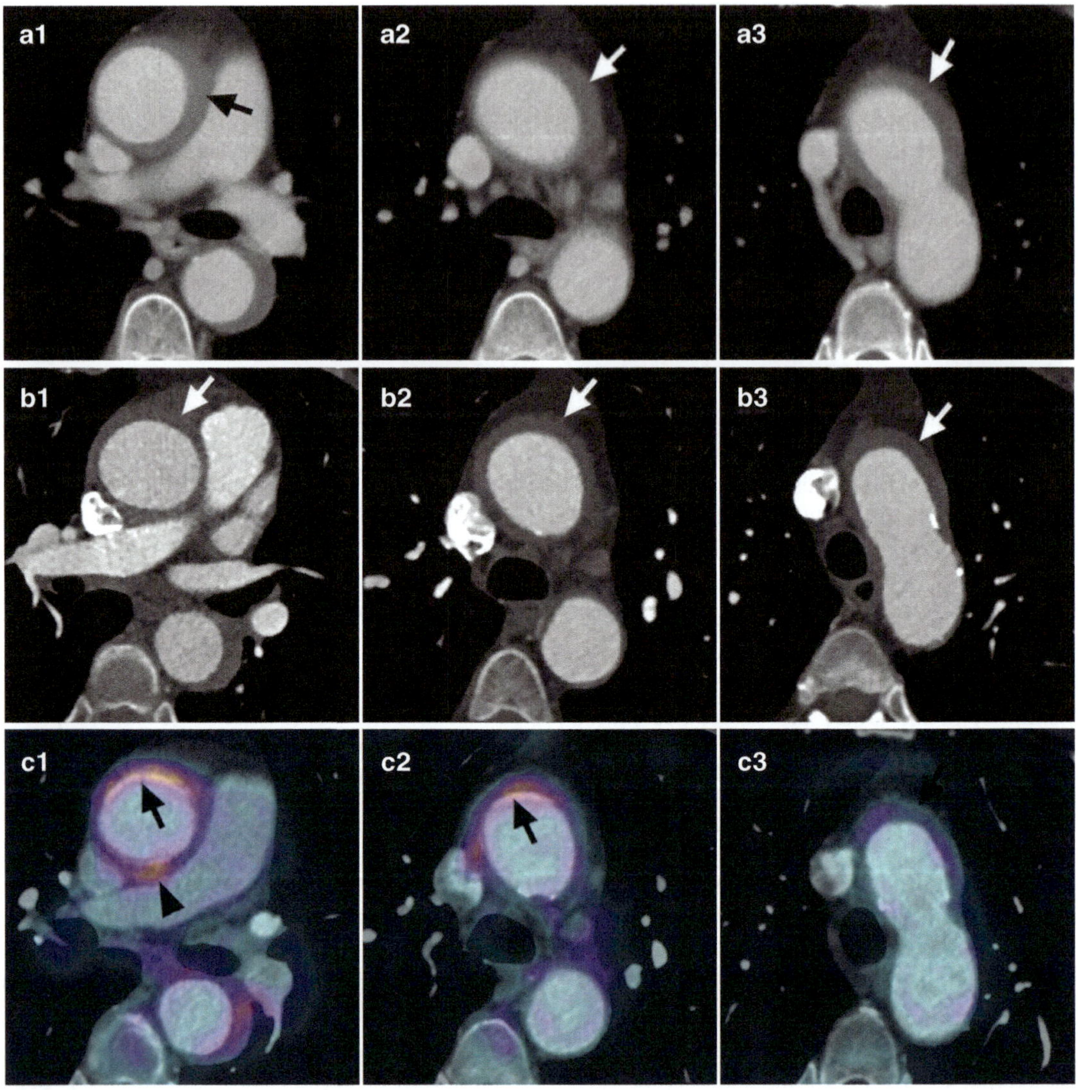

Fig. 13 An example of aortitis evolution over time. A 65-year-old woman affected by Takayasu arteritis underwent a CTA of the thoracic aorta (**a1**–**a3**) that showed an important thickening of the aortic wall especially of the left lateral wall of the ascending aorta (arrows). Two years later, a new CTA (**b1**–**b3**) showed increasing thickening of the wall of the ascending aorta, including its anterior part (arrows). Three years later, an additional follow-up exam, this time combining CTA and PET acquisitions (**c1**–**c3**) showed strong metabolic activity at the level of the anterior wall of the proximal ascending aorta (**c1** and **c2**, arrows) but also of the posterior wall at the level of the pulmonary trunk (**c1**, arrowhead), a region where the thickening of the wall had remained about constant over the years. Furthermore, the metabolism of the anterior wall just before the aortic arch (**c3**, arrow) was milder while the increase in thickening of the wall in this area had been important, highlighting how the thickening of the wall cannot be reliably considered as a perfect mirror of the underlying inflammation

aorta but employed to assess valvular function will be discussed in the appropriate chapter regarding valves.

Hemodynamic parameters of the aorta in different pathologies have been the object of numerous studies.

However, due to the many assumptions and to the required accurate definition of geometrical and physiological boundary conditions to compute values, the clinical applications of these parameters as derived from 4D flow sequences remain very limited (Dyverfeldt et al. 2015).

5.2.1 Dissection

Non-invasive 4D-flow analysis of true and false lumen hemodynamics showed that the true lumen has higher total flow per cardiac cycle and peak flow while the false lumen has higher retrograde flow (François et al. 2013).

The potential clinical role of 4D-flow has been assessed for type B dissections to help predict their progressive dilation. Rapid aortic growth was found to be associated with higher percentage of flow diverted to the false lumen as well as lower entry tear peak velocity and increased time-averaged wall shear stress experienced by the aortic wall (Shang et al. 2015; Burris et al. 2020).

5.2.2 Bicuspid Aortic Valve (BAV)

In patients with BAV, even in those without significant valvular pathology, the flow in the ascending aorta is more helical as compared to the laminal flow in patients with tricuspid aortic valves. This results in through-plane velocity, circumferential WSS, and net WSS being increased at the proximal ascending aorta while axial WSS is decreased (Papaioannou and Stefanadis 2005; Potthast et al. 2010).

Differences have been found also among different BAV types. The flow is altered and eccentric impinging at the right-anterior walls for right-left BAV and right-posterior walls for right-non coronary BAV compared to controls in the aortic root (Rodríguez-Palomares et al. 2018; Meierhofer et al. 2013) followed by a more pronounced rotational movement in the ascending aorta for the right-non coronary BAV (Rodríguez-Palomares et al. 2018).

The altered flow pattern and shear distribution have been hypothesized to influence aortopathy on a molecular basis as well as the aortic dilation pattern in BAV patients (Della Corte et al. 2008; Rodríguez-Palomares et al. 2018).

5.2.3 Coarctation

4D flow has been assessed as a promising non-invasive tool to determine hemodynamic characteristics of the aorta in patients with coarctation, especially after repair. Indeed, a more turbulent flow has been found at the level of stenosis in operated patients and especially in post-stenotic dilatations (Frydrychowicz et al. 2011; Hope et al. 2010). However, several confounding factors, including similar findings in the presence of a steeply angled aortic arch (the so-called gothic arch), and the lack of validation in a large cohort of patients as well as the lack of precise cutoff values, limit the use of these preliminary findings.

References

Abdel-Wahab M, Mehilli J, Frerker C et al (2014) Comparison of balloon-expandable vs self-expandable valves in patients undergoing transcatheter aortic valve replacement: the CHOICE randomized clinical trial. JAMA 311:1503–1514

Achenbach S, Delgado V, Hausleiter J, Schoenhagen P, Min JK, Leipsic JA (2012) SCCT expert consensus document on computed tomography imaging before transcatheter aortic valve implantation (TAVI)/transcatheter aortic valve replacement (TAVR). J Cardiovasc Comput Tomogr 6:366–380

Aluquin VPR, Albano SA, Chan F, Sandborg C, Pitlick PT (2002) Magnetic resonance imaging in the diagnosis and follow up of Takayasu's arteritis in children. Ann Rheum Dis 61:526–529

Baumgartner H, Falk V, Bax JJ et al (2017) 2017 ESC/EACTS guidelines for the management of valvular heart disease. Eur Heart J 38:2739. https://doi.org/10.1093/eurheartj/ehx391

Blanke P, Weir-McCall JR, Achenbach S et al (2019) Computed tomography imaging in the context of transcatheter aortic valve implantation (TAVI)/transcatheter aortic valve replacement (TAVR): an expert consensus document of the Society of Cardiovascular Computed Tomography. JACC Cardiovasc Imaging 12:1–24

Boccalini S, Bons LR, van den Hoven AT, van den Bosch AE, Krestin GP, Roos-Hesselink J, Budde RPJ (2021a) Bicuspid aortic valve annulus: assessment of geometry and size changes during the cardiac cycle as measured with a standardized method to define the annular plane. Eur Radiol 31:8116–8129

Boccalini S, Si-Mohamed SA, Lacombe H et al (2021b) First in-human results of computed tomography angiography for coronary stent assessment with a spectral photon counting computed tomography. Invest Radiol 57(4):212–221

Bons LR, Duijnhouwer AL, Boccalini S et al (2019) Intermodality variation of aortic dimensions: how, where and when to measure the ascending aorta. Int J Cardiol 276:230–235

Borger MA, Fedak PWM, Stephens EH et al (2018) The American Association for Thoracic Surgery consensus guidelines on bicuspid aortic valve–related aortopathy: full online-only version. J Thorac Cardiovasc Surg 156:e41–e74

Burris NS, Nordsletten DA, Nordsletten DA et al (2020) False lumen ejection fraction predicts growth in type B aortic dissection: preliminary results. Eur J Cardiothoracic Surg 57:896–903

Callaghan FM, Grieve SM (2018) Translational physiology: normal patterns of thoracic aortic wall shear stress measured using four-dimensional flow MRI in a large population. Am J Physiol Heart Circ Physiol 315:H1174–H1181

Choe YH, Kim DK, Koh EM, Do YS, Lee WR (1999) Takayasu arteritis: diagnosis with MR imaging and MR angiography in acute and chronic active stages. J Magn Reson Imaging 10:751–757

Clouse WD, Hallett JW, Schaff HV, Gayari MM, Ilstrup DM, Melton LJ (1998) Improved prognosis of thoracic aortic aneurysms. A population-based study. JAMA 280:1926–1929

De Heer LM, Budde RPJ, Van Prehn J, Mali WPTM, Bartels LW, Stella PR, Van Herwerden LA, Kluin J, Vincken KL (2012) Pulsatile distention of the nondiseased and stenotic aortic valve annulus: analysis with electrocardiogram-gated computed tomography. Ann Thorac Surg 93:516–522

Dejaco C, Ramiro S, Duftner C et al (2018) EULAR recommendations for the use of imaging in large vessel vasculitis in clinical practice. Ann Rheum Dis 77:636–643

Della Corte A, Quarto C, Bancone C et al (2008) Spatiotemporal patterns of smooth muscle cell changes in ascending aortic dilatation with bicuspid and tricuspid aortic valve stenosis: focus on cell-matrix signaling. J Thorac Cardiovasc Surg 135:1–4

Devereux RB, de Simone G, Arnett DK et al (2012) Normal limits in relation to age, body size and gender of two-dimensional echocardiographic aortic root dimensions in persons ≥15 years of age. Am J Cardiol 110:1189–1194

Dyverfeldt P, Bissell M, Barker AJ et al (2015) 4D flow cardiovascular magnetic resonance consensus statement. J Cardiovasc Magn Reson 17:1–19

Elattar M, Wiegerinck E, van Kesteren F, Dubois L, Planken N, Vanbavel E, Baan J, Marquering H (2016) Automatic aortic root landmark detection in CTA images for preprocedural planning of transcatheter aortic valve implantation. Int J Cardiovasc Imaging 32:501–511

Erbel R, Aboyans V, Boileau C et al (2014) 2014 ESC guidelines on the diagnosis and treatment of aortic diseases: document covering acute and chronic aortic diseases of the thoracic and abdominal aorta of the adult. The task force for the diagnosis and treatment of aortic diseases of the European. Eur Heart J 35:2873–2926

Evangelista A, Dominguez R, Sebastia C, Salas A, Permanyer-Miralda G, Avegliano G, Elorz C, Gonzalez-Alujas T, Del Castillo HG, Soler-Soler J (2003) Long-term follow-up of aortic intramural hematoma: predictors of outcome. Circulation 108:583–589

Evangelista A, Dominguez R, Sebastia C, Salas A, Permanyer-Miralda G, Avegliano G, Gomez-Bosh Z, Gonzalez-Alujas T, Garcia Del Castillo H, Soler-Soler J (2004) Prognostic value of clinical and morphologic findings in short-term evolution of aortic intramural haematoma: therapeutic implications. Eur Heart J 25:81–87

Evangelista A, Czerny M, Nienaber C, Schepens M, Rousseau H, Cao P, Moral S, Fattori R (2014) Interdisciplinary expert consensus on management of type B intramural haematoma and penetrating aortic ulcer. Eur J Cardiothorac Surg 47:209–217

Evangelista A, Isselbacher EM, Bossone E et al (2018) Insights from the international registry of acute aortic dissection: a 20-year experience of collaborative clinical research. Circulation 137:1846–1860 .

François CJ, Markl M, Schiebler ML, Niespodzany E, Landgraf BR, Schlensak C, Frydrychowicz A (2013) Four-dimensional, flow-sensitive magnetic resonance imaging of blood flow patterns in thoracic aortic dissections. J Thorac Cardiovasc Surg 145:1359–1366

Francone M, Budde RPJ, Bremerich J et al (2020) CT and MR imaging prior to transcatheter aortic valve implantation: standardisation of scanning protocols, measurements and reporting—a consensus document by the European Society of Cardiovascular Radiology (ESCR). Eur Radiol 30:2627–2650

Frangieh AH, Michel J, Deutsch O, Joner M, Pellegrini C, Rheude T, Bleiziffer S, Kasel AM (2019) Aortic annulus sizing in stenotic bicommissural non-raphe-type bicuspid aortic valves: reconstructing a three-dimensional structure using only two hinge points. Clin Res Cardiol 108:6–15

Frydrychowicz A, Markl M, Hirtler D, Harloff A, Schlensak C, Geiger J, Stiller B, Arnold R (2011)

Aortic hemodynamics in patients with and without repair of aortic coarctation. Invest Radiol 46:317–325
Garcia J, Barker AJ, Markl M (2019) The role of imaging of flow patterns by 4D flow MRI in aortic stenosis. JACC Cardiovasc Imaging 12:252–266
Gautier M, Detaint D, Fermanian C et al (2010) Nomograms for aortic root diameters in children using two-dimensional echocardiography. Am J Cardiol 105:888–894
Goldstein SA, Evangelista A, Abbara S et al (2015) Multimodality imaging of diseases of the thoracic aorta in adults: from the American Society of Echocardiography and the European Association of Cardiovascular Imaging. J Am Soc Echocardiogr 28:119–182
Haensig M (2019) Type B intramural hematoma: focus on reasons for development and overlapping clinical disease. Ann Cardiothorac Surg 8:494–496
Hamdan A, Guetta V, Konen E et al (2012) Deformation dynamics and mechanical properties of the aortic annulus by 4-dimensional computed tomography: insights into the functional anatomy of the aortic valve complex and implications for transcatheter aortic valve therapy. J Am Coll Cardiol 59:119–127
Hiratzka LF, Bakris GL, Beckman JA et al (2010) 2010 ACCF/AHA/AATS/ACR/ASA/SCA/SCAI/SIR/STS/SVM guidelines for the diagnosis and management of patients with thoracic aortic disease: a report of the American College of Cardiology Foundation/American Heart Association Task Force on Practice Guidelines. Circulation 121:e266–e369
Hope MD, Meadows AK, Hope TA, Ordovas KG, Saloner D, Reddy GP, Alley MT, Higgins CB (2010) Clinical evaluation of aortic coarctation with 4D flow MR imaging. J Magn Reson Imaging 31:711–718
Kim W-K, Renker M, Rolf A et al (2019) Annular versus supra-annular sizing for TAVI in bicuspid aortic valve stenosis. EuroIntervention 15:e231–e238
Lin FY, Devereux RB, Roman MJ et al (2008) Assessment of the thoracic aorta by multidetector computed tomography: age- and sex-specific reference values in adults without evident cardiovascular disease. J Cardiovasc Comput Tomogr 2:298–308
Lu TLC, Huber CH, Rizzo E, Dehmeshki J, von Segesser LK, Qanadli SD (2009) Ascending aorta measurements as assessed by ECG-gated multi-detector computed tomography: a pilot study to establish normative values for transcatheter therapies. Eur Radiol 19:664–669
Mahtta D, Elgendy IY, Bavry AA (2017) From CoreValve to Evolut PRO: reviewing the journey of self-expanding transcatheter aortic valves. Cardiol Ther 6:183–192
Mao SS, Ahmadi N, Shah B, Beckmann D, Chen A, Ngo L, Flores FR, Gao YL, Budoff MJ (2008) Normal thoracic aorta diameter on cardiac computed tomography in healthy asymptomatic adults. Acad Radiol 15:827–834
Markl M, Frydrychowicz A, Kozerke S, Hope M, Wieben O (2012) 4D flow MRI. J Magn Reson Imaging 36:1015–1036
Matsunaga N, Hayashi K, Sakamoto I, Ogawa Y, Matsumoto T (1997) Takayasu arteritis: protean radiologic manifestations and diagnosis. Radiographics 17:579–594
Meierhofer C, Schneider EP, Lyko C, Hutter A, Martinoff S, Markl M, Hager A, Hess J, Stern H, Fratz S (2013) Wall shear stress and flow patterns in the ascending aorta in patients with bicuspid aortic valves differ significantly from tricuspid aortic valves: a prospective study. Eur Heart J Cardiovasc Imaging 14:797–804
Müller-Eschner M, Rengier F, Partovi S, Weber TF, Kopp-Schneider A, Geisbüsch P, Kauczor HU, Von Tengg-Kobligk H (2013) Accuracy and variability of semiautomatic centerline analysis versus manual aortic measurement techniques for TEVAR. Eur J Vasc Endovasc Surg 45:241–247
Nayak KS, Nielsen JF, Bernstein MA et al (2015) Cardiovascular magnetic resonance phase contrast imaging. J Cardiovasc Magn Reson 17:1–26
Papaioannou TG, Stefanadis C (2005) Vascular wall shear stress: basic principles and methods. Hellenic J Cardiol 46:9–15
Potthast S, Mitsumori L, Stanescu LA, Richardson ML, Branch K, Dubinsky TJ, Maki JH (2010) Measuring aortic diameter with different MR techniques: comparison of three-dimensional (3D) navigated steady-state free-precession (SSFP), 3D contrast-enhanced magnetic resonance angiography (CE-MRA), 2D T2 black blood, and 2D cine SSFP. J Magn Reson Imaging 31:177–184
Puppo C, Massollo M, Paparo F, Camellino D, Piccardo A, Shoushtari Zadeh Naseri M, Villavecchia G, Rollandi GA, Cimmino MA (2014) Giant cell arteritis: a systematic review of the qualitative and semiquantitative methods to assess vasculitis with 18F-fluorodeoxyglucose positron emission tomography. Biomed Res Int 2014:1–11
Quint LE, Liu PS, Booher AM, Watcharotone K, Myles JD (2013) Proximal thoracic aortic diameter measurements at CT: repeatability and reproducibility according to measurement method. Int J Cardiovasc Imaging 29:479–488
Rampoldi V, Trimarchi S, Eagle KA et al (2007) Simple risk models to predict surgical mortality in acute type A aortic dissection: the International Registry of Acute Aortic Dissection Score. Ann Thorac Surg 83:55–61
Rengier F, Weber TF, Partovi S, Müller-Eschner M, Böckler D, Kauczor H-U, von Tengg-Kobligk H (2011) Reliability of semiautomatic centerline analysis versus manual aortic measurement techniques for TEVAR among non-experts. Eur J Vasc Endovasc Surg 42:324–331
Rodríguez-Palomares JF, Dux-Santoy L, Guala A et al (2018) Aortic flow patterns and wall shear stress maps by 4D-flow cardiovascular magnetic resonance in the

assessment of aortic dilatation in bicuspid aortic valve disease. J Cardiovasc Magn Reson 20:28
Rogers IS, Massaro JM, Truong QA, Mahabadi AA, Kriegel MF, Fox CS, Thanassoulis G, Isselbacher EM, Hoffmann U, O'Donnell CJ (2013) Distribution, determinants, and normal reference values of thoracic and abdominal aortic diameters by computed tomography (from the Framingham Heart Study). Am J Cardiol 111:1510–1516
Sampson UKA, Norman PE, Fowkes FGR et al (2014) Global and regional burden of aortic dissection and aneurysms: mortality trends in 21 world regions, 1990 to 2010. Glob Heart 9:171–180
Shang EK, Nathan DP, Fairman RM, Bavaria JE, Gorman RC, Gorman JH, Jackson BM (2015) Use of computational fluid dynamics studies in predicting aneurysmal degeneration of acute type B aortic dissections. J Vasc Surg 62:279–284
Sheil MLK, Jenkins O, Sholler GF (1995) Echocardiographic assessment of aortic root dimensions in normal children based on measurement of a new ratio of aortic size independent of growth. Am J Cardiol 75:711–715
Sievers HH, Schmidtke C (2007) A classification system for the bicuspid aortic valve from 304 surgical specimens. J Thorac Cardiovasc Surg 133:1226–1233
Sigovan M, Hope MD, Dyverfeldt P, Saloner D (2011) Comparison of four-dimensional flow parameters for quantification of flow eccentricity in the ascending aorta. J Magn Reson Imaging 34:1226–1230
Si-Mohamed SA, Boccalini S, Lacombe H et al (2022) Coronary CT angiography with photon-counting CT: first-in-human results. Radiology 303:303. https://doi.org/10.1148/radiol.211780
Suchá D, Tuncay V, Prakken NHJ, Leiner T, Van Ooijen PMA, Oudkerk M, Budde RPJ (2015) Does the aortic annulus undergo conformational change throughout the cardiac cycle? A systematic review. Eur Heart J Cardiovasc Imaging 16:1307–1317
Sueyoshi E, Imada T, Sakamoto I, Matsuoka Y, Hayashi K (2002) Analysis of predictive factors for progression of type B aortic intramural hematoma with computed tomography. J Vasc Surg 35:1179–1183
Tchetche D, De Biase C, Van Gils L et al (2019) Bicuspid aortic valve anatomy and relationship with devices: the BAVARD multicenter Registry: a European picture of contemporary multidetector computed tomography sizing for bicuspid valves. Circ Cardiovasc Interv 12:1–10
Thiele H, Kurz T, Feistritzer HJ et al (2020) Comparison of newer generation self-expandable vs. balloon-expandable valves in transcatheter aortic valve implantation: the randomized SOLVE-TAVI trial. Eur Heart J 41:1890–1899
Trimarchi S, Jonker FHW, van Bogerijen GHW, Tolenaar JL, Moll FL, Czerny M, Patel HJ (2014) Predicting aortic enlargement in type B aortic dissection. Ann Cardiothorac Surg 3:285–291
Turkbey EB, Jain A, Johnson C et al (2014) Determinants and normal values of ascending aortic diameter by age, gender, and race/ethnicity in the Multi-Ethnic Study of Atherosclerosis (MESA). J Magn Reson Imaging 39:360–368
Williams DM, Lee DY, Hamilton BH, Marx MV, Narasimham DL, Kazanjian SN, Prince MR, Andrews JC, Cho KJ, Deeb GM (1997) The dissected aorta: Part III. Anatomy and radiologic diagnosis of branch-vessel compromise. Radiology 203:37–44
Wolak A, Gransar H, Thomson LEJ et al (2008) Aortic size assessment by noncontrast cardiac computed tomography: normal limits by age, gender, and body surface area. JACC Cardiovasc Imaging 1:200–209
Yang S, Li X, Chao B et al (2014) Abdominal aortic intimal flap motion characterization in acute aortic dissection: assessed with retrospective ECG-gated thoracoabdominal aorta dual-source CT angiography. PLoS One 9:1–9

Vascular Measurements for Thoracic Interventional Radiology

Antoine Khalil, Waqaas Mohammad, Marie-Pierre Debray, and Augustin Gaudemer

Contents

A. Khalil (✉) · W. Mohammad · M.-P. Debray · A. Gaudemer
Service d'Imagerie Médicale diagnostique et interventionnelle, CHU Bichat-Claude Bernard, Paris, France

Université Paris-Cité, UMR Inserm 1149, Paris, France
e-mail: antoine.khalil@aphp.fr

The field of interventional radiology in the thorax is broad and includes both percutaneous and endovascular interventions. Measurements are primarily dedicated to endovascular intervention. Endovascular interventional radiology involves the right (superior vena cava (SVC) and pulmonary arteries) or left (bronchial and non-bronchial systemic arteries) circulation. A major purpose of this chapter is to clarify the normal and abnormal size of these vascular structures from the perspective of the interventional radiologist. The aorta will be treated in a separate chapter (see Chapter by Sara Boccallini).

1 Superior Vena Cava

The SVC is the confluence of the right and left brachiocephalic veins and carries blood from the upper body (head, neck, and upper extremities) to the right atrium, while also carrying blood from the postero-inferior part of the body via the azygos system. The maximum diameter of the SVC is 2.1 cm ± 0.7 cm (Mahlon and Yoon 2007). Lin et al. (2009), in a CT series using cardiac gating, suggest that the largest diameter of the SVC ranges from 1.5 to 2.8 cm and the smallest diameter ranges from 1 to 2.4 cm. There are anatomical variants to be aware of, such as a double SVC (a right and a

Med Radiol Diagn Imaging (2026)
https://doi.org/10.1007/174_2025_678,
Published Online: 01 January 2026

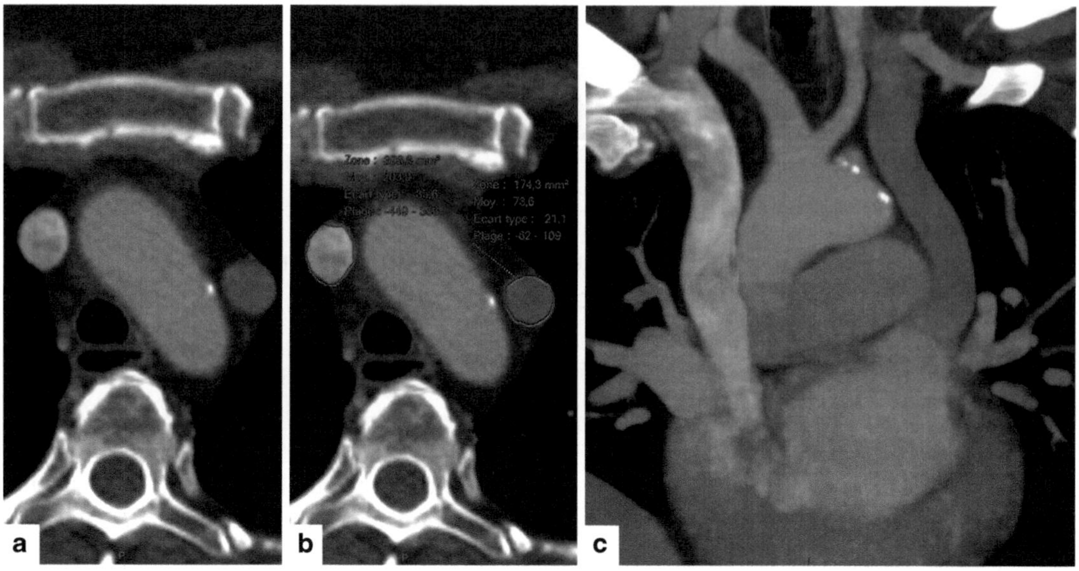

Fig. 1 Bilateral superior vena cava. A CT-angiography was performed as part of the pre-implantation evaluation for a cardiac pacemaker. (**a**, **b**) Axial images demonstrate two rounded structures on either side of the aortic arch, consistent with a double superior vena cava. The left superior vena cava drains into the right atrium via the coronary sinus. The cross-sectional areas of the right and left superior vena cava measure 204 mm^2 and 174 mm^2, respectively. (**c**) Coronal reconstruction clearly delineating the course of both superior vena cava, the left one passing behind the left atrium. Note the absence of left brachiocephalic vein

left SVC, with or without a left brachiocephalic vein) or a unique left superior vena cava (Fig. 1). In most cases, the left SVC drains into the coronary sinus, which terminates in the right atrium, but it can drain into the left atrium or a pulmonary vein, creating a right-left shunt with its attendant potential complications (Fig. 2). Obstruction (tumoral invasion of the lumen), compression (by a tumor or mediastinal fibrosis), or stenosis (secondary to a malpositioned central catheter) of SVC are responsible for the reduction in its luminal diameter (Fig. 3). The stenosis becomes hemodynamically significant when the patent area of SVC is less than 1.07 cm^2 (Lin et al. 2009; Sonavane et al. 2015).

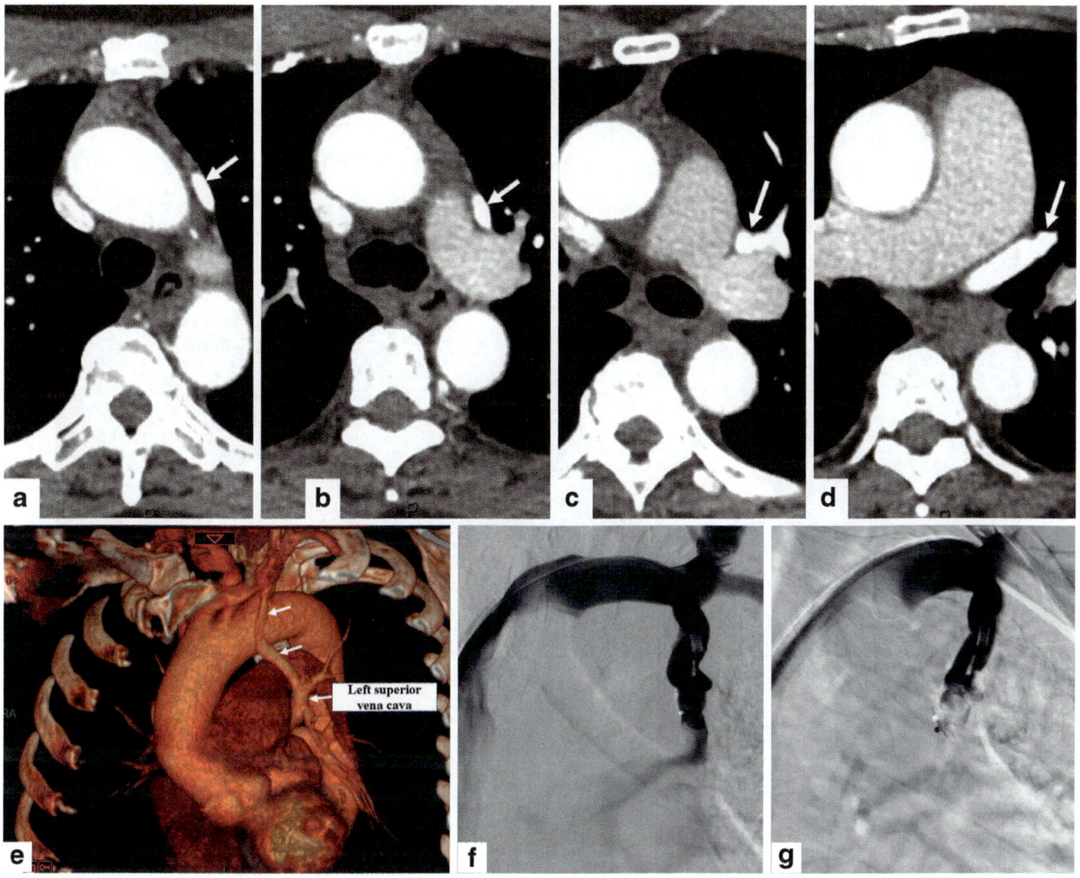

Fig. 2 Right-to-left shunt with "left superior vena cava" draining into the left superior pulmonary vein. Actually, such a vein should be called a *vertical vein* corresponding to a persistent patent anterior cardinal vein. A 75-year-old woman was admitted for an acute ischemic stroke. Contrast echocardiography with a bubble study, performed via a left arm venous injection, demonstrated direct passage of microbubbles into the left cardiac chambers through an aberrant drainage of the superior vena cava. (**a–d**) Contrast-enhanced CT-angiography depicts an anomalous left superior vena cava (arrows; 5 × 10 mm) draining into the left superior pulmonary vein, accounting for the right-to-left shunt. (**e**) Three-dimensional Volume-Rendered Technique left lateral view clearly delineates the course of the anomalous vessel (arrows) and its connection to the left superior pulmonary vein. The diameter of the left superior vena cava at the junction with the left superior pulmonary vein measures 7 × 5 mm. (**f**, **g**) Left superior vena cava angiogram confirms its drainage into the left superior pulmonary vein and demonstrates the post-occlusion control image following endovascular closure of the vessel with a 10 mm vascular plug. The occlusion device was oversized by approximately 40–50% based on CT measurements

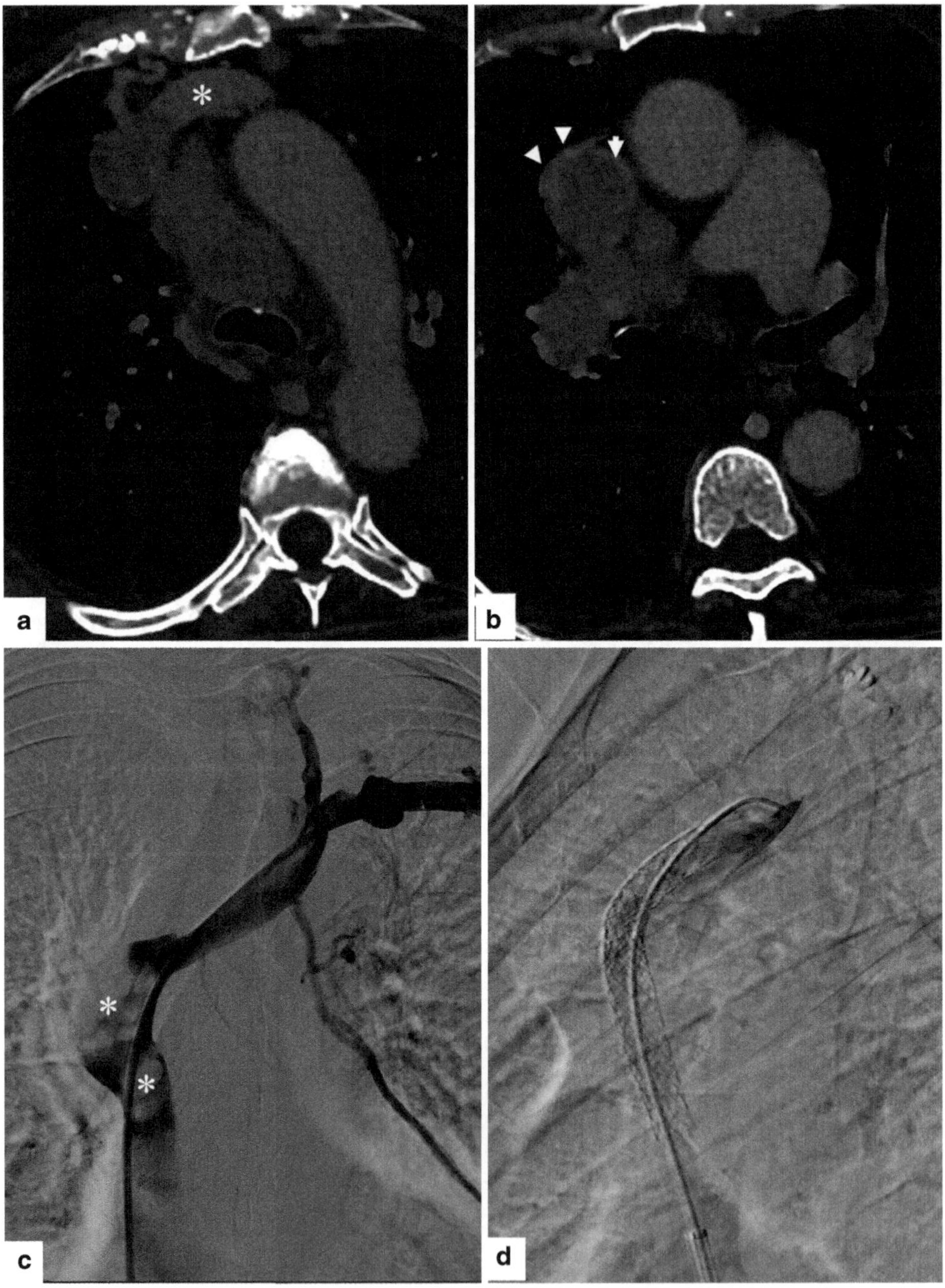

Fig. 3 Superior vena cava syndrome. A 65-year-old patient was hospitalized for a superior vena cava syndrome, which revealed a pulmonary adenocarcinoma with mediastinal lymphadenopathy. (**a, b**) Axial contrast-enhanced CT images (portal venous phase) demonstrate a patent left brachiocephalic vein (*) and a soft-tissue mass within the superior vena cava suggestive of venous tumor involvement. A thin rim of contrast enhancement persists around the mass within the SVC (arrowheads). (**c**) Superior vena cava angiogram shows collateral drainage via the left pericardial vein and a tumoral thrombus (*) partially obstructing the SVC lumen. (**d**) Immediate post-procedural angiography following placement of a double 12-mm covered stent shows the stent patency and the disappearance of the collateral drainage. The choice of diameter in cases of thrombosis or stenosis aims to ensure adequate lumen opening for contrast agent passage without risk of rupture; the residual lumen should be greater than 10 mm. (**e–g**) Follow-up CT-angiography at 3 months demonstrates patency of the covered stent (*) along with marked improvement of the superior vena cava syndrome. Note a small apposition thrombus along the posterolateral wall of the stent

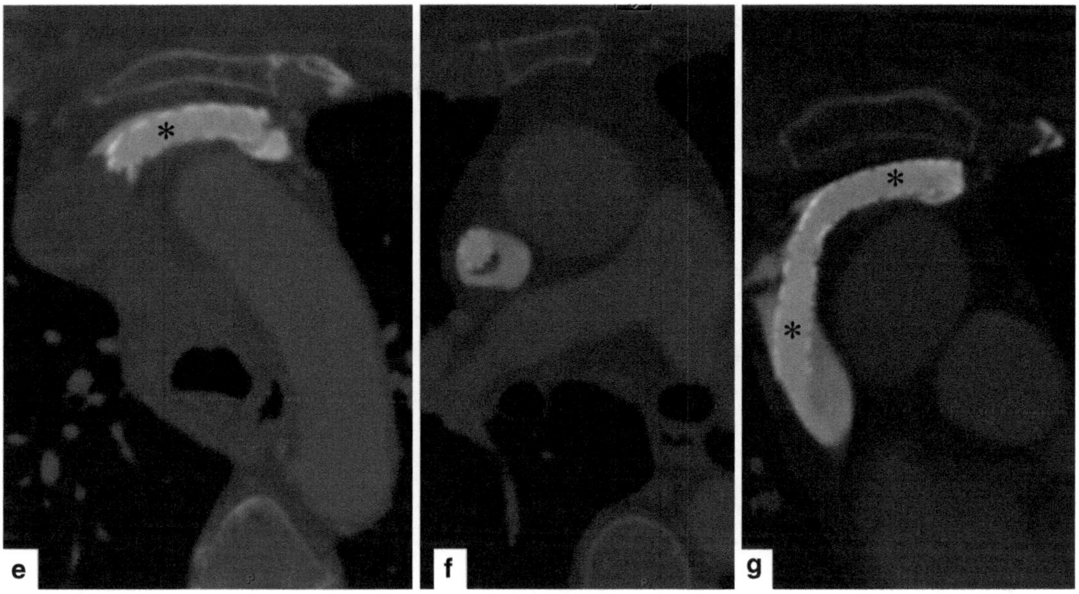

Fig. 3 (continued)

2 Pulmonary Artery

Several studies have reported normal measurements of the trunk of the main pulmonary artery, as well as that of the right and left pulmonary arteries (see Chapter by Galea et al.).

In interventional radiology, measurement of the main pulmonary artery is of particular interest in cases of erosion (by tumor or infectious process) or stenosis (by tumor or mediastinal fibrosis) in order to adjust stent size (Fig. 4) (Khalil et al. 2008).

Concerning pulmonary arteriovenous malformations (PAVMs), the draining pulmonary vein is often larger than the feeding pulmonary artery(ies) that is(are) also enlarged (Faughnan et al. 2020) (Fig. 5). Current guidelines for the management of PAVMs provide specific recommendations regarding the diameter of the feeding pulmonary artery(ies) suitable for embolization/vaso-occlusion (Faughnan et al. 2020). According to the Hereditary hemorrhagic telangiectasia (HHT) Foundation and international consensus:

- Traditional threshold: Feeding arteries ≥3 mm in diameter are generally considered as indication for embolization, even in asymptomatic PAVMs.
- Small PAVMs (<2–3 mm): These lesions are typically monitored with periodic CT imaging and are not embolized unless they become symptomatic or demonstrate rapid growth.
- Recent recommendations: Some centers now advocate treatment for feeding arteries ≥2 mm when appropriate microcatheters, microcoils, or plugs are available, particularly in patients at high risk of paradoxical embolism.

The occlusion material (coils, plugs, or stent graft) is adapted with an oversize of 30–40%. Therefore, prior knowledge of the feeding pulmonary artery(-ies) size is essential to appropriately tailor the sizing of occlusion materials to each feeding artery of the PAVM.

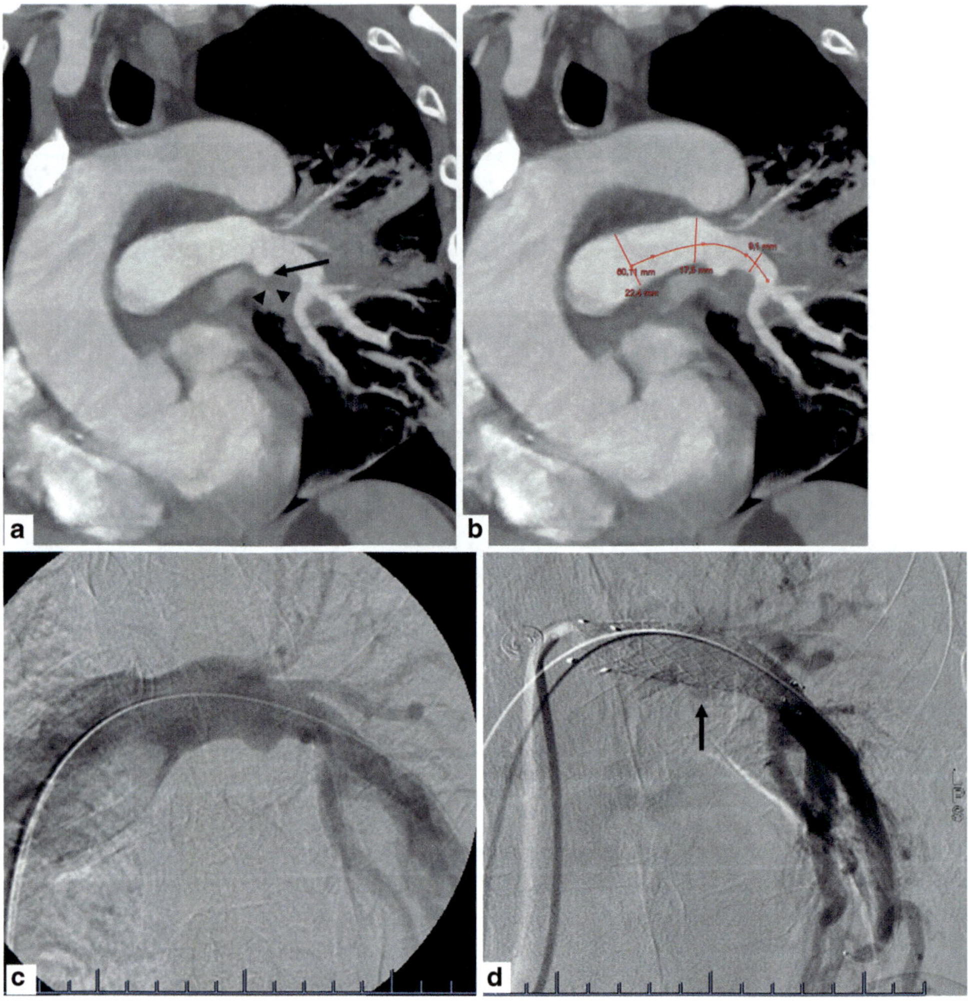

Fig. 4 Stent grafting of proximal pulmonary artery false aneurysm. A 55-year-old man with proximal lung cancer, hemoptysis of 100 mL leading to a CT-angiography. (**a**) Sagittal oblique reconstruction showing a false aneurysm (arrow) of the left main pulmonary artery within tumoral necrosis (arrowhead). (**b**) The stent graft is planned to have a proximal and distal diameter of 22 and 9 mm respectively, making it ideally to use a conical stent which is not commercially available. (**c**) Left antero-lateral view angiogram shows the good correlation with CT-angiography. (**d**) A stent graft of 14 mm in diameter and 6 cm long is placed to cover the aneurysm and the area of necrosis. A control angiogram shows good stent coverage of the distal part of the pulmonary artery, and a remaining opacification of the false aneurysm (arrow) due to non-coverage of the proximal part of the pulmonary artery. (**e**) Control after filling with coils the void between the pulmonary artery wall and the stent graft. (**f**) CT-angiography 10 days later shows absence of recurrence of the false aneurysm and patency of left inferior lobar artery

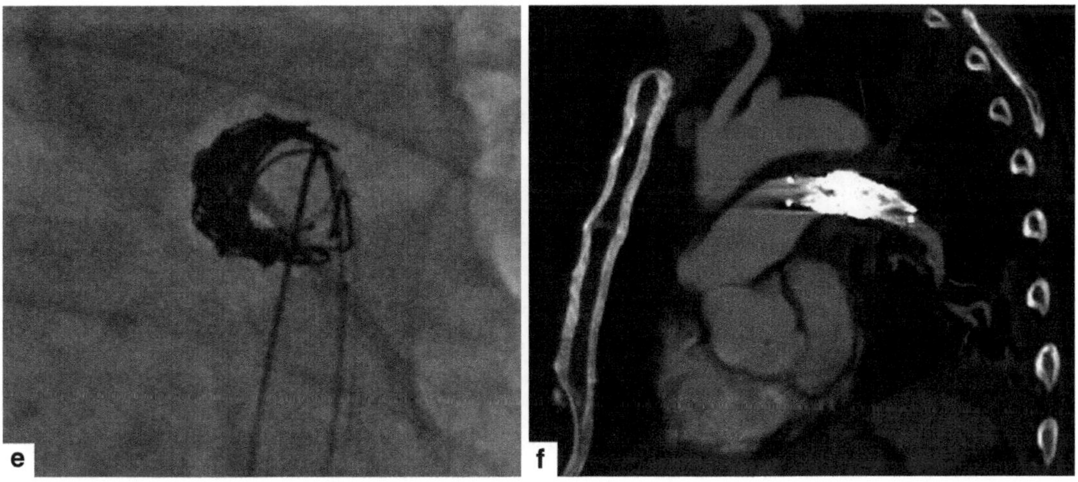

Fig. 4 (continued)

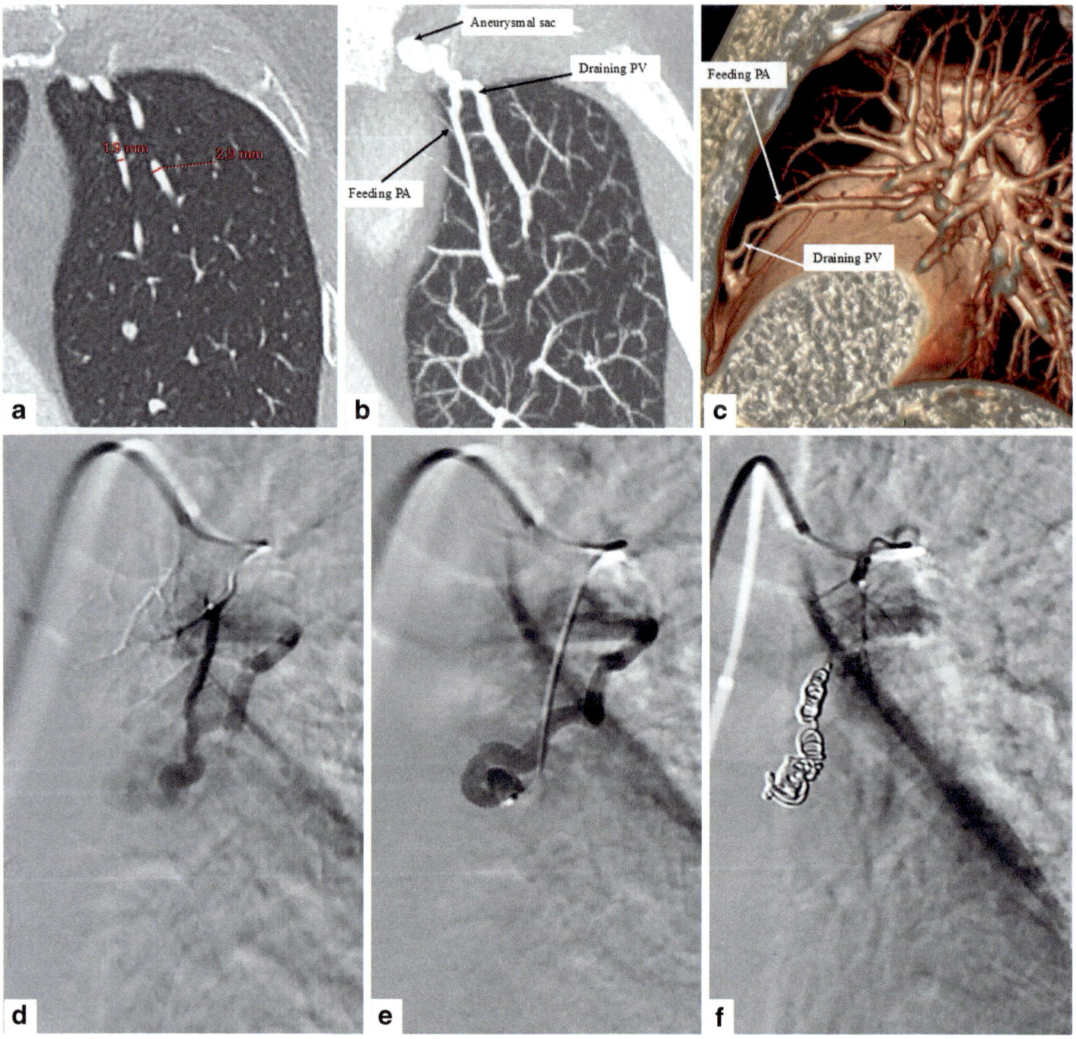

Fig. 5 Pulmonary arteriovenous malformation revealed by an ischemic stroke. 46-year-old woman hospitalized for an ischemic stroke. Cardiac ultrasound with bubble test revealed a bubble passage at 4 cardiac cycles confirming an intrapulmonary shunt. Chest CT scan revealed a lingular and a right inferior lobar pulmonary arteriovenous malformations (PAVM). (**a**) Oblique CT axial-section shows the feeding pulmonary artery (measured at 2 mm) and the draining pulmonary vein (measured at 3 mm) of the lingular PAVM. (**b**) Maximum Intensity Projection reconstruction showing the connection between artery and vein via an aneurysmal sac. (**c**) Left lateral view with Volume-Rendering Technique showing the PAVM in contact with the heart. (**d**) Angiogram of the PAVM opacified via the feeding pulmonary artery, clearly showing the difference in size between the artery and the draining vein. (**e**) Selective opacification of the feeding pulmonary artery close to the PAVM sac. (**f**) Control angiogram after occlusion of the feeding artery with coils (4 mm diameter), showing the absence of opacification of the treated PAVM

3 Bronchial Arteries

On angiography, the usual origin of the orthotopic bronchial arteries (BAs) is projected between two lines formed above by the lower limit of the aortic arch and below by the left main bronchus, namely, between T5 and T6–T7, with a preponderance of their origin at the level of the projection of the left main bronchus lucency. BAs originating outside this region are called ectopic BA. The superior right BA arises in 70–80% of cases from the first or second right intercostal artery, forming a right broncho-intercostal trunk (Bruzzi et al. 2006; Remy-Jardin et al. 2004). With over 30 years' personal experience of bronchial arteries embolization, for practical reasons, we prefer to use the term *atypic origin* for BA arising from the floor or wall of the aortic arch. Indeed, this origin is present in over 40% of patients (Khalil et al. 2015).

In adults, the diameter of BAs is 1.5 mm from the mediastinum to the hilum, then decreases further to 0.75 to 0.5 mm during lobar division (Deffebach et al. 1987). Normal-sized BAs are hardly visible in the pulmonary hilum on CT. The term "BA hypertrophy or enlargement" is used with confidence when BAs reach a diameter of 2 mm or more in the mediastinum and/or when BAs are visible in the pulmonary hilum (Fig. 6). BAs follow a mediastinal path to reach the bronchial tree and follow bronchi into the pulmonary hilum (Fig. 7). On the other hand, the non-bronchial systemic arteries typically pass through the pleura (Yoon et al. 2003), except for the inferior triangular ligament artery, which supplies the lungs by coursing through the mediastinal recess beneath the inferior pulmonary vein. The transpleural pathway requires prior pleural symphysis and therefore chronic pleural disease (Fig. 8). During their mediastinal course, the BAs have a rich anastomotic network with other vessels vascularizing mediastinal structures (esophagus, lymphatic chains, and vagus nerve). This anastomotic network, often not visible on CT and rarely visible on angiography, prevents us from occluding these vessels proximally. The development of anastomotic connections between

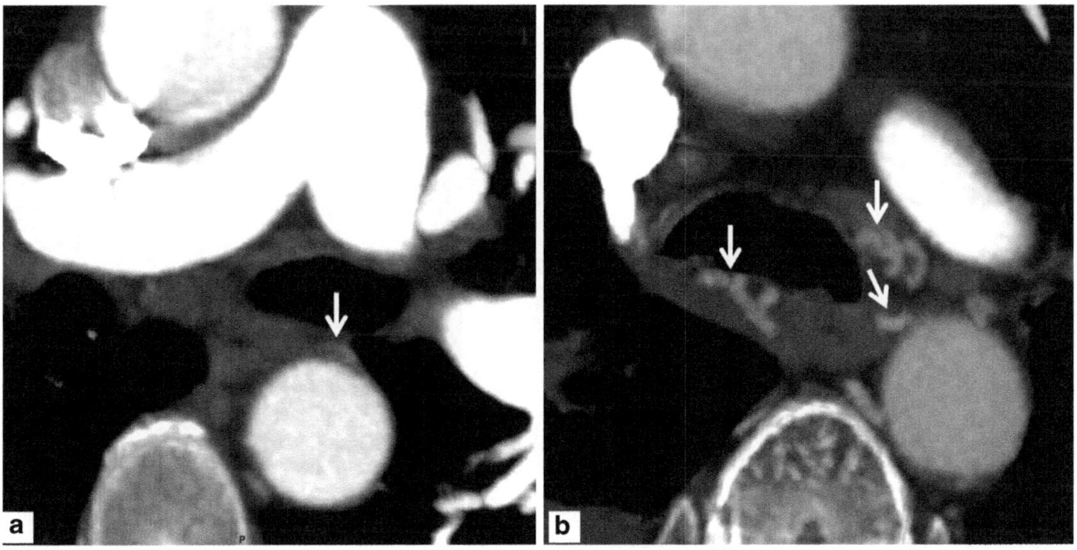

Fig. 6 Bronchial artery anatomy. Bronchial arteries in two different patients. (**a**) CT angiography view performed for chest pain shows a normal bronchial artery (arrow) arising from the anterior wall of the aorta at the level of the left main bronchus, with a diameter of 1 mm. (**b**) CT angiography view performed for hemoptysis in a patient with bronchiectasis shows hypertrophied (3 mm in diameter) and tortuous bronchial arteries (arrows)

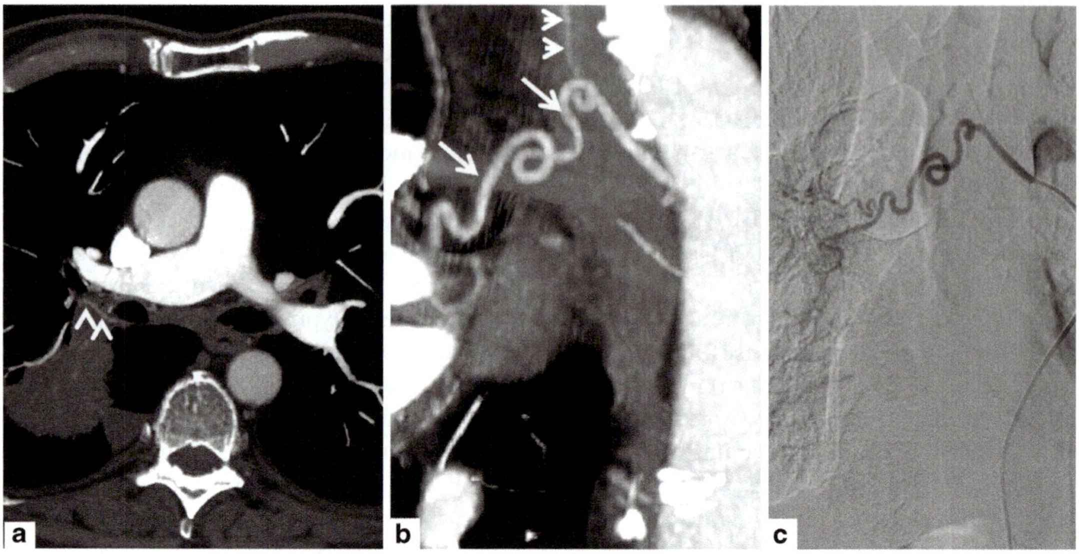

Fig. 7 Hemoptysis with bronchial artery enlargement. A 65-year-old patient hospitalized for hemoptysis due to bronchiectasis. (**a**) CT axial slice shows a hypertrophied bronchial artery (3 mm in diameter) visible in the hilum (arrowheads). (**b**) Oblique coronal MIP reconstruction shows the image of a right bronchointercostal trunk, with a right intercostal artery (arrowhead) and a hypertrophied right bronchial artery (arrows). (**c**) Angiogram of the right broncho-intercostal trunk shows good correlation between CT and angiography

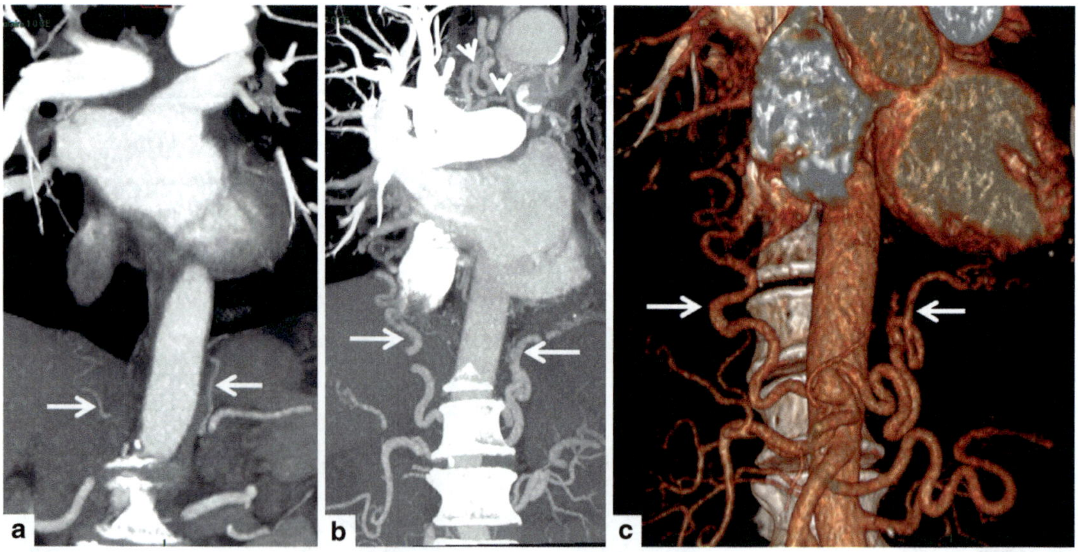

Fig. 8 Enlargement of non-bronchial systemic arteries (inferior phrenic arteries). Normal and enlarged appearance of the inferior phrenic artery on coronal views in two patients. (**a**) Normal aspect of the inferior phrenic arteries (arrows) in a patient evaluated for chest pain. (**b**) Marked hypertrophy of the inferior phrenic arteries (arrows) and the bronchial arteries (4 mm) (arrowheads) in a patient with bronchiectasis on a CT angiography. (**c**) Coronal VRT reconstruction clearly shows the hypertrophied inferior phrenic arteries (arrows) in the same patient

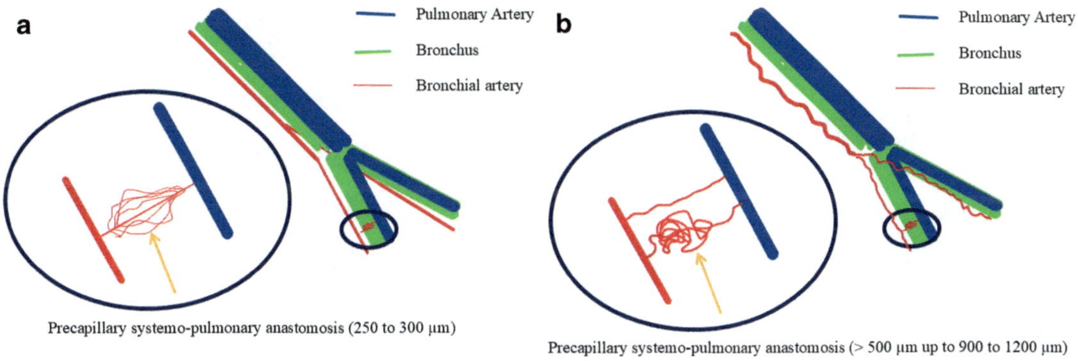

Fig. 9 Schematic representation of precapillary anastomoses between the bronchial arteries and the pulmonary arteries. (**a**) The bronchial arteries follow the course of the bronchi and show precapillary anastomoses with the pulmonary artery, which also lies along the bronchus. The normal size of these anastomoses is about 250–300 µm. (**b**) In cases of chronic inflammatory disease or chronic pulmonary embolism, systemic-to-pulmonary arteries anastomoses may enlarge, and the systemic arterial diameter can reach 1200 µm. This diameter changes guide adjustment of the size of the embolization material

the distal segments of BAs (in the setting of proximal occlusion) and adjacent systemic arteries considered at risk can be observed. Such proximal occlusion indeed entails the possibility of distal revascularization of the BAs through collateral supply arising from other vascular territories, including the coronary, esophageal, or intercostal arteries. Catheterization or embolization of these anastomotic pathways through such collateral vessels may be hazardous, as inadvertent embolization of the territories supplied by these arteries could occur.

There are also anastomoses between BAs and its arteries (precapillary anastomoses), whose maximum diameter in normal condition is 250–300 µm (Fig. 9). These anastomoses may be enlarged, together with enlargement of the BAs, in some chronic infectious diseases (tuberculosis and especially its sequelae, chronic cavitary aspergillosis, etc.), bronchiectasis, or disease with occlusion or stenosis of the proximal pulmonary arteries (thromboembolic diseases such as chronic pulmonary embolism or post-embolic pulmonary hypertension, Takayasu's disease, compression by a tumor process or mediastinal fibrosis, etc.). Knowing the presence and size of these precapillary anastomoses in a normal or pathological situation helps us to select the appropriate particle size to use. Thus, the minimum particle size is 400–500 µm and 700–1300 µm in the presence of a shunt visible on angiography (Figs. 9 and 10).

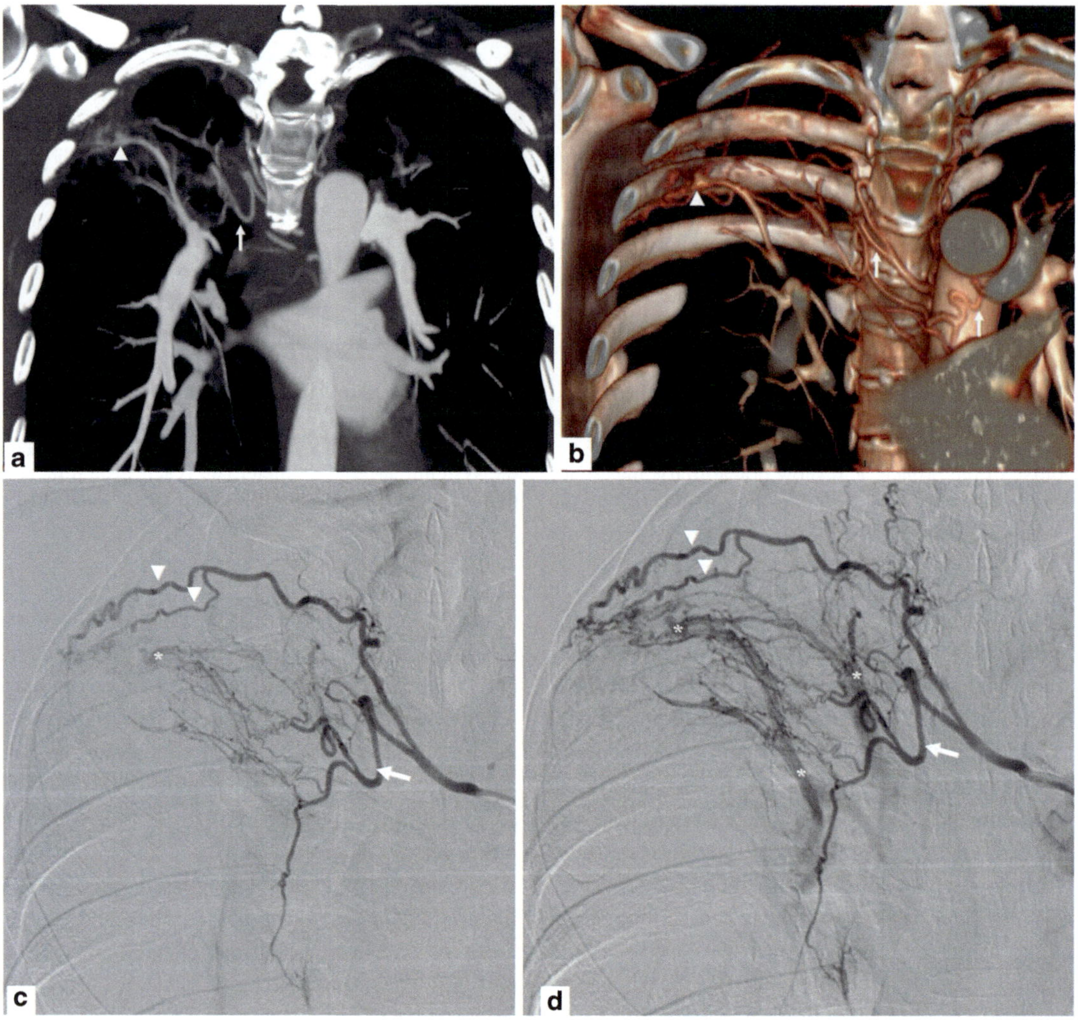

Fig. 10 Hemoptysis with Rassmussen aneurysm and systemic arteries enlargement. A 48-year-old male patient followed for right apical sequelae of tuberculosis is hospitalized for hemoptysis. (**a**, **b**) Coronal view reconstructions in 8 mm MIP (**a**) and 25 mm VRT (**b**) show opacification of hypertrophied bronchial arteries (arrows; 2.2 mm in diameter) with a distal pulmonary arterial aneurysm (arrowhead). (**c**, **d**) Subsequent angiogram showing hypertrophy of the bronchial systemic arteries (arrows) and non-bronchial arteries (intercostal arteries, arrowheads; 2.4 mm in diameter) with retrograde opacification of the branches of the pulmonary artery (*)

4 Intercostal Arteries

The caliber of the intercostal arteries shows considerable variation depending on their anatomical location and origin. The posterior segments originating from the descending thoracic aorta exhibit a larger diameter compared with the anterior segments located near the sternum. The diameter generally increases from the first to the fifth intercostal artery, with the fifth artery representing the largest among those evaluated, whereas the sixth intercostal artery shows a slight reduction in caliber. The remaining distal intercostal arteries have not been assessed in detail because of their short course and limited relevance as potential vascular graft.

Histomorphometric data from cadaveric studies have reported a mean diameter of approxi-

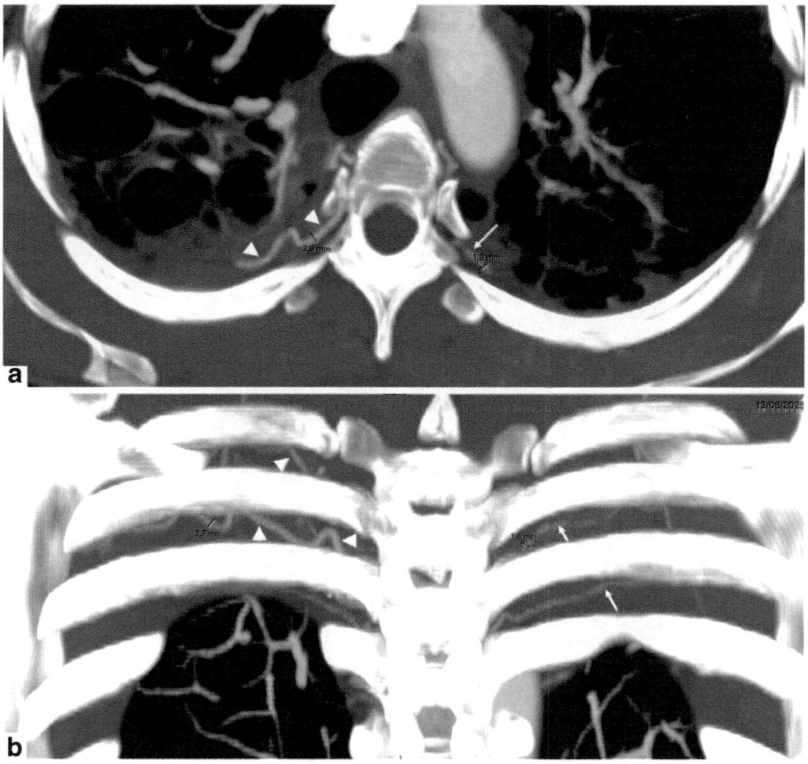

Fig. 11 Enlargement of the intercostal arteries in the right upper lobe in a patient with sequelae of tuberculosis. (**a**) Axial 15 mm maximum intensity projection (MIP) view of CT angiography shows a tortuous and enlarged right intercostal artery (arrowheads; 2.9 mm in diameter), compared with a normal left intercostal artery (arrow; 1.9 mm in diameter). (**b**) Coronal 20 mm MIP view of CT angiography shows a tortuous and enlarged right intercostal artery (arrowheads; 2.7 mm in diameter), compared with a normal left intercostal artery (arrow; 1.8 mm in diameter). The difference in measured diameters between axial and coronal reconstructions is related to the measurement location along the intercostal artery from its origin

mately 1.4 ± 0.3 mm at the origin of the fifth intercostal artery and 0.9 ± 0.2 mm at a distance of 30 cm from its origin (Van Son et al. 1993; Kuhlman et al. 2015). These measurements are consistent with the small caliber typically observed on CT angiography in asymptomatic individuals.

An intercostal artery is generally considered hypertrophied or pathological when its diameter exceeds 2 mm, regardless of its anatomical position (Figs. 10 and 11). Such enlargement is most frequently associated with systemic-to-pulmonary shunts, arteriovenous fistulas, aortic coarctation, or intercostal tumoral involvement. Recognition of these variations and potential hypertrophic changes is essential in interventional radiology procedures, particularly during thoracic embolization or biopsy, to avoid inadvertent vascular injury or non-target embolization.

5 Internal Thoracic Artery

The mean diameter of the internal thoracic arteries varies according to the level of intercostal space and is consistently larger on the right than on the left side. These findings are consistent with previous anatomical studies. Amez et al. (Arnez et al. 1995) reported mean diameters of 2.8 mm, 2.6 mm, and 2.6 mm for the internal thoracic artery in cadaveric specimens at the third, fourth, and fifth intercostal spaces, respectively. On CT angiography (Cook et al. 2016), the mean

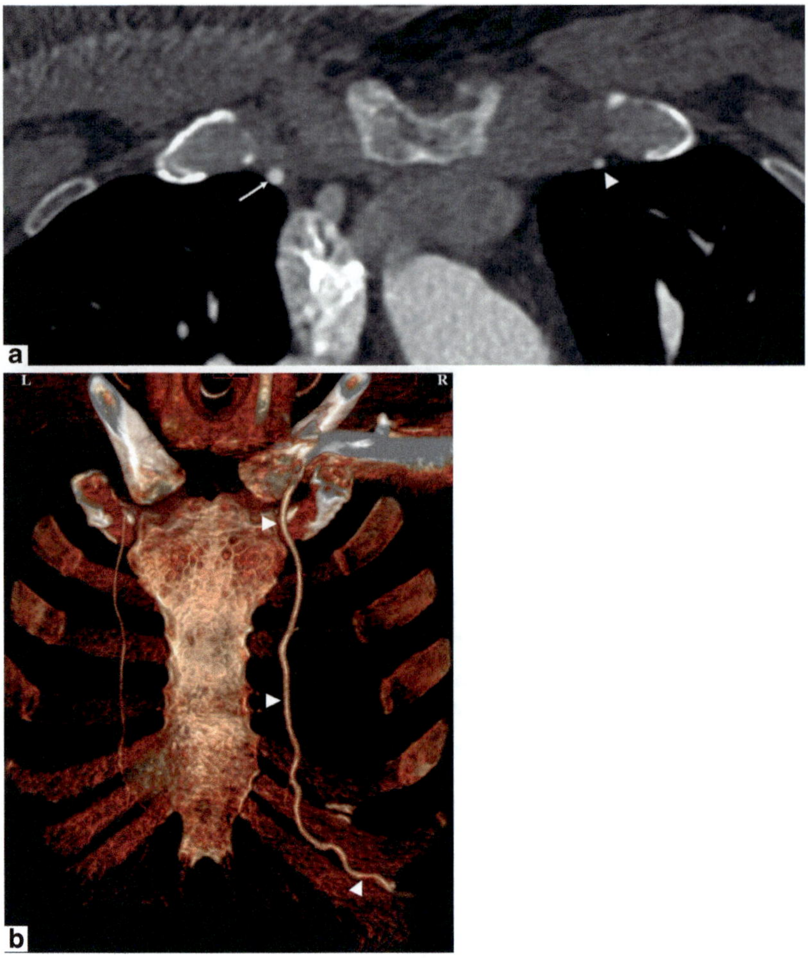

Fig. 12 Enlargement of the right internal thoracic artery secondary to systemic-to-pulmonary fistulae. (**a**) Axial CT angiography shows enlargement of the right internal thoracic artery (arrow; 5.1 mm in diameter) and a normal left internal thoracic artery (arrowhead; 2.3 mm). (**b**) Postero-anterior coronal view of VRT reconstruction clearly demonstrates the enlargement of the right internal thoracic artery (arrowheads)

diameters measured at the second, third, and fourth intercostal spaces were 3.0 ± 0.5 mm, 2.9 ± 0.4 mm, and 2.5 ± 0.4 mm, respectively, which are slightly higher than those observed on anatomical specimens, likely reflecting in vivo vascular distension.

An internal thoracic artery is generally considered hypertrophied when its diameter exceeds 4 mm (Fig. 12). This enlargement is most commonly associated with the presence of systemic-to-pulmonary shunts, arteriovenous fistulas, coarctation, or tumoral processes. Recognition of such hypertrophy on CT angiography is essential, as it may indicate underlying pathological vascular recruitment and can have important implications for planning interventional radiology or surgical procedures.

6 Bronchopulmonary Sequestration

Bronchopulmonary sequestration is a congenital anomaly of lung development that may involve both vascular and bronchial structures. It is classically subdivided into intralobar and extralobar forms. From a vascular standpoint, this malformation is defined by the replacement of the pulmonary arterial vascularization of a lung area by a systemic artery and is associated with a variable degree of bronchial developmental abnormality (Hou et al. 2017; Gabelloni et al. 2021).

The intralobar form, which is the most frequently encountered, is characterized by a common pleura with the normal lung and by venous drainage occurring predominantly into the pulmonary veins. By contrast, the extralobar form is distinguished by the presence of a separate own pleura and venous drainage directed predominantly toward the azygos system or the vena cava.

Furthermore, intralobar bronchopulmonary sequestration is the only form that may, under certain circumstances, be amenable to treatment by interventional radiology. The Pryce classification distinguishes three different types of sequestration, all of which share the presence of a systemic artery replacing a segment of a pulmonary artery:

- Type I: absence of bronchial developmental anomaly
- Type II: partial bronchial developmental anomaly
- Type III: complete separation between the normal bronchial tree and that of the sequestered pulmonary segment

The anomalous systemic artery most often arises directly from the thoracic aorta or from aorta at the thoracoabdominal junction. More rarely, the origin may be from other arterial branches like the celiac trunk or the subclavian artery. Only intralobar sequestration classified as Pryce type 1 can be treated curatively by embolization (Fig. 13) in case of hemoptysis (Szablics et al. 2025; Bi et al. 2021). In the other subgroups, Pryce types 2 and 3, where a congenital bronchial anomaly is present, embolization may serve as an emergency treatment for hemoptysis (Fig. 14), but surgery remains the definitive therapy. The size of the systemic feeding artery is variable, ranging from 3 to 14 mm with a median diameter of 8 mm, and cases have been reported with a feeding artery measuring up to 25 mm. Of note, the size of the anomalous artery may be irregular and increase in its intraparenchymal course. Regardless of the size of the feeding artery, the indication for treatment is determined by the presence of hemoptysis or associated symptoms. The size of the artery guides the preparation of endovascular treatment, including the choice of embolization materials or the size of coils, vascular plugs, or, more rarely, covered stents.

In conclusion, accurate knowledge of thoracic vessel dimensions is essential for optimizing interventional radiological procedures, while also looking at their morphology and anatomical location. While most vessels can be assessed using cross-sectional imaging (CT and/or MR), some may require dynamic contrast opacification in the angiography suite for adequate visualization.

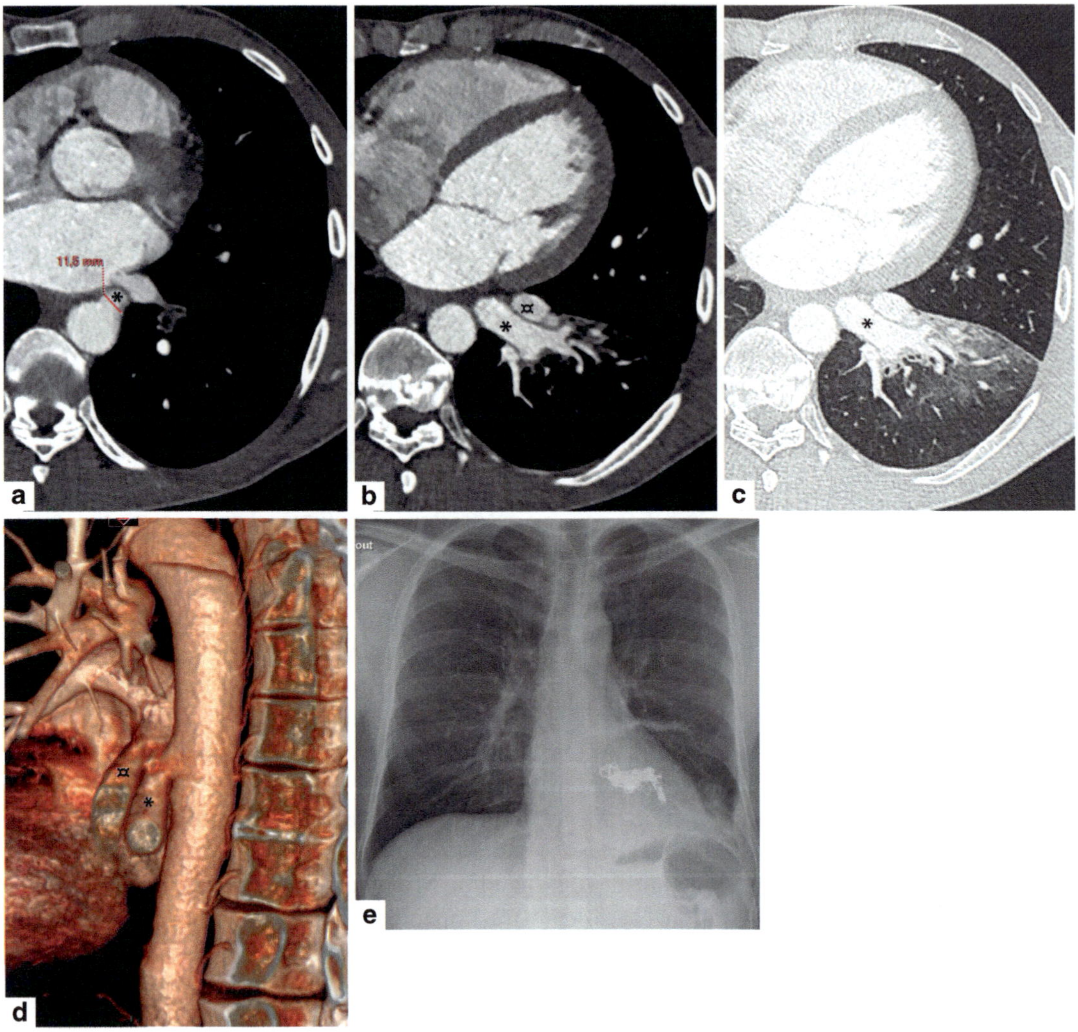

Fig. 13 Pryce type 1 intralobar bronchopulmonary sequestration with hemoptysis. A 28-year-old man presented with hemoptysis, leading to the diagnosis of a Pryce type 1 intralobar bronchopulmonary sequestration. (**a**, **b**) Axial CT angiography shows the feeding systemic artery of the intralobar bronchopulmonary sequestration arising from the right anterolateral aortic wall, measuring 11.5 mm in diameter and presenting with a descending course. Its diameter increases to 12.5 mm along its intraparenchymal course (*) posterior to the left inferior pulmonary vein (¤). (**c**) Axial lung-window CT shows pulmonary consolidation consistent with alveolar flooding by blood related to hemoptysis, without other parenchymal abnormalities. (**d**) Oblique sagittal VRT reconstruction clearly demonstrates the feeding artery (*) located just posterior to the left inferior pulmonary vein (¤). (**e**) Frontal chest radiograph obtained 24 h after embolization shows the micro-coils, measuring 8–18 mm in diameter

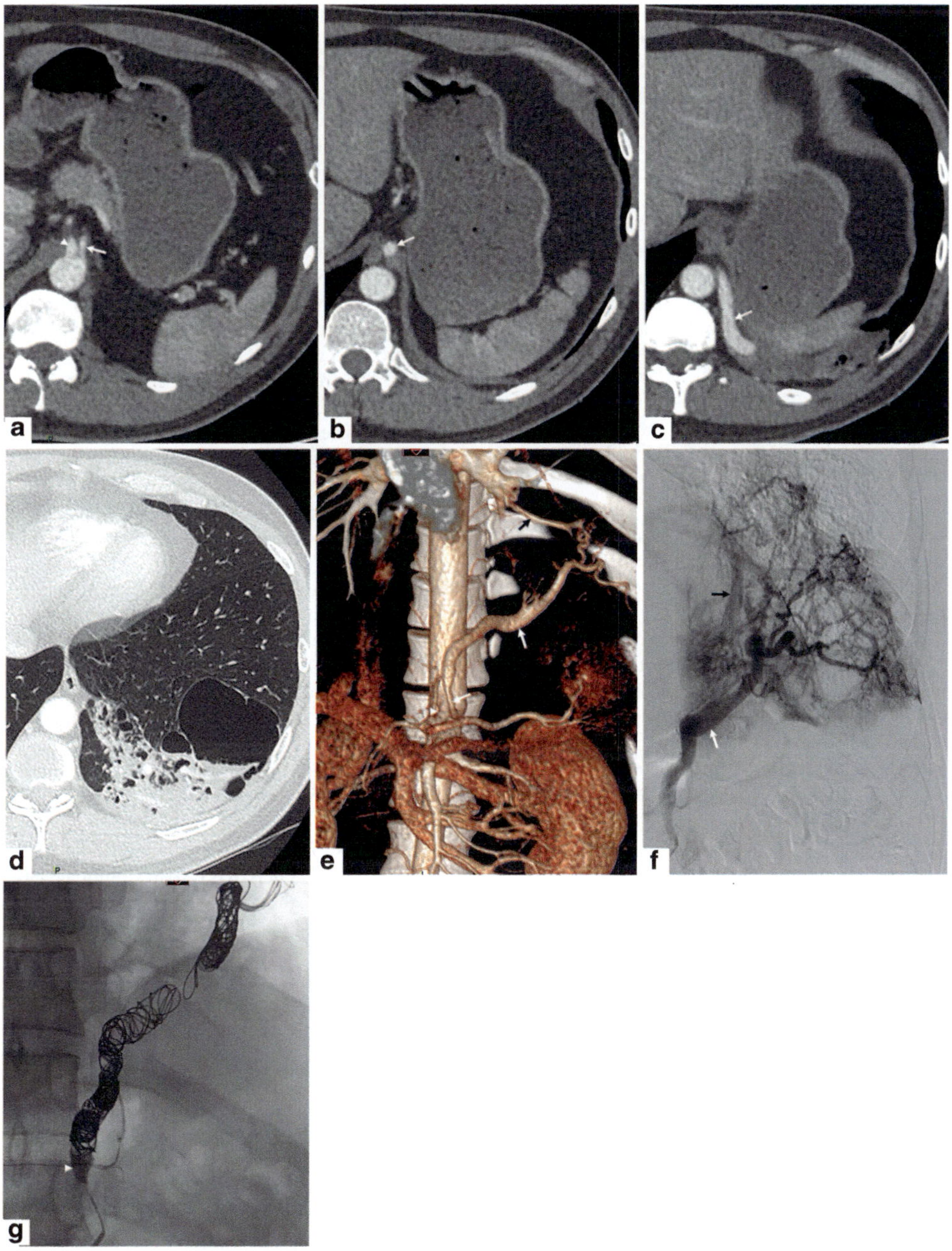

Fig. 14 Pryce type 3 intralobar bronchopulmonary sequestration with hemoptysis. A 36-year-old man was treated for recurrent infections of the left lower lobe with recent episodes of hemoptysis. (**a**–**c**) Axial CT angiography shows the feeding systemic artery (3 mm) (arrow in **a**) of the intralobar bronchopulmonary sequestration arising just next to the origin of the celiac trunk (arrowhead), and then coursing through the diaphragm toward the left hemithorax where it enlarges to 9 mm (arrow in **c**). (**d**) Axial lung-window CT shows pulmonary consolidation and cystic changes corresponding to parenchymal abnormalities secondary to associated congenital pulmonary airway malformation (CPAM), repeated infections, and hemoptysis. (**e**) Coronal VRT reconstruction clearly shows the feeding systemic artery (white arrow) of the bronchopulmonary sequestration arising adjacent to the origin of the celiac trunk (arrowhead), along with venous drainage (black arrow) into the left inferior pulmonary vein. (**f**) Angiography of the systemic arterial supply to the bronchopulmonary sequestration (white arrowhead) demonstrates the vascularization of the abnormal pulmonary parenchyma and venous drainage into the left inferior pulmonary vein (black arrow). (**g**) Final control after occlusion of the feeding artery using micro-coils (12–14 mm) followed by embolization with a liquid agent (Onyx®, arrowhead). The patient received a two-week course of antibiotics, had no recurrence of hemoptysis, and subsequently underwent an elective left lower lobectomy

Disclaimer All measurements in this book have been obtained from peer-reviewed papers and guidelines from professional organizations, unless explicitly stated otherwise. While the authors, editors, and publisher have gone through a rigorous process to establish their correct reproduction from the original source, each measurement must be interpreted in the correct clinical context, this along with an accurate way of measurement, and taking into account all technical variables, this including follow-up exams with various equipment or software. Neither the authors, the editors, nor the publisher can accept any legal responsibility for any improper application or interpretation of these measurements as well as their potential consequences.

References

Arnez ZM, Valdatta L, Tyler MP, Planinšek F (1995) Anatomy of the internal mammary veins and their use in free TRAM flap breast reconstruction. Br J Plast Surg 48(8):540–545

Bi Y, Li J, Yi M, Ren J, Han X (2021) Clinical outcomes of transarterial embolization in the treatment of pulmonary sequestration. Cardiovasc Intervent Radiol 44(9):1491–1496

Bruzzi JF, Rémy-Jardin M, Delhaye D, Teisseire A, Khalil C, Rémy J (2006) Multi-detector row CT of hemoptysis. Radiographics 26(1):3–22. https://doi.org/10.1148/rg.261045726

Cook JA, Tholpady SS, Momeni A, Chu MW (2016) Predictors of internal mammary vessel diameter: a computed tomographic angiography-assisted anatomic analysis. J Plast Reconstr Aesthet Surg 69(10):1340–1348

Deffebach ME, Charan NB, Lakshminarayan S, Butler J (1987) The bronchial circulation: small, but a vital attribute of the lung. Am Rev Respir Dis 135(2):463–481

Faughnan ME, Mager JJ, Hetts SW, Palda VA, Lang-Robertson K, Buscarini E et al (2020) Second international guidelines for the diagnosis and management of hereditary hemorrhagic telangiectasia. Ann Intern Med 173(12):989–1001. https://doi.org/10.7326/M20-1443

Gabelloni M, Faggioni L, Accogli S, Aringhieri G, Neri E (2021) Pulmonary sequestration: what the radiologist should know. Clin Imaging 73:61–72. https://doi.org/10.1016/j.clinimag.2020.11.040

Hou X, Li J, Li J, Cai B (2017) Anomalous systemic arterial supply of pulmonary sequestration in adult patients. Ann Thorac Med 12(1):46–50

Khalil A, Parrot A, Nedelcu C, Fartoukh M, Marsault C, Carette MF (2008) Severe hemoptysis of pulmonary arterial origin: signs and role of multidetector row CT angiography. Chest 133(1):212–219

Khalil A, Fedida B, Parrot A, Haddad S, Fartoukh M, Carette MF (2015) Severe hemoptysis: from diagnosis to embolization. Diagn Interv Imaging 96(7–8):775–788

Kuhlman DR, Khuder SA, Lane RD (2015) Factors influencing the diameter of human anterior and posterior intercostal arteries. Clin Anat 28(2):219–226

Lin FY, Devereux RB, Roman MJ, Meng J, Jow VM, Simprini L, Jacobs A, Weinsaft JW, Shaw LJ, Berman DS, Callister TQ, Min JK (2009) The right sided great vessels by cardiac multidetector computed tomography: normative reference values among healthy adults free of cardiopulmonary disease, hypertension, and obesity. Acad Radiol 16(8):981–987. https://doi.org/10.1016/j.acra.2009.03.016

Mahlon MA, Yoon HC (2007) CT angiography of the superior vena cava: normative values and implications for central venous catheter position. J Vasc Interv Radiol 18(9):1106–1110. https://doi.org/10.1016/j.jvir.2007.06.002

Remy-Jardin M, Bouaziz N, Dumont P, Brillet PY, Bruzzi J, Remy J (2004) Bronchial and nonbronchial systemic arteries at multi-detector row CT angiography: comparison with conventional angiography. Radiology 233(3):741–749

Sonavane SK, Milner DM, Singh SP, Abdel Aal AK, Shahir KS, Chaturvedi A (2015) Comprehensive imaging review of the superior vena cava. Radiographics 35(7):1873–1892. https://doi.org/10.1148/rg.2015150056

Szablics FÉ, Bérczi Á, Nyárády BB, Philippovich M, Szőnyi Á, Dósa E (2025) Pulmonary sequestration in adults: endovascular and hybrid treatment strategies—a systematic review. J Clin Med 14(21):7493. https://doi.org/10.3390/jcm14217493

Van Son JAM, Smedts F, Korving J, Guyt A, de Kok LB (1993) Intercostal artery: histomorphometric study to assess its suitability as a coronary bypass graft. Ann Thorac Surg 56(5):1078–1081

Yoon W, Kim YH, Kim JK, Kim YC, Park JG, Kang HK (2003) Massive hemoptysis: prediction of nonbronchial systemic arterial supply with chest CT. Radiology 227(1):232–238

Part IV
Clinical Part - Heart

Imaging of the Coronary Arteries: Normal Dimensions and Measurements

Haroun El-Addouli, Luca Saba, Niels R. Van der Werf, Ricardo P. J. Budde, Riccardo Cau, Richard A. P. Takx, and Rodrigo Salgado

Contents

H. El-Addouli
Department of Radiology, AZ Monica, Antwerp, Belgium
e-mail: haroun.el.addouli@azmonica.be

L. Saba · R. Cau
Department of Radiology, Azienda Ospedaliero Universitaria, University of Cagliari, Cagliari, Italy

N. R. Van der Werf
Erasmus University Medical Center, Rotterdam, The Netherlands
e-mail: Niels.vander.Werf@philips.com

R. P. J. Budde
Department of Radiology and Nuclear Medicine, Erasmus MC, Rotterdam, The Netherlands
e-mail: r.budde@erasmusmc.nl

R. A. P. Takx
Department of Radiology, Amsterdam University Medical Center, Amsterdam, The Netherlands

R. Salgado (✉)
Department of Radiology, University Hospital of Antwerp, Edegem, Belgium

Faculty of Medicine and Health Sciences, University of Antwerp, Wilrijk, Belgium

Department of Radiology, Holy Heart Hospital, Lier, Belgium
e-mail: Rodrigo.salgado@uza.be

Med Radiol Diagn Imaging (2026)
https://doi.org/10.1007/174_2024_503,
Published Online: 06 September 2024

1 Normal Coronary Artery Diameters

1.1 Introduction

The coronary artery diameter is influenced by gender, age, anatomic variation, and certain physiological and pathological processes (Yang et al. 2006; Zhou et al. 2017). Tables 1 and 2 summarizes the average coronary diameters for coronary segments in a healthy population measured with coronary angiography (Dodge et al. 2018). Several papers state a good correlation of coronary lumen diameter measurements of CT and coronary arteriography, especially for the proximal and midsegments (Sinha et al. 2006). Therefore, the coronary diameters mentioned can be used interchangeably between these imaging techniques. Because of the caliber of the IVUS probe, measurements can only be obtained in the proximal and midsegments of the coronary arteries, and diameter measurements may be influenced due to vasospasm related to vessel manipulation (Dickerson et al. 2010).

1.2 CT Viewing Options

A CT examination of the coronary arteries is routinely evaluated on a workstation, most of which offer different options to analyze the acquired dataset. As the different ways to look at the dataset may also influence performed measurements, we will now briefly summarize the most common options, with their advantages and disadvantages (Fig. 1).

Table 1 Normal coronary artery diameters in men and women as derived from conventional angiography

	Normal men (mm)	Normal women (mm)
Left main		
Middle	4.5 ± 0.5	3.9 ± 0.4
LAD		
Proximal	3.6 ± 0.5	3.2 ± 0.5
Mid	2.5 ± 0.5	2.4 ± 0.4
Distal	1.7 ± 0.5	1.6 ± 0.4
LCX		
Proximal	3.4 ± 0.5	2.9 ± 0.6
Mid	2.8 ± 0.6	3.1 ± 0.4
Distal	1.6 ± 0.6	1.4 ± 0.6
RCA		
Proximal	3.9 ± 0.6	3.3 ± 0.6
Mid	3.4 ± 0.5	3.0 ± 0.5
Distal	3.1 ± 0.5	2.8 ± 0.5

1.2.1 Native Axial Images

Every evaluation of a cardiac CT examination should start by reviewing the native axial images. The reader will then quickly obtain an overall assessment of image quality, degree of atherosclerosis and can identify segments that need further detailed exploration. This initial evaluation can also be used to identify the most appropriate cardiac phase in which different coronary arteries can be best visualized. As the speed of motion of the three coronary arteries is not uniform, in some instances, a different cardiac phase can be required for reliable evaluation of, e.g., RCA vs. LAD.

1.2.2 Multiplanar Reformations

The process of reformatting image data acquired in a certain plane into another plane with dedicated software is called multiplanar reformation (MPR). In the case of CT imaging, the acquired imaging plane is usually the axial plane (Fig. 1a),

Table 2 Normal coronary artery diameters as derived from conventional angiography, also considering coronary artery dominance

	Lumen diameter		
	RCA dominant (diameter in mm)	Balanced dominance (diameter in mm)	Left dominant (diameter in mm)
Left main			
Middle	4.5 ± 0.5	4.4 ± 0.4	4.6 ± 0.4
LAD			
Proximal	3.6 ± 0.5	3.6 ± 0.4	3.7 ± 0.2
Mid	2.5 ± 0.5	2.5 ± 0.4	2.8 ± 0.4
Distal	1.7 ± 0.5	1.8 ± 0.4	2.0 ± 0.3
LCX			
Proximal	3.4 ± 0.5	3.4 ± 0.5	4.2 ± 0.6
Mid	2.8 ± 0.6	3.2 ± 0.4	3.4 ± 0.6
Distal	1.6 ± 0.6	2.5 ± 0.5	3.2 ± 0.5
RCA			
Proximal	3.9 ± 0.6	3.0 ± 0.5	2.8 ± 0.5
Mid	3.4 ± 0.5	2.7 ± 0.4	2.2 ± 0.3
Distal	3.1 ± 0.5	2.0 ± 0.6	1.1 ± 0.4

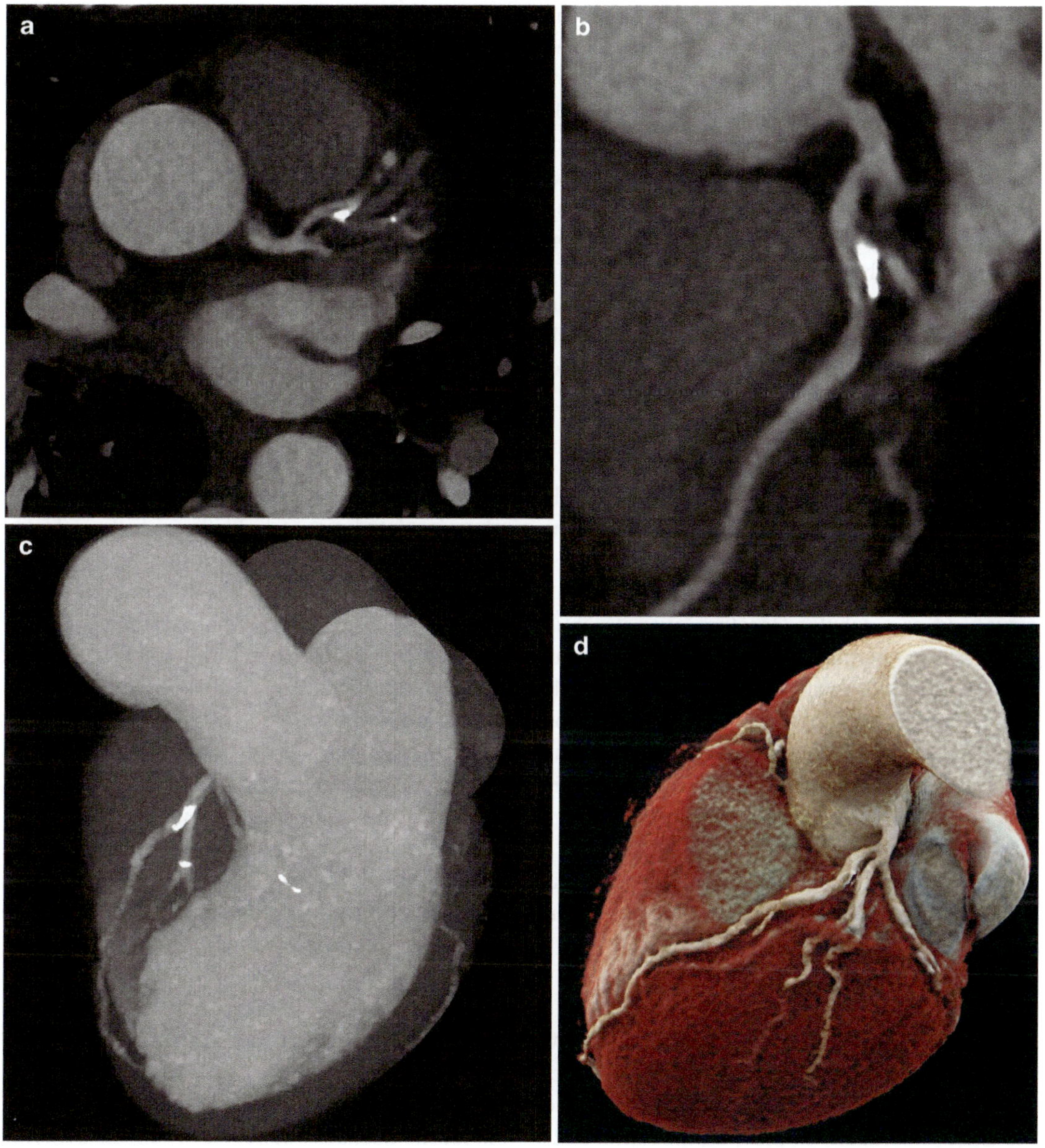

Fig. 1 This figure illustrates the importance of the chosen imaging mode for evaluation of coronary stenosis. A standard axial MPR image will show you the calcified plaque against the LAD, but unless properly reformatted in a double-oblique way, it will not accurately reflect the impact on the lumen (**a**). The curved MPR image conversely nicely illustrated the relation of the plaque with the lumen, revealing the presence of positive remodeling and only limited effect on luminal stenosis (**b**). The MIP image will overemphasize the size of the calcified plaque, and given that its nature is a projection technique, it is not useful to assess the degree of luminal stenosis (**c**). Finally, the VR image gives an accurate 3D image of the heart and coronary arteries, but is less suitable for the assessment of cross-sectional luminal narrowing as this information is not directly provided with the same detail as on an MPR image (**d**). *MPR* multiplanar reformation, *MIP* maximum intensity projection, *VR* volume rendering, *LAD* left anterior descending

but it can be accomplished with imaging data from any other plane. Primordial for the success of this process is the acquisition of isometric voxels in a volumetric fashion in order to have the same spatial resolution in all directions. If not, image blurring can occur in some reformed planes, with image quality becoming insufficient to perform accurate measurements. While conflicting data has been reported regarding the diagnostic accuracy of various software manipulations (Budoff et al. 2006), in our experience, this technique offers the most robust diagnostic accuracy for measuring coronary stenosis.

1.2.3 Curved MPR

Curved multiplanar reformation (cMPR) is the result of another software manipulation. This method uses software to trace a vessel of interest. After defining the vessel centerline, the vessel is visualized as a tubular structure over its entire length within one single image (Fig. 1b). Software manipulation can rotate this vessel to assess the vessel lumen over 360°. cMPR is a valuable tool for detecting coronary stenosis, on condition that the vessel is evaluated in multiple angles. While this technique has according to some authors a slightly lower diagnostic accuracy compared to MPR for measuring coronary stenosis (Fishman et al. 2006), in our experience, it remains a robust post-processing technique.

1.2.4 Maximum Intensity Projection

Maximum intensity projection (MIP) is a software manipulation which projects the voxels with the highest attenuation value along lines of the slices included in the volume onto a 2D image. This method highlights high-density structures, as bone or contrast-filled vessels, whereas low-density structures, e.g., lung or fat, are more suppressed. MIP is a good method to assess the global size and location of the coronary arteries, but measuring vessels is more troublesome and is not recommended, given that it remains a projection technique (Fig. 1c). An important limitation of this visualization is that the presence of other high-attenuation structures can conceal vascular structures; therefore, evaluation of atherosclerotic vessels with extensive calcifications poses a serious problem with this technique. A second significant limitation is the loss of 3D information as a 3D structure is projected onto a two-dimensional image (Fishman et al. 2006). Finally, small variations in window and level settings can inflate measurement errors.

1.2.5 Volume Rendering

Volume rendering (VR) is another software manipulation that uses a computer algorithm used to transform axial acquired images into a 3D image. To perform volume rendering, one must execute three steps: volume definition, classification, and projection. In the final step, the projection step, the user selects the preferred orientation of a simulated ray of light through the selected and classified volume. As a result, the algorithm produces an image with 3D information, which can be displayed on a computer screen (Fig. 1d). As atherosclerotic plaque formation is mostly not circular, significant stenosis can be missed when only one viewing angle is considered, so evaluation of multiple viewing angles is needed to ensure adequate stenosis detection. Furthermore, given the small caliber of coronary arteries, a significant margin of error is seen in measuring coronary arteries (Mahnken et al. 2003). As such, it is not recommended to use this technique for the evaluation of coronary artery stenosis.

1.3 Confounding Factors

1.3.1 Body Habitus

In recent decades, there has been an evolving trend in the average body shape of patients, as obesity is becoming more common in the general population. Body shape significantly affects image quality, with more noise in images of patients with higher body mass index (BMI). This increased noise makes it more challenging to detect and characterize plaques.

1.3.2 Coronary Dominance

The coronary dominance is described by the vessel which supplies the posterior portion of the interventricular septum and gives rise to the posterior descending artery (PDA). Thus, the PDA rises from the right coronary artery (RCA) in a right dominant system (80–85%) and from the left circumflex artery (LCX) in a left dominant system (≈8%). A codominant circulation (≈7%) of the posterior interventricular septum is shared by the RCA and LCX. The coronary dominance has a great impact on the diameter of the RCA and LCX, as Table 2 clearly demonstrates. In contrary, the diameter of the left anterior descending artery (LAD) is only slightly influenced by the dominance (Dodge et al. 2018). This is in line of what one might expect given the differences in distribution of blood flow in the different distribution variants.

1.3.3 Pharmacology

Several pharmacological agents have an influence on the coronary diameter.

Nitroglycerine, either administered as a spray or in tablet form, is frequently used in cardiac CT examinations due to its vasodilating effects on the coronary arteries without significant influence on heart rate or blood pressure (Feldman et al. 1979). As such, it has a proven benefit in evaluating coronary arteries with CT, increasing the number of visualized branches, image quality of small branches, and diagnostic accuracy (Takx et al. 2015). While the effect on the diameter of the coronary arteries varies depending on the dose and timing of administration and the location of branches, a meta-analysis reported a mean increase in vessel diameter between 8% and 30% (Feldman et al. 1979). The relative increase in diameter has been reported to be larger in distal segments (Okada et al. 2015).

However, the vasodilatory effect seems to be different between healthy and diseased vessel segments, varying between 20% and 40% in normal segments and just 5% and 10% in diseased segments (Hoffmann et al. 2006). Therefore, conventional angiography studies have reported an overestimation of 8% (Conti et al. 1983). Nevertheless, how this number translates to CT examinations is not known, as CT has a three-dimensional approach to stenosis evaluation compared with the 2D projection technique of conventional angiography.

2 Quantification of Coronary Calcium

2.1 Background

The coronary artery calcium score (CACS) measures the amount of calcification in the coronary arteries as determined by a non-contrast-enhanced CT scan. The CACS has proven to strongly predict future cardiovascular events (Budoff et al. 2006). Moreover, the absence of coronary calcifications (i.e., a CACS of zero) is associated with a very low rate of future cardiovascular events (Blaha et al. 2016). Absence of coronary calcifications gives patients a "warranty period" of 3.4–7.1 years of being free from cardiovascular events (Dzaye et al. 2021). CACS is therefore a potential biomarker to be used in cardiovascular disease prevention. Although the presence of coronary calcifications, indicated by a CACS >0, does not provide details regarding the potential degree of stenosis, their location, or the causal relationship between coronary calcifications and luminal stenoses, some studies have utilized CACS in diagnostic evaluations of patients with stable chest pain. Specifically, a CACS of 0 may indicate the absence of significant coronary stenosis, enabling physicians to avoid the need for further testing with a coronary CT angiography (CCTA) (Lubbers et al. 2016).

2.2 Types of CAC Scores and How They Are Measured

Clinically, Agatston et al.'s method for quantifying coronary artery calcium, which was described in 1990, is considered the current reference standard and remains the most employed methodology in clinical practice today (Agatston et al. 1990). Despite having excellent prognostic value, the suboptimal reproducibility of this scoring method has nevertheless led to the introduction of alternative CACS methods (Detrano et al. 2005; Hong et al. 2003a; Willemink et al. 2019). These methods include the volume and mass score, which both measure physical characteristics of the calcifications (Callister et al. 1998; McCollough et al. 2007). Below, the most important literature characteristics of these three CACS are described. CT vendors have implemented these characteristics in their own CACS software with vendor-specific parameters (van Praagh et al. 2021).

2.2.1 Agatston Score

The Agatston score is calculated by defining all groups of voxels in the coronary arteries that have a Hounsfield unit (HU) value of 130 or higher and cover an area of more than 1 mm^2 on each of the axial slices. The total area of a calcification per slice is multiplied by a weighting factor that depends on the peak HU value within the calcified lesion (factor 1 for HU 130–199; 2 for HU 200–299; 3 for HU 300–399; and 4 for HU ≥400) to calculate the lesion score. To calculate the total Agatston score, the scores of all the lesions in every slice are added together.

2.2.2 Mass Score

For the mass score, the mean CT number of a calcification (again HU >130) is multiplied by its volume. To obtain absolute values, a mass calibration factor is needed to convert CT numbers to mass. For this, a known calcium calibration object containing a known amount of hydroxyapatite needs to be scanned and its HU value measured (McCollough et al. 2007). Ideally, this calibration object is included in the same scan acquisition as the patient to adjust for any deviations in HU values in the specific scan. Alternatively, post-processing software packages may use predefined correction factors for specific scan acquisition settings.

The mass score can then be calculated by multiplying the mean HU value of a calcification (HU_{mean}) by the volume (V) of the calcification on that image and the calibration factor (c). The overall mass values for all lesions in all slices are summed to obtain the total mass score (M):

$$M = \Sigma\left(\mathrm{HU}_{\mathrm{mean}} \cdot V \cdot c\right)$$

2.2.3 Volume Score

Callister et al. described the volume score, which measures the total volume of a calcification in cubic millimeters (Callister et al. 1998). For this, again all voxels which exceed the CACS threshold of 130 HU are summed and multiplied by the volume of a single voxel. However, for the volume score, datasets are interpolated to obtain isotropic voxels, i.e., equal voxel sizes both in- and through-plane.

2.3 Reporting of CACS

The Agatston calcium score can be reported as the absolute number only, but a percentile score based on normal reference values in age-, sex-, and race-matched individuals is often added. Several reference populations and studies can be used of which the MESA study is the most widely used (McClelland et al. 2006). The percentile scores can easily be calculated using the online calculator that requires entering the patient's age, gender and race (https://www.mesa-nhlbi.org/Calcium/input.aspx) (Fig. 2). It should be noted that no reference values are available for individ-

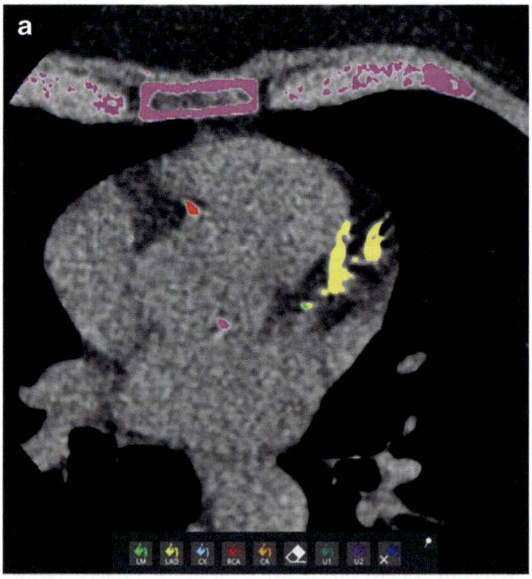

Fig. 2 Extensive coronary calcification in a 63-year-old woman with nonspecific chest pain. The software color codes the coronary calcifications according to the different coronary arteries (**a**) and provides a per-coronary and total Agatston score of calcium burden (**b**). This total score is then used to calculate the percentile according to age and gender, in this case using the MESA study reference values (**c**). This patient is well above the 95th percentile (red circle in panel **c**), with a calculated coronary age of >84 years. Note that both calcium volume and Agatston score are given in panel (**b**), but only the Agatston score is used to calculate the percentile using the MESA study data. *MESA* Multi-Ethnic Study of Atherosclerosis

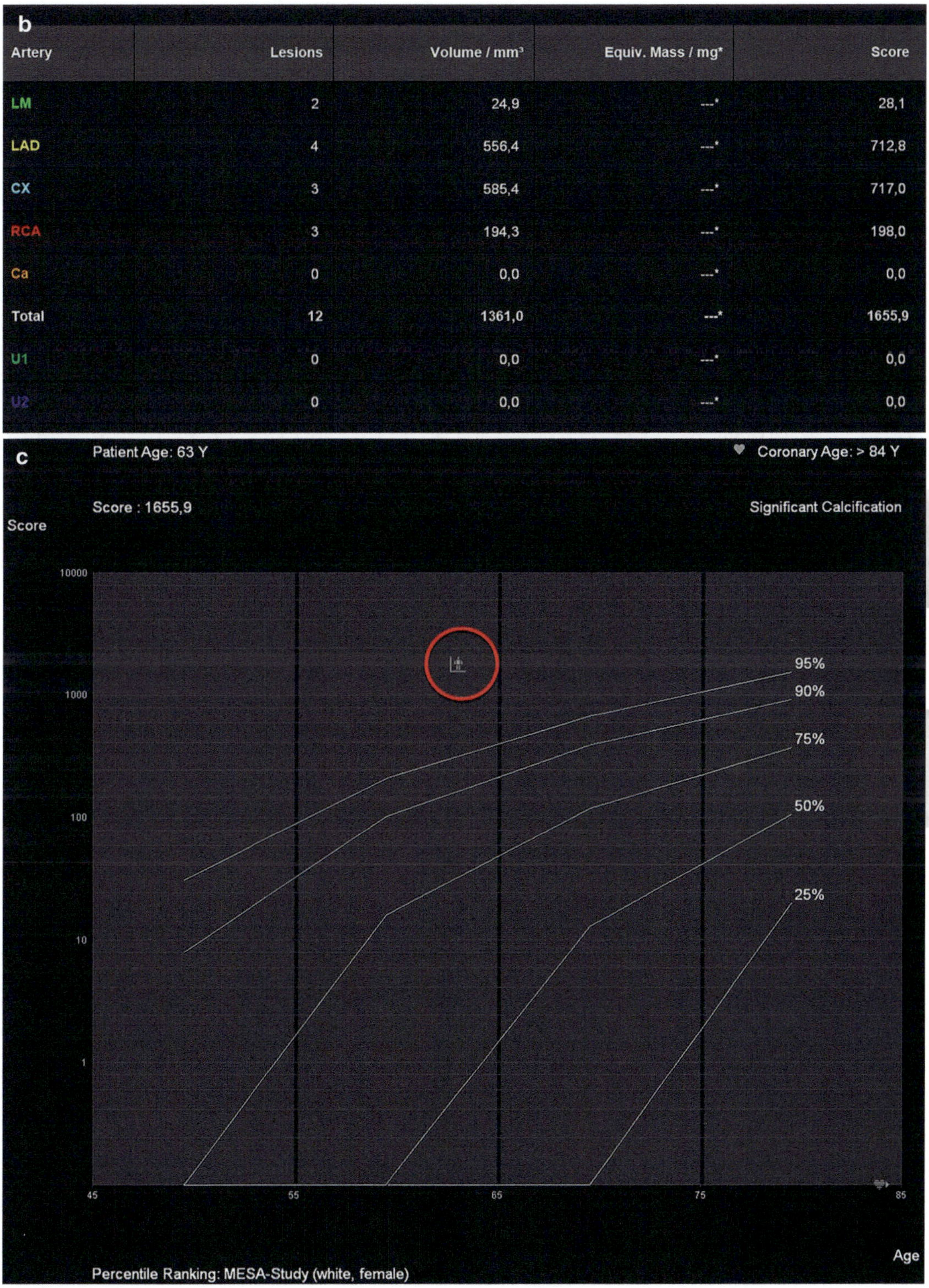

Artery	Lesions	Volume / mm³	Equiv. Mass / mg*	Score
LM	2	24,9	---*	28,1
LAD	4	556,4	---*	712,8
CX	3	585,4	---*	717,0
RCA	3	194,3	---*	198,0
Ca	0	0,0	---*	0,0
Total	12	1361,0	---*	1655,9
U1	0	0,0	---*	0,0
U2	0	0,0	---*	0,0

Fig. 2 (continued)

uals younger than 45 years. In addition, the MESA site offers the possibility to calculate an "arterial age" by combining the Agatston CAC with age, gender, cholesterol, systolic blood pressure, smoking status, and use of medication for hypertension (www.mesa-nhlbi.org/Calcium/ArterialAge.aspx).

2.4 CT Scan Acquisition and Reconstruction

The first description of the CACS by Agatston was based on images obtained on electron beam CT scanners that are now no longer used (Agatston et al. 1990). The reference Agatston scores used for the MESA database were acquired on both EBCT and multislice CT scanners (McClelland et al. 2006).

Given the importance of reference values, the CAC score acquisition protocol still adheres to the same parameters that were used for the validation studies. This implies the use of a tube potential equal to 120 kV peak (kVp). Images should be acquired ECG-gated or triggered and reconstructed at 3 mm thick axial slices using filtered back projection and vendor-specific reconstruction kernels/filters. Images can be acquired in systolic or diastolic phases of the cardiac cycle depending on the heart rate (Husmann et al. 2007). Whereas in the past a rod with a known hydroxyapatite density had to be included in the scanned region for calibration purposes to calculate the mass score, modern post-processing software use embedded predefined calibration factors.

2.5 Factors Affecting the CACS

The fact that CACS provides a single quantitative number makes it an appealing score for clinical use. One should keep in mind, however, that many factors influence the CACS and can lead to substantial variation in the CACS (up to 50% in Agatston score) and patient classification. These factors include patient size (Willemink et al. 2015), heart rate (Funabashi et al. 2006; Groen et al. 2007), coronary vessel displacement and vessel trajectory (Tigges et al. 2012) (1), CT system (Greuter et al. 2007), CT detector technology (Kopp et al. 2002), spectral beam shaping (Tesche et al. 2017; Vonder et al. 2018), spiral or sequential modes, scan starting position (Rutten et al. 2008a) (2), cardiac phase (Rutten et al. 2008b), reconstruction technique (3–5), slice increments (Schlosser et al. 2007), slice thickness (Groen et al. 2007), CAC scoring software (van Praagh et al. 2021; Weininger et al. 2012), and CAC quantification parameters (Hong et al. 2003a, b).

In general, Agatston scores are a function of the number of voxels which exceed the CAC scoring threshold (conventionally 130 HU) and the maximum CT number of these voxels. The above mentioned factors influence either or both of these parameters. For increased heart rates, for example, the number of voxels of a CAC increases due to motion blur. For low-density CAC, motion blurring results in less voxels exceeding the CAC scoring threshold of 130 Hounsfield units (HU), thereby decreasing the Agatston score, while the opposite is true for high-density CAC. Motion artifacts can also decrease this maximum number, thereby decreasing the resulting Agatston score. If, for example, the maximum CT number was 201 HU without coronary artery motion and 198 HU with coronary artery motion, this would result in a reduction of the Agatston score by a factor of 2 (Agatston et al. 1990; Alluri et al. 2015).

Also, the relative X-ray spectrum influences the number of voxels which exceed the CAC threshold, as well as the maximum CT number within each lesion. For large patients, for example, the X-ray beam is attenuated more. This influences the resulting CT numbers, and therefore the resulting Agatston scores. The same is true for different CT systems, with different X-ray tube filters or for the application of spectral beam-shaping filters.

Patient size affects the CACS, and larger body sizes are associated with an underestimation of the CACS even when using weight-adjusted acquisition settings (Willemink et al. 2015). Presumably larger body sizes usually result in more noise in the CT images leading to the underestimation.

2.6 Post-processing Software to Calculate CAC

Many different software packages are commercially available that can be used for (semi)automatic CAC calculation. The minimum size (connected number of voxels) which is included in the analysis can be software specific and differs from the literature standard of ≥1 mm^2 (van Praagh et al. 2021). Nowadays, various software packages include artificial intelligence algorithms that already automatically select the lesions with an HU value of more than 130 that are located in the coronary arteries and highlight them. The person reporting the scan only needs to check the correctness of the segmentation and include any calcification that was missed or delete segmented calcifications outside the coronary arteries (e.g., calcifications in the mitral valve annulus that may be easily mistaken for calcifications in the circumflex coronary artery).

2.7 New Developments

Given the tremendous development in CT imaging in the last two decades which saw a variety of new techniques being introduced, there is a huge potential to reduce the patient radiation exposure associated with coronary calcium score scans as well as improve image quality and measurement accuracy. However, we are currently limited by the strict acquisition requirements (most notably the need for using 120 kV) and the 3 mm thick slice thickness that were used in the initial large cohort validation studies and need to be enforced up to this day for reproducible measurements and meaningful use of the percentile scores.

Reducing the tube potential—which increases calcium contrast—and reducing the slice thickness—which reduces partial volume effects—both increase coronary artery calcium detectability (van Praagh et al. 2022). This increase in calcium detection subsequently increases CACS robustness. For the Agatston score, an increase in robustness can further increase the negative predictive value of a zero Agatston score for adverse cardiovascular events. This is especially true for small but high-density calcifications or large but low-density calcifications. For current protocols, partial volume and blooming effects may lead to an erroneous zero Agatston score.

New image reconstruction kernels/filters have been introduced that allow for 120 kV-like reconstructions of images acquired at different kVp (Booij et al. 2020; van der Werf et al. 2021).

For current state-of-the-art energy-integrating CT systems, Van Praagh et al. described a new CACS protocol utilizing a reduced tube potential of 100 kV together with small slice thickness reconstructions of 1 mm (van Praagh et al. 2021). For phantom measurements, this resulted in a radiation dose reduction of 25% with increased reproducibility.

The advent of dual-layer detector systems with spectral reconstructions allows for reconstruction of virtual non-contrast images from CTA datasets. The calcium score can be derived "for free" using these images. Although the obtained CAC correlates well with those derived from true non-contrast-enhanced acquisitions, they are systematically underestimated (Gassert et al. 2021).

For novel photon-counting CT (PCCT) systems, reduced detector pixel element size results in inherent increased spatial resolution in comparison with conventional energy-integrating detector systems. With this, smaller calcifications could be detected, further increasing CACS robustness (Symons et al. 2019). Also, PCCT allows for reconstruction of virtual non-contrast images similar to those described above. It remains to be determined if they underestimate the CAC to a similar extent.

The interpretation of CAC changes over time may change due to new insights in plaque dynamics, especially after putting patients on statin medication. Interestingly, the PARADIGM study showed that patients on statins demonstrated a larger change in coronary plaque composition from noncalcified to calcified compared to patients not on statins. Hence, this will result in a larger increase in calcium score over time but may represent a smaller increase in risk as noncalcified plaques are considered more prone to rupture. More data is needed however to confirm these findings (Lee et al. 2018; Motoyama et al. 2009).

2.8 Conclusion

The coronary calcium score is a strong independent predictor for future cardiovascular events. Currently, image acquisition needs to be performed using strict acquisition parameters that are based on outdated scan acquisition techniques. There is an urgent need for a "recalibration" of the calcium score using contemporary image acquisition techniques that allow for substantial dose reduction and reduction in intraindividual CAC scores, which will contribute to even more widespread use and make CAC a robust parameter.

3 Coronary Stenosis Measurement

3.1 CT vs. Conventional Angiography

CT has become a leading imaging tool in the last decade for evaluating patients with low to intermediate pretest probability of disease who may have obstructive coronary artery disease but which cannot be ruled out by other noninvasive methods (Knuuti et al. 2019). CT's main strength is its high negative predictive value, confirming with high confidence the absence of significant coronary artery disease. Therefore, a detailed quantification of the degree of coronary stenosis has never been the purpose of a CT examination, a task in practice given to conventional coronary angiography given its higher temporal and spatial resolution. Nevertheless, it is customary to assess the degree of luminal narrowing with CT, which helps identify patients in whom potentially significant stenosis cannot be ruled out and need further testing.

Conventional coronary angiography remains the gold standard for the evaluation of coronary artery stenosis. However, CT-derived measurements do not always correlate well with conventional angiography-derived stenosis quantification. This discrepancy is partly due to the different physical nature of these imaging modalities and some inherent technical issues associated with CT imaging. However, new artificial intelligence-based methods are delivering promising results, narrowing the gap in stenosis quantification between CT and quantitative conventional angiography (Dundas et al. 2023). While CT has the benefit of being a true 3D imaging modality, its image quality can be compromised by both patient- and technical-related factors. Also, it is less suited to evaluate coronary arteries with extensive calcifications, often leading to overestimation of stenosis compared with conventional angiography (Fig. 3).

However, CT imaging can assess both luminal narrowing and the underlying atherosclerotic plaque. It provides an evaluation of luminal patency and plaque composition analysis for the presence of high-risk features, as well as an estimation of global plaque burden (Fig. 4). This is important, as an appropriate assessment of not only focal coronary artery disease but also global atherosclerotic burden is an important element in establishing the most proper course of action, both regarding the treatment of current disease and establishing effective preventive measures.

Finally, CT has a significant advantage over conventional angiography in that viewing angles of a stenotic lesion can be optimized after the data acquisition, while quantitative coronary angiography remains limited to the images obtained during the examination. This can be useful when evaluating complex lesions with noncircular geometry.

Table 3 provides a comparison between both imaging modalities.

3.2 Methods for CT-Derived Luminal Stenosis Determination

Various CT techniques are available to evaluate coronary artery luminal stenosis. Most commonly, the degree of luminal diameter stenosis

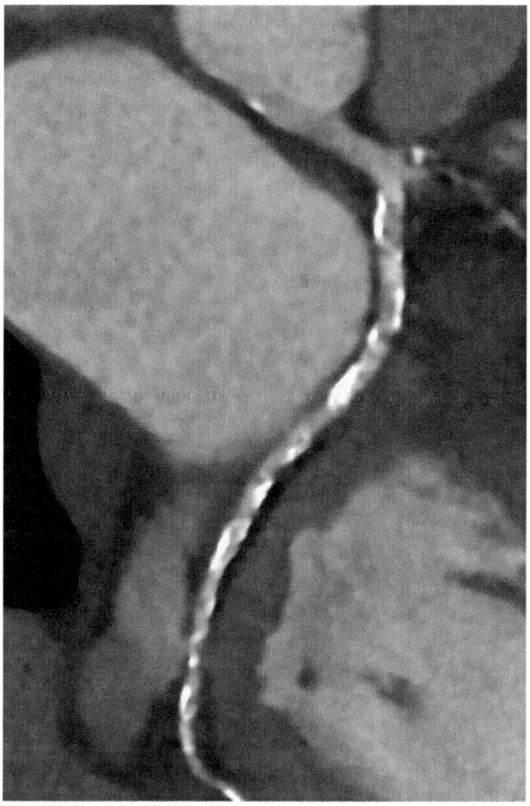

Fig. 3 A 67-year-old man with extensive coronary calcifications in the circumflex artery. While CT is excellent to rule out obstructive coronary artery disease, it is less suited to evaluate the stenotic effect of calcified plaques, especially when prominent as in this case. When calcifications are extensive, most observers tend to overestimate the degree of stenosis compared with conventional angiography. As such, these patients should be referred for further testing as obstructive coronary artery disease cannot be ruled out by CT alone

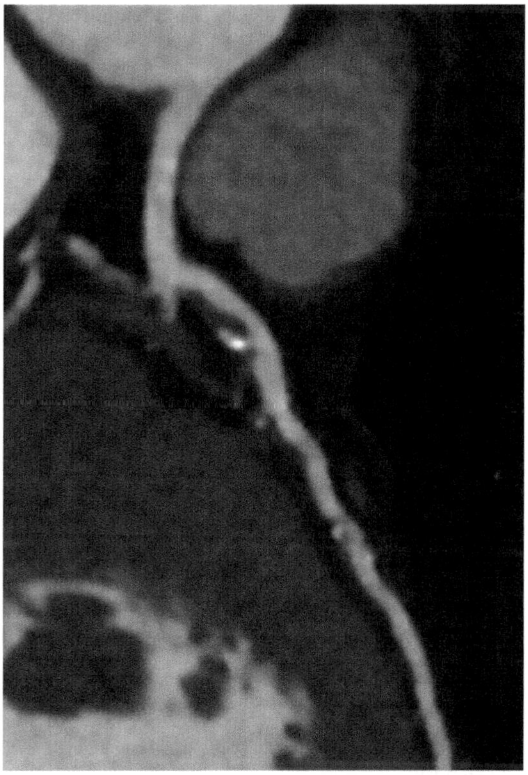

Fig. 4 A 52-year-old man with a large plaque in the proximal LAD, mainly composed of noncalcified components, with positive remodeling, an eccentric calcification, and a slightly irregular contour of the luminal plaque border. While the luminal stenosis is only moderate, the several high-risk features of this plaque provide additional prognostic information not provided by conventional angiography. Therefore, a correct report must not only include an assessment of luminal stenosis but also address plaque features

can be determined by comparing a segment of luminal narrowing either visually or (semi-) quantitatively with a chosen reference diameter. Other less commonly used methods include area stenosis, minimum lumen diameter (MLD), or minimum lumen area (MLA). Although each method has its advantages, visually CT-derived diameter stenosis is the preferred method in practice due to its pragmatic nature and widespread use in all major clinical studies and trials that validate the clinical application of coronary artery CT.

3.2.1 Diameter-Based Coronary Artery Luminal Stenosis

There are two common CT-derived coronary artery stenosis evaluation approaches: visual estimation vs. quantitative calculation, the latter either manually or using dedicated software tools.

Visual stenosis estimation is, as stated, most common due to its convenience and speed. The methodology is straightforward. Using a workstation that allows analysis of the full volumetric dataset, the coronary arteries are evaluated for the presence of plaque and its effects on the luminal

Table 3 A comparison of the main similarities and differences of conventional angiography and coronary CT angiography

	Conventional coronary angiography	Coronary CT angiography
Assessment method	Direct visualization of contrast-filled lumen	Visualization of both lumen and vessel wall using volumetric data, different imaging modes, and post-processing options available
Measurement techniques	Visual estimation and quantitative coronary angiography	Visual estimation and semiautomatic software tools available, but visual estimation reported in ranges of stenosis is mostly common
Accuracy	High spatial and temporal resolution, gold standard for stenosis measurement	Lower spatial and temporal resolution compared to angiography, but improving over scan generations. Heart rate control remains a critical factor for optimal image quality
Plaque assessment	Limited to the lumen, cannot visualize plaque morphology	Visualizes both lumen and plaque, including calcified and noncalcified plaques. Can visualize positive remodeling
Radiation exposure	Lower per procedure, but cumulative dose can be high due to repeated procedures in complex cases	Modern systems can provide examinations at very low radiation exposure levels, depending on body habitus and heart rate
Invasiveness	Invasive, requiring catheter placement	Noninvasive
Image quality factors	Affected by patient movement and technical expertise	Affected by technical (e.g., motion artifacts, heart rate, and image noise) and patient-related (e.g., body habitus) factors
Common confounding factors for stenosis measurement	Vessel overlap and projection angles due to 2D nature	Calcifications causing blooming artifacts Motion artifacts Vessel tortuosity Partial volume effects and difficulty assessing small arteries
Clinical use	Primarily used for diagnosis and intervention and suitable for all clinical settings (acute and stable chest pain)	Mainly used for diagnostic purposes in patients with low to intermediate risk in which obstructive coronary artery disease cannot be ruled out

diameter. Once a particular coronary segment of interest has been identified, the MLD is visually evaluated by correctly aligning the imaging planes. The estimated diameter is then visually compared to a reference diameter, commonly located in a normal arterial segment in close proximity to the target lesion. Ideally, no side branch vessels should be present between the site of MLD and the reference segment. The visually estimated ratio between the MLD and the reference diameter is then reported as the estimated degree of stenosis (Fig. 5).

As the degree of stenosis is a visual estimation, the reported stenosis severity is not an exact number. As proposed by guideline publications from expert societies, two characteristics are commonly reported: a qualitative description of the degree of stenosis and a visual estimation of the actual luminal narrowing expressed as a range correlating with degrees of severity (Leipsic et al. 2014). This manner of reporting, together with the description of the plaque characteristics and other particular anatomical features (e.g., location at a bifurcation), will help the referring clinician in selecting which patients may benefit from further investigation (Table 4). This means that the lack of a detailed degree of stenosis measurement does not interfere with the clinical role of cardiac CT, which is selecting which patient may benefit most from further testing.

Quantitative stenosis estimation can be done manually or semiautomatically using dedicated

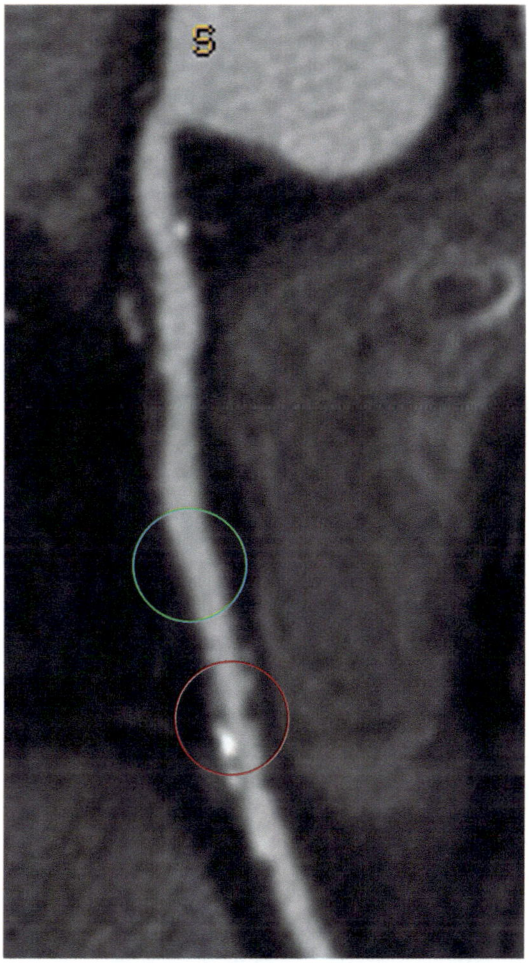

Fig. 5 A 60-year-old man with a coronary plaque of mixed composition in the right coronary artery. On this curved MPR image, the site of the most prominent stenosis is visually identified (red circle) and visually compared with an adjacent normal segment (green circle). The visually estimated stenosis was reported as ±50% diameter stenosis, subsequently confirmed with conventional angiography

software solutions. The manual method follows the same principle as the visual estimation explained before, with the addition of a manual measurement of the lumen at the reference location and the site of MLD on a correctly reformatted double-oblique cross-sectional image. In the semiautomatic process, the user usually indicates a segment of a coronary artery to be analyzed, followed by a proposition of the software package for the location of MLD and reference diameter, both of which can be manually adjusted (Fig. 6).

Table 4 Proposed visually determined reporting scale for luminal stenosis and plaque burden (from Leipsic et al. 2014)

Grading scale for stenosis severity	
Degree of luminal diameter stenosis	Terminology
0%	No visible stenosis
1–24%	Minimal stenosis
25–49%	Mild stenosis
50–69%	Moderate stenosis
70–99%	Severe stenosis
100%	Occluded
Grading scale for plaque burden (visually estimated)	
Mild amount of plaque	
Moderate amount of plaque	
Severe amount of plaque	
Extensive amount of plaque	

3.2.2 Area-Based Coronary Artery Luminal Stenosis

An area-based approach to luminal stenosis has several advantages over a diameter-based stenosis assessment. It is better suited to reflect the impact of irregular luminal contours and noncircular stenosis, adhering more closely to indices of hemodynamic significance than a single lumen diameter. Also, it is less dependent on the choice of reference site, especially when using an absolute value for MLD and MLA (Plank et al. 2016). However, despite these theoretical benefits, area measurement of coronary artery stenosis remains in practice impractical due to often inadequate contour tracing of software modules, requiring manual editing and making the whole process more time-consuming. Furthermore, guidelines for further intervention are currently based on diameter-derived stenosis, with the gold standard remaining to be conventional angiography.

As software algorithms continue to improve, area stenosis may become more feasible in the future, but currently an increase in their widespread application is not expected. At this moment, area-based stenosis is mostly investigated in a research setting.

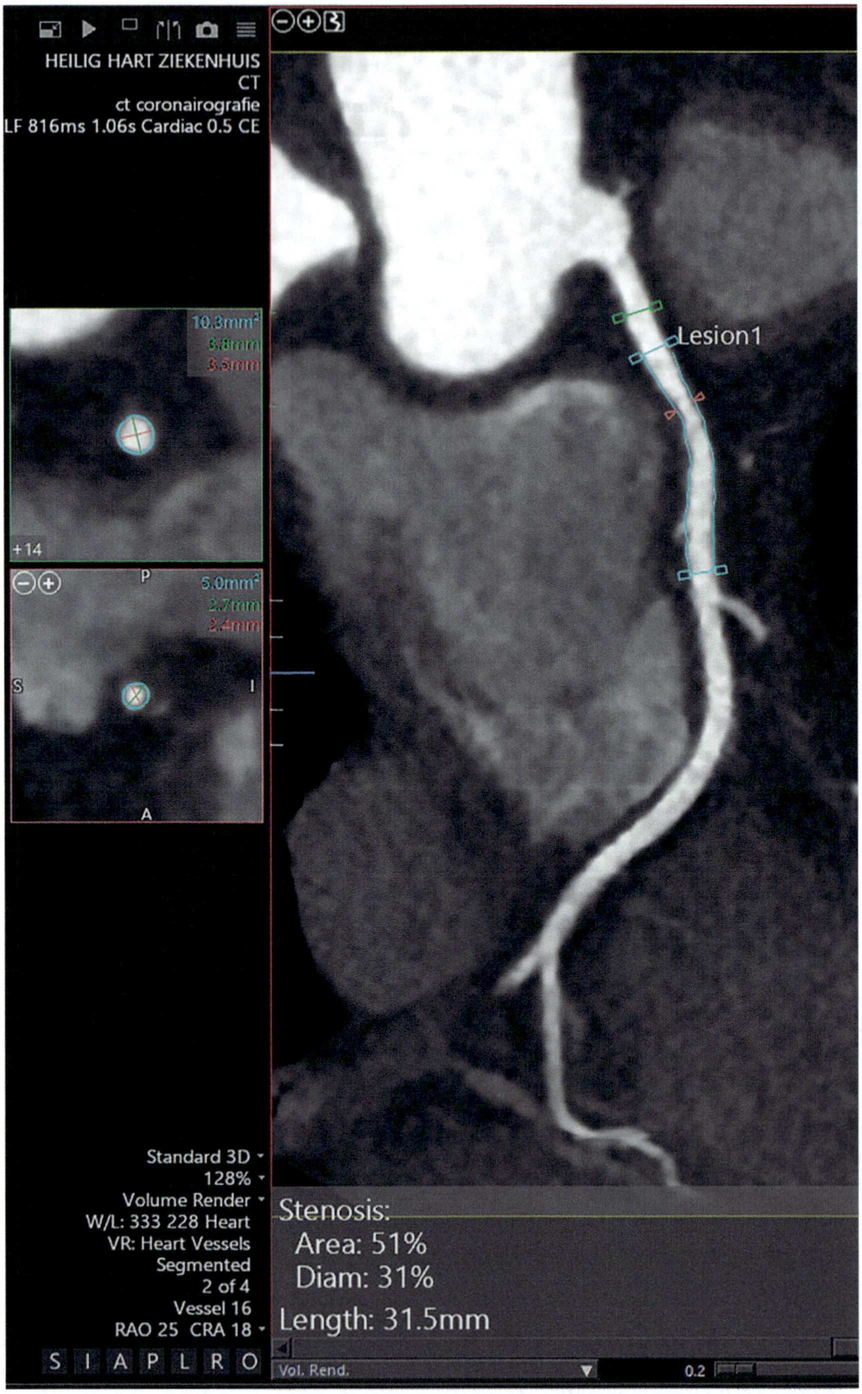

Fig. 6 Semiautomatic quantification of a coronary stenosis. The blue lines indicate the segment of interest, in which a site of minimal luminal diameter is proposed (red arrows). This is compared to a proposed proximal reference segment (green line). The proposed luminal contours are also given on the left side of the image and are user-adjustable. If approved by the user, the measurements in this case correspond to a diameter stenosis of 51% and area stenosis of 31%. Caution should be given not to report these results too literally, using them more as an indication to further refine a visual estimation of stenosis

3.3 Confounding Factors for Coronary Luminal Stenosis Evaluation

Several confounding factors may influence the accuracy of the measurement.

All approaches are significantly influenced by image quality. Suboptimal image quality, especially in segments with smaller vessel diameter, quickly complicates the exact determination of the luminal borders, leading to an often overestimation of stenosis severity. Image quality can be degraded by a combination of decreased signal-to-noise ratio, motion artifacts due to insufficient temporal resolution or patient motion, inappropriate choice of cardiac phase, or suboptimal arterial opacification. A more detailed description of all factors contributing to image quality and measures that can be taken is given in the chapter "Technical Aspects of Cardiac CT."

The presence of calcifications is also a known confounding factor for both methods, as lumen visibility decreases due to blooming artifacts (Fig. 3). Manual adjustment to a more appropriate window level and width, as the use of a sharper kernel, may help in a more reliable assessment of luminal contours. While some authors have suggested not to perform a CT angiography above a certain level of coronary calcifications (e.g., Agatston score >400), this approach is not universally followed. A high Agatston score can also be the result of many small calcifications that do not affect luminal evaluation (Fig. 7), while a single large calcification in a specific segment may pose a very local diagnostic problem.

Some vendors have provided varying methods for obtaining a dataset in which calcified plaques have been subtracted. While the resulting image has a visual quality that more closely matches that of conventional angiography, this approach is seldom used to increase the accuracy of luminal stenosis.

Vessel size is also a confounding factor, as measurements performed in small vessels and at arterial bifurcations will more often underestimate the degree of stenosis. Therefore, it is mandatory to use all available information on a workstation, reformatting the different imaging planes in order to obtain the most appropriate view for evaluation.

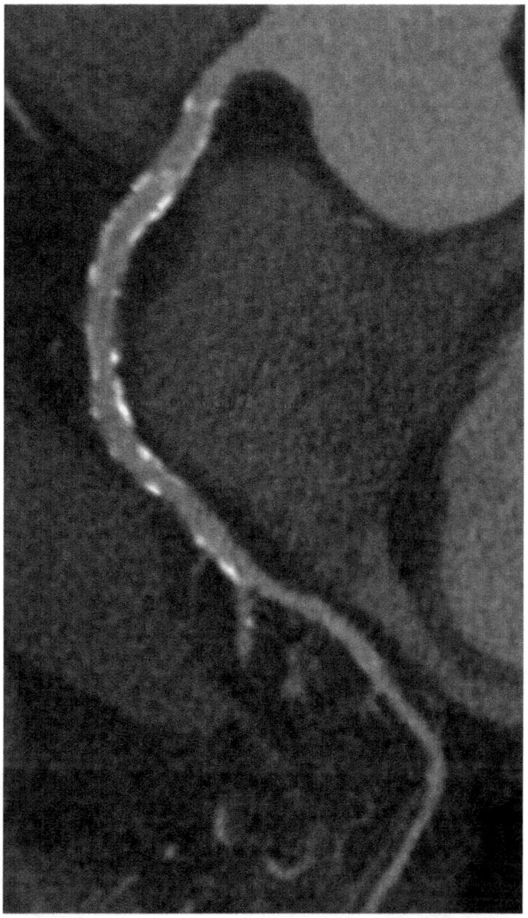

Fig. 7 Extensive coronary calcification in a 72-year-old man with an Agatston score of 823. Nevertheless, the calcifications are small and excentric. Together with good image quality, this allows to exclude significant coronary artery disease, despite the prominent amount of calcifications. As such, we do not recommend a fixed threshold of Agatston score value as a criterion to not proceed with CT angiography, but consider each patient on a case-by-case basis

The presence of arterial remodeling is an important plaque feature that must be assessed and reported, as it complements the degree of luminal stenosis with important prognostic information. Positive arterial remodeling refers to the phenomenon where a plaque does not grow inward but instead expands outward, increasing the total diameter of the affected vessel segment but not necessarily resulting in a significant luminal narrowing (Fig. 8). As such, the degree of luminal narrowing does not reflect the amount of local atherosclerosis, leading to underestimation of the severity of the disease. Also, the presence of positive remodeling is considered a high-risk plaque feature, increasing the risk of plaque rupture independently of other factors. To calculate the amount of positive remodeling, one must first measure the maximum outer vessel diameter, followed by calculating the ratio of this diameter with either (1) the outer diameter of a normal proximal reference or (2) the average outer diameter of the proximal and distal vessel segment. A ratio >1.1 indicates positive remodeling (Gauss et al. 2011). Positive remodeling can also be calculated as the vessel cross-sectional area at the level of the maximal stenosis divided by the average of the proximal and distal reference sites' cross-sectional areas (Achenbach et al. 2004).

Despite advances in software development, semiautomated quantification of coronary artery stenosis remains not standard practice in most centers. Despite the visually appealing presentation and stenosis quantification, the accurate delineation of the lumen contour must always be visually validated and manually corrected when necessary. Therefore, while this software-based approach has the potential to minimize inter- and intraobserver variations, in practice, it is often more time-consuming than a visual estimation and therefore not routinely performed. It is also important to remember that the primary goal of CT in patients with chronic coronary syndrome is to exclude obstructive CAD, and not the correct quantification for stenosis severity. When the stenosis degree cannot reliably be assessed, further investigation should be recommended.

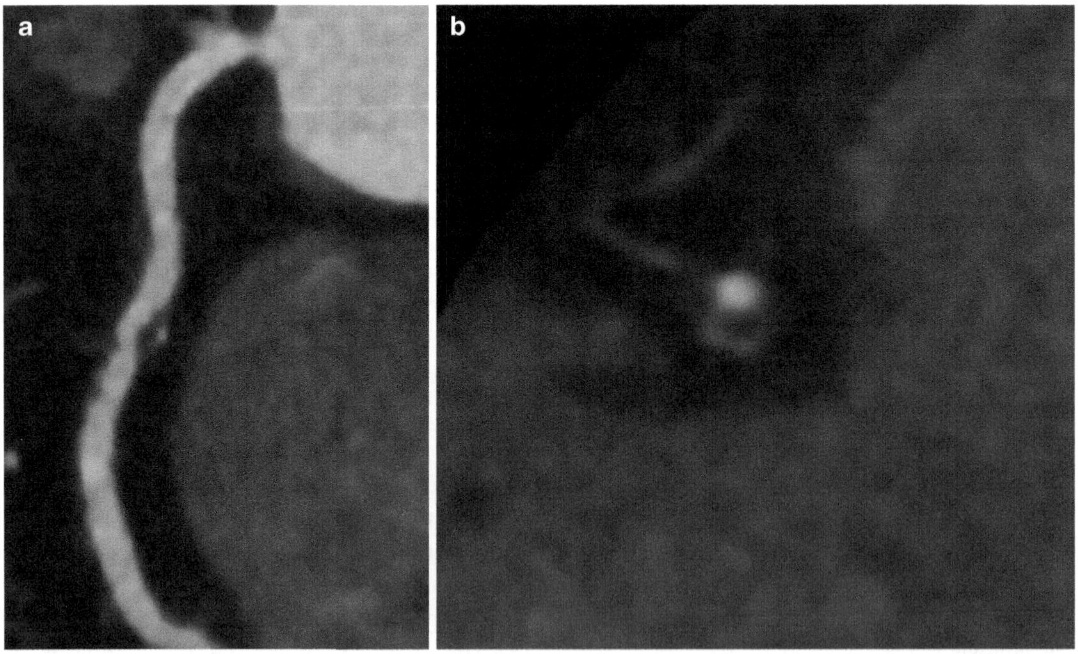

Fig. 8 A 63-year-old man with a mostly noncalcified plaque in the proximal RCA, extending outward. As such, luminal repercussion remains limited (**a**). The cross-sectional image further illustrates the outward extension (**b**). Even though the effect of the luminal diameter is limited, this plaque characteristic is considered a high-risk feature and must be reported

4 Evaluation of Plaque Composition

4.1 Identification of Plaque Components

Atherosclerotic plaque composition has been identified as an important determinant of cardiovascular risk. In practice, plaque composition is described as making a simple descriptive distinction between calcified, noncalcified, and mixed plaques (containing both calcified and noncalcified components). This approach works well, as it discriminates between calcified lesions that are considered stable and plaque that contains a soft tissue component and other morphological features, which makes them potentially more susceptible to plaque rupture. Other high-risk plaque features have been reported (Motoyama et al. 2009), which include the presence of spotty calcification, positive remodeling, and low-attenuation plaque density with extrinsic density (possible calcification). Currently, no specific measurements are required in the further workup of these high-risk plaque features.

CT has nevertheless the potential to provide a more detailed analysis of the histology of different plaque components based on their density measured in Hounsfield units (HU), which have been correlated with IVUS or pathology examinations. Several ranges have been reported which have been associated with different plaque components (Chang et al. 2018). The HU range for necrotic core is typically defined as −30 to 30 HU. However, an alternate HU range of −30 to 75 HU has also been proposed, with improved correlative findings with virtual histology IVUS (Brodoefel et al. 2008). Fibrofatty plaque is characterized by an HU range of 30–130 HU, while fibrous plaque has an HU range of 130–350 HU.

Calcified plaque is defined as having an HU value greater than 350. Recent reports further categorize calcified plaque as low (351–699 HU), medium (700–999 HU), and high (>1000 HU) density (van Rosendael et al. 2020).

4.2 Confounding Factors

Despite this potential for further plaque characterization by means of a simple measurement of density, it is important to note that the HU range for intravenous contrast (100–500 HU) is broad and overlaps with the HU ranges for atherosclerotic plaque components, complicating reliable measurements in what in practice are already small lesions.

Furthermore, the described fixed thresholding HU ranges to categorize plaque components do not consider individual variations in luminal attenuation, and there is a considerable overlap in HU density ranges between different plaque components (Bienstock et al. 2023). An alternative approach, known as adaptive thresholding, uses scan-specific classification of atherosclerotic plaque composition, automatically derived from the luminal attenuation of "normal blood pool" as measured in the aorta (Dey et al. 2009).

To date, comparative analysis has not definitively established the superiority of one thresholding approach over the other. However, adaptive thresholding techniques that consider scan-specific details may overcome the limitations associated with fixed thresholding (Bienstock et al. 2023). Nevertheless, it is safe to state that detailed plaque composition has not reached the level of accuracy required to be used routinely in clinical practice for now.

5 Evaluation of Global Coronary Plaque Burden

One of the main benefits of cardiac CT over conventional angiography is its ability to visualize both the lumen and coronary plaques in the vessel wall. This implies that, while a subject may not have significant obstructive CAD, the global atherosclerotic burden of the coronary arteries can still be significant. Also, specific plaque features are associated with an increased risk for rupture and hence acute coronary events, regardless of their degree of luminal stenosis.

Table 5 Scoring systems for assessing global plaque burden. Note that the CAD-RADS is different as it is more a structured reporting system, combining the highest degree of luminal stenosis in a coronary artery with several modifiers to provide a more complete assessment of coronary plaque burden

Score	Calculation method
Segment involved score (SIS)	Counts the number of coronary artery segments with any degree of plaque (typically based on a 16- or 17-segment model). Each segment with a plaque scores 1 point
Segment Stenosis Score (SSS)	Assesses the severity of stenosis in each segment. Scores range from 0 to 4 based on the degree of stenosis: 0 (0%), 1 (1–49%), 2 (50–69%), 3 (70–99%), 4 (100%). The sum of all segment scores gives the total SSS
CT Leaman Score (CLS)	Evaluates both the extent and severity of coronary atherosclerosis, considering segment location, plaque burden, and degree of stenosis. A weighted sum of scores from individual segments, accounting for factors like left main involvement and proximal segment stenosis
Multivessel Aggregate Score (MVAS)	Combines the number of vessels with significant stenosis (usually >50%) and their respective segments. The score increases with the number of affected vessels and the severity of their stenosis
CAD-RADS 2.0 Score (CR2.0)	Provides a standardized reporting system for coronary CT angiography findings. Scores range from CAD-RADS 0 (no plaque or stenosis) to CAD-RADS 5 (severe stenosis ≥70% in at least one segment), with modifiers for high-risk plaque and prior coronary artery bypass grafts (CABG) or stenting

CAD-RADS Coronary Artery Disease-Reporting and Data System

The use of semiquantitative scores for evaluation of atherosclerotic burden by coronary artery CT is not widespread. One of the main reasons for their lack of diffusion in mainstream practices is the sometimes significant additionally generated workload to obtain such a score and the lack of guidelines on how to convert a score into a concrete clinical treatment plan (with the exception of the CAD-RADS score). Table 5 provides an overview on how these different scores are calculated. However, several studies have shown their clear prognostic value (Maclean et al. 2023).

It is important to note the differences in the nature of these scores. The Segment Involvement Score (SIS) focuses on the presence of any coronary plaque, while the Segment Stenosis Score (SSS) is based on the severity of stenosis within segments. The CT Leaman score (CLS) is a more complex score considering both the extent and location/severity of atherosclerosis. The Coronary Artery Disease-Reporting and Data System (CAD-RADS) 2.0 is more a clinical reporting system that standardizes the assessment and communication of findings (Cury et al. 2022). It is based on the highest degree of stenosis found in the CT evaluation, but incorporates several modifiers to account for the contribution of high-risk plaque features but also functional information derived from FFR-CT and myocardial perfusion. Finally, it provides recommendations for further management of these patients based on the obtained score, both in patients with acute and stable chest pain.

6 FFR-CT and Transluminal Gradient

While establishing the degree of coronary artery stenosis remains one of the main parameters to establish a possible therapeutical intervention, the degree of luminal stenosis and its hemodynamic repercussions do not always correlate well. Technological innovations have paved the way for the mainstream introduction of techniques that can provide more insight into the functional effects of a specific plaque, providing a better selection of patients who might benefit from a coronary revascularization. The two main methods for functional assessment using CT are fractional flow reserve (FFR) measurement with CT and myocardial perfusion. The latter is explained in detail in the chapter “Hemodynamic Assessment of Coronary Flow: Myocardial Perfusion Using CT/MR.” In the following chapters, we will discuss FFR-CT and a third method named transluminal attenuation gradient.

6.1 Invasive FFR

Angiography is used to guide the decision to perform percutaneous coronary intervention (PCI), such as balloon angioplasty or stenting. During invasive coronary angiography (ICA), the stenosis degree is visually scored and categorized into mild, moderate, or severe. Especially in case of moderate stenosis, it is challenging to select those who would benefit from revascularization. Over the last decade, the treatment of coronary artery disease (CAD) has radically changed. The landmark FAME and COURAGE trials caused a shift from revascularization based on anatomic stenosis degree to one guided by hemodynamic significance of the stenosis (Pijls et al. 2010; Shaw et al. 2008). Fractional flow reserve (FFR) allows for the assessment of hemodynamic significance (Pijls et al. 1996). The European Society of Cardiology guideline recommends the use of FFR in stenosis grade between 40% and 90%, without evidence of ischemia in noninvasive testing, or in patients with multivessel disease (Neumann et al. 2019a). FFR is quantified per lesion during ICA using a pressure wire. It is calculated as the ratio between the post-stenotic and pre-stenotic coronary artery pressure during adenosine-induced hyperemia (de Bruyne and Sarma 2008). FFR has a "gray zone" ischemic threshold value between 0.75 and 0.80. The measurement is unaffected by changes in heart rate, blood pressure, and myocardial contractility (de Bruyne et al. 1996; Pijls et al. 1995). Several studies demonstrated that FFR-guided revascularization reduces the rate of death, myocardial infarction, or urgent revascularization (Xaplanteris et al. 2018). Currently, FFR is regarded as the reference standard for evaluating hemodynamic significance of coronary artery (Neumann et al. 2019b).

6.2 FFR-CT

6.2.1 Principle of FFR-CT

Similar to ICA, the hemodynamic significance of moderate stenoses on CTA is difficult to assess. Advances in computational fluid dynamics allow for the computation of FFR-CT using coronary CTA images, without the administration of adenosine or the need for additional CT scans (Table 6). Coronary blood flow response to adenosine is modeled, and the FFR value is calculated using the Navier-Stokes equations, while taking microcirculatory resistance into account (Taylor et al. 2013). HeartFlow (Redwood City, California, USA) was the first to provide offsite FFR-CT analysis (CTA datasets are sent to HeartFlow for analysis). In case of HeartFlow, a standard coronary CTA can be used, which should meet the minimum requirements set by the SSCT (Abbara et al. 2016). This means the scan should be performed on ≥64-slice CT scanner with cardiac gating capability, and adequate premedication such as beta-blockers and nitroglycerin should be administrated (Takx et al. 2015; Abbara et al. 2016). In addition, the scans should meet minimum quality requirements for HeartFlow evaluation (i.e., ≥8 out of 10 consecutive cases should pass initial quality check) (NICE 2021). The images are uploaded to HeartFlow servers. Algorithms using artificial intelligence segment the coronaries, after which

Table 6 Comparison between invasive FFR and CT-derived FFR

	Invasive FFR	FFR_{CT}
Additional hyperemia medication	Yes	NA
Measurement	Quantitative flow ratio based on pressure	Modeled using the Navier-stokes equations
Materials	Pressure monitoring guidewire	Software algorithm
Spatial resolution	0.1 mm	0.5 mm
Temporal resolution	4–8 ms	66 ms
Additional radiation burden	4 mSv	NA
Additional procedural time	9 min	NA
Additional contrast	50 mL	NA

References for estimates (Funabashi et al. 2006; Groen et al. 2007)

analysts make further adjustments when needed (HeartFlow 2022). Finally, blood flow is modeled and FFR-CT values are generated for the entire coronary arterial tree. Turnaround of these analyses is ≤5 h for more than 50% of cases (HeartFlow 2022). The results are represented per vessel, and the report is available as pdf, which can be incorporated in the medical file of the patient (Fig. 9). Others have developed applications for onsite FFR-CT analysis, which requires the individual institution to adjust the automatically generated vessel segmentation, which can take between 30 min and 2 h (Asher et al. 2018). Onsite software uses a reduced model, calculating values only in stenotic regions (Taylor et al. 2013). HeartFlow FFR-CT received regulatory approval in the United States, the United Kingdom, and Japan. The PLATFORM study demonstrated the clinical utility of FFR-CT to guide therapy (Fig. 10). FFR-CT reduced the number of ICA by 60% and significantly reduced ICA showing non-obstructive CAD (Douglas et al. 2015).

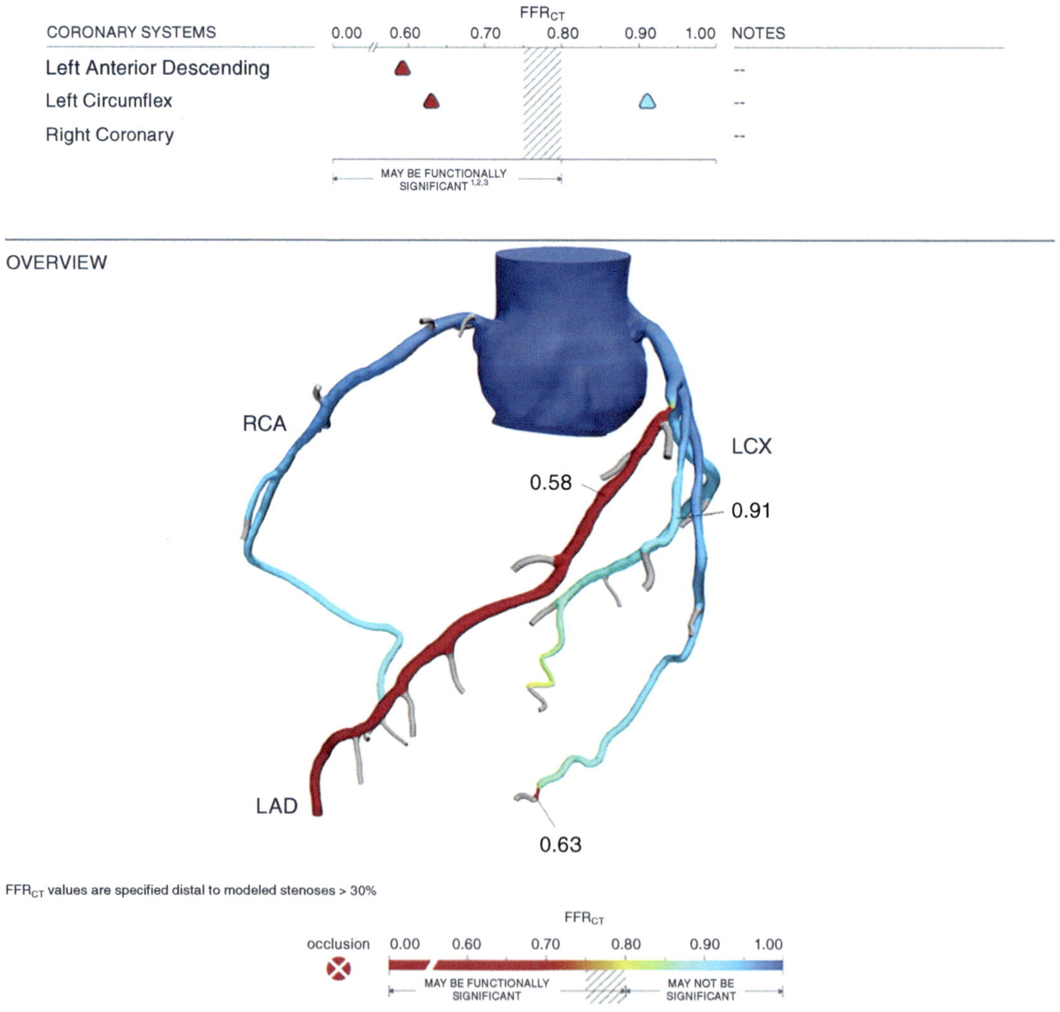

Fig. 9 FFR-CT report as provided by HeartFlow. A coronary tree is illustrated with numerical values indicating the calculated CT-derived FFR value in different coronary arteries. A color coding is also used to reflect calculated FFR values. In this case, low calculated FFR values in the LAD and distal LCX indicate a hemodynamically significant stenosis

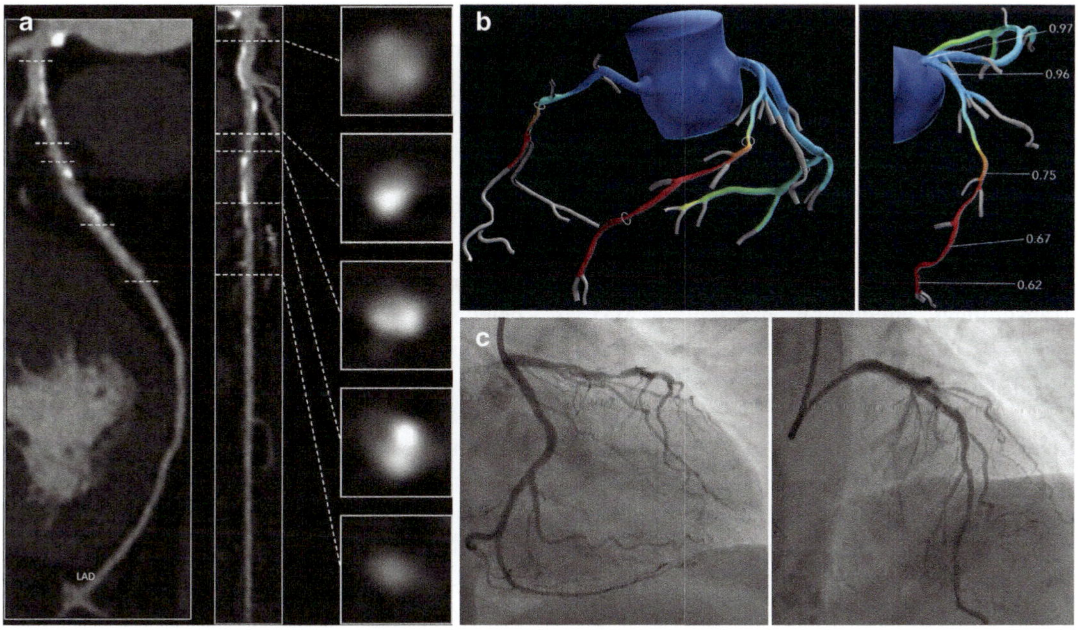

Fig. 10 A 69-year-old woman with several cardiovascular risk factors underwent CCTA prior to major non-cardiovascular surgery. CCTA showed diffuse calcifications with severe stenosis (70%) in the middle segment of LAD (**a**). FFR-CT (HeartFlow) confirmed the hemodynamic significance of the stenosis (**b**), revealing a significant flow reduction (FFR = 0.62) in the distal segment of the vessel. ICA was successfully performed with the implantation of three stents in the LAD (**c**). *CCTA* cardiac computed tomography angiography, *LAD* left anterior descending artery, *FFR-CT* fractional flow reserve, *ICA* invasive coronary angiography. (Case courtesy of Federica Catapano MD, PhD, and Marco Francone MD, PhD, Humanitas University, Milan, Italy)

6.2.2 Diagnostic Accuracy of FFR-CT

The diagnostic performance of several CT techniques was evaluated in a meta-analysis for the detection of hemodynamically significant CAD (Celeng et al. 2019). FFR_{CT} showed in 2432 vessels a sensitivity of 85% (95% CI 82–87%) and specificity of 78% (95% CI 72–83%), which mainly showed an improvement in specificity over coronary CTA (61% [95% CI 54–68%], sensitivity was 87% [95% CI 84–91%]). FFR_{CT} performed similar to CT perfusion without the need for additional image acquisitions or pharmacological stress agents. In addition, the results also indicated that the performance of on-site FFR_{CT} algorithms was similar to off-site FFR_{CT} (Celeng et al. 2019).

6.2.3 Confounding Factors of FFR-CT

An important limitation of FFR_{CT} is that not all coronary CTA exams are suitable for FFR_{CT} calculation. Heart rate control and administration of nitroglycerin are pivotal. In a cohort of 10,621 clinical patients, the FFR_{CT} rejection rate was 8.4% (Pontone et al. 2019). Most commonly, this is due to motion artifacts (81.4%) and image noise (22.1%; please note that more than one reason for rejection is possible) (Pontone et al. 2019). Also, the presence of a stent, CABG, or cardiac device is a common cause of rejection (16.2%) (Pontone et al. 2019). FFR_{CT} analysis seems feasible in the presence of severe calcification, which results in blooming and beam hardening (Norgaard et al. 2015).

HeartFlow currently does not calculate FFR_{CT} values for vessels with diameters less than 1.8 mm. Also, FFR_{CT} values have not been validated in vessels with metallic stents. A certain degree of variation between modeling (FFR_{CT}) and invasively measured FFR is expected, especially when a strict (binary) threshold is used. Nevertheless, some variation is also observed for repeated measures of invasive FFR (Petraco et al.

2013). In order to improve successful FFR_{CT} assessment, HeartFlow provides recommendations per vendor for acquisition and reconstruction settings (HeartFlow 2022).

6.3 Transluminal Attenuation Gradient (TAG)

Transluminal attenuation gradient (TAG) is another technique that uses CTA images for detection of hemodynamically significant CAD. TAG is quantified using contrast opacification in the coronaries and is measured manually or (semi)automatically in Hounsfield units in a series of evenly spaced regions of interest (Fig. 11) (Einstein 2013). Data points in regions with motion or blooming artifacts from luminal calcium should be excluded. TAG is expressed as a regression coefficient of the line fitting the contrast opacification of the ROI at the respective distance from the coronary ostium (Einstein 2013). In theory, the opacification should diminish more in case of a hemodynamically significant stenosis, and the cutoff point is dependent on hardware and contrast protocol.

6.3.1 Diagnostic Accuracy of TAG

Only a limited number of studies investigated the diagnostic performance of TAG. In the previously mentioned meta-analysis, TAG was investigated in 726 vessels (Celeng et al. 2019). Sensitivity of TAG was moderate (59% [95% CI 46–72%]), whereas specificity differed substantially at vessel vs. patient level (77% vs. 39%) (Celeng et al. 2019). Discrepancies could be dependent on the acquisition technique and scanner hardware. Ideally, CTA images are acquired on modern scanners equipped with a high number of detector rows (256-slice and 320-detector row scanners), which allows for up to 16 cm *Z*-axis coverage and thus coverage of the heart in a single rotation, thus avoiding stair-step artifacts.

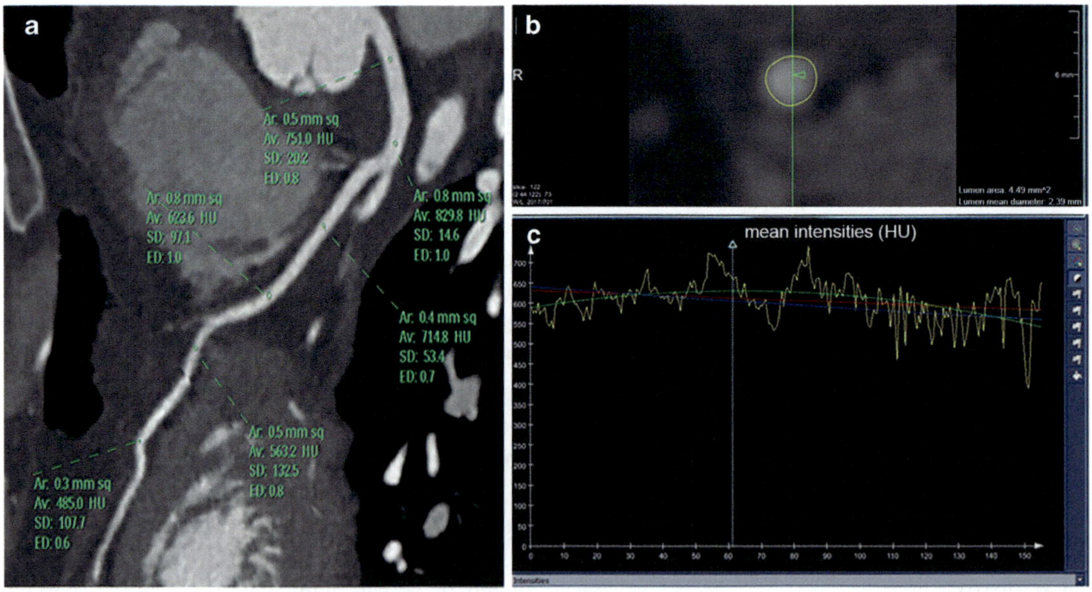

Fig. 11 Measurement of TAG in a vessel without stenosis. HU values are manually recorded in the left anterior descending artery (LAD) from the proximal to the distal part (**a**). Panels (**b**) and (**c**) illustrate semiautomatic TAG measurement. Panel (**b**) shows the cross section of the lumen. Panel (**c**) shows the semiautomatically measured HU values in the LAD on *y*-axis and the length from the origin on the *x*-axis with adjusted slopes

6.3.2 Confounding Factors of TAG

Optimal contrast opacification is a prerequisite for the use of TAG. TAG depends on the time-density curve of the contrast agent and scanning time. Additionally, contrast dilution due to different rates of coronary inflow, coronary branching, and coronary lesions can influence the results (Gould et al. 2019). Scanners with only 4 cm coverage require acquisition over multiple heartbeats. Thus, contrast opacification along the vessels will not be at a single time point, which could reduce the diagnostic performance of TAG (Einstein 2013). To correct for the time-dependent variation of contrast due to imaging of multiple heartbeats, TAG with corrected coronary opacification (TAG-CCO) has been introduced (Choi et al. 2011). Park et al. (2016) showed that TAG decreases with diminution of vessel diameter, which implies that TAG values might be driven by differences in diameters. Finally, in a study by Bom et al. (2019), TAG did not provide incremental diagnostic value over coronary CTA alone for the identification of ischemia as defined by $[^{15}O]H_2O$ PET and/or invasive FFR.

6.4 Conclusion

FFR_{CT} could, in case of intermediate stenosis, refine the referral of patients to ICA. Both on-site and off-site algorithms show good performance. Nevertheless, CT image quality has to be sufficient, and small vessels and stents are not validated. For the clinical use of TAG, there is currently insufficient evidence.

7 Conclusion

In summary, coronary calcium quantification, exclusion of significant stenosis with CT, and potential of FFR-CT have greatly enhanced diagnostic and prognostic capabilities in cardiology. Coronary calcium quantification accurately measures calcified plaque, allowing for patient risk stratification and preventive measures. CT-based exclusion of significant stenosis has revolutionized the evaluation of suspected coronary artery disease, reducing the need for invasive procedures. FFR-CT, a continuously evolving technology, enables functional assessment of coronary lesions, identifying patients who would benefit most from revascularization. This optimizes resource utilization and improves patient outcomes by reducing unnecessary invasive angiograms and minimizing complications. The synergistic application of these advanced imaging techniques will continue to reshape the diagnostic and prognostic landscape in noninvasive cardiac imaging. Other techniques like transluminal attenuation gradient have conversely faded from clinical practice, failing to meet the required balance between practical use, evidence-based support, and clinical dissemination.

References

Abbara S, Blanke P, Maroules CD et al (2016) SCCT guidelines for the performance and acquisition of coronary computed tomographic angiography: a report of the society of Cardiovascular Computed Tomography Guidelines Committee Endorsed by the North American Society for Cardiovascular Imaging (NASCI). J Cardiovasc Comput Tomogr 10:435–449

Achenbach S, Ropers D, Hoffmann U et al (2004) Assessment of coronary remodeling in stenotic and nonstenotic coronary atherosclerotic lesions by multidetector spiral computed tomography. J Am Coll Cardiol 43:842–847

Agatston AS, Janowitz WR, Hildner FJ et al (1990) Quantification of coronary artery calcium using

ultrafast computed tomography. J Am Coll Cardiol 15:827–832
Alluri K, Joshi PH, Henry TS et al (2015) Scoring of coronary artery calcium scans: history, assumptions, current limitations, and future directions. Atherosclerosis 239:109–117
Asher A, Singhal A, Thornton G et al (2018) FFRCT derived from computed tomography angiography: the experience in the UK. Expert Rev Cardiovasc Ther 16:919–929
Bienstock S, Lin F, Blankstein R et al (2023) Advances in coronary computed tomographic angiographic imaging of atherosclerosis for risk stratification and preventive care. JACC Cardiovasc Imaging 16:1099–1115
Blaha MJ, Cainzos-Achirica M, Greenland P et al (2016) Role of coronary artery calcium score of zero and other negative risk markers for cardiovascular disease: the Multi-Ethnic Study of Atherosclerosis (MESA). Circulation 133:849–858
Bom MJ, Driessen RS, Stuijfzand WJ et al (2019) Diagnostic value of transluminal attenuation gradient for the presence of ischemia as defined by fractional flow reserve and quantitative positron emission tomography. JACC Cardiovasc Imaging Imaging 12:323–333
Booij R, van der Werf NR, Budde RPJ et al (2020) Dose reduction for CT coronary calcium scoring with a calcium-aware image reconstruction technique: a phantom study. Eur Radiol 30:3346–3355
Brodoefel H, Reimann A, Heuschmid M et al (2008) Characterization of coronary atherosclerosis by dual-source computed tomography and HU-based color mapping: a pilot study. Eur Radiol 18:2466–2474
Budoff MJ, Achenbach S, Blumenthal RS et al (2006) Assessment of coronary artery disease by cardiac computed tomography: a scientific statement from the American Heart Association Committee on Cardiovascular Imaging and Intervention, Council on Cardiovascular Radiology and Intervention, and Committee on Cardiac Imaging, Council on Clinical Cardiology. Circulation 114:1761–1791
Callister TQ, Cooil B, Raya SP et al (1998) Coronary artery disease: improved reproducibility of calcium scoring with an electron-beam CT volumetric method. Radiology 208:807–814
Celeng C, Leiner T, Maurovich-Horvat P et al (2019) Anatomical and functional computed tomography for diagnosing hemodynamically significant coronary artery disease: a meta-analysis. JACC Cardiovasc Imaging 12:1316–1325
Chang H-J, Lin FY, Lee S-E et al (2018) Coronary atherosclerotic precursors of acute coronary syndromes. J Am Coll Cardiol 71:2511–2522
Choi JH, Min JK, Labounty TM et al (2011) Intracoronary transluminal attenuation gradient in coronary CT angiography for determining coronary artery stenosis. JACC Cardiovasc Imaging 4:1149–1157
Conti CR, Feldman RL, Repine CJ et al (1983) Effect of glyceryl trinitrate on coronary and systemic hemodynamics in man. Am J Med 74:28–32
Cury RC, Leipsic J, Abbara S et al (2022) CAD-RADSTM 2.0-2022 coronary artery disease-reporting and data system an expert consensus document of the Society of Cardiovascular Computed Tomography (SCCT), the American College of Cardiology (ACC), the American College of Radiology (ACR), and the North America Society of Cardiovascular Imaging (NASCI). J Cardiovasc Comput 16:536–557
de Bruyne BD, Sarma J (2008) Fractional flow reserve: a review: invasive imaging. Heart 94:949–959
de Bruyne B, Bartunek J, Sys SU et al (1996) Simultaneous coronary pressure and flow velocity measurements in humans: feasibility, reproducibility, and hemodynamic dependence of coronary flow velocity reserve, hyperemic flow versus pressure slope index, and fractional flow reserve. Circulation 94:1842–1849
Detrano RC, Anderson M, Nelson J et al (2005) Coronary calcium measurements: effect of CT scanner type and calcium measure on rescan reproducibility—MESA study. Radiology 236:477–484
Dey D, Cheng VY, Slomka PJ et al (2009) Automated 3-dimensional quantification of noncalcified and calcified coronary plaque from coronary CT angiography. J Cardiovasc Comput Tomogr 3:372–382
Dickerson JA, Nagaraja HN, Raman SV (2010) Gender-related differences in coronary artery dimensions: a volumetric analysis. Clin Cardiol 33:E44–E49
Dodge JT Jr, Brown BG, Bolson EL et al (2018) Lumen diameter of normal human coronary arteries. Influence of age, sex, anatomic variation, and left ventricular hypertrophy or dilation. Circulation 86:232–246
Douglas PS, Pontone G, Hlatky MA et al (2015) Clinical outcomes of fractional flow reserve by computed tomographic angiography-guided diagnostic strategies vs. usual care in patients with suspected coronary artery disease: the prospective longitudinal trial of FFR(CT): outcome and resource impacts study. Eur Heart J 36:3359–3367
Dundas J, Leipsic JA, Sellers S et al (2023) Artificial intelligence-based coronary stenosis quantification at coronary CT angiography versus quantitative coronary angiography. Radiol Cardiothorac Imaging 5:e230124
Dzaye O, Dardari ZA, Cainzos-Achirica M et al (2021) Warranty period of a calcium score of zero: comprehensive analysis from MESA. JACC Cardiovasc Imaging 14:990–1002
Einstein AJ (2013) TAG-is it it?: improving coronary computed tomography angiography with the isotemporal transluminal contrast attenuation gradient. J Am Coll Cardiol 61:1280–1282
Feldman RL, Pepine CJ, Curry RC et al (1979) Coronary arterial responses to graded doses of nitroglycerin. Am J Cardiol 43:91–97

Fishman EK, Ney DR, Heath DG et al (2006) Volume rendering versus maximum intensity projection in CT angiography: what works best, when, and why. Radiographics 26:905–922

Funabashi N, Koide K, Mizuno N et al (2006) Influence of heart rate on the detectability and reproducibility of multislice computed tomography for measuring coronary calcium score using a pulsating calcified mock-vessel in comparison with electron beam tomography. Int J Cardiol 113:113–117

Gassert FG, Schacky CE, Muller-Leisse C et al (2021) Calcium scoring using virtual non-contrast images from a dual-layer spectral detector CT: comparison to true non-contrast data and evaluation of proportionality factor in a large patient collective. Eur Radiol 31:6193–6199

Gauss S, Achenbach S, Pflederer T et al (2011) Assessment of coronary artery remodelling by dual-source CT: a head-to-head comparison with intravascular ultrasound. Heart 97:991

Gould KL, Johnson NP, Kirkeeide R (2019) TAG, you're out. JACC Cardiovasc Imaging 12:334–337

Greuter MJ, Dijkstra H, Groen JM et al (2007) 64 slice MDCT generally underestimates coronary calcium scores as compared to EBT: a phantom study. Med Phys 34:3510–3519

Groen JM, Greuter MJ, Schmidt B et al (2007) The influence of heart rate, slice thickness, and calcification density on calcium scores using 64-slice multidetector computed tomography: a systematic phantom study. Investig Radiol 42:848–855

HeartFlow (2022). https://www.heartflow.com/education/ccta-resources/

Hoffmann U, Ferencik M, Cury RC et al (2006) Coronary CT angiography. J Nucl Med 47:797–806

Hong C, Bae KT, Pilgram TK (2003a) Coronary artery calcium: accuracy and reproducibility of measurements with multi-detector row CT—assessment of effects of different thresholds and quantification methods. Radiology 227:795–801

Hong C, Bae KT, Pilgram TK et al (2003b) Coronary artery calcium quantification at multi-detector row CT: influence of heart rate and measurement methods on interacquisition variability initial experience. Radiology 228:95–100

Husmann L, Leschka S, Desbiolles L et al (2007) Coronary artery motion and cardiac phases: dependency on heart rate—implications for CT image reconstruction. Radiology 245:567–576

Knuuti J, Wijns W, Saraste A et al (2019) ESC guidelines for the diagnosis and management of chronic coronary syndromes. The task force for the diagnosis and management of chronic coronary syndromes of the European Society of Cardiology (ESC). Eur Heart J. Epub ahead of print. https://doi.org/10.1093/eurheartj/ehz425

Kopp AF, Ohnesorge B, Becker C et al (2002) Reproducibility and accuracy of coronary calcium measurements with multi-detector row versus electron-beam CT. Radiology 225:113–119

Lee SE, Chang HJ, Sung JM et al (2018) Effects of statins on coronary atherosclerotic plaques: the PARADIGM study. JACC Cardiovasc Imaging 11:1475–1484

Leipsic J, Abbara S, Achenbach S et al (2014) SCCT guidelines for the interpretation and reporting of coronary CT angiography: a report of the Society of Cardiovascular Computed Tomography Guidelines Committee. J Cardiovasc Comput Tomogr 8:342–358

Lubbers M, Dedic A, Coenen A et al (2016) Calcium imaging and selective computed tomography angiography in comparison to functional testing for suspected coronary artery disease: the multicentre, randomized CRESCENT trial. Eur Heart J 37:1232–1243

Maclean E, Cronshaw R, Newby DE et al (2023. Epub ahead of print) Prognostic utility of semi-quantitative coronary computed tomography angiography scores in the SCOT-HEART trial. J Cardiovasc Comput Tomogr. https://doi.org/10.1016/j.jcct.2023.08.009

Mahnken AH, Wildberger JE, Sinha AM et al (2003) Value of 3D-volume rendering in the assessment of coronary arteries with retrospectively ECG-gated multislice spiral CT. Acta Radiol 44:302–309

McClelland RL, Chung H, Detrano R et al (2006) Distribution of coronary artery calcium by race, gender, and age: results from the Multi-Ethnic Study of Atherosclerosis (MESA). Circulation 113:30–37

McCollough CH, Ulzheimer S, Halliburton SS et al (2007) Coronary artery calcium: a multi-institutional, multimanufacturer international standard for quantification at cardiac CT. Radiology 243:527–538

Motoyama S, Sarai M, Harigaya H et al (2009) Computed tomographic angiography characteristics of atherosclerotic plaques subsequently resulting in acute coronary syndrome. J Am Coll Cardiol 54:49–57

Neumann FJ, Sousa-Uva M, Ahlsson A et al (2019a) 2018 ESC/EACTS guidelines on myocardial revascularization. J Am Coll Cardiol 40:87–165

Neumann F-J, Sousa-Uva M, Ahlsson A et al (2019b) 2018 ESC/EACTS guidelines on myocardial revascularization. Eur Heart J 40:87–165

NICE (2021) HeartFlow FFRCT for estimating fractional flow reserve from coronary CT angiography. https://www.nice.org.uk/guidance/mtg32/resources/adoption-support-resource-insights-from-the-nhs-4363972813/chapter/5-How-to-implement-NICEs-guidance-on-HeartFlow-FFRCT

Norgaard BL, Gaur S, Leipsic J et al (2015) Influence of coronary calcification on the diagnostic performance of CT angiography derived FFR in coronary artery disease: a substudy of the NXT trial. JACC Cardiovasc Imaging 8:1045–1055

Okada M, Nakashima Y, Nomura T et al (2015) Coronary vasodilation by the use of sublingual nitroglycerin using 64-slice dual-source coronary computed tomography angiography. J Cardiol 65:230–236

Park EA, Lee W, Park SJ et al (2016) Influence of coronary artery diameter on intracoronary transluminal attenuation gradient during CT angiography. JACC Cardiovasc Imaging 9:1074–1083

Petraco R, Sen S, Nijjer S et al (2013) Fractional flow reserve-guided revascularization: practical implications of a diagnostic gray zone and measurement variability on clinical decisions. JACC Cardiovasc Interv 6:222–225

Pijls NH, Gelder BV, der Voort PV et al (1995) Fractional flow reserve. A useful index to evaluate the influence of an epicardial coronary stenosis on myocardial blood flow. Circulation 92:3183–3193

Pijls NHJ, de Bruyne B, Peels K et al (1996) Measurement of fractional flow reserve to assess the functional severity of coronary-artery stenoses. N Engl J Med 334:1703–1708

Pijls NH, Fearon WF, Tonino PA et al (2010) Fractional flow reserve versus angiography for guiding percutaneous coronary intervention in patients with multivessel coronary artery disease: 2-year follow-up of the FAME (Fractional Flow Reserve Versus Angiography for Multivessel Evaluation) study. J Am Coll Cardiol 56:177–184

Plank F, Burghard P, Friedrich G et al (2016) Quantitative coronary CT angiography: absolute lumen sizing rather than % stenosis predicts hemodynamically relevant stenosis. Eur Radiol 26:3781–3789

Pontone G, Weir-McCall JR, Baggiano A et al (2019) Determinants of rejection rate for coronary CT angiography fractional flow reserve analysis. Radiology 292:597–605

Rutten A, Isgum I, Prokop M (2008a) Coronary calcification: effect of small variation of scan starting position on Agatston, volume, and mass scores. Radiology 246:90–98

Rutten A, Krul SP, Meijs MF et al (2008b) Variability of coronary calcium scores throughout the cardiac cycle: implications for the appropriate use of electrocardiogram-dose modulation with retrospectively gated computed tomography. Investig Radiol 43:187–194

Schlosser T, Hunold P, Voigtlander T et al (2007) Coronary artery calcium scoring: influence of reconstruction interval and reconstruction increment using 64-MDCT. AJR Am J Roentgenol 188:1063–1068

Shaw LJ, Berman DS, Maron DJ et al (2008) Optimal medical therapy with or without percutaneous coronary intervention to reduce ischemic burden. Circulation 117:1283–1291

Sinha A-M, Mahnken AH, Borghans A et al (2006) Multidetector-row computed tomography vs. angiography and intravascular ultrasound for the evaluation of the diameter of proximal coronary arteries. Int J Cardiol 110:40–45

Symons R, Sandfort V, Mallek M et al (2019) Coronary artery calcium scoring with photon-counting CT: first in vivo human experience. Int J Cardiovasc Imaging 35:733–739

Takx RAP, Suchá D, Park J et al (2015) Sublingual nitroglycerin administration in coronary computed tomography angiography: a systematic review. Eur Radiol 25:3536–3542

Taylor CA, Fonte TA, Min JK (2013) Computational fluid dynamics applied to cardiac computed tomography for noninvasive quantification of fractional flow reserve scientific basis. J Am Coll Cardiol 61:2233–2241

Tesche C, Cecco CND, Schoepf UJ et al (2017) CT coronary calcium scoring with tin filtration using iterative beam-hardening calcium correction reconstruction. Eur J Radiol 91:29–34

Tigges S, Arepalli CD, Tridandapani S et al (2012) A phantom study of the effect of heart rate, coronary artery displacement and vessel trajectory on coronary artery calcium score: potential for risk misclassification. J Cardiovasc Comput Tomogr 6:260–267

van der Werf NR, Booij R, Schmidt B et al (2021) Evaluating a calcium-aware kernel for CT CAC scoring with varying surrounding materials and heart rates: a dynamic phantom study. Eur Radiol 31:9211–9220

van Praagh GD, van der Werf NR, Wang J et al (2021) Fully automated quantification method (FQM) of coronary calcium in an anthropomorphic phantom. Med Phys 48:3730–3740

van Praagh GD, Wang J, van der Werf NR et al (2022) Coronary artery calcium scoring. Investig Radiol 57:13–22

van Rosendael AR, Narula J, Lin FY et al (2020) Association of high-density calcified 1K plaque with risk of acute coronary syndrome. JAMA Cardiol 5:282–290

Vonder M, van der Werf NR, Leiner T et al (2018) The impact of dose reduction on the quantification of coronary artery calcifications and risk categorization: a systematic review. J Cardiovasc Comput Tomogr 12:352–363

Weininger M, Ritz KS, Schoepf UJ et al (2012) Interplatform reproducibility of CT coronary calcium scoring software. Radiology 265:70–77

Willemink MJ, Abramiuc B, den Harder AM et al (2015) Coronary calcium scores are systematically underestimated at a large chest size: a multivendor phantom study. J Cardiovasc Comput Tomogr 9:415–421

Willemink MJ, van der Werf NR, Nieman K et al (2019) Coronary artery calcium: a technical argument for a new scoring method. J Cardiovasc Comput Tomogr 13:347–352

Xaplanteris P, Fournier S, Pijls NHJ et al (2018) Five-year outcomes with PCI guided by fractional flow reserve. N Engl J Med 379:250–259

Yang F, Minutello RM, Bhagan S et al (2006) The impact of gender on vessel size in patients with angiographically normal coronary arteries. J Interv Cardiol 19:340–344

Zhou F-F, Liu Y, Ge P-C et al (2017) Coronary artery diameter is inversely associated with the severity of coronary lesions in patients undergoing coronary angiography. Cell Physiol Biochem 43:1247–1257

Hemodynamic Assessment of Coronary Flow: Myocardial Perfusion Using CT/MR

Olivier Ghekiere, Marly van Assen,
and Alain Nchimi

Contents

O. Ghekiere
Department of Radiology, Jessa Ziekenhuis, Hasselt, Belgium

Faculty of Medicine and Life Sciences, Hasselt University, Hasselt, Belgium

M. van Assen
Translational Lab for Cardiothoracic Imaging and Artificial Intelligence, Department of Radiology and Imaging Sciences, Emory University, Atlanta, GA, USA

A. Nchimi (✉)
Medical Imaging Department, Centre Hospitalier de Luxembourg, Luxembourg, Luxembourg

1 Introduction

Despite a downward trend in cardiovascular disease (CVD) incidence, they remain the leading cause of mortality and morbidity worldwide. One of their most lethal manifestations is coronary artery disease (CAD), in which alteration of the blood supply to the myocardium may cause transitory or definitive loss of function (Amini et al. 2021). To tackle the burden of cardiovascular disease, research has been driven toward finding appropriate techniques to assess coronary flow. Early techniques required placement of a catheter in the coronary arteries. While they currently remain the modality of choice for real-time flow or pressure measurement, they are increasingly challenged by newer less invasive diagnostic imaging techniques (Neumann et al. 2019). Isotopic imaging techniques, including single-photon emission computed tomography (SPECT) and later positron emission tomography (PET), were the first to build on the insight that the myocardial uptake of an intravenously injected tracer can provide valuable information that could replace that obtained by invasive coronary flow assessment (Flotats et al. 2011). Furthermore, contrast-enhanced computed tomography (CT) and magnetic resonance imaging (MRI) have contrast enhancement kinetics largely similar to that of radioisotopes and microspheres. Also, recent software and hardware developments in CT and MRI have enabled the rapid consecutive acquisition of (dynamic) volumetric or sequential

Med Radiol Diagn Imaging (2026)

https://doi.org/10.1007/174_2024_484,
Published Online: 06 September 2024

datasets with higher spatial and temporal resolution as compared to isotopic imaging (Coelho-Filho et al. 2013; Dewey et al. 2020). The prospect of extracting clinically useful information from the kinetic information of a bolus of contrast would further improve the overall morphological and functional evaluation of the major coronary arteries. However, challenges remain posed by the contribution to the disease process of the distal coronary arteries, subject to the same obstructive process or compensatory vasodilatation. Despite ongoing progress (Hsu et al. 2018), challenges posed by the reproducibility of the processing of dynamic CT/MRI examination and the less widespread availability of platforms providing quantitative perfusion from these data in clinical practice currently restrict these approaches to research centers. In this chapter, we will briefly describe diagnostic approaches to the evaluation of myocardial perfusion from dynamic CT and MRI and discuss their clinical usefulness.

2 Coronary Flow Regulation

Tissue perfusion can be defined as a volume of fluid flowing per unit of time through a tissue. Myocardial perfusion is conventionally defined as the blood flow (myocardial blood flow (MBF); mL/min) through 100 g of myocardium (MBF/100 g). Assessing myocardial blood flow in vivo is challenging given the inherent coronary anatomy and physiology complexity, as well as the limitations of the measuring techniques. Some imaging techniques allow measurements directly on the epicardial coronary arteries, whereas in other techniques, measurements can only be done on the myocardium (thus the myocardial microvasculature).

The coronary vasculature consists of coronary arteries serving as large conductance and resistance vessels, the latter typically less than 100 μm in diameter (= microcirculation), which distribute and regulate myocardial blood flow. The blood flow across the capillaries depends on the interaction between intracoronary driving pressure and microvascular resistance in a relationship defined as "coronary autoregulation" (Fig. 1). At rest, the myocardial oxygen extraction is almost maximal; therefore, an increase of the coronary flow via dilatation of the microvasculature occurs in response to higher myocardial oxygen demands. This regulation of coronary vascular resistance has been exploited for the diagnosis and characterization of impaired blood supply to the myocardium (Schelbert 2010; Heusch 2008). In case of proximal (epicardial) coronary stenosis, the distal flow at rest may be kept constant by the relaxation of the microvascular vascular smooth muscle until very tight stenoses (around 90% diameter reduction) occur. However, a condition of maximal hyperemia annihilates this reserve of compensation, with flow decreasing with lesser severity of stenoses, around 50% diameter reduction (Fig. 1) (Gould et al. 1974). The difference (or the ratio) between the resting and maximal vasodilatation (or exercise) coronary flows is termed the coronary flow reserve (CFR), which represents the amount of microvascular resistance that can be lifted (or inversely, the amount of additional flow that can be provided) to support any flow demand on top of the resting state. Lastly, given constraints posed by the ventricular systolic pressure, peak flow in the coronary arteries occurs during ventricular diastole, in contrast to other organs. The contractile workload is not uniformly distributed in the myocardium, as the subendocardium has the higher contribution. The myocardial perfusion mirrors this distribution, with a net transmural gradient from the subendocardium through the subepicardium.

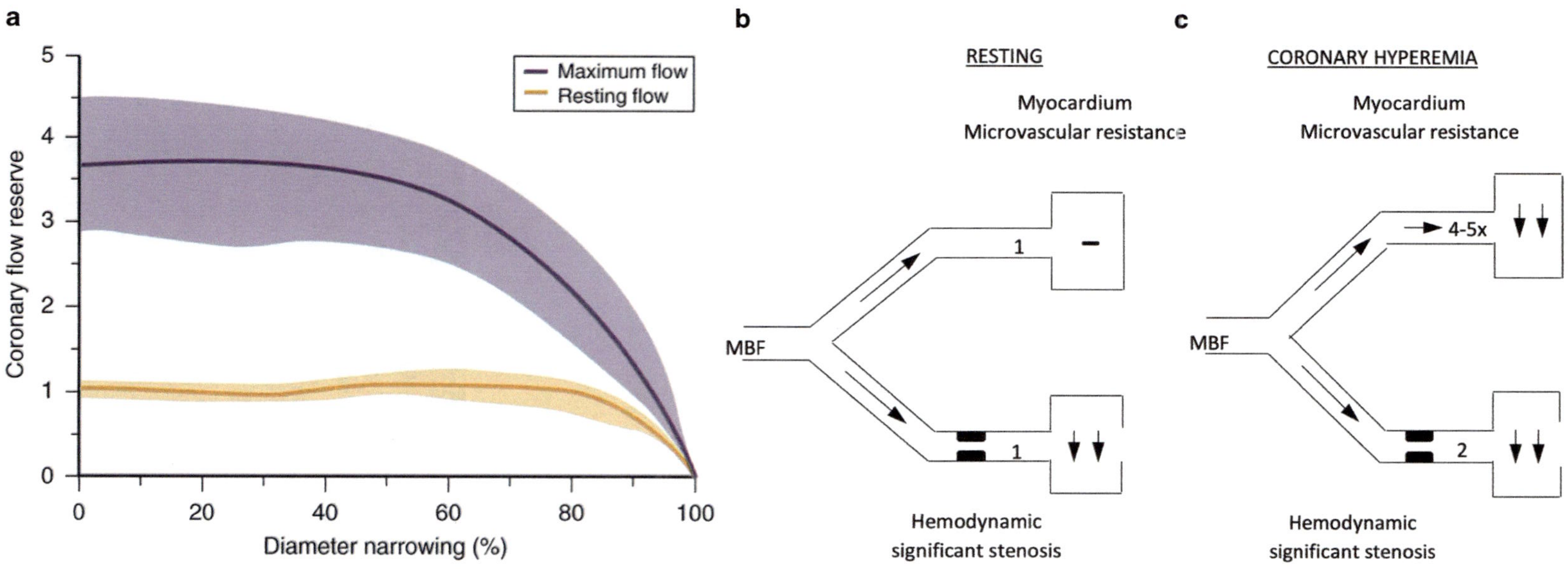

Fig. 1 Principles of myocardial flow regulation and hyperemia stress testing. Resting myocardial blood flow can be kept constant with increasing degree of coronary stenoses until up to 80–90% diameter reduction. When the same experiment is carried out under maximal vasodilatation, the blood flow enhances up to four times but cannot be kept constant above around 50% diameter coronary (**a**) (adapted from Gould et al. 1974). Right panel schematically represents the flow in a myocardial segment supplied by an artery with flow-limiting stenosis and a segment with a normal supply. The flow is similar in the two segments at rest due to the microvascular reserve (**b**), whereas upon maximal vasodilatation, the exhausted reserve fails to compensate for the flow difference between the two segments (**c**)

3 Definitions

In practice, CFR is the ratio of either coronary flow myocardial perfusion or any of their derivatives at maximal hyperemia versus their respective values at rest (Gould et al. 1990). As such, CFR is highly sensitive to coronary vascular disease, and a value <2 indicates a flow-reducing or functionally significant coronary vascular disease (Young et al. 1977). Relative CFR (rCFR) is a "normalized" value of the CFR, which is defined as the ratio of either hyperemic coronary flow, myocardial blood flow, or any of their derivatives, measured in a coronary territory, versus the respective values in another territory (Stuijfzand et al. 2015), which minimizes the impact of both the collateral flow and the diffuse/microvascular coronary disease in the assessment of focal coronary artery disease (Meuwissen et al. 2001). rCFR is measured invasively through a pressure-sensitive coronary catheter. Fractional flow reserve (FFR) is defined as the ratio of the mean distal coronary pressure distal to a coronary stenosis to that in the aorta during maximal hyperemia (De Bruyne et al. 1994). FFR measurement is highly recommended for the management of coronary stenoses, according to contemporary revascularization guidelines (Fig. 2) (Neumann et al. 2019). In clinical practice, a cutoff FFR value of 0.80 is used to guide revascularization. However, a "gray zone" with uncertain clinical significance exists between 0.75 and 0.80 (Johnson et al. 2014). In summary, FFR <0.75 identifies inducible ischemia requiring coronary

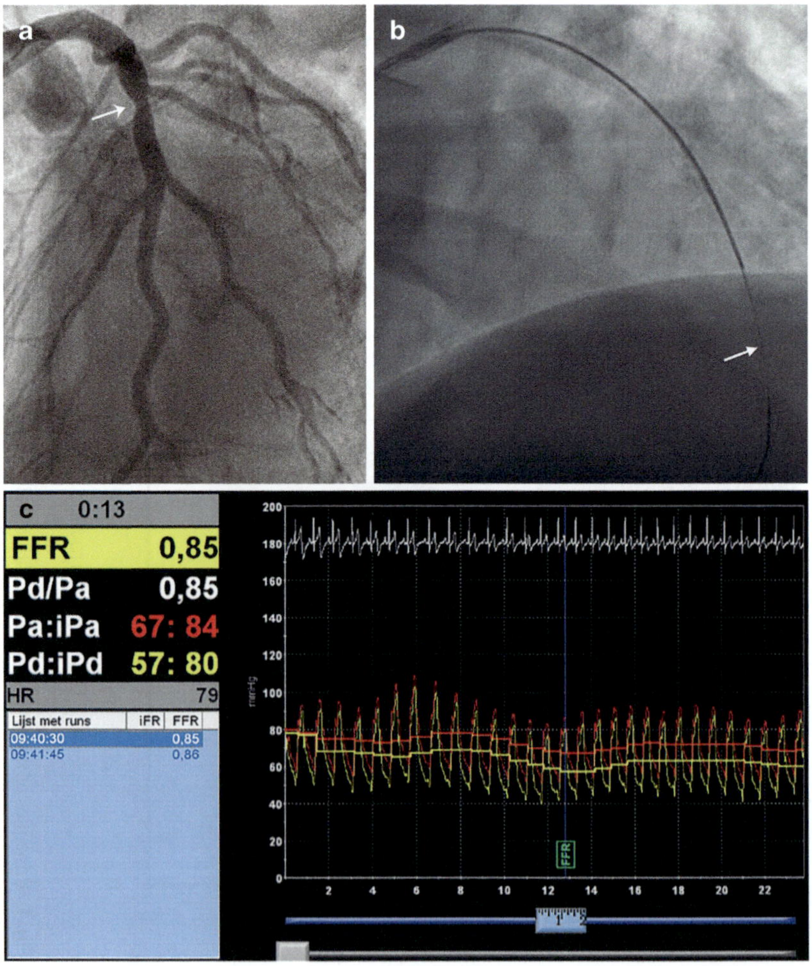

Fig. 2 Fractional flow reserve assessment. A pressure-sensitive catheter is inserted distal to a stenosis of the midportion of the left anterior descending artery (arrow in **a**) on catheter coronary angiography in a 56-year-old patient after vasodilatation (200 μg intracoronary adenosine). The ratio between the peak pressures distal to the stenosis (arrow in **b**) and the aorta (FFR) is 0.85 (**c**)

revascularization (Zimmermann et al. 2015), whereas FFR >0.80 reliably excludes myocardial ischemia (De Bruyne et al. 2012).

Instantaneous wave-free ratio (IFR) is a recently described invasive alternative to FFR that requires no hyperemia but uses the same pressure wires. IFR is the ratio of the distal coronary artery pressure to that of the aortic outflow tract (Pa) during a period of diastole known as the "wave-free period" in which competing blood flow altering these pressures is negligible. With IFR, the cutoff for flow limitation is 0.89, and the "gray zone" is between 0.86 and 0.93 (Götberg et al. 2017).

4 Perfusion Imaging Protocols

4.1 General Requirements

As FFR and IFR are invasive and expensive methods requiring intravenous contrast and ionizing radiation and carry risks of procedural complications such as coronary spasm, dissection, or perforation, several noninvasive imaging techniques have been developed for the evaluation of myocardial perfusion, each with its respective strengths and weaknesses (Driessen et al. 2022). Dynamic CT and MRI perfusion are based on the principle of acquiring (a set of consecutive) images during the first pass of an intravenous bolus of, respectively, 0.3–0.6 g/kg of iodinated and 0.075–0.1 mmol/kg of a gadolinium chelate contrast agents. Consequently, patient preparation for perfusion cardiac CT or MRI starts by checking the respective contraindications for both examinations' contrast agents. In addition, there are several common and technique-specific points to consider in patient preparation and perfusion examination realization.

4.1.1 Stressor Agent

Patients should refrain from caffeinated meals and drinks (coffee, tea, chocolate, etc.) at least 24 h before the examination, given the interfering effects of caffeine on the effectiveness of the pharmacological stressor agent used to achieve maximal hyperemia. Studies have reported that 5–15% of perfusion MRI examinations result in false-negative results, in many cases due to drug interactions and subsequent insufficient hyperemia (Greenwood et al. 2012; Kidambi et al. 2016).

Caffeine, e.g., interacts with the stressor agent in multiple ways, hampering the induction of hyperemia and, as such, possibly resulting in false-negative examinations. First, caffeine interacts with the same receptors as adenosine. Caffeine induces capillary de-recruitment by increasing sympathetic nerve activity, both resulting in a reduced difference in perfusion between healthy and impaired tissue (Schelbert 2010). Conversely, adenosine causes unwanted short-term side effects such as bronchial constriction. This is especially relevant in patients with reactive airway disease, which constitutes a contraindication to adenosine. These diseases include asthma and chronic obstructive pulmonary disease (COPD), a frequent comorbidity in patients with CAD. Although adenosine requires continuous intravenous administration and weight-based dosing, its short half-life allows for the rapid resolution of harmful side effects upon discontinuation of contrast medium administration (Faulds et al. 1991).

Another stressor agent being increasingly used is regadenoson, a potent and selective coronary vasodilator with a rapid onset of action and a longer half-life compared to adenosine (Al Jaroudi and Iskandrian 2009). Therefore, regadenoson can be administered as a fixed-dose bolus without weight adjustments. Furthermore, given its selectivity, there are fewer side effects making it suitable even for COPD patients. In addition, studies have shown that regadenoson is less sensitive to the competing effects of caffeine than adenosine (van Dijk et al. 2017a; Kuijpers et al. 2018). However, some studies also report negative effects of the use of regadenoson, which includes higher incidence of arrhythmias and increased need for application of the rescue agent aminophylline (Brink et al. 2015).

Appropriate coronary vasodilatation stress requires the administration of adenosine for

2–5 min at a rate of 140 μg/min/kg, or a single injection of 0.4 mg of regadenoson. Other vasodilators exist but are not suitable for CT/MRI because of their (too long or too short) half-life time.

4.1.2 Coverage

Although the minimal requirements for perfusion MRI include only three short-axis slices, the accuracy of the examination depends on the heart coverage. Therefore, efforts are undertaken by some scanner manufacturers to perform myocardial perfusion MRI via 3D approaches, which is already the case with CT. Indeed, large-bore multidetector CT scanners (256–320 detector rows) cover the full left ventricle without table movement, whereas the dual-source CT (DSCT) scanners use the shuttle mode to achieve the same because of their limited *z*-axis coverage. The shuttle mode consists of back-and-forth table movements (Assen et al. 2020). A problem introduced by the moving table positions is the possibility of motion artifacts, especially in high heart rates and contrast differences between two table positions (Ghekiere et al. 2017).

4.1.3 Temporal Resolution

Precise contrast agent kinetics is mandatory for dynamic perfusion CT/MRI. The ability to capture two events occurring in distinct moments defines the temporal resolution of this technique. The temporal resolution of dynamic perfusion CT/MRI should exceed the time window of the fastest process observed, which is typically the vascular transit time. The temporal resolution of CT/MRI is often in the range of 1–4 s, which is sufficient to sample the vascular transit time without major underestimation (Ishida et al. 2016). Nevertheless, depending on the scanner type and the patient's heart rate, a lower temporal sampling rate may occur, especially on CT with heart rate restrictions imposed by ECG gating. For example, the shuttle mode with DCST may allow acquiring images every second heartbeat for low heart rates, up to one every 4 heartbeats at higher heart rates (which are common in stress situations) (Ishida et al. 2016; Mahnken et al. 2010; Bindschadler et al. 2014).

4.1.4 Cardiac Phase for Image Acquisition

Image acquisition is possible in the systolic or diastolic phase. Despite studies reporting higher stress MBF on images acquired in diastole as compared to a systole acquisition (Nchimi et al. 2014a; Motwani et al. 2012, 2014), similar diagnostic accuracy for myocardial ischemia was observed in both phases (Motwani et al. 2012, 2014). As such, several important advantages exist for an acquisition in the systolic phase. First, the heart is contracted during systole, with maximal contraction at end systole, resulting in a smaller total heart volume and a shorter basal-apical length. Thus, the range that needs to be covered for visualizing the entire heart within one scan cycle is reduced. Because of this maximal contraction, the myocardium is thicker in systole and allows for easier delineation during analysis. Secondly, although the systolic phase is shorter than the diastolic phase, the systolic phase has a constant duration (200 ms approximately) independent of heart rate and is less sensitive to arrhythmia. Finally, image acquisition during the systolic phase results in a lower contrast dose in the left ventricle and thus dark-rim artifacts (Motwani et al. 2012, 2014; Caruso et al. 2016; Rossi et al. 2014).

4.2 Issues and Requirements Specific to MRI

4.2.1 Sequence

Contrast agent free perfusion MRI techniques such as arterial spin labeling or blood oxygen level-dependent imaging remain currently reserved for research. In practice, the currently most used sequences are T1-weighted sequences to take advantage of the T1-shortening effect of gadolinium chelate bolus passing through the hyperemic myocardial vasculature. Different types of readouts can be chosen to optimally capture myocardial perfusion, including echoplanar, gradient echo, and steady-state free precession (Kellman and Arai 2007). While pulse sequences for perfusion assessment can vary in terms of readout and in terms of acceleration, all are acceptable as long as they meet the following characteristics: high spatial resolution (1.2–1.5 × 1.2–1.5 mm), a sufficient temporal resolution to acquire each stack of images every 1–2 heartbeats, enough coverage to acquire 3–5 slices over the left ventricle per heartbeat, and a high dynamic signal response to ensure a minimal signal increase of 250–300% over pre-contrast baseline tissue signal (van Assen et al. 2020; Schulz-Menger et al. 2020).

4.2.2 Field Strength

Most of the MRI perfusion examinations are performed using either 1.5 or 3.0 Tesla (T) systems, which have respective strengths and weaknesses. While 3T can provide higher signal-to-noise and contrast-to-noise ratios, it is also associated with more magnetic field ($B1$ and $B0$) inhomogeneities rendering the 3T approach more susceptible to artifacts hampering the analysis of perfusion defects. The use of 3T systems also results in a quadruple increase in RF power absorption, which impedes the application of some of the 1.5T perfusion sequences (Ferreira et al. 2013). Lastly, at 3T, the magnetohydrodynamic distortion of the ECG signal is increased, resulting in more difficulties with triggering, leading to an increase in cardiac motion artifacts.

4.3 Issues and Requirements Specific to CT

4.3.1 Order of Acquisition of Angiography and Perfusion

In most cases, CT perfusion is performed in association with coronary CT angiography (CCTA) that may require administration of beta-blockers to lower the heart rate to optimize image quality (Ghekiere et al. 2017). The use of beta-blockers and sublingual nitrates may have a negative effect on the detection of myocardial ischemia by increasing the diastolic perfusion time (Zoghbi et al. 2008). These constraints and the likelihood of CAD determine the sequences of acquisition of the respective CCTA and perfusion CT examinations. In patients with a high probability for or known CAD or in patients with stents or bypasses, myocardial ischemia is deemed likely. Therefore, functional evaluation is more important than anatomical evaluation. Thus, stress CT perfusion imaging should be performed first, eliminating the effect of contrast contamination and the suppressing effect of beta-blockers and nitroglycerin on myocardial ischemia (Assen et al. 2020; Zoghbi et al. 2008; Machecourt et al. 1994). In patients with a low to intermediate probability for CAD, it is preferable to start with CCTA to avoid unneeded CT perfusion testing in case of no obstructive CAD. An important factor for successful multi-acquisition imaging is to allow sufficient time between each examination to allow clearance of both the contrast agent and the stressor agent for the subsequent acquisition.

4.3.2 Static Versus Dynamic Myocardial Perfusion

There are currently two main methods of CT myocardial perfusion imaging (MPI), namely, static (sMPI) and dynamic (dMPI). sMPI, the most researched technique, consists of a single electrocardiogram (ECG)-gated, iodinated contrast-enhanced CT acquisition of the heart. sMPI can be performed using either single- or dual-energy (SECT or DECT) settings. sMPI imaging indirectly evaluates myocardial perfusion by showing the distribution of contrast (SECT) or iodine concentrations (DECT) throughout the myocardium at a *single* time point. Therefore, scan timing is an important factor. Acquisition should be timed to coincide with the early arterial phase, at the peak of the tissue contrast enhancement. Acquiring the images too early will lead to the presence of coronary artery enhancement without myocardial enhancement, while acquiring the images too late will decrease the enhancement differences between diseased and normal myocardium. The timing of the peak can be estimated using a test bolus or bolus tracking technique, with optimal time delays for subsequent sMPI varying between 2 and 4 s, depending on the measurement location (ascending or descending aorta) of the test bolus and on the enhancement threshold (150 or 250 HU) triggering the acquisition (Assen et al. 2020; Pelgrim et al. 2017).

dMPI is done through acquisition of multiple consecutive volumes over the needed time to cover the entire myocardial in- and outflow of contrast medium. dMPI can be performed by using rest- and stress-phase acquisitions to discriminate myocardial ischemia from infarction. Ischemic defects are only present on stress images, while infarcted defects are found on both rest and stress images. Whereas for sMPI the rest-phase acquisition is similar to the CCTA and can be performed using the standard CCTA protocol (Assen et al. 2020), with dMPI, CCTA must be acquired separately due to the dynamic nature of the whole acquisition. As performing rest and stress acquisitions in a dynamic fashion results in high radiation doses, several studies with dMPI report only a stress acquisition.

4.3.3 Radiation Dose

sMPI can be performed at a radiation dose similar to that of CCTA that ranges between 2 and 9 mSv for combined rest-stress examinations (Pelgrim et al. 2015; Varga-Szemes et al. 2015; Williams and Newby 2016). DECT imaging from a dual source and that from SECT are not statistically different at 120 kV (Henzler et al. 2012). The radiation dose of dMPI is obviously higher than that of sMPI due to the higher number of acquisitions. The reported doses of dMPI range between 5 and 13 mSv (Assen et al. 2020; Caruso et al. 2016; Williams and Newby 2016), with recent studies done with newer scanners reporting doses as low as 5–9 mSv (Pontone et al. 2019a; Coenen et al. 2017). dMPI radiation doses are expected to drop further with new techniques requiring only a limited number of optimally timed acquisitions including the one that could be used for CCTA (Hubbard et al. 2019). Radiation exposure can be reduced by using lower kV levels (100 kV instead of 120 kV) while maintaining optimal image quality in high-end systems. Additionally, some manufacturers offer the use of a tin (Sn) filter to block low-energy photons resulting in a dose reduction and optimized image quality at the interface between soft tissue and air while also reducing beam-hardening effects.

5 Data Analysis

Assessment of myocardial perfusion can be performed qualitatively, semiquantitatively, or quantitatively. Qualitative analysis refers to visual detection of inducible myocardial perfusion defects (low signal intensity or density) distal to a coronary stenosis. Myocardial perfusion can be assessed on a segment, territory, or patient basis. Assessing whether a patient has myocardial ischemia determines the need for revascularization. For this reason, per-patient analysis is clinically the most important, whereas segment and territory analysis is mostly used for communication or research. The 16-segment American Heart Association model is recommended for segmental analysis (Cerqueira et al. 2002). This segmentation uses three imaging slices at basal, mid-cavity, and apical level. The basal and mid-cavity slices are each divided into six equal segments, whereas the apical slice is divided into four equal segments. The apex (segment 17) is often not taken into account for perfusion analysis because the limited scan width of most scanners does not allow the apex to be imaged on MRI (Cerqueira et al. 2002). Analysis of vessel territories is based on a three-vessel division, namely, the right coronary artery (RCA) and both the left anterior descending (LAD) and circumflex (LCx) arteries' territories. Perfusion parameters are calculated per segment, after which multiple segments are averaged to represent a territory. Segments 1, 2, 7, 8, 13, and 14 are assigned to the LAD; segments 3, 4, 9, 10, and 15 are assigned to RCA; and segments 5, 6, 11, 12, and 16 are generally assigned to the LCx, depending on coronary dominance and anatomic variations (Klocke et al. 2003). Segmental and territory analyses can be additionally used to compare different methods that analyze CAD severity.

5.1 Artifacts and Qualitative Analyses

Perfusion analyses may be complicated by the presence of imaging artifacts. Artifacts are often easily recognizable upon proper analysis. Motion artifacts caused by mis-triggering or respiratory or non-respiratory patient motion are frequent and common to both CT and MRI. Other frequent artifacts specific to MRI include wraparound artifacts that occur from phase undersampling, whereas insufficient spatial resolution typically manifests as dark subendocardial zones during the contrast first pass. These artifacts typically appear in subjects with thin myocardial walls (Kwong et al. 2019), in the phase-encoding direction and last for a few images only (Nchimi et al. 2014a; Ferreira et al. 2013). While cumbersome, this "dark-rim" artifact (Gibbs ringing artifact) is becoming less of a concern with advances in MRI hardware and software. As all artifacts can impede or prevent myocardial perfusion assessment, the easiest way to limit their presence on MRI is to run "testing" sequences without contrast medium, to identify and fix artifacts on MRI before proceeding to the true hyperemic perfusion acquisition (Nchimi et al. 2014b).

For consistent and reproducible reading, standardized windowing and leveling are important. A combined analysis of stress perfusion and late gadolinium enhancement (LGE) images should always be performed when assessing inducible perfusion defects. First, LGE images are evaluated to discriminate scars and viable myocardium. In a second step, only viable segments are considered for further evaluation. A perfusion defect is most commonly defined as low-enhancing myocardial segment including at least the subendocardium that lasts for ≥6 heart beats (≥3 frames if the slice is acquired every other heartbeat) and involves ≥1/3 of the LV wall thickness (i.e., >1 pixel) (Fig. 3). Hypo-enhanced areas that do not meet these criteria are most likely artifacts, scars, or noncoronary myocardial disease (van Assen et al. 2020).

For MRI, the "splenic switch-off sign" is a useful marker of the maximal vasodilatation response after adenosine administration, detecting splenic blood flow attenuation during stress perfusion (spleen appears dark). An absent splenic switch-off represents a failure of the stressor to induce maximal vasodilatation and thus a risk for false-negative ischemia testing (Manisty et al. 2015).

For CT interpretation, the biggest issues are beam-hardening artifacts. Beam hardening is a well-known artifact caused by high-density objects that absorb the lower energy photons from the X-ray source. Beam-hardening artifacts lead to hypo-enhanced areas and can be misinterpreted as false-positive perfusion defects. This misinterpretation most commonly occurs in areas close to high contrast concentrations. For example, the basal inferolateral wall, adjacent to the descending aorta and the left ventricle, is often affected by these artifacts (Patel et al. 2020). As a result, beam-hardening correction algorithms are emerging (Machida et al. 2015; Stenner et al. 2010; Rodriguez-Granillo et al. 2015).

It is recommended that the interpretation of CCTA and myocardial perfusion images is performed concomitantly. Software used for visual analysis requires at least the ability to facilitate all conventional reconstruction formats for CCTA analysis including axial and multiplanar reformations (MPRs), maximum intensity projections (MIPs), minimal intensity projections (MinIPs), and average projections. For the analysis of dMPI, a temporal representation of myocardial enhancement is required (Patel et al. 2020).

CT perfusion can be analyzed using both systolic and diastolic images, depending on acquisition parameters. Reviewing images at multiple phases increases confidence for the discrimination of artifacts and true perfusion defects. Images can be viewed in the standard orthogonal views—the short axis, vertical long axis, and horizontal long axis. As with MRI, windowing is an important step of visual analysis, and the following window levels are recommended: window width of 200–300 and level setting of 100–150 with an average slice thickness of 5–8 mm. Virtual monoenergetic images (VMIs) can be created from DECT sMPI. DECT offers the advantages of reconstruction at multiple energy levels by using different percentages of the low and high energy data. Low-energy reconstruction (e.g., below 80 kV) will lead to an increase in contrast attenuation exceeding the increase in noise level. These images can be used to assess patients who cannot receive the normal dose of contrast agent or when the contrast bolus

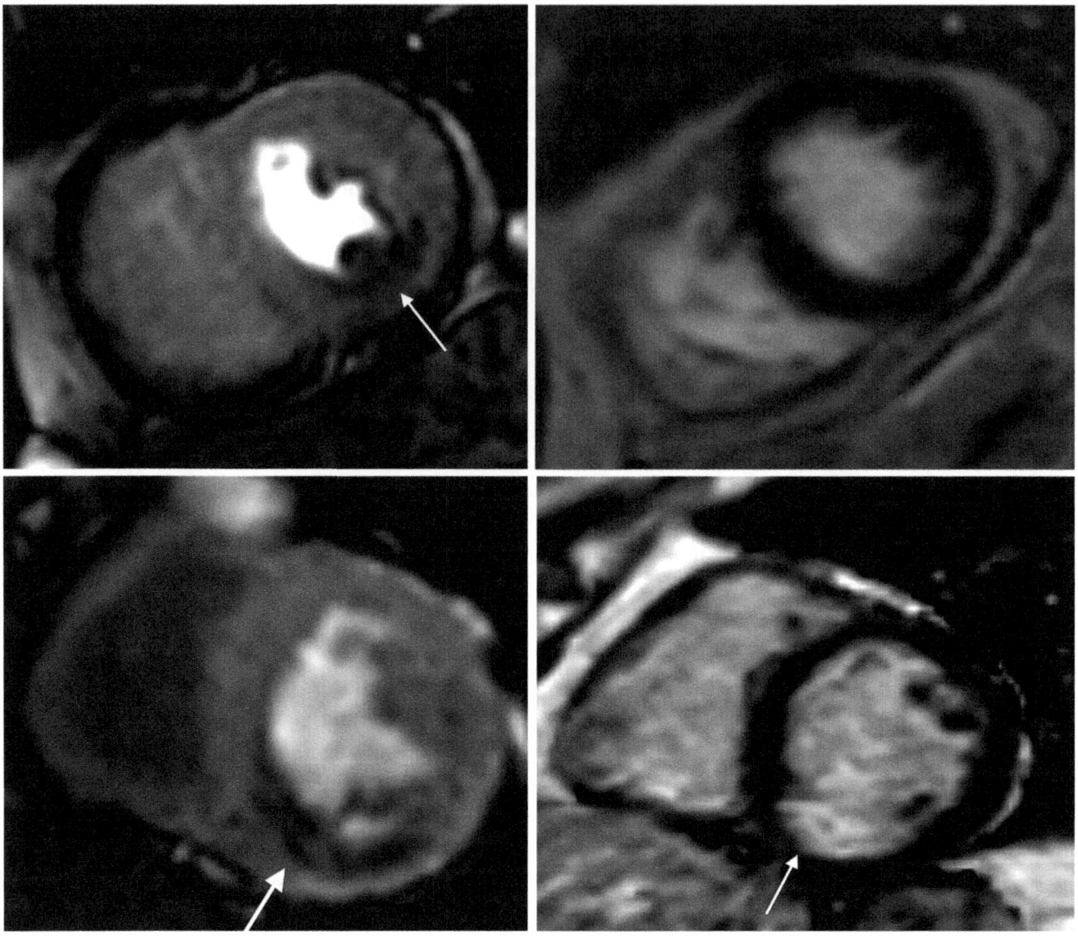

Fig. 3 Visual interpretation of myocardial perfusion MRI. The top row is an example of ischemic perfusion defect, where the early enhancement image at stress shows a hypo-enhancing segment in the inferior LV wall (white arrow), whereas the late gadolinium enhancement (LGE) image at the same level is normal (right image). The bottom row shows an infarct-related perfusion defect (arrow) on both stress perfusion (left image, hypo-enhancing tissue) and LGE (right image, hyper-enhancing tissue with a subendocardial basis)

is suboptimal (Rogers et al. 2010; Beeres et al. 2016). High-energy reconstructions (e.g., 110 kV and higher) can be used to reduce blooming artifacts or metal artifacts, enhancing the ability to analyze severely calcified plaques or stents (Albrecht et al. 2016; Secchi et al. 2015).

5.2 Quantitative and Semiquantitative Analysis

For quantitative and semiquantitative assessment, the contrast medium kinetics during the first pass of a bolus is a function of two time-intensity curves, namely, the tissue attenuation curve (TAC) which describes the concentration of contrast medium in the myocardium over time and the arterial input function (AIF) which describes the concentration of contrast medium in the supplying artery (the aorta or the left ventricle) over the same timescale as the TAC. Considering that the contrast media used for MRI (gadolinium chelate) and CT (iodine) behaves according to the same kinetic principles, the same approach can be used on both techniques (Ingrisch and Sourbron 2013; Pelgrim et al. 2016). Quantitative perfusion can be divided into two phases. First, the signal-time curves (AIF and TAC) should be transformed into contrast concentration-time curves (Ingrisch and Sourbron 2013; George et al. 2007). This conversion step is easier on CT as compared to MRI, as the relationship between Hounsfield unit value and iodine concentration is linear (George et al. 2007), whereas on MRI, there is an effect of signal saturation with higher concentrations of gadolinium (Utz et al. 2007; Hsu et al. 2008). On MRI, the contrast dose required for qualitative analyses should be reduced by more than half when performing quantitative analysis to avoid saturation. Dual-bolus techniques and, in particular, dual-pulse sequence approach help solving this issue by providing lookup tables taking into account the specific pulse sequence features and contrast medium types and doses (Coenen et al. 2017; Hubbard et al. 2019). In a second step, the myocardial perfusion is estimated from the interdependence of these time-concentration curves where contrast medium concentration in the myocardium over time is related to that in the supplying artery and an impulse response function (IRF) (Fig. 4) via the following generic equation (Assen et al. 2020; Ishida et al. 2016; Ingrisch and Sourbron 2013; Pelgrim et al. 2016):

$$\mathrm{TAC}(t) = \mathrm{MBF} * \mathrm{AIF}(t) \otimes \mathrm{IRF}(t) \quad (1)$$

where TAC(t) is the function of the tissue concentration curve over time, MBF is the myocardial blood flow, AIF(t) is the function of the arterial input function, and IRF(t) is the impulse response function over time. It is useful to consider the arterial input as a sequence of impulses whose amplitudes follow that of the observed arterial input. Each of these impulses generates a corresponding impulse response in the myocardium that is scaled and delayed according to the corresponding arterial impulse. IRF thus represents the residue function (i.e., the amount of the tracer decaying from the tissue for each impulse). When IRF(t) is known, the TAC can be obtained as a summation of adjusted IRFs from each impulse in a mathematical operation called convolution integral, represented in Eq. (1) by ⊗. Herein, AIF and TAC are measured from the perfusion images, whereas IRF(t) is the unknown parameter, which implies to reverse the above process by an operation called deconvolution. Once determined, IRF(t) leads to estimates of myocardial perfusion via model-independent approaches where the area under IRF(t) curve represents the mean transit time. However, the main issue with a deconvolution integral approach is that in contrast to forward processes like convolution, deconvolution cannot give a unique solution because there are multiple IRF(t) estimations possible that would result in the same TAC(t) or even a better approximation of the TAC(t). This problem is solved in model-dependent deconvolution by determining a generic model to represent the IRF(t) and setting predefined boundaries for the estimated parameters describing this model (Assen et al. 2020). In this method, a tracer kinetic model is assumed to represent IRF(t), after which the model parameters can be optimized to best fit Eq. (1) to the measured TAC data (Ingrisch and Sourbron 2013; Pelgrim et al. 2016). With these models, observing a fountain helps understanding the relation between the maximal impulse response (or residue) and MBF. Indeed, water describes a mathematical function (flow = $F(t)$) as it flows from a fountain until its landing point (Fig. 5). If $F(t)$ is known, solving its equation at $t = 0$ gives the initial flow. MBF is thus the solution of the IRF(t) equation when the t is zero. Obviously, noise in either the AIF or the TAC, caused for example by imaging artifacts, can influence the model optimization and result in an unstable solution for IRF(t) and incorrect MBF values (Gamel et al. 1973). Similarly, reducing artifacts is therefore an important challenge for quantitative analyses.

Because of the above-described technical and theoretical challenges, the quantitative approaches are used to approach the MBF using CT, MRI, and PET in experimental settings, whereas visual analyses make the bulk of the clinical value of these examinations. When the visual analysis is doubtful or when a quick and broadly available quantification method of the perfusion is needed, semiquantitative parameters can be derived from the TAC curves. These parameters include the peak enhancement, time to peak, and area under the curve of the TAC (Fig. 4). From these semiquantitative parameters,

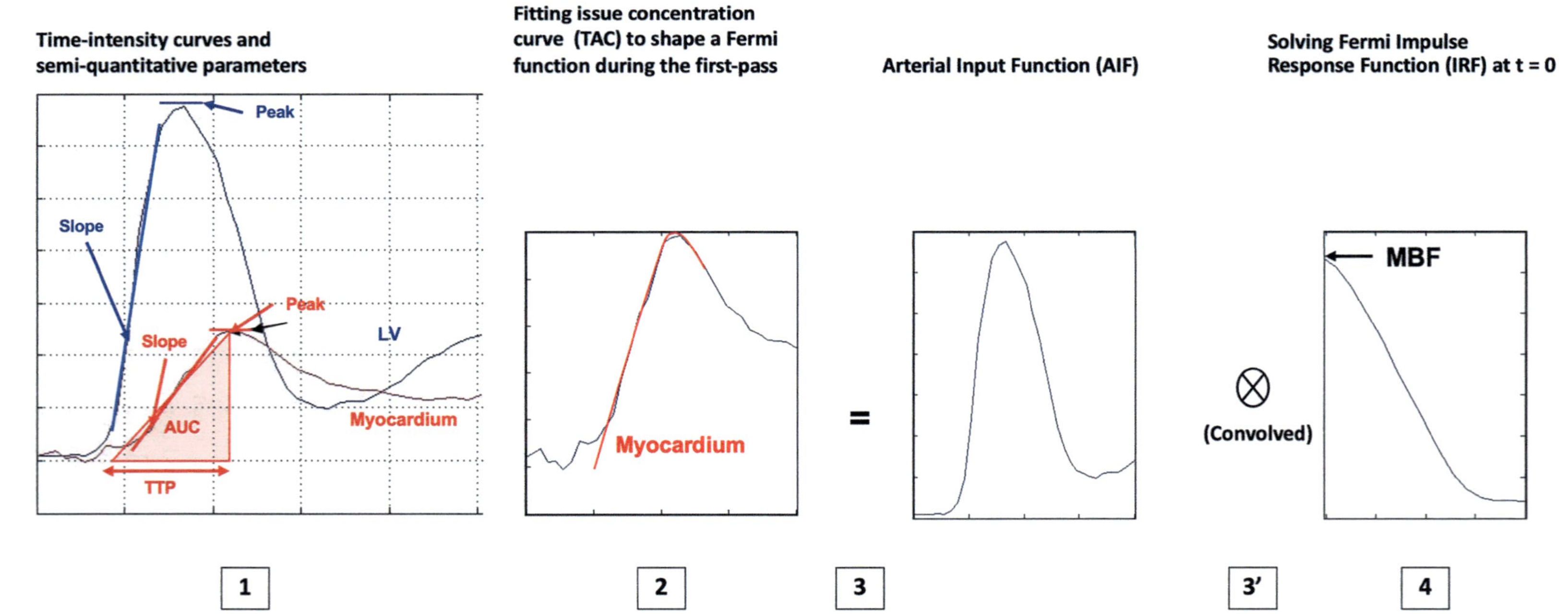

Fig. 4 Main steps for quantitative assessment of myocardial blood flow (MBF) from dynamic imaging. The left graph (1) displays the raw time-signal curves of the myocardium and the left ventricle cavity during the pass of a bolus of contrast, along with semiquantitative parameters defining these curves. After translation of these curves in time concentration, the first-pass myocardial curve is fitted to a function in a model-based approach (most often a Fermi function) (2) and used along with the left ventricle cavity curve (3) over the same time to fit the best impulse function (3′) by deconvolution. The solution at $t = 0$ of the impulse function gives the myocardial blood flow (MBF) (4)

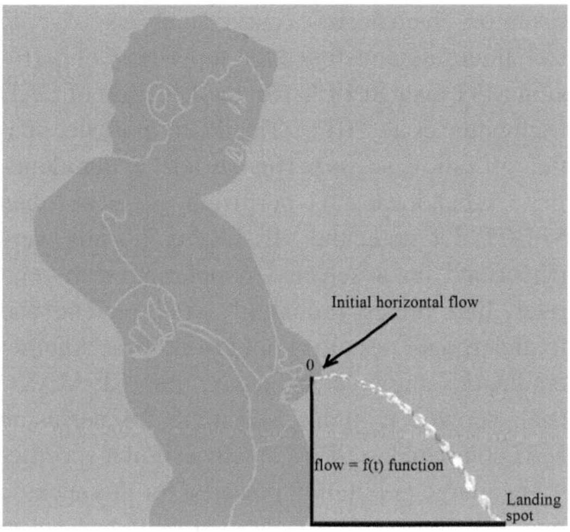

Fig. 5 The initial value of a decay function. In a famous Brussels water fountain (Manneken Pis), the water jet describes a mathematical function (flow = $F(t)$) as it flows until its landing point, which is characterized by a progressive decay of its horizontal value. If $F(t)$ is known, solving its equation at $t = 0$ would determine the initial horizontal flow

the upslope is the most commonly used in semiquantitative analysis of myocardial perfusion (Assen et al. 2020; Ingrisch and Sourbron 2013; Pelgrim et al. 2016) (Table 1).

Stress MBF estimates from quantitative and semiquantitative analyses can be interpreted as lone values or divided by the resting values to represent the CFR. In practice, quantitative and semiquantitative perfusion MRI considers stress-only or stress-to-rest maximum upslopes (myocardial perfusion reserve) for the diagnosis of inducible perfusion defects. Other reported methods of semiquantitative analysis consist of evaluating the transmural flow gradient (i.e., the ratio between subendocardial and subepicardial MBF) (Chiribiri et al. 2013) and the relative CFR or relative perfusion index, which is similar to the FFR principle (i.e., the ratio of stress maximum upslope in an artery with stenosis to stress maximum upslope in a normally perfused myocardial segment) (Ghekiere et al. 2019; Yang et al. 2020).

Table 1 Step-by-step buildup of semiquantitative myocardial perfusion parameters based on the slope of the myocardial time-tissue concentration curve (TAC)

Problem	Solution	Parameter	Comparator
Raw myocardial enhancement upslope depends on sampling resolution	Improve sampling's temporal resolution	NA	NA
Raw myocardial enhancement upslope depends on the arterial input	Divide by the arterial input function (i.e., the ventricular enhancement upslope)	Normalized myocardial enhancement upslope (SL)	NA
Myocardial enhancement upslope is prone to averaging errors	Change to maximal enhancement upslope	Max enhancement slope (SL_{MAX})	MBF
Stress and rest enhancement kinetics are interdependent	Compare stress to rest values	Stress/rest ratio (${}^{S}SL_{MAX}/{}^{R}SL_{MAX}$)	CFR
Myocardial vasculature is inhomogeneous	Compare to "normal control" values	Ratio (stress SL_{MAX} (1)/stress SL_{MAX} (2))	rCFR
There is a myocardial transmural flow gradient	Compare endocardial and epicardial values	TPI ratio (${}^{END}SL_{MAX}/{}^{EPI}SL_{MAX}$)	None

MBF myocardial blood flow, *CFR* coronary flow reserve, *rCFR* relative CFR, *END* endocardium, *EPI* epicardium, *R* rest, *S* stress, *NA* not applicable. Similar approaches, with slightly different inconveniences and adjustments, can be proposed with other components of the myocardial TAC than slope (e.g., time to peak, peak, area under the curve) (Fig. 4)

6 Results

6.1 Clinical Interest

Noninvasive stress imaging for the detection of myocardial ischemia can be performed during pharmacological vasodilatation in patients who cannot exercise to an adequate cardiac workload (>85% of target heart rate). A significant number of patients (at least 25% of outpatients and 50% of hospitalization patients) are unable or contraindicated to exercise because of physical limitations or baseline ECG abnormalities, such as left bundle branch block, pre-excitation syndromes, repolarization abnormalities due to left ventricle hypertrophy, and digoxin use (Klocke et al. 2003). In these patients, non-exercise stress testing with pharmacologic agents (e.g., dipyridamole, adenosine, regadenoson, dobutamine, or one of their derivates) is the optimal examination (Cury et al. 2014). Compared with exercise testing, a similar increased coronary flow response during maximal vasodilation with pharmacologic agents can be obtained (Duncker and Bache 2008).

6.2 Diagnostic Value

6.2.1 Perfusion MRI

One of the earliest multislice approach studies on stress perfusion MRI in an unselected population showed a sensitivity and specificity of 0.91 and 0.94 for the detection of CAD defined by PET, and a sensitivity and specificity of 0.87 and 0.85 for the detection of CAD as defined by quantitative coronary angiography (QCA) (diameter stenosis >50%) (Schwitter et al. 2001). These results were an early indicator that perfusion MRI provides information about the ischemic burden and identifies patients with CAD, like other perfusion imaging modalities. The MR-IMPACT-II trial investigated the diagnostic performance of stress perfusion MRI and SPECT (which is still one of the most used perfusion modalities, especially in the United States) for the detection of CAD using CCA as the reference standard. The receiver-operator characteristic curve analyses of both techniques demonstrated the superiority of perfusion MRI over SPECT for the detection of CAD (Schwitter et al. 2013). Thanks to a greater spatial resolution, stress perfusion MRI better identifies subendocardial perfusion defects than SPECT. Of note, the MR-IMPACT trials were performed on a selected population with relatively high pretest probability as all patients had to undergo all tests to avoid testing bias. Another landmark single-center study, the CE-MARC trial, showed a higher sensitivity of perfusion MRI compared to SPECT with a similar specificity in a large population powered for this specific purpose (Greenwood et al. 2012). Based on an anatomical standard of reference (QCA) for diagnosing significant obstructive CAD, an initial meta-analysis evaluating adenosine perfusion MRI reported a sensitivity of 0.90 and a specificity 0.81 (Hamon et al. 2010).

Several meta-analyses evaluated the diagnostic accuracy of stress perfusion MRI using FFR, a relative perfusion index, as gold standard, with respective sensitivities and specificities ranging between 0.89–0.90 and 0.85–0.87 on a patient level (Li et al. 2014; Desai and Jha 2013; Takx et al. 2015) (Table 2). The prospective PACIFIC II study, including patients with prior myocardial infarction and/or PCI, and new symptoms of ischemic CAD, compared diagnostic accuracy of qualitative perfusion MRI, ^{99m}Tc-tetrofosmin SPECT, and [^{15}O]H_2O PET to identify FFR $\leq$0.80 and FFR <0.75 coronary stenoses with diagnostic accuracy for MRI of 64% and 71%, respectively (Driessen et al. 2022). The added value of noninvasive imaging in this high-risk population is questionable and may be explained by the discordances observed between FFR and the qualitative evaluation of noninvasive imaging methods.

Besides patient selection, part of the heterogeneity of the diagnostic value of stress perfusion MRI comes from the standard of reference. On the one hand, there is a fundamental difference between the morphologic appearance of a coronary stenosis and its hemodynamic repercussions. On the other hand, there is an intrinsic

Table 2 Diagnostic value of perfusion MR to diagnose the functional significance of coronary artery stenoses

Study	Pretest	Sensitivity	Specificity	Gold standard
Schwitter (2001)—(Schwitter et al. 2001)	Suspected CAD referred for ICA	91%	94%	PET
		87%	85%	QCA: diameter stenosis >50%
Schwitter (2013)—MR-IMPACT-II (Schwitter et al. 2013)	High pretest probability	67%	61%	ICA: diameter stenosis ≥50%
Greenwoord (2012)—CE-MARC (Greenwood et al. 2012)	Suspected angina pectoris and at least one cardiovascular risk factor	86.5% (81.8–90.1)	83.4% (79.5–86.7)	ICA: diameter stenosis ≥50%
Hammon (2010)—Meta-analysis (Hamon et al. 2010)	Unselected population	90% (88–91)	81% (78–83)	QCA: diameter stenosis >50% or >70%
Driessen (2022)—PACIFIC II (Driessen et al. 2022)	Prior myocardial infarct and/or PCI; symptoms of ischemic CAD	66% (56–75)	65% (49–74)	FFR ≤0.80 FFR ≤0.75
Li (2014)—Meta-analysis (Li et al. 2014)	No history of PCI or bypass graft surgery	90% (86–93)	87% (82–90)	FFR ≤0.75 or FFR ≤0.80
Dessai (2013)—Meta-analysis (Desai and Jha 2013)	Stable CAD	89.1% (84–93)	84.9% (76.6–91.1)	FFR <0.75 or FFR <0.80
Takx (2015)—Meta-analysis (Takx et al. 2015)	Patients with suspected or known CAD	89% (86–92)	87% (83–90)	FFR ≤0.75 or FFR ≤0.80

95% confidence interval in parentheses, *PET* positron emission tomography, *ICA* invasive coronary angiography, *QCA* quantitative coronary angiography, *FFR* fractional flow reserve, *MR* magnetic resonance, *PCI* percutaneous coronary intervention, *CAD* coronary artery disease

difference between FFR, validated as a relative perfusion index (ratio of hyperemic flow pressure in a stenotic coronary artery to the hyperemic flow pressure in a normal coronary artery), and perfusion MRI quantitative and semiquantitative indices. In contrast to the FFR value, myocardial perfusion MRI may be affected not only by epicardial stenoses, but also by the influence of microvascular resistance and collateral flow. The relative myocardial perfusion index, similar to the FFR principle, was the best semiquantitative MRI perfusion parameter to predict FFR-defined inducible coronary ischemia (Ghekiere et al. 2019). As a result, the only meta-analysis that collected (semi-) quantitative perfusion MRI also found considerable heterogeneity of its diagnostic value (van Dijk et al. 2017b). While the FFR value remains the gold standard to define stenosis-specific ischemia and the most acknowledged determinant of cardiovascular events and survival (Zimmermann et al. 2015; De Bruyne et al. 2012), the current use of a 0.80 FFR cutoff value to determine the need for revascularization is debated (Johnson et al. 2014).

6.2.2 Perfusion CT

None of the other noninvasive perfusion imaging techniques allow simultaneous anatomical and functional evaluation of coronary artery disease (CAD) like CT does. Coronary CT angiography (CCTA) yields a very high sensitivity and negative predictive value for significant (>50% diameter reduction) CAD (Menke and Kowalski 2016; Yang et al. 2014). Myocardial perfusion CT adds important functional information to CCTA. The CORE320 study is the largest study to date with sMPI, including 381 patients and reporting an accuracy of 0.93, with respective sensitivity and specificity of 0.80 and 0.74 when using the combination of SPECT and CCA as reference (George et al. 2011, 2015; Rochitte et al. 2014; Magalhaes et al. 2015). Another multicenter study performed by Cury et al., who included 110 patients, investigated the accuracy of static perfusion CT compared to SPECT and showed a slightly higher sensitivity and specificity of 0.90 and 0.84 with an overall accuracy of 0.87 (Cury et al. 2015). Meta-analysis on static perfusion CT showed that the average sensitivity and specificity ranged between 0.75–0.84 and 0.78–0.95 for a variety of image protocols and reference standards used (Pelgrim et al. 2015; Tashakkor et al. 2012). A limited number of studies have been performed on the quantitative analysis of static perfusion CT using DECT. They showed that a rest acquisition is needed to discriminate between ischemic and infarcted myocardium (Delgado Sánchez-Gracián et al. 2016; van Assen et al. 2019a).

For dMPI, similar accuracies have been reported as with sMPI, with an average sensitivity and specificity ranging between 0.76–1.00 and 0.74–1.00, respectively, for inducible perfusion defects (Assen et al. 2020; Caruso et al. 2016; Pelgrim et al. 2015; Varga-Szemes et al. 2015; van Assen et al. 2019b) (Figs. 6 and 7). MBF threshold to discriminate ischemic from normal myocardium ranged between 75 and 136 mL/min/100 g (Assen et al. 2020; Caruso et al. 2016; Pelgrim et al. 2015; Varga-Szemes et al. 2015; van Assen et al. 2019b). Table 3 shows a selection of studies using ICA/FFR as reference standard for static dual- and single-energy perfusion and dynamic CT perfusion, with corresponding sensitivities and specificities.

6.3 Prognostic Value and Cost-Effectiveness

Reliable information on patient outcome after testing is needed for proper CAD management. There is growing evidence of the prognostic power of stress perfusion MRI. Recently, the large multicenter MR-INFORM study compared stress perfusion MRI and catheter FFR in 918 patients with stable angina and risk factors for CAD. Stress perfusion MRI was associated with

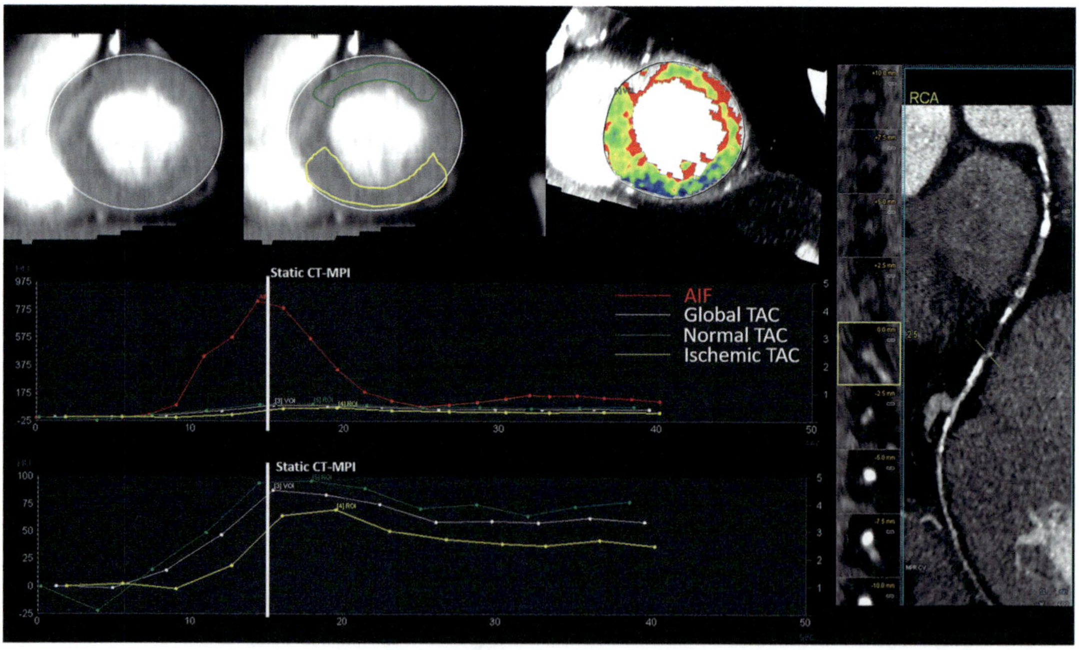

Fig. 6 Overview of myocardial CT perfusion (MPI) principles in a patient with severe right coronary artery (RCA) disease (right panel). The upper graph shows the range of dynamic MPI being acquired over multiple timepoints, while the white vertical line indicates the approximation of the static MPI acquisition. The top left image shows a mid-ventricular short-axis slice with the ROIs used to create the graphs, while the third image shows the dynamic MPI. Top middle images represent myocardial blood flow (MBF) maps (red color represents high values, whereas blue color represents low values) in four-chamber and short-axis planes, indicating a perfusion defect in the inferior wall

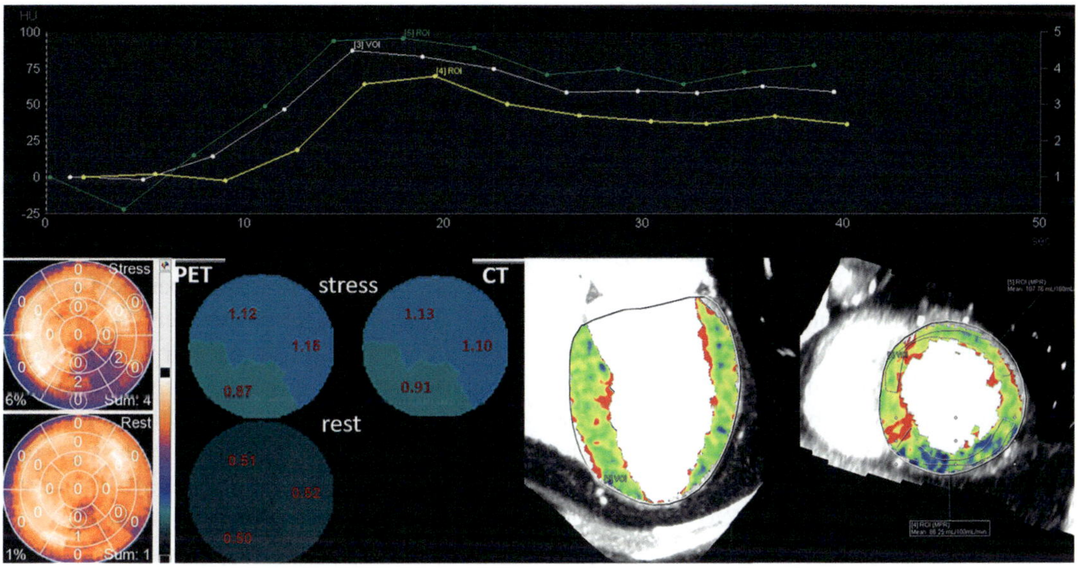

Fig. 7 Comparison of myocardial perfusion CT (MPI) and positron emission tomography (PET) in a patient with severe right coronary artery (RCA) disease (right panel). The top graph shows the tissue curves of normal (green) and ischemic myocardium (yellow); the corresponding myocardial blood flow (MBF) maps are provided for PET (left) and dynamic MPI (right) (red color represents high values, whereas blue color represents low values). The middle image of the bottom row displays the quantitative MBF from both the PET (rest and stress) and CT (stress) images, showing a high degree of similarity

Table 3 Diagnostic value of perfusion CT to diagnose the functional significance of coronary artery stenoses using ICA/FFR as standard (selection)

Study first author and approach to CT perfusion	Pretest	Sensitivity	Specificity	Gold standard
Rossi (2017)—Dynamic (Rossi et al. 2017)	Stable angina patients	89% (76–96)	73% (59–83)	ICA/FFR ≤0.80
Pontone (2019)—Dynamic (Pontone et al. 2019a)	Symptomatic patients scheduled for ICA	73% (63–83)	86% (81–91)	ICA/FFR
Nishiyama (2019)—Dynamic (Nishiyama et al. 2019)	Effort or resting angina, relief of symptoms with nitroglycerin administration, or multiple coronary risk factors	83% (68–98)	93% (88–98)	ICA/FFR ≤0.75
Bettencourt (2013)—Static (Bettencourt et al. 2013)	Intermediate to high pretest probability	71% (62–79)	90% (87–92)	ICA/FFR ≤0.80
Pontone (2018)—Static (Pontone et al. 2019b)	Intermediate to high-risk pretest probability	92% (87–97)	95% (92–97)	ICA/FFR
Ko (2012)—Dual-energy static (Ko et al. 2012)	Intermediate to high-risk pretest probability	89%	74%	ICA

95% confidence interval in parentheses, *ICA* invasive coronary angiography, *FFR* fractional flow reserve, *CAD* coronary artery disease

a lower incidence of revascularization than FFR and was equivalent to FFR in predicting major adverse cardiac events (Nagel et al. 2019). In 9404 patients, obtained by pooling studies including >1000 patients, the mean event rate (for cardiac death and nonfatal myocardial infarction) in the patients with a normal stress perfusion MRI is as low as 0.68%/year (Kwong et al. 2019;

Vincenti et al. 2017; Moschetti et al. 2016; Krittayaphong et al. 2011; Buckert et al. 2013). Strong evidence, therefore, is available that stress perfusion MRI not only excludes prognostically relevant CAD but also identifies patients which can be safely deferred from further testing. On the other hand, an abnormal stress perfusion was strongly associated with patient mortality in a multicenter study of 9151 patients followed up for up to 10 years (Heitner et al. 2019).

Comparisons of stress perfusion MRI with several alternative noninvasive methods repeatedly demonstrated a better cost-effectiveness (Walker et al. 2013; Pletscher et al. 2016). The EuroCMR-registry cost minimization study on 3647 patients with suspected CAD (59 centers from 18 countries) compared an initial stress perfusion MRI, with follow-up CCA only in case of ischemia, with the combined use of CCA and FFR. It showed that the use of stress perfusion MRI reduced costs by 14–34% in the German, UK, Swiss, and US contexts. Costs were reduced even more (59–71%) compared to the use of CCA alone (Moschetti et al. 2016).

For stress CT perfusion, there is limited information about the prognostic value. There are a few studies showing that MPI can add additional value not only for the diagnosis of ischemia but also in the prognosis of adverse cardiac events. A study by Meinel et al. showed in 144 patients that myocardial perfusion CT has incremental predictive value over clinical risk factors and detection of coronary artery stenosis with CCTA for the prediction of MACE using qualitative analysis of dynamic CT-MPI images (Meinel et al. 2017a). Another study by Meinel et al. also showed that global quantification of left ventricular MBF using dMPI may have incremental predictive value for future MACE over clinical risk factors and assessment of stenosis on CCTA (Meinel et al. 2017b). This was confirmed by van Assen et al. who showed that CT-MBF has the highest prognostic value as compared to CCTA and CT-FFR. In multivariate analysis, including clinical factors, CCTA, CT-FFR, and CT-MBF, only CT-MBF significantly contributed to the risk of MACE (HR 10.1), unlike CCTA (HR 1.2) and CT-FFR (HR 2.2) (van Assen et al. 2019b). A study by Nakamura confirmed that CT-MBF has an incremental prognostic value over CCTA. The addition of dynamic CTP to CCTA allows improved risk stratification of patients with CCTA-detected stenosis (Nakamura et al. 2019). Another more recent study from 2021 using a static CT-MPI and CCTA combination compared to SPECT among patients presenting with acute chest pain to the emergency department showed that CT-MBF/CCTA both shorten the length of stay by 28% (20 h [IQR: 16, 37] vs. 30 h [IQR: 19, 44.5]) and the direct costs by 44% ($1750 [IQR: 1474, 2114] vs. $2837 [IQR: 2491, 3554]) (Grandhi et al. 2021). However, the lack of standardized clinical practice for CT-MBF makes it difficult to perform accurate cost analysis.

The CTP-PRO study, impact of stress Cardiac computed Tomography myocardial Perfusion on downstream resources and PROgnosis in patients with suspected or known coronary artery disease, is a multicenter international study that should provide more information on both cost-effectiveness and prognostication of CT-MPI in a prospective trial aiming to include 2000 patients from multiple countries (Pontone et al. 2019c).

7 Current Recommendations

The 2019 ESC guidelines state that unless obstructive CAD can be excluded based on clinical evaluation alone, either noninvasive functional testing or anatomical CCTA evaluation may be used to rule out or establish CAD (Saraste and Knuuti 2020). The choice of noninvasive test modality for this purpose is based on the pretest probability (PTP) of the test's performance in ruling in or ruling out obstructive CAD, patient characteristics, local expertise, and availability of the test, as stated in the ESC guidelines (Saraste and Knuuti 2020). The PTP for noninvasive imaging testing is lowered in comparison with past, recommending testing for PTP >15%, and for PTP of 5–15% if additional "modulators of risk" are present such as classical risk factors, but also changes on resting ECG (Q waves, ST-T alterations), left ventricular dysfunction, pathological stress ECG, and coronary calcifications on CT (if performed) (van Assen et al. 2020; Saraste and Knuuti 2020).

Perfusion MRI is recommended as a class I indication (evidence level B). Perfusion MRI is also recommended as a class I, if CCTA has shown CAD of uncertain functional significance or is nondiagnostic (van Assen et al. 2020; Saraste and Knuuti 2020; Knuuti et al. 2020). CT perfusion is currently not specifically mentioned in the guidelines but could be categorized under additional functional testing.

8 Conclusion

Myocardial perfusion imaging of the heart represents an important advancement in cardiac diagnostics, offering valuable functional insights beyond traditional morphological imaging. This technique can be applied using both CT and MR imaging modalities, making it versatile and widely applicable. Notably, stress perfusion imaging extends its utility by providing real-life situational data, aiding in the assessment of cardiac function under duress. Presently, qualitative assessment remains the predominant approach in clinical practice, but the potential for further expansion of quantitative evaluation of perfusion defects holds promise for the future. Ongoing advancements in software technology are poised to facilitate the quantitative analysis of perfusion data, further enhancing the diagnostic and prognostic capabilities of this imaging technique.

Disclaimer All measurements in this book have been obtained from peer-reviewed papers and guidelines from professional organizations, unless explicitly stated otherwise. While the authors, editors, and publisher have gone through a rigorous process to establish their correct reproduction from the original source, each measurement must be interpreted in the correct clinical context, this along with an accurate way of measurement, and taking into account all technical variables, this including follow-up exams with various equipment or software. Neither the authors, the editors, nor the publisher can accept any legal responsibility for any improper application or interpretation of these measurements as well as their potential consequences.

References

Al Jaroudi W, Iskandrian AE (2009) Regadenoson: a new myocardial stress agent. J Am Coll Cardiol 54(13):1123–1130

Albrecht MH, Scholtz JE, Hüsers K, Beeres M, Bucher AM, Kaup M et al (2016) Advanced image-based virtual monoenergetic dual-energy CT angiography of the abdomen: optimization of kiloelectron volt settings to improve image contrast. Eur Radiol 26(6):1863–1870

Amini M, Zayeri F, Salehi M (2021) Trend analysis of cardiovascular disease mortality, incidence, and mortality-to-incidence ratio: results from global burden of disease study 2017. BMC Public Health 21(1):401

Assen MV, Vonder M, Pelgrim GJ, Von Knebel Doeberitz PL, Vliegenthart R (2020) Computed tomography for myocardial characterization in ischemic heart disease: a state-of-the-art review. Eur Radiol Exp 4(1):36

Beeres M, Trommer J, Frellesen C, Nour-Eldin NE, Scholtz JE, Herrmann E et al (2016) Evaluation of different keV-settings in dual-energy CT angiography of the aorta using advanced image-based virtual monoenergetic imaging. Int J Cardiovasc Imaging 32(1):137–144

Bettencourt N, Chiribiri A, Schuster A, Ferreira N, Sampaio F, Pires-Morais G et al (2013) Direct comparison of cardiac magnetic resonance and multidetector computed tomography stress-rest perfusion imaging for detection of coronary artery disease. J Am Coll Cardiol 61(10):1099–1107

Bindschadler M, Modgil D, Branch KR, La Riviere PJ, Alessio AM (2014) Comparison of blood flow models and acquisitions for quantitative myocardial perfusion estimation from dynamic CT. Phys Med Biol 59(7):1533–1556

Brink HL, Dickerson JA, Stephens JA, Pickworth KK (2015) Comparison of the safety of adenosine and regadenoson in patients undergoing outpatient cardiac stress testing. Pharmacotherapy 35(12):1117–1123

Buckert D, Dewes P, Walcher T, Rottbauer W, Bernhardt P (2013) Intermediate-term prognostic value of reversible perfusion deficit diagnosed by adenosine CMR: a prospective follow-up study in a consecutive patient population. JACC Cardiovasc Imaging 6(1): 56–63

Caruso D, Eid M, Schoepf UJ, Jin KN, Varga-Szemes A, Tesche C et al (2016) Dynamic CT myocardial perfusion imaging. Eur J Radiol 85(10):1893–1899

Cerqueira MD, Weissman NJ, Dilsizian V, Jacobs AK, Kaul S, Laskey WK et al (2002) Standardized myocardial segmentation and nomenclature for tomographic imaging of the heart. A statement for healthcare professionals from the Cardiac Imaging Committee of the Council on Clinical Cardiology of the American Heart Association. Circulation 105(4):539–542

Chiribiri A, Hautvast GL, Lockie T, Schuster A, Bigalke B, Olivotti L et al (2013) Assessment of coronary artery stenosis severity and location: quantitative analysis of transmural perfusion gradients by high-resolution MRI versus FFR. JACC Cardiovasc Imaging 6(5):600–609

Coelho-Filho OR, Rickers C, Kwong RY, Jerosch-Herold M (2013) MR myocardial perfusion imaging. Radiology 266(3):701–715

Coenen A, Rossi A, Lubbers MM, Kurata A, Kono AK, Chelu RG et al (2017) Integrating CT myocardial perfusion and CT-FFR in the work-up of coronary artery disease. JACC Cardiovasc Imaging 10(7):760–770

Cury RC, Kitt TM, Feaheny K, Akin J, George RT (2014) Regadenoson-stress myocardial CT perfusion and single-photon emission CT: rationale, design, and acquisition methods of a prospective, multicenter, multivendor comparison. J Cardiovasc Comput Tomogr 8(1):2–12

Cury RC, Kitt TM, Feaheny K, Blankstein R, Ghoshhajra BB, Budoff MJ et al (2015) A randomized, multicenter, multivendor study of myocardial perfusion imaging with regadenoson CT perfusion vs single photon emission CT. J Cardiovasc Comput Tomogr 9(2):103–12.e1–2

De Bruyne B, Baudhuin T, Melin JA, Pijls NH, Sys SU, Bol A et al (1994) Coronary flow reserve calculated from pressure measurements in humans. Validation with positron emission tomography. Circulation 89(3):1013–1022

De Bruyne B, Pijls NH, Kalesan B, Barbato E, Tonino PA, Piroth Z et al (2012) Fractional flow reserve-guided PCI versus medical therapy in stable coronary disease. N Engl J Med 367(11):991–1001

Delgado Sánchez-Gracián C, Oca Pernas R, Trinidad López C, Santos Armentia E, Vaamonde Liste A, Vázquez Caamaño M, Tardáguila de la Fuente G (2016) Quantitative myocardial perfusion with stress dual-energy CT: iodine concentration differences between normal and ischemic or necrotic myocardium. Initial experience. Eur Radiol 26(9):3199–3207

Desai RR, Jha S (2013) Diagnostic performance of cardiac stress perfusion MRI in the detection of coronary artery disease using fractional flow reserve as the reference standard: a meta-analysis. AJR Am J Roentgenol 201(2):W245–W252

Dewey M, Siebes M, Kachelrieß M, Kofoed KF, Maurovich-Horvat P, Nikolaou K et al (2020) Clinical quantitative cardiac imaging for the assessment of myocardial ischaemia. Nat Rev Cardiol 17(7):427–450

Driessen RS, van Diemen PA, Raijmakers PG, Knuuti J, Maaniitty T, Underwood SR et al (2022) Functional stress imaging to predict abnormal coronary fractional flow reserve: the PACIFIC 2 study. Eur Heart J 43:3118

Duncker DJ, Bache RJ (2008) Regulation of coronary blood flow during exercise. Physiol Rev 88(3):1009–1086

Faulds D, Chrisp P, Buckley MM (1991) Adenosine. An evaluation of its use in cardiac diagnostic procedures, and in the treatment of paroxysmal supraventricular tachycardia. Drugs 41(4):596–624

Ferreira PF, Gatehouse PD, Mohiaddin RH, Firmin DN (2013) Cardiovascular magnetic resonance artefacts. J Cardiovasc Magn Reson 15(1):41

Flotats A, Knuuti J, Gutberlet M, Marcassa C, Bengel FM, Kaufmann PA et al (2011) Hybrid cardiac imaging: SPECT/CT and PET/CT. A joint position statement by the European Association of Nuclear Medicine (EANM), the European Society of Cardiac Radiology (ESCR) and the European Council of Nuclear Cardiology (ECNC). Eur J Nucl Med Mol Imaging 38(1):201–212

Gamel J, Rousseau WF, Katholi CR, Mesel E (1973) Pitfalls in digital computation of the impulse response of vascular beds from indicator-dilution curves. Circ Res 32(4):516–523

George RT, Jerosch-Herold M, Silva C, Kitagawa K, Bluemke DA, Lima JA, Lardo AC (2007) Quantification of myocardial perfusion using dynamic 64-detector computed tomography. Investig Radiol 42(12):815–822

George RT, Arbab-Zadeh A, Cerci RJ, Vavere AL, Kitagawa K, Dewey M et al (2011) Diagnostic performance of combined noninvasive coronary angiography and myocardial perfusion imaging using 320-MDCT: the CT angiography and perfusion methods of the CORE320 multicenter multinational diagnostic study. AJR Am J Roentgenol 197(4):829–837

George RT, Mehra VC, Chen MY, Kitagawa K, Arbab-Zadeh A, Miller JM et al (2015) Myocardial CT perfusion imaging and SPECT for the diagnosis of coronary artery disease: a head-to-head comparison from the CORE320 multicenter diagnostic performance study. Radiology 274(2):626

Ghekiere O, Salgado R, Buls N, Leiner T, Mancini I, Vanhoenacker P et al (2017) Image quality in coronary CT angiography: challenges and technical solutions. Br J Radiol 90(1072):20160567

Ghekiere O, Dacher JN, Dewilde W, Mancini I, Cools W, Vanhoenacker PK et al (2019) Value of relative myocardial perfusion at MRI for fractional flow reserve-defined ischemia: a pilot study. AJR Am J Roentgenol 212:1002

Götberg M, Christiansen EH, Gudmundsdottir IJ, Sandhall L, Danielewicz M, Jakobsen L et al (2017) Instantaneous wave-free ratio versus fractional flow reserve to guide PCI. N Engl J Med 376(19):1813–1823

Gould KL, Lipscomb K, Hamilton GW (1974) Physiologic basis for assessing critical coronary stenosis. Instantaneous flow response and regional distribution during coronary hyperemia as measures of coronary flow reserve. Am J Cardiol 33(1):87–94

Gould KL, Kirkeeide RL, Buchi M (1990) Coronary flow reserve as a physiologic measure of stenosis severity. J Am Coll Cardiol 15(2):459–474

Grandhi GR, Batlle JC, Maroules CD, Janowitz W, Peña CS, Ziffer JA et al (2021) Combined stress myocardial CT perfusion and coronary CT angiography as a feasible strategy among patients presenting with acute chest pain to the emergency department. J Cardiovasc Comput Tomogr 15(2):129–136

Greenwood JP, Maredia N, Younger JF, Brown JM, Nixon J, Everett CC et al (2012) Cardiovascular magnetic resonance and single-photon emission computed tomography for diagnosis of coronary heart disease (CE-MARC): a prospective trial. Lancet 379(9814):453–460

Hamon M, Fau G, Née G, Ehtisham J, Morello R, Hamon M (2010) Meta-analysis of the diagnostic performance of stress perfusion cardiovascular magnetic resonance for detection of coronary artery disease. J Cardiovasc Magn Reson 12(1):29

Heitner JF, Kim RJ, Kim HW, Klem I, Shah DJ, Debs D et al (2019) Prognostic value of vasodilator stress cardiac magnetic resonance imaging: a multicenter study with 48 000 patient-years of follow-up. JAMA Cardiol 4(3):256–264

Henzler T, Fink C, Schoenberg SO, Schoepf UJ (2012) Dual-energy CT: radiation dose aspects. AJR Am J Roentgenol 199(5 Suppl):S16–S25

Heusch G (2008) Heart rate in the pathophysiology of coronary blood flow and myocardial ischaemia: benefit from selective bradycardic agents. Br J Pharmacol 153(8):1589–1601

Hsu LY, Kellman P, Arai AE (2008) Nonlinear myocardial signal intensity correction improves quantification of contrast-enhanced first-pass MR perfusion in humans. J Magn Reson Imaging 27(4):793–801

Hsu LY, Jacobs M, Benovoy M, Ta AD, Conn HM, Winkler S et al (2018) Diagnostic performance of fully automated pixel-wise quantitative myocardial perfusion imaging by cardiovascular magnetic resonance. JACC Cardiovasc Imaging 11(5):697–707

Hubbard L, Malkasian S, Zhao Y, Abbona P, Molloi S (2019) Timing optimization of low-dose first-pass analysis dynamic CT myocardial perfusion measurement: validation in a swine model. Eur Radiol Exp 3(1):16

Ingrisch M, Sourbron S (2013) Tracer-kinetic modeling of dynamic contrast-enhanced MRI and CT: a primer. J Pharmacokinet Pharmacodyn 40(3):281–300

Ishida M, Kitagawa K, Ichihara T, Natsume T, Nakayama R, Nagasawa N et al (2016) Underestimation of myocardial blood flow by dynamic perfusion CT: explanations by two-compartment model analysis and limited temporal sampling of dynamic CT. J Cardiovasc Comput Tomogr 10(3):207–214

Johnson NP, Toth GG, Lai D, Zhu H, Acar G, Agostoni P et al (2014) Prognostic value of fractional flow reserve: linking physiologic severity to clinical outcomes. J Am Coll Cardiol 64(16):1641–1654

Kellman P, Arai AE (2007) Imaging sequences for first pass perfusion—a review. J Cardiovasc Magn Reson 9(3):525–537

Kidambi A, Sourbron S, Maredia N, Motwani M, Brown JM, Nixon J et al (2016) Factors associated with false-negative cardiovascular magnetic resonance perfusion studies: a clinical evaluation of magnetic resonance imaging in coronary artery disease (CE-MARC) substudy. J Magn Reson Imaging 43(3):566–573

Klocke FJ, Baird MG, Lorell BH, Bateman TM, Messer JV, Berman DS et al (2003) ACC/AHA/ASNC guidelines for the clinical use of cardiac radionuclide imaging—executive summary: a report of the American College of Cardiology/American Heart Association Task Force on Practice Guidelines (ACC/AHA/ASNC Committee to Revise the 1995 Guidelines for the Clinical Use of Cardiac Radionuclide Imaging). J Am Coll Cardiol 42(7):1318–1333

Knuuti J, Wijns W, Saraste A, Capodanno D, Barbato E, Funck-Brentano C et al (2020) 2019 ESC guidelines for the diagnosis and management of chronic coronary syndromes. Eur Heart J 41(3):407–477

Ko SM, Choi JW, Hwang HK, Song MG, Shin JK, Chee HK (2012) Diagnostic performance of combined noninvasive anatomic and functional assessment with dual-source CT and adenosine-induced stress dual-energy CT for detection of significant coronary stenosis. AJR Am J Roentgenol 198(3):512–520

Krittayaphong R, Chaithiraphan V, Maneesai A, Udompanturak S (2011) Prognostic value of combined magnetic resonance myocardial perfusion imaging and late gadolinium enhancement. Int J Cardiovasc Imaging 27(5):705–714

Kuijpers D, van Dijk R, van Assen M, Kaandorp TAM, van Dijkman PRM, Vliegenthart R et al (2018) Disagreement between splenic switch-off and myocardial T1-mapping after caffeine intake. Int J Cardiovasc Imaging 34(4):625–632

Kwong RY, Ge Y, Steel K, Bingham S, Abdullah S, Fujikura K et al (2019) Cardiac magnetic resonance stress perfusion imaging for evaluation of patients with chest pain. J Am Coll Cardiol 74(14):1741–1755

Li M, Zhou T, Yang LF, Peng ZH, Ding J, Sun G (2014) Diagnostic accuracy of myocardial magnetic resonance perfusion to diagnose ischemic stenosis with fractional flow reserve as reference: systematic review and meta-analysis. JACC Cardiovasc Imaging 7(11):1098–1105

Machecourt J, Longere P, Fagret D, Vanzetto G, Wolf JE, Polidori C et al (1994) Prognostic value of thallium-201 single-photon emission computed tomographic myocardial perfusion imaging according to extent of myocardial defect. Study in 1,926 patients with follow-up at 33 months. J Am Coll Cardiol 23(5):1096–1106

Machida H, Tanaka I, Fukui R, Shen Y, Ishikawa T, Tate E, Ueno E (2015) Current and novel imaging techniques in coronary CT. Radiographics 35(4):991–1010

Magalhaes TA, Kishi S, George RT, Arbab-Zadeh A, Vavere AL, Cox C et al (2015) Combined coronary angiography and myocardial perfusion by computed tomography in the identification of flow-limiting stenosis—the CORE320 study: an integrated analysis of CT coronary angiography and myocardial perfusion. J Cardiovasc Comput Tomogr 9(5):438–445

Mahnken AH, Klotz E, Pietsch H, Schmidt B, Allmendinger T, Haberland U et al (2010) Quantitative whole heart stress perfusion CT imaging as noninvasive assessment of hemodynamics in coronary artery stenosis: preliminary animal experience. Investig Radiol 45(6):298–305

Manisty C, Ripley DP, Herrey AS, Captur G, Wong TC, Petersen SE et al (2015) Splenic switch-off: a tool to assess stress adequacy in adenosine perfusion cardiac MR imaging. Radiology 276(3):732–740

Meinel FG, Pugliese F, Schoepf UJ, Ebersberger U, Wichmann JL, Lo GG et al (2017a) Prognostic value of stress dynamic myocardial perfusion CT in a multicenter population with known or suspected coronary artery disease. AJR Am J Roentgenol 208(4):761–769

Meinel FG, Wichmann JL, Schoepf UJ, Pugliese F, Ebersberger U, Lo GG et al (2017b) Global quantification of left ventricular myocardial perfusion at dynamic CT imaging: prognostic value. J Cardiovasc Comput Tomogr 11(1):16–24

Menke J, Kowalski J (2016) Diagnostic accuracy and utility of coronary CT angiography with consideration of unevaluable results: a systematic review and multivariate Bayesian random-effects meta-analysis with intention to diagnose. Eur Radiol 26(2):451–458

Meuwissen M, Chamuleau SA, Siebes M, Schotborgh CE, Koch KT, de Winter RJ et al (2001) Role of variability in microvascular resistance on fractional flow reserve and coronary blood flow velocity reserve in intermediate coronary lesions. Circulation 103(2): 184–187

Moschetti K, Petersen SE, Pilz G, Kwong RY, Wasserfallen JB, Lombardi M et al (2016) Cost-minimization analysis of three decision strategies for cardiac revascularization: results of the "suspected CAD" cohort of the European cardiovascular magnetic resonance registry. J Cardiovasc Magn Reson 18:3

Motwani M, Fairbairn TA, Larghat A, Mather AN, Biglands JD, Radjenovic A et al (2012) Systolic versus diastolic acquisition in myocardial perfusion MR imaging. Radiology 262(3):816–823

Motwani M, Kidambi A, Sourbron S, Fairbairn TA, Uddin A, Kozerke S et al (2014) Quantitative three-dimensional cardiovascular magnetic resonance myocardial perfusion imaging in systole and diastole. J Cardiovasc Magn Reson 16:19

Nagel E, Greenwood JP, McCann GP, Bettencourt N, Shah AM, Hussain ST et al (2019) Magnetic resonance perfusion or fractional flow reserve in coronary disease. N Engl J Med 380(25):2418–2428

Nakamura S, Kitagawa K, Goto Y, Omori T, Kurita T, Yamada A et al (2019) Incremental prognostic value of myocardial blood flow quantified with stress dynamic computed tomography perfusion imaging. JACC Cardiovasc Imaging 12(7 Pt 2):1379–1387

Nchimi A, Mancini I, Broussaud TK (2014a) Influence of the cardiac cycle on time-intensity curves using multislice dynamic magnetic resonance perfusion. Int J Cardiovasc Imaging 30(7):1347–1355

Nchimi A, Djekic J, Raskinet B, Morar A, Mancini I, Broussaud TK, Ghekiere O (2014b) Myocardial dynamic contrast-enhanced Mr: vascular diseases and beyond. JBR-BTR 97(1):3–10

Neumann FJ, Sousa-Uva M, Ahlsson A, Alfonso F, Banning AP, Benedetto U et al (2019) 2018 ESC/EACTS Guidelines on myocardial revascularization. Eur Heart J 40(2):87–165

Nishiyama H, Tanabe Y, Kido T, Kurata A, Uetani T, Kido T et al (2019) Incremental diagnostic value of whole-heart dynamic computed tomography perfusion imaging for detecting obstructive coronary artery disease. J Cardiol 73(5):425–431

Patel AR, Bamberg F, Branch K, Carrascosa P, Chen M, Cury RC et al (2020) Society of cardiovascular computed tomography expert consensus document on myocardial computed tomography perfusion imaging. J Cardiovasc Comput Tomogr 14(1):87–100

Pelgrim GJ, Dorrius M, Xie X, den Dekker MA, Schoepf UJ, Henzler T et al (2015) The dream of a one-stop-shop: meta-analysis on myocardial perfusion CT. Eur J Radiol 84(12):2411–2420

Pelgrim GJ, Handayani A, Dijkstra H, Prakken NH, Slart RH, Oudkerk M et al (2016) Quantitative myocardial perfusion with dynamic contrast-enhanced imaging in MRI and CT: theoretical models and current implementation. Biomed Res Int 2016:1734190

Pelgrim GJ, Nieuwenhuis ER, Duguay TM, van der Geest RJ, Varga-Szemes A, Slump CH et al (2017) Optimal timing of image acquisition for arterial first pass CT myocardial perfusion imaging. Eur J Radiol 86:227–233

Pletscher M, Walker S, Moschetti K, Pinget C, Wasserfallen JB, Greenwood JP et al (2016) Cost-effectiveness of functional cardiac imaging in the diagnostic work-up of coronary heart disease. Eur Heart J Qual Care Clin Outcomes 2(3):201–207

Pontone G, Baggiano A, Andreini D, Guaricci AI, Guglielmo M, Muscogiuri G et al (2019a) Dynamic stress computed tomography perfusion with a whole-heart coverage scanner in addition to coronary computed tomography angiography and fractional flow reserve computed tomography derived. JACC Cardiovasc Imaging 12(12):2460–2471

Pontone G, Andreini D, Guaricci AI, Baggiano A, Fazzari F, Guglielmo M et al (2019b) Incremental diagnostic value of stress computed tomography myocardial perfusion with whole-heart coverage CT scanner in intermediate- to high-risk symptomatic patients suspected of coronary artery disease. JACC Cardiovasc Imaging 12(2):338–349

Pontone G, De Cecco C, Baggiano A, Guaricci AI, Guglielmo M, Leiner T et al (2019c) Design of CTP-PRO study (impact of stress cardiac computed tomography myocardial perfusion on downstream resources and PROgnosis in patients with suspected or known coronary artery disease: a multicenter international study). Int J Cardiol 292:253–257

Rochitte CE, George RT, Chen MY, Arbab-Zadeh A, Dewey M, Miller JM et al (2014) Computed tomography angiography and perfusion to assess coronary artery stenosis causing perfusion defects by single photon emission computed tomography: the CORE320 study. Eur Heart J 35(17):1120–1130

Rodriguez-Granillo GA, Carrascosa P, Cipriano S, De Zan M, Deviggiano A, Capunay C, Cury RC (2015) Beam hardening artifact reduction using dual energy computed tomography: implications for myocardial perfusion studies. Cardiovasc Diagn Ther 5(1):79–85

Rogers IS, Cury RC, Blankstein R, Shapiro MD, Nieman K, Hoffmann U et al (2010) Comparison of postprocessing techniques for the detection of perfusion defects by cardiac computed tomography in patients presenting with acute ST-segment elevation myocardial infarction. J Cardiovasc Comput Tomogr 4(4):258–266

Rossi A, Merkus D, Klotz E, Mollet N, de Feyter PJ, Krestin GP (2014) Stress myocardial perfusion: imaging with multidetector CT. Radiology 270(1):25–46

Rossi A, Wragg A, Klotz E, Pirro F, Moon JC, Nieman K, Pugliese F (2017) Dynamic computed tomography myocardial perfusion imaging: comparison of clinical analysis methods for the detection of vessel-specific ischemia. Circ Cardiovasc Imaging 10(4):e005505

Saraste A, Knuuti J (2020) ESC 2019 guidelines for the diagnosis and management of chronic coronary syndromes: recommendations for cardiovascular imaging. Herz 45(5):409–420

Schelbert HR (2010) Anatomy and physiology of coronary blood flow. J Nucl Cardiol 17(4):545–554

Schulz-Menger J, Bluemke DA, Bremerich J, Flamm SD, Fogel MA, Friedrich MG et al (2020) Standardized image interpretation and post-processing in cardiovascular magnetic resonance—2020 update: Society for Cardiovascular Magnetic Resonance (SCMR): Board of Trustees Task Force on Standardized Post-Processing. J Cardiovasc Magn Reson 22(1):19

Schwitter J, Nanz D, Kneifel S, Bertschinger K, Büchi M, Knüsel PR et al (2001) Assessment of myocardial perfusion in coronary artery disease by magnetic resonance: a comparison with positron emission tomography and coronary angiography. Circulation 103(18):2230–2235

Schwitter J, Wacker CM, Wilke N, Al-Saadi N, Sauer E, Huettle K et al (2013) MR-IMPACT II: magnetic resonance imaging for myocardial perfusion assessment in coronary artery disease trial: perfusion-cardiac magnetic resonance vs. single-photon emission computed tomography for the detection of coronary artery disease: a comparative multicentre, multivendor trial. Eur Heart J 34(10):775–781

Secchi F, De Cecco CN, Spearman JV, Silverman JR, Ebersberger U, Sardanelli F, Schoepf UJ (2015) Monoenergetic extrapolation of cardiac dual energy CT for artifact reduction. Acta Radiol 56(4):413–418

Stenner P, Schmidt B, Allmendinger T, Flohr T, Kachelrie M (2010) Dynamic iterative beam hardening correction (DIBHC) in myocardial perfusion imaging using contrast-enhanced computed tomography. Investig Radiol 45(6):314–323

Stuijfzand WJ, Uusitalo V, Kero T, Danad I, Rijnierse MT, Saraste A et al (2015) Relative flow reserve derived from quantitative perfusion imaging may not outperform stress myocardial blood flow for identification of hemodynamically significant coronary artery disease. Circ Cardiovasc Imaging 8(1):e002400

Takx RA, Blomberg BA, El Aidi H, Habets J, de Jong PA, Nagel E et al (2015) Diagnostic accuracy of stress myocardial perfusion imaging compared to invasive coronary angiography with fractional flow reserve meta-analysis. Circ Cardiovasc Imaging 8(1):e002666

Tashakkor AY, Nicolaou S, Leipsic J, Mancini GB (2012) The emerging role of cardiac computed tomography for the assessment of coronary perfusion: a systematic review and meta-analysis. Can J Cardiol 28(4):413–422

Utz W, Niendorf T, Wassmuth R, Messroghli D, Dietz R, Schulz-Menger J (2007) Contrast-dose relation in first-pass myocardial MR perfusion imaging. J Magn Reson Imaging 25(6):1131–1135

van Assen M, Lavra F, Schoepf UJ, Jacobs BE, Williams BT, Thompson ZM et al (2019a) Iodine quantification based on rest/stress perfusion dual energy CT to differentiate ischemic, infarcted and normal myocardium. Eur J Radiol 112:136–143

van Assen M, De Cecco CN, Eid M, von Knebel Doeberitz P, Scarabello M, Lavra F et al (2019b) Prognostic value of CT myocardial perfusion imaging and CT-derived fractional flow reserve for major adverse cardiac events in patients with coronary artery disease. J Cardiovasc Comput Tomogr 13(3):26–33

van Assen M, Kuijpers DJ, Schwitter J (2020) MRI perfusion in patients with stable chest-pain. Br J Radiol 93(1113):20190881

van Dijk R, Kuijpers D, Kaandorp TAM, van Dijkman PRM, Vliegenthart R, van der Harst P, Oudkerk M (2017a) Effects of caffeine intake prior to stress cardiac magnetic resonance perfusion imaging on regadenoson- versus adenosine-induced hyperemia as measured by T1 mapping. Int J Cardiovasc Imaging 33(11):1753–1759

van Dijk R, van Assen M, Vliegenthart R, de Bock GH, van der Harst P, Oudkerk M (2017b) Diagnostic performance of semi-quantitative and quantitative stress CMR perfusion analysis: a meta-analysis. J Cardiovasc Magn Reson 19(1):92

Varga-Szemes A, Meinel FG, De Cecco CN, Fuller SR, Bayer RR 2nd, Schoepf UJ (2015) CT myocardial perfusion imaging. AJR Am J Roentgenol 204(3):487–497

Vincenti G, Masci PG, Monney P, Rutz T, Hugelshofer S, Gaxherri M et al (2017) Stress perfusion CMR in patients with known and suspected CAD: prognostic value and optimal ischemic threshold for revascularization. JACC Cardiovasc Imaging 10(5): 526–537

Walker S, Girardin F, McKenna C, Ball SG, Nixon J, Plein S et al (2013) Cost-effectiveness of cardiovascular magnetic resonance in the diagnosis of coronary heart disease: an economic evaluation using data from the CE-MARC study. Heart 99(12):873–881

Williams MC, Newby DE (2016) CT myocardial perfusion imaging: current status and future directions. Clin Radiol 71(8):739–749

Yang L, Zhou T, Zhang R, Xu L, Peng Z, Ding J et al (2014) Meta-analysis: diagnostic accuracy of coronary CT angiography with prospective ECG gating based on step-and-shoot, flash and volume modes for detection of coronary artery disease. Eur Radiol 24(10):2345–2352

Yang J, Dou G, He B, Jin Q, Chen Z, Jing J et al (2020) Stress myocardial blood flow ratio by dynamic CT perfusion identifies hemodynamically significant CAD. JACC Cardiovasc Imaging 13(4): 966–976

Young DF, Cholvin NR, Kirkeeide RL, Roth AC (1977) Hemodynamics of arterial stenoses at elevated flow rates. Circ Res 41(1):99–107

Zimmermann FM, Ferrara A, Johnson NP, van Nunen LX, Escaned J, Albertsson P et al (2015) Deferral vs. performance of percutaneous coronary intervention of functionally non-significant coronary stenosis: 15-year follow-up of the DEFER trial. Eur Heart J 36(45):3182–3188

Zoghbi GJ, Dorfman TA, Iskandrian AE (2008) The effects of medications on myocardial perfusion. J Am Coll Cardiol 52(6):401–416

Heart Chambers

Farah Cadour and Jean-Nicolas Dacher

Contents

F. Cadour · J.-N. Dacher (✉)
Department of Radiology and Medical Imaging (Cardiac Imaging Unit), CHU de Rouen Normandie—Hôpital Charles Nicolle, University of Rouen Normandie, Rouen, France
e-mail: Jean-Nicolas.Dacher@chu-rouen.fr

Abstract

Knowledge of the anatomy of the six chambers of the heart is paramount to a comprehensive reading of a cardiac imaging exam. From the extensively studied left ventricle to the less known right atrial appendage, each cavity comes with its own particularity and normal parameters. Standard cardiac anatomical planes should be well known for understanding and applying reference values.

The aim of this chapter is to remind the characteristics and anatomy of the different heart chambers but also to emphasize on the parameters derived from the various measurements of each chamber and their application in routine cardiology.

1 Introduction

Contrary to traditional concepts, the heart comprises six cavities instead of four: two atria with their respective appendages and two ventricles. In recent years, ECG-gated cardiac MRI and CT have proven to be effective in the metric, volumetric, and functional assessment of these heart cavities, establishing both techniques as the gold standard. The full anatomical volumetric coverage is a shared advantage between these two methods compared to echocardiography, with the latter retaining its undisputed superiority in tem-

Med Radiol Diagn Imaging (2026)
https://doi.org/10.1007/174_2023_453,
Published Online: 06 September 2024

poral resolution. CT's main advantage is volumetric acquisition, while its primary limitation is exposure to ionizing radiation, especially in younger individuals and females.

The objective of this chapter is to equip general radiologists with a foundational understanding of assessing heart dimensions using conventional and ECG-gated examinations.

Measurements indexed to body surface area (BSA) are extremely important in routine cardiology. Consequently, patients should be weighed and measured before undergoing imaging. Height and weight reported by patients should be treated with caution and must not be used for precise follow-up purposes, such as evaluating treatment efficacy.

By definition, heart chamber measurements should be drawn from ECG-gated acquisitions although reasonable approximations can be derived from conventional CT imaging.

In this chapter, our focus will be restricted to modal heart cavities; complex scenarios that may arise in the context of congenital heart disease will not be addressed.

2 Cardiac Anatomic Planes

Optimal measurement of cardiac cavities requires a good knowledge of conventional cardiac planes that are either directly acquired in MRI or secondarily reformatted from axial slices on CT.

Let us choose CT (Fig. 1) as an example:

- First, on the axial view passing through the middle of the heart chambers, the operator draws a line passing through the apex of the left ventricle, the middle of the mitral valve, and the posterior aspect of the left atrium. This plane provides a vertical long-axis (VLA) view (also called two-chamber view, 2C).
- On the VLA view, the operator draws a line joining the middle of the posterior left atrial wall, the center of the mitral valve, and the LV apex to obtain a pseudo-four-chamber (4C) view.
- A line perpendicular to the great axis of the LV is then drawn on both VLA and pseudo-4C view; the short-axis (SA) view is obtained. The SA plane can then be moved from the basis to the apex of the two ventricles.

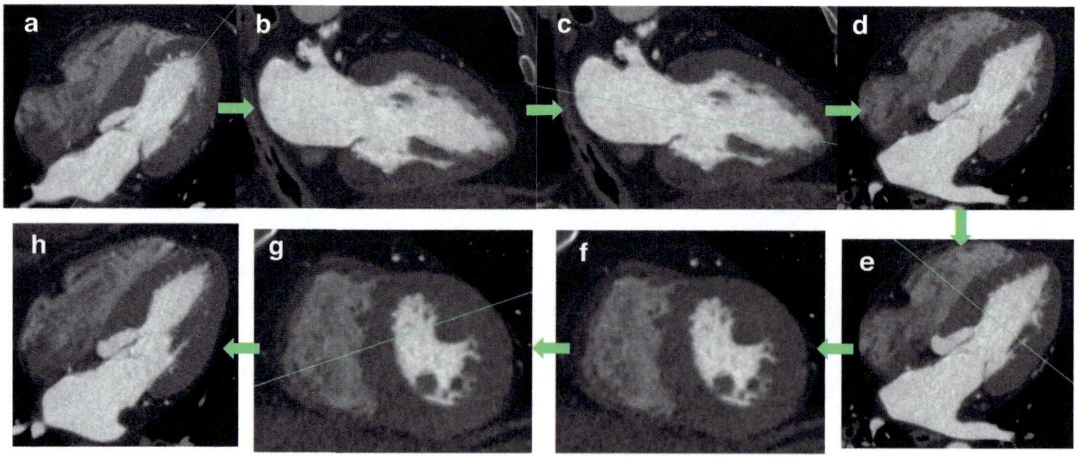

Fig. 1 Standard cardiac anatomical planes. (**a**) Native axial CT scanner: line shows how to get the 2C view; (**b**) 2C view; (**c**) 2C view: line shows how to get the pseudo-4C view; (**d**) pseudo-4C view; (**e**) pseudo-4C view: line shows how to get the SA view (plane to be also orthogonally placed on 2C view); (**f**) SA view; (**g**) SA view: line shows how to get the 4C view; (**h**) 4C view

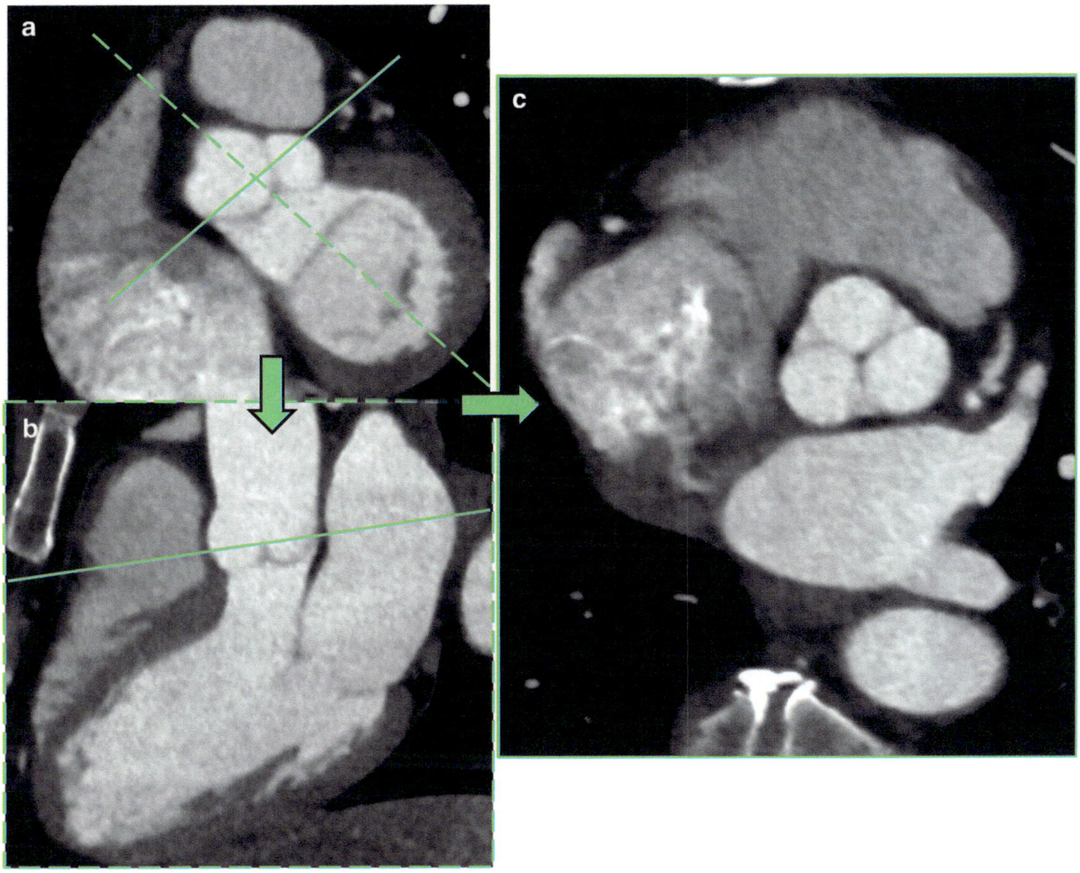

Fig. 2 Dashed green line (**a**) passing through the mid-aorta, 90° to 4C plane provides the left ventricular outflow tract view (LVOT) (**b**). Double obliquity reformatting results (by translation) in the plane of aortic valve, annulus, and sinotubular junction (sinus of Valsalva is shown in **c**)

- Then, a line is drawn on the mid-ventricle SA slice joining the anterior papillary muscle to the angle formed between the inferior and free wall of the right ventricle (RV). This results in the true 4C view (also called horizontal long-axis view).
- In the short axis and at the base of the LV, another line can be drawn in the great axis of the ascending aorta (perpendicular to the 4C plane) (Fig. 2) (between the center of the aorta and the center of the mitral valve) to build the three-chamber (3C) view (an equivalent to the parasagittal long-axis view of echocardiography).
- Finally, the aortic valve and sinus of Valsalva can be defined from the last two slices to define aortic valve cuspidity and measure the aortic root including (caudal to cephalad) the left ventricular outflow tract (LVOT), the aortic annulus (a virtual ovoid joining the three hinge points of the aortic valve), the sinus of Valsalva, and finally the sinotubular junction.

3 Left Ventricle (LV)

3.1 LV Volume and Ejection Fraction

The LV is a cone-shaped cavity limited by four walls: septal, lateral, inferior, and anterior. The mitral ring located at its base is an important landmark to reliably assess LV parameters. The mitral valve is attached to the papillary muscles (when modal, anterior and posterior) by the chordae tendineae.

Assessing the LV volumes, mass, and ejection fraction (EF) represents one of the major objectives of any cardiac evaluation. Many automated or semiautomated tools are available. However, all of them are based on the same principle. Manual, automated (using machine learning), or semiautomated endocardial and epicardial contours are drawn in the SA from the base to the apex of the LV at the end-diastolic and end-systolic phase. The mitral valve needs to be pinpointed in two orthogonal planes (typically 2C and 4C views) as well as the cephalic and caudal LV-right ventricle (RV) junctions and the apex of both ventricles. On MRI, this evaluation is drawn from a stack of cine slices (steady-state free precession) covering the whole LV in the short axis. The same operation can be performed on CT provided that temporal coverage encompasses diastole and systole.

While available software is generally effective in handling standard situations, operators should always verify and validate the results. Any form of remodeling or irregular heart rate can introduce errors and necessitate manual adjustments. Particular attention should be given to contouring and identifying end-diastolic and end-systolic phases. It is important to note that end-systolic volumes may be overestimated (resulting in underestimation of ejection fraction) in cases of arrhythmia (Schulz-Menger et al. 2020).

Special attention should be given to the LV basal slices, as decisions regarding their partial or complete inclusion or exclusion from contouring can be challenging due to their proximity to the left atrium (LA) and the systolic descent of the mitral valve. The geometry of the LV explains why errors in basal slice segmentation can significantly impact LVEF and LV volume (Caudron et al. 2012). We recommend simultaneously displaying SA, 2C, and 4C views for cross-referencing. If this display is not available, the left atrial appendage (LAA) can serve as a landmark for the LA. Moreover, the most basal slice should be contoured if at least 50% of the blood volume is encircled by LV myocardium. Lastly, the LVOT should be included as part of the LV blood volume up to the level of the aortic valve cusps.

The papillary muscles represent a significant part of the LV myocardial mass. There is no consensus on the inclusion of papillary muscles either in the LV mass or in the LV volume. Reproducibility of measurements seems improved when papillary muscles are included in the blood volume. The SCMR guidelines recommend to consistently include the papillary muscles in the LV mass (preferred) or in the LV volume, but not in both, and to stipulate one's choice (Schulz-Menger et al. 2020).

Estimation of LV volumes can be achieved using the standard volume formula applied to long-axis planes (preferably two, but at least one):

$$\text{Volume} = 0.85 \times \frac{\text{Cavity area 1} \times \text{Cavity area 2}}{\text{Cavity length}}.$$

It is important to note that this formula includes two cavity areas, indicating that the estimation is based on both the 2C and 4C views, but it could be calculated using only one long-axis plane. The cavity length is measured in both planes, and the shorter of the two is used in the formula.

An approximation of LV diameter can be obtained by measuring the maximal LV diameter at end diastole, with the measurement located at the base of the cavity and basal to the tips of the papillary muscles, either in the 4C or in the LVOT plane. In adults, it is generally considered that the LV is dilated when this distance exceeds 52 mm (Puntmann et al. 2013).

Finally, comparing the LV maximal diameter to its equivalent for the RV on the same slice (rarely at slightly different levels) can be particularly useful, especially in emergency situations. In a normal heart, the RV diameter is approximately one-third of the LV diameter. Moreover, an RV/LV ratio ≥ 1 is always considered abnormal (Konstantinides et al. 2020). In the context of pulmonary embolism, this increased ratio reflects acute RV dysfunction and eliminates the need for additional transthoracic echocardiography. In chronic situations, an elevated RV/LV ratio can be observed in a variety of conditions including atrial septal defect (Fig. 3), pulmonary hypertension, and arrhythmogenic cardiomyopathy.

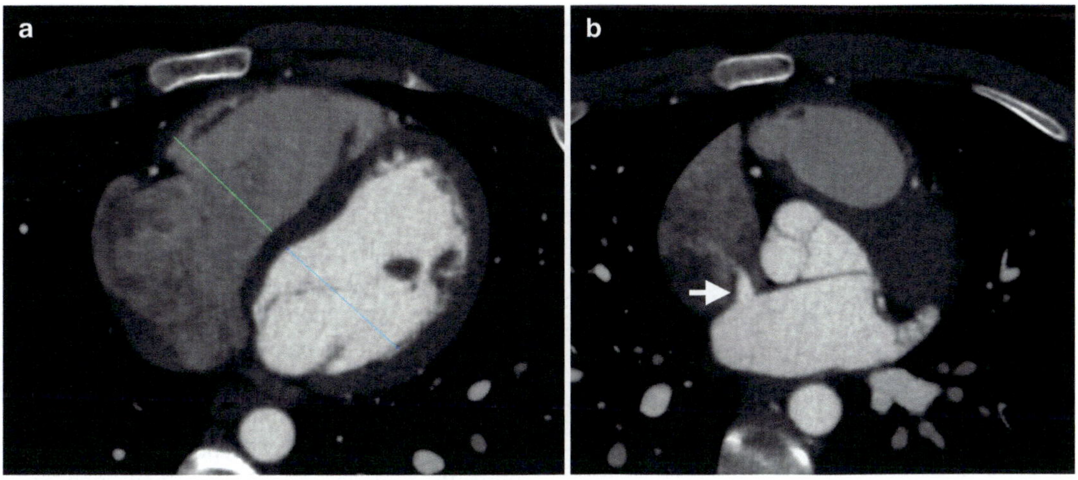

Fig. 3 Measurement of RV/LV ratio (green/blue diameter = 0.92) on axial slice (**a**) of a cardiac CT disclosing a moderately dilated right ventricle (LV is normal sized). In the present case, ostium secundum atrial septal defect was diagnosed with an obvious left-to-right shunt (arrow) (**b**)

Table 1 Left ventricle normal values

Left ventricle	Male	Female	Athlete male	Athlete female
EF (%)	64 ± 8	66 ± 7	56 ± 5	57 ± 6
SV (mL)	103 ± 21	83 ± 16	144 ± 28	112 ± 23
ED vol (mL)	155 ± 30	123 ± 22	256 ± 35	197 ± 29
ES vol (mL)	55 ± 15	43 ± 11	112 ± 22	85 ± 17
Mass (g)	121 ± 28	83 ± 21	132 ± 25	88 ± 16
SV_i (mL/m^2)	52 ± 10	49 ± 8	71 ± 13	60 ± 11
ED vol_i (mL/m^2)	79 ± 15	73 ± 12	126 ± 15	107 ± 14
ES vol_i (mL/m^2)	29 ± 9	25 ± 7	55 ± 10	47 ± 9
$LVMass_i$ (g/m^2)	62 ± 11	49 ± 10	66 ± 12	48 ± 8

Results are presented as mean ± standard deviation
Note that LV absolute and normalized values decrease with age in a continuous manner. For more details, please see Kawel-Boehm et al. (2020). Male and female athlete values are based on the mean values between regular (9–18-h sport activity per week) and elite (>18 h/week) athletes according to references (Kawel-Boehm et al. 2020; Prakken et al. 2010) with SV being the difference between ED and ES volumes
EF ejection fraction, *ED/ES vol* absolute end-diastolic/systolic volumes, *ED/ES* vol_i indexed end-diastolic/systolic volumes, *SV/SV*$_i$ absolute and indexed stroke volumes

Left ventricular normal values are given in Table 1. Note that global and regional deformation of the myocardium (circumferential, radial, and longitudinal strain) can be assessed by cine MRI based on feature tracking (Kawel-Boehm et al. 2020).

3.2 LV Myocardial Thickness

Detection of any kind of hypertrophy (e.g., sarcomeric hypertrophic cardiomyopathy, infiltrative or hypertensive heart disease) is possible using CT or MRI. However, such diagnoses rely on ECG gating. The end-diastolic phase should be chosen for reference thickness measurements (Fig. 4), although maximal thickening at end systole may also be provided for prognostic purposes. Misdiagnosis of hypertrophy can occur when measurements are performed on non-synchronized or systolic phase images. Papillary muscles, myocardial trabeculations, and septomarginal trabeculation should not be included in myocardial thickness calculations. Measurements

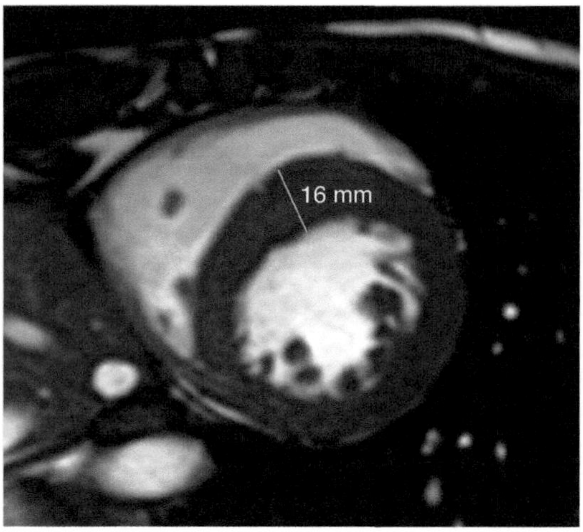

Fig. 4 CMR diagnosis of hypertrophic cardiomyopathy with 16 mm septal basal thickness as indicated

Table 2 Myocardial hypertrophy—normal values at end diastole (echo standards) according to Dayal and Müller (2017)

	Normal values	Mild HT	Moderate HT	Severe HT
Male (mm)	6–10	11–13	14–16	>16
Female (mm)	6–9	10–12	13–15	>15

Note that hypertrophic cardiomyopathy is defined on cardiac MRI as a myocardial thickness ≥15 mm (≥13 mm in case of family history or positive genetic test)
HT hypertrophy

should always be performed orthogonally to the myocardium, as oblique measurements can lead to overestimation. The apex is one accepted exception, where long-axis views should be used.

Severity of hypertrophy can be determined according to measurements provided in Table 2. In adults, hypertrophic cardiomyopathy (HCM) is defined as a thickness ≥15 mm anywhere in the LV in the absence of another cause of hypertrophy and >13 mm with a family history of HCM or a positive genetic test (Ommen et al. 2020). In cases with ≥30 mm myocardial thickness, an increased risk of sudden death has been demonstrated, and the implantation of an implantable cardioverter-defibrillator for primary prevention should be considered (North American model) (Veselka et al. 2017).

It is important to note that athletes (typically engaging in >10 h of sports activity per week) may exhibit a physiological adaptation to training, leading to an expected increase in myocardial thickness ranging from 13 to 16 mm and moderate and balanced dilation of all four heart chambers. The thickening will generally be symmetrical and decrease after detraining, which can help differentiate it from HCM (Pelliccia et al. 2018). Any suspicion of hypertrophy should be correlated with the patient's sport activity status.

A mean ratio of septal/lateral thickness >1.5 is characteristic of asymmetric septal HCM compared to concentric LV hypertrophy (which is typically seen in pressure overload such as in arterial hypertension).

LV non-compaction is not an easy diagnosis. It can be suggested when the ratio of trabeculated to compact myocardium thickness is >2.3 (Petersen et al. 2005), with some authors even suggesting higher ratios (Kawel et al. 2012).

Abnormal thinning of the myocardium can also be detected using CT and MRI; this is often the result of a chronic myocardial infarction, which may be associated with an intraventricular thrombus. It is generally considered that a myocardial segment is nonviable when measured at less than 6 mm (Cwajg et al. 2000; Garcia et al. 2020). However, this threshold is debated, with the extent of late gadolinium enhancement being the most critical predictive factor (Shah et al. 2013). It is essential to remember that CT or MRI is much more effective than echocardiography for ruling out thrombus, particularly when located at the LV/RV apex.

4 Left Atrium (LA)

The LA is the most posterior and superior cardiac cavity. By convention, the LA volume (or surface) should be measured at end systole, just before the opening of the mitral valve. The LAA and pulmonary vein connections should be excluded from the LA volume calculation. Both CT and MRI can be used, provided that ECG synchronization was performed and the systolic phase is available. A dilated LA is a marker of diastolic dysfunction (Caudron et al. 2011a) and increased left ventricular filling pressures when confounding factors, such as atrial fibrillation (AF) and mitral valve disease, have been excluded.

There are at least three methods for measuring the LA:

1. The simplest method involves measuring the LA area in the 4C view. This area should not exceed 24 cm^2 or 15 cm^2/m^2 in adults (Petersen et al. 2019). This measurement can be sufficient in patients with normal-sized LAs.
2. For a more precise measurement (e.g., in the follow-up of a patient with restrictive/infiltrative disease), the biplane area-length method (Nacif et al. 2013) can be employed. This method can be performed either manually or automatically. The LA area is measured in both 4C and 2C views. The minimal length of the cavity is also recorded in both planes (Fig. 5).The LA volume is derived from the formula mentioned earlier for the LV volume. This technique is quite efficient in CT, as volume acquisition allows the operator to define maximal areas in both planes. In MRI, success depends on an accurate positioning of 4C and 2C slices and minimal variations in the patient's breath-holding.
3. Finally, the Simpson's method can provide LA volumes and EF based on the same principles as for the LV. Although this technique can be routinely applied in conventional cardiac MR, it requires extensive temporal synchronization in CT to incorporate both diastolic and systolic phases, resulting in an increased radiation exposure. While Simpson's method is considered the reference, we routinely use the biplane area-length method due to its simplicity and reproducibility (Nacif et al. 2013).

The left atrium is considered dilated when >50 mL/m^2 in adults (Petersen et al. 2019).

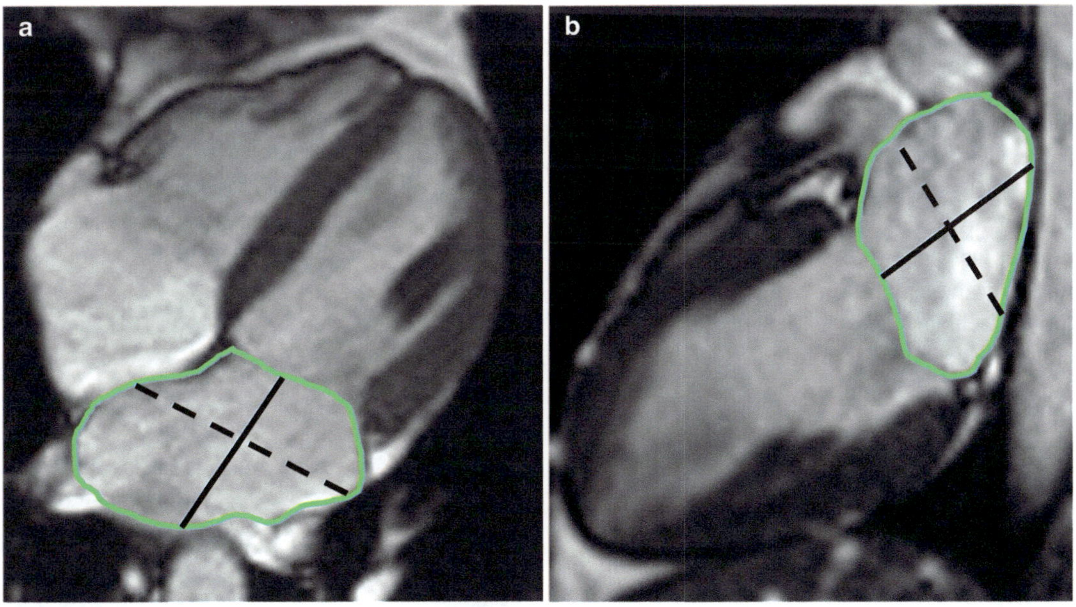

Fig. 5 Measurement of left atrial volume based on the biplane area-length method. Panel **a** depicts left atrial area in 4C view. Panel **b** shows the left atrial area in 2C view. Minimal length of the left atrial (full black line) is used to calculate the left atrial volume (see formula in Sect. 3.1)

5 Left Atrial Appendage (LAA)

In recent years, imaging of the previously largely ignored LAA has gained interest due to the development of percutaneous closure devices. These devices are designed to be placed in the LAA to prevent ischemic events in elderly patients with contraindications to anticoagulants. The goal of those devices is to exclude the LAA, a cul-de-sac with slow flow, from the circulation and to prevent as such thrombus formation. The measurement of LAA is beyond the scope of this chapter, and we invite the interested readers to consult the paper by Tacher et al. (2021). The morphology of the LAA (cactus, chicken wing, windsock, cauliflower) should be described as some specific shapes (e.g., chicken wing) have been shown to be less associated with embolic events in patients with AF (Di Biase et al. 2012).

6 Right Ventricle (RV)

The right ventricle (RV), the most anterior cardiac cavity, appears triangular in its long axis. At its base, the tricuspid valve inserts into the septum more anteriorly and apically than the mitral valve. The RV comprises three portions (Sanz et al. 2019): (1) the inlet, which includes the tricuspid valve, subvalvular apparatus, chordae tendineae, and papillary muscles (notably, these insert on the septum, in contrast to the LV); (2) the trabeculated apex, which includes the moderator band; and (3) the outlet, which includes the pulmonary infundibulum (or conus) and the pulmonary valve.

The geometry of the RV is more complex than that of the LV. Segmentation in the axial (transverse) plane has been demonstrated to be more reliable and accurate than in the SA plane (Alfakih et al. 2003; Atalay et al. 2013). However, axial plane multislice acquisition is not commonly performed in MRI, as it increases examination time. The most convenient approach is to segment the RV in the SA plane after identifying the tricuspid valve in two planes using the same principle as for the LV (SA, 4C, and RV vertical long-axis are used for cross-referencing). It is worth noting that an SA view displaying the coronary sinus crosses the RA and should not be included in the RV volume. Manual corrections are often more necessary than for the LV, particularly for the infundibulum, considering the poor visibility of the normal pulmonary valve. If the pulmonary valve is visible, the contours should be included up to it, but not beyond this level (Schulz-Menger et al. 2020). In common practice, endocardium tracing is sufficient considering the thinness (~3 mm) of the RV wall.

When RV mass evaluation is required (e.g., in the context of pulmonary stenosis/regurgitation such as in Fallot patients), both endo- and epicardial contours can be performed. Cardiac infiltration (Fig. 6) or pulmonary hypertension can also cause RV wall thickening.

Note that RV trabeculations should be included in the RV volume for reproducibility reasons (Kawel-Boehm et al. 2020). Normal values are presented in Table 3.

Tricuspid annular plane systolic excursion (TAPSE) is widely used in echocardiography (Seemann et al. 2017; Sepúlveda-Martínez et al. 2021) due to the predominantly longitudinal shortening of the RV. It is considered abnormal if <17 mm (Rudski et al. 2010). Although TAPSE can easily be recorded by MRI or CT, its diagnostic value is subject to debate (Lee et al. 2018).

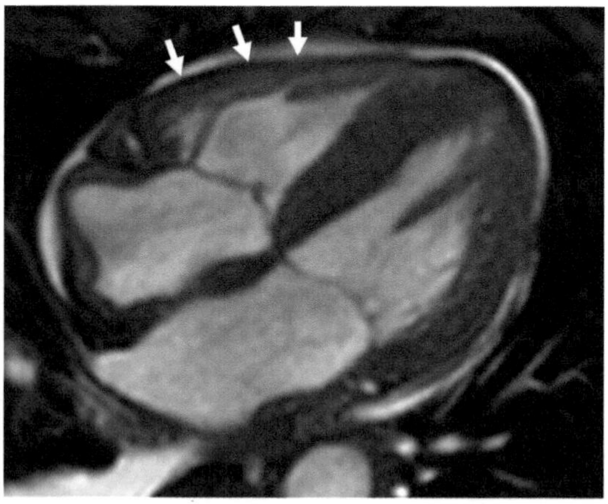

Fig. 6 Hypertrophy of the right ventricle free wall (arrows) in a patient with cardiac amyloidosis

Table 3 Right ventricle normal values

Right ventricle	Male	Female	Athlete male	Athlete female
EF (%)	66 ± 7	66 ± 7	50 ± 4	52 ± 5
SV (mL)	106 ± 18	83 ± 13	143 ± 34	112 ± 26
ED vol (mL)	163 ± 27	127 ± 24	284 ± 42	214 ± 32
ES vol (mL)	57 ± 17	44 ± 15	141 ± 27	102 ± 20
SV_i (mL/m^2)	54 ± 8	48 ± 7	71 ± 15	60 ± 14
ED vol_i (mL/m^2)	83 ± 13	74 ± 12	140 ± 18	116 ± 16
ES vol_i (mL/m^2)	29 ± 9	26 ± 8	69 ± 12	56 ± 13

Results presented as mean ± standard deviation
For more details, please see Kawel-Boehm et al. (2020). Male and female athlete values are based on the mean values between regular (9–18-h sport activity per week) and elite (>18 h/week) athletes according to references (Kawel-Boehm et al. 2020; Prakken et al. 2010) with SV being the difference between ED and ES volumes
EF ejection fraction, *ED/ES vol/vol$_i$* absolute/indexed end-diastolic/systolic volumes, *SV/SV$_i$* absolute and index stroke volumes

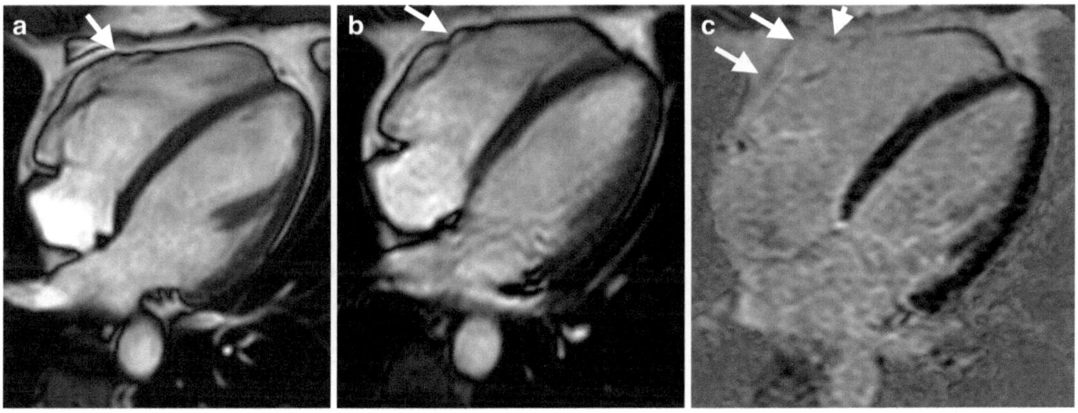

Fig. 7 Cardiac MRI of a patient with arrhythmogenic cardiomyopathy. (**a** and **b**) Subtle accordion sign of the RV free wall. (**c**) Late gadolinium enhancement of the RV myocardium on PSIR sequence. *PSIR* phase-sensitive inversion recovery

Another quick and more precise RV function parameter is the RV fractional area change (RVFAC). The RVFAC accounts for both longitudinal and transversal components of RV contraction. It is calculated as the difference between end-diastolic and end-systolic RV areas (on 4C views) divided by the end-diastolic area. An RVFAC of <41% accurately predicts an RVEF of <45% (Caudron et al. 2011b). If there is any clinical suspicion of altered RV function, a precise evaluation of the RV using the short-axis disk method is recommended.

It is worth noting that to confirm RV functional parameters, a comparison of RV stroke volume to LV stroke volume can be performed. Indeed, in the absence of shunt or valvular regurgitation, RV and LV stroke volumes should be similar.

A basal RV diameter >42 mm suggests dilatation in adults (Rudski et al. 2010). In children, RV dilatation is suggested when the end-systolic area is >10.5 cm^2/m^2 and end-diastolic area is >8.5 cm^2/m^2 (Barczuk-Falęcka et al. 2018).

The association of a decreased TAPSE, dilated RV, a "crinkled" appearance of the RVOT, and subtricuspid region (also known as the "accordion sign") with dyskinesia (Dalal et al. 2009) should suggest arrhythmogenic cardiomyopathy (Fig. 7). Confirmation of a reduced RVEF (≤40%) and a dilated RV (≥100 mL/m^2 in men, ≥90 mL/m^2 in women) through segmentation on short axis (as mentioned above) are criteria (respectively, major and minor) that can contribute to the diagnosis (Towbin et al. 2019).

7 Right Atrium (RA)

By convention and similarly to the LA, RA volume (or surface) measurements should be performed when the RA displays its maximal volume, e.g., just before the opening of the tricuspid valve.

Methods to evaluate the RA are relatively similar to those for the LA (Sievers et al. 2007) and are based on the biplane area-length method. Right atrium size is, in part, determined by factors affecting RV filling. Therefore, RA volume may be a sign of RV diastolic dysfunction (Maceira et al. 2013). An RA surface >16 cm^2/m^2 or a longitudinal diameter in 2C view >3.5 cm/m^2 (Maceira et al. 2013) could indicate RA enlargement. The right atrial appendage should be excluded, as well as the confluence of the superior and inferior vena cava.

8 Right Atrial Appendage (RAA)

The RAA is a prolongation of the RA, located at its anterosuperior part and showing a wider neck compared to the LAA (Subramaniam et al. 2006). No specific dimensions have been published for the RAA. Although rare, thrombi can form in the RAA, carrying an increased risk of pulmonary embolism especially in case of AF (Anfinogenova et al. 2020).

9 Conclusion

Heart chamber measurements require a good understanding of cardiac anatomy and standard CT and MR reference planes. Here are some important points to keep in mind:

1. Cardiac MRI, including a stack of cine short-axis views, remains the gold standard for evaluating ejection fraction, mass, and volumes.
2. Assessing RVEF is more challenging than evaluating LVEF due to the complex morphology of the RV.
3. An altered atrioventricular plane displacement may indicate systolic ventricular dysfunction.
4. Volume estimation of LA/RA can be easily done in routine practice using the biplane area-length method.
5. Dilated LA/RA may indicate diastolic dysfunction, which can precede systolic dysfunction.
6. The LA and LAA are common locations for thrombi, especially in patients with atrial fibrillation.

Disclaimer All measurements in this book have been obtained from peer-reviewed papers and guidelines from professional organizations, unless explicitly stated otherwise. While the authors, editors, and publisher have gone through a rigorous process to establish their correct reproduction from the original source, each measurement must be interpreted in the correct clinical context, this along with an accurate way of measurement, and taking into account all technical variables, this including follow-up exams with various equipment or software. Neither the authors, the editors, nor the publisher can accept any legal responsibility for any improper application or interpretation of these measurements as well as their potential consequences.

References

Alfakih K, Plein S, Bloomer T, Jones T, Ridgway J, Sivananthan M (2003) Comparison of right ventricular volume measurements between axial and short axis orientation using steady-state free precession magnetic resonance imaging. J Magn Reson Imaging 18(1):25–32. https://doi.org/10.1002/jmri.10329

Anfinogenova ND, Vasiltseva OY, Vrublevsky AV, Vorozhtsova IN, Popov SV, Smorgon AV, Mochula OV, Ussov WY (2020) Right atrial thrombosis and pulmonary embolism: a narrative review. Semin Thromb Hemost 46(8):895–907. https://doi.org/10.1055/s-0040-1718399

Atalay MK, Chang KJ, Grand DJ, Haji-Momenian S, Machan JT, Sheehan FH (2013) The transaxial orientation is superior to both the short axis and horizontal long axis orientations for determining right ventricular volume and ejection fraction using Simpson's method with cardiac magnetic resonance. ISRN Cardiol 2013:268697. https://doi.org/10.1155/2013/268697

Barczuk-Falęcka M, Małek ŁA, Roik D, Werys K, Werner B, Brzewski M (2018) Right ventricular end-systolic

area as a simple first-line marker predicting right ventricular enlargement and decreased systolic function in children referred for cardiac magnetic resonance imaging. Clin Radiol 73(6):592.e9–592.e14. https://doi.org/10.1016/j.crad.2018.01.020
Caudron J, Fares J, Bauer F, Dacher J-N (2011a) Evaluation of left ventricular diastolic function with cardiac MR imaging. Radiographics 31(1):239–259. https://doi.org/10.1148/rg.311105049
Caudron J, Fares J, Vivier P-H, Lefebvre V, Petitjean C, Dacher J-N (2011b) Diagnostic accuracy and variability of three semi-quantitative methods for assessing right ventricular systolic function from cardiac MRI in patients with acquired heart disease. Eur Radiol 21(10):2111–2120. https://doi.org/10.1007/s00330-011-2152-0
Caudron J, Fares J, Lefebvre V, Vivier P-H, Petitjean C, Dacher J-N (2012) Cardiac MRI assessment of right ventricular function in acquired heart disease: factors of variability. Acad Radiol 19(8):991–1002. https://doi.org/10.1016/j.acra.2012.03.022
Cwajg JM, Cwajg E, Nagueh SF, He ZX, Qureshi U, Olmos LI, Quinones MA, Verani MS, Winters WL, Zoghbi WA (2000) End-diastolic wall thickness as a predictor of recovery of function in myocardial hibernation: relation to rest-redistribution T1-201 tomography and dobutamine stress echocardiography. J Am Coll Cardiol 35(5):1152–1161. https://doi.org/10.1016/s0735-1097(00)00525-8
Dalal D, Tandri H, Judge DP, Amat N, Macedo R, Jain R, Tichnell C, Daly A, James C, Russell SD, Abraham T, Bluemke DA, Calkins H (2009) Morphologic variants of familial arrhythmogenic right ventricular dysplasia/cardiomyopathy a genetics-magnetic resonance imaging correlation study. J Am Coll Cardiol 53(15):1289–1299. https://doi.org/10.1016/j.jacc.2008.12.045
Dayal NB, Müller H (2017) Discovery of left ventricular hypertrophy during adult echocardiography. Rev Med Suisse 13(564):1106–1112
Di Biase L, Santangeli P, Anselmino M, Mohanty P, Salvetti I, Gili S, Horton R, Sanchez JE, Bai R, Mohanty S, Pump A, Cereceda Brantes M, Gallinghouse GJ, Burkhardt JD, Cesarani F, Scaglione M, Natale A, Gaita F (2012) Does the left atrial appendage morphology correlate with the risk of stroke in patients with atrial fibrillation? Results from a multicenter study. J Am Coll Cardiol 60(6):531–538. https://doi.org/10.1016/j.jacc.2012.04.032
Garcia MJ, Kwong RY, Scherrer-Crosbie M, Taub CC, Blankstein R, Lima J, Bonow RO, Eshtehardi P, Bois JP, American Heart Association Council on Cardiovascular Radiology and Intervention and Council on Clinical Cardiology (2020) State of the art: imaging for myocardial viability: a scientific statement from the American Heart Association. Circ Cardiovasc Imaging 13(7):e000053. https://doi.org/10.1161/HCI.0000000000000053
Kawel N, Nacif M, Arai AE, Gomes AS, Hundley WG, Johnson WC, Prince MR, Stacey RB, Lima JAC, Bluemke DA (2012) Trabeculated (noncompacted) and compact myocardium in adults: the multi-ethnic study of atherosclerosis. Circ Cardiovasc Imaging 5(3):357–366. https://doi.org/10.1161/CIRCIMAGING.111.971713
Kawel-Boehm N, Hetzel SJ, Ambale-Venkatesh B, Captur G, Francois CJ, Jerosch-Herold M, Salerno M, Teague SD, Valsangiacomo-Buechel E, van der Geest RJ, Bluemke DA (2020) Reference ranges ("normal values") for cardiovascular magnetic resonance (CMR) in adults and children: 2020 update. J Cardiovasc Magn Reson 22(1):87. https://doi.org/10.1186/s12968-020-00683-3
Konstantinides SV, Meyer G, Becattini C, Bueno H, Geersing G-J, Harjola V-P, Huisman MV, Humbert M, Jennings CS, Jiménez D, Kucher N, Lang IM, Lankeit M, Lorusso R, Mazzolai L, Meneveau N, Ní Áinle F, Prandoni P, Pruszczyk P et al (2020) 2019 ESC guidelines for the diagnosis and management of acute pulmonary embolism developed in collaboration with the European Respiratory Society (ERS). Eur Heart J 41(4):543–603. https://doi.org/10.1093/eurheartj/ehz405
Lee JZ, Low S-W, Pasha AK, Howe CL, Lee KS, Suryanarayana PG (2018) Comparison of tricuspid annular plane systolic excursion with fractional area change for the evaluation of right ventricular systolic function: a meta-analysis. Open Heart 5(1):e000667. https://doi.org/10.1136/openhrt-2017-000667
Maceira AM, Cosín-Sales J, Roughton M, Prasad SK, Pennell DJ (2013) Reference right atrial dimensions and volume estimation by steady state free precession cardiovascular magnetic resonance. J Cardiovasc Magn Reson 15(1):29. https://doi.org/10.1186/1532-429X-15-29
Nacif MS, Barranhas AD, Türkbey E, Marchiori E, Kawel N, Mello RAF, Falcão RO, Oliveira AC, Rochitte CE (2013) Left atrial volume quantification using cardiac MRI in atrial fibrillation: comparison of the Simpson's method with biplane area-length, ellipse, and three-dimensional methods. Diagn Interv Radiol (Ankara, Turkey) 19(3):213–220. https://doi.org/10.5152/dir.2012.002
Ommen SR, Mital S, Burke MA, Day SM, Deswal A, Elliott P, Evanovich LL, Hung J, Joglar JA, Kantor P, Kimmelstiel C, Kittleson M, Link MS, Maron MS, Martinez MW, Miyake CY, Schaff HV, Semsarian C, Sorajja P (2020) 2020 AHA/ACC guideline for the diagnosis and treatment of patients with hypertrophic cardiomyopathy: a report of the American College of Cardiology/American Heart Association Joint Committee on Clinical Practice Guidelines. Circulation 142(25):e558–e631. https://doi.org/10.1161/CIR.0000000000000937
Pelliccia A, Caselli S, Sharma S, Basso C, Bax JJ, Corrado D, D'Andrea A, D'Ascenzi F, Di Paolo FM, Edvardsen T, Gati S, Galderisi M, Heidbuchel H, Nchimi A, Nieman K, Papadakis M, Pisicchio C, Schmied C, Popescu BA, et al. Internal reviewers for EAPC and EACVI (2018) European Association of Preventive

Cardiology (EAPC) and European Association of Cardiovascular Imaging (EACVI) joint position statement: recommendations for the indication and interpretation of cardiovascular imaging in the evaluation of the athlete's heart. Eur Heart J 39(21):1949–1969. https://doi.org/10.1093/eurheartj/ehx532

Petersen SE, Selvanayagam JB, Wiesmann F, Robson MD, Francis JM, Anderson RH, Watkins H, Neubauer S (2005) Left ventricular non-compaction: insights from cardiovascular magnetic resonance imaging. J Am Coll Cardiol 46(1):101–105. https://doi.org/10.1016/j.jacc.2005.03.045

Petersen SE, Khanji MY, Plein S, Lancellotti P, Bucciarelli-Ducci C (2019) European Association of Cardiovascular Imaging expert consensus paper: a comprehensive review of cardiovascular magnetic resonance normal values of cardiac chamber size and aortic root in adults and recommendations for grading severity. Eur Heart J Cardiovasc Imaging 20(12):1321–1331. https://doi.org/10.1093/ehjci/jez232

Prakken NH, Velthuis BK, Teske AJ, Mosterd A, Mali WP, Cramer MJ (2010) Cardiac MRI reference values for athletes and nonathletes corrected for body surface area, training hours/week and sex. Eur J Cardiovasc Prev Rehabil 17(2):198–203. https://doi.org/10.1097/HJR.0b013e3283347fdb

Puntmann VO, Gebker R, Duckett S, Mirelis J, Schnackenburg B, Graefe M, Razavi R, Fleck E, Nagel E (2013) Left ventricular chamber dimensions and wall thickness by cardiovascular magnetic resonance: comparison with transthoracic echocardiography. Eur Heart J Cardiovasc Imaging 14(3):240–246. https://doi.org/10.1093/ehjci/jes145

Rudski LG, Lai WW, Afilalo J, Hua L, Handschumacher MD, Chandrasekaran K, Solomon SD, Louie EK, Schiller NB (2010) Guidelines for the echocardiographic assessment of the right heart in adults: a report from the American Society of Echocardiography endorsed by the European Association of Echocardiography, a registered branch of the European Society of Cardiology, and the Canadian Society of Echocardiography. J Am Soc Echocardiogr 23(7):685–713; quiz 786–788. https://doi.org/10.1016/j.echo.2010.05.010

Sanz J, Sánchez-Quintana D, Bossone E, Bogaard HJ, Naeije R (2019) Anatomy, function, and dysfunction of the right ventricle: JACC state-of-the-art review. J Am Coll Cardiol 73(12):1463–1482. https://doi.org/10.1016/j.jacc.2018.12.076

Schulz-Menger J, Bluemke DA, Bremerich J, Flamm SD, Fogel MA, Friedrich MG, Kim RJ, von Knobelsdorff-Brenkenhoff F, Kramer CM, Pennell DJ, Plein S, Nagel E (2020) Standardized image interpretation and post-processing in cardiovascular magnetic resonance - 2020 update: Society for Cardiovascular Magnetic Resonance (SCMR): Board of Trustees Task Force on Standardized Post-Processing. J Cardiovasc Magn Reson 22(1):19. https://doi.org/10.1186/s12968-020-00610-6

Seemann F, Pahlm U, Steding-Ehrenborg K, Ostenfeld E, Erlinge D, Dubois-Rande J-L, Jensen SE, Atar D, Arheden H, Carlsson M, Heiberg E (2017) Time-resolved tracking of the atrioventricular plane displacement in cardiovascular magnetic resonance (CMR) images. BMC Med Imaging 17:19. https://doi.org/10.1186/s12880-017-0189-5

Sepúlveda-Martínez A, Steding-Ehrenborg K, Rodríguez-López M, Ostenfeld E, Valenzuela-Alcaráz B, Heiberg E, Gratacós E, Prat-González S, Crispi F, Hedström E (2021) Atrioventricular plane displacement versus mitral and tricuspid annular plane systolic excursion: a comparison between cardiac magnetic resonance and M-mode echocardiography. Clin Physiol Funct Imaging 41(3):262–270. https://doi.org/10.1111/cpf.12693

Shah DJ, Kim HW, James O, Parker M, Wu E, Bonow RO, Judd RM, Kim RJ (2013) Prevalence of regional myocardial thinning and relationship with myocardial scarring in patients with coronary artery disease. JAMA 309(9):909–918. https://doi.org/10.1001/jama.2013.1381

Sievers B, Addo M, Breuckmann F, Barkhausen J, Erbel R (2007) Reference right atrial function determined by steady-state free precession cardiovascular magnetic resonance. J Cardiovasc Magn Reson 9(5):807–814. https://doi.org/10.1080/10976640701545552

Subramaniam B, Riley MF, Panzica PJ, Manning WJ (2006) Transesophageal echocardiographic assessment of right atrial appendage anatomy and function: comparison with the left atrial appendage and implications for local thrombus formation. J Am Soc Echocardiogr 19(4):429–433. https://doi.org/10.1016/j.echo.2005.10.013

Tacher V, Sifaoui I, Kharrat R, Dacher J-N, Chevance V, Gallet R, Teiger E, Kobeiter H, Le Pennec V, Jacquier A, Mandry D, Macron L, Derbel H, Deux J-F (2021) The use of cardiac computed tomography angiography in the assessment of percutaneous left atrial appendage closure—review and experts recommendations endorsed by the Société française d'imagerie cardiaque et vasculaire diagnostique et interventionnelle. Diagn Interv Imaging 102(10):586–592. https://doi.org/10.1016/j.diii.2021.05.010

Towbin JA, McKenna WJ, Abrams DJ, Ackerman MJ, Calkins H, Darrieux FCC, Daubert JP, de Chillou C, DePasquale EC, Desai MY, Estes NAM, Hua W, Indik JH, Ingles J, James CA, John RM, Judge DP, Keegan R, Krahn AD et al (2019) 2019 HRS expert consensus statement on evaluation, risk stratification, and management of arrhythmogenic cardiomyopathy. Heart Rhythm 16(11):e301–e372. https://doi.org/10.1016/j.hrthm.2019.05.007

Veselka J, Anavekar NS, Charron P (2017) Hypertrophic obstructive cardiomyopathy. Lancet (London, England) 389(10075):1253–1267. https://doi.org/10.1016/S0140-6736(16)31321-6

Valvular Flow

Savine C. S. Minderhoud and Alexander Hirsch

Contents

Abstract

Noninvasive evaluation of valve function is key in the diagnosis and choice of treatment in valvular disease. Echocardiography is the first choice to diagnose and to assess the mechanism, severity and prognosis of valvular disease. Cardiovascular magnetic resonance is used when there is inadequate quality or discrepant results with echocardiography. This chapter provides an overview on how to measure valvular flow accurately and when valvular flow can be used in clinical practice using cardiovascular magnetic resonance.

1 Pathophysiological Background

The primary function of cardiac valves is to ensure that blood flows in only one direction and, hence, prevent backward flow of blood. Pressure gradients are the driving forces behind blood flow, allowing blood to flow from regions with higher pressures to regions with lower pressures, but also regulate valve opening and closure. Cardiac valves open passively when upstream pressure exceeds downstream pressure and close passively when downstream pressure exceeds upstream pressure (Silverthorn et al. 2010). Each valve is anchored by a fibrous ring, the annulus, which is interconnected and forms together the cardiac skeleton (Fig. 1) (Dahou et al. 2019).

S. C. S. Minderhoud · A. Hirsch (✉)
Department of Cardiology and Radiology and Nuclear Medicine, Erasmus MC, University Medical Center Rotterdam, Rotterdam, The Netherlands
e-mail: s.minderhoud@erasmusmc.nl; a.hirsch@erasmusmc.nl

Med Radiol Diagn Imaging (2026)

https://doi.org/10.1007/174_2023_451,
Published Online: 06 September 2024

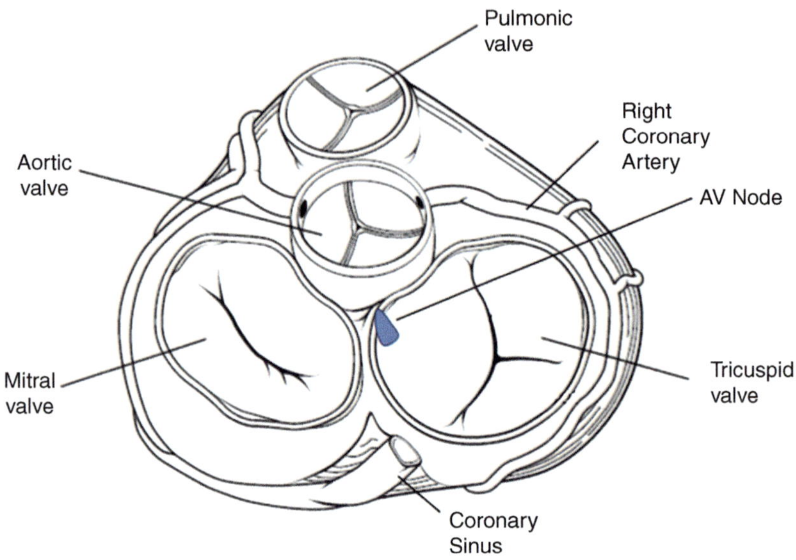

Fig. 1 The four cardiac valves of the heart. (Adapted from Dahou et al. 2019). *AV* atrioventricular

Both leakage and stenosis of each valve can occur. Regurgitation leads to a volume overload of the affected cardiac chamber, while stenosis leads to a pressure overload. Acute lesions can cause acute symptoms, whereas chronic valvular disease is generally compensated and therefore well tolerated for longer periods of time, with cardiac function as such often remaining preserved for years.

The mitral valve and tricuspid valve are the atrioventricular valves and separate the atria from the ventricles. Regurgitation, a key malfunction of these valves, can be divided into two primary categories. *Primary regurgitation* is typically precipitated by a malfunction of the valve leaflets or the subvalvular apparatus. This type of defect often emerges secondary to degenerative valve disease, endocarditis, or papillary muscle rupture resulting from acute myocardial infarction. *Secondary regurgitation*, on the other hand, arises due to the dilatation of the annulus, atria, or ventricles. Such expansion may prevent complete coaptation of the leaflets, leading to this form of regurgitation. Conversely, *valvular stenosis*, although less common in these valves, is predominantly instigated by rheumatic heart disease, which stands as the principal causative agent of atrioventricular valve stenosis (Baumgartner et al. 2021; Horstkotte et al. 1991; Vahanian et al. 2022).

Semilunar valves separate the ventricles from the great arteries: the aortic valve located between the left ventricle (LV) and aorta and the pulmonary valve between the right ventricle (RV) and the main pulmonary artery.

Aortic regurgitation results from dilation of the aortic root or abnormalities of the aortic valve leaflets caused by atherosclerotic degeneration, infective endocarditis, rheumatic disease, or a different morphology as in bicuspid aortic valves (Bekeredjian and Grayburn 2005).

Underlying mechanisms of *aortic stenosis* are most commonly degenerative thickening and calcification in the elderly, but also include rheumatic and bicuspid aortic valve disease. Besides at the valvular level, flow obstruction can also occur due to congenital defects at the sub- or supravalvular level. LV outflow tract obstruction can also occur in case of hypertrophic cardiomyopathy and may also lead to systolic anterior motion of the anterior mitral valve leaflet and mitral regurgitation.

Pulmonary stenosis is usually of congenital origin, and the stenosis can present at the sub-, supra-, or valvular level. In general, a surgical or endovascular intervention is required during childhood to (sometimes temporarily) restore valvular function, for example in children born with tetralogy of Fallot. Nevertheless, this intervention will often be the most common cause of *pulmonary regurgitation* later in life, for which close monitoring and eventually a reintervention may be required.

The most important parameters to assess valvular function are the transvalvular flow and velocity of the blood. In cardiovascular physiology, the term "flow" is commonly imprecisely used. Flow is often used to indicate flow rate, the volume of blood which passes per unit time. As such, flow rate actually measures *how much* blood passes through a point during a given unit of time, while velocity measures *how fast* blood passes through that same point. The relationship between flow rate (Q), velocity (v), and area (A) is established by the formula $v = Q/A$. This implicates that as area decreases in, e.g., a stenotic valve, transvalvular velocity must increase to continue to deliver the same amount of flow. Therefore, *peak blood velocity* is an important marker to quantify the degree of stenosis. Conversely, the relative amount of backward flow/retrograde volume compared to forward flow/antegrade volume quantifies the severity of valvular regurgitation. Finally, when correctly measured, a difference between aortic and pulmonary flow measurements indicates the presence of an intra- or extracardiac shunt.

2 Imaging Modalities to Visualize and Quantify Flow

Valvular heart disease is primarily assessed with Doppler echocardiography. This technique is excellent to measure blood flow velocities given its high temporal resolution and is routinely used due to its wide availability, portability, relatively low costs, and lack of contraindications. However, it is limited by its interobserver variability and acoustic windows and can only assess velocities accurately if flow is parallel to the transducer. Due to these limitations, imaging of right-sided heart valves can be difficult with echocardiography, especially the pulmonary valve in adults.

Computed tomography provides a fast three-dimensional (3D) scan with excellent spatial resolution; however, it has limited value measuring blood flow velocity and is as such not used for this indication. Therefore, in this chapter on valvular flow, only the application of cardiovascular magnetic resonance (CMR) will be discussed. For the quantification of valvular leaflet calcifications in patients with aortic valve stenosis, we refer to the chapter "Coronary Calcium Quantification."

In general, valvular assessment using CMR is indicated if echocardiographic quality is inadequate or measurements are borderline or ambiguous (Baumgartner et al. 2021; Otto et al. 2021; Stout et al. 2019; Vahanian et al. 2022). CMR is a noninvasive and nonionizing imaging technique that can be used to assess the severity of valvular lesions, particularly regurgitant lesions. However, one of its strengths is that it additionally assesses ventricular volumes and function, abnormalities of the great vessels, and myocardial tissue characterization including myocardial fibrosis and viability during one single imaging session (Myerson 2021). CMR is the gold standard imaging method for quantification of RV volumes and systolic function and is, therefore, particularly useful to evaluate the consequences of tricuspid and pulmonary regurgitation. It also has an incremental value for assessing the severity of aortic and mitral regurgitation and quantifying shunt ratios in congenital heart disease (Baumgartner et al. 2021; Stout et al. 2019). Finally, given unrestricted image planes, CMR can provide a complete overview of all four valves.

2.1 CMR Image Acquisition

CMR has the unique property to simultaneously register blood velocity and morphological data. With phase-contrast (PC) imaging, the MRI signal is used to visualize and quantify velocity. With this so-called PC method, spins that move along the magnetic field gradient acquire a shift in their phase of rotation that is different in comparison to stationary spins (Wymer et al. 2020). This phase shift is proportional to the velocity of the blood. Anatomical information is visualized on the magnitude images and resembles a normal bright-blood image. On the phase images, the gray value of each pixel represents the velocity information in that voxel. Stationary tissue is being displayed as mid-gray, with velocities in forward (positive) and reverse (negative) directions being represented as higher (toward white) and lower (toward black) pixel intensities (Biglands et al. 2012). Traditionally, PC data is acquired in a two-dimension plane (2D), and velocity information is mea-

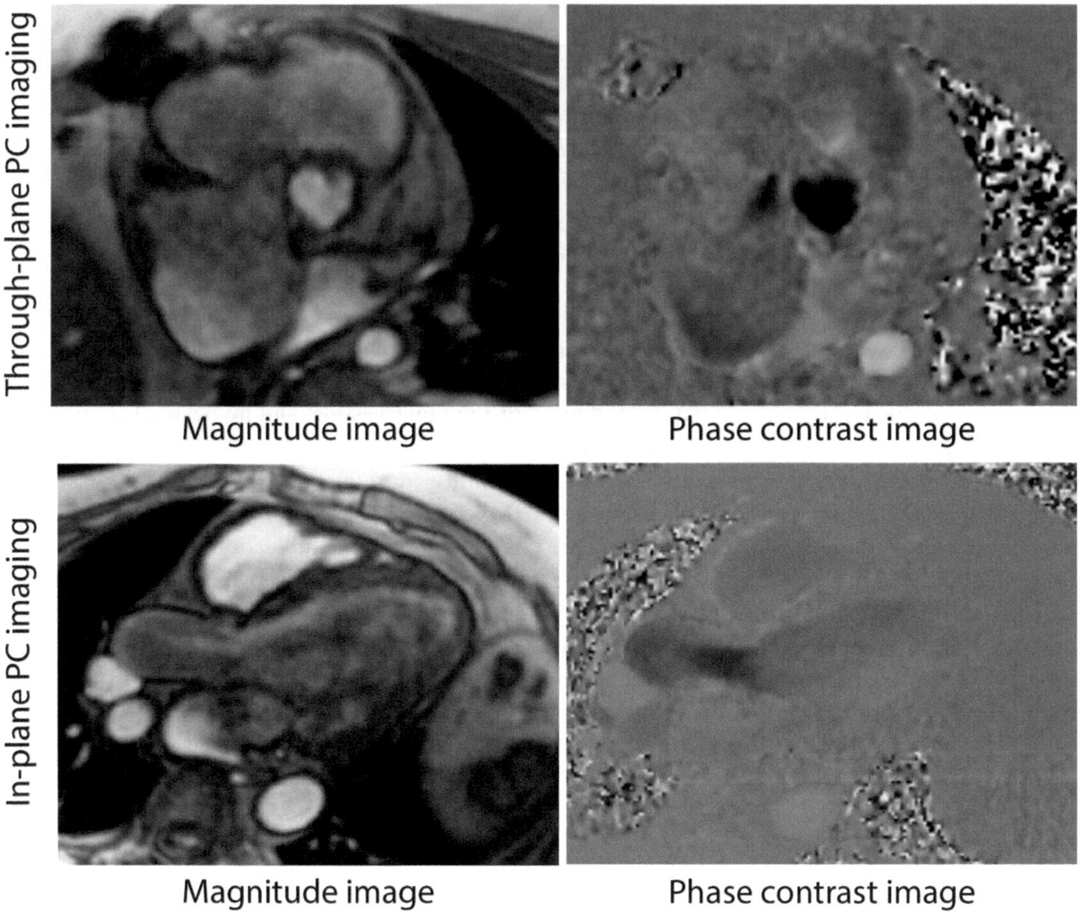

Fig. 2 (Top) Through-plane flow measurement at the level of the aortic valve. (Bottom) In-plane flow measurement of the aortic valve with measurement of velocity in left-right orientation

sured in one direction during the cardiac cycle. This can be "through-plane" or "in-plane" (Fig. 2). In the latter case, the velocity is measured in either anterior-posterior or left-right direction. With 2D PC CMR, the regurgitation fraction of the aortic and pulmonary valve can be directly quantified. Tricuspid and mitral valve regurgitation can be assessed indirectly, as described later in detail.

Due to technical advances, it is currently also possible to acquire PC data of a 3D volume during the entire cardiac cycle in a reasonable amount time. This is called 4D flow CMR and refers to PC CMR with flow encoding in all three spatial directions that is resolved relative to all three dimensions of space and to the dimension of time along the cardiac cycle (3D + time = 4D) (Dyverfeldt et al. 2015). With this technique, it is therefore possible to assess the function of all four cardiac valves using a single acquisition.

Table 1 summarizes the recommendations concerning acquisition, analysis, and measurements of 2D and 4D flow PC imaging.

Cine imaging with a balanced steady-state free precession (bSSFP) sequence is the preferred sequence to assess cardiac anatomy, volumes, and function because it provides high signal-to-noise ratio and excellent contrast between myocardium and blood pool. These cine images are acquired in standard LV long-axis (two-, three-, and four-chamber) and short-axis (stack from base to apex) views. In case of right-sided heart disease, additional views can be

Table 1 Summary of acquisition, analysis, and measurements of 2D and 4D flow phase-contrast imaging

	2D flow	4D flow
Acquisition	• One-direction, through-plane phase-contrast imaging orthogonally to the expected main blood flow or maximum velocity • In-plane resolution ≥10 pixels per vessel • Slice thickness 5–8 mm • Temporal resolution ≤50 ms • VENC ≥ expected peak velocity (in case of normal systemic flow 150 cm/s and normal pulmonary flow 100 cm/s) • Retrospective or prospective ECG gating • Breath-hold or free breathing with multiple signal averages in patients with limited breath-holding capabilities or in specific congenital conditions	• 3D volume coverage including valves and vessels of interest • Spatial resolution typically between 1.5 × 1.5 × 1.5 and 3.0 × 3.0 × 3.0 mm • Temporal resolution ≤40 ms • VENC ≥ expected peak velocity of the vessel or valve of interest • Retrospective or prospective ECG gating • Free breathing with or without respiratory gating (navigator, bellows, self-gating)
Phase-offset correction[a]	• No correction of phase-offset errors • Stationary tissue correction • Static phantom correction	• Stationary tissue correction
Analysis	• Semiautomatic contour detection of vessel/valve of interest with manual adaptation of individual cardiac phases • Review phase and magnitude images side by side • Exclude the noise outside the vessel	• During post-processing, orientation of planes can be chosen. Similar planes can be used as 2D flow planes (i.e., aortic valve, main pulmonary artery, left and right pulmonary artery) • Flow measurements in multiplane reconstructions • Flow measurements using (semi) automated valve tracking
Outcome parameters	• Antegrade flow, retrograde flow, net flow • Regurgitation fraction • Cardiac output and index • Peak and mean velocity • Q_p/Q_s ratio	• Antegrade flow, retrograde flow, net flow • Regurgitation fraction • Cardiac output and index • Peak and mean velocity • Q_p/Q_s ratio

Q_p pulmonary flow, Q_s systemic flow

[a]Currently, there is no evidence on which method is appropriate and should be recommended to correct for phase-offset errors

acquired including two-chamber RV, RV outflow tract, and a stack of axial images (Kramer et al. 2020). bSSFP sequences normally produce images with a "bright-blood" appearance. In the presence of flow jets, however, a signal void is often seen at the location of the jet. However this is less pronounced in bSSFP images compared to images acquired by spoiled gradient-echo pulse sequences, which are sometimes still used in higher-field-strength 3 Tesla systems or in patients with cardiac devices (Biglands et al. 2012). With cine imaging, location and direction of the regurgitation or stenotic flow jets can be assessed. In general, small leaks have narrow jets, which are more striking on cine images, while a more severe regurgitation is harder to see, especially at the pulmonary valve due to lower pressure gradient (Fig. 3). Qualitative assessment of these flow jets must be done with caution, as the size of the signal void depends on the pulse sequence type, the echo time, and a number of other parameters that affect the imaging gradient strength and duration (Biglands et al. 2012).

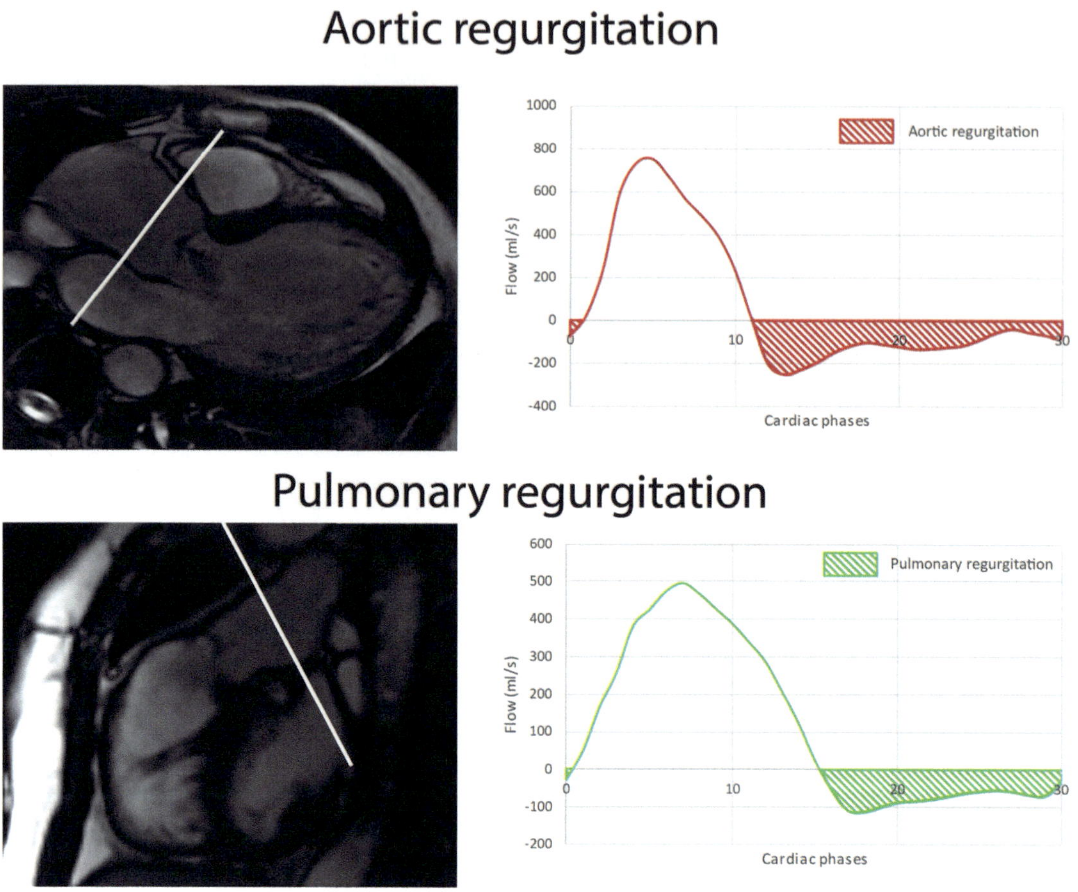

Fig. 3 Left panels depict balanced steady-state free precession (bSSFP) images. The white lines show the plane of the flow measurement, top aorta, and bottom pulmonary artery. Right panels show the corresponding flow versus time curves. Regurgitation fraction is calculated by dividing the retrograde flow by antegrade flow × 100%. Top panel: bicuspid aortic valve patient with severe aortic regurgitation with a regurgitation fraction of 51%. Bottom panel: tetralogy of Fallot patient with moderate pulmonary regurgitation with a regurgitation fraction of 24%

2.1.1 2D Flow Phase-Contrast Imaging

Valvular disease is still commonly assessed with 2D PC imaging using a velocity-encoded spoiled gradient-echo pulse sequence. With through-plane PC imaging, antegrade flow, retrograde flow, net flow, regurgitation fraction, and mean and maximum velocities can be quantified (Fig. 3). With in-plane PC, the location and extent of a stenosis or regurgitant jet flow can be visualized, but this should not be used for estimation of flow.

The vessel or valve of interest is by preference positioned in the magnetic isocenter of the scanner and in the center of the planned acquisition to minimize phase offset errors. Slice thickness is advised to be between 5 and 8 mm, and an in-plane resolution of at least 1/10th of the vessel diameter is advised (Kramer et al. 2020). When the voxel size is too large, because of the partial volume effects, velocities are averaged out, flow can be underestimated, and flow jets may not be visualized.

A temporal resolution of ≤50 ms between phases is advised. For example, in patients with a heart rate of 60 beats per minute, at least 20 scanned cardiac phases are required. Often, the temporal resolution is artificially increased by creating extra phases using image interpolation. When the temporal resolution is too low, highest velocities are not registered and maximum velocities can be underestimated (Fig. 4) (Lotz et al. 2002). Number of views per segment should then be decreased to increase temporal resolution. Temporal resolution with standard PC imaging remains low compared to echocardiography and, therefore, CMR-based flow velocities are sometimes underestimated compared to Doppler echocardiography. Overall, the correct balance between spatial, temporal resolution and scan time should be found, as for example increasing the temporal resolution will require to decrease the spatial resolution or to prolong scan time.

Scans can be performed during breath-hold or free breathing. A typical breath-hold PC scan takes about 12–15 s during which a sufficiently high temporal and spatial resolution can be achieved for accurate flow measurements. However, this is not always feasible in some populations like patients with limited breath-holding capabilities or young children. Free-breathing acquisition with multiple signal averages can then be a good alternative, although acquisition time is substantially prolonged. Also, in some specific patient populations, it is important to acquire flow data during free breathing, for example in patients with a Fontan circulation.

Velocity encoding sensitivity (VENC) is a setting that changes the strength of the bipolar gradients; therefore, it sets the range across which the velocities are acquired. A VENC set too low causes wrapping around of velocity information within a voxel, causing a mosaic pattern on the image, called aliasing (Fig. 5). As a result, flow

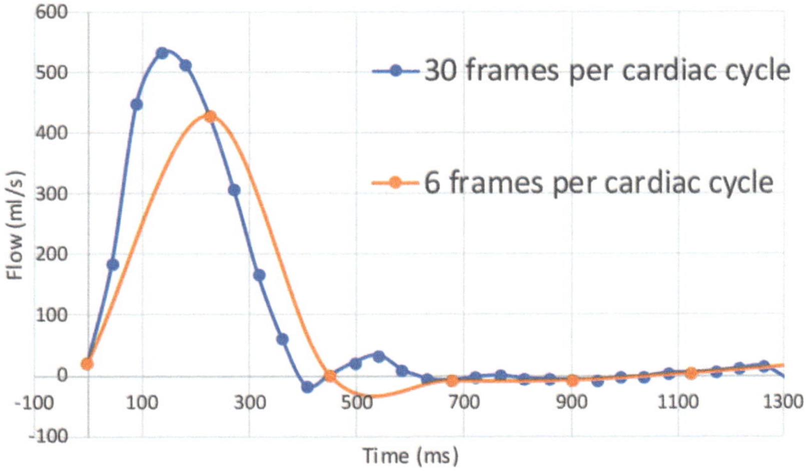

Fig. 4 Two flow curves during the cardiac cycle with different temporal resolution. If temporal resolution is too low, this can lead to underestimation of peak velocity and flow. Optimal temporal resolution is depending on the heart rate but should be at least <50 ms and approximately 25–30 phases per cardiac cycle

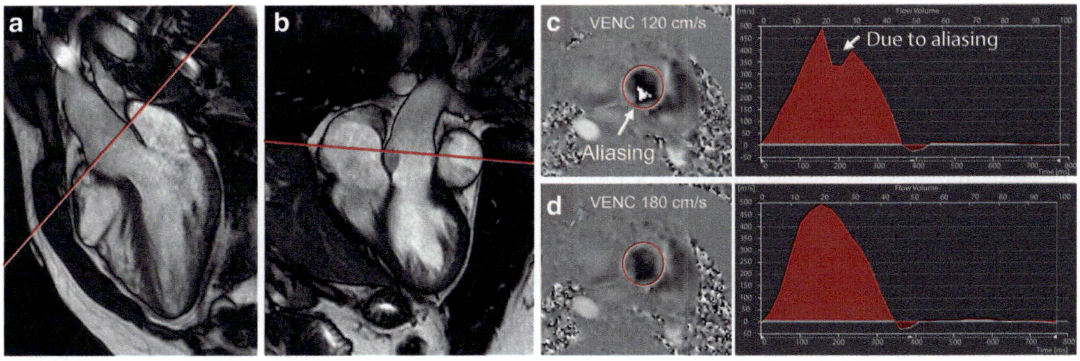

Fig. 5 Example of aliasing when measuring aortic valvular flow. (**a, b**) Demonstrate the planning of the valvular measurement at the tips of aortic valve leaflets (red lines). (**c**) Aliasing occurs using a VENC of 120 cm/s, and corresponding flow curve is showing a typical dip in the curve at maximum flow. (**d**) By increasing the VENC to 180 cm/s, aliasing has disappeared and the flow curve is normalized

analysis is unreliable. Although aliasing correction is available in several post-processing software packages, it is only possible to correct this to a certain degree. Preferably, the acquisition is repeated with a higher VENC until no aliasing occurs. Conversely, the VENC which is set too high will cause signal-to-noise ratio to decrease, with the increased noise subsequently affecting or masking flow jets and especially peak velocities (Lotz et al. 2002). Therefore, it is good practice to start with the lowest expected velocity without aliasing, and when aliasing does occur, the VENC should be increased accordingly. If it is difficult to know what the maximum velocity will be, an in-plane acquisition could be helpful to measure the peak velocity. Also, a "VENC scout" or "flow scout" can be performed to assess the appropriate velocity, although currently not all vendors provide this sequence. For normal systemic flow, a VENC of 150 cm/s is advised and 100 cm/s for right-sided flow. Finally, echo time should be set as short as possible, in particular when stenoses are imaged (Kramer et al. 2020).

PC imaging can be performed with prospective or retrospective ECG gating. With prospective ECG gating, the scanner collects k-space lines for each cardiac time frame, and its timing is based on R-wave detection. A limitation is that no data is collected in the late-diastolic phase, which is especially important when assessing the inflow of the mitral and tricuspid valve and regurgitation of the aorta and pulmonary valve. However, it has advantages in patients with continuously variable R-R intervals, as in, e.g., atrial fibrillation, in which prospective ECG gating would be a better option than retrospective gating.

With retrospective ECG gating, the entire cardiac cycle is measured and is therefore in general the preferred method. It also leads to a higher effective temporal resolution. In patients with a limited number of premature ventricular or atrial beats, retrospective ECG gating with arrythmia rejection is a possibility. Arrythmia rejection is a method to reject irregular R-R intervals. However, this can lead to very long breath-holds.

Also, real-time flow imaging can provide a solution to overcome the problem of averaging cardiac cycles of different lengths in patients with arrhythmias but also shows the physiological change per cardiac cycle. However, this sequence is currently not widely available, limiting its practical application and diffusion.

Finally, presence of metal-containing material may lead to signal loss and will be seen as an artifact. This can occur in patients after cardiac surgery and stent placement or in patients with implanted cardiac devices or previous valve replacement. Careful planning and assessment of the PC images should be done to assess if accurate measurements can be obtained. In patients after valve replacement, flow measurements should be planned distally from the valve.

In Table 2, a summary of sources of errors in flow measurements, implications, and possible solutions is presented.

2.1.2 4D Flow CMR

For a 4D flow CMR acquisition, the whole heart should be covered and scanning in the transversal plane is preferred (Zhong et al. 2019). 4D flow CMR is still time consuming and can take up to 15 min depending on spatial coverage and acceleration, limiting its usage in daily clinical practice. To speed this up, acceleration approaches such as parallel imaging, compressed sensing, and non-Cartesian trajectory techniques have been developed. Administration of a contrast agent improves the signal-to-noise ratio, but research so far indicates that there is no effect on the measurements itself, specifically intervalvular consistency (Juffermans et al. 2021). Spatial resolution should be at least $3.0 \times 3.0 \times 3.0$ mm^3 and temporal resolution $\leq$40 ms for intracardiac analysis (Dyverfeldt et al. 2015). Shortest echo and repetition time are preferred (Zhong et al. 2019). Retrospective gating is preferred over prospective, since then the entire cardiac cycle is covered. Respiratory motion suppression is important, and compensation for respiratory-related artifacts is achieved with bellow reading, navigator gating of the diaphragm motion, or self-gating techniques (Demirkiran et al. 2021). The VENC should be set 10% higher than the maximum expected velocity (Dyverfeldt et al. 2015). A 2D flow scout can help to set the correct VENC. Setting the VENC can be challenging if both very high and low veloci-

Table 2 Sources of errors in flow measurements, implications, and possible solutions

Factor	Effect	Implications	Possible solution
Eddy currents	Background phase-offset errors	Unreliable flow and velocity measurements	• Vessel of interest at isocenter of scanner • Phantom scan for correction • Consider other correction methods (i.e., stationary tissue correction)
Deviation of image plane (2D flow)	Smaller velocities detected	Underestimation of the maximum velocity and flow	• Use two orthogonal views to plan flow sequence perpendicular to the direction of flow • For maximum velocity measurement, plan acquisition perpendicular to flow direction
Inadequate spatial resolution	Partial volume effects leading to averaging out of peak velocities	Lower maximum velocities	• Slice thickness ≤7 mm • For small vessels in plane resolution, minimum 4–6 pixels per vessel diameter; however, ≥10 pixels preferred
Inadequate temporal resolution	Insufficient timepoints with information are collected	Lower maximum velocities and flow are measured	• Temporal resolution <50 ms • If breath-hold too long, consider free breathing
Too low VENC	Aliasing, where velocity information is wrapped around within a voxel	Unreliable measurement, acquisition should be repeated	• Increase VENC • To a certain extent, unwrap possible during post-processing
Too high VENC	Noise increases with higher VENCs. The maximum velocity can be masked	Underestimation of maximum velocities/ unreliable flow measurements	• Decrease VENC with optimal within 10–25% of the true peak velocity
Arrhythmias	Images are not averaged with the correct phase of the cardiac cycle	Unreliable flow and velocity measurements	• Rescan • Arrythmia rejection • Prospective triggering
Turbulence	Signal loss and backward and forward flow are averaged per cardiac phase	Precision of flow measurement declines	• Different acquisition plane (i.e., at the valve, measuring left and right pulmonary arteries separately instead of main pulmonary artery)

VENC velocity encoding sensitivity

ties need to be measured. For analyses of the valves, two orthogonally orientated cine images of each individual valve are recommended if retrospective valvular tracking will be performed (Fig. 6) (Juffermans et al. 2021).

With 4D flow CMR, all components of the velocity direction are known, and no underestimation of velocity can occur due to inaccurate planning. Therefore, 4D flow CMR is superior to 2D flow for quantification and identification of peak flow velocities (Adriaans et al. 2020). In general, with 4D flow CMR, velocity information of a large 3D volume is collected, and therefore, retrospectively, flow parameters can be assessed at multiple levels and orientations. However, 4D flow scanning takes longer as previously stated, and a final quality assessment can only take place after reconstruction of all images has been completed. If quality is suboptimal, i.e., due to artifacts, or VENC was set too low, no backup sequences are available as with multiple 2D PC image acquisitions.

2.1.3 Measurement Errors

Influences intrinsic to an MRI system, such as an elevated slew rate and larger gradient amplitude, contribute to the escalation of eddy currents (Rolf et al. 2011). Nevertheless, these eddy currents are constrained at the magnetic isocenter. The combination of eddy currents, Maxwell fields, and nonlinear magnetic field gradients induces phase-offset inaccuracies. Adjustments for Maxwell

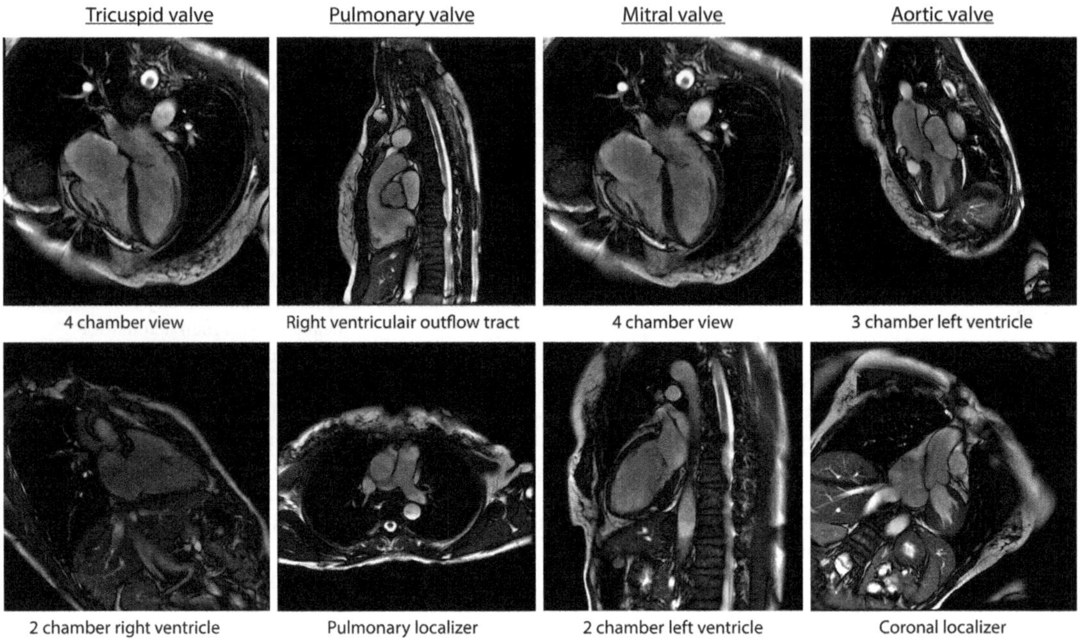

Fig. 6 Planning of valvular flow. Two acquisitions per valve are recommended in order to plan the flow sequence perpendicular to the vessel or valve of interest. For 4D flow analysis, retrospective valve tracking can be used, and therefore, these two orthogonal views per valve are also recommended

field and nonlinear magnetic field gradients can be applied during the image reconstruction stage, but rectifying eddy currents proves challenging. Positioning the subject vessel or valve at the magnetic isocenter and making phase-offset corrections during post-processing could mitigate the impact of phase-offset errors on flow assessments. While peak velocity remains relatively unaffected by minor background phase offsets, volume measurements are considerably sensitive to even slight background phase offsets due to the compounding effect of spatial and temporal integration (Schulz-Menger et al. 2020). The susceptibility to phase-offset errors varies with scanner characteristics; some scanners exhibit a higher tendency toward these errors (Gatehouse et al. 2010).

Stationary tissue correction and static phantom correction have been suggested as potential rectification methods (Fig. 7). Stationary tissue correction approximates the phase-offset error using linear (first order), tilted (second order), or curved (third order) interpolation at the vessel of interest, utilizing surrounding stationary tissue. However, phase offset does not typically follow a predictable pattern and may vary substantially across different scanners. Hence, this method could potentially amplify, rather than reduce, your error margin, especially in 2D PC imaging, where stationary tissue may be scarce (Minderhoud et al. 2020).

Alternatively, scanning a static phantom using identical sequence parameters allows for pixel-by-pixel background subtraction, often regarded as the standard method. However, this approach has its limitations, such as the additional scanning time required for the phantom, and due to temporal instability, phase-offset patterns may vary between patient and phantom scans. In conclusion, a meticulous evaluation of phase-offset errors for each individual scanner is paramount in deciding whether routine implementation of phantom correction is necessary.

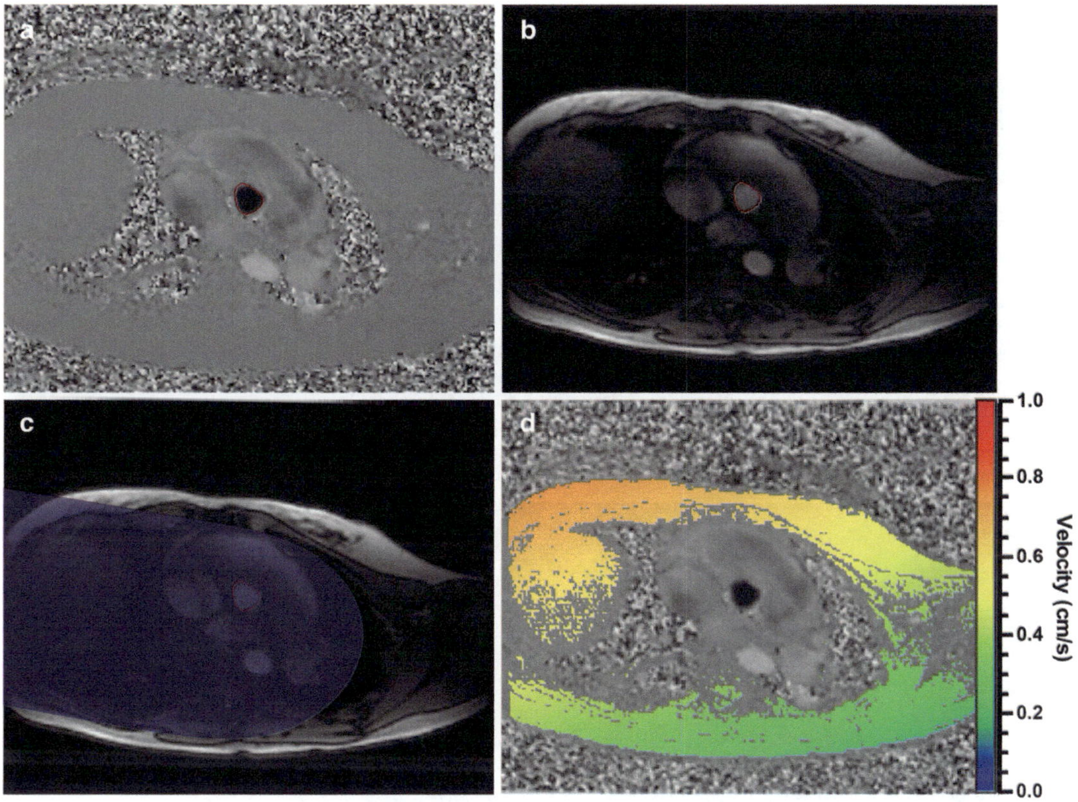

Fig. 7 Example of phase-contrast imaging with (**a**) phase-contrast image, (**b**) magnitude image, (**c**) magnitude image with overprojection of static phantom acquired directly after the patient was taken out the bore with exactly the same scan parameters, and (**d**) stationary tissue detection used for phase-offset correction

2.2 Planning of Valvular Flow in 2D PC Imaging

The most accurate flow results with through-plane 2D PC imaging are obtained when the acquisition is planned orthogonally to the expected main blood flow or perpendicular to the flow jet in case the parameter of interest is the maximum velocity. If the plane is not orthogonally placed to the vessel and flow direction, velocity vectors in the encoded direction are smaller. Significant underestimation of the velocity occurs when there is more than 15° of deviation of the image plane from the true flow.

To correctly plan the PC sequence, first two localizer images in two different directions should be acquired (Fig. 6). For the aortic valve, a coronal localizer should be acquired perpendicular on the three-chamber view through the aortic valve. For the pulmonary valve, an RV outflow tract cine is acquired and a second view perpendicular to this plane. For the mitral valve, a standard long-axis two-chamber and four-chamber can be used, and for the tricuspid valve, a standard four-chamber and a two-chamber cine of the RV (planned perpendicular on the four-chamber through the tricuspid valve) is required.

For assessing maximum velocities over the aortic and pulmonary valve, the image plane should be planned just distally from the valve leaflet tips in systole. A breath-hold sequence is preferred over free breathing due to more through-plane motion close to the valve during free breathing. A more accurate measurement of peak velocities can be made with a breath-hold sequence. For flow measurements, the acquisition plane can be more distally from the valve. Planning of the aortic and pulmonary flow is shown in Fig. 8. For the aortic valve, the image plane can be either planned at the valve coaptation or above. If flow is measured at the sinotubular junction or above, it should be noted that coronary flow is missed, which is about

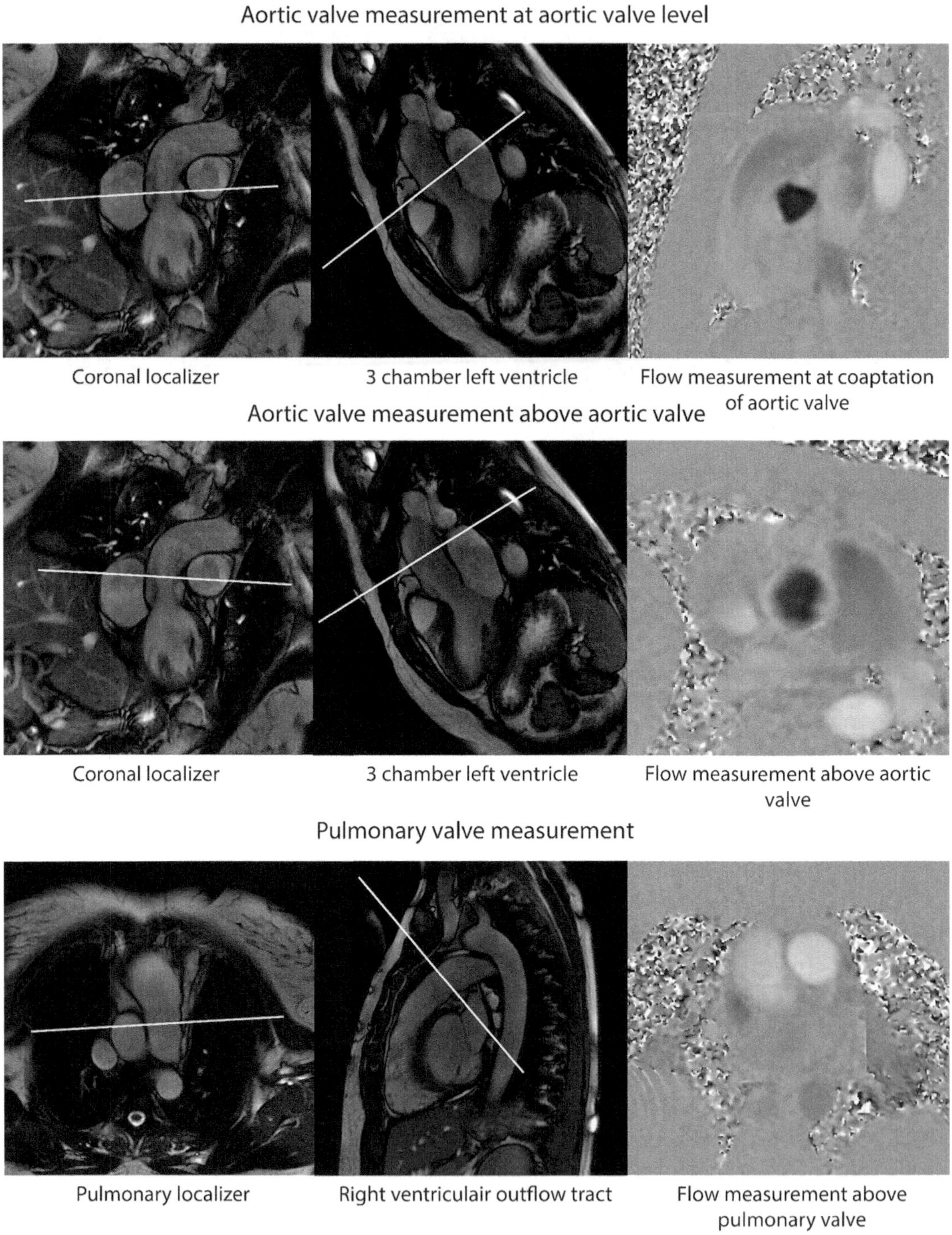

Fig. 8 Planning of aortic and pulmonary flow measurements. Top row: planning of through-plane aortic flow at tips of aortic valve leaflets; middle row: measurement of flow at the level of the ascending aorta; bottom row: planning of through-plane flow of the main pulmonary artery between the valve and pulmonary bifurcation

5% of the cardiac output. Flow in the pulmonary artery is commonly measured about 1–2 cm distally from the valve level and proximal to the pulmonary bifurcation. While planning the level of the acquisition, attention should be paid to the dynamic motion of the valve annulus across the cardiac cycle.

It is important to plan the acquisition at a position where the flow is laminar to reduce the influence of turbulent flow. In case of turbulence, there is both forward and backward flow within the scanned vessel during the same cardiac phase. Commonly, in post-processing software packages, the velocity information per cardiac phase is averaged, meaning that forward and backward flow during turbulence is also averaged (Fig. 9). During analysis, attention should be paid if turbulence is present, and the results should then be

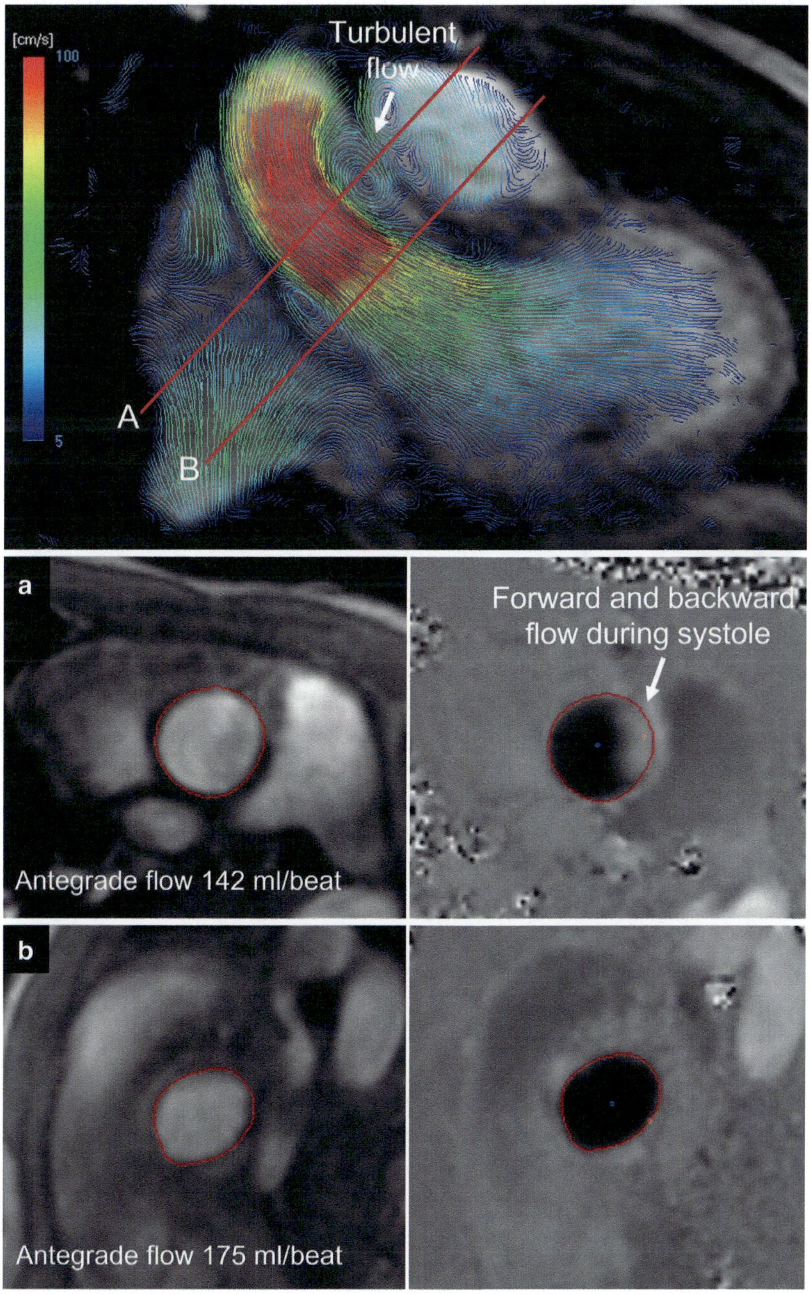

Fig. 9 Patient with turbulent flow in the ascending aorta. Top panel: 4D flow image showing turbulent flow just above the sinotubular junction. (**a**) Flow measurement at the level of turbulence leads to underestimation of the antegrade flow. (**b**) Flow measurement below the level of turbulence results in a higher measured antegrade flow

interpreted appropriately. In valves with both turbulent stenotic and regurgitant jets, no single slice position can estimate both forward and backward flow accurately and it is advised to perform PC images at multiple levels and orientations and perhaps with different VENCs in order to obtain a complete assessment as possible.

For the mitral and tricuspid valve, the transvalvular flow measurement is planned on the long-axis cine views as described in Fig. 6. However, direct measurement of regurgitation volume is not accurate on these 2D PC images due to the movement of the valvular plane.

2.3 Quantification of Valvular Flow

Several commercial software packages are available to analyze the 2D PC images. It is advised to review the phase and magnitude images side by side. The first step is to decide if phase-offset error correction should be done (see paragraph about measurement errors above). If a phantom has been scanned, preferable background subtraction using a static phantom should be applied. Then, automatic contour detection of the vessel of interest is used as a starting point, but contours should always be manually reviewed. Contours should be checked on the phase images, since the area of the flow on the phase images might be slightly larger than the anatomical area on the magnitude images due to partial volume effects and significant movement of the vessel (Lotz et al. 2002; Schulz-Menger et al. 2020). Also, presence of aliasing should be checked, and, if necessary, aliasing correction to a certain extent can be applied in most software packages.

Also, for 4D flow CMR analysis, several software packages (with or without valve tracking) are available. However, these are still under development and analysis is less straightforward as for 2D PC imaging. Analysis should start by evaluating the quality of the images. If phase wrapping is present, correct for aliasing or do not measure at a level where aliasing is present. Stationary tissue correction can be applied in most software packages.

If valve tracking is not used during postprocessing, similar planes as for 2D PC imaging are commonly used (i.e., ascending aorta, main pulmonary artery, left and right pulmonary artery) and analysis is in general similar to 2D PC imaging analysis.

If cine images are used for anatomical information and valve tracking, attention should be kept on misalignment between cine and 4D flow acquisition, and if necessary, this should be corrected (Fig. 10) (Juffermans et al. 2021). All four valves are separately analyzed. Software with (automatic) valve tracking is advised as valve tracking considers the movement of the valvular plane and increases the accuracy of the measurement (Kamphuis et al. 2019). Manually, the contours of all four valves are adjusted separately per phase. Due to the turbulent nature of a regurgitation jet, artifacts can occur in the valvular plane. Regurgitation flow could be assessed in a plane with the maximum flow subvalvular in a region without turbulence perpendicular to the flow jet, rather than aligning with the anatomical valve. Measurements can still be very challenging with eccentric or multiple regurgitation jets.

Regarding peak velocities, in general, 2D PC imaging underestimates the peak velocity compared to echocardiography. Doppler echocardiography measurements correlate excellent with invasively measured pressures but tend to overestimate the peak velocity. While 4D flow measurements have no significant bias, the correlation is good, but not excellent compared with invasive measurements (Archer et al. 2020; Grafton-Clarke et al. 2022). In cases of eccentric and multiple jets, 4D flow is preferred as it allows retrospective measurement at any location covered by the 4D flow.

The flow per heartbeat is calculated by integration of the velocity over time per heartbeat and taking a second integral over the cross-sectional area. Depending on the direction of the velocity sign, antegrade (forward) and retrograde (backward) volume can be distinguished. Subtraction of antegrade and retrograde volume of all cardiac phases gives the net volume (Schulz-Menger et al. 2020). Net volume (in mL) multiplied by heart rate and divided by 1000

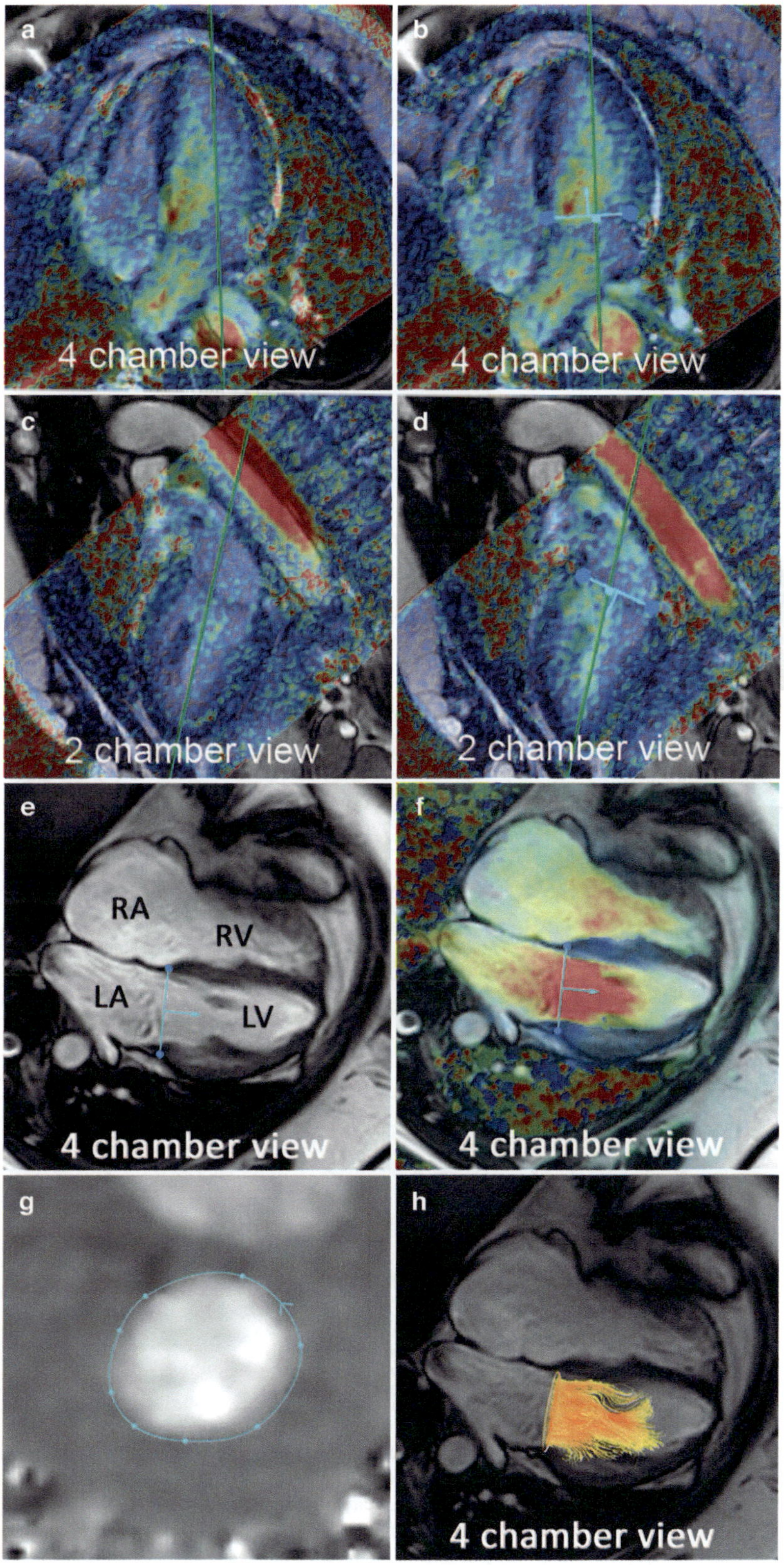

Fig. 10 A stepwise approach for mitral valve assessment with automated valve tracking on 4D flow. Start with visual inspection of cine views with projected 4D flow CMR-derived through-valve velocity maps. (**a**) Misalignment in four-chamber view, (**b**) correction of misalignment in four-chamber view. Misalignment should be checked in two directions: (**c**) misalignment in two-chamber view, (**d**) correction of misalignment in two-chamber view. (**e**) Automated valve tracking of the annular plane in four-chamber view (two-chamber view not shown here), (**f**) visual inspection of cine view with projected 4D flow CMR-derived through-valve velocity maps. (**g**) Delineation of the valve in each cardiac phase and (**h**) streamline visualization of the 4D flow CMR-derived transvalvular velocity (Adapted from Juffermans et al. 2021)

gives the cardiac output in liter per minute. Regurgitation fraction is calculated by dividing the retrograde volume over the antegrade volume times 100%. This method is often used to estimate the degree of regurgitation of the semilunar valves. In case of a large, dilated aorta, the quantification of aortic regurgitation volume might be inaccurate. Alternatively, the net pulmonary artery flow or the sum of the caval return can be subtracted from the aortic forward flow in the absence of any aortic and pulmonary collateral flow (Schulz-Menger et al. 2020). Regurgitation of the atrioventricular valves can be measured by direct measurement of the diastolic flow across the valve and subtraction of the systolic forward flow of the associated semilunar valve. However, most often, an indirect measurement is performed. Indirectly, the regurgitation volume is quantified by measurement of the stroke volume of the adjacent ventricle and subtraction of the forward flow across the associated semilunar valve. The regurgitation fraction is then calculated by dividing the regurgitation volume from the stroke volume of the adjacent ventricle (Fig. 11). Other indirect ways are also shown in Fig. 11. With 4D flow, automatic valve tracking improves the measurement as it considers the movement of the valvular plane. This is especially important when assessing the tricuspid or mitral valve (Westenberg et al. 2008). Furthermore, the regional flow distribution to the pulmonary arteries can be calculated by measuring the flow in both left and right pulmonary arteries separately, and this can also be used as an internal check for consistency of the measurements in the main pulmonary artery. Finally, valvular measurement can be used to estimate the size of a shunt by subtracting the pulmonary artery net flow (Q_p) by the aortic, systemic, net flow (Q_s) giving the Q_p/Q_s ratio.

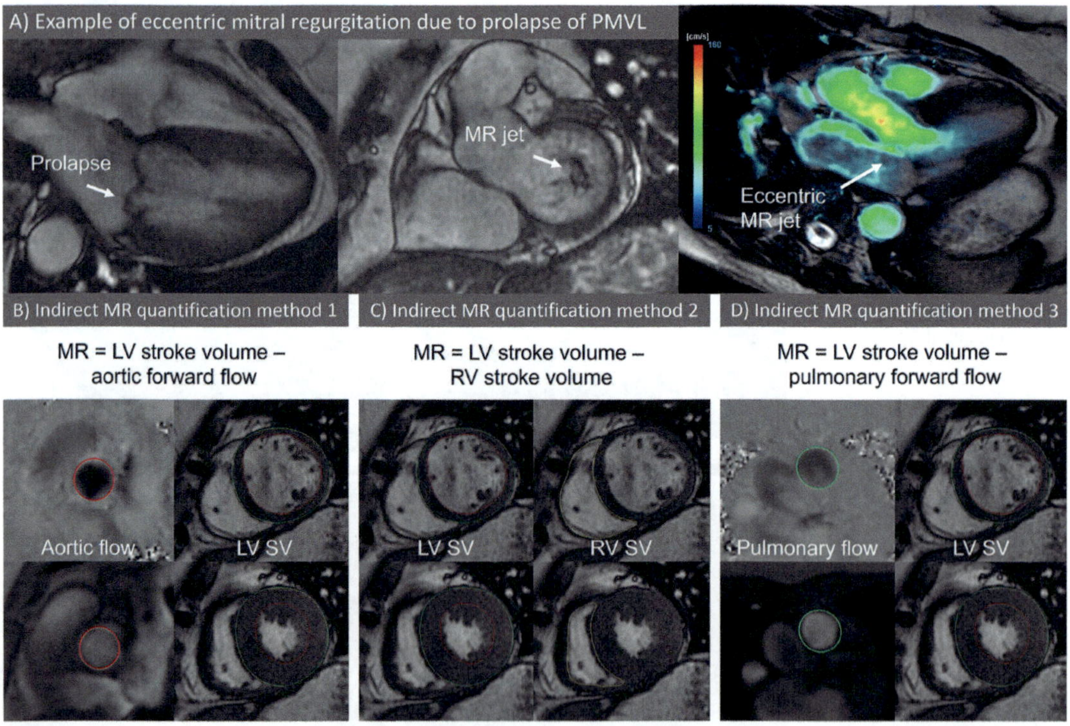

Fig. 11 (**a**) Example of an eccentric mitral regurgitation due to prolapse of posterior mitral valve leaflet (PMVL). Mitral valve regurgitation (MR) volume (mL) can be measured using three different indirect methods. (**b**) Subtracting left ventricular (LV) stroke volume (SV) by aortic forward flow (i.e., not valid in the presence of ventricular septum defect). (**c**) Subtracting LV stroke volume by right ventricular (RV) stroke volume (only valid in single-valve disease). (**d**) Subtracting LV stroke volume by pulmonary forward flow. Mitral valve regurgitation fraction is calculated by dividing the regurgitation volume by LV stroke volume times 100%

2.4 Valvular Stenosis

As discussed in the previous paragraph, the mean and maximum velocity can be assessed using through-plane and in-plane PC imaging and used as parameters for stenosis severity. This technique can also be used for example in LV outflow tract obstruction in hypertrophic cardiomyopathy to assess where flow acceleration occurs.

Regarding valvular stenosis, direct measurement of the valve area is also possible using planimetry. Therefore, a stack of thin-sliced cine images without inter-slice gap is planned parallel to the valve. The valve area can then be measured at the valve tips in systole for the semilunar valves and in diastole for the atrioventricular valves. An example of aortic valve stenosis and aortic valve area (AVA) measurement is presented in Fig. 12.

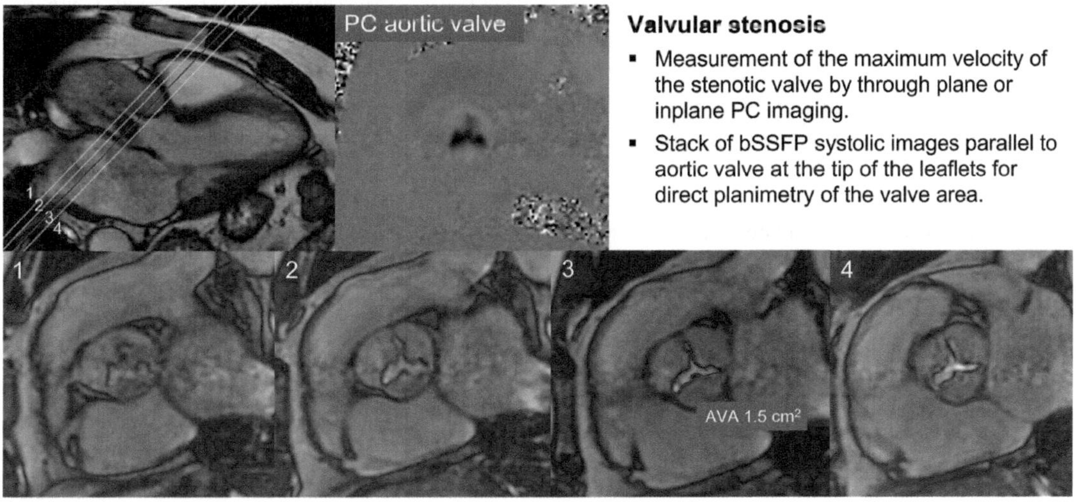

Fig. 12 Measurements in a patient with aortic stenosis. Top: maximal velocity is assessed using phase-contrast (PC) imaging in a plane orthogonal to the aortic stenosis jet. Bottom: aortic valve area planimetry. A stack of balanced steady-state free precession (bSSFP) images during systole is acquired at multiple levels using a thin slice thickness (~4–5 mm) without an inter-slice gap. During systole, the level which exactly recorded the valve opening with the smallest aortic valve area (AVA) is determined and measured

2.5 Classification of Valvular Disease Severity

Currently, reference values do not exist for assessment of valvular regurgitation and stenoses. Both pathologies are generally categorized into no/trace, mild, moderate, or severe pathology, and this categorization is largely based on echocardiographic guidelines. However, several studies suggest that CMR-determined thresholds for regurgitation might be more appropriate (Myerson et al. 2012, 2016; Uretsky et al. 2015). Table 3 gives an overview of how regurgitation and stenosis could be classified per valve (Garg et al. 2020; Myerson 2021; Zoghbi et al. 2017). Well-validated thresholds are still required, ideally based on outcome data (Garg et al. 2020). Reproducibility of PC imaging is high for retrograde volume and regurgitant fraction ($r > 0.97$), if patients have similar loading conditions (Dulce et al. 1992; Globits et al. 1996). Excellent correlations between invasive and PC imaging-based regurgitation quantification have been reported (Hundley et al. 1995). Strong correlations are found between Doppler echocardiography and PC imaging (Kizilbash et al. 1998). For velocities, reproducibility using PC imaging was good ($r > 0.97$, aortic valve level). However, CMR has the tendency to underestimate especially higher velocities compared to echocardiography, but the correlation is otherwise strong between the two modalities (Caruthers et al. 2003).

Table 3 Proposed CMR-based thresholds for valvular stenosis and regurgitation grade and shunt measurements

Proposed CMR thresholds for stenosis severity based on peak velocity (m/s)				
	None	*Mild*	*Moderate*	*Severe*
Pulmonary	–	<3	3–4	>4
Aortic	–	<3	3–4	>4
Proposed CMR thresholds for regurgitation severity based on regurgitation fraction (%)[a]				
	None	*Mild*	*Moderate*	*Severe*
Tricuspid	0–5%	5–20%	20–40%	>40%
Pulmonary	0–5%	5–20%	20–40%	>40%
Mitral	0–5%	5–20%	20–40%	>40%
Aortic	0–5%	5–20%	20–33%	>33%
Shunt	*Lower limit*		*Upper limit*	
Q_p/Q_s	<0.8		>1.2	
Hemodynamically significant shunt	–		>1.5	

Q_p pulmonary flow, Q_s systemic flow

[a] These thresholds are not definite and all are study based. Good validated thresholds are still required, ideally on the basis of outcome data (Garg et al. 2020)

3 Clinical Implementation

3.1 Aortic and Pulmonary Valve Disease

In aortic stenotic disease, CMR is especially useful and indicated when the acoustic window with echocardiography is inadequate or incoherence exists between the AVA and valvular gradient. However, CMR is inferior in terms of temporal resolution, turbulence can lead to flow artifacts, and partial-volume effects of 2D flow imaging in the *z*-direction can lead to underestimation of the maximal velocity. Nevertheless, an advantage of CMR is that a direct AVA measurement by planimetry can be performed. Furthermore, aortic valve morphology and concomitant aortopathy can be assessed, and the impact of the valve disease on the myocardium can be determined by measuring ventricular volumes, function, mass, and fibrosis during the same examination. Underlying pathologies of LV hypertrophy can be distinguished like cardiac amyloidosis (Singh and McCann 2019). Myocardial fibrosis can be assessed with late gadolinium enhancement, which is associated with a worse prognosis and more diffuse fibrosis with T1 mapping (Musa et al. 2018). In patients with hypertrophic cardiomyopathy with systolic anterior motion of the anterior mitral valve leaflet and in patients with a subvalvular fibrotic ridge below the valve, the severity and location of the left ventricular outflow tract obstruction can be assessed with in- and through-plane PC acquisitions, although this is only possible in rest.

Assessment of aortic regurgitation with CMR is accurate and gives a good quantitative measurement of the regurgitation fraction. During the same examination, the mechanism of aortic valve regurgitation, aortic valve morphology, information on aortic pathology, and a comprehensive assessment of LV function and volumes can be done.

Pulmonary valve stenosis assessment is done similarly as aortic valve stenosis assessment. CMR can help to distinguish between RV outflow tract obstruction caused by aberrant muscular band in a double-chamber RV and a subvalvular stenosis. With CMR, RV hypertrophy and dysfunction can be measured and additional levels of stenoses in the pulmonary arteries can be evaluated with contrast or non-contrast magnetic resonance angiography. One of the most important indications for valvular assessment with CMR is pulmonary valve regurgitation and concomitant quantification of RV volumes and function and evaluation of the pulmonary branches. These results are used for timing of surgical interventions, for example in patients after repaired tetralogy of Fallot.

3.2 Mitral and Tricuspid Valve Disease

With regard to mitral and tricuspid valve stenosis, echocardiography is the preferred imaging method. However, using cine imaging, a valve area can directly be measured by planimetry. In mitral valve regurgitation disease, CMR can be used for further quantification of the regurgitant volume and fraction. However, CMR is a second-line noninvasive test. There might be more than one defect, or the regurgitation jet is eccentric as it could be in case of mitral valve prolapse, tethering of a leaflet, or scallop. When echocardiographic assessment is unsatisfactory and discrepancy between echo-based measurements exists, CMR is indicated. A contiguous stack of cine slice gives a comprehensive coverage of all scallops of the mitral valve and helps to assess the leaflet morphology and the mechanism of mitral valve regurgitation. Again, this can be combined with a comprehensive analysis of the LV including late gadolinium enhancement in, for example, patients with mitral valve prolapse and mitral annular disjunction and also in patients with secondary mitral valve regurgitation due to ischemic heart disease for viability assessment. Due to the limited spatial and temporal resolution, CMR is not recommend for the assessment of valve lesions like vegetation in patients with suspected infective endocarditis.

Tricuspid regurgitation assessment with CMR is not well established, and severity grading has not been validated. Direct assessment with 2D flow PC is problematic because of substantial through-plane motion of the valve similar to the mitral valve. Therefore, a contiguous stack of cine images is advised to assess tricuspid valve morphology. Through-plane velocity measurements can be used to determine the size and shape of tricuspid regurgitation orifice. Indirect methods allow quantification of regurgitation volume by subtracting the pulmonary forward volume from the RV stroke volume. However, it is important to notice that the measurement error for RV volumes is higher than for the LV. 4D flow CMR using valve tracking is a promising new technique; however, it should be further validated especially in more complex congenital patients like those with Ebstein anomaly. Also, cardiac devices like pacemakers or implantable cardiac defibrillator can hamper reliable measurements.

3.3 Prosthetic Valves

The vast majority of the mechanical valves are safe in 1.5 T and 3 T scanners. Velocity mapping is often unreliable close to the mechanical valve due to local artifacts (Fig. 13). This assessment can be done distally from the mechanical valve, and regurgitation volume and fraction can be assessed in these patients. Transcatheter aortic valve implantation has evolved into a widely used therapy in patients with severe aortic stenosis. Aortic regurgitation due to paravalvular leak is an important complication of this procedure and can accurately be quantified with through-plane PC imaging. CMR is also useful to assess the aortic root for postoperative dissection or false aneurysms.

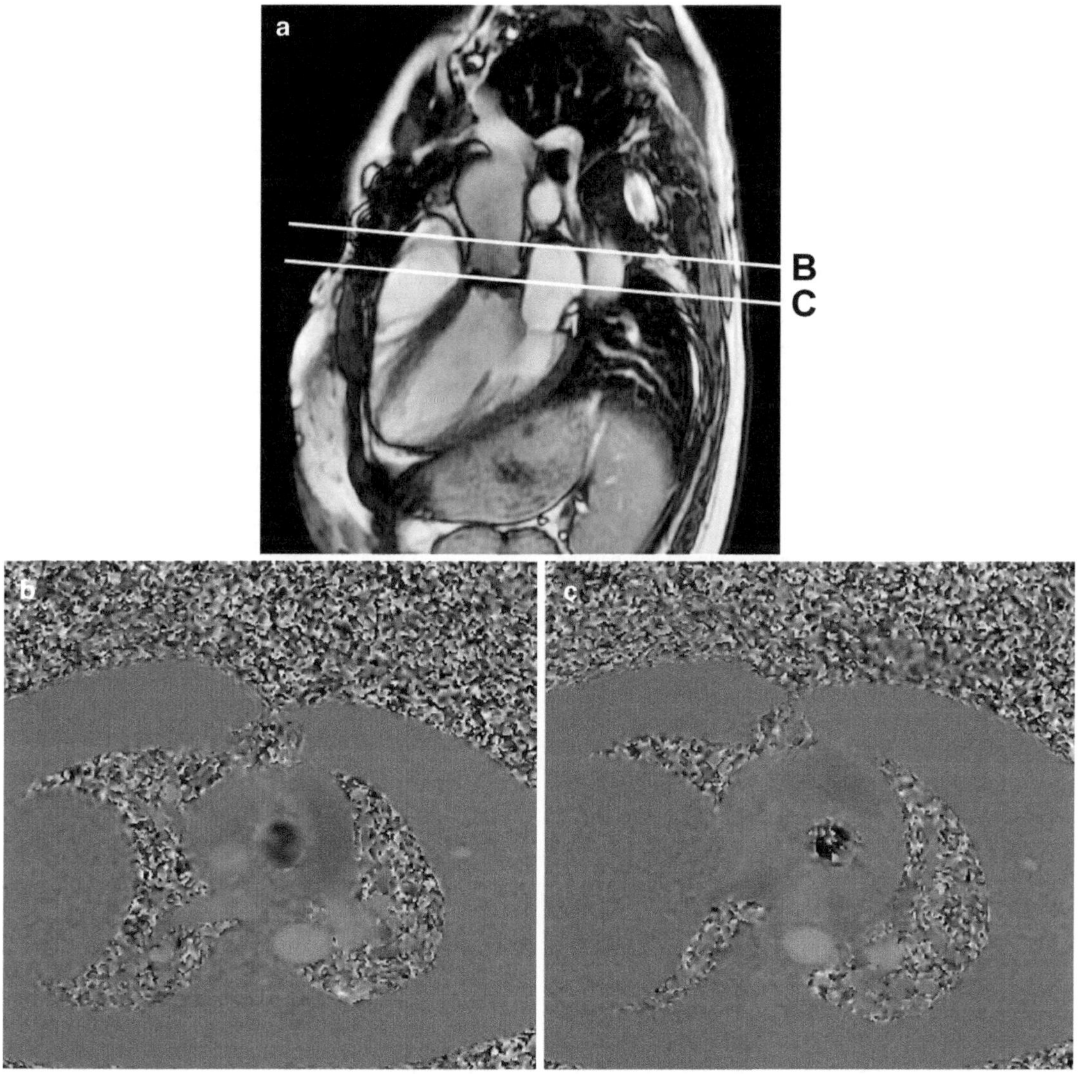

Fig. 13 (**a**) Three-chamber view of a patient with a mechanical valve in aortic position. (**b**) Phase-contrast image above valvular level. (**c**) Phase-contrast image at valvular level with clear artifacts. Due to distortion of the magnetic field, flow needs to be measured above or below the mechanic valve

Disclaimer All measurements in this book have been obtained from peer-reviewed papers and guidelines from professional organizations, unless explicitly stated otherwise. While the authors, editors, and publisher have gone through a rigorous process to establish their correct reproduction from the original source, each measurement must be interpreted in the correct clinical context, this along with an accurate way of measurement, and taking into account all technical variables, this including follow-up exams with various equipment or software. Neither the authors, the editors, nor the publisher can accept any legal responsibility for any improper application or interpretation of these measurements as well as their potential consequences.

References

Adriaans BP, Westenberg JJM, van Cauteren YJM et al (2020) Clinical assessment of aortic valve stenosis: comparison between 4D flow MRI and transthoracic echocardiography. J Magn Reson Imaging 51:472–480

Archer GT, Elhawaz A, Barker N et al (2020) Validation of four-dimensional flow cardiovascular magnetic resonance for aortic stenosis assessment. Sci Rep 10:10569

Baumgartner H, De Backer J, Babu-Narayan SV et al (2021) 2020 ESC Guidelines for the management of adult congenital heart disease. Eur Heart J 42:563–645

Bekeredjian R, Grayburn PA (2005) Valvular heart disease: aortic regurgitation. Circulation 112:125–134

Biglands JD, Radjenovic A, Ridgway JP (2012) Cardiovascular magnetic resonance physics for clinicians: part II. J Cardiovasc Magn Reson 14

Caruthers SD, Lin SJ, Brown P et al (2003) Practical value of cardiac magnetic resonance imaging for clinical quantification of aortic valve stenosis: comparison with echocardiography. Circulation 108:2236–2243

Dahou A, Levin D, Reisman M, Hahn RT (2019) Anatomy and physiology of the tricuspid valve. JACC Cardiovasc Imaging 12:458–468

Demirkiran A, van Ooij P, Westenberg JJM et al (2021) Clinical intra-cardiac 4D flow CMR: acquisition, analysis, and clinical applications. Eur Heart J Cardiovasc Imaging 23:154–165

Dulce MC, Mostbeck GH, O'Sullivan M et al (1992) Severity of aortic regurgitation: interstudy reproducibility of measurements with velocity-encoded cine MR imaging. Radiology 185:235–240

Dyverfeldt P, Bissell M, Barker AJ et al (2015) 4D flow cardiovascular magnetic resonance consensus statement. J Cardiovasc Magn Reson 17:1–19

Garg P, Swift AJ, Zhong L et al (2020) Assessment of mitral valve regurgitation by cardiovascular magnetic resonance imaging. Nat Rev Cardiol 17:298–312

Gatehouse P, Rolf M, Graves M et al (2010) Flow measurement by cardiovascular magnetic resonance: a multi-centre multi-vendor study of background phase offset errors that can compromise the accuracy of derived regurgitant or shunt flow measurements. J Cardiovasc Magn Reson 12:5

Globits S, Blake L, Bourne M et al (1996) Assessment of hemodynamic effects of angiotensin-converting enzyme inhibitor therapy in chronic aortic regurgitation by using velocity-encoded cine magnetic resonance imaging. Am Heart J 131:289–293

Grafton-Clarke C, Njoku P, Aben JP et al (2022) Validation of aortic valve pressure gradient quantification using semi-automated 4D flow CMR pipeline. BMC Res Notes 15:151

Horstkotte D, Niehues R, Strauer BE (1991) Pathomorphological aspects, aetiology and natural history of acquired mitral valve stenosis. Eur Heart J 12:55–60

Hundley WG, Li HF, Willard JE et al (1995) Magnetic resonance imaging assessment of the severity of mitral regurgitation: comparison with invasive techniques. Circulation 92:1151–1158

Juffermans JF, Minderhoud SCS, Wittgren J et al (2021) Multicenter consistency assessment of valvular flow quantification with automated valve tracking in 4D flow CMR. JACC Cardiovasc Imaging 14:1354–1366

Kamphuis VP, Roest AAW, Marsan NA et al (2019) Automated cardiac valve tracking for flow quantification with four-dimensional flow MRI. Radiology 290:70–78

Kizilbash AM, Hundley WG, Willett DWL et al (1998) Comparison of quantitative doppler with magnetic resonance imaging for assessment of the severity of mitral regurgitation. Am J Cardiol 81:792–795

Kramer CM, Barkhausen J, Bucciarelli-Ducci C et al (2020) Standardized cardiovascular magnetic resonance imaging (CMR) protocols: 2020 update. J Cardiovasc Magn Reson 22:1–18

Lotz J, Meier C, Leppert A, Galanski M (2002) Cardiovascular flow measurement with phase-contrast MR imaging: basic facts and implementation. Radiographics 22:651–671

Minderhoud SCS, van der Velde N, Wentzel JJ et al (2020) The clinical impact of phase offset errors and different correction methods in cardiovascular magnetic resonance phase contrast imaging: a multi-scanner study. J Cardiovasc Magn Reson 22:68

Musa TA, Treibel TA, Vassiliou VS et al (2018) Myocardial scar and mortality in severe aortic stenosis: data from the BSCMR valve consortium. Circulation 138:1935–1947

Myerson SG (2021) CMR in evaluating valvular heart disease: diagnosis, severity, and outcomes. JACC Cardiovasc Imaging 14:2020–2032

Myerson SG, Arcy J, Christiansen JP et al (2016) Valvular heart disease determination of clinical outcome in mitral regurgitation with cardiovascular magnetic resonance quantification. Circulation 133: 2287–2296

Myerson SG, D'arcy J, Mohiaddin R et al (2012) Aortic regurgitation quantification using cardiovascular magnetic resonance: association with clinical outcome. Circulation 126:1452–1460

Otto CM, Nishimura RA, Bonow RO et al (2021) 2020 ACC/AHA guideline for the management of patients with valvular heart disease: a report of the American College of Cardiology/American Heart Association Joint Committee on Clinical Practice Guidelines. J Am Coll Cardiol 77:e25–e197

Rolf MP, Hofman MBM, Gatehouse PD et al (2011) Sequence optimization to reduce velocity offsets in cardiovascular magnetic resonance volume flow quantification - a multi-vendor study. J Cardiovasc Magn Reson 13:18

Schulz-Menger J, Bluemke DA, Bremerich J et al (2020) Standardized image interpretation and post-processing in cardiovascular magnetic resonance - 2020 update: Society for Cardiovascular Magnetic Resonance (SCMR): Board of Trustees Task Force on Standardized Post-Processing. J Cardiovasc Magn Reson 22:19

Silverthorn DU, Johnson BR, Ober WC et al (2010) Human physiology an integrated approach. Fifth, Pearson Education, Boston

Singh A, McCann GP (2019) Cardiac magnetic resonance imaging for the assessment of aortic stenosis. Heart 105:489–497

Stout KK, Daniels CJ, Aboulhosn JA et al (2019) 2018 AHA/ACC guideline for the management of adults with congenital heart disease: a report of the American College of Cardiology/American Heart Association Task Force on Clinical Practice Guidelines. J Am Coll Cardiol 73:e81–e192

Uretsky S, Gillam L, Lang R et al (2015) Discordance between echocardiography and MRI in the assessment of mitral regurgitation severity. J Am Coll Cardiol 65:1079–1088

Vahanian A, Beyersdorf F, Praz F et al (2022) 2021 ESC/EACTS Guidelines for the management of valvular heart disease. Eur Heart J 43:561–632

Westenberg JJM, Roes SD, Marsan NA et al (2008) Mitral valve and tricuspid valve blood flow: accurate quantification with 3D velocity-encoded MR imaging with retrospective valve tracking. Radiology 249:792–800

Wymer DT, Patel KP, Burke WF, Bhatia VK (2020) Phase-contrast MRI: physics, techniques, and clinical applications. Radiographics 40:122–140

Zhong L, Schrauben EM, Garcia J et al (2019) Intracardiac 4D flow MRI in congenital heart disease: recommendations on behalf of the ISMRM Flow & Motion Study Group. J Magn Reson Imaging 50:677–681

Zoghbi WA, Adams D, Bonow RO et al (2017) Recommendations for noninvasive evaluation of native valvular regurgitation: a report from the American Society of Echocardiography Developed in Collaboration with the Society for Cardiovascular Magnetic Resonance. J Am Soc Echocardiogr 30:303–371

Myocardial Tissue Characterization

Nadine Kawel-Boehm

Contents

N. Kawel-Boehm (✉)
Department of Radiology, Kantonsspital Graubuenden, Chur, Switzerland
e-mail: nadine.kawel-boehm@ksgr.ch

1 Replacement Fibrosis: Delayed Enhancement in CT/MR

1.1 (Patho)Physiological and Technical Background

The normal left ventricular human myocardium is a composition of different structural elements. Cardiomyocytes account for about 75% of the normal human myocardial volume. The reminder 25% are allotted to the interstitium or extracellular volume (ECV), which contains blood vessels, nerves, various cells including fibroblasts, a gel-like ground substance composed of glycosaminoglycans and glycoproteins, and fibrillar connective tissue (Mewton et al. 2011; Weber 1989). The fibrillar connective tissue predominantly contains type I and III collagen and is also termed (extracellular) collagen matrix (Weber 1989) accounting for about 2–4% of the total myocardial volume of the left ventricle (Mewton et al. 2011). The collagen fibers provide a scaffolding for the cellular components and blood vessels and play an important role for the even transmission of the contractile force generated by myocytes (Weber 1989; Kong et al. 2014). About 85% of the total collagen is type I collagen, mainly associated with thick fibers that confer tensile strength (Weber 1989; Kong et al. 2014). Type III collagen, representing about 11% of the total collagen, is associated with thin fibers that confer resilience (Weber 1989; Kong et al. 2014).

Med Radiol Diagn Imaging (2026)

https://doi.org/10.1007/174_2023_403,
Published Online: 06 September 2024

Although myocytes account for 75% of the myocardial volume, they represent only 25% of the number of cells in the healthy heart (Jugdutt 2003). Seventy-five percent of the cells in the myocardium are nonmyocytes, of which the vast majority are fibroblasts (Jugdutt 2003). In the healthy heart, fibroblasts are responsible for the regulation of collagen turnover.

Acute myocardial injury characterized by myocyte death, e.g., due to myocardial infarction, induces an inflammatory response leading to an activation of the fibroblasts and ultimately to a focal replacement of the dead myocytes by fibrous tissue, mainly type I collagen (Kong et al. 2014). This focal type of replacement fibrosis or myocardial scarring is not only characteristic for myocardial infarction but it also occurs, e.g., in myocarditis, sarcoidosis, and hypertrophic cardiomyopathy (Mewton et al. 2011).

Cardiac magnetic resonance (CMR) imaging enables visualization of focal myocardial scar by means of late-gadolinium enhancement (LGE) imaging (Kellman and Arai 2012). LGE imaging is based on the intravenous application of a gadolinium-based contrast agent (GBCA) that shortens the T1-relaxation time. T1 shortening is greater in regions with a higher GBCA concentration (Kellman and Arai 2012). Visualization of a focal myocardial scar is related to differences in GBCA distribution and wash-in and wash-out kinetics of injured myocardium compared to normal myocardium.

In normal myocardium, the GBCA used for LGE imaging cannot cross the cell membrane of myocytes. After intravenous injection, the contrast agent and gadolinium molecules, respectively, diffuse from the intravascular in the relatively small extracellular space till an equilibrium is reached (Vohringer et al. 2007). As described above, in chronic myocardial injury, dead myocytes are replaced by a collagenous scar leading to an increase of the extracellular space. Thus, the volume of distribution for the gadolinium molecules is enlarged compared to normal myocardium (Vohringer et al. 2007).

The volume of distribution is also enlarged in acute myocardial injury, e.g., due to acute myocardial infarction. Acute myocardial injury is characterized by rupture of the cell membranes of the myocytes, enabling gadolinium molecules to distribute in the intracellular space. Further, in acute myocardial injury, the volume of distribution is also enlarged due to edema leading to an expansion of the extracellular volume (Kellman and Arai 2012).

The effect in acute and chronic myocardial injury is similar; due to enlargement of the volume of distribution, the concentration of GBCA is higher in areas of focal myocardial injury compared to normal myocardium.

Further, the wash-in and wash-out kinetics of the gadolinium-based contrast agent is different in normal myocardium compared to acute myocyte damage and chronic collagenous scar (Kellman and Arai 2012). It takes some minutes till the gadolinium molecules diffuse into the area of necrosis or scar and also to be washed out again, while the processes are faster in normal myocardium with intact vascular supply.

A special finding that can occur in the central necrotic region of subacute myocardial infarction is the "no-reflow" phenomenon. Due to delayed contrast penetration related to capillary plugging and subsequent hypoperfusion, the subendocardium or central core in the region of a bright subacute infarct remains black on LGE imaging (Vohringer et al. 2007). Due to prolongated arrival of the contrast, the area of microvascular obstruction (MVO) appears smaller with time after contrast administration (Vohringer et al. 2007).

Due to similar kinetics of gadolinium and iodine-based contrast agents, late-enhancement imaging has also been shown to be feasible by means of computed tomography (CT) (Gerber et al. 2006). Similar to the GBCA, the non-ionic iodinated contrast agents used for CT imaging are also extracellular and are not metabolized and excreted by the kidneys (Scully et al. 2018). In analogy to LGE imaging by CMR, where the T1-relaxation time varies by the concentration of the GBCA due to a linear relationship between the relaxation rate of the longitudinal magnetization and the change in contrast agent concentration, in CT late-enhancement imaging, the signal density values (Hounsfield units) are directly related to the attenuation of the X-ray beam by iodine molecules (Kellman and Arai 2012; Rodriguez-Granillo 2017). Further, a slow wash-in and slow wash-out of an iodine-based contrast medium in regions of myocardial infarction have been described, resulting in late enhancement between 4 and 20 min after intravenous contrast injection (Gerber et al. 2006). Similar to MR, late enhancement in CT is a result of the accumulation of iodine and delayed wash-out in areas of focal myocardial injury.

In patients with myocardial infarction, a good agreement was found between areas of late enhancement by contrast enhanced CT and areas of LGE by contrast enhanced MR (Gerber et al. 2006).

1.2 Image Acquisition and Analysis

1.2.1 Acquisition of Late Gadolinium Enhancement (LGE) Images by CMR

LGE images are acquired between 10 and 30 min after intravenous administration of GBCA at a dose of 0.15–0.2 mmol/kg body weight (Kellman and Arai 2012; Jimenez Juan et al. 2015). Late image acquisition is performed due to the mechanisms described above; the contrast agent will be washed out already from normal myocardium while it is still present in injured myocardium leading to differences in T1-relaxation time. For assessment of the left ventricle, images are acquired in a vertical long-axis view (2-chamber view), left ventricular outflow tract view (3-chamber view), horizontal long-axis view (4-chamber view), and a stack of short-axis images covering the entire left ventricle. The typical slice thickness varies between 6 and 8 mm, and the images of the short-axis stack are frequently acquired with a gap of 2–4 mm. Particularly for quantification of the LGE extent, slices of the LGE short-axis stack are acquired continuously without a gap. Image acquisition is usually performed during mid to late diastole to minimize cardiac motion (Kellman and Arai 2012). Generally, inversion recovery or phase sensitive inversion recovery (PSIR) T1-weighted sequences are used for LGE imaging (Kellman and Arai 2012). In clinical practice, mainly 2-dimensional (2D) inversion recovery gradient echo (GRE) or steady-state free precession (SSFP) techniques are used (Jimenez Juan et al. 2015). For patients short of breath, 2D single-shot inversion recovery SSFP sequences can be applied during free breathing but with limited spatial resolution (Jimenez Juan et al. 2015). If a high spatial resolution is required, 3D respiratory-gated inversion recovery sequences can be obtained, requiring a long acquisition time (Jimenez Juan et al. 2015).

To optimally identify focal myocardial injury by means of LGE imaging, a high contrast between normal myocardium and focal scar or necrosis is desired. Normal myocardium should appear black on the resulting image while scar/necrosis is bright due to the higher gadolinium concentration. The optimal contrast is achieved when the inversion recovery time (TI) is chosen to null the normal myocardium (Kellman and Arai 2012). To avoid measurement errors, image acquisition at the correct TI is particularly important for LGE quantification. There are different ways to determine the optimal TI (Kellman and Arai 2012): First, on a trial and error basis by acquiring the same image with different TIs to identify the optimal TI by the best resulting image with normal myocardium appearing black. Second, by means of a "TI-scout," that acquires several images during one breath hold at different cardiac phases with varying TIs. And third, to calculate TI by means of T1 mapping using the following formula: $TI = T1 \ln(2) = 0.69\ T1$, where T1 is the measured myocardial T1-relaxation time and ln the natural logarithm (Kellman and Arai 2012). If the inversion time was set too short, the normal myocardium will not be "nulled," which means that a positive signal is generated and the remote myocardium will not appear black on the resulting image (Finn et al. 2006).

For LGE imaging of the left atrium, three-dimensional sequences with respiratory navigation and ECG-gating acquired 15–25 min after contrast administration are preferred due to the high spatial resolution enabling visualization of the thin left atrial wall (Zghaib and Nazarian 2018). Images are acquired during atrial diastole with an inversion time chosen to null the left atrial myocardium.

1.2.2 Quantification of CMR Late-Gadolinium Enhancement (LGE)

Beside visual assessment and identification of different LGE patterns characteristic for ischemic and non-ischemic cardiomyopathies, the amount of LGE can be quantified in different ways (Table 1). In myocardial infarction, the transmural extent of the infarct can be measured and quantified as percent in relation to the total thickness of the left ventricular myocardial wall (Choi et al. 2001). Further, LGE extent can be quantified as the number of myocardial segments involved based on the 17-segment model of the American Heart Association (Cerqueira et al. 2002). The total amount of LGE can also be quantified as mass in gram, volume in milliliter, or percent of the total myocardial mass or volume.

While it is fast and easy to measure transmural extent or to count the number of segments affected by LGE, quantification of the total amount of LGE requires dedicated software, is a time-consuming process, complicated by different techniques available and influenced by several confounding factors.

Table 1 Techniques for the quantification of CMR late-gadolinium enhancement

Technique	Description
Manual planimetry	Manual contouring of areas of LGE based on visual identification of LGE.
Manual adjustment of signal intensity threshold	Segmentation of LGE by manual adjustment of the signal intensity threshold based on visual identification of LGE.
Signal Threshold versus Reference Mean (STRM)	Semiautomatic grayscale threshold technique. LGE defined as signal intensity with 2, 3, 4, 5, 6, 7, 8, 9, or 10 standard deviations above the mean signal intensity of normal myocardium.
Full Width at Half Maximum (FWHM)	Semiautomatic. LGE defined as signal intensity exceeding 50% of the maximum signal intensity of visual apparent LGE.
Otsu Auto Threshold (OAT) technique	(Semi)-automatic. LGE defined as signal intensity by automatic division of a signal intensity histogram.

LGE late-gadolinium enhancement

Different manual and semiautomatic segmentation techniques have been described for the quantification of the total amount of LGE. The semiautomatic methods can be divided into threshold-based methods (Flett et al. 2011; Vermes et al. 2013), learning methods (Positano et al. 2005; O'Donnell et al. 2003), and comprehensive methods (Hsu et al. 2006; Tao et al. 2010; Heiberg et al. 2005). Missing boundary information leading to false inclusion of regions due to noise has been described as disadvantage of the threshold-based methods and learning methods (Lu et al. 2012). To overcome this problem, boundary information was included in the comprehensive methods. However, due to the ease of use and commercial availability of the threshold-based methods, they were applied in most studies. Thus, this chapter focusses on the description of the threshold-based methods.

The short-axis stack is analyzed for LGE segmentation. LGE images with motion artifacts and improper setting of the inversion time should not be used for LGE quantification.

For all manual and semiautomatic threshold-based techniques, LGE segmentation starts with manual tracing of the endocardial and epicardial left ventricular myocardial borders of each short-axis slice, avoiding inclusion of the adjacent blood pool and tissue.

For the manual approach of LGE quantification, areas of LGE can be either traced manually or marked by manual adjustment of the signal intensity threshold that discriminates between normal myocardium and LGE. LGE mass in grams is calculated by summing the volume of LGE in all short-axis slices multiplied by 1.05 g/mL (specific gravity of myocardium).

The semiautomatic techniques of LGE segmentation that are commercially available by different vendors of CMR analysis software include Signal Threshold versus Reference Mean (STRM) (Harrigan et al. 2011), Full Width at Half Maximum (FWHM) (Amado et al. 2004), and the Otsu Auto Threshold (OAT) technique (Vermes et al. 2013).

The STRM technique is a semiautomatic grayscale threshold technique. Areas of LGE are segmented with a signal intensity of 2, 3, 4, 5, 6, 7, 8, 9, or 10 standard deviations (SD) above the mean signal intensity of remote myocardium (Harrigan et al. 2011). Normal myocardium is identified visually and marked by a manually drawn region of interest (ROI).

For the FWHM technique, a ROI is manually drawn in an area of LGE. The maximum signal intensity inside the region is determined automatically, and LGE is defined by a signal intensity exceeding 50% of the maximum signal intensity of the ROI (Amado et al. 2004).

For the OAT technique, no region of interest is required. The optimal threshold that discriminates between normal myocardium and LGE is defined automatically by division of a signal intensity histogram based on a search for values that minimize the intraclass variance between two populations of signal intensities (Vermes et al. 2013).

Finally, all semiautomatic methods can be complemented by manual adjustment.

1.2.3 Acquisition of Late-Enhancement Images by CT

For late-enhancement imaging by CT, different acquisition protocols have been published in clinical studies (Rodriguez-Granillo 2017; Bastarrika et al. 2010; Bettencourt et al. 2013; Esposito et al. 2016; George et al. 2012; Goetti et al. 2011; Jacquier et al. 2008; Mahnken et al. 2005; Meinel et al. 2014; Wichmann et al. 2013). In most studies, image acquisition is performed 5–15 min after intravenous application of an iodine-based contrast agent with a concentration of 350 mg/mL, 370 mg/mL or 400 mg/mL. Total contrast volume varies between 120 and 180 mL. Different types of CT scanners have been used, including 16-, 64-, and 320-slice multidetector CT scanners as well as dual-source and dual-energy techniques. Prospective and retrospective ECG-gating have been reported. To increase signal to noise and reduce dose, slice thickness can be increased (e.g., 1.5 mm) (Gerber et al. 2006; Blankstein et al. 2009). Tube voltages of 80, 100, and 120 kV for the single source scanners and 140/100 and 80/140 kV for dual-energy scanners have been applied in different studies. However, delineation of late enhancement has been shown to be improved at a lower energy level (Rodriguez-Granillo 2017).

1.2.4 Quantification of CT Late Enhancement

While in early contrast-enhanced CT during the arterial phase, injured myocardium appears hypodense compared to the remote myocardium, it is hyperdense on delayed images (Blankstein et al. 2009). For quantification of late enhancement, CT images are reconstructed at a soft kernel (Rodriguez-Granillo 2017; Zhao et al. 2014). In analogy to LGE-CMR, CT late-enhancement images can be reformatted as a stack of 5–10 mm thick short-axis images (Rodriguez-Granillo 2017; Zhao et al. 2014).

Segmentation of CT late enhancement can be performed by manual contouring (Zhao et al. 2014). Other techniques for quantification of late enhancement in CT have not been published yet.

1.3 Expected Result and Range of Normal Values

In general, late enhancement should not be present in the normal human myocardium and is characteristic for different types of ischemic and non-ischemic cardiomyopathies (Vohringer et al. 2007). Clinical significance of incidentally detected non-ischemic late enhancement remains unknown (Turkbey et al. 2015). In certain cardiac diseases, the extent of late enhancement has been identified as prognostic factor. Some studies present cutoff values with respect to the amount of LGE, that have been identified as indicator for a certain outcome. These values are presented for each disease separately in Sect. 1.5.

1.4 Confounding Factors

Several factors related to image acquisition and image evaluation have been assessed regarding their potential effect on the amount of LGE quantified by CMR imaging (Table 2). While there has been extensive evaluation of the confounding factors of LGE quantification in CMR imaging, these factors have not been assessed in detail regarding quantification of late enhancement by CT. Thus, this paragraph focusses on the confounding factors related to LGE segmentation by CMR.

1.4.1 LGE Segmentation Technique

The amount of CMR-LGE has been shown to vary substantially by the method used for segmentation (Amado et al. 2004). Reported values of LGE mass measured by two different quantification techniques can differ by a factor of 5 or more (Harrigan et al. 2011).

Despite several publications comparing the different quantification techniques, there is still no consensus which method to use for quantification of LGE due to discordant results (Flett et al. 2011; Vermes et al. 2013; Harrigan et al. 2011; Amado et al. 2004; Grani et al. 2019a; Khan et al. 2015; Mikami et al. 2014). The varying designs of these studies might explain the different results. Some studies compared the accuracy of different techniques for LGE quantification using different standards of reference, e.g., visual quantification of LGE or histological quantification of focal fibrosis. Other studies had a clinical focus and assessed the association with cardiac events (Flett et al. 2011; Vermes et al. 2013; Harrigan et al. 2011; Amado et al. 2004; Grani et al. 2019a; Khan et al. 2015; Mikami et al. 2014). And yet other studies focused on the assessment of the reproducibility of the different methods for LGE segmentation (Flett et al. 2011; Vermes et al. 2013; Harrigan et al. 2011; Grani et al. 2019a;

Table 2 Confounding factors in LGE quantification by CMR

Factor	Effect	Implications for clinical practice
Segmentation technique	LGE extent significantly different depending on the method used for quantification	No uniform recommendation for quantification method; method should be chosen with respect to availability, desired performance regarding accuracy, reproducibility, association with outcome measures, and the cardiac disease which will be assessed
Inversion time	Incorrect selection of inversion time can lead to false high amounts of LGE	Only LGE images with correct "nulling" of normal myocardium should be used for LGE quantification
Contrast delay	LGE extent in acute myocardial infarction larger early after contrast administration (EGE) compared to late imaging (LGE); no difference between 10 and 30 min after contrast administration	Extent of acute myocardial infarction larger with EGE compared to LGE, revealing area at risk
Contrast agent	LGE extent significantly higher for GBCA with higher relaxivity	GBCA of identical relaxivity should be used for follow-up studies
Contouring	Incorrect contouring of myocardial borders and LGE can lead to over- and underestimation of total myocardial mass/volume and LGE extent	Precise contouring is mandatory
Microvascular obstruction	Areas of microvascular obstruction in subacute myocardial infarction excluded from LGE extent when a threshold-based technique is used for quantification leading to underestimation of the LGE extent	Areas of microvascular obstruction have to be added manually to the LGE extent when a threshold-based technique is used for LGE quantification
Acute versus chronic disease	LGE extent substantially larger in acute disease (e.g., in myocardial infarction)	No general recommendation whether infarct size should be measured at acute or chronic stage. Depends on clinical or research question

LGE late-gadolinium enhancement, *EGE* early-gadolinium enhancement, *GBCA* gadolinium-based contrast agent

Khan et al. 2015; Mikami et al. 2014). Finally, the optimal technique for LGE quantification might vary depending on the cardiac disease which is quantified and the related differences in LGE distribution and intensity (Flett et al. 2011; Kim et al. 2009). Examples of different study designs and results are listed below.

Amado et al. correlated infarct size quantified by the STRM method with standard deviations (SD) of 1, 2, 3, 4, 5, 6, and 7 and by the FWHM technique with histologically measured infarct size in dogs and found the best correlation for the FWHM technique (Amado et al. 2004). Vermes et al. compared accuracy and reproducibility of the STRM method (2, 3, and 5 SD), the FWHM and the OAT technique for quantification of LGE in patients with acute myocardial infarction and acute myocarditis to manual segmentation as standard of reference (Vermes et al. 2013). Compared to manual segmentation, LGE mass was overestimated with the STRM method at thresholds of 2 and 3 SD and underestimated using the FWHM technique while no difference was found between LGE mass quantified by the OAT technique in comparison to manual quantification. Reproducibility was best for the OAT and FWHM technique.

Khan et al. measured infarct size in LGE images using the STRM technique at a threshold of 5, 6, 7, and 8 SD, the FWHM and the OAT technique and compared to manual quantification as reference standard (Khan et al. 2015). Best correlation with manual segmentation was found for the FWHM technique and STRM with 8 SD, while infarct size was overestimated with the OAT technique.

Graeni et al. assessed the association of LGE quantified by STRM at a threshold of 2, 3, 4, 5, 6, and 7 SD, FWHM technique and a visual presence score, based on the presence or absence of LGE in each segment, with major adverse cardiovascular events (MACE) in 670 patients with suspected myocarditis over a median follow-up of 4.7 years (Grani et al. 2019a). In a multivariable model adjusted for age, sex, BMI, and left ventricular ejection fraction LGE quantified by the FWHM technique, STRM at 3 SD and the visual presence score were significantly associated with MACE.

Flett et al. compared the reproducibility of measurements of the LGE extent in different cardiac diseases including acute and chronic myocardial infarction and hypertrophic cardiomyopathy (HCM), obtained by the STRM method with 2, 3, 4, 5, and 6 SD and the FWHM method (Flett et al. 2011). The FWHM method showed the highest reproducibility. However, for all quantification techniques, reproducibility was worse for HCM compared to acute and chronic myocardial infarction.

Particularly, in HCM there is no consensus regarding the appropriate technique for LGE quantification. The presence of replacement fibrosis and interstitial fibrosis that is characteristic for HCM leads to LGE of different signal intensities, where low-intensity LGE predominates (Naeger et al. 2015). There is no consensus whether areas of low-signal intensity ("gray zone") LGE should be included in the total LGE extent (Naeger et al. 2015; Maron 2013). The different methods available for LGE quantification lead to significantly different results particularly in HCM related to the exclusion or inclusion of low-intensity LGE at a different extent (Fig. 1).

Mikami et al. assessed accuracy and reproducibility of different techniques for LGE quantification, including STRM with a threshold at 2, 3, 4, 5, and 6 SD above the mean signal intensity of normal myocardium, the FWHM and the OAT technique in 76 patient with HCM (Mikami et al. 2014). The FWHM technique showed the highest reproducibility but underestimated LGE volume compared to manual segmentation. Greatest accuracy was achieved by the STRM technique with a threshold set at 3 SD. In a similar study in 33 patients with HCM, the authors found the best agreement with manual segmentation for the STRM technique at 6 SD (Spiewak et al. 2010).

Moravsky et al. assessed the correlation between different LGE quantification techniques (STRM with a threshold at 2, 4, 5, 6, and 10 SD and FWHM) with histological quantification of interstitial and replacement fibrosis of specimens after septal myectomy in 29 patients with HCM (Moravsky et al. 2013). While LGE quantified with the STRM method at 10 SD correlated best with replacement fibrosis, the STRM method at 5

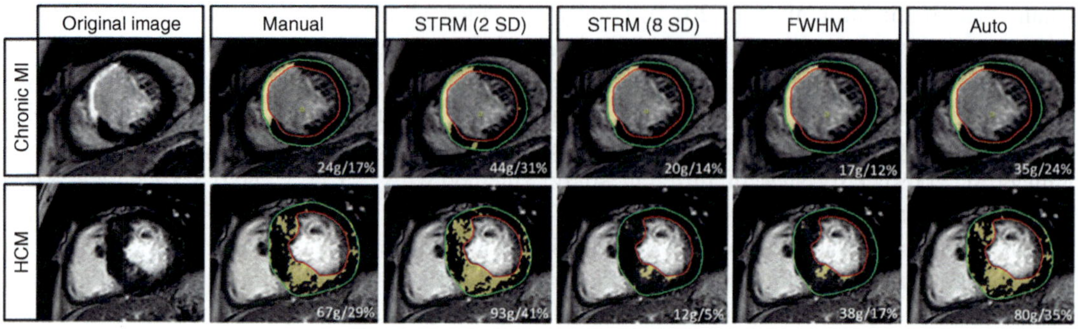

Fig. 1 Quantification of late-gadolinium enhancement (LGE) with five different methods: manual threshold adjustment (manual), signal threshold versus reference mean (STRM) with 2 SD and 8 SD, respectively, above the mean, Full Width at Half Maximum (FWHM), and auto threshold (auto). The top row shows an exemplary slice of the entire short-axis stack of LGE quantification in a case of chronic myocardial infarction (chronic MI). The bottom row shows an exemplary slice of the entire short-axis stack of a case of hypertrophic cardiomyopathy (HCM). The numbers in the lower right corner of each image indicate the amount of LGE in g and in percent of the entire myocardial mass obtained with each method. There is substantial variation in the amount of LGE calculated with the different methods. However, there is less variation of the segmentation of the high intensity LGE in myocardial infarction (12–31%) compared to the low-intensity LGE in HCM (5–41%)

SD showed the strongest correlation with the total fibrosis (combined interstitial and replacement fibrosis).

The results suggest that different cardiac diseases might require different techniques for optimal LGE quantification. According to the current literature, there is no consensus regarding the best method for LGE quantification. The current guidelines by the Society for Cardiovascular Magnetic Resonance (SCMR) on standardized post processing do not include dedicated recommendations for LGE quantification (Schulz-Menger et al. 2020). The method should be chosen with respect to availability, the desired performance regarding accuracy, reproducibility, association with outcome measures, and the cardiac disease which will be assessed. With respect to the future, first publications of automated LGE quantification methods based on artificial intelligence and convolutional neural networks show promising results that require further assessment and validation (Fahmy et al. 2018, 2020).

1.4.2 Inversion Time

Incorrect selection of the inversion time results in LGE images where the normal myocardium does not appear black but with a low-intensity bright signal instead, surrounded by a thin dark rim. Marking the slightly hyperintense myocardium as remote myocardium in threshold-based techniques will lead to underestimation of the LGE extent (Moravsky et al. 2013). Therefore, image acquisition with the correct inversion time to "null" the normal myocardium is mandatory.

1.4.3 Contrast Delay

Amado et al. showed that LGE size quantified by the FWHM technique did not differ with the delay after contrast injection in 13 animals in acute myocardial infarction between 6 and 30 min after contrast injection (Amado et al. 2004). In another animal study, it was shown that LGE extent in acute myocardial infarction changed between 3 min (early-gadolinium enhancement) and 10–15 min (LGE), revealing the area at risk (Hammer-Hansen et al. 2017).

1.4.4 Contrast Agent

It has been shown that LGE extent varies significantly with the relaxivity of the GBCA used for LGE imaging. Liu et al. scanned 30 patients with hypertrophic cardiomyopathy twice, using gadobutrol and gadopentetate dimeglumine and quantified LGE manually based on visual assessment, by means of the STRM technique with thresholds at 2, 5, and 6 SD and the FWHM technique (Liu et al. 2017a). LGE volume was significantly higher with gadobutrol compared to gadopentetate dimeglumine for all quantification techniques. Similarly, Rudolf et al. compared LGE mass quantified in 15 patients with hypertrophic cardiomyopathy, who were scanned twice using gadopentetate dimeglumine and gadobenate dimeglumine, respectively (Rudolph et al. 2014). LGE mass was higher with gadobenate dimeglumine, which has a higher relaxivity compared to gadopentetate dimeglumine.

1.4.5 Contouring of the Myocardium and LGE

Not only for manual but also for semiautomatic threshold-based LGE quantification techniques, delineation of the epicardial and endocardial contours of the entire short-axis stack of LGE images is performed manually. Also the region of interest required for the STRM and FWHM techniques is drawn manually and placed in a location based on visual assessment. Klem et al. demonstrated that the subjective delineation of endo- and epicardial borders is source of variability in LGE quantification (Klem et al. 2017). False placement of contours can lead to an over- or underestimation of total myocardial volume/mass and also of the volume/mass of LGE. Inclusion of the blood pool or epicardial fat leads to a false high amount of LGE. Therefore, careful contouring and placement of ROI are mandatory for LGE quantification.

Placement of the ROI to define normal myocardium for the STRM method or enhanced myocardium for the FWHM technique can also be source of error. Inclusion of areas of low-intensity LGE in the ROI, that should define remote myocardium for the STRM method, leads to underestimation of the true LGE extent. If LGE is patchy, e.g., in myocarditis or sarcoidosis, it might be difficult to place the ROI including the region of maximum signal for the FWHM technique.

1.4.6 Microvascular Obstruction (MVO)

The area of no-reflow that might occur as black subendocardial border or central core in subacute myocardial infarction is excluded from LGE segmentation using semiautomatic threshold-based techniques due to a signal intensity below the threshold (Fig. 2). To avoid underestimation of the infarct size, areas of MVO have to be added manually to the infarct mass and volume, respectively (Klem et al. 2017).

1.4.7 Acute Versus Chronic Disease

Particularly in myocardial infarction, it has been shown that the extent of LGE varies between the acute and chronic stage. In the early stage (≤10 days), infarct size is larger due to edema and cellular elements while it may shrink to 25% of the initial volume when the necrotic tissue is replaced by scar (Kim et al. 2009). There is no general recommendation regarding the time point when infarct size should be measured. It should be chosen with respect to the clinical or research question (Kim et al. 2009).

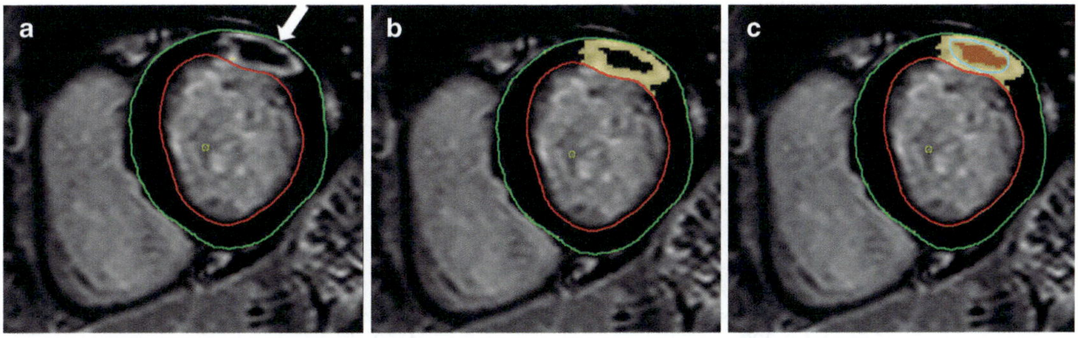

Fig. 2 Quantification of late-gadolinium enhancement (LGE) in subacute myocardial infarction with "no reflow." Small transmural infarct anterolateral showing as LGE with hypointense central core due to microvascular obstruction (arrow in **a**). With all semiautomatic segmentation methods, the hypointense core will not be included in the infarct mass (**b**) and has to be added manually (**c**) to avoid underestimation of the infarct size

1.5 Clinical Implementation

In clinical practice, late-enhancement images are mainly assessed visually to identify LGE patterns, characteristic for ischemic or non-ischemic cardiomyopathies (Vohringer et al. 2007). However, quantitative analysis of the extent of late enhancement has been shown to have important prognostic clinical implications in several cardiac diseases. The primary clinical indications for quantification of late enhancement are acute and chronic myocardial infarction and hypertrophic cardiomyopathy. However, quantitative analysis of LGE has also been shown to have prognostic value in cardiac sarcoidosis (Murtagh et al. 2016; Crawford et al. 2014), myocarditis (Grani et al. 2017), and non-ischemic dilated cardiomyopathy (Gulati et al. 2013).

Table 3 lists selected studies providing thresholds of LGE quantification that might be helpful in guiding clinical decisions and patient management.

1.5.1 Myocardial Infarction

The relationship between the extent of myocardial infarction, measured as the transmural extent or the number of myocardial segments involved, and the likelihood of improvement in myocardial contractility after revascularization was assessed in several studies (Choi et al. 2001; Schvartzman et al. 2003; Pegg et al. 2010; Kim et al. 1999; Selvanayagam et al. 2004). Kim et al. demonstrated in 50 patients after elective revascularization that reversible myocardial dysfunction is related to the transmural extent of myocardial infarction measured on CMR-LGE imaging (Kim et al. 1999). Contractility increased post-revascularization in 78% of myocardial segments without LGE but in only 2% of segments with LGE of a transmural extent of >75%. The result

Table 3 Prognostic implications of LGE quantification based on previous publications

Disease	Measurement	Prognostic implications
Myocardial infarction	Transmural extent of infarct of <50% and/or 10 viable segments	Indicate high likelihood of functional recovery after revascularization (Choi et al. 2001; Pegg et al. 2010; Kim et al. 1999; Selvanayagam et al. 2004)
	Infarct size ≥18.5% of the total LV myocardial volume	Significant predictor of adverse outcome: death, recurrent myocardial infarction, heart failure (Wu et al. 2008)
	Infarct size ≥23% of the total LV myocardial volume	Predictor of late LV dysfunction (Larose et al. 2010)
Hypertrophic cardiomyopathy	LGE extent of ≥15% of the total LV mass in HCM patients considered low-risk according to conventional risk stratification	Independent predictor of sudden death; might be helpful to identify patients for ICD therapy (Chan et al. 2014)
Sarcoidosis	LGE extent of ≥9 left and/or right ventricular segments LGE extent of >6% of the total LV mass	Increased risk to develop ventricular tachycardia or fibrillation; might be helpful to identify patients for ICD therapy (Crawford et al. 2014)
	LGE extent of >5.7% of the total LV mass	Increased risk of death or ventricular tachycardia; might be helpful to identify patients for ICD therapy (Murtagh et al. 2016)
Atrial fibrillation	Pre-ablation LGE extent (%) of the total LA wall volume: Stage 1, <10% Stage 2, ≥10% <20% Stage 3, ≥20% <30% Stage 4, ≥30%	Indicative for recurrence after ablation; cumulative incidence: Stage 1, 15.3% Stage 2, 35.8% Stage 3, 45.9% Stage 4, 69.4% Might be helpful for patient selection and to plan ablation strategy (Marrouche et al. 2014)
	Post-ablation LGE extent >23% of the LA wall volume	Low likelihood of recurrence (McGann et al. 2008)

LGE late-gadolinium enhancement, *LV* left ventricular, *ICD* implantable cardioverter defibrillator, *LA* left atria was supported in a study by Selvanayagam et al. who assessed the improvement in myocardial contractility in 56 patients with coronary artery disease after elective coronary artery bypass graft (Selvanayagam et al. 2004). In this study, regional function improved in 86% of myocardial segments without LGE but in only 4% of segments with a transmural extent of LGE >76%. According to a study by Choi et al., the best predictor of improvement of global function measured as ejection fraction was the extent of dysfunctional myocardium that was not infarcted or with infarction of a transmural extent of <25% (Choi et al. 2001). Pegg et al. could demonstrate that the improvement in ejection fraction in 33 patients with coronary artery disease 6 month after revascularization was best predicted by ≥10 viable and normal segments (defined as a mural extent of LGE <50%) (Pegg et al. 2010).

Based on the results of these publications, it became routine practice to consider revascularization in patients after myocardial infarction with a transmural extent of <50% and/or >10 viable segments (Jimenez Juan et al. 2015; Child and Das 2012).

Further, it has been shown in several studies that infarct size measured as transmural extent or total amount of LGE is a stronger predictor of outcome than left ventricular ejection fraction and left ventricular volumes (Roes et al. 2007; Wu et al. 2008; Kwon et al. 2009).

Wu et al. demonstrated that the infarct size quantified by manual planimetry on LGE images in % of the total myocardial volume was an independent predictor of adverse outcome (death, recurrent myocardial infarction, and heart failure) (Wu et al. 2008). According to a study by Larose et al., infarct volume, quantified by the FWHM method early after primary angioplasty in 103 patients with acute myocardial infarction, was a stronger predictor of LV dysfunction compared to infarct transmurality (Larose et al. 2010). A LGE volume of ≥23% predicted late LV dysfunction with a sensitivity of 89% and a specificity of 74%.

However, despite these promising results, quantification of total infarct volume or mass has not become routine clinical practice yet.

It has been demonstrated that not only total infarct size but also infarct morphology assessed by LGE imaging is an important prognostic indicator. Based on differences in signal intensity, a peri-infarct zone can be identified which is less intense compared to the infarct core (Schmidt et al. 2007; Yan et al. 2006). The peri-infarct zone is thought to be composed of viable myocytes and nonviable fibrotic tissue, providing a potentially arrhythmogenic substrate (Haghbayan et al. 2019). It has been shown to be associated with ventricular tachyarrhythmia and with cardiovascular mortality in patients with ischemic cardiomyopathy (Schmidt et al. 2007; Yan et al. 2006; Demirel et al. 2014).

Quantification of the peri-infarct zone is not routinely performed in current clinical practice. However, there is evidence that it might be a valuable tool, e.g., to identify patients appropriate for implantable-defibrillator therapy (Gao et al. 2012).

In a recent meta-analysis with respect to the prognostic value of quantification of the peri-infarct zone, the extent of the peri-infarct zone was a predictor of all-cause mortality, appropriate implantable-defibrillator therapy, and inducibility of ventricular tachycardia on electrophysiological study (Haghbayan et al. 2019). According to the meta-analysis, that included 20 studies, mainly two techniques were used for separation and quantification, respectively, of the infarct core and the peri-infarct zone. Using the FWHM method, the infarct core was defined as ≥50% of the maximal detected signal intensity and the peri-infarct zone as the surrounding area measuring either 35–50% of the maximal signal intensity or a signal intensity higher than the peak signal intensity of the remote myocardium. In other studies, the STRM method was applied with different signal intensity thresholds between 2 SD and 6 SD to separate between infarct core and peri-infarct zone (Haghbayan et al. 2019).

1.5.2 Hypertrophic Cardiomyopathy (HCM)

More than 50% of patients with HCM present with LGE at CMR imaging (Weng et al. 2016).

Presence and extent of LGE in patients with HCM have been shown to be an important indicator for cardiovascular events and help to identify candidates for ICD implantation (Weng et al. 2016; Maron and Maron 2016). According to the results of a multicenter prospective study that followed 1293 patients with HCM for more than 3 years, an LGE extent of ≥15% of the left ventricular mass was an independent predictor of sudden death (Chan et al. 2014). Beyond conventional risk markers, LGE-CMR provides the opportunity to identify subjects with extensive LGE that might benefit from an ICD therapy (Maron and Maron 2016).

In a recently published meta-analysis evaluating the prognostic value of LGE in patients with HCM, that included five studies with a total of 2993 patients followed for a median of ~37 month, the extent of LGE was associated with an increased risk for sudden cardiac death, heart failure death, all-cause mortality, and cardiovascular mortality (Weng et al. 2016). The extent of LGE remained associated with the risk of sudden cardiac death after adjustment for baseline characteristics (Weng et al. 2016).

All of the five individual studies included in the meta-analysis used different methods for LGE quantification. Some authors used a semiautomatic method for LGE quantification, including Bruder et al. who applied the STRM method with a signal intensity threshold of 2 standard deviations (Bruder et al. 2010) and Ismail et al. who used the FWHM technique (Ismail et al. 2014) while others preferred a manual approach by either adjusting a grayscale threshold slider (Chan et al. 2014) or manual tracing areas of LGE (Rubinshtein et al. 2010). For quantification of LGE, Hen et al. counted the number of segments with LGE (Hen et al. 2014). Thus, in some studies low-intensity ("gray zone") LGE was included in the total amount of LGE and excluded in other studies. In yet other studies, the handling of low-intensity LGE is not described (Rubinshtein et al. 2010; Hen et al. 2014).

The different methods used for LGE quantification reflect the current situation without uniform recommendations regarding inclusion or exclusion of low-intensity LGE or a specific quantification method.

1.5.3 Other Non-ischemic Cardiomyopathies and Myocarditis

Although not routinely performed in clinical practice yet, quantitative analysis of LGE has been identified as independent risk factor in several non-ischemic cardiac diseases suggesting to incorporate LGE quantification also in clinical practice. However, further studies are required to identify cutoff values indicating certain clinical consequences.

Graeni et al. assessed the event rate of 670 patients with suspected myocarditis over a median follow-up of 4.7 years. A 10% increase in the LGE extent quantified by the FWHM method corresponded to a 79% increase in the risk to develop major adverse cardiovascular events (all-cause death, heart failure decompensation, heart transplantation, documented sustained ventricular arrhythmia, and recurrent acute myocarditis) (Grani et al. 2017).

Ventricular arrhythmias and sudden death are known complications in patients with cardiac sarcoidosis. It has been shown in some studies that quantification of CMR-LGE helps to identify subjects at risk who might benefit from ICD therapy. Crawford et al. followed 51 patients with cardiac sarcoidosis and a left ventricular ejection fraction of >35 for a mean of 48 month (Crawford et al. 2014). Using a cutoff of ≥9 left and/or right ventricular segments with LGE enabled differentiation between patients who developed ventricular tachycardia or ventricular fibrillation from patients who did not, with a sensitivity of 92% and specificity of 88%. Further, a LGE extent of more than 6% of the left ventricular mass quantified by the FWHM method identified patients who developed ventricular tachycardia or ventricular fibrillation with a sensitivity of 75% and a specificity of 82%. Similarly, in the 41 LGE-positive patients of a study including 205 patients with extracardiac sarcoidosis and a left ventricular ejection fraction of >50%, total amount of LGE (quantified by the STRM method with a cutoff at >5 SD) was the best predictor of adverse events (all-cause death, sustained ventricular arrhythmia, or appropriate ICD shock) during a mean follow-up of 36 month (Murtagh et al. 2016). Patients with an LGE extent of >5.7% of the total left ventricular mass could be classified as high risk of death or ventricular tachycardia with a sensitivity of 87% and a specificity of 62%.

Another example for the prognostic value of LGE quantification is related to patients with non-ischemic dilated cardiomyopathy (NIDCM) who typically present with mid-wall LGE due to replacement fibrosis. Gulati et al. demonstrated that in 472 patients with NIDCM followed over a median of 5.3 years, the extent of the mid-wall LGE was independently associated with adverse events (Gulati et al. 2013).

1.5.4 Atrial Fibrillation

Atrial fibrillation is the most common cardia arrhythmia that can be treated by pulmonary vein antrum isolation by means of radiofrequency ablation. Atrial fibrillation is associated with fibrotic changes of the left atrial wall (Burstein and Nattel 2008) resulting in areas of hyperintense signal in LGE imaging (Zghaib and Nazarian 2018). Left atrial LGE imaging has been used for the quantification of pre-ablation fibrosis as well as post-ablation scar. It has been shown that left atrial LGE correlates with low-voltage areas on electroanatomical mapping and that the extent of pre-ablation left atrial fibrosis is a predictor of successful ablation (Oakes et al. 2009). In a multicenter prospective cohort study including 260 patients with paroxysmal and persistent atrial fibrillation, left atrial LGE was quantified and classified in four different stages depending on the LGE extent in % LGE of the total left atrial wall volume: stage 1, <10%; stage 2, ≥10% <20%; stage 3, ≥20% <30%; stage 4, ≥30% (Marrouche et al. 2014). The extent of left atrial LGE was indicative for recurrent atrial fibrillation with a cumulative incidence of recurrent arrhythmia of 15.3% at stage 1, 35.8% at stage 2, 45.9% at stage 3, and 69.4% at stage 4. Thus, quantification of left atrial LGE might be helpful for patient selection with respect to treatment with pulmonary vein isolation and to plan ablation strategy.

Further, the extent of post-ablation scar was able to predict outcome. In a study by McGann et al. arrhythmia recurrence 3 month after pulmonary vein antrum ablation correlated with the degree of LGE. No recurrence was detected in patients with ablation related scar of >23% of the LA wall volume (McGann et al. 2008).

2 Interstitial Fibrosis: T1-Mapping and Extracellular Volume

2.1 (Patho)Physiological and Technical Background

This paragraph continues the previous paragraph related to the pathophysiological background of replacement fibrosis, where the composition of the left ventricular myocardium, the fraction and function of each component, and the contrast distribution and kinetics are described in detail.

The cardiac interstitium or extracellular volume (ECV), that accounts for 25% of the total myocardial volume, is a composition of blood vessels, nerves, various cells, and collagen fibers. The latter accounting for about 2–4% of the total myocardial left ventricular volume of the healthy heart (Mewton et al. 2011). While in replacement fibrosis, dead myocytes are focally replaced by a collagenous scar, in interstitial fibrosis an increased amount of collagen fibers is diffusely distributed in the interstitium between the myocytes and also perivascular leading to an expansion of the extracellular volume (Mewton et al. 2011; Weber 1989).

Interstitial fibrosis occurs in various cardiac diseases including hypertensive heart disease, hypertrophic cardiomyopathy, dilated cardiomyopathy, diabetes mellitus, valvular disorders, and in the normal aging process of the heart and has been related to diastolic and systolic dysfunction (Mewton et al. 2011; Weber 1989).

While LGE imaging is the method of choice for the assessment of focal replacement fibrosis related to regional differences in the accumulation of gadolinium as described above, the evaluation of diffuse interstitial fibrosis by LGE imaging is limited in cases where the entire myocardium is involved and no reference region of remote myocardium is present.

The T1 longitudinal relaxation time (T1) is the time constant that represents how fast the nuclear spin magnetization returns to its equilibrium after a radiofrequency pulse was applied. Due to characteristic differences between T1 time of various tissues, it is an important component of soft tissue contrast in MRI. Also myocardium has a characteristic T1 time, which might be altered in different cardiac pathologies including diffuse interstitial myocardial fibrosis. Therefore, quantification of myocardial T1 time by means of T1 mapping has the potential to detect/assess diffuse interstitial fibrosis.

Compared to normal myocardium, the expansion of the extracellular space leads to a prolongation of the longitudinal T1 relaxation time (T1) of the myocardium that can be measured by means of CMR T1 mapping sequences in the absence of GBCA (Radenkovic et al. 2017). After contrast injection, the gadolinium molecules distribute between the intravascular and the interstitial space till an equilibrium is reached (Wong et al. 2012). The larger volume of distribution for the GBCA in diffuse interstitial fibrosis compared to healthy myocardium results in a higher amount of gadolinium molecules and a greater shortening of myocardial T1 time after contrast administration. Related to contrast wash-out, myocardial T1 time increases with time after contrast administration (Mewton et al. 2011). The concentration of gadolinium is directly related to the differences between pre- and postcontrast reciprocal values of T1 time (Messroghli et al. 2011). Thus, estimation of T1 time by means of T1 mapping enables quantification of the concentration of gadolinium in the myocardium and in the blood pool. The extent of the extracellular volume fraction can be calculated by the following formula (Messroghli et al. 2011):

$$\frac{(1/T1_{\text{myocardium post contrast}} - 1/T1_{\text{myocardium pre contrast}})}{(1/T1_{\text{blood post contrast}} - 1/T1_{\text{blood pre contrast}})} \times (1 - \text{hematocrit})$$

Based on these relationships, native T1 time and ECV, respectively, may serve as surrogate for diffuse myocardial fibrosis. In several studies, a good correlation has been shown between native T1 time and ECV, respectively, with diffuse myocardial fibrosis quantified histologically (Diao et al. 2016). While myocardial T1 time is a composite measure of the entire myocardium including myocytes and the interstitial space, calculation of the ECV reflects the extent of the interstitial space. In diffuse interstitial fibrosis, the interstitial space is enlarged compared to healthy myocardium resulting in a higher ECV value (Wong et al. 2012).

Calculation of ECV has also been shown to be feasible by means of cardiac CT with a good correlation with CMR derived ECV and with histological measures of fibrosis (Nacif et al. 2012; Bandula et al. 2013). In analogy to CMR derived ECV, ECV obtained by CT can be calculated by the following formula:

$$\frac{(HU_{\text{myocardium post contrast}} - HU_{\text{myocardium pre contrast}})}{(HU_{\text{blood post contrast}} - HU_{\text{blood pre contrast}})} \times (1 - \text{hematocrit})$$

2.2 Image Acquisition and Analysis

2.2.1 Acquisition of T1 Maps by CMR

The basic principle of parametric mapping in general can be summarized as the acquisition of multiple images with different weighting regarding the parameter of interest followed by a fitting procedure of the signal intensities of the individual images for calculation of a parametric map, which is a single image of the fitted relaxation parameters (Salerno and Kramer 2013). Different techniques have been developed for T1 mapping. Current T1 mapping sequences, acquired during a single breath hold, consist of a T1 magnetization preparation pulse followed by the acquisition of several images at different time points during T1 recovery acquired at the same anatomic location and the same time point of the cardiac cycle. Co-registration of each pixel enables fitting of an exponential recovery curve of the longitudinal magnetization (Radenkovic et al. 2017; Puntmann et al. 2016a). The T1 time corresponds to the time when T1 recovery is 63% complete. For T1 mapping, the inversion recovery (IR) and saturation recovery (SR) techniques can be distinguished based on differences in the magnetization preparation prepulse (Puntmann et al. 2016a). For the inversion recovery techniques such as the MOdified Look-Locker Inversion Recovery (MOLLI) sequence, a 180° preparation pulse is applied that inverts the magnetization in the *z* direction while for the saturation recovery techniques (e.g., SAturation recovery single SHot Acquisition [SASHA]) a 90° saturation preparation prepulse is used that tips the magnetization into the transverse plane. For the IR techniques, some heart beats are used for image acquisition at different inversion times and some to allow for full signal recovery after the 180° prepulse (recovery beats). Different variants of MOLLI have been described with varying numbers of acquired images and recovery beats. In T1 mapping sequences based on the IR technique, an image is acquired after every 90° prepulse and during every heartbeat, respectively.

Compared to the T1 values obtained with a T1 turbo spin echo (TSE) sequence, which is considered the gold standard T1 mapping technique but impractical for clinical practice due to multiple long breath holds, the T1 values obtained with the inversion recovery techniques are less accurate but more precise while the saturation recovery techniques tend to be more accurate but less precise (Puntmann et al. 2016a). A combined IR-SR sequence is also available (SAturation Pulse-Prepared Heart rate-independent Inversion REcovery [SAPPHIRE]). Table 4 lists the sequences commonly used for T1 mapping according to (Radenkovic et al. 2017; Taylor et al. 2016).

The current consensus statement by the Society for Cardiovascular Magnetic Resonance (SCMR) gives detailed recommendation regarding the implementation of the T1 mapping technique (Messroghli et al. 2017). T1 mapping can be performed at MR scanners with a field strength of 1.5 or 3 T using a commercially available pulse sequence. According to the guidelines, for the assessment of diffuse disease T1 maps should be acquired in short-axis view at the basal and mid-ventricular level and an optional long-axis view. However, in clinical practice and in several publications frequently only a single short-axis slice at the mid-ventricular level is obtained. Native T1 maps and the ECV can be used for the assessment of diffuse

Table 4 Common T1 mapping sequences

Sequence	T1 preparation	Imaging readout	No of heartbeats; Acquisition scheme[a]	Strength	Limitations
Original MOLLI	IR	Single-shot end-diastolic bSSFP	17 HB; 3(3)3(3)5	High SNR High spatial resolution High precision	Less accurate Long breath hold
MOLLI variant	IR	Single-shot end-diastolic bSSFP	11 HB; 5(3)3	High SNR High spatial resolution High precision	Less accurate
ShMOLLI	IR	Single-shot end-diastolic bSSFP	9 HB; 5(1)1(1)1	High SNR High spatial resolution High precision Short breath hold	Less accurate Low number of images for fitting
SASHA	SR	Single-shot bSSFP	11 HB; every heartbeat	High accuracy Low blood-myocardial contrast	Less precise
SAPPHIRE	SR/IR	Single-shot bSSFP	9 HB; every heartbeat	High accuracy Improved precision compared to SASHA Short breath hold	Less precise compared to MOLLI Low SNR

[a] Number or images acquired after each inversion, numbers in parentheses represent the number of recovery heartbeats; *HB* heart beat, *MOLLI* MOdified Look-Locker Inversion Recovery, *IR* inversion recovery, *bSSFP* balanced Steady-State Free Precession, *SNR* signal to noise ratio, *ShMOLLI* shortened MOLLI, *SASHA* SAturation Recovery Single SHot Acquisition, *SR* saturation recovery, *SAPPHIRE* SAturation Pulse-Prepared Heart Rate Independent Inversion REcovery Sequence

interstitial fibrosis. The calculation of ECV requires additional acquisition of a postcontrast T1 map, that should be acquired at the same position and cardiac phase as the precontrast T1 map. Some vendors offer optimized acquisition schemes for the acquisition of pre and postcontrast T1 maps. Postcontrast T1 maps should be acquired between 10 and 30 min after intravenous administration of an extracellular contrast agent at a dose between 0.1 and 0.2 mmol/kg. Images are usually acquired in diastole, however, acquisition in systole is feasible with good image quality and might be advantageous in patients with arrhythmia or very thin myocardium (Fig. 3) (Messroghli et al. 2017; Kawel et al. 2012a).

The hematocrit, required for ECV calculation, should be obtained within 24 h of scanning (Messroghli et al. 2017). However, since the hematocrit shows a significant diurnal, postural, and postprandial variation and changes with hydration and exercise, the blood sample should be ideally taken immediately before or after the scan (Bluemke and Kawel-Boehm 2016). Taking the blood sample after the scan has the advantage that it can be decided during or immediately after the scan if calculation of ECV is required; avoiding an unnecessary lab test in cases where the hematocrit is not needed.

2.2.2 Evaluation of CMR T1 Maps

Maps can be displayed in color or grayscale. T1 maps of impaired quality should not be used for calculation of T1 time and ECV, respectively. In diffuse disease T1 time can be calculated by drawing an ROI in the interventricular septum or by an ROI that includes the entire LV myocardium of a T1 map acquired at mid-ventricular short axis. For calculation of global T1 time, ROIs are drawn to encompass the entire LV myocardium of T1 maps acquired in short axis at the basal, mid-ventricular, and apical level. When drawing the ROI, care has to be taken to avoid inclusion of the adjacent blood and tissue. In focal disease, additional ROIs can be drawn to include visually abnormal areas (Messroghli et al. 2017). This however requires acquisition of an entire stack of short-axis T1 maps to enable visual detection of areas of focal disease. For calculation of ECV by the formula given in the previous paragraph, T1 time has to be quantified in the myocardium and the blood pool on pre- and postcontrast T1 maps.

2.2.3 CT Image Acquisition and Calculation of CT ECV

Since ECV calculation based on cardiac CT is not performed in routine clinical practice there is no standard protocol for image acquisition.

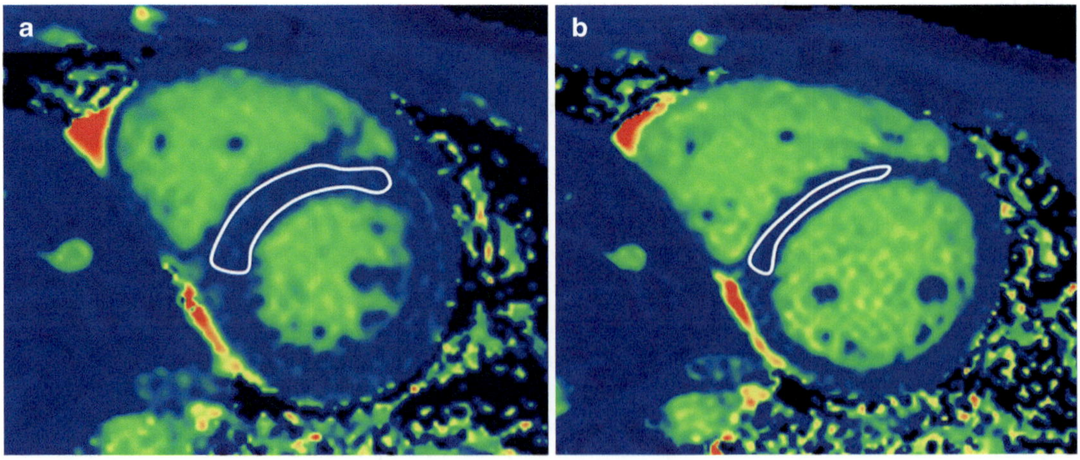

Fig. 3 T1 map acquired at systole (**a**) and diastole (**b**). At systole, the myocardium is thicker allowing to draw a larger region of interest without inclusion of adjacent blood to measure myocardial T1 relaxation time

Regarding contrast administration, in previous publications, a single bolus approach and an equilibrium technique have been described (Nacif et al. 2012; Bandula et al. 2013).

For the native CT scan, Nacif et al. acquired images similar to calcium scoring using prospective ECG-gating at a tube voltage of 120 kV, a tube current of 300 mA, and a section thickness of 3 mm at a 320-detector row CT scanner, covering the entire heart with a single gantry rotation in a single cardiac phase (Nacif et al. 2012). The postcontrast CT images were acquired 10 min after a bolus infusion of 125 ± 24 mL of iodinated contrast material at a rate of 4–5 mL/s using the same parameters as for the precontrast scan. CT attenuation values of the myocardium and the blood were measured on the pre- and postcontrast images that were reformatted to the short-axis plane.

Bandula et al. acquired images by means of a 64-detector row CT scanner and retrospective ECG-gating at a tube voltage of 120 kV, a tube current-time product of 160 mAs and a section thickness of 1.2 mm (Bandula et al. 2013). Images were acquired before and 25 min after intravenous injection of a contrast bolus of 1 mg per kg body weight at a rate of 3 mL/s followed by and infusion of 1.88 mL/kg per hour to achieve a steady state of the contrast material concentration.

Regarding the ideal delay for postcontrast image acquisition using the equilibrium technique, Treibel et al. found a stronger correlation for CT derived ECV with MR derived ECV for 5-min postcontrast images compared to 15-min images (Treibel et al. 2015).

The protocol also depends on the CT scanner available with dual-energy CT scanners obviating separate acquisition of a native scan. Instead, for calculation of ECV, two sets of images are generated with different tube voltages (Lee et al. 2016). Lee et al. acquired images on a dual-source CT scanner using retrospective ECG-gating 12 min after contrast injection at tube voltages of 140/100 kV (Lee et al. 2016).

2.3 Expected Result and Range of Normal Values

In contrast to other quantitative parameters that can be obtained by CMR such as chamber volumes and ejection fraction, universal reference ranges do not exist for normal myocardial T1 time and ECV. Further, cutoff values to differentiate between healthy myocardium and different myocardial diseases were not established. Due to a number of factors including technical and acquisition related parameters as well as physiologic/patient related confounders, there is large variation in reported values of normal native myocardial T1 time and ECV, which has been demonstrated in a recent meta-analysis (Gottbrecht et al. 2019).

Therefore, according to the current guidelines, every site has to establish their own site/scanner specific reference ranges for normal native myocardial T1 time (Messroghli et al. 2017). To establish an individual T1 reference range that enables detection of small changes characteristic for diffuse myocardial fibrosis, values of 50 gender and age adjusted healthy subjects are required. The lower and upper limits of normal can be calculated as the mean T1 value of these reference subjects plus and minus 2 standard deviations (Messroghli et al. 2017). Since there is variation related to the MR scanner, separate reference ranges have to be evaluated for individual scanners used for CMR imaging at the same institution. Phantom-based control is required after each change to the CMR system such as a software update (Messroghli et al. 2017).

According to the current guidelines, with respect to ECV published reference ranges using the same CMR system and pulse sequence may be acceptable (Messroghli et al. 2017). However, comparison of published references ranges for ECV obtained with the same pulse sequence at the same MR scanner shows substantial variation (Gottbrecht et al. 2019), indicating the need of a site/scanner specific reference range also for ECV.

Pooled weighted mean values as well as upper and lower limits of native myocardial T1 time and ECV can be found in the recent "CMR normal value review" (Kawel-Boehm et al. 2020). However, these values can just serve as orientation but do not replace calculation of site-specific normal values. To enable comparison of native T1 values obtained with different CMR systems, *Z*-score transformation of the numerical results is recommended (Messroghli et al. 2017). The *Z*-score can be calculated as follows: *Z*-score = (T1 − mean)/SD, where T1 is the measured native myocardial T1 time of an individual subject and mean and SD are the mean and standard deviation of native myocardial T1 time obtained from the reference group of healthy subjects as described above (Kranzusch et al. 2020).

2.4 Confounding Factors

Confounding factors related to T1 mapping by means of CMR have been assessed extensively including technical factors regarding the MR system and the pulse sequence, factors related to image acquisition and evaluation as well as the contrast agent and administration and also physiologic/patient related factors and caveats regarding the interpretation of the results. Confounding factors and related implications for clinical practice are listed in Table 5.

2.4.1 CMR System

Native T1 time varies by field strength with about 28% higher values obtained at MR scanners with a field strength of 3 T compared to 1.5 T while

Table 5 Confounding factors of T1 mapping by CMR

Factor	Effect	Implications for clinical practice
CMR system	Substantial variation of native T1 time and ECV even between scanners of the same manufacturer and type and for the same pulse sequence	Institution/scanner specific reference ranges required
Field strength	Myocardial T1 time higher at 3 T compared to 1.5 T	Absolute values cannot be compared between 1.5 and 3 T. *Z*-score transformation could be performed alternatively
B_0 and B_1 inhomogeneities	Contributes to heterogeneity of published reference ranges	Volume-selective B_0 shimming at 1.5 T and 3 T and B_1 volume shimming at 3 T is recommended
Pulse sequence	Substantial difference of T1 times and ECV obtained with different sequences	Absolute values cannot be compared between different sequences. *Z*-score transformation could be performed alternatively
Cardiac cycle	Myocardial T1 time precontrast lower at systole, postcontrast lower at diastole, ECV higher in diastole	Scanning at systole and diastole is feasible. Absolute values cannot be compared between cardiac phases. Patient values should be compared to reference ranges obtained at the same cardiac phase
Arrythmia	Images are not acquired at identical cardiac phase hampering co-registration and leading to measurement errors.	Image acquisition at systole should be considered.
Contrast agent	Contrast agents with protein binding characteristics result in higher postcontrast myocardial T1 time and lower ECV	Extracellular non-protein binding contrast agent should be used for T1 mapping/calculation of ECV
Contrast delay	Small increase in ECV over time	Postcontrast T1 maps should be ideally acquired at the same delay
Contrast dose	Postcontrast myocardial T1 time and ECV decrease with higher contrast dose	An identical contrast dose should be used. Absolute values obtained with different doses cannot be compared
Gender	Conflicting publications. Women might have higher native myocardial T1 and ECV	Gender specific reference ranges should be considered

Table 5 (continued)

Factor	Effect	Implications for clinical practice
Age	Conflicting publications	Reference ranges for different age groups might be considered
Body temperature	T1 time increases by about 1% for every 1 °C	Minor relevance. No consequence
ROI	Regional variation of myocardial T1 time. Inclusion of adjacent tissue/blood results in false high or low T1 times	To assess diffuse myocardial disease, measurements of myocardial T1 time should be obtained in the septum of a mid-cavity short-axis T1 map with an ROI including >20 pixels. If the myocardium is thin, acquisition at systole should be considered if reference ranges for systole are available. Inclusion of papillary muscle and trabeculation should be avoided for measurements of T1 time of blood
Confounding substrates	Native myocardial T1 time and ECV, respectively, are affected by different substrates that can increase or decrease values and can occur concomitantly in the myocardium.	A prolongation of native myocardial T1 time and higher ECV are not specific for diffuse interstitial fibrosis.
Large, overlapping reference ranges	Overlap between T1 time and ECV, respectively measured in different myocardial pathologies characterized by diffuse interstitial fibrosis and also with normal reference range	Complicates diagnosing disease of the individual patient

ECV does not vary by field strength (Kawel et al. 2012a; Gottbrecht et al. 2019).

At 3 T B_0 and B_1 inhomogeneities are confounding factors that might explain the heterogeneity of published reference ranges (Gottbrecht et al. 2019).

Native myocardial T1 time and ECV obtained with different CMR systems vary substantially, even between scanners of the same manufacturer and type and for the same pulse sequence. Therefore scanner specific reference ranges should be established (Gottbrecht et al. 2019).

2.4.2 Mapping Sequence

There is substantial variation of native T1 time and ECV between the different pulse sequences (Gottbrecht et al. 2019; Roujol et al. 2014). The differences are not just statistically significant but also clinically relevant and in the order of changes that are expected to occur between normal and disease. Roujol et al. scanned healthy individuals with four different T1 mapping sequences each using the same MR scanner (Roujol et al. 2014). The largest difference between mean native T1 time was observed between the ShMOLLI sequence (595 ms) and SAPPHIRE (1202 ms). ECV ranged from 0.18 for SASHA to 0.27 for MOLLI.

Both the inversion recovery and saturation recovery techniques tend to overestimate the true T1 time, however, saturation recovery techniques have been shown to be more accurate compared to inversion recovery techniques (Puntmann et al. 2016a).

The different versions of the MOLLI sequence with varying number of inversions, images, and recovery beats result in different myocardial T1 times (Roujol et al. 2014). MOLLI sequences have been shown to have a nonlinear dependency on heart rate for longer T1 values (Lee et al. 2011). MOLLI is further sensitive to magnetization transfer effects, T2, flip angle, and off-resonance, responsible for the lower accuracy (Robson et al. 2013; Kellman and Hansen 2014; Kellman et al. 2013, 2014). Saturation recovery sequences are less sensitive to these effects and therefore more accurate but less precise.

2.4.3 Systole Versus Diastole

Mapping sequences are usually acquired during diastole. However, acquisition during systole results in good image quality and can also be performed routinely (Kawel et al. 2012a). Particularly in subjects with arrhythmia and thin myocardium, it might be advantageous to acquire images during systole (Fig. 3). However, reference ranges need to be adjusted since there are differences in T1 time and ECV between systole and diastole mainly related to changes in myocardial blood volume and less partial-volume effects at systole (Kawel et al. 2012a; Messner et al. 2018; Ferreira et al. 2015; Reiter et al. 2014).

2.4.4 Contrast Agent

Postcontrast T1 time has been shown to vary between contrast agents with different relaxivity (Kawel et al. 2012b). Contrast agents with protein binding characteristics that bind to albumin in the blood are expected to have a different distribution between blood and interstitial space compared to non-protein binding contrast agents explaining differences in ECV (Kawel et al. 2012b).

While postcontrast T1 time increases with time after contrast administration due to contrast excretion, a slight increase over time has also been shown for ECV (11% during 45 min after contrast injection) (Kawel et al. 2012b).

Not only postcontrast T1 time but also ECV has been shown to be dose dependent in a study where subjects were scanned with three different contrast doses of 0.1, 0.15, and 0.2 mmol/kg (Dabir et al. 2014).

2.4.5 Gender

There are conflicting results in publications regarding the relationship of native myocardial T1 time with gender. In a cohort of 1231 subjects of a large multicenter study, women had significantly greater ECV and precontrast myocardial T1 time (Liu et al. 2013). In a cohort of 342 healthy volunteers, women had a significantly longer native myocardial T1 time compared to men up to the age of 45 years (Piechnik et al. 2013). After the age of 45, there was no significant difference in native myocardial T1 time between men and women. In a recent meta-analysis, there was no association between native myocardial T1 time and gender but ECV values were higher in studies including more females (Gottbrecht et al. 2019). Other studies did not show a relationship between native myocardial T1 time and ECV, respectively, with gender (Dabir et al. 2014; von Knobelsdorff-Brenkenhoff et al. 2013).

2.4.6 Age

Also regarding the relationship of native myocardial T1 time and ECV, respectively, with age, study results vary. In the multicenter study already mentioned above, greater precontrast myocardial T1 time and ECV were associated with older age only in men (Liu et al. 2013). Piechnik et al. on the other hand reported a decrease of native myocardial T1 time with age in women (Piechnik et al. 2013). Another study also reported a decrease of native myocardial T1 time with age, while analysis was not performed for men and women separately (von Knobelsdorff-Brenkenhoff et al. 2013). Other studies did not find age-related differences of T1 time and/or ECV (Gottbrecht et al. 2019; Dabir et al. 2014).

2.4.7 Body Temperature

T1 time has been shown to increase with body temperature. However, the effect is small (about 1% for every 1 °C), and patients referred for CMR are typically not affected by fever or hypothermia (Messroghli et al. 2017).

2.4.8 Measurement Technique

T1 time of the myocardium and the blood pool is measured by drawing an ROI. On the one hand, the size of the ROI should not be too small but on the other hand care has to be taken to avoid inclusion of adjacent structures, e.g., the adjacent blood when measuring T1 of the myocardium or a papillary muscle when measuring T1 of blood. Inclusion or exclusion of areas of focal replacement scar will affect the result significantly. Whether a focal scar should be included or excluded depends on the clinical question.

With respect to myocarditis, Dabir et al. compared the diagnostic performance of different measurement approaches of myocardial T1 time and ECV, respectively. Measurements were obtained for the entire (global) LV myocardium (ROI drawn to encompass the entire LV myocardium of three short-axis slices acquired at the basal, mid-ventricular, and apical level), for the entire LV myocardium of a mid-ventricular short-axis slice, for the mid-ventricular septal wall and for the remote myocardium (normokinetic segments with no visual edema or presence of LGE). For all measurement approaches, native T1 time and ECV, respectively, were significantly higher compared to healthy controls. However, the diagnostic performance was best for the global approach (Fig. 4) (Dabir et al. 2019a).

Small regional variations of myocardial T1 time and ECV have been demonstrated between the septal compared to the non-septal myocardium with a slightly longer native myocardial T1 time and higher ECV of the septum (Kawel et al. 2012a).

Von Knobelsdorff-Brenkenhoff described an increase of the precontrast myocardial T1 time from base to apex (von Knobelsdorff-Brenkenhoff et al. 2013) while Messroghli et al. could not detect a significant difference of T1 values between myocardial T1 values measured on short-axis slices acquired at the basal, mid-ventricular, and apical level of the left ventricle (Messroghli et al. 2006).

2.4.9 Confounding Substrates

A prolongation of native myocardial T1 time and higher ECV is not specific for diffuse interstitial fibrosis but is also present in edema and amyloid deposition. Native T1 time and ECV are lower in the presence of lipid (e.g., Anderson-Fabry disease and lipomatous metaplasia in chronic myocardial infarction), iron overload, and hemorrhage (Haaf et al. 2016). Therefore, a prolongation of native myocardial T1 time or enlargement of the ECV alone is not synonymous for diffuse interstitial fibrosis. Further, substrates with an opposing effect on T1 time and ECV such as diffuse fibrosis and lipid might occur concomitantly in the myocardium potentially resulting in a normal T1 time.

2.4.10 Large, Overlapping Reference Ranges

Due to large reference ranges for native myocardial T1 time and ECV, there is substantial overlap between normal values and values measured in various diseases (Gottbrecht et al. 2019; Liu et al. 2017b; Kawel-Boehm et al. 2020). In a typical research scenario, the mean T1 time and/or ECV of a group of patients with a known cardiac disease are compared to a group of healthy control subjects showing a statistical significant difference between the mean values of the two groups. However, in clinical practice, the situation is different; it has to be decided whether a single patient has a disease or not and which disease it is.

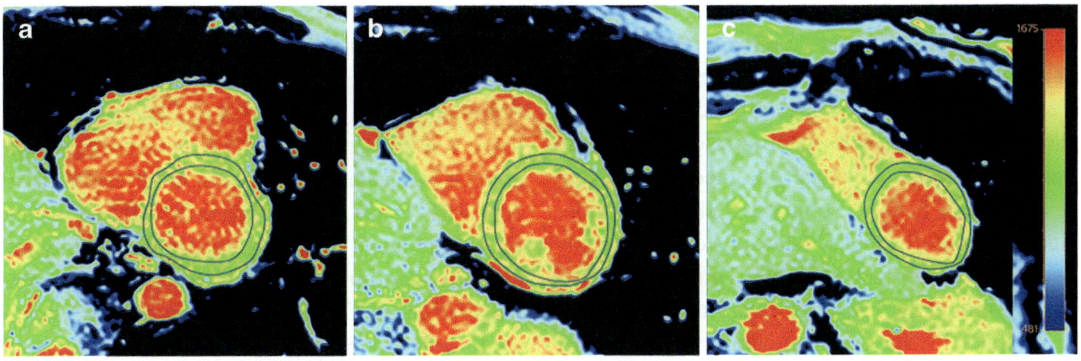

Fig. 4 T1 map acquired in short axis at the basal (**a**), mid-ventricular (**b**), and apical level (**c**). To measure global myocardial T1 relaxation time, a region of interest was drawn on each slice encompassing the entire left ventricular myocardium according to reference (Dabir et al. 2019a)

Liu et al. obtained native myocardial T1 time in 1291 subjects, including 70 control subjects to establish a normal reference range and patients with various cardiac diseases including, e.g., acute and prior myocarditis, hypertrophic and dilated cardiomyopathy, hypertensive heart disease, and aortic stenosis. The authors showed substantial overlap between native myocardial T1 time among the different diseases and also with the normal reference range (Liu et al. 2017b). Only values obtained in iron overload, Anderson-Fabry disease, and amyloid did not overlap with the normal reference range.

Due to large normal ranges of native myocardial T1 time and ECV, pathology might be missed in individual patients. A patient with a T1-time close to the upper limit of normal might have had a baseline value close to the lower limit of normal. However, unless repetitive scanning is performed, the change over time is not detected and larger changes of up to 100 ms might not be evident due to the large range of normal values.

2.5 Clinical Implementation

T1 mapping has been applied to assess different diseases characterized by diffuse interstitial fibrosis of the myocardium, including primary cardiac diseases such as aortic stenosis, non-ischemic dilated cardiomyopathy (DCM) and hypertrophic cardiomyopathy (HCM), and extracardiac diseases with cardiac manifestation, e.g., hypertensive heart disease, diabetes, rheumatoid arthritis, and systemic sclerosis (Radenkovic et al. 2017). However, since T1 mapping is a new CMR technique, that is currently complicated by the requirement of site-specific reference ranges and the overlap of values obtained in different diseases and healthy subjects, dedicated guidelines and cutoff values regarding diagnosis and prognosis are not yet available. Thus, the following paragraphs will give an overview of the current state of the clinical application of T1 mapping and future perspective related to different diseases characterized by interstitial myocardial fibrosis.

2.5.1 Aortic Stenosis

There are conflicting results of studies assessing patients with aortic stenosis by means of cardiac T1 mapping. While some authors reported a significant difference of native myocardial T1 time and ECV, respectively, between patients with aortic stenosis and healthy adults, others did not find a significant difference (Bull et al. 2013; Chin et al. 2014; Singh et al. 2015; Lee et al. 2015). Nadjiri et al. assessed ECV as a predictor of adverse events in subjects after transcatheter aortic valve replacement (TAVR) (Nadjiri et al. 2016). The authors could not demonstrate a significant correlation between ECV and death or congestive heart failure after TAVR. Patients who developed conduction abnormalities post TAVR had, different than expected, statistically lower ECV values compared to those without an event. Everett et al. showed that ECV was associated with cardiovascular mortality and also independently associated with all-cause mortality in 440 patients with severe aortic stenosis after aortic valve intervention (Everett et al. 2020).

Further research is required to assess the prognostic value of T1 mapping for adverse events after postaortic valve intervention and the impact on timing and replacement procedure.

2.5.2 Non-ischemic Dilated Cardiomyopathy (NIDCM)

A strong correlation between ECV and histologically quantified fibrosis has been demonstrated in patients with DCM (aus dem Siepen et al. 2015). In several studies, native myocardial T1 time and ECV have been shown to be significantly different between patients and healthy control subjects (aus dem Siepen et al. 2015; Dass et al. 2012; Puntmann et al. 2013; Cui et al. 2019). However, there is a large overlap of the values obtained in control subjects and patients with DCM (Liu et al. 2017b; aus dem Siepen et al. 2015). Further, measurements of T1 time are complicated by the thin myocardium prone to partial-volume artifacts. Higher ECV has been shown to be associated with adverse outcome in patients with NIDCM indicating that T1 mapping might play a role for risk assessment in NIDM (Barison et al. 2015; Puntmann et al. 2016b).

However, uniform risk categories and clinical recommendations are not yet available.

2.5.3 Myocarditis

In 2018, the original Lake Louis Criteria for the diagnosis of acute myocarditis by CMR were updated, now including T1 mapping as surrogate for edema, hyperemia, necrosis, and fibrosis (Ferreira et al. 2018). Regional or global increase of native myocardial T1 relaxation time and/or ECV compared to local reference ranges indicates myocarditis. The updated Lake Louise Criteria yielded a higher sensitivity at identical specificity compared to the old Criteria (Luetkens et al. 2019).

In terms of risk stratification, in patients with suspected myocarditis Graeni et al. demonstrated a significant association of ECV ≥35% with major adverse cardiac events (composite of all-cause death, heart failure hospitalization, heart transplantation, documented sustained ventricular arrhythmia, recurrent myocarditis) in a multivariable model adjusted for age, LVEF, and LGE size (Grani et al. 2019b).

2.5.4 Hypertrophic Cardiomyopathy (HCM)

Native myocardial T1 time and ECV are elevated in patients with HCM compared to healthy subjects (Dass et al. 2012; Puntmann et al. 2013) even in patients without LGE (Xu et al. 2020). T1 mapping might be useful to differentiate between HCM and hypertrophy in athlete's heart, where native myocardial T1 time and ECV are decreased due to myocyte hypertrophy (Swoboda et al. 2016). Elevated global ECV has been shown to predict sudden cardiac death in patients with HCM indicating the usefulness of ECV to identify patients for ICD therapy (Avanesov et al. 2017).

Similar to NIDCM, further research is required to establish dedicated guidelines based on distinct cutoff values.

2.5.5 Extracardiac Diseases with Cardiac Manifestation

Native myocardial T1 time and ECV were elevated in left ventricular hypertrophy related to hypertensive heart disease (HHD) compared to healthy individuals in some studies (Wu et al. 2017) while other studies could not detect a significant difference between the two groups (von Knobelsdorff-Brenkenhoff et al. 2016). In clinical practice to differentiate hypertrophy related to hypertension from HCM is challenging. Due to the overlap of native myocardial T1 time and ECV, respectively, and the fact that both diseases might be present at different stages, the discriminative ability of T1 mapping alone is limited (Liu et al. 2017b). Radiomic texture analysis of T1 mapping might have the potential to improve discrimination between HHD and HCM compared to T1 mapping alone (Neisius et al. 2019).

In patients with diabetes mellitus (Gao et al. 2019; Al-Badri et al. 2018), rheumatoid arthritis (Ntusi et al. 2015), and systemic sclerosis (Lee et al. 2018), native myocardial T1 time and/or ECV were elevated related to diffuse myocardial fibroses compared to values obtained in healthy subjects indicating a potential for detecting early cardiac involvement and monitor disease progression.

2.5.6 Monitoring Course of Disease

In a large number of studies, native myocardial T1 time and ECV have been identified as imaging biomarker of different diseases characterized by myocardial interstitial fibrosis. The high reproducibility makes T1 mapping a valuable tool to assess the course of disease. Disease progression or response to treatment can be monitored in follow-up examinations guiding therapy and clinical decisions. Since the values obtained by T1 mapping in an individual patient serve as personalized reference, normal values of healthy controls are not required for comparison.

3 T2-Mapping

3.1 (Patho)Physiological and Technical Background

Eighty percent of the normal myocardium consists of water, of which 77% is intracellular and 23% intravascular (Eitel and Friedrich 2011). Acute myocardial injury of ischemic or inflammatory origin is characterized by myocardial edema. Cytotoxic edema which is characterized by an increased intracellular water content and subsequent myocyte swelling can be distinguished from vasogenic edema with fluid accumulation in the interstitial space (Eitel and Friedrich 2011). Edema leads to an increase of myocardial stiffness and decreased compliance.

Myocardial edema can be measured by means of T2 mapping. T2 is a measure of the decay of the transverse magnetization (Messroghli et al. 2017). The more rapidly moving water molecules have a lower tendency to transfer their spin leading to a slower dephasing of the transverse magnetization and therefore have a long T2 decay. Thus, myocardial T2 relaxation time is longer in the presence of myocardial edema, e.g., due to acute myocardial infarction or myocardial inflammation.

To quantify T2 relaxation time by means of T2 mapping, during a single breath hold, several images are acquired at different echo times and fitted to an exponential decay curve (Messroghli et al. 2017). T2 is the time required for the transverse magnetization to decrease to approximately 37% of the original value.

3.2 Image Acquisition and Analysis

T2 mapping can be performed at 1.5 T and 3 T. T2-prepared bSSFP or gradient-echo sequences with at least three source images of different echo times are recommended for T2 mapping acquired prior to contrast administration (Messroghli et al. 2017). T2 maps are usually acquired in a mid-ventricular short-axis orientation, and myocardial T2 time is measured by an ROI in the interventricular septum avoiding inclusion of adjacent blood.

3.3 Expected Result and Range of Normal Values

Also for T2 mapping site/scanner specific reference ranges have to be established in the same way described for T1 mapping in the previous paragraph. For comparison published normal myocardial T2 values can be found here (Kawel-Boehm et al. 2020).

3.4 Confounding Factors

3.4.1 Technical Factors

Similar to T1 mapping, the T2 mapping technique is influenced by several technical factors including sensitivity to T1, off-resonance effects, and the technique used for motion correction (Messroghli et al. 2017; Roujol et al. 2015). T2 is slightly shorter at 3 T compared to 1.5 T and T2 varies by the pulse sequence and the scanner vendor (Kawel-Boehm et al. 2020).

The variation of T2 time by several technical factors indicates the necessity to establish site/scanner specific reference ranges and standardization of protocols and scan parameters.

3.4.2 Regional Variation

A significant increase of left ventricular myocardial T2 relaxation time from the base to the apex was demonstrated in several studies (von Knobelsdorff-Brenkenhoff et al. 2013; Bonner et al. 2015; Granitz et al. 2019).

3.4.3 Gender

Women had longer myocardial T2 compared to men in two studies performed at 1.5 T (Bonner et al. 2015; Granitz et al. 2019), indicating that gender specific reference ranges are required. However, at 3 T gender differences were not confirmed (von Knobelsdorff-Brenkenhoff et al. 2013; Granitz et al. 2019).

3.4.4 Age

While one study revealed an increase of myocardial T2 relaxation time with age (Bonner et al. 2015), other studies could not demonstrate a variation of T2 by age (von Knobelsdorff-Brenkenhoff et al. 2013; Granitz et al. 2019).

3.4.5 Heart Rate

An increase in T2 with increasing heart rate was demonstrated in two studies (von Knobelsdorff-Brenkenhoff et al. 2013; Granitz et al. 2019), while another study could not find a correlation between myocardial T2 and heart rate (Bonner et al. 2015).

3.5 Clinical Implementation

3.5.1 Acute Myocardial Infarction

Myocardial edema occurring in acute myocardial infarction is characterized by an increased free water content and prolongation of T2. T2 mapping can be used to detect myocardial edema and distinguish acute from chronic myocardial infarction, since edema is only present in the acute setting (Giri et al. 2009).

The "area at risk" (AAR) is the myocardial tissue supplied by the culprit lesion in myocardial infarction consisting of irreversibly injured myocardium and viable/salvaged myocardium (Wright et al. 2009). Together with LGE imaging, T2-weighted imaging has been applied to identify myocardial salvage and the success of coronary revascularization therapy (Wright et al. 2009). However, there is controversy regarding this concept (Croisille et al. 2012). Instead of T2-weighted imaging T2 mapping has also been applied for quantification of the AAR (Bulluck et al. 2015). For this approach, T2 maps were acquired in short-axis orientation covering the entire left ventricle. Different thresholding techniques can be applied as described for LGE imaging above. Myocardial areas with elevated T2 but without demarcation of myocardial infarction on LGE imaging correspond to myocardial salvage (Bulluck et al. 2015).

3.5.2 Myocarditis

The updated Lake Louis Criteria for the diagnosis of acute myocarditis by CMR now include T2 mapping for the diagnosis of edema (Ferreira et al. 2018). Regional or global increase of myocardial T2 relaxation time compared to local reference ranges is considered one of several criteria indicating acute myocarditis.

3.5.3 Cardiac Transplant Rejection

Myocardial T2 relaxation time has been shown to be significantly elevated in acute cardiac transplant rejection (Vermes et al. 2018). The authors of one study could show that T2 mapping in combination with ECV quantification enabled diagnosis of transplant rejection in all cases of rejection (7/20 heart transplant recipients) avoiding endomyocardial biopsy (Vermes et al. 2018).

3.5.4 Takotsubo Cardiomyopathy

T2 mapping has also proven to be useful in the diagnosis of edema in Takotsubo cardiomyopathy (Dabir et al. 2019b). The authors of a recent publication obtained T2 maps in short-axis orientation at the basal, mid-ventricular, and apical level (Dabir et al. 2019b). In patients with Takotsubo cardiomyopathy, T2 values were elevated compared to healthy controls and also higher in segments with abnormal wall motion compared to normal wall motion. Interestingly, T2 values were also higher in segments with normal wall motion compared to healthy controls. Further studies are required to assess the potential of T2 relaxation time as a marker of disease progress.

Disclaimer All measurements in this book have been obtained from peer-reviewed papers and guidelines from professional organizations, unless explicitly stated otherwise. While the authors, editors, and publisher have gone through a rigorous process to establish their correct reproduction from the original source, each measurement must be interpreted in the correct clinical context, this along with an accurate way of measurement, and taking into account all technical variables, this including follow-up exams with various equipment or software. Neither the authors, the editors, nor the publisher can accept any legal responsibility for any improper application or interpretation of these measurements as well as their potential consequences.

References

Al-Badri A, Hashmath Z, Oldland GH, Miller R, Javaid K, Syed AA, Ansari B, Gaddam S, Witschey WR, Akers SR, Chirinos JA (2018) Poor glycemic control is associated with increased extracellular volume fraction in diabetes. Diabetes Care 41(9):2019–2025. https://doi.org/10.2337/dc18-0324

Amado LC, Gerber BL, Gupta SN, Rettmann DW, Szarf G, Schock R, Nasir K, Kraitchman DL, Lima JA (2004) Accurate and objective infarct sizing by contrast-enhanced magnetic resonance imaging in a canine myocardial infarction model. J Am Coll Cardiol 44(12):2383–2389. https://doi.org/10.1016/j.jacc.2004.09.020

aus dem Siepen F, Buss SJ, Messroghli D, Andre F, Lossnitzer D, Seitz S, Keller M, Schnabel PA, Giannitsis E, Korosoglou G, Katus HA, Steen H (2015) T1 mapping in dilated cardiomyopathy with cardiac magnetic resonance: quantification of diffuse myocardial fibrosis and comparison with endomyocardial biopsy. Eur Heart J Cardiovasc Imaging 16(2):210–216. https://doi.org/10.1093/ehjci/jeu183

Avanesov M, Munch J, Weinrich J, Well L, Saring D, Stehning C, Tahir E, Bohnen S, Radunski UK, Muellerleile K, Adam G, Patten M, Lund G (2017) Prediction of the estimated 5-year risk of sudden cardiac death and syncope or non-sustained ventricular tachycardia in patients with hypertrophic cardiomyopathy using late gadolinium enhancement and extracellular volume CMR. Eur Radiol 27(12):5136–5145. https://doi.org/10.1007/s00330-017-4869-x

Bandula S, White SK, Flett AS, Lawrence D, Pugliese F, Ashworth MT, Punwani S, Taylor SA, Moon JC (2013) Measurement of myocardial extracellular volume fraction by using equilibrium contrast-enhanced CT: validation against histologic findings. Radiology 269(2):396–403. https://doi.org/10.1148/radiol.13130130

Barison A, Del Torto A, Chiappino S, Aquaro GD, Todiere G, Vergaro G, Passino C, Lombardi M, Emdin M, Masci PG (2015) Prognostic significance of myocardial extracellular volume fraction in nonischaemic dilated cardiomyopathy. J Cardiovasc Med (Hagerstown) 16(10):681–687. https://doi.org/10.2459/JCM.0000000000000275

Bastarrika G, Ramos-Duran L, Rosenblum MA, Kang DK, Rowe GW, Schoepf UJ (2010) Adenosine-stress dynamic myocardial CT perfusion imaging: initial clinical experience. Invest Radiol 45(6):306–313. https://doi.org/10.1097/RLI.0b013e3181dfa2f2

Bettencourt N, Ferreira ND, Leite D, Carvalho M, Ferreira WDS, Schuster A, Chiribiri A, Leite-Moreira A, Silva-Cardoso J, Nagel E, Gama V (2013) CAD detection in patients with intermediate-high pre-test probability: low-dose CT delayed enhancement detects ischemic myocardial scar with moderate accuracy but does not improve performance of a stress-rest CT perfusion protocol. JACC Cardiovasc Imaging 6(10):1062–1071. https://doi.org/10.1016/j.jcmg.2013.04.013

Blankstein R, Rogers IS, Cury RC (2009) Practical tips and tricks in cardiovascular computed tomography: diagnosis of myocardial infarction. J Cardiovasc Comput Tomogr 3(2):104–111. https://doi.org/10.1016/j.jcct.2008.10.014

Bluemke DA, Kawel-Boehm N (2016) Can a MR imaging scanner accurately measure hematocrit to determine ECV fraction? JACC Cardiovasc Imaging 9(1):64–66. https://doi.org/10.1016/j.jcmg.2015.11.009

Bonner F, Janzarik N, Jacoby C, Spieker M, Schnackenburg B, Range F, Butzbach B, Haberkorn S, Westenfeld R, Neizel-Wittke M, Flogel U, Kelm M (2015) Myocardial T2 mapping reveals age- and sex-related differences in volunteers. J Cardiovasc Magn Reson 17(1):9. https://doi.org/10.1186/s12968-015-0118-0

Bruder O, Wagner A, Jensen CJ, Schneider S, Ong P, Kispert EM, Nassenstein K, Schlosser T, Sabin GV, Sechtem U, Mahrholdt H (2010) Myocardial scar visualized by cardiovascular magnetic resonance imaging predicts major adverse events in patients with hypertrophic cardiomyopathy. J Am Coll Cardiol 56(11):875–887. https://doi.org/10.1016/j.jacc.2010.05.007

Bull S, White SK, Piechnik SK, Flett AS, Ferreira VM, Loudon M, Francis JM, Karamitsos TD, Prendergast BD, Robson MD, Neubauer S, Moon JC, Myerson SG (2013) Human non-contrast T1 values and correlation with histology in diffuse fibrosis. Heart 99(13):932–937. https://doi.org/10.1136/heartjnl-2012-303052

Bulluck H, White SK, Rosmini S, Bhuva A, Treibel TA, Fontana M, Abdel-Gadir A, Herrey A, Manisty C, Wan SM, Groves A, Menezes L, Moon JC, Hausenloy DJ (2015) T1 mapping and T2 mapping at 3T for quantifying the area-at-risk in reperfused STEMI patients. J Cardiovasc Magn Reson 17:73. https://doi.org/10.1186/s12968-015-0173-6

Burstein B, Nattel S (2008) Atrial fibrosis: mechanisms and clinical relevance in atrial fibrillation. J Am Coll Cardiol 51(8):802–809. https://doi.org/10.1016/j.jacc.2007.09.064

Cerqueira MD, Weissman NJ, Dilsizian V, Jacobs AK, Kaul S, Laskey WK, Pennell DJ, Rumberger JA, Ryan T, Verani MS, American Heart Association Writing Group on Myocardial Segmentation and Registration for Cardiac Imaging (2002) Standardized myocardial segmentation and nomenclature for tomographic imaging of the heart. A statement for healthcare professionals from the Cardiac Imaging Committee of the Council on Clinical Cardiology of the American Heart Association. Circulation 105(4):539–542. https://doi.org/10.1161/hc0402.102975

Chan RH, Maron BJ, Olivotto I, Pencina MJ, Assenza GE, Haas T, Lesser JR, Gruner C, Crean AM, Rakowski H, Udelson JE, Rowin E, Lombardi M, Cecchi F, Tomberli B, Spirito P, Formisano F, Biagini E, Rapezzi C, De Cecco CN, Autore C, Cook EF, Hong SN, Gibson CM, Manning WJ, Appelbaum E, Maron MS (2014) Prognostic value of quantitative contrast-enhanced cardiovascular magnetic resonance for the evaluation of sudden death risk in patients with hypertrophic cardiomyopathy. Circulation 130(6):484–495. https://doi.org/10.1161/CIRCULATIONAHA.113.007094

Child NM, Das R (2012) Is cardiac magnetic resonance imaging assessment of myocardial viability use-

ful for predicting which patients with impaired ventricles might benefit from revascularization? Interact Cardiovasc Thorac Surg 14(4):395–398. https://doi.org/10.1093/icvts/ivr161
Chin CW, Semple S, Malley T, White AC, Mirsadraee S, Weale PJ, Prasad S, Newby DE, Dweck MR (2014) Optimization and comparison of myocardial T1 techniques at 3T in patients with aortic stenosis. Eur Heart J Cardiovasc Imaging 15(5):556–565. https://doi.org/10.1093/ehjci/jet245
Choi KM, Kim RJ, Gubernikoff G, Vargas JD, Parker M, Judd RM (2001) Transmural extent of acute myocardial infarction predicts long-term improvement in contractile function. Circulation 104(10):1101–1107. https://doi.org/10.1161/hc3501.096798
Crawford T, Mueller G, Sarsam S, Prasitdumrong H, Chaiyen N, Gu X, Schuller J, Kron J, Nour KA, Cheng A, Ji SY, Feinstein S, Gupta S, Ilg K, Sinno M, Abu-Hashish S, Al-Mallah M, Sauer WH, Ellenbogen K, Morady F, Bogun F (2014) Magnetic resonance imaging for identifying patients with cardiac sarcoidosis and preserved or mildly reduced left ventricular function at risk of ventricular arrhythmias. Circ Arrhythm Electrophysiol 7(6):1109–1115. https://doi.org/10.1161/CIRCEP.113.000156
Croisille P, Kim HW, Kim RJ (2012) Controversies in cardiovascular MR imaging: T2-weighted imaging should not be used to delineate the area at risk in ischemic myocardial injury. Radiology 265(1):12–22. https://doi.org/10.1148/radiol.12111769
Cui Y, Chen Y, Cao Y, Liu J, Song J, Zhang S, Kong X, Han P, Shi H (2019) Myocardial extracellular volume fraction measurements with MOLLI 5(3)3 by cardiovascular MRI for the discrimination of healthy volunteers from dilated and hypertrophic cardiomyopathy patients. Clin Radiol 74(9):732.e739–732.e716. https://doi.org/10.1016/j.crad.2019.04.019
Dabir D, Child N, Kalra A, Rogers T, Gebker R, Jabbour A, Plein S, Yu CY, Otton J, Kidambi A, McDiarmid A, Broadbent D, Higgins DM, Schnackenburg B, Foote L, Cummins C, Nagel E, Puntmann VO (2014) Reference values for healthy human myocardium using a T1 mapping methodology: results from the International T1 Multicenter cardiovascular magnetic resonance study. J Cardiovasc Magn Reson 16:69. https://doi.org/10.1186/s12968-014-0069-x
Dabir D, Vollbrecht TM, Luetkens JA, Kuetting DLR, Isaak A, Feisst A, Fimmers R, Sprinkart AM, Schild HH, Thomas D (2019a) Multiparametric cardiovascular magnetic resonance imaging in acute myocarditis: a comparison of different measurement approaches. J Cardiovasc Magn Reson 21(1):54. https://doi.org/10.1186/s12968-019-0568-x
Dabir D, Luetkens J, Kuetting DLR, Feisst A, Isaak A, Schild HH, Thomas D (2019b) Cardiac magnetic resonance including parametric mapping in acute Takotsubo syndrome: preliminary findings. Eur J Radiol 113:217–224. https://doi.org/10.1016/j.ejrad.2019.02.026
Dass S, Suttie JJ, Piechnik SK, Ferreira VM, Holloway CJ, Banerjee R, Mahmod M, Cochlin L, Karamitsos TD, Robson MD, Watkins H, Neubauer S (2012) Myocardial tissue characterization using magnetic resonance noncontrast t1 mapping in hypertrophic and dilated cardiomyopathy. Circ Cardiovasc Imaging 5(6):726–733. https://doi.org/10.1161/CIRCIMAGING.112.976738
Demirel F, Adiyaman A, Timmer JR, Dambrink JH, Kok M, Boeve WJ, Elvan A (2014) Myocardial scar characteristics based on cardiac magnetic resonance imaging is associated with ventricular tachyarrhythmia in patients with ischemic cardiomyopathy. Int J Cardiol 177(2):392–399. https://doi.org/10.1016/j.ijcard.2014.08.132
Diao KY, Yang ZG, Xu HY, Liu X, Zhang Q, Shi K, Jiang L, Xie LJ, Wen LY, Guo YK (2016) Histologic validation of myocardial fibrosis measured by T1 mapping: a systematic review and meta-analysis. J Cardiovasc Magn Reson 18(1):92. https://doi.org/10.1186/s12968-016-0313-7
Eitel I, Friedrich MG (2011) T2-weighted cardiovascular magnetic resonance in acute cardiac disease. J Cardiovasc Magn Reson 13:13. https://doi.org/10.1186/1532-429X-13-13
Esposito A, Palmisano A, Antunes S, Maccabelli G, Colantoni C, Rancoita PMV, Baratto F, Di Serio C, Rizzo G, De Cobelli F, Della Bella P, Del Maschio A (2016) Cardiac CT with delayed enhancement in the characterization of ventricular tachycardia structural substrate: relationship between CT-segmented scar and electro-anatomic mapping. JACC Cardiovasc Imaging 9(7):822–832. https://doi.org/10.1016/j.jcmg.2015.10.024
Everett RJ, Treibel TA, Fukui M, Lee H, Rigolli M, Singh A, Bijsterveld P, Tastet L, Musa TA, Dobson L, Chin C, Captur G, Om SY, Wiesemann S, Ferreira VM, Piechnik SK, Schulz-Menger J, Schelbert EB, Clavel MA, Newby DE, Myerson SG, Pibarot P, Lee S, Cavalcante JL, Lee SP, McCann GP, Greenwood JP, Moon JC, Dweck MR (2020) Extracellular myocardial volume in patients with aortic stenosis. J Am Coll Cardiol 75(3):304–316. https://doi.org/10.1016/j.jacc.2019.11.032
Fahmy AS, Rausch J, Neisius U, Chan RH, Maron MS, Appelbaum E, Menze B, Nezafat R (2018) Automated cardiac MR scar quantification in hypertrophic cardiomyopathy using deep convolutional neural networks. JACC Cardiovasc Imaging 11(12):1917–1918. https://doi.org/10.1016/j.jcmg.2018.04.030
Fahmy AS, Neisius U, Chan RH, Rowin EJ, Manning WJ, Maron MS, Nezafat R (2020) Three-dimensional deep convolutional neural networks for automated myocardial scar quantification in hypertrophic cardiomyopathy: a multicenter multivendor study. Radiology 294(1):52–60. https://doi.org/10.1148/radiol.2019190737
Ferreira VM, Wijesurendra RS, Liu A, Greiser A, Casadei B, Robson MD, Neubauer S, Piechnik SK

(2015) Systolic ShMOLLI myocardial T1-mapping for improved robustness to partial-volume effects and applications in tachyarrhythmias. J Cardiovasc Magn Reson 17:77. https://doi.org/10.1186/s12968-015-0182-5

Ferreira VM, Schulz-Menger J, Holmvang G, Kramer CM, Carbone I, Sechtem U, Kindermann I, Gutberlet M, Cooper LT, Liu P, Friedrich MG (2018) Cardiovascular magnetic resonance in nonischemic myocardial inflammation: expert recommendations. J Am Coll Cardiol 72(24):3158–3176. https://doi.org/10.1016/j.jacc.2018.09.072

Finn JP, Nael K, Deshpande V, Ratib O, Laub G (2006) Cardiac MR imaging: state of the technology. Radiology 241(2):338–354. https://doi.org/10.1148/radiol.2412041866

Flett AS, Hasleton J, Cook C, Hausenloy D, Quarta G, Ariti C, Muthurangu V, Moon JC (2011) Evaluation of techniques for the quantification of myocardial scar of differing etiology using cardiac magnetic resonance. JACC Cardiovasc Imaging 4(2):150–156. https://doi.org/10.1016/j.jcmg.2010.11.015

Gao P, Yee R, Gula L, Krahn AD, Skanes A, Leong-Sit P, Klein GJ, Stirrat J, Fine N, Pallaveshi L, Wisenberg G, Thompson TR, Prato F, Drangova M, White JA (2012) Prediction of arrhythmic events in ischemic and dilated cardiomyopathy patients referred for implantable cardiac defibrillator: evaluation of multiple scar quantification measures for late gadolinium enhancement magnetic resonance imaging. Circ Cardiovasc Imaging 5(4):448–456. https://doi.org/10.1161/CIRCIMAGING.111.971549

Gao Y, Yang ZG, Ren Y, Liu X, Jiang L, Xie LJ, Hu BY, Shen MT, Xu HY, Li ZL, Xia CC, Li YM, Deng LL, Deng MY, Zhou XY, Guo YK (2019) Evaluation of myocardial fibrosis in diabetes with cardiac magnetic resonance T1-mapping: correlation with the high-level hemoglobin A1c. Diabetes Res Clin Pract 150:72–80. https://doi.org/10.1016/j.diabres.2019.03.004

George RT, Arbab-Zadeh A, Miller JM, Vavere AL, Bengel FM, Lardo AC, Lima JA (2012) Computed tomography myocardial perfusion imaging with 320-row detector computed tomography accurately detects myocardial ischemia in patients with obstructive coronary artery disease. Circ Cardiovasc Imaging 5(3):333–340. https://doi.org/10.1161/CIRCIMAGING.111.969303

Gerber BL, Belge B, Legros GJ, Lim P, Poncelet A, Pasquet A, Gisellu G, Coche E, Vanoverschelde JL (2006) Characterization of acute and chronic myocardial infarcts by multidetector computed tomography: comparison with contrast-enhanced magnetic resonance. Circulation 113(6):823–833. https://doi.org/10.1161/CIRCULATIONAHA.104.529511

Giri S, Chung YC, Merchant A, Mihai G, Rajagopalan S, Raman SV, Simonetti OP (2009) T2 quantification for improved detection of myocardial edema. J Cardiovasc Magn Reson 11:56. https://doi.org/10.1186/1532-429X-11-56

Goetti R, Feuchtner G, Stolzmann P, Donati OF, Wieser M, Plass A, Frauenfelder T, Leschka S, Alkadhi H (2011) Delayed enhancement imaging of myocardial viability: low-dose high-pitch CT versus MRI. Eur Radiol 21(10):2091–2099. https://doi.org/10.1007/s00330-011-2149-8

Gottbrecht M, Kramer CM, Salerno M (2019) Native T1 and extracellular volume measurements by cardiac MRI in healthy adults: a meta-analysis. Radiology 290(2):317–326. https://doi.org/10.1148/radiol.2018180226

Grani C, Eichhorn C, Biere L, Murthy VL, Agarwal V, Kaneko K, Cuddy S, Aghayev A, Steigner M, Blankstein R, Jerosch-Herold M, Kwong RY (2017) Prognostic value of cardiac magnetic resonance tissue characterization in risk stratifying patients with suspected myocarditis. J Am Coll Cardiol 70(16):1964–1976. https://doi.org/10.1016/j.jacc.2017.08.050

Grani C, Eichhorn C, Biere L, Kaneko K, Murthy VL, Agarwal V, Aghayev A, Steigner M, Blankstein R, Jerosch-Herold M, Kwong RY (2019a) Comparison of myocardial fibrosis quantification methods by cardiovascular magnetic resonance imaging for risk stratification of patients with suspected myocarditis. J Cardiovasc Magn Reson 21(1):14. https://doi.org/10.1186/s12968-019-0520-0

Grani C, Biere L, Eichhorn C, Kaneko K, Agarwal V, Aghayev A, Steigner M, Blankstein R, Jerosch-Herold M, Kwong RY (2019b) Incremental value of extracellular volume assessment by cardiovascular magnetic resonance imaging in risk stratifying patients with suspected myocarditis. Int J Cardiovasc Imaging 35(6):1067–1078. https://doi.org/10.1007/s10554-019-01552-6

Granitz M, Motloch LJ, Granitz C, Meissnitzer M, Hitzl W, Hergan K, Schlattau A (2019) Comparison of native myocardial T1 and T2 mapping at 1.5T and 3T in healthy volunteers : reference values and clinical implications. Wien Klin Wochenschr 131(7–8):143–155. https://doi.org/10.1007/s00508-018-1411-3

Gulati A, Jabbour A, Ismail TF, Guha K, Khwaja J, Raza S, Morarji K, Brown TD, Ismail NA, Dweck MR, Di Pietro E, Roughton M, Wage R, Daryani Y, O'Hanlon R, Sheppard MN, Alpendurada F, Lyon AR, Cook SA, Cowie MR, Assomull RG, Pennell DJ, Prasad SK (2013) Association of fibrosis with mortality and sudden cardiac death in patients with nonischemic dilated cardiomyopathy. JAMA 309(9):896–908. https://doi.org/10.1001/jama.2013.1363

Haaf P, Garg P, Messroghli DR, Broadbent DA, Greenwood JP, Plein S (2016) Cardiac T1 mapping and extracellular volume (ECV) in clinical practice: a comprehensive review. J Cardiovasc Magn Reson 18(1):89. https://doi.org/10.1186/s12968-016-0308-4

Haghbayan H, Lougheed N, Deva DP, Chan KKW, Lima JAC, Yan AT (2019) Peri-infarct quantification by cardiac magnetic resonance to predict outcomes in ischemic cardiomyopathy: prognostic systematic review and meta-analysis. Circ Cardiovasc Imaging 12(11):e009156. https://doi.org/10.1161/CIRCIMAGING.119.009156

Hammer-Hansen S, Leung SW, Hsu LY, Wilson JR, Taylor J, Greve AM, Thune JJ, Kober L, Kellman P, Arai AE (2017) Early gadolinium enhancement for determination of area at risk: a preclinical validation study. JACC Cardiovasc Imaging 10(2):130–139. https://doi.org/10.1016/j.jcmg.2016.04.009

Harrigan CJ, Peters DC, Gibson CM, Maron BJ, Manning WJ, Maron MS, Appelbaum E (2011) Hypertrophic cardiomyopathy: quantification of late gadolinium enhancement with contrast-enhanced cardiovascular MR imaging. Radiology 258(1):128–133. https://doi.org/10.1148/radiol.10090526

Heiberg E, Engblom H, Engvall J, Hedstrom E, Ugander M, Arheden H (2005) Semi-automatic quantification of myocardial infarction from delayed contrast enhanced magnetic resonance imaging. Scand Cardiovasc J 39(5):267–275. https://doi.org/10.1080/14017430500340543

Hen Y, Iguchi N, Utanohara Y, Takada K, Machida H, Takayama M, Sumiyoshi T (2014) Prognostic value of late gadolinium enhancement on cardiac magnetic resonance imaging in Japanese hypertrophic cardiomyopathy patients. Circ J 78(4):929–937. https://doi.org/10.1253/circj.cj-13-0979

Hsu LY, Natanzon A, Kellman P, Hirsch GA, Aletras AH, Arai AE (2006) Quantitative myocardial infarction on delayed enhancement MRI. Part I: Animal validation of an automated feature analysis and combined thresholding infarct sizing algorithm. J Magn Reson Imaging 23(3):298–308. https://doi.org/10.1002/jmri.20496

Ismail TF, Jabbour A, Gulati A, Mallorie A, Raza S, Cowling TE, Das B, Khwaja J, Alpendurada FD, Wage R, Roughton M, McKenna WJ, Moon JC, Varnava A, Shakespeare C, Cowie MR, Cook SA, Elliott P, O'Hanlon R, Pennell DJ, Prasad SK (2014) Role of late gadolinium enhancement cardiovascular magnetic resonance in the risk stratification of hypertrophic cardiomyopathy. Heart 100(23):1851–1858. https://doi.org/10.1136/heartjnl-2013-305471

Jacquier A, Boussel L, Amabile N, Bartoli JM, Douek P, Moulin G, Paganelli F, Saeed M, Revel D, Croisille P (2008) Multidetector computed tomography in reperfused acute myocardial infarction. Assessment of infarct size and no-reflow in comparison with cardiac magnetic resonance imaging. Invest Radiol 43(11):773–781. https://doi.org/10.1097/RLI.0b013e318181c8dd

Jimenez Juan L, Crean AM, Wintersperger BJ (2015) Late gadolinium enhancement imaging in assessment of myocardial viability: techniques and clinical applications. Radiol Clin North Am 53(2):397–411. https://doi.org/10.1016/j.rcl.2014.11.004

Jugdutt BI (2003) Ventricular remodeling after infarction and the extracellular collagen matrix: when is enough enough? Circulation 108(11):1395–1403. https://doi.org/10.1161/01.CIR.0000085658.98621.49

Kawel N, Nacif M, Zavodni A, Jones J, Liu S, Sibley CT, Bluemke DA (2012a) T1 mapping of the myocardium: intra-individual assessment of the effect of field strength, cardiac cycle and variation by myocardial region. J Cardiovasc Magn Reson 14:27. https://doi.org/10.1186/1532-429X-14-27

Kawel N, Nacif M, Zavodni A, Jones J, Liu S, Sibley CT, Bluemke DA (2012b) T1 mapping of the myocardium: intra-individual assessment of post-contrast T1 time evolution and extracellular volume fraction at 3T for Gd-DTPA and Gd-BOPTA. J Cardiovasc Magn Reson 14:26. https://doi.org/10.1186/1532-429X-14-26

Kawel-Boehm N, Hetzel SJ, Ambale-Venkatesh B, Captur G, Francois CJ, Jerosch-Herold M, Salerno M, Teague SD, Valsangiacomo-Buechel E, van der Geest RJ, Bluemke DA (2020) Reference ranges ("normal values") for cardiovascular magnetic resonance (CMR) in adults and children: 2020 update. J Cardiovasc Magn Reson 22(1):87. https://doi.org/10.1186/s12968-020-00683-3

Kellman P, Arai AE (2012) Cardiac imaging techniques for physicians: late enhancement. J Magn Reson Imaging 36(3):529–542. https://doi.org/10.1002/jmri.23605

Kellman P, Hansen MS (2014) T1-mapping in the heart: accuracy and precision. J Cardiovasc Magn Reson 16:2. https://doi.org/10.1186/1532-429X-16-2

Kellman P, Herzka DA, Arai AE, Hansen MS (2013) Influence of Off-resonance in myocardial T1-mapping using SSFP based MOLLI method. J Cardiovasc Magn Reson 15:63. https://doi.org/10.1186/1532-429X-15-63

Kellman P, Herzka DA, Hansen MS (2014) Adiabatic inversion pulses for myocardial T1 mapping. Magn Reson Med 71(4):1428–1434. https://doi.org/10.1002/mrm.24793

Khan JN, Nazir SA, Horsfield MA, Singh A, Kanagala P, Greenwood JP, Gershlick AH, McCann GP (2015) Comparison of semi-automated methods to quantify infarct size and area at risk by cardiovascular magnetic resonance imaging at 1.5T and 3.0T field strengths. BMC Res Notes 8:52. https://doi.org/10.1186/s13104-015-1007-1

Kim RJ, Fieno DS, Parrish TB, Harris K, Chen EL, Simonetti O, Bundy J, Finn JP, Klocke FJ, Judd RM (1999) Relationship of MRI delayed contrast enhancement to irreversible injury, infarct age, and contractile function. Circulation 100(19):1992–2002. https://doi.org/10.1161/01.cir.100.19.1992

Kim HW, Farzaneh-Far A, Kim RJ (2009) Cardiovascular magnetic resonance in patients with myocardial infarction: current and emerging applications. J Am Coll Cardiol 55(1):1–16. https://doi.org/10.1016/j.jacc.2009.06.059

Klem I, Heiberg E, Van Assche L, Parker MA, Kim HW, Grizzard JD, Arheden H, Kim RJ (2017) Sources of variability in quantification of cardiovascular magnetic resonance infarct size - reproducibility among three core laboratories. J Cardiovasc Magn Reson 19(1):62. https://doi.org/10.1186/s12968-017-0378-y

Kong P, Christia P, Frangogiannis NG (2014) The pathogenesis of cardiac fibrosis. Cell Mol Life Sci 71(4):549–574. https://doi.org/10.1007/s00018-013-1349-6

Kranzusch R, Aus dem Siepen F, Wiesemann S, Zange L, Jeuthe S, Ferreira da Silva T, Kuehne T, Pieske B, Tillmanns C, Friedrich MG, Schulz-Menger J, Messroghli DR (2020) Z-score mapping for standardized analysis and reporting of cardiovascular magnetic resonance modified Look-Locker inversion recovery (MOLLI) T1 data: normal behavior and validation in patients with amyloidosis. J Cardiovasc Magn Reson 22(1):6. https://doi.org/10.1186/s12968-019-0595-7

Kwon DH, Halley CM, Carrigan TP, Zysek V, Popovic ZB, Setser R, Schoenhagen P, Starling RC, Flamm SD, Desai MY (2009) Extent of left ventricular scar predicts outcomes in ischemic cardiomyopathy patients with significantly reduced systolic function: a delayed hyperenhancement cardiac magnetic resonance study. JACC Cardiovasc Imaging 2(1):34–44. https://doi.org/10.1016/j.jcmg.2008.09.010

Larose E, Rodes-Cabau J, Pibarot P, Rinfret S, Proulx G, Nguyen CM, Dery JP, Gleeton O, Roy L, Noel B, Barbeau G, Rouleau J, Boudreault JR, Amyot M, De Larochelliere R, Bertrand OF (2010) Predicting late myocardial recovery and outcomes in the early hours of ST-segment elevation myocardial infarction traditional measures compared with microvascular obstruction, salvaged myocardium, and necrosis characteristics by cardiovascular magnetic resonance. J Am Coll Cardiol 55(22):2459–2469. https://doi.org/10.1016/j.jacc.2010.02.033

Lee JJ, Liu S, Nacif MS, Ugander M, Han J, Kawel N, Sibley CT, Kellman P, Arai AE, Bluemke DA (2011) Myocardial T1 and extracellular volume fraction mapping at 3 tesla. J Cardiovasc Magn Reson 13:75. https://doi.org/10.1186/1532-429X-13-75

Lee SP, Lee W, Lee JM, Park EA, Kim HK, Kim YJ, Sohn DW (2015) Assessment of diffuse myocardial fibrosis by using MR imaging in asymptomatic patients with aortic stenosis. Radiology 274(2):359–369. https://doi.org/10.1148/radiol.14141120

Lee HJ, Im DJ, Youn JC, Chang S, Suh YJ, Hong YJ, Kim YJ, Hur J, Choi BW (2016) Myocardial extracellular volume fraction with dual-energy equilibrium contrast-enhanced cardiac CT in nonischemic cardiomyopathy: a prospective comparison with cardiac MR imaging. Radiology 280(1):49–57. https://doi.org/10.1148/radiol.2016151289

Lee DC, Hinchcliff ME, Sarnari R, Stark MM, Lee J, Koloms K, Hoffmann A, Carns M, Thakrar A, Aren K, Varga J, Aquino A, Carr JC, Benefield BC, Shah SJ (2018) Diffuse cardiac fibrosis quantification in early systemic sclerosis by magnetic resonance imaging and correlation with skin fibrosis. J Scleroderma Relat Disord 3(2):159–169. https://doi.org/10.1177/2397198318762888

Liu CY, Liu YC, Wu C, Armstrong A, Volpe GJ, van der Geest RJ, Liu Y, Hundley WG, Gomes AS, Liu S, Nacif M, Bluemke DA, Lima JAC (2013) Evaluation of age-related interstitial myocardial fibrosis with cardiac magnetic resonance contrast-enhanced T1 mapping: MESA (Multi-Ethnic Study of Atherosclerosis). J Am Coll Cardiol 62(14):1280–1287. https://doi.org/10.1016/j.jacc.2013.05.078

Liu D, Ma X, Liu J, Zhao L, Chen H, Xu L, Sun Z, Fan Z (2017a) Quantitative analysis of late gadolinium enhancement in hypertrophic cardiomyopathy: comparison of diagnostic performance in myocardial fibrosis between gadobutrol and gadopentetate dimeglumine. Int J Cardiovasc Imaging 33(8):1191–1200. https://doi.org/10.1007/s10554-017-1101-7

Liu JM, Liu A, Leal J, McMillan F, Francis J, Greiser A, Rider OJ, Myerson S, Neubauer S, Ferreira VM, Piechnik SK (2017b) Measurement of myocardial native T1 in cardiovascular diseases and norm in 1291 subjects. J Cardiovasc Magn Reson 19(1):74. https://doi.org/10.1186/s12968-017-0386-y

Lu Y, Yang Y, Connelly KA, Wright GA, Radau PE (2012) Automated quantification of myocardial infarction using graph cuts on contrast delayed enhanced magnetic resonance images. Quant Imaging Med Surg 2(2):81–86. https://doi.org/10.3978/j.issn.2223-4292.2012.05.03

Luetkens JA, Faron A, Isaak A, Dabir D, Kuetting D, Feisst A, Schmeel FC, Sprinkart AM, Thomas D (2019) Comparison of original and 2018 Lake Louise criteria for diagnosis of acute myocarditis: results of a validation cohort. Radiol Cardiothorac Imaging 1(3):e190010

Mahnken AH, Koos R, Katoh M, Wildberger JE, Spuentrup E, Buecker A, Gunther RW, Kuhl HP (2005) Assessment of myocardial viability in reperfused acute myocardial infarction using 16-slice computed tomography in comparison to magnetic resonance imaging. J Am Coll Cardiol 45(12):2042–2047. https://doi.org/10.1016/j.jacc.2005.03.035

Maron MS (2013) Contrast-enhanced CMR in HCM: what lies behind the bright light of LGE and why it now matters. JACC Cardiovasc Imaging 6(5):597–599. https://doi.org/10.1016/j.jcmg.2012.10.028

Maron BJ, Maron MS (2016) LGE means better selection of HCM patients for primary prevention implantable defibrillators. JACC Cardiovasc Imaging 9(12):1403–1406. https://doi.org/10.1016/j.jcmg.2016.01.032

Marrouche NF, Wilber D, Hindricks G, Jais P, Akoum N, Marchlinski F, Kholmovski E, Burgon N, Hu N, Mont L, Deneke T, Duytschaever M, Neumann T, Mansour M, Mahnkopf C, Herweg B, Daoud E, Wissner E, Bansmann P, Brachmann J (2014) Association of atrial tissue fibrosis identified by delayed enhancement MRI and atrial fibrillation catheter ablation: the DECAAF study. JAMA 311(5):498–506. https://doi.org/10.1001/jama.2014.3

McGann CJ, Kholmovski EG, Oakes RS, Blauer JJ, Daccarett M, Segerson N, Airey KJ, Akoum N, Fish E, Badger TJ, DiBella EV, Parker D, MacLeod RS, Marrouche NF (2008) New magnetic resonance imaging-based method for defining the extent of left atrial wall injury after the ablation of atrial fibrillation. J Am Coll Cardiol 52(15):1263–1271. https://doi.org/10.1016/j.jacc.2008.05.062

Meinel FG, De Cecco CN, Schoepf UJ, Nance JW Jr, Silverman JR, Flowers BA, Henzler T (2014) First-arterial-pass dual-energy CT for assessment of myocardial blood supply: do we need rest, stress, and delayed acquisition? Comparison with SPECT. Radiology 270(3):708–716. https://doi.org/10.1148/radiol.13131183

Messner NM, Budjan J, Lossnitzer D, Papavassiliu T, Schad LR, Weingartner S, Zollner FG (2018) Saturation-recovery myocardial T1-mapping during systole: accurate and robust quantification in the presence of arrhythmia. Sci Rep 8(1):5251. https://doi.org/10.1038/s41598-018-23506-z

Messroghli DR, Plein S, Higgins DM, Walters K, Jones TR, Ridgway JP, Sivananthan MU (2006) Human myocardium: single-breath-hold MR T1 mapping with high spatial resolution—reproducibility study. Radiology 238(3):1004–1012. https://doi.org/10.1148/radiol.2382041903

Messroghli DR, Nordmeyer S, Dietrich T, Dirsch O, Kaschina E, Savvatis K, Oh-Ici D, Klein C, Berger F, Kuehne T (2011) Assessment of diffuse myocardial fibrosis in rats using small-animal Look-Locker inversion recovery T1 mapping. Circ Cardiovasc Imaging 4(6):636–640. https://doi.org/10.1161/CIRCIMAGING.111.966796

Messroghli DR, Moon JC, Ferreira VM, Grosse-Wortmann L, He T, Kellman P, Mascherbauer J, Nezafat R, Salerno M, Schelbert EB, Taylor AJ, Thompson R, Ugander M, van Heeswijk RB, Friedrich MG (2017) Clinical recommendations for cardiovascular magnetic resonance mapping of T1, T2, T2* and extracellular volume: a consensus statement by the Society for Cardiovascular Magnetic Resonance (SCMR) endorsed by the European Association for Cardiovascular Imaging (EACVI). J Cardiovasc Magn Reson 19(1):75. https://doi.org/10.1186/s12968-017-0389-8

Mewton N, Liu CY, Croisille P, Bluemke D, Lima JA (2011) Assessment of myocardial fibrosis with cardiovascular magnetic resonance. J Am Coll Cardiol 57(8):891–903. https://doi.org/10.1016/j.jacc.2010.11.013

Mikami Y, Kolman L, Joncas SX, Stirrat J, Scholl D, Rajchl M, Lydell CP, Weeks SG, Howarth AG, White JA (2014) Accuracy and reproducibility of semi-automated late gadolinium enhancement quantification techniques in patients with hypertrophic cardiomyopathy. J Cardiovasc Magn Reson 16:85. https://doi.org/10.1186/s12968-014-0085-x

Moravsky G, Ofek E, Rakowski H, Butany J, Williams L, Ralph-Edwards A, Wintersperger BJ, Crean A (2013) Myocardial fibrosis in hypertrophic cardiomyopathy: accurate reflection of histopathological findings by CMR. JACC Cardiovasc Imaging 6(5):587–596. https://doi.org/10.1016/j.jcmg.2012.09.018

Murtagh G, Laffin LJ, Beshai JF, Maffessanti F, Bonham CA, Patel AV, Yu Z, Addetia K, Mor-Avi V, Moss JD, Hogarth DK, Sweiss NJ, Lang RM, Patel AR (2016) Prognosis of myocardial damage in sarcoidosis patients with preserved left ventricular ejection fraction: risk stratification using cardiovascular magnetic resonance. Circ Cardiovasc Imaging 9(1):e003738. https://doi.org/10.1161/CIRCIMAGING.115.003738

Nacif MS, Kawel N, Lee JJ, Chen X, Yao J, Zavodni A, Sibley CT, Lima JA, Liu S, Bluemke DA (2012) Interstitial myocardial fibrosis assessed as extracellular volume fraction with low-radiation-dose cardiac CT. Radiology 264(3):876–883. https://doi.org/10.1148/radiol.12112458

Nadjiri J, Nieberler H, Hendrich E, Will A, Pellegrini C, Husser O, Hengstenberg C, Greiser A, Martinoff S, Hadamitzky M (2016) Prognostic value of T1-mapping in TAVR patients: extra-cellular volume as a possible predictor for peri- and post-TAVR adverse events. Int J Cardiovasc Imaging 32(11):1625–1633. https://doi.org/10.1007/s10554-016-0948-3

Naeger DM, Higgins C, De Marco T, Muzzarelli S, Ordovas KG (2015) Low-intensity late gadolinium enhancement predominates in hypertrophic cardiomyopathy. Clin Imaging 39(3):432–436. https://doi.org/10.1016/j.clinimag.2015.01.001

Neisius U, El-Rewaidy H, Nakamori S, Rodriguez J, Manning WJ, Nezafat R (2019) Radiomic analysis of myocardial native T1 imaging discriminates between hypertensive heart disease and hypertrophic cardiomyopathy. JACC Cardiovasc Imaging 12(10):1946–1954. https://doi.org/10.1016/j.jcmg.2018.11.024

Ntusi NAB, Piechnik SK, Francis JM, Ferreira VM, Matthews PM, Robson MD, Wordsworth PB, Neubauer S, Karamitsos TD (2015) Diffuse myocardial fibrosis and inflammation in rheumatoid arthritis: insights from CMR T1 mapping. JACC Cardiovasc Imaging 8(5):526–536. https://doi.org/10.1016/j.jcmg.2014.12.025

O'Donnell TP, Xu N, Setser RM, White RD (2003) Semi-automatic segmentation of nonviable cardiac tissue using cine and delayed enhancement magnetic resonance images. In: Medical imaging 2003: physiology and function: methods, systems, and applications. International Society for Optics and Photonics, pp 242–251

Oakes RS, Badger TJ, Kholmovski EG, Akoum N, Burgon NS, Fish EN, Blauer JJ, Rao SN, DiBella EV, Segerson NM, Daccarett M, Windfelder J, McGann CJ, Parker D, MacLeod RS, Marrouche NF (2009) Detection and quantification of left atrial structural remodeling with delayed-enhancement magnetic resonance imaging in patients with atrial fibrillation. Circulation 119(13):1758–1767. https://doi.org/10.1161/CIRCULATIONAHA.108.811877

Pegg TJ, Selvanayagam JB, Jennifer J, Francis JM, Karamitsos TD, Dall'Armellina E, Smith KL, Taggart DP, Neubauer S (2010) Prediction of global left ventricular functional recovery in patients with heart failure undergoing surgical revascularisation, based on late gadolinium enhancement cardiovascular magnetic

resonance. J Cardiovasc Magn Reson 12:56. https://doi.org/10.1186/1532-429X-12-56
Piechnik SK, Ferreira VM, Lewandowski AJ, Ntusi NA, Banerjee R, Holloway C, Hofman MB, Sado DM, Maestrini V, White SK, Lazdam M, Karamitsos T, Moon JC, Neubauer S, Leeson P, Robson MD (2013) Normal variation of magnetic resonance T1 relaxation times in the human population at 1.5 T using ShMOLLI. J Cardiovasc Magn Reson 15:13. https://doi.org/10.1186/1532-429X-15-13
Positano V, Pingitore A, Giorgetti A, Favilli B, Santarelli MF, Landini L, Marzullo P, Lombardi M (2005) A fast and effective method to assess myocardial necrosis by means of contrast magnetic resonance imaging. J Cardiovasc Magn Reson 7(2):487–494. https://doi.org/10.1081/jcmr-200053630
Puntmann VO, Voigt T, Chen Z, Mayr M, Karim R, Rhode K, Pastor A, Carr-White G, Razavi R, Schaeffter T, Nagel E (2013) Native T1 mapping in differentiation of normal myocardium from diffuse disease in hypertrophic and dilated cardiomyopathy. JACC Cardiovasc Imaging 6(4):475–484. https://doi.org/10.1016/j.jcmg.2012.08.019
Puntmann VO, Peker E, Chandrashekhar Y, Nagel E (2016a) T1 mapping in characterizing myocardial disease: a comprehensive review. Circ Res 119(2):277–299. https://doi.org/10.1161/CIRCRESAHA.116.307974
Puntmann VO, Carr-White G, Jabbour A, Yu CY, Gebker R, Kelle S, Hinojar R, Doltra A, Varma N, Child N, Rogers T, Suna G, Arroyo Ucar E, Goodman B, Khan S, Dabir D, Herrmann E, Zeiher AM, Nagel E, International TMCMROS (2016b) T1-mapping and outcome in nonischemic cardiomyopathy: all-cause mortality and heart failure. JACC Cardiovasc Imaging 9(1):40–50. https://doi.org/10.1016/j.jcmg.2015.12.001
Radenkovic D, Weingartner S, Ricketts L, Moon JC, Captur G (2017) T1 mapping in cardiac MRI. Heart Fail Rev 22(4):415–430. https://doi.org/10.1007/s10741-017-9627-2
Reiter U, Reiter G, Dorr K, Greiser A, Maderthaner R, Fuchsjager M (2014) Normal diastolic and systolic myocardial T1 values at 1.5-T MR imaging: correlations and blood normalization. Radiology 271(2):365–372. https://doi.org/10.1148/radiol.13131225
Robson MD, Piechnik SK, Tunnicliffe EM, Neubauer S (2013) T1 measurements in the human myocardium: the effects of magnetization transfer on the SASHA and MOLLI sequences. Magn Reson Med 70(3):664–670. https://doi.org/10.1002/mrm.24867
Rodriguez-Granillo GA (2017) Delayed enhancement cardiac computed tomography for the assessment of myocardial infarction: from bench to bedside. Cardiovasc Diagn Ther 7(2):159–170. https://doi.org/10.21037/cdt.2017.03.16
Roes SD, Kelle S, Kaandorp TA, Kokocinski T, Poldermans D, Lamb HJ, Boersma E, van der Wall EE, Fleck E, de Roos A, Nagel E, Bax JJ (2007) Comparison of myocardial infarct size assessed with contrast-enhanced magnetic resonance imaging and left ventricular function and volumes to predict mortality in patients with healed myocardial infarction. Am J Cardiol 100(6):930–936. https://doi.org/10.1016/j.amjcard.2007.04.029
Roujol S, Weingartner S, Foppa M, Chow K, Kawaji K, Ngo LH, Kellman P, Manning WJ, Thompson RB, Nezafat R (2014) Accuracy, precision, and reproducibility of four T1 mapping sequences: a head-to-head comparison of MOLLI, ShMOLLI, SASHA, and SAPPHIRE. Radiology 272(3):683–689. https://doi.org/10.1148/radiol.14140296
Roujol S, Basha TA, Weingartner S, Akcakaya M, Berg S, Manning WJ, Nezafat R (2015) Impact of motion correction on reproducibility and spatial variability of quantitative myocardial T2 mapping. J Cardiovasc Magn Reson 17:46. https://doi.org/10.1186/s12968-015-0141-1
Rubinshtein R, Glockner JF, Ommen SR, Araoz PA, Ackerman MJ, Sorajja P, Bos JM, Tajik AJ, Valeti US, Nishimura RA, Gersh BJ (2010) Characteristics and clinical significance of late gadolinium enhancement by contrast-enhanced magnetic resonance imaging in patients with hypertrophic cardiomyopathy. Circ Heart Fail 3(1):51–58. https://doi.org/10.1161/CIRCHEARTFAILURE.109.854026
Rudolph A, von Knobelsdorff-Brenkenhoff F, Wassmuth R, Prothmann M, Utz W, Schulz-Menger J (2014) Assessment of nonischemic fibrosis in hypertrophic cardiomyopathy: comparison of gadopentetate dimeglumine and gadobenate dimeglumine for enhanced cardiovascular magnetic resonance imaging. J Magn Reson Imaging 39(5):1153–1160. https://doi.org/10.1002/jmri.24264
Salerno M, Kramer CM (2013) Advances in parametric mapping with CMR imaging. JACC Cardiovasc Imaging 6(7):806–822. https://doi.org/10.1016/j.jcmg.2013.05.005
Schmidt A, Azevedo CF, Cheng A, Gupta SN, Bluemke DA, Foo TK, Gerstenblith G, Weiss RG, Marban E, Tomaselli GF, Lima JA, Wu KC (2007) Infarct tissue heterogeneity by magnetic resonance imaging identifies enhanced cardiac arrhythmia susceptibility in patients with left ventricular dysfunction. Circulation 115(15):2006–2014. https://doi.org/10.1161/CIRCULATIONAHA.106.653568
Schulz-Menger J, Bluemke DA, Bremerich J, Flamm SD, Fogel MA, Friedrich MG, Kim RJ, von Knobelsdorff-Brenkenhoff F, Kramer CM, Pennell DJ, Plein S, Nagel E (2020) Standardized image interpretation and post-processing in cardiovascular magnetic resonance - 2020 update : Society for Cardiovascular Magnetic Resonance (SCMR): Board of Trustees Task Force on Standardized Post-Processing. J Cardiovasc Magn Reson 22(1):19. https://doi.org/10.1186/s12968-020-00610-6
Schvartzman PR, Srichai MB, Grimm RA, Obuchowski NA, Hammer DF, McCarthy PM, Kasper JM, White RD (2003) Nonstress delayed-enhancement magnetic resonance imaging of the myocardium predicts

improvement of function after revascularization for chronic ischemic heart disease with left ventricular dysfunction. Am Heart J 146(3):535–541. https://doi.org/10.1016/S0002-8703(03)00318-1
Scully PR, Bastarrika G, Moon JC, Treibel TA (2018) Myocardial extracellular volume quantification by cardiovascular magnetic resonance and computed tomography. Curr Cardiol Rep 20(3):15. https://doi.org/10.1007/s11886-018-0961-3
Selvanayagam JB, Kardos A, Francis JM, Wiesmann F, Petersen SE, Taggart DP, Neubauer S (2004) Value of delayed-enhancement cardiovascular magnetic resonance imaging in predicting myocardial viability after surgical revascularization. Circulation 110(12):1535–1541. https://doi.org/10.1161/01.CIR.0000142045.22628.74
Singh A, Horsfield MA, Bekele S, Khan JN, Greiser A, McCann GP (2015) Myocardial T1 and extracellular volume fraction measurement in asymptomatic patients with aortic stenosis: reproducibility and comparison with age-matched controls. Eur Heart J Cardiovasc Imaging 16(7):763–770. https://doi.org/10.1093/ehjci/jev007
Spiewak M, Malek LA, Misko J, Chojnowska L, Milosz B, Klopotowski M, Petryka J, Dabrowski M, Kepka C, Ruzyllo W (2010) Comparison of different quantification methods of late gadolinium enhancement in patients with hypertrophic cardiomyopathy. Eur J Radiol 74(3):e149–e153. https://doi.org/10.1016/j.ejrad.2009.05.035
Swoboda PP, McDiarmid AK, Erhayiem B, Broadbent DA, Dobson LE, Garg P, Ferguson C, Page SP, Greenwood JP, Plein S (2016) Assessing myocardial extracellular volume by T1 mapping to distinguish hypertrophic cardiomyopathy from athlete's heart. J Am Coll Cardiol 67(18):2189–2190. https://doi.org/10.1016/j.jacc.2016.02.054
Tao Q, Milles J, Zeppenfeld K, Lamb HJ, Bax JJ, Reiber JH, van der Geest RJ (2010) Automated segmentation of myocardial scar in late enhancement MRI using combined intensity and spatial information. Magn Reson Med 64(2):586–594. https://doi.org/10.1002/mrm.22422
Taylor AJ, Salerno M, Dharmakumar R, Jerosch-Herold M (2016) T1 mapping: basic techniques and clinical applications. JACC Cardiovasc Imaging 9(1):67–81. https://doi.org/10.1016/j.jcmg.2015.11.005
Treibel TA, Bandula S, Fontana M, White SK, Gilbertson JA, Herrey AS, Gillmore JD, Punwani S, Hawkins PN, Taylor SA, Moon JC (2015) Extracellular volume quantification by dynamic equilibrium cardiac computed tomography in cardiac amyloidosis. J Cardiovasc Comput Tomogr 9(6):585–592. https://doi.org/10.1016/j.jcct.2015.07.001
Turkbey EB, Nacif MS, Guo M, McClelland RL, Teixeira PB, Bild DE, Barr RG, Shea S, Post W, Burke G, Budoff MJ, Folsom AR, Liu CY, Lima JA, Bluemke DA (2015) Prevalence and correlates of myocardial scar in a US cohort. JAMA 314(18):1945–1954. https://doi.org/10.1001/jama.2015.14849
Vermes E, Childs H, Carbone I, Barckow P, Friedrich MG (2013) Auto-threshold quantification of late gadolinium enhancement in patients with acute heart disease. J Magn Reson Imaging 37(2):382–390. https://doi.org/10.1002/jmri.23814
Vermes E, Pantaleon C, Auvet A, Cazeneuve N, Machet MC, Delhommais A, Bourguignon T, Aupart M, Brunereau L (2018) Cardiovascular magnetic resonance in heart transplant patients: diagnostic value of quantitative tissue markers: T2 mapping and extracellular volume fraction, for acute rejection diagnosis. J Cardiovasc Magn Reson 20(1):59. https://doi.org/10.1186/s12968-018-0480-9
Vohringer M, Mahrholdt H, Yilmaz A, Sechtem U (2007) Significance of late gadolinium enhancement in cardiovascular magnetic resonance imaging (CMR). Herz 32(2):129–137. https://doi.org/10.1007/s00059-007-2972-5
von Knobelsdorff-Brenkenhoff F, Prothmann M, Dieringer MA, Wassmuth R, Greiser A, Schwenke C, Niendorf T, Schulz-Menger J (2013) Myocardial T1 and T2 mapping at 3 T: reference values, influencing factors and implications. J Cardiovasc Magn Reson 15:53. https://doi.org/10.1186/1532-429X-15-53
von Knobelsdorff-Brenkenhoff F, Mueller AK, Prothmann M, Hennig P, Dieringer MA, Schmacht L, Greiser A, Schulz-Menger J (2016) Cardiac fibrosis in aortic stenosis and hypertensive heart disease assessed by magnetic resonance T1 mapping. J Heart Valve Dis 25(5):527–533
Weber KT (1989) Cardiac interstitium in health and disease: the fibrillar collagen network. J Am Coll Cardiol 13(7):1637–1652. https://doi.org/10.1016/0735-1097(89)90360-4
Weng Z, Yao J, Chan RH, He J, Yang X, Zhou Y, He Y (2016) Prognostic value of LGE-CMR in HCM: a meta-analysis. JACC Cardiovasc Imaging 9(12):1392–1402. https://doi.org/10.1016/j.jcmg.2016.02.031
Wichmann JL, Bauer RW, Doss M, Stock W, Lehnert T, Bodelle B, Frellesen C, Vogl TJ, Kerl JM (2013) Diagnostic accuracy of late iodine-enhancement dual-energy computed tomography for the detection of chronic myocardial infarction compared with late gadolinium-enhancement 3-T magnetic resonance imaging. Invest Radiol 48(12):851–856. https://doi.org/10.1097/RLI.0b013e31829d91a8
Wong TC, Piehler K, Meier CG, Testa SM, Klock AM, Aneizi AA, Shakesprere J, Kellman P, Shroff SG, Schwartzman DS, Mulukutla SR, Simon MA, Schelbert EB (2012) Association between extracellular matrix expansion quantified by cardiovascular magnetic resonance and short-term mortality. Circulation 126(10):1206–1216. https://doi.org/10.1161/CIRCULATIONAHA.111.089409
Wright J, Adriaenssens T, Dymarkowski S, Desmet W, Bogaert J (2009) Quantification of myocardial area at risk with T2-weighted CMR: comparison with contrast-enhanced CMR and coronary angiography. JACC Cardiovasc Imaging 2(7):825–831. https://doi.org/10.1016/j.jcmg.2009.02.011

Wu E, Ortiz JT, Tejedor P, Lee DC, Bucciarelli-Ducci C, Kansal P, Carr JC, Holly TA, Lloyd-Jones D, Klocke FJ, Bonow RO (2008) Infarct size by contrast enhanced cardiac magnetic resonance is a stronger predictor of outcomes than left ventricular ejection fraction or end-systolic volume index: prospective cohort study. Heart 94(6):730–736. https://doi.org/10.1136/hrt.2007.122622

Wu LM, Wu R, Ou YR, Chen BH, Yao QY, Lu Q, Hu J, Jiang M, An DA, Xu JR (2017) Fibrosis quantification in hypertensive heart disease with LVH and Non-LVH: findings from T1 mapping and contrast-free cardiac diffusion-weighted imaging. Sci Rep 7(1):559. https://doi.org/10.1038/s41598-017-00627-5

Xu J, Zhuang B, Sirajuddin A, Li S, Huang J, Yin G, Song L, Jiang Y, Zhao S, Lu M (2020) MRI T1 mapping in hypertrophic cardiomyopathy: evaluation in patients without late gadolinium enhancement and hemodynamic obstruction. Radiology 294(2):275–286. https://doi.org/10.1148/radiol.2019190651

Yan AT, Shayne AJ, Brown KA, Gupta SN, Chan CW, Luu TM, Di Carli MF, Reynolds HG, Stevenson WG, Kwong RY (2006) Characterization of the peri-infarct zone by contrast-enhanced cardiac magnetic resonance imaging is a powerful predictor of post-myocardial infarction mortality. Circulation 114(1):32–39. https://doi.org/10.1161/CIRCULATIONAHA.106.613414

Zghaib T, Nazarian S (2018) New insights into the use of cardiac magnetic resonance imaging to guide decision making in atrial fibrillation management. Can J Cardiol 34(11):1461–1470. https://doi.org/10.1016/j.cjca.2018.07.007

Zhao L, Ma X, Feuchtner GM, Zhang C, Fan Z (2014) Quantification of myocardial delayed enhancement and wall thickness in hypertrophic cardiomyopathy: multidetector computed tomography versus magnetic resonance imaging. Eur J Radiol 83(10):1778–1785. https://doi.org/10.1016/j.ejrad.2014.05.035

Measurements in Cardiovascular Imaging: A Blessing and a Curse?

Rodrigo Salgado

Contents

1 Introduction

The well-known proverb "measuring is knowing" holds true in many instances, as it elevates the discussion from a subjective assessment of a particular problem to a more quantitative approach. In practice, this approach has proven to be effective. For example, we use the degree of luminal coronary artery stenosis to guide the need for conventional angiography and potential revascularization. Similarly, we use standardized thresholds for aortic dimensions to determine the need and frequency of follow-up, as well as to help us identify the best possible moment to proceed with an intervention. In these examples, measurements are an essential component of established guidelines, allowing us to make informed decisions and optimize treatment plans.

The ultimate goal, which should always be at the forefront, is to improve patient outcome.

In this book, several experts have provided us with the necessary knowledge on how to perform different measurements using CT and MR scans, highlighting various confounding factors to ensure the correct interpretation of these results. As a closing chapter, we review here a few topics that should always be kept in mind when dealing with measurements in cardiovascular imaging.

2 Comparing Imaging Modalities

It has become evident that different imaging modalities measure different aspects of the same pathology, highlighting various characteristics. For instance, while CT angiography is still inferior to conventional angiography in accurately measuring luminal diameter stenosis, it allows

R. Salgado (✉)
Department of Radiology, Antwerp University Hospital, Edegem, Belgium

Faculty of Medicine and Health Sciences, University of Antwerp, Wilrijk, Belgium

Department of Radiology, Holy Heart Hospital, Lier, Belgium
e-mail: rodrigo.salgado@uza.be

https://doi.org/10.1007/174_2024_498,
Published Online: 06 September 2024

for the visualization of the underlying plaque (Kolossváry et al. 2017). Echocardiography remains the most important imaging modality for the initial evaluation of cardiac function but is less consistent and reliable than cardiac MR (CMR) in providing quantification of functional parameters and has been validated as an essential technique for various conditions (Leiner et al. 2020). Furthermore, both conventional angiography and echocardiography (with the exception of 3D echocardiography, which is not a standard imaging modality) are 2D based, while CT, for example, provides full 3D anatomical coverage.

The lessons to be learned here are twofold. First, one must always exercise caution when comparing measurements between imaging modalities that have a different physical nature. A prime example is the evaluation of the aortic annulus in patients who are candidates for transcatheter aortic valve replacement. While landmark studies used echocardiography for annular sizing, this has now in practice almost completely been replaced/complemented by a CT-based evaluation, providing a more comprehensive evaluation of the anatomy and thus leading to more accurate measurements (Francone et al. 2020). Although echocardiography-derived measurements are not inherently wrong, they often measure in a different plane. Second, imaging modalities are more often complementary than mutually exclusive. When there is a severe discrepancy between measurements performed using different imaging modalities, the measurement method and the quality of the image data should be scrutinized for errors.

Finally, what constitutes a normal value can be updated over time, as post-processing tools become more reliable and consistent, and variations regarding the influence of gender and ethnicity are included in the available reference data (Raisi-Estabragh et al. 2024). We can only hope that this trend will continue, providing us with a more diverse dataset that can be applied to a broader range of patients coming from different ethnic backgrounds.

3 An Exact Number Is a Dangerous Thing

As software development and imaging techniques improve, the number of measurements that are possible and can be delivered with minimal effort is steadily increasing. CMR can now, e.g., provide information derived from the histological composition of the myocardium through parametric imaging, which goes beyond the known detection of myocardial replacement fibrosis using delayed enhancement. These new parameters have proven to be very helpful in practice, aiding in the detection of interstitial fibrosis and myocardial inflammation, which in some patients would have remained invisible using more standard techniques (Cundari et al. 2021). CT-FFR and myocardial perfusion allow us to provide functional information with CT, an imaging modality that was generally perceived as allowing only morphological assessment.

However, the purpose of this book is also to caution the reader against taking these measurements at face value. For example, parametric T1 and T2 values are not always easy to interpret, with normal ranges that are not always strictly defined and vary from scanner to scanner (Reiter et al. 2018, 2020). Other measurements have similar gray zones between normal and abnormal states and may sometimes add more confusion to the differential diagnosis, which takes us one step backward. Finally, every measurement has its margin of error, which may be due to technical, patient-related, and pathology-related causes.

As always, measurements, no matter how advanced they may be or how confidently they may be displayed on computer screens by advanced software packages, are just one component of the complex puzzle of correctly interpreting all imaging findings. It is the task of every clinician, including the radiologist as a central figure in the diagnostic evaluation of a patient, to use common sense, carefully correlating imaging findings with previous medical history and current clinical presentation, and not to be distracted by a false sense of security and certainty that a numerical value of a given parameter may provide.

4 Potential New Biomarkers for the Future and the Rise of AI

The digitalization of modern healthcare equipment, especially medical imaging, makes it particularly suitable for data mining using artificial intelligence systems. This approach allows us to extract more information than before from the same dataset, sometimes without the need to rescan the patient. One of these new biomarkers is the detection of perivascular inflammation surrounding the coronary arteries (Oikonomou et al. 2018; Antoniades et al. 2019). Contemporary knowledge has established inflammation as an important component in the pathophysiology of atherosclerosis, opening avenues for research that would not have been possible a few years ago. The initial results appearing in the literature are nothing short of astonishing and are currently the subject of intense debate and research focus regarding their future use. Other potential biomarkers have also been reported, often the result of technological innovations but invariably limited to specific research projects.

However, these new biomarkers, however grounded they may be in the underlying pathophysiology, must be approached with caution for several reasons.

First, these biomarkers have only been investigated in the controlled environment of a research project, using software tools that are not commonplace and are still being fine-tuned. Additionally, there is a significant difference between detecting an abnormality (e.g., perivascular inflammation), assessing the degree of expression (either visually or quantitatively), and translating these findings into clear clinical guidelines that can be applied to specific patients and positively affect their outcomes. Therefore, despite the potential that new biomarkers represent, they must remain subject to the same rigorous validation process that established parameters (like the Agatston score) have undergone before being allowed to enter mainstream clinical practice.

Finally, availability of imaging techniques remains an issue. Modern techniques like CT-FFR are still not considered standard components of a mainstream radiology practice. While this may change in the future, it is safe to say that many centers currently do not have access to CT-FFR or have little to no practical experience in myocardial perfusion, despite the inclusion of both techniques in guidelines for acute and stable chest pain (Gulati et al. 2021). Therefore, the ability to perform a measurement starts with the available equipment and available expertise, which is not universally the same.

5 Conclusion

Measurements in cardiovascular imaging have significantly helped us establish diagnoses, monitor patients over time, and determine the correct thresholds for possible interventions. However, the interpretation of these measurements is not always straightforward and is influenced by several factors, as detailed in the different chapters of this book.

Therefore, knowledge of the origin of a measurement, the various confounding factors, and, most importantly, the critical step of converting a measurement into a clinical decision will remain the privilege and responsibility of the modern radiologist for a considerable time to come. We hope that this book has provided you with the necessary guidance to help you in this process.

Disclaimer All measurements in this book have been obtained from peer-reviewed papers and guidelines from professional organizations, unless explicitly stated otherwise. While the authors, editors, and publisher have gone through a rigorous process to establish their correct reproduction from the original source, each measurement must be interpreted in the correct clinical context, this along with an accurate way of measurement, and taking into account all technical variables, this including follow-up exams with various equipment or software. Neither the authors, the editors, nor the publisher can accept any legal responsibility for any improper application or interpretation of these measurements as well as their potential consequences.

References

Antoniades C, Kotanidis CP, Berman DS (2019) State-of-the-art review article. Atherosclerosis affecting fat: what can we learn by imaging perivascular adipose tissue? J Cardiovasc Comput Tomogr 13:288–296

Cundari G, Galea N, Rubeis GD, Frustaci A, Cilia F, Mancuso G et al (2021) Use of the new Lake Louise Criteria improves CMR detection of atypical forms of acute myocarditis. Int J Cardiovasc Imaging 37:1395–1404

Francone M, Budde RPJ, Bremerich J, Dacher JN, Loewe C, Wolf F et al (2020) CT and MR imaging prior to transcatheter aortic valve implantation: standardisation of scanning protocols, measurements and reporting—a consensus document by the European Society of Cardiovascular Radiology (ESCR). Eur Radiol 30:2627–2650

Gulati M, Levy PD, Mukherjee D, Amsterdam E, Bhatt DL, Birtcher KK et al (2021) 2021 AHA/ACC/ASE/CHEST/SAEM/SCCT/SCMR guideline for the evaluation and diagnosis of chest pain: a report of the American College of Cardiology/American Heart Association Joint Committee on Clinical Practice Guidelines. Circulation 144:e368–e454

Kolossváry M, Szilveszter B, Merkely B, Maurovich-Horvat P (2017) Plaque imaging with CT—a comprehensive review on coronary CT angiography based risk assessment. Cardiovasc Diagn Ther 7:489–506

Leiner T, Bogaert J, Friedrich MG, Mohiaddin R, Muthurangu V, Myerson S et al (2020) SCMR Position Paper (2020) on clinical indications for cardiovascular magnetic resonance. J Cardiovasc Magn Reson 22:76

Oikonomou EK, Marwan M, Desai MY, Mancio J, Alashi A, Centeno EH et al (2018) Non-invasive detection of coronary inflammation using computed tomography and prediction of residual cardiovascular risk (the CRISP CT study): a post-hoc analysis of prospective outcome data. Lancet 392:929–939

Raisi-Estabragh Z, Szabo L, McCracken C, Bülow R, Aquaro GD, Andre F et al (2024) Cardiovascular magnetic resonance reference ranges from the Healthy Hearts Consortium. JACC Cardiovasc Imaging. https://doi.org/10.1016/j.jcmg.2024.01.009

Reiter G, Reiter C, Kräuter C, Fuchsjäger M, Reiter U (2018) Cardiac magnetic resonance T1 mapping. Part 1: aspects of acquisition and evaluation. Eur J Radiol 109:223–234

Reiter U, Reiter C, Kräuter C, Nizhnikava V, Fuchsjäger M, Reiter G (2020) Quantitative clinical cardiac magnetic resonance imaging. Röfo 192:246–256

Correction to: Thymus

Jeanne B. Ackman

**Correction to:
Chapter 469 in: J. B. Ackman, Med Radiol Diagn Imaging, https://doi.org/10.1007/174_2023_469**

The original version of this chapter was inadvertently published without the disclaimer text shown below, which has now been included.

Disclaimer All measurements in this book have been obtained from peer-reviewed papers and guidelines from professional organizations, unless explicitly stated otherwise. While the authors, editors, and publisher have gone through a rigorous process to establish their correct reproduction from the original source, each measurement must be interpreted in the correct clinical context, this along with an accurate way of measurement, and taking into account all technical variables, this including follow-up exams with various equipment or software. Neither the authors, the editors, nor the publisher can accept any legal responsibility for any improper application or interpretation of these measurements as well as their potential consequences.

The updated version of this chapter can be found at https://doi.org/10.1007/174_2023_469

Med Radiol Diagn Imaging (2026)
https://doi.org/10.1007/174_2025_588,
Published Online: 24 April 2025

GPSR Compliance

The European Union's (EU) General Product Safety Regulation (GPSR) is a set of rules that requires consumer products to be safe and our obligations to ensure this.

If you have any concerns about our products, you can contact us on ProductSafety@springernature.com

In case Publisher is established outside the EU, the EU authorized representative is:

Springer Nature Customer Service Center GmbH
Europaplatz 3
69115 Heidelberg, Germany

Batch number: 10732799

Printed by Printforce, the Netherlands